Wound Care

A Collaborative Practice Manual for Physical Therapists and Nurses

Second Edition

Edited by

Carrie Sussman, PT
Owner and Operator
Sussman Physical Therapy, Inc.
Wound Care Management Services
Torrance, California

Barbara M. Bates-Jensen, PhD, RN, CWOCN
Adjunct Assistant Professor in Residence
Department of Medicine
Division of Geriatrics
UCLA School of Medicine
University of California Los Angeles
Los Angeles, California

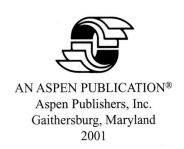

AN ASPEN PUBLICATION®
Aspen Publishers, Inc.
Gaithersburg, Maryland
2001

The author has made every effort to ensure the accuracy of the information herein. However, appropriate information sources should be consulted, especially for new or unfamiliar procedures. It is the responsibility of every practitioner to evaluate the appropriateness of a particular opinion in the context of actual clinical situations and with due consideration to new developments. The author, editors, and the publisher cannot be held responsible for any typographical or other errors found in this book.

Library of Congress Cataloging-in-Publication Data

Sussman, Carrie.
Wound care: a collaborative practice manual for physical therapists and nurses/
Carrie Sussman, Barbara M. Bates-Jensen—2nd ed.
p.; cm
Includes bibliographical references and index.
ISBN 0-8342-1973-5
1. Wounds and injuries—Treatment. 2. Physical therapy. 3. Nursing. I. Bates-Jensen,
Barbara M. II. Title.
[DNLM: 1. Wounds and Injuries—nursing. 2. Wounds and Injuries—rehabilitation.
3. Physical Therapy—methods. 4. Wounds and Injuries—diagnosis. WO700 S964w 2001]
RD93.W683 2001
617.1—dc21
2001033335

Cover Photos:
Top right, Copyright © Nancy Elftman.
Middle, Copyright © Evonne Fowler.
Bottom right, Copyright © B.M. Bates-Jensen.

Orders: (800) 638-8437
Customer Service: (800) 234-1660

About Aspen Publishers • For more than 40 years, Aspen has been a leading professional publisher in a variety of disciplines. Aspen's vast information resources are available in both print and electronic formats. We are committed to providing the highest quality information available in the most appropriate format for our customers. Visit Aspen's Internet site for more information resources, directories, articles, and a searchable version of Aspen's full catalog, including the most recent publications: **www.aspenpublishers.com**
Aspen Publishers, Inc. • The hallmark of quality in publishing
Member of the worldwide Wolters Kluwer group

Editorial Services: Nora McElfish
Library of Congress Catalog Card Number: 2001033335
ISBN: 0-8342-1973-5

Printed in the United States of America

1 2 3 4 5

Table of Contents

Color Plates

Contributors

Barbara M. Bates-Jensen, PhD, RN, CWOCN
Adjunct Assistant Professor in Residence
Department of Medicine
Division of Geriatrics
UCLA School of Medicine
University of California Los Angeles
Los Angeles, California

Nancy N. Byl, PhD, MPH, PT, FAPTA
Professor and Chair
Department of Physical Therapy and Rehabilitation Science
University of California at San Francisco
San Francisco, California

Joan E. Conlan, LVN, CPed
Certified Pedorthotist
Theraped
Mt. Shasta, California

Teresa Conner-Kerr, PhD, PT, CWS(D)
Associate Professor
Department of Physical Therapy
School of Allied Health Sciences
Co-Director of the Collaborative Wound Healing
    Laboratory
Department of Interdisciplinary Studies
Brody School of Medicine
East Carolina University
Greenville, North Carolina

Carlos E. Donayre, MD
Associate Professor of Surgery
Department of Vascular and General Surgery
School of Medicine
Harbor/UCLA Medical Center
University of California Los Angeles
Los Angeles, California

Mary Dyson, PhD, LDH(Hon), FAIUM(Hon),
    FSCP(Hon), CBiol, MIBiol
Retired Director of Tissue Repair Research Unit, UMDS
Emeritus Reader, KCL
Centre for Cardiovascular Biology and Medicine
Guy's Hospital Campus
Kings College
University of London
England, United Kingdom

Joy Edvalson, MSN, RNET, FNP, CWOCN
Advance Practice Nurse, Private Practice
Wound-Ostomy Innovators
North Hills, California

Nancy Elftman, CO, FAAOP, CPed
Certified Orthotist
Certified Pedorthotist
Cosmos Extremity/Hands on Foot, Inc.
LaVerne, California

Evonne Fowler, RN, MN, CNS, CWOCN
Founding President
Association for Advanced Wound Care
Chairperson
Symposium on Advanced Wound Care
Bellflower Kaiser Hospital
Bellflower, California

Dayna E. Gary, OTR, CWS
Occupational Therapist
Certified Wound Specialist
The LAC–USC Regional Burn Center
Los Angeles, California

Mark S. Granick, MD, FACS
Professor of Surgery
Chief of Plastic Surgery
New Jersey Medical School–UMDNJ
Newark, New Jersey

Elizabeth Hiltabidel, RN, MSN, CWOCN
Advance Practice Nurse, Wound and Ostomy Care
Loma Linda University Medical Center
Loma Linda, California

Teresa J. Kelechi, PhDc, MSN, RNCS, CWCN
Clinical Director
University Diagnostic Center Foot Care Clinic
Medical University of South Carolina
Charleston, South Carolina

Bruce A. Kraemer, MD
Associate Professor of Plastic and Reconstructive Surgery
Washington University School of Medicine
St. Louis, Missouri

Diane L. Krasner, PhD, RN, CWOCN, CWS, FAAN
Vice President for Clinical and Educational Services
Dumex Medical
Baltimore, Maryland

Harriett Baugh Loehne, PT, CWS
Clinical Coordinator
Care Program
Archbold Medical Center
Thomasville, Georgia

Gregory K. Patterson, MD, CWS
Partner/General and Vascular Surgery
South Georgia Surgical Associates
Medical Director
Archbold Wound Care Program
Interpreting Physician
Archbold Cardiovascular Laboratory
Thomasville, Georgia

Mary Ellen Posthauer, RD, CD
Registered/Certified Dietitian
President
M.E.P. Healthcare Dietary Services, Inc.
Evansville, Indiana

Laurie M. Rappl, PT, CWS
Clinical Support Manager
Span-American Medical Systems, Inc.
Simpsonville, South Carolina

Susie Seaman, MSN, FNP, CETN
Nurse Practitioner
Grossmont Hospital Wound Healing Center
Sharp HealthCare
San Diego, California

Carrie Sussman, PT
Owner and Operator
Sussman Physical Therapy, Inc.
Wound Care Management Services
Torrance, California

Geoffrey Sussman, JP Ph C, MPS, MSHPA, AFAIPM, MSMA, MAPSA
Director, Wound Education and Research
Department of Pharmacy Practice
Victoria College of Pharmacy
Monash University
Parkville, Victoria, Australia

Paula Tashjian, RN, MSN, CWOCN
Certified Wound, Ostomy, and Continence Nurse
WOC 'N' Consulting
San Diego, California

Nancy Tomaselli, MSN, RN, CS, CRNP, CWOCN
President/CEO
Premier Health Solutions
Cherry Hill, New Jersey

Adela M. Valenzuela, RN, MSN, CWON
Advance Practice Nurse, Wound and Ostomy Care
Loma Linda University Medical Center
Loma Linda, California

R. Scott Ward, PhD, PT
Associate Professor
Division of Physical Therapy
University of Utah
Salt Lake City, Utah

James D. Wethe, MD
Plastic Surgeon
South Bay Plastic Surgery
Torrance, California

Laurel A. Wiersema-Bryant, MSN, RN, CNS
Clinical Nurse Specialist/Adult Nurse Practitioner
Barnes-Jewish Hospital, A Member of BJC Health Care
St. Louis, Missouri

Foreword

Wound Care: A Collaborative Practice Manual for Physical Therapists and Nurses has been updated to reflect current best practices based on the latest research evidence. The second edition continues to provide the reader with a solid foundation of wound knowledge and encourages a holistic patient approach through collaborative interdisciplinary management.

Wound research is continually revealing new ways of explaining and understanding wound healing and validating practice methods. Whether a newcomer or a seasoned wound care specialist, this book will be a valuable resource to access this information. The chapters are written by wound care specialists from many disciplines on the forefront of wound healing practice and research. They have joined together to share their accumulated knowledge base, wisdom, and diverse experiences and expertise in wound management.

These experts have reviewed the research literature, dissected it for the student and clinician, and presented the evidence needed for clinical decision making and best patient outcomes that are the foundation of evidence-based practice.

Welcome to lifelong learning! Most wound care specialists are self-directed learners. We continually educate ourselves in order to change our behavior or practice for the benefit of our clients. By integrating new knowledge gleaned from studying this second edition, practicing the new skills learned, combined with our past experiences (expert knowing), we will advance the field of wound management. *Wound Care: A Collaborative Practice Manual for Physical Therapists and Nurses, Second Edition* provides a living resource for excellence in wound management.

Thank you for making a difference.

Evonne Fowler, RN, MN, CNS, CWOCN
Founding President
Association for Advanced Wound Care
Chairperson
Symposium on Advanced Wound Care
Bellflower Kaiser Hospital
Bellflower, California

A New Edition for the New Millennium

The second edition of *Wound Care: A Collaborative Practice Manual for Physical Therapists and Nurses* has been completely updated to reflect new information and six pertinent chapters, new illustrations, and color plates have been added to the material from the first edition. The organization of the book has not changed but has been expanded to encompass the new materials. Along with new chapters there are new contributors from different disciplines.

THE MULTIDISCIPLINARY COLLABORATIVE TEAM

Writing this book has been a collaborative effort between the two editors and our expert contributors. Early on in the writing, it was recognized that, just as in the real world, the skills and expertise of a multidisciplinary team were needed to provide the scope of information needed for wound management. The writing team represents the disciplines usually found on the wound management team. Our book draws on the expertise of many disciplines including medicine, surgery, nursing, physical therapy, research, orthotics, pharmacy, nutrition and dietetics, and occupational therapy. A number of the chapters are coauthored by representatives from different disciplines. Two authors are from outside the United States. Wound management is a global problem and a multidisciplinary challenge, and collaboration across all borders must be encouraged. Yes, at times, collaborating was challenging, but it has been very rewarding. It seemed very logical that we should prepare this work as a collaborative effort, thus setting the stage for collaborative practice.

ORGANIZATION OF THE BOOK

The book is organized into four parts. Part I, Introduction to Wound Diagnosis, reviews the diagnostic process used by both nurses and physical therapists when evaluating the patient with a wound. Why start with diagnosis? Nurses and physical therapists have extensive education with unique bodies of knowledge and, as professionals, have a level of autonomy and self-regulation. The use of a process to arrive at a diagnosis for the patient with a wound provides clarity in communication and collaborative practice. Clear communication assists with accountability and greater professional autonomy. Historically, nurses and physical therapists have used the medical diagnosis of the patient to describe the focus of their practice. There is better nursing and physical therapy-related terminology to describe the impairments, risk factors, and functional deficits for which nurses and physical therapists intervene. As it turns out, terminologies used by nurses and physical therapists are very similar—all the better to foster communication and collaboration between the two groups.

After presenting the diagnostic process in Chapter 1, the rest of Part I reviews implementation of the diagnostic process and includes the chapters Wound Healing Physiology and Chronic Wound Healing, Nutritional Assessment and Treatment, Assessment of the Skin and Wound, Wound Measurements, Tools To Measure Wound Healing, and Vascular Evaluation. These chapters form the assessment foundation for the patient with a wound.

Part II, Management by Wound Characteristics, describes management of the wound by specific wound characteristics. Recently, the American Physical Therapy Association convened a panel of five integumentary subject matter expert physical therapists to develop proactive patterns for management of integumentary impairments and disabilities. It was the consensus of the panel that wounds and burns are managed similarly and that the factors affecting management of the wound are the depth of the injury (partial versus full thickness and extension into deep tissues) and the wound-associated characteristics of necrosis, edema, and infection. Everything else revolves around management of the wound environment or the factors influencing healing. Chapters include Management of Necrotic Tissue, Management of Exudate and Infection, Management of Edema, Management of the Wound Environment with Dressings and Topical Agents, Management of the Wound Environment with Advanced Therapies, and Management of Scar. Three wound characteristics—necrotic tissue, exudate and infection, and edema—are the wound characteristics that most often drive interventions and cause concerns for clinicians. Management of scar, a consequence of wound healing, is often overlooked unless it is abnormal or there is patient complaint. Each chapter begins with a definition of the characteristic, the significance of the findings, assessment for the characteristic, and basic interventions appropriate for the wound characteristic. Each chapter ends with outcome measures, self-care teaching guidelines, and referral criteria for the specific wound characteristic. Where appropriate, procedures and protocols for interventions are included.

Part III, Management by Wound Etiology, focuses on management of the wound by etiology and includes the chapters Acute Surgical Wound Management, Pressure Ulcers: Pathophysiology and Prevention, Management of Pressure by Therapeutic Positioning, Diagnosis and Management of Vascular Ulcers, Management of the Neuropathic Foot, Management of the Skin and Nails, and Management of Malignant Wounds and Fistulas. The chapters focus on pathophysiology, prevention, classification, and intervention.

Part IV, Management of Wound Healing with Physical Therapy Technologies, applies the diagnostic process to selection of wound treatment interventions with physical therapy technologies. Chapters include Electrical Stimulation for Wound Healing, Pulsed Electromagnetic Fields, Ultraviolet Light and Wound Healing, Therapeutic and Diagnostic Ultrasound, Whirlpool, and Pulsatile Lavage with Suction. Each physical therapy technology chapter begins with a definition of the intervention, the science and theory of the intervention as it relates to wound healing, and application of the diagnostic process to appropriate selection of candidates for treatment. Each chapter includes protocols and expected outcome results for the therapy described, as well as case studies.

Carrie Sussman
Barbara M. Bates-Jensen

ACKNOWLEDGMENTS

We would like to express our appreciation to the many individuals who have made the first and second editions of this book possible:

- The outstanding and dedicated individuals who have contributed their considerable clinical and academic knowledge by authoring the chapters of this book
- Amy Martin, Mary Anne Langdon, Ruth Bloom, Nora McElfish, Laura Smith, Jan Kortkamp, Patricia Messick, and the rest of the staff at Aspen Publishers, Inc. for their help and support in production
- The reviewers and consultants whose suggestions were invaluable during development: Michelle Cameron, PT, OCS, Linda Frankenberger, MS, PT, Deborah Hagler, PT, Robert Kellogg, PhD, PT, Marko Markov, PhD, Gretchen Swanson, MPH, PT, Eleanor Price, PhD, Nancy A. Stotts, EdD, RN, Rebecca Lewthwiate, PhD, and Luther Kloth, MS, PT
- Kris Johnson, Erin McEntyre, and Debbie Denton, who took care of the many details associated with preparation of the manuscript
- The authors, publishers, companies, and colleagues who have allowed us to publish their artwork, photographs, and tables to illustrate the information

To our husbands and children—Robert Sussman and Ronald, Holly, and Thomas Jensen, who have sweated the big and small stuff with us during the years of development and preparation of the manuscript and without whom completion of this project would not have been possible.

Carrie Sussman
Barbara M. Bates-Jensen

The Need for Evidence-Based Collaborative Practice

Carrie Sussman and Barbara M. Bates-Jensen

EVIDENCE-BASED PRACTICE

Evidence-based practice (EBP) had its philosophical origins in Paris in the middle of the nineteenth century.[1] Today, it is a hot topic for clinicians, health care organizations, health care lawyers, payers, policy makers, and consumers. In the last decade, numerous articles have been written and courses presented on the topic. The interpretation of what evidence-based practice entails has evolved and adapted to the realities of clinical practice and research. *Evidence* means "proof" or "confirmation." EBP shifts decisions about providing health care from "what has always been done," or traditions, and "I think this is what should be done," or opinions, to what science demonstrates in an objective fashion should be done. Practice that is based on the best available evidence is increasingly becoming the expectation for clinicians and health care organizations.[2]

Treatments based on outdated knowledge and personal opinions are considered unacceptable in health care today. Difficulties arise because many areas of practice do not have a critical mass of scientific knowledge available for use. So the clinician must rely on the best scientific evidence available until further evidence is gathered. Clinicians must be able to evaluate and weigh the strength of research evidence in order to apply it to practice. It is relevant to begin the second edition of *Wound Care: A Collaborative Practice Manual for Physical Therapists and Nurses* with a brief overview of EBP—what it *is* and what it is *not*. The editors and contributors have tried to incorporate the available scientific knowledge in their writings to facilitate speedy transfer of information on best practices to the clinician to improve patient outcomes.

"Evidence-based medicine is the conscientious, explicit, and judicious use of current best evidence in making decisions about the care of individual patients."[1(p71)] Physicians have been initiators and developers of EBP; however, the methodology has spread and been embraced by many other health care disciplines, including nursing and physical therapy. All health care clinicians are now expected to justify their practices with the best science available. Evidence-based practice requires integration of relevant research evidence into clinical practice, using expertise and judgment to apply it for individual patient management. Scientific evidence provides a framework for clinical decision making but actual use of EBP begins and ends with clinical expertise.[3] Clinical expertise is defined as the proficiency and judgment acquired by an individual clinician through clinical experience and practice.[1]

Outcomes research is tied to EBP by the ease with which outcomes research can be used to support clinical practice and is an important effective means to document the effect of interventions on patient outcomes. Outcomes research focuses on the end results of patient care and includes attention to structures of care (such as elements of organization and administration that affect care), process of care (such as care delivery methods, practice styles, use of guidelines or standards) and outcomes of care (including cost and quality). Outcomes research is typically quasi-experimental or observational in research design. This type of research makes little or no use of experimental control. Therefore, it is most often ranked as a level III or IV type of evidence (see Exhibit I–1). The techniques used in outcomes research emerged from evaluation research and have components of economic analysis and epidemiology, with a strong focus on the quality of care.[2] Outcome studies provide good opportunities for developing sound scientific basis for interventions, and they typically incorporate attention to quality and cost. Outcomes research can provide clinicians with the evidence needed to support EBP.

Other evidence for practice comes from both basic research and applied clinical research. Applied clinical research is generally more useful clinically because it typically involves testing the accuracy and precision of diagnostic tests, prognostic markers, and the efficacy and safety of therapeutic, rehabilitative, and preventive regimens.[1] Important exceptions are where basic science reveals the nature of the cause-effect relationship and, thus, suggests key targets for interventions, even before applied clinical research is available to verify or refute the viability of that "intervention application." Again, some research may be better than none, with appropriate appreciation for the less-than-direct relationship likely for the basic science-application interface. Randomized, controlled clinical trials (RCTs) are only one form of scientific evidence; there is room in EBP for other research approaches and designs. Clinical evidence includes both quantitative and qualitative research approaches, as well as various levels of research. Abstract poster or podium presentations at professional meetings, original research reports in peer-reviewed journals, and metanalyses of findings in one particular area all constitute scientific evidence that may be used as a basis for practice.[4]

EBP is not a substitute for clinical judgment and experience. Relying solely on evidence without clinical expertise to judge the appropriate application of the evidence to an individual patient is unacceptable. Without current best evidence, practice would stagnate and lose relevance, to the detriment of patient care and practice development. EBP is not a "cookbook" approach to practice because it integrates the clinical expertise of the clinician, the research evidence from external sources with choices by the patient.

The information explosion has made it impossible for clinicians to keep up with all new research. EBP is a strategy for handling the rapidly growing volume of medical literature in the context of individual patient problems. It is a process of lifelong self-directed learning. Critical evaluation of the research and synthesis of the results is a labor-intensive process. Clinicians can attempt to do all the steps on their own or to use some judicious shortcuts. Use of systematic reviews of the literature, evidence-based practice databases, evidence-based clinical practice guidelines, and recently published well-referenced textbooks might all be considered shortcuts. To truly practice based on the scientific evidence available requires knowledge and skills in accessing information, based on asking a series of appropriate clinical questions, rather than using a topic or key word. Formulating clear, focused, patient-related questions is a prerequisite to answering them. Straus and Sackett suggest

that four components of an answerable clinical question must be specified:

1. The patient or problem being addressed
2. The intervention under consideration
3. A comparison intervention or an alternative treatment
4. Specific clinical outcomes of interest[5]

Clinical Wisdom: *Steps in Using Evidence in Practice*

1. Find, in the most efficient way, the best evidence to answer a clinically relevant question. Start with evidence to which have been applied experimental controls (eg, systematic reviews of the literature, evidence-based clinical practice guidelines, published research, presented papers and posters).
2. Critically appraise the evidence for its validity (closeness to truth) and usefulness (clinical applicability).
3. Integrate the appraisal of evidence with clinical expertise and apply the results to clinical practice (clinical judgment and patient preferences). Examples of this include: clinical examination, laboratory tests, patient questionnaire, etc.
4. Evaluate your performance.

Source: Reprinted with permission from *The British Medical Journal,* Vol. 317, pp. 339–340, © 1998, The BMJ Publishing Group.

In the course of evaluating a patient, many questions arise. It is critical to successful research utilization to choose questions that are most important to quality of patient care. Factors to consider include: feasibility, clinician interest, generalizability of the question to other patients, and significance of the problem.[5] Types of clinical questions that are typically asked relate to: etiology, intervention(s), diagnosis, prognosis, or clinic management issues—practice/organization management, quality assurance, cost-effectiveness, cost-benefit analysis, ethical matters, etc.

After defining the clinical question, it is important to seek the best resources to provide answers that are research based. The growth of scientific research, improved scientific methods, and the exponential growth of information that has followed has led to new methods for managing access to the data. In the 1990s, four methods emerged to help the clinician access synthesized research information that can be used to deliver improved patient care. These include clinical practice guidelines, access to EBP databases (eg, National Library of Medicine free database of research literature, PubMed, Cumulative Index of Nursing and Allied Health Literature (CINAHAL—proprietary), Physiotherapy Evidence Database (PEDro—appraisals of single articles), Evidence-Based Medicine, and the Cochrane Database of Systematic Reviews. The database list at the end of this introduction gives the Web site addresses. Other major sources of literature synthesis are systematic reviews (SRs). The highest quality SRs are usually quantitative forms of reviews, in contrast to narrative reviews, which introduce the authors' subjective biases while identifying and weighing the evidence summarized. SRs of the literature, including meta-nalysis, which is a statistical summarizing of the results of multiple studies on the same topic, help to cohere conflicting research results and are useful in identifying research gaps.[6] Where appropriate, reference to the strength of evidence and the source of evaluation is provided in this text.

CLINICAL PRACTICE GUIDELINES

Clinical practice guidelines (CPGs) represent a synthesis of practice and research that have been developed to provide health care practitioners with sound strategies presented as recommendations for caring for patients, based on the best available scientific literature and expert opinion with the intent to deliver the best possible health care.[7] A formal definition of clinical practice guidelines was provided by the Institute of Medicine in 1990.[8]

In 1989, the Agency for Health Care Policy and Research (AHCPR), now the Agency for Health Care Research and Quality (AHRQ), was established by the U.S. Congress under the Balanced Budget Act of 1989 to carry out a mission of facilitating development of clinical practice guidelines and disseminating the research findings and guidelines to health care providers, policy makers, and the public. To accomplish this mission, AHCPR convened panels of experts to review the literature and develop clinically appropriate guidelines. Over the next several years, AHCPR commissioned clinical practice guidelines on 19 topics. Techniques developed by AHCPR for evaluating scientific evidence as a basis for clinical practice and health policy are still valid.

Examples of AHCPR clinical practice guidelines related to wounds are guidelines for the prediction, prevention, and treatment of pressure ulcers.[9,10] Subsequently, the AHCPR redefined its role from the organization to fund development of new guidelines to that of facilitator for the development of future guidelines, and changed its name. With AHCPR encouragement, other individuals and professional groups have carried on this mission by issuing new clinical practice guidelines or updating the previous iteration. Some of these include the American Medical Directors Association *Treatment of Pressure Ulcers Guideline*;[11] University of Pennsylvania *Venous Leg Ulcer Guideline*;[12] *Ostomy/Wound Management* special supplement update of diabetic ulcer,

venous leg ulcer, and pressure ulcer guidelines;[13] and the *Pressure Ulcer Prevention and Treatment Following Spinal Cord Injury Clinical Practice* guidelines.[14]

In 1998, the American Association of Health Plans and the American Medical Association, along with AHCPR, developed the National Guideline Clearinghouse Web site, dedicated to enhancing access to evidence-based clinical practice guidelines. Guideline summaries are updated regularly. A broad variety of clinical guidelines are found through this site, and the clinician needs to assess the quality of each guideline and the applicability to the clinical situation. As a result of the high-quality work of the AHCPR and the panels they enlisted, CPGs have developed reputations for quality. Not all clinical practice guidelines have a strong evidence base. In fact, some CPGs have been developed with little systematic effort to find and appraise the relevant literature; these are clinical practice guidelines developed on the basis of clinical opinion only and are not evidence-based. Fortunately, more and more CPGs are developed on the basis of research evidence and clinical judgment, and a few have begun to formally incorporate patient perspectives (in the form of patient focus groups; Europe appears to lead in this category) in their development.[15] On some topics, the best evidence available is level IV nonrandomized case-controlled, nonobjective, nonblinded studies, case series studies, or level V case series and expert opinion. The CPG reader should check the methods described in the CPG report for gathering and appraising research evidence and incorporating it with other clinician or patient sources. Ultimately, it is the thoroughness with which the work is done that requires careful scrutiny.[15]

CPGs are *not* fixed protocols but are intended as a guide for health care professionals and providers to follow. Guidelines are not inclusive or exclusive of all the methods that may be reasonable to treat a specific condition with the desired outcomes. Guidelines cannot replace clinical decision making and must be applied based on the needs of the individual patient, taking into account the variations of clinical settings, resources, and patient characteristics, while always using professional judgment.[16]

Levels of Evidence and Grades of Recommendations

EBP has a strong emphasis on evaluation of the rigors of the research reported. A number of approaches have been published on evaluating the quality of research studies and the evidence presented. The AHCPR clinical practice guidelines were developed based on the existing evidence in particular areas. The evidence in the guidelines was rated as to the strength it provided to support the intervention. Those studies with stronger controls were more powerful and, thus, were awarded higher levels of evidence (see Exhibit I–1). Using some method to rate the strength of the research is

Exhibit I–1 Levels of Evidence and Grades of Recommendations: Quality Ratings

Level of Evidence	Etiology and Intervention Studies*	Diagnosis (Dx)/ Evaluation Studies	Prognosis Studies	Grade of Recommendation for CPG**
I	SR† of multiple RCTs with high power (large Ns; homogeneity of findings within analyses)	SR of multiple Level II diagnostic studies (large Ns; homogeneity of findings)	SR of multiple Level II prognosis studies (with homogeneity of included cohort studies)	A
II	single, well-done RCT	single, well-done, diagnostic/evaluation study in which independent blind comparison is made of patients from an appropriate spectrum of patients who are at risk for the disease/condition, all of whom have undergone both the assessment (test) of interest and the reference standard	single, well-done, prospective cohort study, in which all enrollees are representative of patients with the condition and initially free of the outcomes of interest (entered at a similar point in disease or condition process) and at least 80% are followed to major end points	A
III	• nonrandomized concurrent cohort/comparison study • quasi-experimental/natural experiment • cross-sectional study (prospective/concurrent studies without experimental control)	Dx study in which at least one of the following applies: • independent blind comparison of subjects • set of nonconsecutive patients used or narrow spectrum of study individuals/patients, all of whom have undergone both assessment of interest and reference standard tests • independent blind/objective comparison of appropriate spectrum of subjects, but not all subjects tested with reference standard	• SR (with homogeneity) of retrospective cohort studies or untreated control groups in RCTs • single retrospective cohort study or untreated control groups in RCTs • outcomes research	B
IV	nonrandomized case-control or historical cohort/comparison study (subjects drawn from two or more different time periods; at least partially retrospective)	Dx study in which any of the following applies: • reference standard was unobjective, unblinded, or not independently applied • study was performed in an inappropriate spectrum of individuals (eg, patients with 2 different known dx/conditions)	• case series study • poor-quality prognostic cohort study (biased sampling in favor of patients, who already have target outcome, or measured outcomes in less than 80% of subjects, or outcomes determined in unblinded or nonobjective way, or no correction for confounding factors)	C
V	case series or case report without controls			C

*Note that etiology and intervention studies are rated on the same basis because both are concerned with determining cause-and-effect relationships. Multiple randomized controlled trials, or RCTs, with random assignment of subjects to groups (intervention) or experiments (etiology) are better than single RCTs or experiments, which are, in turn, stronger than comparisons made without experimental controls for confounding variables.
** A recommendation for practice for inclusion in a clinical practice guideline (CPG). Recommendation is made on the bases of available evidence of high to low quality. Recommendations based on higher levels of evidence (eg, Level I) are made with more confidence relative to the external (research) evidence and receive higher grades (eg, A). Research evidence-based recommendations for practice should be integrated with clinical judgment and patient perspectives before application to an individual patient.
† SR = Systematic Review (including metanalysis). Systematic reviews are usually quantitative in nature and follow explicit criteria for study inclusion/exclusion and evidence quality appraisal.
Note: Appraisers should consider downgrading studies (eg, rate as Level IV instead of III) when the research design fits one level but the implementation of the methods is significantly flawed.

Source: Data from C. Ball et al, Levels of Evidence and Grades of Recommendations, Center for Evidence Based Medicine, http://cebm.jr2.ox.ac.uk/docs/levels, 7/31/00, A. Laupacis et al, How to Use an Article About Prognosis, Evidence Base Medicine Working Group, Journal of the American Medical Association, Vol. 272, No. 3, pp.234–237, © 1994, American Medical Association, and Rebecca Lewthwaite, PhD, Rancho Los Amigos National Rehabilitation Center and the University of Southern California.

common in all areas attempting either to prepare practice guidelines or to synthesize findings (such as with the Cochrane reports). Grading systems for research share some similarities. The gold standard for intervention efficacy, effectiveness, and etiology is the RCT because of the power and strength of these types of studies. Other study designs used for these purposes receive lower ratings based on the rigor of the research, and evidence that comes from expert opinion or authority is typically rated the lowest. For studies about diagnosis/evaluation and prognosis, RCTs are not the gold standard; other features must be present.[15] The best available external evidence may include basic research or research "borrowed" from a similar or adjacent diagnosis, assuming that there is no compelling reason to rule out this evidence as applicable. The AHCPR panel recognized this deficit in the evidence-based literature and included animal studies as level II evidence. However, the dearth of high-quality evidence resulted in grading most of the recommendations in the pressure ulcer guidelines as a "C."

Sackett[17] developed a hierarchy of levels of scientific evidence that has evolved over the ensuing years through his efforts and those of others in his group. As a consequence, the present evidence-based medicine hierarchy provides more rigor in categorizing studies from higher to lower levels of evidence, with I the highest level and V the lowest, than was done in the past. Recommendations for clinical practice are then graded A, B, or C, depending on the level of scientific evidence that supports the recommendations. The hierarchy of evidence has become more sophisticated and expanded from the classifications that were used by the panel commissioned by the AHCPR. Exhibit I–2 shows an adaptation of Sackett's level of evidence table and relationship to grade of recommendations by Lewthwaite.[15] This table includes information about the classification of the study as it relates to etiology/intervention, diagnosis/evaluation, and prognosis. The process of evaluating evidence is not static and is expected to continue its evolution.

Systematic reviews have criteria for grading research. For example, the PEDro method of scoring is based on the number of "yes" answers to 10 criteria—the more "yes" answers, the higher the score will be for the study. The 10 items include random and concealed allocation; baseline comparability; blind assessors; blind subjects; blind therapists; adequate follow-up; intention to treat analysis; between-group comparisons; point estimates and variability; and eligibility criteria. Once the research paper is graded, it can be categorized according to the level of evidence hierarchy.

Practical Guidelines for Using EBP

Skepticism about the utility and appropriate use of EBP remains within the medical community.[3,18] There are those who express doubt that the busy clinician faced with a unique

Exhibit I–2 Strength of Evidence Levels Used by the AHCPR in Providing Support for Recommendations in the Clinical Practice Guidelines for Pressure Ulcer Treatment

A. Results of two or more randomized controlled clinical trials on pressure ulcers in humans provide support.
B. Results of two or more controlled clinical trials on pressure ulcers in humans provide support or, when appropriate, results of two or more controlled trials in an animal model provide indirect support.
C. This rating requires one or more of the following: (1) results of one controlled trial; (2) results of at least two case series/descriptive studies on pressure ulcers in humans; or (3) expert opinion.

Source: Reprinted with permission from Bergstrom et al., (1994)Treatment of Pressure Ulcers, *Clinical Practice Guideline, No. 15*, U.S. Department of Health and Human Services: Public Health Service Agency for Health Care Policy and Research, AHCPR Publication No. 95-0652, December 1994.

patient situation will resort to research for "correct" ways to treat patients. The clinician is apt to find that the research will produce contradictory findings regarding the effectiveness of a specific treatment, that there are discrepancies between the patients described in the study literature and the patient being seen, and that there are discrepancies between clinicians about the best treatment approach. Difficulties in research utilization are not new, and the issues remain the same—how best to institute change within an organizational setting. The problems of translating research to clinical practice leads to using inference rather than direct application of research. The translation is based on the judgment of the clinician about the extent of similarity between studies and the patient who receives treatment. As long as inference is required to translate the research to clinical practice, there will be no proof that any treatment plan is absolutely 100% the best or most appropriate choice for the patient.[18]

How, then, should clinicians proceed? Audits in medicine, surgery, psychiatry, and general practice have demonstrated that clinical services that strive to provide evidence-based care can do so for about four-fifths of their patients.[3] Clinicians should not despair about the discrepancies, controversies, and contradictions found in the literature but should use these findings to increase the dialogue about practice, increase research in the area, improve research methods, and, in turn, improve clinical practice. The best approach for EBP is a collaborative approach where each discipline contributes to the organizational culture of research used in practice. It is through collaboration that EBP may be more fully implemented within the realities of the current health care environment.

Evidence-Based Practice and This Book

Wound Care: A Collaborative Practice Manual for Physical Therapists and Nurses editors and contributors are here to help with the process of EBP. Each individual has applied his or her expert clinical judgment to select the pertinent literature, critically appraise the evidence, determine its clinical relevance, classify it, and pare down the information into clinically useful, patient-focused treatment decisions. The chapters are designed to present the evidence needed to narrow the focus of the clinician quickly toward answering pertinent clinical questions. A clinical example of how to research a question using this textbook is presented in Exhibit I–3.

The objectives at the beginning of each chapter and the review questions at the end have been prepared to focus the search for highly relevant information found within the chapter. Many chapters present synthesized pertinent research in matrices that show the elements of the studies at a glance. Where appropriate, matrices are used to show the clinical protocols used in the studies. Case studies, found in most chapters, focus on individual patients and the clinical decision-making expertise used by the case presenter when applying the evidence. The preappraised evidence and clinical decision making can be accessed by busy clinicians in seconds. Thus, both clinicians and students can use this textbook as a tool toward becoming proficient in the EBP process.

COLLABORATION

Physical therapy and nursing are the two health care disciplines most often involved in providing care for the patient with a wound. We believe one key to providing optimal wound care management to individuals with chronic wounds is collaborative practice between the health care disciplines. It has been our experience that, in clinical practice, true collaboration is not the standard, and, in many instances, there exists some level of conflict between disciplines, especially nursing and physical therapy. Conflicts may arise from misconceptions about the "other" discipline's ability, education level, or experience with wounds, from interpersonal differences, or from "turf battles," wherein one discipline is fighting with the other for greater control over the wound care segment of health care. Much of the conflict may be related to simple misunderstanding about the true nature of collaborative practice. True interdisciplinary collaboration does not require that one discipline "give up control" of wound care, nor does it require that clinicians always agree on management options for patients. An environment that supports a collaborative spirit allows clinicians from both disciplines to provide their unique perspectives to best meet the needs for each individual patient with a wound problem.

Exhibit I–3 Evidence-Based Practice Information from Wound Care: A Collaborative Practice Manual for Physical Therapists and Nurses—Clinical Example on How To Research a Question in This Text

> **Case Description:** 35-year-old male with spinal cord injury below T12 × 2 years. Two-month history of pressure ulcer on the right ischial tuberosity. Ulcer size: 8 cm² × 2 cm depth. Foul, copious drainage.
>
> **Initial treatment:** Whirlpool, debridement, and saline-soaked gauze dressings.
>
> **Reason for referral:** Prior treatment interventions have not progressed wound toward healing, and wound now shows clinical signs of infection.
>
> **Clinical Questions: What is etiology? What is the wound diagnosis? How can exudate and infection be managed? What is the prognosis? What interventions are appropriate and expected outcomes?**
> 1. **Etiology and prognosis:** Chapter 15, Pressure Ulcers: Pathophysiology and Prevention
> 2. **Wound Diagnosis:** Chapter 4, Assessment of the Skin and Wound
> 3. **Interventions and Expected Outcomes:**
>   - Chapter 16, Management of Pressure by Therapeutic Positioning
>   - Chapter 9, Management of Exudate and Infection
>   - Chapter 11, Management of the Wound Environment with Dressings and Topical Agents
>   - Chapter 12, Management of the Wound Environment with Advanced Therapies
>   - Chapter 21, Electrical Stimulation for Wound Healing
>   - Chapter 22, Pulsed Electromagnetic Fields
>   - Chapter 23, Ultraviolet Light and Wound Healing
>   - Chapter 25, Whirlpool
>   - Chapter 26, Pulsed Lavage with Suction

Collaboration is challenging. The challenges to collaboration include the wide variety of clinical settings in which patients with wounds are managed, the variety of education and experience of clinicians, and the struggles of each discipline to clarify and better define professional roles. Yet when collaboration is implemented successfully, the rewards to clinicians, payers, health care agencies, and patients are numerous. Clinicians benefit from the free exchange of ideas from differing perspectives and the excitement of working as a team to solve patient problems. Payers and health care settings benefit from fewer duplicated services and better patient outcomes at lower costs. Patients benefit from improved wound healing management, including better wound healing outcomes, as a result of health care service integration. To practice in a collaborative spirit, each discipline must understand the process of wound healing, chronic wound difficulties, and the skills and services offered by each discipline. Each practitioner has areas of knowledge that, by definition, are not shared by others. Yet both physical therapy and nursing practice have many similarities.

The main purpose of this book is to provide basic as well as more advanced information on wound healing and wound care therapies to nurses, physical therapists (PTs), and other health care team members in a user-friendly resource volume for clinicians who deal with wounds on a daily basis and who do not have access to a "wound care expert." A secondary purpose of this manual is to promote collaborative wound management between nurses and PTs by providing a better understanding of the similarities and differences between disciplines. This book is for nurses and PTs in acute care, rehabilitation, long-term care, outpatient care, and home health care settings. The book is formatted for use as a quick reference guide in any clinical setting. The book is designed to appeal to several groups of nurses. Certified wound, ostomy, continence nurses and certified wound care nurses (CWCNs) are often consulted on wound care and have additional education in wound care. CWCNs may find the book a direct aid to their practices and a valuable educational tool for use with other clinicians involved in wound care. Home health care nurses and nurses in long-term care settings, in conjunction with PTs, provide direct wound care in the home and long-term care setting with minimal support or education in new technologies for wound care diagnosis or management. Rehabilitation nurses work with spinal cord-injured patients; these patients are a high-risk group for pressure ulcer wounds, and treatment of pressure ulcers is one of the main points in the book. Advanced practice nurses, nurse practitioners, and clinical nurse specialists, who see large numbers of geriatric patients, will find the book a valuable tool for assessment, diagnosis, and treatment. PTs will find the text valuable as a reference for therapy and as an educational tool for use with other health care professionals. PTs are being asked to do more in the wound care arena, and many feel the need for additional education in this dynamic area. EBP provides an excellent methodology for collaborative practice.

EDUCATION OF NURSES AND PHYSICAL THERAPISTS

Nurses are licensed health care professionals who diagnose and treat human responses to health and illness.[19] The nursing profession is committed to the care and nurturing of both healthy and ill people, individually or in groups and communities. There are four essential features of contemporary nursing practice, as defined by the American Nurses' Association Social Policy Statement: "Attention to the full range of human experiences and responses to health and illness without restriction to a problem-focused orientation, integration of objective data with knowledge gained from an understanding of the patient or group's subjective experience, application of scientific knowledge to the processes of diagnosis and treatment, and provision of a caring relationship that facilitates health and healing."[20(p6)] The difference between professional and technical nurses is the depth and breadth of clinical nursing practice, based on the knowledge foundation of the nurse, the nurse's role, and the type of patient service.[21] Nurses study biologic, physical, and social sciences, in addition to nursing theory and the science of nursing practice. Nurses acquire knowledge in anatomy, physiology, pathophysiology, pharmacology, microbiology, chemistry, and statistics, as well as nursing science. Nursing education includes the traditional focus on illness and acute care clinical practice and the more pressing current focus on health promotion and community nursing.

Nurses practice at a variety of educational levels. The vocational or practical nurse education programs are located in technical or vocational schools. The vocational nurse education program is typically 1 year in length and leads to a certificate of completion and eligibility to take the state licensure examination to be designated as a licensed vocational nurse (LVN) or a licensed practical nurse (LPN). LPNs and LVNs are prepared to work with and be supervised by registered nurses (RNs). The purpose of the vocational nurse programs is to prepare assistant licensed nurse workers.[22] These programs generally do not articulate well with collegiate nursing programs, although LPNs/LVNs may receive advanced placement in collegiate programs.

The first formal nursing education in the United States was in diploma programs. Diploma programs are typically hospital based and were the predominant model for nursing education in this country. Diploma programs are usually 2–3 years in length, and many include summer sessions. Graduates of diploma programs are eligible to take the RN licensure examination. The purpose of the diploma programs is to prepare clinically competent bedside nurses.[22] Some diploma programs have now aligned with other academic institutions, and many now offer an associate degree in nursing—ADN or AA.[23] Associate degree programs are community or junior college based, and the nursing portion is 2 years in length. The purpose of the associate degree nursing programs is to prepare competent technical bedside nurses for secondary care settings.[22] Many nurses enter associate degree programs with future intentions of continuing their education in nursing at the baccalaureate level.[23] Some 4-year university programs also offer combination degree programs to allow flexibility.

Baccalaureate programs in nursing are 4 years in length, with the nursing curriculum typically concentrated at the upper division. Graduates of baccalaureate programs are prepared as nurse generalists to practice nursing in beginning leadership positions in a variety of settings. In 1965, the American Nurses' Association designated the baccalaureate degree as the entry level for professional nursing practice. The majority of programs admit both prelicensure students and RNs who are graduates of diploma or associate degree programs. The general education requirements are the same for all students, and those with prior nursing education or experience are allowed to progress through the nursing curriculum by designs that capitalize on prior learning.

Master's degree education in nursing is typically 2 years in length and builds on the baccalaureate nursing major. Program content usually includes a group of core graduate-level courses, research course work, and specialty nursing courses. Master's-prepared nurses function at an advanced practice level and include nurse anesthetists, nurse midwives, nurse practitioners, and clinical nurse specialists. The degree most often awarded on completion of a master's program is the MSN (master of science in nursing) or the MN (master of nursing) degree. The purpose of master's education in nursing is to prepare advanced practice nurses in a specialty area, such as adult nurse practitioners, psychiatric mental health nursing, or nursing management.[23] In addition, advanced practice nurses serve as mentors, consultants, and educators of nurses in basic practice. They conduct research to expand the knowledge base of nursing practice, provide leadership for practice changes, and contribute to the advancement of the profession, health care, and society in general.[20]

Doctoral programs in nursing range from 3 to 5 years of full-time study. Doctoral programs include advanced content in concept development, theoretical analysis, research, statistics, advanced nursing, and supporting cognates or electives. Doctoral programs prepare leaders for programs in education, administration, clinical practice, and research.

In addition to formal education programs, many nurses are specialty certified. The need for specialization in nursing developed as technologic advances in health care occurred over the last 10 years. Specialty programs are varied in scope, length of time, and requirements. Most specialty programs prepare RNs to take a certification examination as a part of credentialing in the specialty area. Certification requirements vary, depending on the specialty area, and may include completion of an education or training program, as well as clinical experience requirements. National certification examinations are offered through professional organizations in a variety of specialties, including wound care and enterostomal therapy nursing. In most states, RNs are required to maintain currency in their practice by completing specified amounts of continuing education.

PTs are licensed health care professionals who evaluate and treat people with health problems resulting from disease or injury. The American Physical Therapy Association (APTA) is the national organization representing the physical therapy profession, which accredits education programs for PTs and PT assistants (PTAs). Professional education required for PTs includes a minimum of 4 years of college or university level training, resulting in a baccalaureate degree in physical therapy from an accredited professional education program. After 2002, a post-baccalaureate degree will be required for entry level. The information explosion in the health-related sciences has led to current requirements that most therapists enter the profession as master's level-prepared clinicians. Now there is a trend toward entry-level and postclinical doctoral education. Nearly half of the physical therapist education programs have either developed or indicated an interest in developing such education. This is in keeping with the APTA vision 2020 goal to have PT services provided by doctors of PT in 2020.[24]

Following graduation, PTs must pass a national licensing examination to qualify for state licensure. Like nurses, PTs may be specialty certified in a variety of areas of practice. Although there is no current specialty certification for wound care, instruction in wound management skills is a requirement for accreditation of PT and PTA programs. The requirements for continuing education for relicensure by PTs varies by state. The fact is that most PTs seek continuing education so as to be at the cutting edge of practice, even though it may not be a mandated requirement. The Wound Management Special Interest Group within the Section on Clinical Electrophysiology of the APTA was formed to bring together PTs and PTAs from many practice settings who have special interest in wound management.

PTAs are trained and licensed paraprofessionals with 2 years of educational training in an approved PTA program or who have worked as a physical therapy aide for a specific period of time and have then passed a qualifying examination. The PTA provides services under the supervision of a PT. The PTA can perform various tests and measures for which the assistant is trained, such as wound measurements, tissue attribute recording, and provision of treatment services with physical agents and electrotherapeutic modalities. Both PTs and PTAs are qualified to apply topical agents and dressings to wounds; however, only PTs should perform sharp wound debridement.

Many individuals are surprised that the PT is included in the wound management team. Reports of wound management, including burn and wound interventions, by PTs have appeared in the physical therapy literature for more than three decades. By education and training, PTs learn anatomy, physiology, and pathophysiology related to body systems responsible for repair and regeneration of soft tissue. For example, human cadaver dissection is part of the basic anatomy education of the PT and provides a foundation for the skills needed in sharp debridement of nonviable tissue.

Courses in cardiopulmonary and vascular system physiology are required. These two systems are critical to wound healing. Neuropathy plays an important part in development of chronic wounds. PTs take courses in neurology and learn neurologic testing and effects of insensitivity on the integumentary system. The PT is expected to examine the integument as part of an overall evaluation. Postsurgical wounds are routinely seen and evaluated by the PT as part of the rehabilitation service. For example, dehiscence of a wound on an amputated limb requires wound management before prosthetic training is initiated. PTs also are skilled in the use of physical agents (heat, light, sound, and water), electrotherapeutic modalities, and therapeutic exercise, all of which are used in wound healing strategies. The PT can manage the wound, as well as the prosthetic training and an exercise program to achieve the desired outcomes. PTs are interested in evidence-based health care choices, and many research studies by PTs on wound healing that demonstrate treatment efficacy are cited in this book.

Physical therapy represents the care and services provided by or under the direct supervision of a PT.[25] Services provided by others using technologies generically referred to as physical therapy should not be confused with the services of a PT. Outcomes research studies show that expected outcomes may not be equivalent.[26] PTs are important players in the provision of primary care, defined as "integrated accessible health care services by clinicians who are accountable for addressing a large majority of personal health care need, developing a sustained partnership with patients and practicing in the context of family and community."[27(p712)] In 30 states, direct access to physical therapy services from a licensed PT is part of the practice acts. PTs play major roles in secondary and tertiary care, as well. For example, patients with wounds are often seen initially by another health care practitioner, then referred to the PT. PTs provide tertiary care in highly specialized, complex, and technologically advanced settings. In such situations, a patient may have a traumatic wound, surgical wound, or burn plus complicating medical problems, and the PT is called upon to manage the wound, as well as the other aspects of patient rehabilitation.

WOUND SPECIALIST CERTIFICATION

In October 1999, the first American Academy of Wound Management (AAWM) board certification examination was held. The examination consists of 150 multiple-choice questions. Multiple references are used in the question development process, including *Wound Care: A Collaborative Practice Manual for Physical Therapists and Nurses*. Three levels of certification are available, depending on the level of academic training. Levels 2 (Fellow) and 3 (Diplomat) certification require at least 2 years of clinical or research experience in

wound care. Level 1 (Clinical Associate level) requires 5 years of clinical or research experience and licensure in the related health discipline. AAWM was founded and incorporated in 1995 as a voluntary not-for-profit organization and is dedicated to the multidisciplinary team approach in promoting the science of prevention, care, and treatment of acute and chronic wounds.[28] The purpose of the certification is to recognize competence in the field of wound management and research. By 2000, nearly 1,300 individuals from many disciplines were certified as wound specialists.[29]

DATABASES

The National Guideline Clearinghouse
www.guideline.gov/index.asp contains a large database of evidence-based clinical practice guidelines. The mission of the clearinghouse is to encourage the dissemination, implementation, and use of clinical practice guidelines.

Cochrane Library of Systematic Reviews
www.update-software.com/cochrane/cochrane-frame.html

National Library of Medicine: PubMed
www.ncbi.nlm.nih.gov/PubMed

Cumulative Index of Nursing and Allied Health Literature (CINAHL—proprietary)

Physiotherapy Evidence Database (PEDro)
www.cchs.usyd.edu.au/pedro

Center for Evidence-Based Medicine
http://cebm.jr2.ox.ac.uk

RESOURCES

Wound Ostomy and Continence Nurses Society (WOCN)
1550 S. Coast Highway, Suite 201
Laguna Beach, CA 92651
Phone: (888) 224-WOCN
http://www.wocn.org

American Physical Therapy Association (APTA)
1111 North Fairfax St.
Alexandria, VA 22314-1488
Phone: (800) 999-APTA
http://www.apta.org

APTA Clinical Electrophysiology Section/Wound Management Special Interest Group
http://www.aptasce.com

American Academy of Wound Management (AAWM)
1255 23rd St., NW
Washington, DC 20037
Phone: (202) 521-0368, FAX (202) 833-3636
http://www.aawm.org
e-mail: woundnet@aawm.org

REFERENCES

1. Sackett D, Rosenberg W, Muir-Gray J, et al. Evidence based medicine: What it is and what it isn't. *Br Med J.* 1996;312(13 January):71–72.

2. Burns N, Grove S, eds. *Outcomes Research. In the Practice of Nursing Research: Conduct, Critique, and Utilization.* 4th ed. Philadelphia: WB Saunders; 2001:287–329.

3. Straus S, Sackett D. Using research findings in clinical practice. *Br Med J.* 1999;318(30 January):332–333.

4. Levi S. Evidenced-based practice. *Gerinotes.* 2000;7(5):11–12, 23.

5. Straus S, Sackett D. Using research findings in clinical practice. *Br Med J.* 1998;317(1 August):339–342.

6. Bero L, Ar J. How consumers and policymakers can use systematic reviews for decision making. *Ann Int Med.* 1997;127:37–42.

7. Garrard J. Introduction. In: *Health Sciences Literature Review Made Easy.* Gaithersburg, MD: Aspen Publishers; 1999:4–20.

8. Field M, Lohr K, eds. *Institute of Medicine. Clinical Practice Guidelines: Directions for a New Program.* Washington, DC: National Academy Press; 1990:39.

9. Bergstrom N, Allman RM, Carlson CE, et al. *Pressure Ulcers in Adults: Prediction and Preventions.* Rockville, MD: U.S. Department of Health and Human Services (DHHS); 1992.

10. Bergstrom N, Allman RM, Carlson CE, et al. *Clinical Practice Guideline: Treatment of Pressure Ulcers.* Rockville, MD: DHHS, U.S. Public Health Service (PHS), Agency for Health Care Research and Quality (AHRQ), formerly known as the Agency for Health Care Policy and Research (AHCPR); 1994.

11. Taler G, Bauman T, Breeding C, et al. *Pressure Ulcers: Clinical Practice Guideline.* Columbia, MD: American Medical Directors Association; 1996:1–14.

12. Beitz JM, Burton CS, Kerstein MD, et al. *Venous Leg Ulcer Guideline.* Philadelphia: University of Pennsylvania; 1997:45.

13. Krasner D, Sibbald G. Moving beyond the AHCPR guidelines: Wound care evolution over the last five years. *Ostomy/Wound Manage.* 1999;45(1A Suppl):6S–118S.

14. Garber SL, Biddle AK, Click CN, et al. *Pressure Ulcer Prevention and Treatment following Spinal Cord Injury: A Clinical Practice Guideline for Health-Care Professionals.* Jackson Heights, NY: Paralyzed Veterans of America; 2000:12–14.

15. Lethwaite R. *Levels of Evidence and Grades of Recommendations: Quality Ratings.* Los Angeles: Rancho Los Amigos Rehabilitation Center and the University of Southern California; 2001.

16. *National Guideline Clearinghouse.* 1999. http://www.guideline.gov/index.asp. Rockville, MD.

17. Sackett D. Rules of evidence and clinical recommendations on the use of antithrombotic agents. *Chest.* 1989;95(2):2s–4s.

18. Fabio RP. Myth of evidence-based practice. *J Orthop Sports Phys Ther.* 1999;29(11):632–34.

19. American Nurses' Association. *Nursing: A Social Policy Statement.* Kansas City, MO; 1980.

20. American Nurses' Association. *Nursing's Social Policy Statement.* Washington, DC; 1995.

21. American Nurses' Association. *Facts about Nursing.* Kansas City, MO; 1987.

22. Hart SE. Pathways of nursing education. In: Creasia JL, Parker B, eds. *Conceptual Foundations of Professional Nursing Practice.* 2nd ed. St. Louis, MO: CV Mosby; 1996:26–45.

23. Kozier B, Erb G, Blais K. *Professional Nursing Practice: Concepts and Perspectives.* 3rd ed. Menlo Park, CA: Addison-Wesley; 1997:2–27.

24. DPT Programs on Rise. *PT Bulletin Online.* 2001;2(13). Accessed March 23, 2001.

25. American Physical Therapy Association. A guide to physical therapist practice. I: A description of patient management. *Phys Ther.* 1995;75:707–764.

26. American Physical Therapy Association. *Outcomes Effectiveness of Physical Therapy: An Annotated Bibliography.* Alexandria, VA; 1994.

27. Donaldson M, Yordy K, Vanselow N. *Defining Primary Care: An Interim Report.* Washington, DC: National Academy Press; 1994.

28. Evans C. History of the American Academy of Wound Management. *Adv Skin Wound Care.* 1999;12(6):310–311.

29. American Academy of Wound Management, http://www.aawm.org. Accessed March 2001.

SUGGESTED READING

Bury T, Mead J. *Evidence-Based Healthcare: A Practical Guide for Therapists.* Boston: Butterworth Heinemann; 1998.

Garrard J. *Health Sciences Literature Review Made Easy.* Gaithersburg, MD: Aspen Publishers; 1999.

Sackett DL, Richardson WS, Rosenberg W, Haynes RB. *Evidence-Based Medicine: How To Practice and Teach EBM.* New York: Churchill-Livingstone; 1997.

COLOR PLATES

PROGRESSION THROUGH THREE PHASES OF WOUND HEALING
Plates 1–6

The patient is a 97-year-old nursing home resident with Stage IV pressure ulcers in the bilateral rib cage and sacral area.

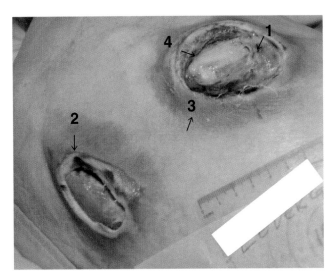

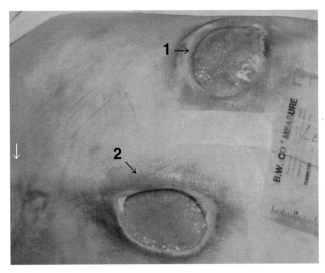

1. Chronic wound converted to acute inflammatory phase.
   (1) Yellow, stringy slough;
   (2) Edema;
   (3) Skin color changes (red), erythema;
   (4) Rib bone noted in superior ulcer.
   Wound healing phase diagnosis: acute inflammatory phase.
   Wound severity diagnosis: Impaired integumentary integrity secondary to skin involvement extending into fascia, muscle, bone. (Stage IV pressure ulcer.)
   Source: Reprinted with permission, copyright © C. Sussman.

2. Same wound as in Plate 1.
   (1) Rolled epidermal ridge around granulation base;
   (2) Brown hemosiderin staining (hemosiderosis).
   Wound healing phase: proliferative phase.
   Source: Reprinted with permission, copyright © C. Sussman.

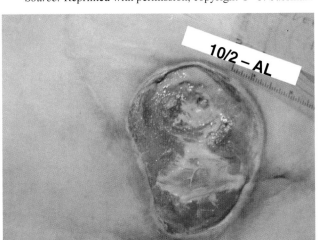

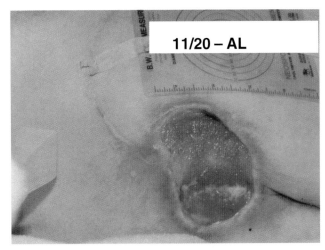

3. Same patient as in Plate 1. Chronic wound: converted to acute proliferative phase. This is a sacral wound with stringy, yellow slough evident. Note example of epidermal ridge formation. Predominant wound healing phase diagnosis: Proliferative phase. Wound severity diagnosis: same as in Plate 1.
   Source: Reprinted with permission, copyright © C. Sussman.

4. Same wound as Plate 3 progressing through the proliferative phase of healing. Wound contracting and proliferating. Note change in size, shape, depth, and new healthy granulation tissue compared to Plate 3.
   Source: Reprinted with permission, copyright © C. Sussman.

1

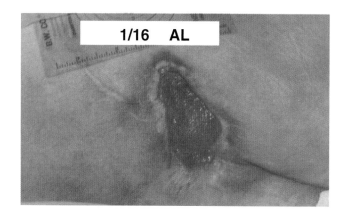

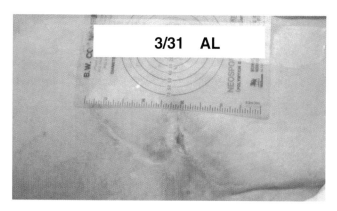

5. Note sustained wound contraction evident between Plates 4 and 5. Note epithelialization (light pink) along wound edges. Wound is in both epithelialization and proliferative phases.
Source: Reprinted with permission, copyright © C. Sussman.

6. The wound is completely resurfaced. It is in the remodeling phase.
Source: Reprinted with permission, copyright © C. Sussman.

PROGRESSION THROUGH PROLIFERATIVE PHASE
Plates 7–9

Plates 7 to 9 show a sacral pressure ulcer progressing from chronic inflammatory phase through the proliferative phase of wound healing. In Plates 8 and 9 the wound edges demonstrate epithelial migration with new epidermis clearly visible as bright pink in this dark-skinned patient in Plates 7 to 9.

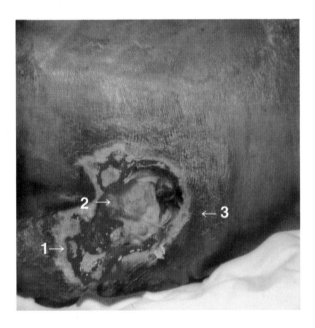

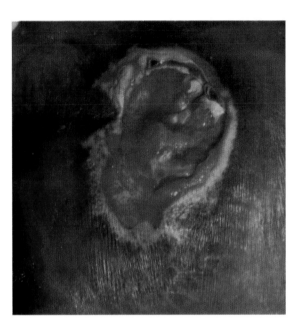

7. Chronic inflammatory phase. Note the following wound characteristics:
   (1) Sanguineous drainage;
   (2) Muscle exposure;
   (3) Hemosiderin staining surrounding the wound.
   Source: Reprinted with permission, copyright © B.M. Bates-Jensen.

8. Acute proliferative phase. Note the attached wound edges from the 12-o'clock to 6-o'clock positions and how well vascularized granulation tissue fills up one side of the ulcer. New pink border of epithelium surrounds the granulation tissue.
   Source: Reprinted with permission, copyright © B.M. Bates-Jensen.

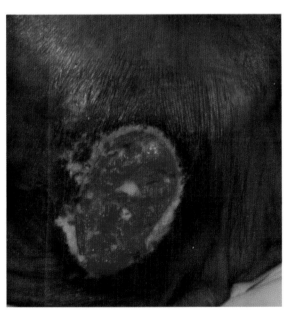

9. All of the wound edges are now attached to wound base. Note the presence of fibrin (yellow) within the granulation tissue. Ready for epithelialization phase.
   Source: Reprinted with permission, copyright © B.M. Bates-Jensen.

ABNORMAL PROLIFERATIVE PHASE
Plates 10 and 11

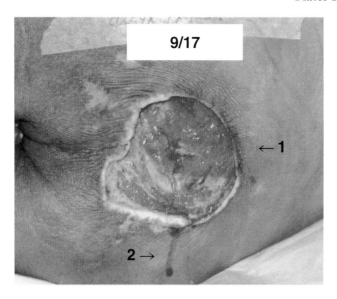

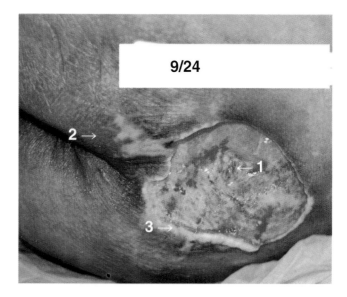

10. Acute proliferative phase.
    (1) Hemosiderin staining;
    (2) Sanguineous drainage.
    Source: Reprinted with permission, copyright © B.M. Bates-Jensen.

11. Chronic proliferative phase with attributes of infection.
    (1) Hemorrhagic area of trauma;
    (2) Hypopigmentation;
    (3) Dull pink granulation tissue.
    Source: Reprinted with permission, copyright © B.M. Bates-Jensen.

WOUND IN REMODELING PHASE
Plate 12

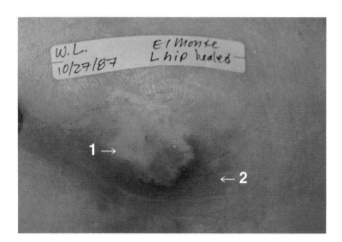

12. An example of a wound in the remodeling phase of wound healing.
    (1) New epithelium (scar);
    (2) Hyperpigmentation (Hemosiderin-staining).
    Source: Reprinted with permission, copyright © B.M. Bates-Jensen.

ANATOMY OF SOFT TISSUE
Plate 13

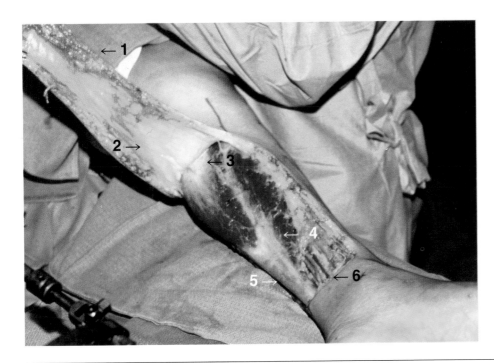

13. Full-thickness skin resected from calf.
(1) Vascularized dermis;
(2) Yellow healthy fat tissue;
(3) White fibrous fascia;
(4) Dark red muscle tissue;
(5) Tendon covered with peritenon;
(6) Blood vessel.
Source: Reprinted with permission, copyright © J. Wethe.

WOUNDING OF THE SKIN
Plates 14–18

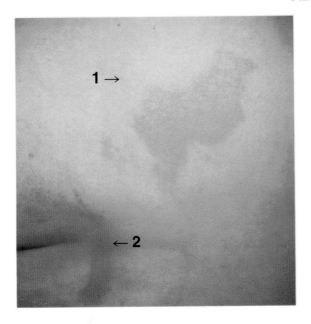

14. Superficial wounding of skin.
(1) This wound would be classified as a stage I pressure ulcer;
(2) This wound is perineal dermatitis. Note location over rectum.
Source: Reprinted with permission, copyright © B.M. Bates-Jensen.

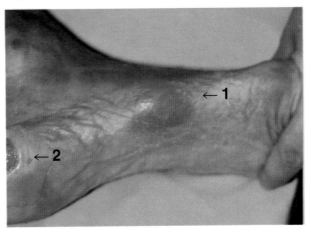

15. (1) Intact skin with subcutaneous microvascular bleeding (unblanchable erythema) suggesting deeper trauma located over a bony surface, and would be classified as a stage I pressure ulcer;
(2) Maceration of periwound skin.
Source: Reprinted with permission, copyright © B.M. Bates-Jensen.

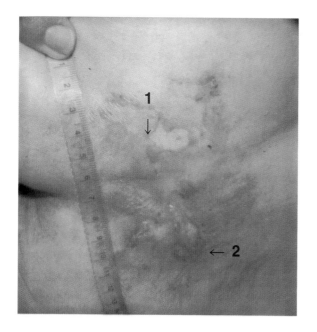

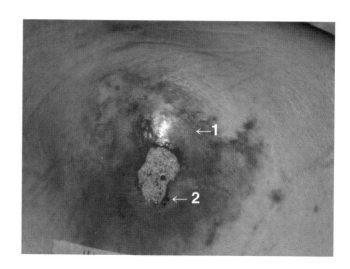

16. Perineal dermatitis with classic differentiating characteristics of diffuse erythema across buttocks and perineal area and partial-thickness skin loss. This wound is in the acute inflammatory phase and was not staged.
(1)   Multiple, partial-thickness lesions with irregular borders;
(2)   Lesions occur across area singly and in groups and may or may not be over a bony prominence.
Source: Reprinted with permission, copyright © B.M. Bates-Jensen.

17. Acute inflammatory phase, partial thickness stage II pressure ulcer located over bony prominence.
(1)   Erythema and edema;
(2)   Reticular layer of dermis.
Source: Reprinted with permission, copyright © B.M. Bates-Jensen.

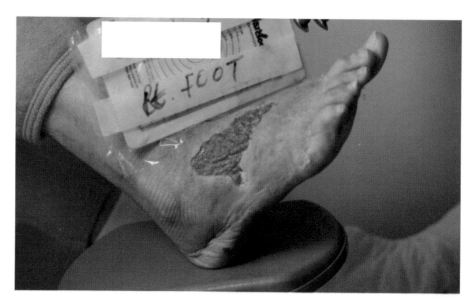

18. Full-thickness skin loss in the acute proliferative phase. The wound was not due to pressure and was not staged. Wound edges are soft and flexible to touch.
Source: Reprinted with permission, copyright © C. Sussman.

ASSESSMENT OF DARKLY PIGMENTED SKIN
Plates 19–22

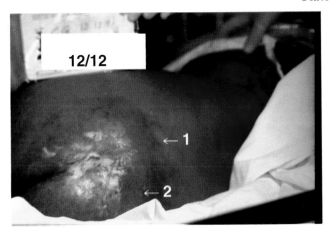

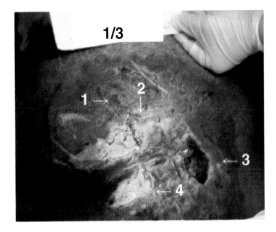

19. Pressure ulceration with multiple, small, stage II open areas. Wound is in acute inflammatory phase. Note onset date 12/12.
    (1) There is a clear line of dermarcation between healthy tissues and inflamed tissue;
    (2) Evidence of discoloration, edema, and induration suggest underlying tissue death. Assess tissue temperature and pain.
    Source: Reprinted with permission, copyright © C. Sussman.

20. Same pressure ulceration as in Plate 19. Three weeks later the skin now shows evidence of the severe tissue destruction that occurred at the time of trauma. Note delayed manifestation of injury at the skin level. The date was 1/3.
    (1) Continued demarcation of inflamed tissue;
    (2) Irregular diffuse wound edges;
    (3) Eschar, black, and adherent;
    (4) Partial-thickness skin loss. There is enlargement of stage II ulcers compared with those in Plate 19.
    The correct staging for this sacrococcygeal pressure ulcer is at minimum a stage III. Once eschar is removed, true depth of tissue loss can be determined. Documentation should reflect a combined area of wounding, including all three visible ulcers and the area of inflammation. This is the overall size estimate for the pressure ulcer. Inflammation now chronic.
    Source: Reprinted with permission, copyright © C. Sussman.

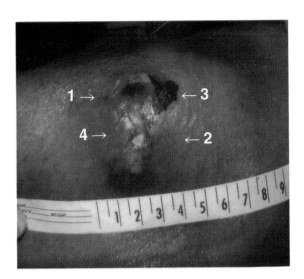

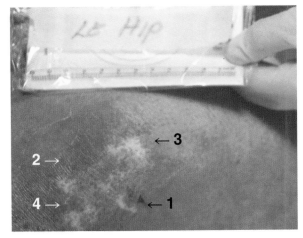

21. Assessment of inflammatory phase attributes in darkly pigmented skin.
    (1) Erythema gives skin a reddish brown glow;
    (2) Hemorrhage of microvasculature gives skin purplish gray hue;
    (3) Eschar—note tissue texture change to hard black;
    (4) Use skin color of adjacent skin for reference of normal skin tones.
    Source: Reprinted with permission, copyright © B.M. Bates-Jensen.

22. Assessment of epithelialization and remodeling attributes in darkly pigmented skin.
    (1) New epithelial tissue that is light red;
    (2) New scar tissue that lacks melanin and is bright pink;
    (3) Old scar tissue that lacks melanin and is silvery white;
    (4) Residual hemosiderin staining.
    Source: Reprinted with permission, copyright © C. Sussman.

ABNORMAL WOUND ATTRIBUTES
Plates 23–25

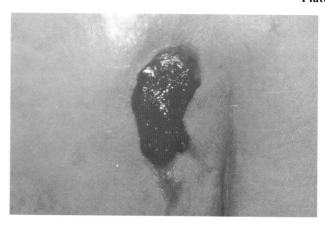

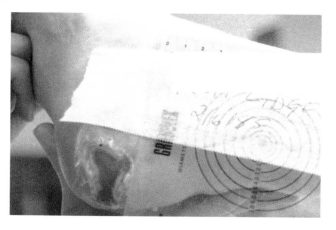

23. Wound is in chronic proliferative phase. Hypergranulation tissue; absence of epithelialization phase.
Source: Reprinted with permission, copyright © B.M. Bates-Jensen.

24. There is an absence of epithelialization phase. Hyperkeratosis on heel ulcer of a 100-year-old woman.
Source: Reprinted with permission, copyright © C. Sussman.

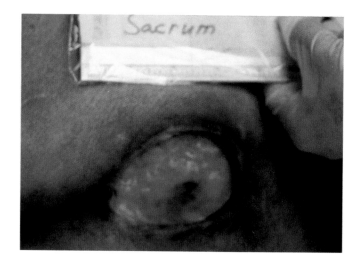

25. Wound is in chronic proliferative phase
    (1) Trauma to granulation tissue caused hemorrhagic spot that may go on to necrose.
    (2) Hemosiderin staining from prior bleeding surrounds ulcer. Wound is in chronic proliferative phase.
Source: Reprinted with permission, copyright © C. Sussman.

NECROTIC TISSUE TYPES
Plates 26–32

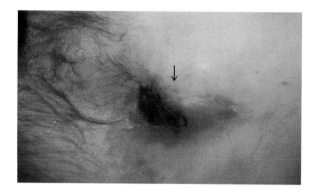

26. Hard, leathery eschar in the chronic inflammatory phase. Notice how the eschar looks similar to a scab.
Source: Reprinted with permission, copyright © B.M. Bates-Jensen.

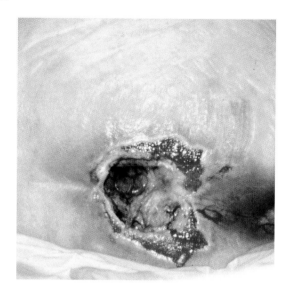

27. Soft, soggy, black eschar in the absence of inflammatory phase.
Source: Reprinted with permission, copyright © B.M. Bates-Jensen.

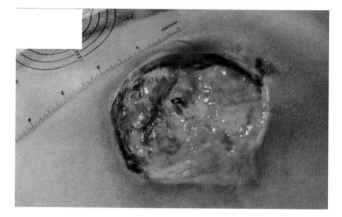

28. Chronic wound converted to acute inflammatory phase with yellow, mucinous slough.
Source: Reprinted with permission, copyright © C. Sussman.

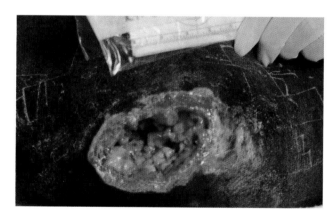

29. Necrotic fatty tissue.
Source: Reprinted with permission, copyright © C. Sussman.

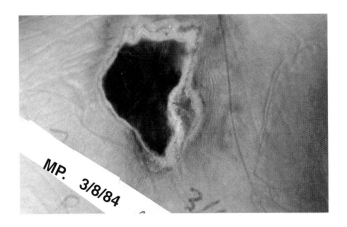

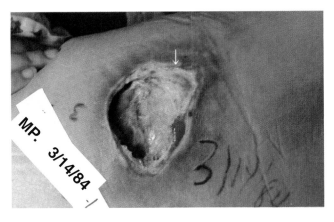

30. Eschar before debridement. Absence of inflammatory phase and proliferative phase.
Source: Reprinted with permission, copyright © C. Sussman.

31. Eschar after debridement. Necrotic fat and fascia often called slough. Restart of inflammatory phase. Absence of proliferative phase.
Source: Reprinted with permission, copyright © C. Sussman.

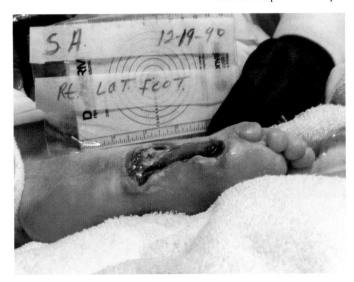

32. Soft soggy necrosis and bruising often referred to as "purple" ulcer. Foot shows signs of cellulitis and edema. Acute inflammatory phase.
Source: Reprinted with permission, copyright © C. Sussman.

WOUND EDGES
Plates 33–36

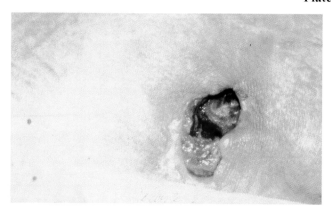

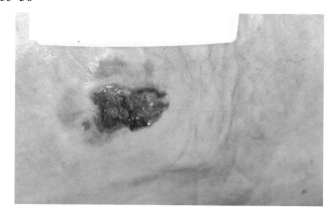

33. Absence of proliferative phase. Wound with no epithelialization present. The wound is clean, but nonprofilerating.
Source: Reprinted with permission, copyright © B.M. Bates-Jensen.

34. Same wound as in Plate 33. Wound is in acute proliferative phase with evidence of new epithelial migration.
Source: Reprinted with permission, copyright © B.M. Bates-Jensen.

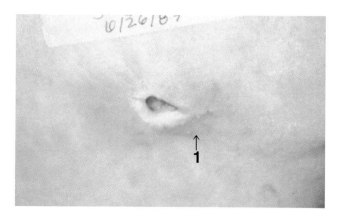

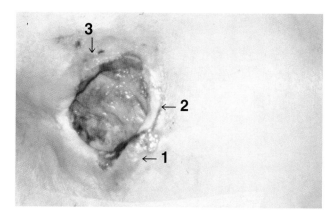

35. There is an absence of epithelialization phase.
 (1) Wound lacking epithelialization due to chronic fibrosis and scarring at wound edge. Edges achieve unique, grayish hue in both dark and lightly pigmented skin. Note rolled and thickened attributes. Chronic proliferative phase.
Source: Reprinted with permission, copyright © B.M. Bates-Jensen.

36. An example of knowledge gained from careful examination of the wound edge. This is an example of a chronic deep ulcer that does not bleed easily. Wound is in chronic proliferative phase.
 (1) New pressure-induced damage (hemorrhage);
 (2) Maceration from wound fluid;
 (3) Friction injury with signs of inflammation.
Source: Reprinted with permission, copyright © B.M. Bates-Jensen.

SURGICAL DISSECTION FOR TUNNELING
Plates 37 and 38

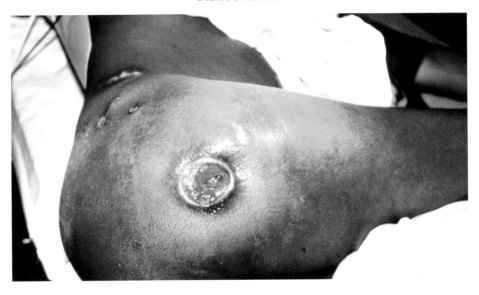

37. Unobservable tunneling.
Source: Reprinted with permission, copyright © J. Wethe.

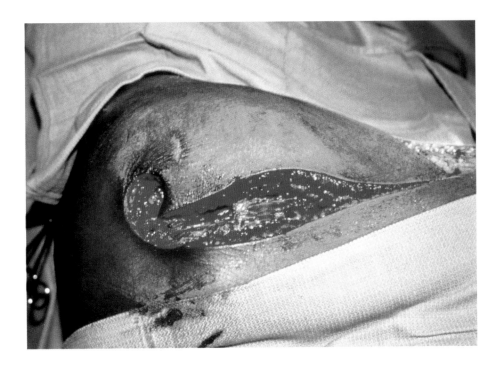

38. Same wound as Plate 37 with surgical dissection demonstrating the extent of the tunneling process, forming a sinus tract.
Source: Reprinted with permission, copyright © J. Wethe.

UNDERMINING AND TUNNELING
Plates 39–41

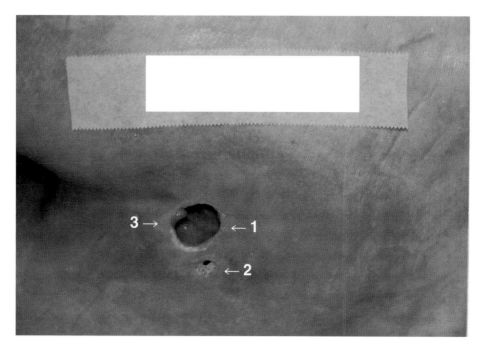

39. Wound with tunneling before insertion of a cotton-tipped applicator.
(1) Ulcer reoccurrence at site of old scar tissue;
(2) Skin bridge between two open ulcers;
(3) Surrounding skin has unblanchable erythema. Wound edges rolled under demonstrate chronic inflammatory phase;
(4) Absence of proliferative phase.
Source: Reprinted with permission, copyright © B.M. Bates-Jensen.

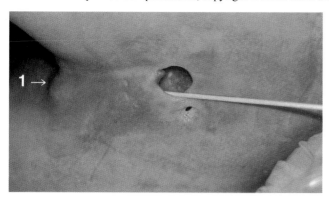

40. Same wound as in Plate 39. The wound overall size is much larger than the surface open area. Tunneling is present.
(1) Note bulge from end of cotton-tipped applicator.
Source: Reprinted with permission, copyright © B.M. Bates-Jensen.

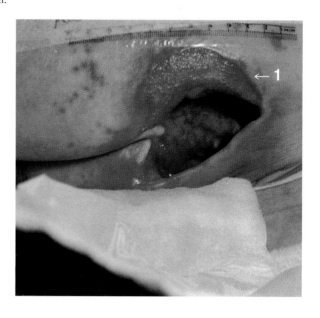

41. Undermined wound.
(1) Note shelf.
Source: Reprinted with permission, copyright © C. Sussman.

READING THE DRESSING: WOUND EXUDATE ASSESSMENT
Plates 42–47

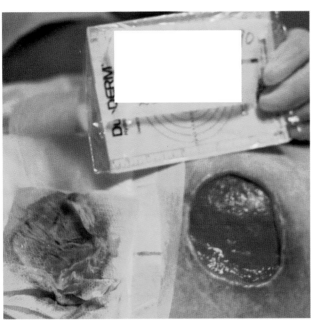

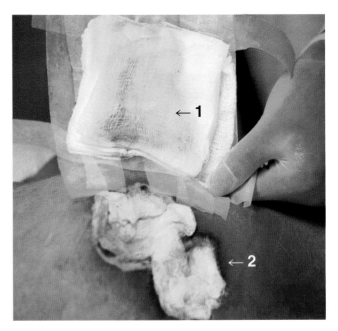

42. Wound appears "clean" but is in chronic proliferative phase. The quantity of exudate is determined by the amount of dressing saturated by the drainage.
(1) Moderate to large amount of sanguineous exudate;
(2) Moderate to large amount of purulent exudate;
(3) Evaluate for infection.
Source: Reprinted with permission, copyright © C. Sussman.

43. Wound with packing still present.
(1) Moderate amount of serous exudate on dressing;
(2) Green color of exudate suggests possible infection.
Source: Reprinted with permission, copyright © C. Sussman.

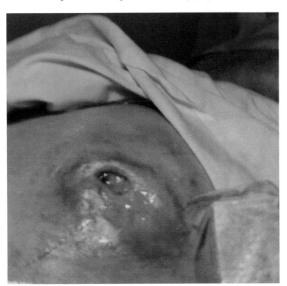

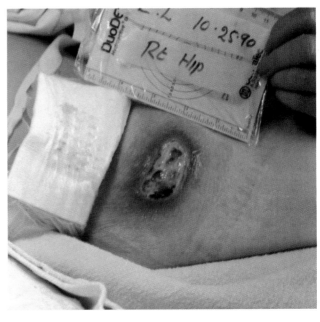

44. Wound with composite dressing. Dressing shows moderate amount of serosanguineous exudate. The wound bed shows gelatinous mass that may be gelatinous edema. Evaluate for trauma. Bright pink skin is scar tissue.
Source: Reprinted with permission, copyright © C. Sussman.

45. Wound with composite dressing shows scant amount of serous exudate. Wound is in chronic inflammatory phase. There is an absence of proliferative phase. Wound is Stage III pressure ulcer.
Source: Reprinted with permission, copyright © C. Sussman.

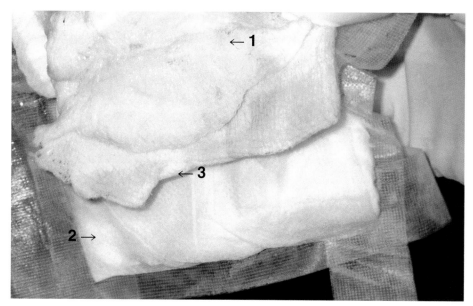

46. (1) Large amount of serous drainage;

(2) Note how drainage flows into secondary dressing;

(3) Note green tinge to edges of dressing, suggesting anaerobic infection (eg, pseudomonas). Monitor for a degenerative change in exudate type from present serous to purulent (eg, greener, thicker, and more opaque).

Source: Reprinted with permission, copyright © C. Sussman.

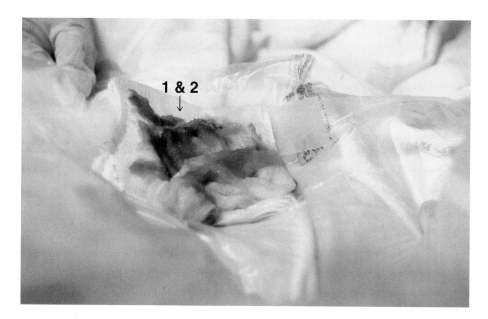

47. Large amount of purulent exudate.

(1) Thick, opaque cloudy appearance;

(2) Note green color. Assess for odor.

Source: Reprinted with permission, copyright © C. Sussman.

SCAR ATTRIBUTES
Plates 48–51

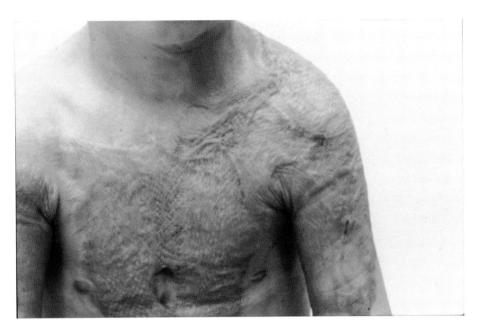

48. Hypertrophic scar.
Source: Copyright © 2001, R. Scott Ward, PT, PhD.

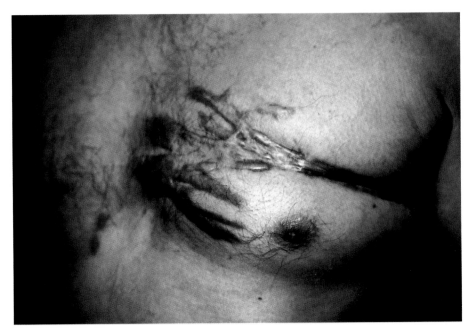

49. Immature keloid scar.
Source: Copyright © 2001, R. Scott Ward, PT, PhD.

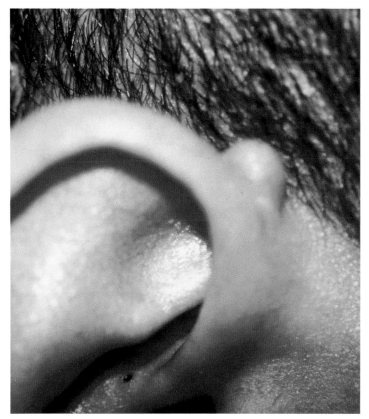

50. Keloid scar.
Source: Copyright © 2001, R. Scott Ward, PT, PhD.

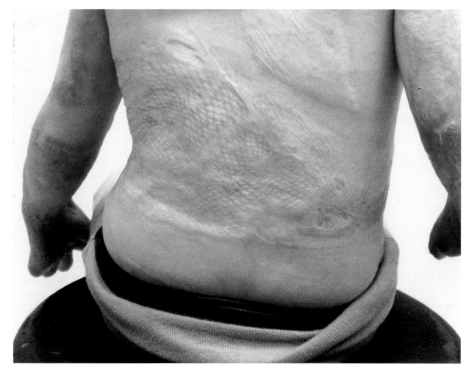

51. Maturing keloid scar.
Source: Copyright © 2001, R. Scott Ward, PT, PhD.

ARTERIAL ISCHEMIC WOUNDS
Plates 52–54

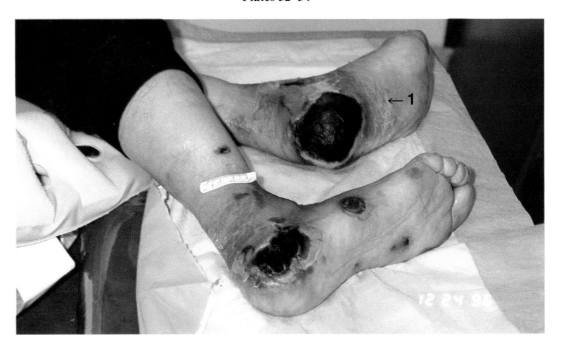

52. Severe arterial ischemic disease with multiple ischemic ulcers below the ankle bilaterally. Wounds are in absence of inflammatory phase with hard, dry, black eschar covering. Do not debride.

(1)   Note trophic changes on foot, evidence of scaling.

Source: Reprinted with permission, copyright © E. Fowler.

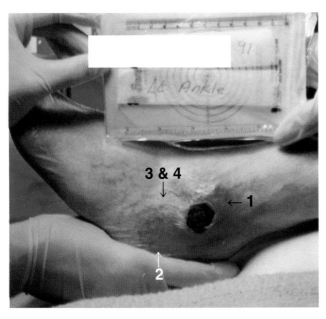

53. Classic ischemic ulcer. Note:
(1)   Chronic inflammation with cellulitis;
(2)   Punched-out ulcer edges;
(3)   Covering of dry, black eschar;
(4)   Location over lateral malleolus.
Source: Reprinted with permission, copyright © C. Sussman.

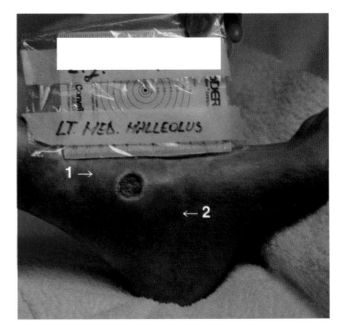

54. Ischemic ulcer in chronic proliferative phase and absence of epithelialization phase. Note:
(1)   Punched-out ulcer appearance with rolled wound edges;
(2)   Dependent rubor.
Source: Reprinted with permission, copyright © C. Sussman.

VENOUS DISEASE
Plates 55–60

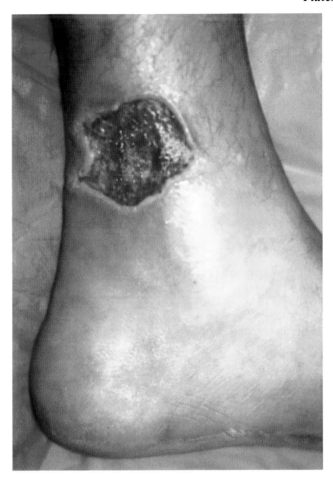

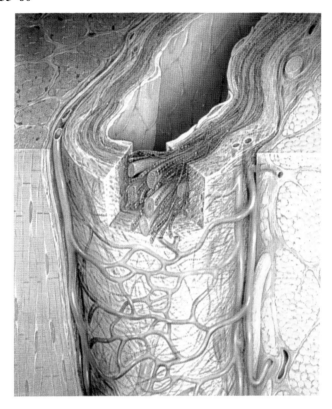

56. Structure of the venous wall. Cross-section of a venous branch of lower extremity reveals a relative standard wall structure. The intima is covered by uninterrupted endothelium which is connected to a thin connective tissue layer. The media is structured much more loosely than corresponding arteries, and is composed of distinct layers of collagenous and elastic fibers between which narrow strips of smooth muscle are found.
Source: Reprinted with permission, copyright © C. Donayre.

55. Ischemic ulcer in a 55-year-old male smoker with a 4-month history of having "blistered" his ankle with the subsequent formation of a painful ulcer. He was diagnosed as having a venous stasis ulcer and was treated with wet-to-dry dressing changes three times per day. Despite good compliance his ulcer failed to improve. The physical exam revealed absent femoral, popliteal, and pedal pulses with an ABI of 0.35. The ulcer edge was irregular, but the base was clean and had adequate granulation tissue. Even though the ulcer was located proximal to the medial malleolus, the typical location of chronic venous stasis ulcers, this patient did not exhibit any of the physical signs of chronic venous insufficiency such as brawny edema, hyperpigmentation, or stasis dermatitis. See Chapter 17, Diagnosis and Management of Vascular Ulcers, for photos of angiogram on same patient (Figure 17–4).
Source: Reprinted with permission, copyright © C. Donayre.

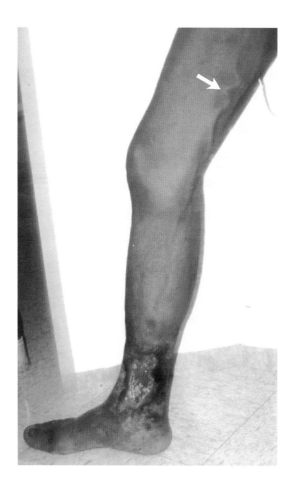

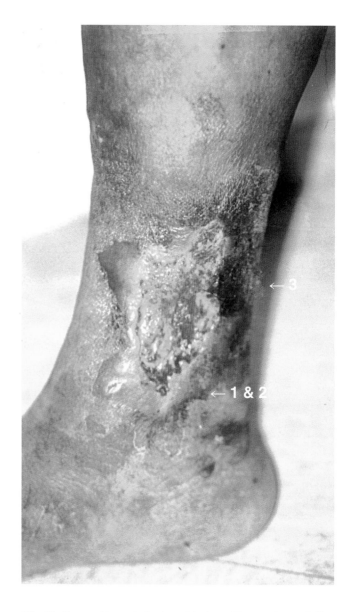

57. Venous stasis ulceration. This 49-year-old male with a 3-year history of recurrent venous ulceration was being treated with Unna boot changes once a week. Physical exam revealed patent femoral, popliteal, and pedal pulses. An enlarged, dilated, and tortuous greater saphenous vein was easily visualized with the patient in a standing position (white arrow). A duplex scan confirmed isolated greater saphenous vein incompetence, with a normal deep and perforator vein system.
Source: Reprinted with permission, copyright © C. Donayre.

58. Shallow and irregularly shaped lesion with a good granulating base and the associated physical signs of chronic venous insufficiency such as hyperpigmentation, chronic scarring, and skin contraction in the ankle region are readily identified. Note the classic characteristics of venous disease:
   (1) Irregular edges;
   (2) Shallow ulcer;
   (3) Evidence of hyperpigmentation (hemosiderin staining) surrounding ulcer;
   (4) Location above the medial malleolus.
Source: Reprinted with permission, copyright © C. Donayre.

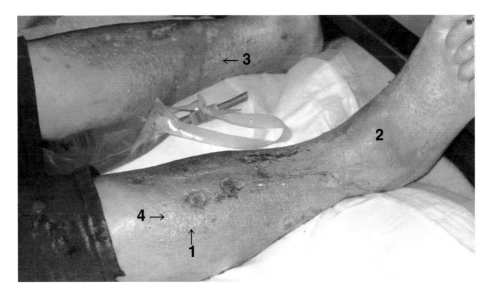

59. Stasis dermatitis. There is an absence of epithelialization phase. Evidence of:
  (1) Brawny edema;
  (2) Trophic skin changes;
  (3) Hemosiderin staining (hyperpigmentation);
  (4) Multiple shallow ulcers.
Source: Reprinted with permission, copyright © B.M. Bates-Jensen.

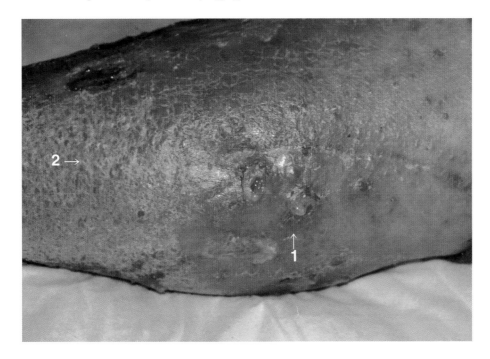

60. Close-up view of same leg as in Plate 59 and shows evidence of:
  (1) Edema leakage through wounds;
  (2) Scaling and crusting (trophic changes) due to lipodermatosclerosis.
Source: Reprinted with permission, copyright © B.M. Bates-Jensen.

MALIGNANT CUTANEOUS WOUNDS
Plates 61–63

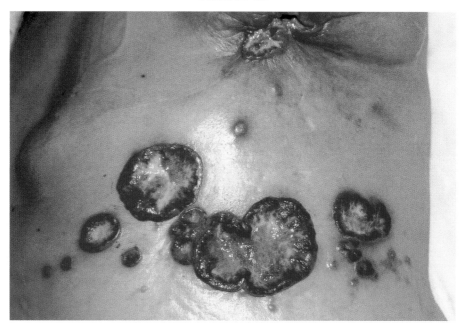

61. Status post left mastectomy with subsequent cutaneous metastasis. Lesions are very friable.
Courtesy of Susie Seaman, MSN, FNP, CETN.

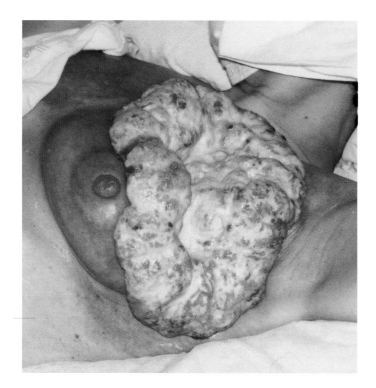

62. Local cutaneous invasion of breast cancer in a patient that refused any surgery or treatment.
Courtesy of Susie Seaman, MSN, FNP, CETN.

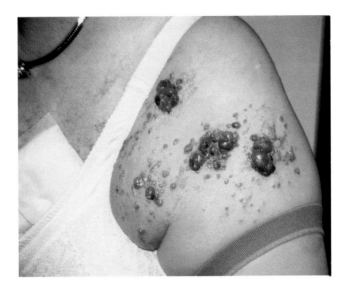

63. Status post left mastectomy with subsequent cutaneous metastasis and significant left arm edema.
Courtesy of Susie Seaman, MSN, FNP, CETN.

WOUND HEALING WITH ELECTRICAL STIMULATION—CHAPTER 21
Plates 64 and 65

Patient with vascular ulcer treated with ED and HVPC (see Chapter 21 for details).

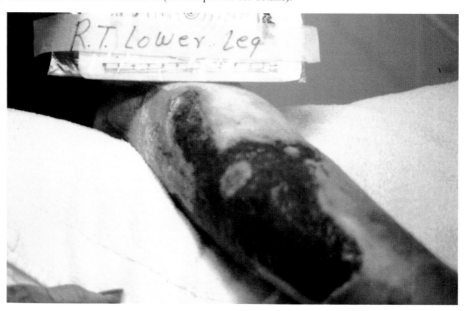

64. Note beefy red granulation tissue and island of epidermal tissue in full thickness wound. The wound is in acute proliferative phase on 12/28.
Source: Reprinted with permission, copyright © C. Sussman.

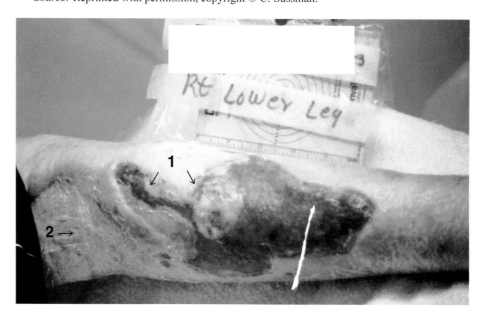

65. Same wound as in Plate 64. Note epidermal migration from wound edges, island, and wound shape changes.
(1)   It had progressed to the acute epithelialization phase by 2/17;
(2)   Note hyperkeratotic skin changes due to old burn wounds and poor circulation.
Source: Reprinted with permission, copyright © C. Sussman.

WOUND HEALING WITH PULSED SHORT WAVE DIATHERMY
CASE STUDY 1—CHAPTER 22
Plates 66–68

Patient with pressure ulcers treated with PSWD (see Chapter 22 for details).

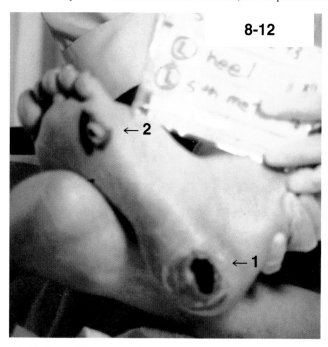

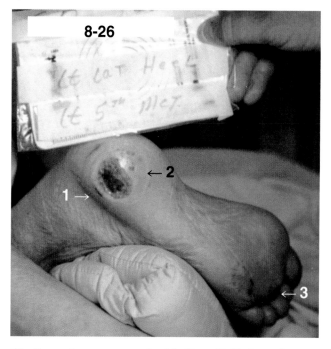

66. Patient with pressure ulcers. PSWD was started on 8/16.
(1) Black eschar on heel wound surrounded by partial-thickness skin loss. There is an absence of inflammatory phase;
(2) Black eschar over the 5th metatarsal head. There is an absence of inflammatory phase.
Source: Reprinted with permission, copyright © C. Sussman.

67. Same ulcer as seen on heel in Plate 66 10 days after start of PSWD.
(1) Eschar removed to soft necrosis;
(2) Reepithelialization of partial-thickness skin loss;
(3) Eschar removed 5th matatarsal. Wound healed.
Source: Reprinted with permission, copyright © C. Sussman.

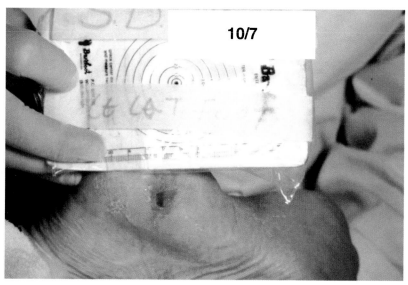

68. Same heel ulcer as in Plates 66 and 67 (10/7). The ulcer healed and is shown in the remodeling phase.
Source: Reprinted with permission, copyright © C. Sussman.

**WOUND HEALING WITH PULSED RADIO FREQUENCY STIMULATION
CASE STUDY 2—CHAPTER 22
Plates 69 and 70**

Patient with incisional wound treated with PRFS (see Chapter 22 for details).

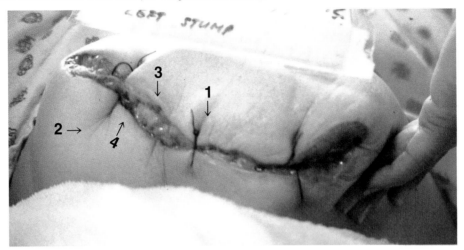

69. Patient with an incision from an above-the-knee amputation left open for delayed primary intention healing. Wound is in acute inflammatory phase. Start of treatment with PRFS 8/3.
    (1)   Sutures placed;
    (2)   Edema;
    (3)   Erythema and tissue tension;
    (4)   Yellow mucinous slough in incision line.
    Source: Reprinted with permission, copyright © C. Sussman.

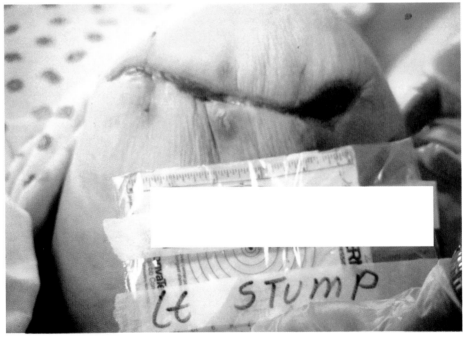

70. Same incision wound as in Plate 69 on 8/17 (14 days later). Note good outcomes: edema free, necrosis free, wound contraction, and granulation. The wound is in acute proliferative phase and epithelialization phase.
    Source: Reprinted with permission, copyright © C. Sussman.

HIGH RESOLUTION ULTRASOUND SCANS
Plates 71–73

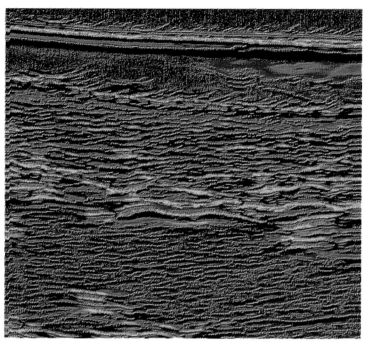

71. High resolution ultrasound B-scan of intact skin on the volar aspect of the forearm. *Source:* Copyright © Paul Wilson.

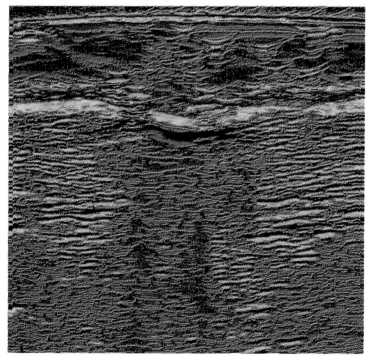

72. High resolution ultrasound B-scan of a full-thickness 4 mm diameter biopsy wound 7 days after wounding. The wound was made through the skin on the volar aspect of the forearm. The superficial eschar overlying the blood clot can be identified; deep to the blood clot is granulation tissue. On either side of the wound is intact skin (see *Color Plate 71*).
Source: Copyright © Paul Wilson.

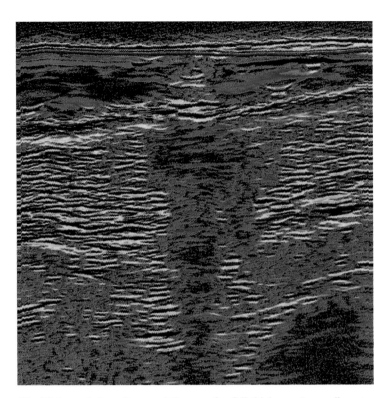

73. High resolution ultrasound B-scan of a full-thickness 4 mm diameter biopsy wound 14 days after wounding. In comparison with color plate 72, the granulation tissue is reduced in width, indicating that wound contraction, associated with the proliferative phase, has occurred. *Source:* Copyright © Paul Wilson.

WOUND HEALING WITH ULTRASOUND
CASE STUDY 1—CHAPTER 24
Plates 74–76

Patient with a venous ulcer 24 hours after onset. (See Chapter 24 for details.)

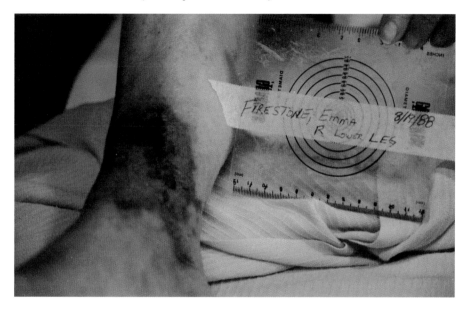

74. Wound is in acute inflammatory phase and shows subcutaneous hemorrhage (ecchymosis) associated with venous disease.
Source: Reprinted with permission, copyright © C. Sussman.

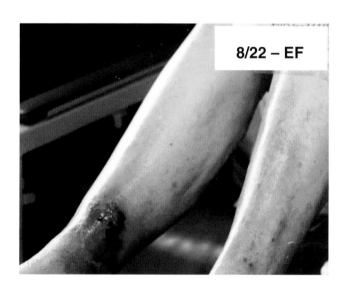

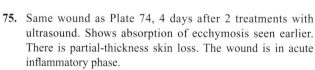

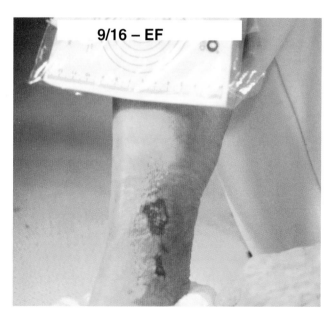

75. Same wound as Plate 74, 4 days after 2 treatments with ultrasound. Shows absorption of ecchymosis seen earlier. There is partial-thickness skin loss. The wound is in acute inflammatory phase.
Source: Reprinted with permission, copyright © C. Sussman.

76. Same ulcer as in Plates 74 and 75, 4 weeks after start of ultrasound. Note wound contraction compared with that in Plate 75. There are soft irregular wound edges and new epithelization. The wound is in epithelialization phase.
Source: Reprinted with permission, copyright © C. Sussman.

WOUND HEALING WITH ULTRASOUND
CASE STUDY 2—CHAPTER 24
Plates 77–80

Patient with blood blister on heel secondary to pressure, treated with ultrasound (US).

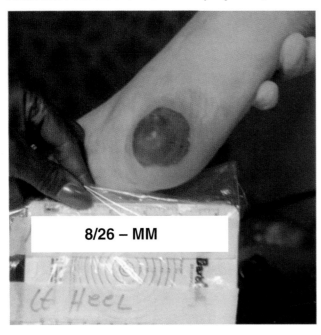

77. Acute inflammatory phase. Blister with bloody fluid at day of identification.
Source: Reprinted with permission, copyright © C. Sussman.

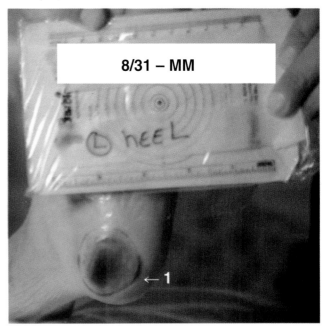

78. Same wound as Plate 77 without blister roof. The periwound skin was treated with daily US for 4 days prior.
(1) Note area of apparent necrosis, hematoma. There is an absence of inflammatory phase.
Source: Reprinted with permission, copyright © C. Sussman.

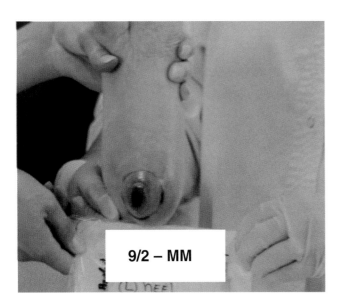

79. Same wound as Plates 77 and 78 after 2 additional periwound US treatments. Note absorption of hematoma by reduced size of necrotic area and mild erythema surrounding the area of necrosis. The wound is in acute inflammatory phase.
Source: Reprinted with permission, copyright © C. Sussman.

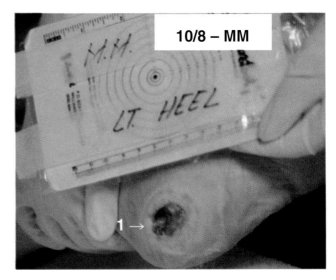

80. Same wound as Plates 77, 78, and 80.
(1) Note focal area of necrosis. Time of change in treatment to ES and sharp debridement. The wound shows the start of proliferative phase.
Source: Reprinted with permission, copyright © C. Sussman.

WOUND HEALING WITH PULSATILE LAVAGE WITH SUCTION—CHAPTER 26
Plates 81–83

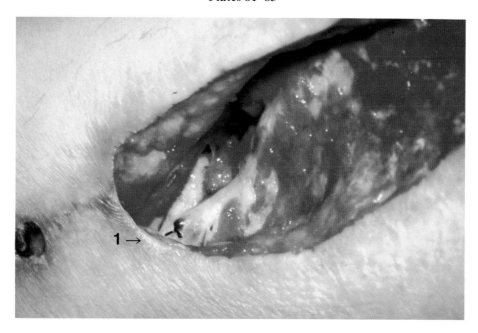

81. (1) Exposed artery in infected bypass graft donor site in lower leg.
Source: Reprinted with permission, copyright © H. Loehne.

Case Study

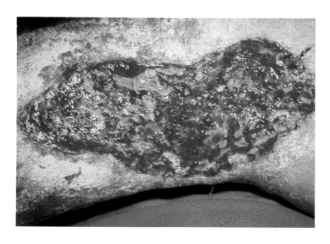

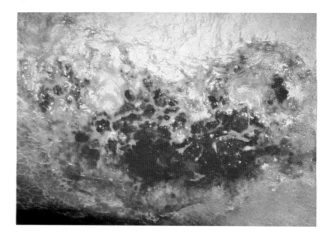

82. Pyoderma gangrenosum ulcer on medial lower leg of 8 years' duration. Chronic epithelialization phase.
Source: Reprinted with permission, copyright © H. Loehne.

83. Pyoderma gangrenosum ulcer (same ulcer as Plate 82) on medial lower leg after 2 weeks of treatment with Pulsavac® System. Note epitheliazation progressing to cover wound surface.
Source: Reprinted with permission, copyright © H. Loehne.

Introduction to Wound Diagnosis

Carrie Sussman

Development of diagnoses to direct and guide treatment by nurses and physical therapists has grown over the last 15 to 20 years. Both disciplines recognize that use of a diagnostic process applies the skills and knowledge of the professional nurse and physical therapist to the appropriate treatment of client situations they can and should treat legally and independently. The role of diagnostician is unfamiliar to many, and practice experience in the area of diagnosis varies from nonexistent to full-practice integration for many years. Because the incorporation of diagnosis into the health care professions is still in its infancy, there is much variance in understanding of the process. Therefore, there are a number of questions that need to be clarified as the process begins:

- What does a diagnosis really mean?
- What kind of information needs to be collected to yield a diagnosis?
- How are diagnoses differentiated from each other?
- How is a diagnosis tailored to the patient's functional problem or human response to health or illness?
- How does diagnosis relate to prognosis and outcomes?
- How does the nursing or physical therapy diagnosis direct interventions?

Advanced clinicians who are more familiar with classification systems and diagnostic methods will have other types of questions:

- Can and should the medical diagnosis be part of the physical therapy diagnostic statement?
- What kind of functional diagnostic statement should be written for a person at risk for wounds?
- What is the difference between diagnosis and classification?

Part I begins with an introduction to the diagnostic process. It seeks to answer these questions, including specifics about wound diagnosis. Guidelines for writing functional diagnoses that are meaningful and related to the prognosis and treatment interventions are included for both disciplines. One issue that became clear to the authors as Chapter 1 was crafted is that the diagnostic process and the terms of the diagnosis of the nurse and physical therapist are very similar. Both incorporate functional impairment and disability into the diagnostic process. For example, the nurse determines the client's response to health or illness as positive functioning, altered functioning, or at risk for altered functioning.[1] Nurses use a diagnosis that incorporates risk that could work equally well for the physical therapist. Nursing diagnosis specifically identifies collaborative problems, then, the health care practitioner needed for joint management. The most appropriate joint manager for wounds may be the dietitian, the physician, or the physical therapist. Nurses already have taxomony for *impaired tissue integrity* and *impaired skin integrity*. Physical therapists use disablement terminology, including the terms *impairment*, *disability*, and *handicap* in their management model.[2]

Functional diagnosis requires understanding of functional impairment. Functional impairment differs from the pathogenesis or etiology of the problem and describes a functional change as physiologic, anatomic, structural, or functional at the tissue, organ, or body system level.[3] Functional impairments are the system or organ impairments that prevent normal function.[4] In impaired wound healing there is a functional impairment of wound healing that occurs at a system, organ, or tissue level in the body. Chapter 2 is devoted to describing acute wound healing physiology and chronic wound healing factors as well as intrinsic, extrinsic, and iatrogenic factors that may influence chronic wound healing.

Assessment, examinations, tests, and measurements are an integral part of establishing a diagnosis. Chapters 3, 4, 5, 6, and 7 describe methods and procedures for collecting information and interpretation of the findings.

At the conclusion of Part I, clinicians will be able to understand acute and chronic wound healing physiology. They will be able to perform the required tests and measures necessary to determine a functional wound diagnosis, develop a prognosis, select appropriate interventions, and document the diagnostic process and the findings with a functional outcomes report. The clinician will then be ready to review Parts II, III, and IV to learn the management skills for different wound-related problems and appropriate interventions.

REFERENCES

1. Carpenito LJ. *Nursing Diagnosis: Application to Clinical Practice.* 6th ed. Philadelphia: J.B. Lippincott; 1994.
2. American Physical Therapy Association. A guide to physical therapy practice, I: a description of patient management. *Phys Ther.* 1995;75:707–764.
3. World Health Organization. *International Classification of Impairments, Disabilities, and Handicaps.* Geneva, Switzerland: WHO Publications Centre USA; 1980.
4. Jette AM. Physical disablement concepts for physical therapy research and practice. *Phys Ther.* 1994;74:380–386.

CHAPTER 1

The Diagnostic Process

Carrie Sussman and Barbara M. Bates-Jensen

CHAPTER OBJECTIVES

At the completion of this chapter, the reader will be able to:

1. Describe each step in the diagnostic process
2. Identify key data to collect during the assessment process
3. Differentiate between behavioral and functional outcomes
4. Explain the importance of determining prognosis during the diagnostic process
5. Describe the process of evaluation using outcomes

This chapter describes the diagnostic process for management of patients with chronic wounds. Nurses and physical therapists use essentially the same decision-making process in diagnosing patient problems, although the terms used to describe the process may differ slightly. Nurses use the nursing process and nursing diagnosis as the framework for planning and evaluating patient care. The nursing process includes the following steps: assessment, diagnosis, goals, interventions, and evaluation. Physical therapy uses a process that includes the steps of assessment, examination, diagnosis, prognosis, and outcomes. To simplify and guide the reader, the diagnostic process has been broken into four steps, each with two or three parts. Step I, assessment, includes review of the reason for referral, history, systems review/physical assessment, and wound assessment. Step II, diagnosis, includes examination strategy, evaluation, and diagnosis. Step III, goals, includes prognosis, goals, outcomes and evaluation of progress. Step IV, intervention, is described in subsequent chapters. Examinations and specific measurements, as well as special test procedures, are found in Chapters 3, 4, 5, and 7, as well as in others.

STEP I: ASSESSMENT PROCESS

The assessment process assists in clinical decision making by avoiding undirected care and inappropriate treatment. Assessment is done for all patients before determining the need for special testing examinations and interventions. For nurses, this process begins when the patient is admitted to the agency. For physical therapists, this process begins with the reason for referral, which is part of the patient history. The assessment process involves gathering data from the patient history and physical examination. The patient history determines which relevant systems reviews are needed in the physical examination. For physical therapists, the history and systems review determine the candidacy or noncandidacy for services; for nurses, the history and systems review determine the direction for the treatment plan. Many physical therapists retain the belief that all referrals automatically show candidacy for wound care. The reality is that not all patients are appropriately referred for physical therapy. To some physical therapists, this will sound like heresy, but proper utilization management is mandatory in today's health care environment.

Utilization management is part of the process of prospective management and is designed to ensure that only medically necessary, reasonable, and appropriate services are provided. Utilization management attempts to influence the treatment pathway and therefore to ensure optimal clinical outcomes.[1] For nurses, the assessment process provides the framework for planning comprehensive wound care, incorporating utilization management and possibly making a referral for physical therapy.

Utilization management for the patient with a wound and with comorbidities and coimpairment is separate but related. Collaborative interdisciplinary management of comorbidities and coimpairments will reduce iatrogenic effects from inappropriate selection of interventions or handling of the wound and will lessen extrinsic and intrinsic complications (see Chapter 2). The interdisciplinary nature inherent in caring for the patient with a wound requires clinicians to determine candidacy for services carefully before initiating referral or treatment. For example, the physical therapist may determine that the patient is not a candidate for whirl-pool therapy as ordered by the physician and may send the findings with an alternative recommendation to the referring physician. The use of standardized forms is the best method of collecting assessment data quickly and efficiently, thus ensuring that important information is not lost. Use of a form that the clinician completes and a form that the patient completes ensures data maintenance from the interview. Partnering or engaging the patient in his or her own care from the beginning is essential to achieving mutually satis-factory outcomes. A self-administered patient history form helps the clinician to focus the interview and can save time. Samples of an assessment form for a self-administered his-tory and an interview form for physical therapists and nurses are presented in Appendixes 1–A and 1–B. Some informa-tion will be found in the patient's medical record, but many times, the patient or significant other can provide additional insights and information not otherwise available.

Review of Admission/Referral

It is essential for a physical therapist to know the reason why a patient is referred. This referral is the first step in documenting patient history. The initial referral for wound care management is usually to the nurse; if the nurse deter-mines a need for physical therapy services, the physical therapist is brought into the team. It is critical for nurses to know expectations and projected outcomes from a physi-cal therapy referral in order to refer appropriately. In some health care settings, a wound care team decides the services necessary for wound management and makes the appropriate referrals. The patient referred to the physical therapist for wound healing is usually an individual who has not shown signs of normal wound repair. Most often, other treatment interventions are in use or have been tried with limited or no success. Physical therapy services usually involve an additional fee.

The referral to physical therapy is regarded as an attempt to maximize and enhance wound repair. However, referral may be for reasons beyond improved wound healing. For example, the patient may be referred for help in cleaning and debriding a necrotic wound, for enhancement of the inflam-matory process, to reinitiate wound repair, or for recurrent infection. For the patient who presents with factors that impair wound healing, the reason for referral is to achieve a clean, stable wound that can be managed easily by the nurse

or caregiver at home. Pain management may be the reason for referral, with physical agents and electrotherapeutic modalities prescribed to help control pain. For both the nurse and the physical therapist, wound closure may not be the highest priority. Both nurses and physical therapists must understand the reason for the referral and the expected outcomes. There must be a match between selected inter-vention and expected outcomes to meet the referral objec-tives. For example, the patient with a foot ulcer secondary to pressure and insensitivity is fearful of amputation and loss of ability to walk. The patient's main concern is limb sal-vage, and expectations are high. In contrast, the family of a debilitated nursing home patient may desire only comfort for their family member, with no expectations of wound closure. Family and caregiver perceptions of various inter-ventions may differ from the clinician's view. What are perceived by one to be heroic and painful measures may, in truth, be normal procedures. The nurse must address these issues before a referral to physical therapy is made.

Patient History

Patient history information is commonly collected by an interview process with the patient, family, significant others, and caregivers; by consultation with other health care practitioners; and by reviewing the medical record. Ideally, in the continuum of care, the information about the patient history will be transmitted with the patient. Unfortunately, this is not always the case. The clinician may have to piece together the history from the many sources listed above. If only a limited amount of medical and social information is available, the clinician may have to choose diagnostic op-tions based on available data. It is easier to plan appropriate care with a complete history.

Clinical Wisdom: *Patient History Needed To Determine Care Direction*

- Reason for admission or referral
- Expectations and perceptions about wound heal-ing
- Psychosocial-cultural-economic history
- Present medical comorbidities
- Current wound status

Remember that one of the primary goals during the patient interview is to begin to develop a therapeutic relationship with the patient and family. The history taking allows the clinician to assess and diagnose patient problems and to place the problem within the context of the individual patient's life. The skills used by clinicians during the patient history are those of listening, observing, and asking questions.

Chief Complaint and Health History

Begin the patient history by finding out the patient's chief complaint or major reason for seeking care and the duration of the problem. Find out why the patient is seeking help at this time. It may be as simple as convenience or it may be that the wound problem is worsening and the patient feels that treatment is needed at this time. Investigate other agendas that the patient may have, other than the obvious problem, by asking a question such as, How did you hope I could help you today? Explore the meaning of the wound with the patient. Questions such as What do you think caused your wound? and Why do you think it started when it did? and How long do you think the wound will last? help to reveal the patient's level of understanding of the health problem. Based on answers obtained, care can be planned that is sensitive to the patient's needs and level of understanding. The clinician seeks a complete understanding of the patient's symptoms (symptoms are the subjective feelings of the patient) during the interview. Seven criteria can be used to describe symptoms: location, character, severity, timing, setting in which the symptom occurs, antecedents and consequences of the symptom, and other associated symptoms.

Clinical Wisdom:
Questions To Ask To Elicit Extent of Wound Symptoms

- *Location:* Where do you feel the wound? Do you feel it anywhere else? Show me where it hurts.
- *Character:* What does it feel like?
- *Severity:* On a scale of 0–10, with 10 being the worst pain you could imagine, how would you rate the discomfort you have now? How does the wound interfere with your usual activities? How bad is it?
- *Timing/Duration:* When did you first notice the wound? How often have you had wounds?
- *Setting:* Does the wound occur in a certain place or under certain circumstances? Is it associated with any specific activity?
- *Antecedents and consequences:* What makes it better? What makes it worse?
- *Other associated symptoms:* Have you noticed any other changes?

During the patient interview, answers to these questions should provide a thorough understanding of the patient's wound symptoms. Review the patient's present health and present illness status. This provides information relevant to the patient's reasons for seeking care. Describe the patient's usual health, then focus on the present problem, investigating the chief complaint thoroughly, as described above. For interpretation and analysis of the patient's problem, it is helpful to document the chief complaint data in chronologic order.

Next, review the patient's past health history. Information about management of and response to past problems provides an indication of the patient's potential response to current treatment of the problem. Much of this information may be available in the patient's medical record. If not available, the following information should be obtained: past general health, childhood illnesses, accidents or injuries with any associated disabilities, hospitalizations, surgeries, major acute or chronic illnesses, immunizations, medications and transfusions, and allergies. Current health information includes allergies, habits, medications, and sleep and exercise patterns, all of which provide information on the patient's health habits. Investigate environmental, food, drug, animal, or other allergies. Specific allergies may have a bearing on interventions chosen for the patient's wound care regimen. Allergic reactions usually affect the gastrointestinal tract, the respiratory tract, and the skin. Some products used for wound care can contribute to an allergic reaction. One is latex that is found in dressings, gloves, and plastic tubing. Tape is another notorious culprit often associated with skin allergies. Sulfonamide is a common drug allergen, and silver sulfadiazine (Silvadene) is a common topical therapy for wound care that contains sulfonamide, so the clinician would need to choose another topical agent to accomplish the goals for that patient. The clinician also should be aware of warning signs and take necessary measures to control an offending allergen. Evaluate current and past habits relevant to the health of the patient, including alcohol, tobacco, substance, drug, and caffeine use. Alcohol, tobacco, and substance use, in particular, present significant problems for tissue perfusion and nutrition for wound healing. Complete a full medication profile, including both prescription and over-the-counter medications, names, dosages, frequency, intended effect, and compliance with the regimen. Many medications interfere with wound healing or may interact with wound therapy.

Evaluate the patient's usual routine for patterns of physical and sedentary activities. Ask the patient to describe a usual day's activities. Exercise patterns influence healing in several wound types, such as venous disease ulcers. Finally, describe the patient's sleep pattern and whether the patient perceives the sleep to be adequate and satisfactory. Ask the patient where he or she usually sleeps. Patients with severe arterial insufficiency may sleep sitting up in recliner chairs because of the pain associated with the disease. Likewise, patients with chronic obstructive pulmonary disease (COPD) may sleep sitting up because of difficulty breathing in the supine position.

The family health history provides information about the general health of the patient's relatives and family. Family health information is helpful in the identification of genetic, familial, or environmental illnesses. Specific areas to target are diabetes mellitus, heart disease, and stroke. Each of these diseases can impair wound healing in an existing wound and is a risk factor for further wounding. If the patient has a family history of these diseases, he or she may have early signs of the disease as yet undiagnosed and is at higher risk of eventual disease development.

Sociologic History

Diagnosis and management of the patient's wound problem is best accomplished within the context of the whole person. It is important to gather information about the patient's sociologic, psychologic, and nutritional status. Sociologic data fall into seven areas: relationships with family and significant others, environment, occupational history, economic status and resources, educational level, daily life, and patterns of health care.

Relationships with family and significant others include gathering information on the patient's position and role in the family, the persons living with the patient, the persons to whom the patient relates, and any recent family changes or crises. The role of the patient within the family may dictate treatment decisions. For example, the grandmother with venous disease ulcers may also be the prime caregiver of young grandchildren; thus, it is unrealistic to expect compliance with a therapeutic regimen that includes frequent periods of elevating lower extremities. The family support system may be a critical component when determining wound care management programs, and answers to questions such as Who will change the wound dressing and perform procedures? Who prepares meals? and Who will transport the patient to the clinic? may influence treatment options. Environment plays a significant role in the health and illness of individuals. Ask questions about the home, community, and work environments. Home care patients present challenging environments for wound repair. For example, the elderly woman living alone with four cats in a two-room trailer with minimal bathroom facilities will require different management strategies than will the middle-aged man living with a spouse and family in a three-bedroom house in the suburbs. The community environment may provide additional resources for the patient, such as senior citizens' centers, health fairs, or the neighborhood grocery store that delivers to the home. The work environment, along with the occupational history, provides information on the ability of the patient to eliminate certain risk factors for impaired healing. For example, the grocery clerk with a venous disease ulcer will need help with work adjustment of a job when standing for long periods of time is required. Occupational history can pinpoint health-risk jobs, such as those that require prolonged standing.

Economic status and resources are important to determine adequacy for therapy compliance. It is not necessary to know the patient's exact income; instead, ask whether the patient feels the income is adequate, and elicit the source of the income. It is important to identify patients with inadequate resources and to make appropriate referrals for financial assistance. Include an assessment of the patient's health insurance resources. If the expectation is prolonged wound healing, a discussion of financial reserves may be desirable. The economic history needs to include not only the patient's payer source for insurance coverage, but also the resources the patient has available to obtain necessary dressing supplies. Some patients have insurance coverage that pays for all dressing supplies, other patients have insurance coverage that pays for only certain types of supplies (gauze, but not tape), and yet other patients have no coverage for supplies at all. The economic history is also needed to determine whether the patient has adequate resources available to pay for a caregiver, if one is needed to come in to help with caregiving or changing dressings.

The educational level of the patient and judgment of age-appropriateness of intellect is helpful in planning future education on self-care of the wound. Ask the patient to describe a typical day and to identify any differences on the weekend. The daily profile allows the clinician to perceive the whole patient. Answers to questions about the social and recreational activities of the patient, as well as typical daily routines, provide valuable insights into the patient's lifestyle and possible health risks. Evaluation of previous health care access and use assists with clinical judgment of past health promotion and prevention activities, and whether the patient's care has had continuity.

Psychologic History

The psychologic history includes an assessment of the patient's cognitive abilities (including learning style, memory, comprehension), responses to illness (coping patterns, reaction to illness), response to care (compliance), and cultural implications for care. Usually, at this point, the clinician has some idea of the patient's comprehension, memory, and overall cognitive status. If mental function is still unclear, the clinician may want to administer a mental status examination, such as the mini-mental status exam. Previous coping patterns and reactions to illness provide insight to possible reactions to the current situation. Has the patient had difficulties with wound healing in the past? Is there a history of chronic wounds? How has the patient responded to previous chronic wounds? Response to previous care and compliance with other therapy regimens may indicate potential adherence difficulties with the current treatment plan.

Cultural History

People come from different walks of life and often have belief systems significantly different from those of the clinician. It is, therefore, very important to take nothing for granted and to assess the patient's and caregiver's values and beliefs about health and wellness. As clinicians, we need to be particularly sensitive in our assessment of the patient's culture and values. As more information is available about the influence of one's culture and values on health and illness, it becomes essential that each patient's views on health and illness be explored prior to determining goals of care and the overall treatment plan.

Nutritional History

Nutrition plays a major role in wound healing (see Chapter 3). During the patient interview, determine the patient's usual daily food intake, risk for malnutrition, and specific nutritional deficiencies. Evaluate the patient's weight in comparison with the usual weight of the patient. Ask the patient to recall all foods eaten in the past 24 hours and determine whether this is a normal pattern for the patient.

Systems Review and Physical Assessment

The systems review portion of the patient history and the physical assessment of each system provide information on comorbidities that may impair wound healing. The individual's capacity to heal may be limited by specific disease effects on tissue integrity and perfusion, patient mobility, compliance, nutrition, and risk for wound infection. Throughout the patient history, systems review, and physical assessment, the clinician should consider host factors that affect wound healing.

Respiratory System

The respiratory system is critical for delivery of oxygen and nutrients to the tissues to promote wound healing and control infection. Pulmonary disease may be progressive in conditions such as cystic fibrosis, COPD, and lung cancer. Nonprogressive disease states to consider are pneumonia, postcardiac or postthoracic surgery, and traumatic injury.

Chronic Obstructive Pulmonary Disease. Patients with COPD have problems concerning pulmonary secretion retention, in which pulmonary secretion fills alveolar sacks and reduces the surface area for transference of oxygen through the alveolar membrane into the bloodstream. Assessment includes evaluation of pulse oximetry, pulmonary function tests, and mode and amount of oxygen delivery. Transcutaneous oxygen transport measurements are also helpful (see Chapter 7). If noninvasive vascular test results are not available, they should be considered as part of the examination strategy for patients with COPD. Oxygen delivery is severely reduced when the body is in the horizontal position. In the supine position, the diaphragm has reduced excursion space that decreases the thoracic expansion and tidal volume of air into the lungs. Elevating the head of the bed and placing the patient in semi-Fowler's position may improve airflow into the lungs. However, skin over the sacrococcygeal area will be at risk for pressure ulcer formation because of shearing and friction forces present in the typical semi-Fowler's position. Decreased mobility is often an additional complication of COPD because of poor endurance, deconditioning, and difficulty of breathing during activity.

Pneumonia. The patient most at risk for pneumonia is the elderly, frail, institutionalized patient with multiple health deficits. The stress of the illness and the related signs and symptoms lead to impaired wound healing. Wounds will generally plateau, fail to continue healing, or deteriorate until the pneumonia is resolved. Wound repair may not be an option for this patient until the underlying disease is under control. Maintaining current wound status and preparing the wound for healing may be goals for this time frame.

Asthma. Asthma is a collection of respiratory symptoms caused by infections, hypersensitivity to irritants (pollutants, allergens), psychologic stress, cold air, exercise, or drug use. Asthma may be symptom-controlled with medications, including steroids such as prednisone. Inquire about the time of onset of the asthma and the start of steroid therapy. Some individuals have a long history of steroid use, and this will affect ability to heal. Steroids repress the inflammatory response, and without inflammation, wound healing will not progress. The effects of steroids can be mitigated by use of oral or topical vitamin A. The physician should be contacted with recommendations for vitamin A administration as soon as possible.

Cardiovascular System

Patients with cardiac disease have poor pump function. There may be dysfunction of the coronary arteries, the valves, or the cardiac electrical conduction system. In general, any dysfunction of the cardiac system poses significant difficulties related to wound healing. The heart is responsible for pumping oxygenated blood through the circulatory system to all body tissues. Thus, if the heart is not functional, all body tissues suffer. Specific pathology with concerns for wound patients include coronary artery disease and congestive heart failure (CHF).

Clinical Wisdom:
Pacemaker Caution for Physical Therapists

Some patients have pacemaker implants to support or replace the dysfunction of the cardiac system. This is important information for physical therapists when selecting a treatment intervention with electrotherapeutic agents.

Coronary Artery Disease. In coronary artery disease, blood vessels may become clogged, producing signs and symptoms of angina pectoris or myocardial infarction. In either case, the effect is to shunt blood flow away from the periphery of the body. This impedes circulation to the tissues, which reduces oxygen and nutrients available to them.

Congestive Heart Failure. Congestive heart failure is the heart's inability to pump enough blood for body functioning. In CHF, the right or left side of the heart can fail. Either case generally involves the other side, and symptoms of both right- and left-sided failure relate to fluid overload. Diuretic therapy is commonly prescribed to assist in fluid balance, decrease the burden on the heart, and thus improve heart pumping action. In evaluation of the patient with CHF and concomitant lower leg ulcers and lower extremity edema, it is essential to differentiate the edema associated with CHF from edema associated with venous disease. Treatment for the edema in the patient with both CHF and venous disease may differ from treatment for the patient with edema related to venous disease only.

Gastrointestinal System

The anatomy of the gastrointestinal (GI) tract includes the esophagus, stomach, small intestine, and large intestine. The GI system is responsible for digestion and absorption of nutrients and fluids. Specific disorders of concern for patients with wounds include GI bleeding or problems with digestion and absorption of nutrients. Gastrointestinal bleeding weakens the patient and decreases blood supply. Any disease causing GI malfunctioning leads to poor absorption of nutrients and fluids for the patient. Patients with gastrostomy tubes receive enteral nutrition directly into the stomach, bypassing the mouth. Tube feedings may be accompanied by loose stools, which can irritate skin and seep into wounds in the pelvic area, resulting in wound contamination. A dietary consultation would be helpful in the optimal management of patients with GI tube feedings or malnutrition related to GI pathology.

Clinical Wisdom: *Diarrhea with GI Tube Feedings*

Diarrhea associated with tube feedings requires investigation. Sometimes, slowing the rate of the feeding infusion, diluting the formula, or using a formula-containing fiber may help to decrease or eliminate the diarrhea. Wound therapy choices for patients with diarrhea from tube feedings include attention to dressings that protect the wound area from fecal contamination.

Nutrition and Hydration. Nutritional screening is an important component of assessment because of the relationship among malnutrition, pressure ulcer development, and impaired wound healing. Nutritional data may be found in the medical record as a single assessment or as pieces of information that the clinician must bring together. A sample nutritional assessment guide and diagram can be found in Chapter 3. If no standardized nutrition assessment form exists within the agency or setting, the clinician should evaluate the following: current weight; prior weight; weight change; and percentage of change in weight, height, and body mass index. Body weight is a commonly used indicator of nutrition. An involuntary increase or decrease in weight of 5% is predictive of a drop in serum albumin.[2] Serum albumin is a measure of protein available for healing; a normal level is greater than 3.5 mg/dL. Other laboratory tests to evaluate include prealbumin levels and total lymphocyte count.

Hydration status can be determined by interpreting intake and output sheets. Intake and output sheets are often kept in the patient's room and may be completed by nurses or nursing assistants, depending on the health care setting. Signs of dehydration include thirst, tongue dryness in nonmouth breathers, and decreased skin turgor. Dehydration affects wound healing by reducing the blood volume available to transport oxygen and nutrients to healing tissues. The state of hydration affects weight and albumin levels.

Case Study: *Malnutrition and Wound Management in End-Stage Illness*

A malnourished patient with a pressure ulcer on the coccyx is in the end stage of life. The patient and family refuse tube feedings and understand the consequences of the minimally nourished and dehydrated condition. In this case, palliative and prevention treatment is indicated. The wound can be kept clean, dressed to control drainage and odor, and managed for pain. Yet the patient is also a candidate for a pressure-relief mattress replacement or specialty bed for prevention of additional skin breakdown. A turning schedule and training of the caregivers is also part of the prevention intervention strategy.

Genitourinary System

The genitourinary system is divided into the upper tract (kidneys and ureters) and the lower tract (bladder, sphincters, and urethra). Patients with kidney failure may require treatment involving some form of dialysis and a special diet that may impair wound healing. The patient with kidney failure often has multiple system failure. Evaluation for other diseases, such as diabetes and hypertension, is warranted because they often coincide with kidney dysfunction.

<table>
<tr><td>

Case Study:
Cognitively Impaired Patient with Leg Ulcers

A patient who was cognitively impaired with a history of venous disease and recurrent ulceration of her legs can demonstrate how the change in nutritional status affected her recurrent ulcers. Emma was an elderly nursing home patient with a diagnosis of Alzheimer's disease and was confined for her safety to a secure medical unit. She was labeled "Mrs. Houdini" because she could undo any restraint, including climbing the bedrails. Emma walked all day long with negative consequences on her venous disease. Compression stockings were out of the question. She would not tolerate putting them on or wearing them. Emma was hyperactive and a very poor eater.

The director of nurses decided to investigate her nutritional status. She reviewed Emma's weight status and found progressive loss of weight over the previous 3–4 months. Consultation with the physician led to further evaluation and revealed a low albumin level of 2.5 mg/dL. Evaluation by the speech pathologist demonstrated delayed swallowing response and resulted in a recommendation for a videofluoroscopic examination.

The nutritional assessment with the resultant recommendation for gastrostomy tube placement was shared with the family. Emma tolerated the procedure well. A benefit of the gastrostomy tube placement for Emma was that it could be covered by her clothing and was out of sight and, therefore, out of mind for this individual, so she left it alone.

In a couple of weeks, the nutrition added to her diet made her much less irritable and hyperactive. Emma could be placed in a gerichair with a restraint tray and her legs were elevated part of the day. She walked with assistance a couple of times a day. She was transferred from the secure unit to the long-term care custodial area of the facility and had more social interaction. She gained weight and had no further episodes of venous dermatitis or ulceration during the next year.

</td></tr>
</table>

Urinary Incontinence. Bladder dysfunction, outlet problems, or sphincter dysfunction can cause urinary incontinence. Urinary incontinence has implications for skin damage, including maceration from moisture on the skin, softening and separating of the epidermal layers, and irritation related to increased friction and shearing. Wound contamination is also an issue for patients with sacrococcygeal wounds and concomitant incontinence.

Peripheral Vascular System

The peripheral vascular system includes the venous, arterial, and lymphatic circulatory systems. Chapter 17 describes the pathogenesis and differential diagnosis of peripheral vascular disease (PVD). The clinician should pay particular attention to all medical chart notations or comments by and questions asked of the patient or family about vascular disorders, including history of hypertension, deep vein thrombosis, claudication, cold feet, and chronic swelling of the lower extremities. Patients with PVD are at high risk for development of chronic wounds and resultant impaired wound healing. The diagnosis of PVD guides the clinician's examination strategy for observational and noninvasive vascular testing. The important observations and testing procedures for patients with PVD are outlined in Chapter 7, Vascular Testing.

Neurologic and Musculoskeletal System

An imbalance or insufficient movement of body segments, limbs, or the whole body, due to impairment or disability of the neurologic or musculoskeletal system, are known factors for predicting certain wound development, such as pressure ulcers and neuropathic ulcers. Neurologic disorders and dysfunction of the musculoskeletal system include a broad range of medical diagnoses, such as spinal cord injury, cerebrovascular accidents, Parkinson's disease, arthritis, and multiple sclerosis. See Chapters 15, 16, and 18 for more information about the impact of movement disability on pathogenesis of pressure ulcers, pressure ulcer prevention, therapeutic positioning, and problems of the neuropathic foot. The neurologic or musculoskeletal deficit guides examination strategies for the clinician. For example, the nurse caring for a patient with limited body movements and neurologic deficits performs a pressure ulcer risk assessment to evaluate risk factors for pressure ulcer development, which may trigger referrals for therapeutic positioning evaluation by a physical therapist and a nutritional consultation. In another example, patients who have had a cerebrovascular accident or stroke may have decreased activity and mobility, increasing their risk for pressure ulcer development or reducing the healing capacity of current wounds.

Cerebrovascular Accident. Cerebrovascular accidents or strokes are caused by disruption in blood flow to the brain. They usually affect one hemisphere of the brain, causing deficits on the contralateral side of the body. Stroke can result in impaired ability to walk, impaired ability to use an upper limb, and inability to communicate, think, or see adequately. The patient's limited ability to move body parts places the patient at risk of developing pressure ulcers, skin tears, or friction and shearing injury.

Arthritis.   Arthritic disorders affect the joints of the body. The two main types are rheumatoid arthritis and osteoarthritis. Osteoarthritis affects older adults and is associated with painful joints, particularly knees, ankles, and hips (weight-bearing joints). Evaluation of the wound patient with arthritis may be more difficult because of pain on positioning for adequate view of the wound. Treatment of arthritis commonly includes nonsteroidal antiinflammatory drugs and steroids, both of which can impair or slow wound healing. Rheumatoid arthritis affects the joints of the hands and fingers, making self-care of wounds difficult or impossible.

Hematologic System

Disease processes such as anemia, fluid and electrolyte imbalance, or other blood dyscrasia associated with medication side effects or disease pathology affect wound healing capacity. Evaluation of laboratory values to rule out anemia, electrolyte imbalance, or infections is the key to hematologic system assessment.

Endocrine System

The endocrine system includes numerous glands that secrete body-regulating hormones. One of those glands is the pancreas, which controls insulin levels in the body. Diabetes mellitus is the disease of most concern in the endocrine system. Diabetes impairs wound healing and poses significant risk for wound development. Glucose levels alter wound healing and immune system functioning to control infection. Check for a diagnosis of diabetes mellitus. Is it type I insulin-dependent or type II non–insulin-dependent? The type of diabetes signals whether the patient will use insulin or diet and exercise to control glucose. Type I diabetics require insulin for glucose management. Type II diabetics manage glucose control initially with diet and exercise, then, if unsuccessful, with oral hypoglycemic agents or insulin.

Normal glucose level is 80 mg/dL. Levels of 180–250 mg/dL or greater are indicators that glucose levels are out of control. Levels of greater than 200 mg/dL are known to have an impact on wound healing.[3] Review of laboratory values is prudent to determine level of diabetic control. Look specifically for a fasting blood glucose level < 140 mg/dL and a glycosylated hemoglobin (HbA_{1c}) of less than 7%. The HbA_{1c} helps to determine the level of glucose control the patient has had over the last 2–3 months. Complications from diabetes generally occur with the length of time the patient has had the disease. Patients with relatively new onset of diabetes may not exhibit neuropathic or vascular complications related to diabetes. Patients with diabetes over longer periods of time and those with type I diabetes are more at risk for complications associated with the disease, such as neuropathy, retinopathy, and vascular changes. The diabetic with a wound should trigger examination of sensa-

tion in the feet and vision testing. Patients with diabetic neuropathy may present with ulcers on the soles of the feet, and care should be taken to examine the plantar surfaces for callus formation, cracking, and bony deformities. Additional information on management of the patient with vascular and neuropathic disabilities related to diabetes is discussed in Chapters 17 and 18.

Although this review of systems with physical assessment guidelines is not inclusive, it provides a framework of those areas of most concern to the clinician managing patients with wounds. A complete history and physical examination provides the context for the wound itself. After completing the history and physical examination, the clinician can turn attention to planning interventions. If the information is very limited, the clinician will have to make a clinical decision about the appropriateness of the referral from the reason for referral, expected outcomes, and personal observations of the patient. Clinicians can complete the general history, systems review, and physical assessment in about 30–40 minutes for a single wound. An experienced clinician can perform a basic physical assessment in 10–15 minutes. Typically, not all information is gathered at the same time. Portions of the history and physical assessment may be gathered over a period of several days after several clinic visits or home visits.

Wound Assessment

Wound assessment involves evaluation of a composite of wound characteristics, including location, shape, size, depth, edges, undermining and tunneling, necrotic tissue characteristics, exudate characteristics, surrounding skin color, peripheral tissue edema and induration, and the presence of granulation tissue and epithelialization (see Chapter 4 on wound assessment, Chapter 5 on wound measurement, and Chapter 6 on tools).

Wound History

The next questions are directed toward acquiring information about the history of the wound. How long has the wound been present? Is there a history of previous wounds? What interventions have been used, and have they been successful? What disciplines have been involved in the management of the wound? For instance, if the patient has been seen by many disciplines and has had multiple interventions without successful progress toward healing, the patient's candidacy for more aggressive intervention is questionable. Previous therapy and response to therapy must be carefully examined to avoid repeating unsuccessful intervention. Some patients may not heal. However, evaluation of past interventions with attention to appropriateness of topical wound care, prevention strategies, risk factor and comorbidity management, and use of adjunct therapy, such as a whirlpool or electrical stimulation, may reveal inconsistencies in treatment approach.

Patient Candidacy for Physical Therapy Services

During the assessment process, the clinician focuses on how the medical history and systems review will affect the candidacy of the patient. Physical therapists may determine the candidacy of the patient for services; with nursing, the option of determining candidacy for nursing services does not exist. The nurse usually has no choice in determining whether or not to provide nursing services to the patient. However, the nurse does have the option of assisting in determination of appropriate therapy for the patient involving other disciplines. The medical history and systems review findings may suggest to the clinician that the patient's problem requires consultation; that it is outside the scope of the clinician's knowledge, experience, or expertise; or that the intervention originally suggested is inappropriate. In physical therapy, the patient is then identified as a noncandidate for the referred physical therapy service. It then becomes the responsibility of the clinician to refer to another practitioner who is more skilled, more knowledgeable, or better able to manage the identified problem or recommend an alternative treatment and management strategy. Below are examples of some criteria that would trigger a referral:

- Vascular testing should be considered if assessment findings include hair loss, skin pallor or cyanosis, and cold temperature of the feet.
- Callus and hemorrhagic spots on the callus are indicators of deeper tissue damage and a need for further assessment for high pressure.
- Toenail abnormalities, if not an area of expertise of the examiner, should be referred.
- Assessment of an abscess in a tunnel or sinus tract requires immediate referral for surgical management.
- Undermining or tunneling, that is, a black hole without a bottom, should be immediately referred for surgical management.
- Signs of granulation tissue infection (superficial bridging, friable tissue, bleeding on contact, pain in the wound, or regression of healing) need medical intervention.

STEP II: DIAGNOSIS

Examination Strategy

The risk factors for impaired healing are identified at this point in the examination, based on data collected during the history and systems review. Because the information about the patient determines the examination strategy, *not* all patients will receive the same examination.

Examination: Part I

There are two parts to the examination. Part I includes testing for factors related to the physiologic or anatomic status of the comorbidities, such as vascular impairment or sensory impairment, that impair healing. These tests have significant weight in the prediction of healing and development of the prognosis. For example, a low ankle-brachial index score indicates severe occlusive disease and is a predictor of failure to heal without reperfusion. Loss of protective sensation in the feet is an indicator of high risk for ulceration of the feet from pressure or trauma and leads to the intervention strategy. The patient with a low ankle-brachial index would not be considered a candidate for physical therapy services or aggressive wound healing interventions because of the severity of the vascular system impairment. The nurse would manage the patient's wound and refer the patient to the vascular surgeon. The patient with the insensitive foot due to neuropathy would be a candidate for physical therapy because this would constitute a medical necessity, requiring the skills of a physical therapist. The physical therapist would predict a functional outcome of risk reduction following interventions of pressure elimination and stimulation, leading to healing. In both cases, the ulcerations are related to underlying medical pathology. In the former case, the ulcer would not be expected to respond unless the underlying pathology was addressed. In the second case, the ulcer management would be appropriate, along with risk reduction management. The interpretation of the data from the history and physical examinations sets the stage for the functional diagnosis and allows triage of cases that should be referred or managed conservatively.

Examination: Part II

Part II of the examination strategy is to look at four key features of the wound assessment. The four key features are: evaluation of the surrounding skin, assessment of the wound tissue, observation of wound drainage, and size measurements.

Sequencing the examination will depend on visual observation and palpation of the impaired tissues. The examiner chooses those tests and measures specific to the wound situation. For example, temperature testing may be the best way to distinguish the presence of inflammatory processes in a pressure ulcer in persons with darkly pigmented skin. A wound tracing may be the best method to measure the irregular shape of a venous ulcer. After completing the examination part of the diagnostic process, the clinician interprets the physiologic and anatomic systems information and wound assessment data. The clinician brings all the data together like the pieces of a puzzle to develop functional diagnosis.[4]

Evaluation and Diagnosis

The evaluation aspect of the diagnostic process includes evaluation and analysis of findings collected previously and leads to clinical judgments. Diagnosis includes the process and is also the conclusion reached after the evaluation data have been organized.[5] Physical therapists are expected to use the diagnostic process to establish a diagnosis for the specific conditions requiring attention. If the findings of the diagnostic process are such that the management of the patient is outside the physical therapist's knowledge, experience, or expertise, the patient should be referred to the appropriate practitioner.[5] The nurse may reach a diagnostic conclusion that a referral to another practitioner is needed, but, as mentioned previously, the nurse usually cannot bow out while waiting for a referral and is required to provide a plan of care for the patient in the interim. The purpose of data analysis is to draw conclusions about a patient's specific problems or needs so that effective interventions can be implemented. Problem identification is a process of diagnostic reasoning in which judgments, decisions, and conclusions are made about the meaning of the data collected to determine whether or not intervention is needed.[6] Diagnosis involves forming a clinical judgment by identifying a disease/condition or human response through scientific evaluation of signs and symptoms, history, and diagnostic studies. In many respects, a diagnosis is analogous to a research hypothesis. For example, a research hypothesis directs the research study, and a diagnosis directs the patient's care plan. Both a research hypothesis and a diagnosis are chosen based on available data and information, and both research hypotheses and diagnoses may be proven correct or incorrect as the study or care plan progresses.

Physical therapy diagnosis is defined as "a label encompassing a cluster of signs, symptoms, syndromes, or categories."[5(p715)] The purpose of a diagnosis is to guide the clinician in determining the most appropriate intervention strategy for the individual. In the event that the diagnostic process does not provide adequate information, intervention may be based on alleviation of symptoms and remediation of deficits.

Nursing diagnoses identify specific human responses to existing or potential health problems. Health problems may be physical, sociologic, or psychologic. Both nurses and physical therapists make diagnoses based on the symptoms or the sequelae of the injurious process, such as impaired wound healing. Physical therapists evaluate the functional implications of impairments and disabilities leading to a functional diagnosis. Impairment is loss or abnormality of psychologic, physiologic, or anatomic structure or function.[7] Impairment describes the loss of function of a body system or organ, due to illness or injury.[8] An example is loss of function of the skin and underlying soft tissue, due to

wounding or underlying pathology. Additional impairment characteristics include the effect of pathology/disease without attributing cause or the loss of a body part, such as by amputation. Underlying pathology creates the susceptibility to loss of function, eg, "undue susceptibility to pressure ulcers" and "undue insensitivity to pain."[8]

The definition of a disability is any restriction or lack (resulting from an impairment) of ability to perform an activity in the manner or within the range considered normal for a human being. Disability may result from impairment or be caused by the person's response to the impairment. Disability may be permanent, reversible, or irreversible. Disability reflects a deviation in performance or behavior within a task or activity.[8] Examples are the disabled person who has musculoskeletal disablement leading to difficulty walking or moving, or integumentary disablement related to the inability of the body to progress from the inflammatory phase of healing to the proliferative phase.

Functional Diagnosis

Functional diagnosis is defined as an assessment of the related impairments and associated disabilities that affect wound status and its ability to heal. Examples of functional diagnosis are the following:

- Impaired sensation (inability to detect pressure or light touch)
- Impaired circulation (Ankle-Brachial Index below 0.8) of lower extremities
- Impaired lower extremity strength and joint range of motion (including manual muscle test and range of motion) resulting in persistent pressure to buttocks
- Impaired healing associated with chronic inflammation phase.

Physical therapists use functional diagnosis to describe the consequence of disease and as a justification of medical necessity, requiring the skills of the physical therapist. With respect to wounds, the wound healing phase can be used as a functional diagnosis to describe the status of wound healing (see wound healing phases described in Chapter 2).

Each phase of healing can be impaired. Impaired wound healing can be described as prolonged, chronic, or failure to occur, meaning absent. For example, a wound with prolonged or chronic inflammation has impaired functioning of the body system(s) needed to progress to the next phase of repair. The particular phase of wound healing that is dysfunctional helps to predict the interventions needed to restart the repair process.[9]

The impairments in wound healing can be labeled with a diagnosis. The *wound healing phase diagnosis* is a diagnosis of impaired status regarding the biologic phase of wound healing. Examples are presented in Exhibit 1–1.

Exhibit 1–1 12 Possible Wound Healing Phase Diagnoses

1. Chronic inflammation
2. Inflammation
3. Absence of inflammation
4. Chronic proliferation
5. Proliferation
6. Absence of proliferation
7. Chronic epithelialization
8. Epithelialization
9. Absence of epithelialization
10. Chronic remodeling
11. Remodeling
12. Absence of remodeling

The wound healing phase diagnosis describes the biologic phase of repair observed by examination of the wound. Wounds become chronic and lacking in the function necessary to progress to the next phase of repair. This can occur in any of the phases of healing. For example, when wound edges curl in and become fibrotic, the wound demonstrates absence of epithelialization, due to impairment in the epithelialization process. Wounds can become "stuck" in the proliferative phase when infection is present and impairs the proliferative process, thus demonstrating chronic proliferation. Wounds can become chronically inflamed when tissue trauma is prolonged. The wound healing phase diagnosis describes the current status of the wound and can be used to predict how the wound healing should progress. This is logical because wound healing is an orderly series of events. A wound in one phase should progress to and through each successive phase. (See Chapter 2 for information about biologic cascade of healing.)

A question frequently asked is how to state the wound healing phase diagnosis of a wound in transition from one phase to another. The transition is usually gradual, and, because phases overlap, it is appropriate to describe the change by using a ratio of the *dominant phase* to the *recessive phase*. *Dominant* refers to the most active phase observed. *Recessive* refers to the less active phase. A ratio is simply a relationship between two variables—in this case, the relationship between two phases of healing. The way it can be used to describe a wound with the dominant phase active inflammation and the recessive phase active proliferation is to write the description as followings: "The wound healing phase diagnosis is INFLAMMATION/proliferation." The use of capital letters for the dominant phase emphasizes its dominance. Small letters show the relationship of the recessive phase. If the two phases are equal, they can both be capitalized (e.g., INFLAMMATION/PROLIFERATION). The prognosis is that the wound healing phase will progress from inflammation to proliferation.

STEP III: PROGNOSIS AND GOALS

Once the diagnosis is established, the clinician predicts, or prognoses, the expected outcome goals and selects an intervention. Prediction is a useful tool for goal setting. Prediction of the maximal improvement expected from an intervention and how long it will take is the *prognosis*. Prognosis may include prediction of *improvement* at different intervals during treatment.[5] Many clinicians are intimidated by the idea of predicting outcomes. The clinician must be familiar with treatment effects of the interventions he or she prescribes and administers. If the clinician cannot predict the effects of an intervention, who can? Why would a patient want to expose himself or herself to the intervention with unpredictable results? Why should a payer reimburse for services with unexpected benefit and indefinite cost? The successful clinician is able to predict the patient outcomes. In the current health care environment, familiarity with prognosis and outcomes is important for both nurses and physical therapists.

Wound Prognosis Options

For wounds, the prognosis options are limited. One system for evaluating secondary intention wound healing defines healing as minimally, acceptably, or ideally healed. An ideally healed wound results in return of the fully restored dermis and epidermis with intact barrier function. An acceptably healed wound has a resurfaced epithelium capable of sustained functional integrity during activities of daily living. A minimally healed wound is characterized by reepithelialization but does not establish a sustained functional result and may recur. In all of these definitions of healing, complete closure of the wound is expected.[10]

For some individuals and some wounds, closure is not an option. The best prognosis that can be made is for a change in the wound healing phase from an impaired or early phase of repair to a more advanced phase of repair. For example, a wound that is chronically inflamed is impaired from progressing to more advanced phases of healing, and the predicted outcome is that the chronic inflammation will progress to acute inflammation. An acutely inflamed wound prognosis is progression to a proliferative phase. Some wounds progress to the proliferative phase, and it is not expected—nor is it preferred—for the wound to close by secondary intention; the prognosis is a clean and stable wound or a wound prepared for surgical closure. A change in phase is a functional outcome prediction. This method monitors a real change in the organ function of the skin and soft tissues, which is a measure of reduced functional impairment.

A prognosis that the wound is not expected to improve based on the results of the diagnostic process may determine referral for other management. Nurses may be expected to care for the wound, but the patient may not be a candidate for physical therapy intervention. Prognosis is not an option for physical therapists; it is a requirement. Medicare has mandated that a functional outcome prediction be established by the physical therapist at the start of care. This is part of utilization management of medical services.

Goals

Nurses' Goals

In determining goals for the patient, the nurse must set priorities, establish the goals, and identify the desired outcomes. Goals are important because they assist in determining outcomes of care and effectiveness of intervention. Goals must be measurable, objective, and based on the prioritized needs of the patient.

Short-term goals are usually actions that must be met before the patient is discharged or moved to another level of care. Long-term goals may require continued attention by the patient and the caregiver long after discharge. Short-term goals should move the patient toward the long-term goal.

Physical Therapists' Goals

Physical therapists also have a historical requirement to document short- and long-term goals. Physical therapists' goals are expected to be measurable, objective, and functional. Goals used by physical therapists must be very specific. Traditionally, a short-term goal has been one that will be achieved in 30 days or less and usually corresponds to the end of the billing period or length of stay. Long-term goals are those predicted to be attainable by the time of discharge. With the shift to short lengths of stay in different care settings, the time frames have also changed to correspond to the setting. Currently, there is a terminology shift away from using the term *goal* and replacing it with *expected outcome*. A goal is a desired or expected result of an intervention. An outcome is the result or status after the intervention. Completing the diagnostic process with recommendations is one outcome of the services of the physical therapist. The physical therapist is able to target specific, measurable outcomes for specific interventions. To make them functional outcomes, they must meet the criteria described below. Target outcomes are short-term specific expectations of change in impairment status. *Prognosis* is the expected outcome after a course of care and is the long-term goal. Examples of wound healing prognoses are the following:

1. Ideally healed closure
2. Acceptably healed closure
3. Minimally healed closure
4. Clean and stable open wound
5. Ready for surgical closure
6. Not expected to improve

Evaluation of Progress and Outcomes

An *outcome* is the result of what is done and is patient- or wound-focused. The intervention or activity that is done to achieve the result is the *process* to achieve an outcome. How are outcomes measured? Performance indicators are objective measurements that are used to benchmark change as a result of an intervention. Providers, payers, regulators, and clinicians are all working toward establishing reliable performance indicators that are useful for reporting clinical outcomes. Exhibit 1–2 lists examples of some wound-related performance indicators, wound outcomes, and functional outcomes for each. Assessing patient outcomes provides the nurse and physical therapist with a means of assessing how the intervention altered the problem. Two types of outcomes are behavioral and functional. Payer groups have an interest in both the behavioral and functional outcomes.[11]

Reporting Outcomes

The reporting of outcomes is frequently confused with process. There has been much discussion about outcomes, but what is being reported is mainly process. This section will discuss some commonly misused terms and the appropriate way to report an outcome.

Prevention is often the target of an intervention. Prevention is the process to reduce or buffer risk. Risk factors usually exist prior to or at the onset of a problem (eg, immobility, deformities, smoking). Buffers are those attempts to reduce or intervene so as to alter the progression of an impairment, disability, or handicap (eg, take pressure off of a diabetic ulcer).[7] There are many reliable performance indicators that measure risk and intervention-related changes used by both nurses and physical therapists. As part of the initial assessment, apply instruments with performance indicators to test the current status, then retest status after applying the chosen intervention to measure achievement of the predicted outcome. For example, instead of saying the prognosis is "prevention of pressure ulcers" or "minimized risk of pressure ulcers," it would be more appropriate to say "risk of pressure ulcers will be reduced from high to moderate, based on the Braden Scale." The Braden Scale (see Chapter 15) is used to measure risk for development of pressure ulcers. Mobility is one portion of the Braden Scale. If a patient on admission has a low mobility score on the Braden Scale, indicating complete immobility, the patient is judged at high risk for development of a pressure ulcer. The patient receives an intervention for mobility training, and the mobility score improves. Now the patient is slightly limited in mobility and makes frequent changes in body position. There has

Exhibit 1–2 Examples of Performance Indicators, Wound Outcomes, and Functional Wound Outcomes

Performance Indicators	Wound Outcomes	Functional Outcome
1. Change in wound and surrounding skin attributes 2. Reduced severity of wound: depth, size 3. Change in wound exudate characteristics, or undermining 4. Closure	Progression through the phases of wound healing (inflammation, proliferation, epithelialization)	1. Clean stable wound ready for surgical closure 2. Dressing changes needed biweekly instead of daily 3. Exudate managed; patient returns to work 4. Return to work/leisure activities
1. Temperature comparison 2. Transcutaneous partial pressure of oxygen level 3. Laser Doppler	Oxygenation or perfusion of tissue	1. Progress to next wound healing phase 2. Pain level no longer interferes with ADL
1. Girth measurements 2. Volume meter measurements 3. Palpation grading system	Edema reduction or controlled	1. Patient able to don compression hose 2. Leg ulcers are smaller, require less frequent dressing changes
1. Wound exudate characteristics 2. Wound and surrounding skin attributes 3. Culture	Infection controlled	1. Wound exudate odor controlled, able to return to community 2. Pain alleviated, patient resumes walking
1. Necrosis free 2. Proliferation phase tissue attributes 3. Change in depth or size	Clean, stable wound	1. Frequency of visits reduced 2. Physical therapy intervention no longer required 3. Patient can now manage wound dressing changes
1. Braden Scale score 2. Functional activities performance 3. Comprehension testing	Reduced risk of pressure ulceration	1. Repositions self in bed 2. Patient performs self-care activities while in wheelchair 3. Patient demonstrates use of hand mirror to monitor skin
1. Wound closure 2. Functional activities performed related to use of scar tissue	Acceptably healed scar	1. Patient identifies risk factors for reulceration 2. Patient uses protective equipment correctly under scar tissue to perform functional activities in wheelchair

been a functional change in the mobility of the patient. The functional outcome is improved mobility status, which leads to the consequence of reduced risk of pressure ulceration.

Another topic of confusion is about *reduced* risk of infection. This is not an outcome. Infection-free or reduction in exudate, odor, or culture results are measurable outcomes. In order for any of these outcomes to be functional outcomes, they must change the way the body system functions. Freedom from infection may be an outcome of wound cleansing, and it becomes a functional outcome if the wound healing progresses to the next phase of repair. The written functional outcome should be stated as "the wound is infection free and the wound healing has progressed from the inflammatory phase to the proliferative phase."

A troublesome word in health care is *maintained*. Maintained is a process that implies no change. *Controlled* should not be mistaken for *maintained*. If the edema is fluctuating, for instance, from treatment to treatment, then stabilizes as a result of intervention, the outcome is edema controlled. A functional outcome for controlled edema would be stated as "the edema in the tissues surrounding the wound is controlled, and the wound is epithelializing." The functional outcome of control of the edema is that the wound progresses to the next phase of healing.

Maximized and *minimized* are similarly confused with outcomes. For example, "maximized participation in activities of daily living" is not about the functional outcome of an intervention with an orthotic device. A functional outcome reports the result of the intervention, such as "the patient performs activities of daily living wearing/using orthotic equipment, has returned to work and/or resumed leisure activities." An example of misuse of *minimized* as an outcome is "minimized stresses precipitating or perpetuating injury." Correct use is: "Functional outcome—patient/caregiver identified stress-reduction methods to minimize risk or injury."

Improved is defined as to make better or enhance in value. Improved is a subjective measure, not a measurable outcome. An outcome reports the objective result of improvement. For example, increased vital capacity measured in liters (performance indicator) is a measurable change in the pulmonary system, with a result of increased oxygenation of tissues for wound healing. The functional outcome is "wound progresses to next phase of healing."

Provided is sometimes confused with an outcome. This is an action by the clinician, not the outcome of the intervention. An example of improper use is "provided electrical stimulation to enhance circulation." This describes the rationale for the intervention, not the outcome. *Promoted* is another inappropriately used word. "Promoted angiogenesis" is a process. Angiogenesis is an expected outcome from treatment and represents an attribute of wound healing. The performance indicators of angiogenesis are change in wound attributes, phase, or size. The outcome is wound progression through proliferative phase.

Behavioral Outcomes.

Behavioral outcomes include behaviors or items that can be observed or monitored to determine whether an acceptable or positive outcome is achieved within the desired time frame. Outcomes must be specific, realistic, time-oriented, objective, patient-centered, and measurable. Write outcomes by listing behaviors or items that can be observed or monitored to determine whether an acceptable or positive outcome is achieved within the desired time frame. The outcome then serves as the evaluation tool.

Use measurable action verbs to describe behavioral outcomes. For example, the verb *understand* is not measurable; we cannot measure a person's understanding. But the verb *identify* is measurable; the patient can be tested to determine whether or not he or she can identify. Other action verbs include *list, record, name, state, describe, explain, demonstrate, use, schedule, differentiate, compare, relate, design, prepare, formulate, select, choose, increase, decrease, stand, walk,* and *participate*. Contrast these action verbs with the verbs *understand, feel, learn, know,* and *accept,* all of which are not measurable. Examples of expected behavioral outcomes for a wound patient are the following: "The patient will describe the signs of wound infection and identify correct action within 24 hours, the patient will demonstrate wound dressing application within 2 days." Documenting that the target outcome was met would include a statement: "Patient is able to describe the signs of infection and list the steps for corrective action. Patient is able to demonstrate correct wound dressing application."

Functional Outcomes.

A functional outcome helps to communicate the change in function to the patient, caregiver, or payer. Physical therapists usually deal with patients who have loss of functional abilities and use functional tests that measure physical attributes to predict the function that the patient is expected to achieve after a course of treatment. What is *function*? Function in this context refers to those activities or actions that are meaningful to the patient or caregiver. Meaningful function is determined while completing the reason for referral portion of the assessment. To be a functional outcome, the results must meet three criteria:[12]

1. Is the result meaningful?
2. Is the result practical?
3. Will the result be sustained outside the treatment setting?

Meaningful is defined as of value to the patient, caregiver, or both. *Practical* means that the outcome is applicable to the patient's life situation. *Sustainable over time* refers to functional abilities achieved through the intervention maintained by the patient or caregiver outside the clinical setting (eg, patient demonstrated ability to apply dressing and stocking during two follow-up visits).[13]

Standardized tests and measurement tools are quite useful to monitor and track change over time. The Pressure Sore Status Tool (PSST) and the Sussman Wound Healing Tool (SWHT) are described in Chapter 6 and can be used to document outcomes of change in wound attributes by change in test scores, then applied to function. For instance, if the PSST is used to monitor exudate amounts, there would be a change in score on that test item from 4 (moderate exudate) to 2 (scant exudate), indicating reduced drainage.

This outcome is measurable, objective, and meets all the criteria listed for a valid outcome, but this information alone is not a functional outcome. To interpret this score as a functional outcome, a statement is needed that connects the findings with meaning to the patient, practical effect, and sustainable result. A resulting statement of functional outcomes is: "Wound exudate PSST score has reduced from 4 (moderate) to 2 (scant) exudate, patient demonstrates ability to monitor for signs of infection and action to take, patient is now able to return to work and will be seen for intermittent follow-up."

Functional outcomes should be documented throughout the course of care, not just at discharge. Statements that can be used to demonstrate intermittent functional change include change in patient lifestyle, change in patient safety, or adaptation to impairment or disability. These statements should be patient-centered and measurable (Exhibit 1–3).

Change in wound tissue attributes and size can also be used as functional outcome (Exhibit 1–4): "Necrosis free, reduced risk of infection, and size reduced 50%, wound is clean and stable, decreased frequency of visits required."

THE FUNCTIONAL OUTCOME REPORT

This chapter has described three of the four steps needed to complete the diagnostic process. The functional outcome report (FOR) developed by Swanson, described below, is a written report describing the diagnostic process.[4] Swanson's FOR helps the therapist to project clinical reasoning that is clear, logical, and understandable to the reader. As previously explained, payers want to know about functional outcomes, not wound measurements and tissue color. The FOR process helps to communicate treatment strategies to justify the intervention and lead to a predictable functional outcome.[13] Exhibit 1–5 is a completed example of the report.

Exhibit 1–3 Example of Functional Outcomes Documented Throughout Course of Care

- *Initial statement:* Patient is unable to sit in wheelchair without trauma to integument.
- *Initial target outcome:* Patient is sitting for 2 hours in adaptive seating system in 2 weeks.
- *Interim outcome after 1 week:* Patient sits for 1 hour in adaptive seating system.
- *Discharge statement:* Patient sits in adaptive seating system for 2 hours without disruption of integumentary integrity. Change in wound tissue attributes and size can also be used as functional outcome: Necrosis free, reduced risk of infection, and size reduced 50%, wound is clean and stable, decreased frequency of visits required.

Exhibit 1–4 How To Write Outcome Statements and Functional Outcomes

When reporting outcomes, use the following guidelines:

1. An outcome expresses the *result* of an intervention—not the intervention or the process—to reach an outcome (eg, wound resurfacing/closure).
2. A behavioral outcome may be learned information (eg, demonstrates application of wound dressing). This outcome would follow an intervention of instruction.
3. Coordination, communication, and documentation are behavioral outcomes used to ensure proper utilization management.

Functional outcomes are written to describe function results of treatment and include three parts:

1. A functional outcome statement describes a meaningful functional change to a body system (eg, progression through the phases of healing).
2. A functional outcome statement describes a practical result of the change in the body system (eg, wound is minimally exudative).
3. A functional outcome statement describes the sustainable result or change in the impairment status or disability resulting from the intervention (eg, pressure elimination allows the patient to sit up in wheelchair 2 hours twice a day).

There are additional examples of the FOR in Chapter 16 and in the case studies in Part IV.

The FOR document has six parts. Part I, Patient History and Medical History, begins with the *reason for referral.* Here, the clinician establishes patient needs. The report will read in one of the following manners:

- Patient/family seek services for . . .
- The patient/family reports . . .
- The following medical problems are associated with this request for service . . .

It is not unusual that, following a course of therapy, there will be residual impairments and disabilities in conjunction with a meaningful functional outcome that is important to the patient (eg, a clean, edema-free wound). This may be the most important goal and the reason for the referral because it is meaningful to the patient.

Part II, Systems Review, is an analysis of *functional limitations.* Function refers to many different activities or actions. With respect to wounds, this includes identification

Exhibit 1–5 Sample FOR

Patient ID: J.J.   **AGE:** 59

Part I

Patient History:

Reason for Referral:

Patient/family seeks services for: Return to social activities and concern about a pressure ulcer on a heel.
Caregiver's report: Less time is now spent out of bed, and patient has episodes of confusion. Patient is usually alert and oriented and has adequate communication skills to make needs, wants, and discomforts known.

Medical History:

Medical Impairments, Taken from Medical History:

- Limited respiratory capacity due to chronic obstructive pulmonary disease.
- Requires continuous oxygen from a concentrator.

Part II

Systems Review:

The Following Systems Are Impaired:

Cardiopulmonary System:

- Pulse oximetry: 98%—good oxygen saturation achieved with supplemental oxygen.

Musculoskeletal System:

- Contracted to 90° at hips and knees and has limited bed mobility.

Vascular System:

- Impaired circulation of the lower extremities: coldness, pallor, absence of hair, and poor pulses.

Integumentary System:

- Skin intact but impaired by eschar over a pressure ulcer on the right heel.

Part III

Evaluation (Clinical Assessment or Diagnosis):

1. Specific functional losses causing the patient's need for service are: loss of wound healing capacity.
2. Patient's functional loss is due to
   - Respiratory impairment and circulatory impairment.
   - Mechanical impairments of the lower extremities (contractures of hips and knees).
   - Motor impairment (unable to reposition in bed and unable to transfer to wheelchair).

Part IV

Functional Diagnosis:

The loss of function causes the following:
- Undue susceptibility for pressure wound on lower feet.
- Inability to heal without integumentary intervention.

Part V

Prognosis:

Patient has improvement potential; will heal following intervention but will continue to be at risk for pressure ulceration.

Part VI

Treatment Plan:

1. Pressure relief to heel.
2. Instruct caregiver in exercise program.
3. Ankle brachial index to guide treatment.
4. Electrical stimulation to heel for increased micro-circulation and autolysis.

---

and analysis of the functional limits of the local tissues to perform the activities necessary to initiate repair. Function also implies that the body systems have the ability to perform the repair. For instance, the current status of the tissue assessment identifies tissue activity (eg, inflammation phase) and the circulatory system response to injury (eg, erythema, edema, pain, and heat).

An impaired circulatory system function will impair the healing process. The clinician writes the report with the following leads:

- The specific functional items that are causing the patient's need for service are (eg, impaired healing response)

- Patient's functional loss of healing is due to (eg, impairment of the circulatory system)
- The loss of function causes the following (eg, inability to progress through the phases of repair without intervention)
- Patient has improvement potential (eg, patient has improvement potential but remains at risk for ischemic ulceration)

In Part III, Evaluation, *clinical assessment or diagnosis* is the clinical impression, based on the results of the tests and measures selected by the clinician. The clinician chooses tests and measures that have performance indicators for wounds. This is defined differently from the medical diagnosis because it focuses on the functional consequence of the disease, rather than on the etiology. See the section on functional diagnosis described earlier.

Part IV, Functional Diagnosis, is the justification of *need for skilled service for the therapy problem*. Utilization management requires that there be an identification of the specific elements that will be changed as a result of the intervention and, once changed, will improve the patient's functional status. An example of a wound problem that can be expected to change as a result of an intervention is a change in the phase of wound healing as a result of an intervention (eg, whirlpool). Change can also be expected in the wound symptoms (eg, erythema free, pain free), which will demonstrate improved functional status of the tissues.

In Part V, Prognosis, *prediction of a functional outcome* is expected because clinicians have a responsibility to know the effect of the selected treatment interventions. Patients and referral sources have a right to this information when they expose themselves to an episode of care. Prediction is not new. Previously, prediction was known as short- and long-term goals. A short-term goal usually referred to a 2- to 4-week period of care, and a long-term goal was what would be achieved at discharge. The functional outcome section of the report has three components related to the predicted functional outcome: the activity that would occur, the performance expected, and the due date. For example, with respect to wounds, the "activity" may be erythema free, the "performance" change to proliferative phase, and the "due date" 2–4 weeks. This segment of the report promotes continuity of care when different or multiple clinicians are involved in the patient's care.

In Part VI, the final step in the FOR is to present the *treatment plan with rationale*. Subsequent chapters will provide the rationale for many different interventions, based on established theory and science. This is the place where the clinician reveals the clinical judgment used to select a treatment plan. For example, the clinician writes that the wound is in a chronic inflammatory phase related to a large amount of necrotic tissue, has failed to respond to prior treatment interventions, and requires debridement to initiate the healing process. This becomes the rationale for selecting the treatment strategy (eg, pulsatile lavage with suction) to clean up the necrotic debris.

Applying FOR to Form HCFA-700

To become familiar with the diagnostic process and the FOR method, review the sample case in Exhibit 1–5. Physical therapists are accustomed to using the Form HCFA-700 (11-91) for documentation (see Appendix 1–C). The HCFA-700 and the FOR method of reporting were designed to work together. A template added to the HCFA-700 (Appendix 1–D) guides the physical therapist through documentation of the diagnostic process and FOR methodology. Appendix 1–E is a sample case report on the HCFA-700, using FOR methodology.

Clinical Wisdom: *HCFA-700 on Computer*

Some facilities have the HCFA-700 form on computer. If a template can be added to the form with the items as listed formatted to fit the computer field, it would help the physical therapist to complete the documentation in an orderly and consistent manner. For those using a hard copy of HCFA-700, a template can still be useful to ensure that all items are recorded following the format.

Evaluation of Progress

Once the target outcomes and goals have been determined, the reevaluation process is really quite simple. The clinician uses performance indicators to measure the patient's progress toward the outcome within the desired time frame. For example, if the target outcome is "patient's wound will demonstrate 25% reduction in size within 2 weeks," the clinician simply monitors wound size over the 2-week period of time, then determines whether the wound has reduced surface area size by 25% at the end of week 2. If the wound has decreased in size more than 25%, the outcome has been exceeded. If the wound has decreased in size by just 25%, the outcome has been acceptably met. If the wound has failed to decrease in size by 25%, the outcome has not been met, and the goals must be adjusted and interventions reviewed. Failure to achieve goals may be related to change in the patient's overall condition, ineffective therapy, or inadequate adherence to the treatment regimen. Reevaluation is an ongoing dynamic process that will recur on a regular basis following reexamination of the effects of treatment. At that time, goals and outcomes may be adjusted, new goals developed, and interventions modified.

Because utilization management attempts to influence the clinical path from the beginning, so as to reduce deviation from an expected course and to produce optimal outcomes, the adjustment of goals and expected outcomes should be minimal. Multiple approximations to reach the target outcome will not be tolerated by patients or third-party payers. For example, the *APTA Guide to PT Practice*[14] lists wound management guidelines regarding range of visits and length of episodic care by physical therapists for patients with wounds. This range represents the lower and upper limits of services that an anticipated 80% of the patients/clients with such wounds will need to achieve in order to reach the predicted goals and outcomes (prognosis) listed. Multiple factors may modify the duration of the episode of care, frequency, and number of visits. Wounds extending into fascia, muscle, or bone (integumentary pattern E), for instance, will require 4–16 weeks (12–112 visits) for an episode of care (all types of etiologies included). The prognosis for wounds of this severity is that, over the course of 4–16 weeks of care by the physical therapist, one of the following will occur:

- Wound will be clean and stable.
- Wound will be prepared for closure.

- Wound will be closed.
- Immature scar will be evident.[14]

CONCLUSION

The diagnostic process described in this chapter is intended as a framework for clinicians working with patients with wounds. The information may or may not be new, but there are times when review of material may be helpful. This chapter is meant to assist those clinicians new to the diagnostic process or unfamiliar with its use. Use of clinical judgment with diagnostic reasoning is one of the essential practice tools that nurses and physical therapists use with the patients they serve.

REVIEW QUESTIONS

1. What are the steps in the diagnostic process?
2. What is the difference between a behavioral and a functional outcome?
3. What are five areas for data collection during the assessment phase?

REFERENCES

1. Clifton DW. Utilization management: Whose job is it? *Rehab Manage.* June/July 1996;38:44.
2. Bergstrom N, Bennett MA, Carlson C, et al. Treatment of pressure ulcers. *Clinical Practice Guideline.* No. 15. Rockville, MD: US Department of Health and Human Services (DHHS), AHCPR Publication No. 95-0652, December 1994.
3. Hisch IB, White PF. Medical management of surgical patients with diabetes. In: Levin ME, O'Neal LW, Bowker JH, eds. *The Diabetic Foot.* Chicago: CV Mosby; 1993.
4. Swanson G. *The Guide to Physical Therapist Practice.* Vol 1. Presented at California chapter, APTA, October 1995; San Diego, CA.
5. American Physical Therapy Association. A guide to physical therapy practice, I: a description of patient management. *Phys Ther.* 1995;75:707–764.
6. Doenges MD, Moorhouse MF, Burley JT. *Application of Nursing Process and Nursing Diagnosis.* 2nd ed. Philadelphia: FA Davis; 1995.
7. Jette AM. Physical disablement concepts for physical therapy research and practice. *Phys Ther.* 1994;74:380–386.
8. Swanson G. *The IDH Guidebook for Physical Therapy.* Long Beach, CA: Swanson and Company; 1995.
9. Sussman C. Case presentation: patient with a pressure ulcer on the coccyx. Paper presented at APTA Scientific Meeting and Exposition, June 1996; Minneapolis, MN.
10. Lazarus GS, Cooper DM, Knighton DR, et al. Definitions and guidelines for assessment of wounds and evaluation of healing. *Arch Dermatol.* 1994;130:489–493.
11. Swanson G. What is an outcome? And what does it mean to you? *Ultra/sounds.* (California Private Practice Special Interest Group—California APTA). 1995;94(51):7.
12. Swanson G. Functional outcome report: The next generation in physical therapy reporting in documenting physical therapy outcomes. In: Stuart D, Ablen S, eds. *Documenting Physical Therapy Outcomes.* Chicago: CV Mosby; 1993:101–134.
13. Staley M, Richard R, et al. Functional outcomes for the patient with burn injuries. *J Burn Care Rehab.* 1996;17(4):362–367.
14. Guide to physical therapist practice. *Phys Ther.* 1997;77:1593–1605.

Appendix 1–A: Patient History Form

Medical Record #_____ Name_____

Street Address _____

City, State, Zip _____

Telephone Number (_____)_____

Sex: M/F_____Height: _____ Weight: _____

Religious Preference: _____

What is your primary reason for seeking wound care today? _____

_____

How long has your wound existed? _____

_____

Who referred you here? _____

Who has been treating you before today? _____

Can you describe what you have been using on your wound? _____

_____

Who has been helping you with your wound care? _____

How have you been paying for your supplies? _____

Have you ever had surgery? _____ Type: _____

Do you have any allergies? Medications (Sulfa, Penicillin) _____ Other? _____

Do you smoke? _____Packs per day: _____ # of years: _____

How often do you use recreational or illicit drugs? _____

How often do you drink alcohol? _____

Do you have any pain? _____

On a scale of 0–10 (0 = No Pain, 10 = Severe Pain), what is your pain level now? 0 - 1 - 2 - 3 - 4 - 5 - 6 - 7 - 8 - 9 - 10

What over-the-counter medications are you taking (Tylenol, aspirin, antacids, vitamins, etc.): _____

_____

What prescription medications are you taking? Please include drug, dose, and frequency: _____

_____

Have you ever been told you had or do you currently have any of the following:

	Past	Present		Past	Present
Stroke:			Hypertension:		
Gangrene:			Cancer:		
Problems with circulation:			Chemotherapy:		
Arterial:			Radiation therapy:		
Venous:			Alternative treatments:		
Diabetes:			Swollen glands:		
Parkinson's:			Muscle spasms:		
Alzheimer's:			Polio or post-polio syndrome:		
Congestive heart failure:			Quadriplegia/paraplegia:		
Problems sleeping:			Myelomeningocele:		
Emphysema:			Decreased sensation:		
Bronchitis:			Arthritis:		
Chronic obstructive pulmonary disease:			Decreased activity:		
Problems controlling urine:			HIV or AIDS:		
Problems controlling bowels:			Hepatitis B:		
Atherosclerosis/arteriosclerosis:			Decreased appetite:		
Malnutrition:			Problems with mobility:		
Dehydration:			Changes in weight greater than 10 pounds:		
Thyroid disorder:			Pacemaker:		

21

Appendix 1–B: Focused Assessment for Wounds

Medical Record # _____ Name _____

Attending Physician: _____

Referral Source: _____MD _____Nurse _____Other

Site: __Office ___Acute Hospital ___Subacute Center ___Nursing Home ___Assisted Living ___Home __Other

  Facility Name / Address / Pts. bed #: _____

Physical Exam: _____year-old M F acquired non-healing wound(s) on   /   /   .

Prior wound management includes:

_____

Past Medical History is positive for the following:

Allergies _____	Alcoholism _____
CVA _____	NIDDM _____
Gangrene _____	Complications of DM _____
PVD _____	Weakness _____
Arterial insufficiency _____	Paraplegia/quadriplegia _____
CAD _____	Immobility/contractures _____
IDDM _____	Parkinson's _____

Vitals: T/P/R _____ BP: L/R_____(sit/stand/lying)

Braden Scale:

Sensory/MS	1. totally limited	2. very limited	3. slightly limited	4. no impairment
Moisture	1. constantly moist	2. very moist	3. occasionally moist	4. dry
Activity	1. bedfast	2. chairfast	3. walks w/assist	4. walks frequently
Mobility	1. 100% immobile	2. very limited	3. slightly limited	4. full mobility
Nutrition	1. very poor	2. < 1/2 daily portion	3. most of portion	4. eats everything
Friction/Shear	1. frequent sliding	2. feeble corrections	3. independent correction	

Braden Scale Total: _____

Mental Status: Alert & Oriented X 3 : Other _____

Skin: (moist, dry, flaky, scaly, condition of nails): _____ Turgor: good / med / poor
  Rubor, cyanosis, atrophy, dermatitis, hair loss, rash, erythema.

EENT (Eyes sunken, swollen lymph nodes): _____ Mucous Membranes Moist: _____

Neuro (Cranial nerves, sensation): _____

Endocrine (Blood sugar/other): _____

Respiratory: Lungs Clear: Other: _____

Cardiac: Regular Rate & Rhythm: Other: _____

Abdomen: G-Tube: Soft/Supple/Without Masses or Tenderness: Other: _____

Perineal: Skin intact _____   Other: _____

Lower Extremities: Ankle Brachial Index: L:_____ R:_____

  Pulses Palpable: Dorsalis Pedis _____ Posterior Tibial _____ Popliteal _____

  Pulse Quality: Bounding _____ Strong _____ Weak _____ Barely Palpable _____

  Doppler: L + _____ : R + _____

  Edema_____ Circumference: (L) _____ : (R) _____

Functional Assessment: ADLs: Independent _____ Minimal Assist _____ Mod Assist _____ Total Assist _____

Labs/Nutrition: Hct: _____% TP: _____ Alb: _____ Prealbumin: _____ Other: _____

       WBC:_____ % O_2 Sat:_____ Lytes: _____

Suggested Tests/Examinations: _____

Source: Adapted with permission of Dean P. Kane, MD, FACS, PA.

Appendix 1–C: Form HCFA-700

Department of Health and Human Services
Health Care Financing Administration

Medicare Part ❏ A ❏ B

FORM APPROVED

PLAN OF TREATMENT FOR OUTPATIENT REHABILITATION *(COMPLETE FOR INITIAL CLAIMS ONLY)*

1. PATIENT'S LAST NAME FIRST NAME M.I.	2. PROVIDER NO.	3. HICN

4. PROVIDER NAME	5. MEDICAL RECORD NO. *(Optional)*	6. ONSET DATE	7. SOC. DATE

8. TYPE:	9. PRIMARY DIAGNOSIS *(Pertinent Medical DX.)*	10. TREATMENT DIAGNOSIS	11. VISITS FROM SOC.

12. PLAN OF TREATMENT FUNCTIONAL GOALS	PLAN
OUTCOME *(Long Term)*	

13. SIGNATURE *(professional established POC including prof. designation)*	14. FREQ/DURATION *(eg, 3 wk–4 wk)*

I CERTIFY THE NEED FOR THESE SERVICES FURNISHED UNDER THIS PLAN OF TREATMENT AND	17. CERTIFICATION FROM THROUGH ❏ N/A
15. PHYSICIAN SIGNATURE 16. DATE	18. ON FILE *(Print/type physician's name)* ❏

20. INITIAL ASSESSMENT *(History, medical complications, level of function at start of care. Reason for referral)*	19. PRIOR HOSPITALIZATION FROM TO ❏ N/A

21. FUNCTIONAL LEVEL *(End of billing period)*   PROGRESS REPORT   ❏ CONTINUE SERVICES *OR*   ❏ DC SERVICES

22. SERVICE DATES FROM   THROUGH

FORM HCFA-700 (11-91)

Source: Reprinted from Form HCFA-700 (11-91), Department of Health and Human Services, Health Care Financing Administration.

Appendix 1–D: HCFA-700 Form with FOR Template To Guide Documentation in Italics

Department of Health and Human Services
Health Care Financing Administration   MEDICARE PART ☒A   ☐ B   OMB NO. 09380227

PLAN OF TREATMENT FOR OUTPATIENT REHABILITATION *(COMPLETE FOR INITIAL CLAIMS ONLY)*

1. PATIENT'S LAST NAME FIRST NAME M.I.	2. PROVIDER NO.	3. HICN
4. PROVIDER NAME 5. MEDICAL RECORD NO. *(Optional)*	6. ONSET DATE	7. SOC. DATE
8. TYPE 9. PRIMARY DIAGNOSIS *(Pertinent Medical Dx)*	10. TREATMENT DIAGNOSIS *(Functional Dx)*	11. VISITS FROM SOC.

12. PLAN OF TREATMENT FUNCTIONAL GOALS GOALS (Short-Term) *(Target Outcomes)* Outcomes (Long-Term) *(Prognosis)*	PLAN (Need for skilled services)
13. SIGNATURE (professional established POC including prof. designation)	14. FREQ/DURATION (eg, 3/wk–4 wk) *(Due Date)*

I CERTIFY THE NEED FOR THESE SERVICES FURNISHED UNDER THIS PLAN OF TREATMENT AND WHILE UNDER MY CARE ☒ N/A	17. CERTIFICATION ☐ N/A FROM THROUGH
15. PHYSICIAN SIGNATURE	16. DATE	18. ON FILE (Print/type physician's name) ☒

| 20. INITIAL ASSESSMENT (History, medical complications, level of function at start of care. Reason for referral) | 19. PRIOR HOSPITALIZATION   ☐ N/A
FROM   TO |

Reason for Referral:

Hx:

Systems Review:

Results of Test and Measures:

Wound Healing Tissue Assessment:

Wound Size:

21. FUNCTIONAL LEVEL *(End of billing period)*   PROGRESS REPORT *(Verify functional outcomes):*
☐ CONTINUE SERVICES or   ☐ DC SERVICES

Change in Wound Functional Status:

Change in Mobility Functional Status:

| 22. Service Dates: FROM   THROUGH |

Source: Reprinted from Form HCFA-700 (11-91), Department of Health and Human Services, Health Care Financing Administration.

Appendix 1–E: Sample Case Report Using HCFA-700

Department of Health and Human Services
Health Care Financing Administration

MEDICARE PART ☒ A   ☐ B

OMB NO. 09380227

PLAN OF TREATMENT FOR OUTPATIENT REHABILITATION (COMPLETE FOR INITIAL CLAIMS ONLY)

1. PATIENT'S LAST NAME	FIRST NAME	M.I.	2. PROVIDER NO.	3. HICN
Luck	George			

4. PROVIDER NAME	5. MEDICAL RECORD NO. *(Optional)*	6. ONSET DATE	7. SOC. DATE
		10/09/01	11/27/01

8. TYPE	9. PRIMARY DIAGNOSIS *(Pertinent Medical Dx)*	10. TREATMENT DIAGNOSIS *(Functional Dx)*	11. VISITS FROM SOC.
	CHF, COPD, multiple decubitus, weakness, debility	2 wounds with impaired wound healing secondary to eschar and chronic inflammatory phase. Impaired mobility, transfers, gait (707; 710.7)	15

12. PLAN OF TREATMENT FUNCTIONAL GOALS

GOALS (Short-Term) *(Target Outcomes)*

Tissue Attribute changes expected:
Necrosis free and wound healing progression to Proliferative
phase Wound #1 & 2   21 days
Reduce risk of pressure ulcers (Reduce Braden score to 19/22)   15 days
Transfers and Gait with FWW to bathroom SBA   15 days

Outcomes (Long-term goals-prognosis of Functional Outcomes)

Target Performance Status:
Patient has improvement potential: Wounds will heal following intervention. Functional independent bed

mobility, transfer and gait with assist device will be restored to enable patient to return to prior living situation in 6 weeks.

PLAN *(Need for skilled PT services)*
1. Wound not improving with routine dressing changes, pressure relief & enzymatic debridement
2. Wounds #1 & 2 require a) sharp debride b) HVPC (electrical stimulation) to stimulate cells of repair and circulation for healing
3. Ther ex., balance, gait training to reduce risk of pressure ulcers and enhance circulation for healing current ulcers

13. SIGNATURE (professional established POC including prof. designation)	14. FREQ/DURATION (Due Date)
	6x/wk daily × 6 wks (36 days)

I CERTIFY THE NEED FOR THESE SERVICES FURNISHED UNDER THIS PLAN OF TREATMENT AND WHILE UNDER MY CARE   ☒ N/A

15. PHYSICIAN SIGNATURE	16. DATE

17. CERTIFICATION   ☒ N/A
FROM   THROUGH

18. ON FILE (Print/type physician's name)
☒

20. INITIAL ASSESSMENT (History, medical complications, level of function at start of care. Reason for referral)	19. PRIOR HOSPITALIZATION ☐ N/A
	FROM 10/08/01 TO 11/26/01

Reason for Referral: Loss of mobility (eg, unable to reposition in bed, or ambulate); necrotic pressure ulcers R upper back and coccyx. Wants to regain prior level of indep. Gait with cane. Heal pressure ulcers for return to retirement home.
Hx: Mild dementia, indep. in gait w/cane; fell in shower and was unable to move; sustained pressure ulcers R upper back and coccyx, CHF, COPD.

Systems Review: 1) Cardiopulmonary system disabilities affect oxygen transport to tissues for repair. 2) Musculoskeletal impairments due to weakness (MMS BLE 3-/5 limit bed mobility, inability to transfer or ambulate without assist of 2 w/4ww × few feet. Diminished balance. 3) Neuromuscular impairment due to reduced cerebral oxygen causes mild functional loss of mentation, impaired mobility and awareness of need to reposition. Risk of Pressure ulcers is moderate (Braden Risk score 17/23). *Results of test and measures:* Wound Severity Dx (stage) delayed until both wounds are debrided. *Wound healing tissue assessment:* 1) R upper Back: presence of tissue attributes "good for healing"; adherence of wound edges; and "not good for healing": necrosis and depth of 0.2cm; 2) coccyx: presence of attributes "not for healing": erythema, necrosis, absence of attributes "good for healing." *Wound Size:* R Up Back: 17.7cm² Coccyx: 4.3cm² .depth >0.2

21. FUNCTIONAL LEVEL PROGRESS REPORT *(End of billing period) (Verify functional outcomes):* ☐ CONTINUE   ☐ DC Services
1) *Change in Wound Status:* a) R upper back: progressed to proliferative phase of healing. Wound is erythema free, necrosis free and has factors "good for healing": Contraction sustained × 2 weeks, edges are adhered. Wound is reduced in size from 17.5cm² to 12.3cm² (decreased 25%), b) Coccyx: increased size and extent from 34.4cm² to 37.41cm² after debriding. Severity Dx: Stage IV Pressure ulcer. Tissue attributes present: "not good for healing" include: Undermining at 9:00 position, necrosis and erythema; good for healing attributes include: granulation-significant reduction in depth from 2.0 cm to 1.5 cm, appearance of contraction and sustained wound contraction for 2 weeks (reduced size). Wound is at end of acute inflammatory phase and progressing to proliferative phase. 2) *Change in Mobility Status:* a) Braden risk score 19/23; b) Performs transfers and gait with min-assist using FWW for 15 feet; c) *Change in Balance* improved from fair to fair+ with functional change. Reduced risk of falling and pressure ulcers.

22. Service Dates: FROM 11/27/01   THROUGH 11/30/01

Source: Reprinted from Department of Health and Human Services, Health Care Financing Administration.

CHAPTER 2

Wound Healing Physiology and Chronic Wound Healing

Carrie Sussman and Barbara M. Bates-Jensen

CHAPTER OBJECTIVES

At the completion of this chapter, the reader will be able to:

1. Define and discuss three models of acute wound healing and chronic wound healing.
2. Describe four phases of acute wound healing physiology and the causative factors that interrupt acute wound healing for each phase of repair.
3. Understand the intrinsic, extrinsic, and iatrogenic factors that may impact the healing process.

Wound healing is a complex process that is well organized and controlled by the interplay of cellular and biochemical events. This chapter reviews three basic wound healing models, chronic wound healing, the physiology of acute wound healing, causative factors that interrupt acute wound healing leading to chronicity, fetal wound healing, and factors that may impact the healing process. To provide optimal wound management, the clinician must first understand normal acute wound healing physiology, be able to recognize the current status of the wound, diagnose abnormal wound healing, and evaluate the benefits of products and outcomes.

WOUND HEALING MODELS

Five basic wound healing models for acute wounds are discussed in this book: (1) superficial wound healing, (2) primary intention wound healing, (3) delayed primary intention wound healing, (4) partial-thickness wound healing, and (5) full-thickness/secondary intention healing (see Table 2–1). Similarities exist in all five. This chapter discusses three of them: superficial, partial-, and full-thickness/secondary

intention healing. Chapter 14 provides discussion on primary and delayed primary intention healing.

Superficial Wound Healing

An alteration in the superficial skin, such as by pressure (stage I pressure ulcers), first-degree burns, and contusion, produces an inflammatory repair process that is comparable to that of open wounds.[1] Superficial skin involvement may be an indicator of deeper soft tissue trauma and needs to be investigated for changes in skin color, temperature (warmth, followed by coolness, indicating tissue devitalization), tension or swelling of tissues, and sensation indicating tissue congestion. If deep tissue death occurs a few days after first observation, the tissues may rupture and become a deep cavity. This often occurs in stage I pressure ulcers and is referred to as the *erupting volcano* effect. *Color Plates 19 and 20* show a pressure ulcer with superficial and partial-thickness (stages I and II) pressure ulcers that manifest the true degree of involvement 3 weeks after first diagnosed. In superficial wound healing, the soft tissues usually heal by themselves over time, but intervention at this stage may hasten return to functional activities, such as work and homemaking. For instance, athletes are seen and treated immediately for superficial soft tissue injuries, with reduced loss of playing time, less pain, and less tissue swelling from congestion in the tissues, which often limits functional activities, resulting in diminished mobility and placing the individual at risk for further wounding. Part IV of this book, "Management of Wound Healing with Physical Therapy Technologies," points out benefits from intervention for superficial wounds (eg, reabsorption of hematoma for faster healing, including stage I pressure ulcers, "purple ulcers," and grade I neuropathic ulcers). *Color Plates 74–76* il-

Table 2–1 Principal Mechanisms of Healing

Healing Method	Mechanisms in Order of Significance
Primary Intention	1. Connective tissue 3-remodeling deposition 2. Epithelialization 3. Remodeling
Secondary Intention	1. Contraction 2. Angiogenesis 3. Connective tissue deposition 4. Epithelialization 5. Remodeling

Source: Reprinted with permission from M.D. Kerstein et al., *The Physiology of Wound Healing*, p.7, © 1998, The Oxford Institute for Continuing Education and Allegheny University of Health Sciences.

lustrate how early intervention reduces hematoma (purple ulceration) and hastens repair. Case studies are described in Chapter 24, "Therapeutic and Diagnostic Ultrasound."

Partial-Thickness Wound Healing

Wounds that have partial-thickness loss of the dermis heal principally by epithelialization, which is the resurfacing of the wound by new epithelial cells that are mostly keratinocytes. Epithelialization is the body's attempt to protect itself from invasion or debris by beginning the process of closing the wound that begins immediately following injury. Epithelial cells at the wound edges, as well as from the dermal appendages—sebaceous glands, sweat glands, and hair follicles—provide a supply of intact epithelial cells to assist in resurfacing the wound by lateral migration.[2,3] If the dermal appendages are present, islands of epidermis may appear throughout the wound surface and speed the resurfacing process. The resulting epithelium is often indistinguishable from the surrounding skin, and the normal function of the skin is restored. Examples of partial-thickness wounds are abrasions, skin tears, stage II pressure ulcers, and second-degree burns.

Full-Thickness Secondary Intention Healing

Full-thickness/secondary intention healing is the chosen method of healing when the wound extends through all layers of the skin and/or if it extends into underlying tissues. For instance, when a large amount of tissue is removed or destroyed and a gap occurs, the wound edges cannot be approximated, or there are nonviable wound margins, it is left to close by secondary intention (see *Color Plates 18, 38, and 81*). Wounds with a high microorganism count, debris, or skin necrosis are also left to close by secondary intention. Full-thickness secondary intention healing is principally by contraction.

Repair of tissue by secondary intention involves scar tissue formation. In this process, the anatomic structure of the scar tissue does not replicate the tissue replaced (eg, muscles, tendons, and nerves). In addition, the surface tissue will not be equal in elasticity or tensile strength to the original.[2]

Sometimes, there is a defect that is too small to close by primary intention, and healing by secondary intention is preferred. Some wounds are incompletely covered by split-thickness skin grafts and are best healed by secondary intention. If a wound is in an area where contraction will produce disfiguring or nonfunctional deformities, the process of healing by secondary intention may be allowed to develop a good, healthy wound bed. Then it may be interrupted and a split-thickness skin graft placed on the granulating wound bed. Full-thickness wound healing involves a process that is nominally divided into four overlapping phases of repair: inflammation, epithelialization, proliferation, and remodeling.

Chronic Wound Healing

Secondary intention is the mechanism for healing associated with chronic wounds.[4] Lazarus defines chronic wounds as those that have "failed to proceed through an orderly and timely process to produce anatomic and functional integrity, or proceeded through the repair process without establishing a sustained anatomic and functional result."[4(p181)] Orderly refers to the orderly progression of the wound through the biological sequences that comprise the phases of repair described under Wound Healing Physiology. Orderliness may be interrupted during any of the phases of healing, but only recently are the causative factors for these interruptions being identified. Causative factors that have been identified as affecting the orderly progression of the healing process are presented for each phase of wound healing. Timeliness relates to the progression of the phases of repair proceeding in a manner that will heal the wound expeditiously. Timeliness is determined by the nature of the wound pathology, the medical status of the patient with the wound, and environmental factors.[4] Those wounds that *do not* repair themselves in an orderly and timely manner are classified as chronic wounds; those that do are classified as acute wounds.

WOUND HEALING PHYSIOLOGY

The physiological process of acute wound healing by different phases has been described by Hunt et al[5] as a cascade of overlapping events that occur in a reasonably predictable fashion. Even though the events overlap, the series of events can be divided into phases. A diagram by Hunt and Van Winkle[6] (Figure 2–1) shows inflammation—the central activity of wound healing—located in the center of the diagram. On either side are the concurrent events that occur as a consequence of injury, proliferation, and epithelialization.

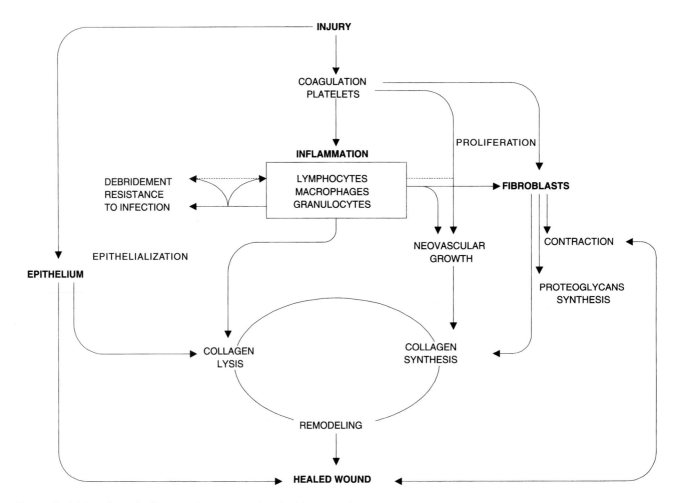

Figure 2–1 Wound repair diagram. *Source:* Reprinted with permission from TK Hunt and W Van Winkle, *Fundamentals of Wound Management in Surgery, Wound Healing: Normal Repair*, p. 1e, © 1976, South Plainfield, NJ: Chirurgecom, Inc.

The lower portion of the diagram represents the coming together of the phases, leading to the remodeling phase of wound healing. The interpretation of the diagram is that four phases—inflammation, epithelialization, proliferation, and remodeling—occur in an orderly, overlapping fashion. The literature describes the phases of repair as either three or four phases, depending on whether epithelialization is included as part of proliferation or as a separate phase. The wound healing model used in this text is based on four phases. The biologic repair process is the same for all wounds, open and closed, regardless of etiology. However, the sequence of repair is completed more quickly in primary healing and when there is superficial and partial-thickness skin involvement. Slower healing occurs when there is full-thickness skin loss extending into and through subcutaneous tissue.[5] Table 2–2 has definitions of the terminology associated with wound healing physiology.

Attributes that distinguish the healing of chronic wounds from acute wound healing are only just being identified. After the process of normal wound healing by phase is explained, attributes and processes that may be responsible for chronic wound healing in each phase are presented. Table 2–3 is a summary of factors that contribute to chronic wound healing during each phase of repair.

INFLAMMATORY PHASE

The classic observable signs and symptoms of inflammation are change in color from surrounding skin (red, blue, purple), temperature (heat), turgor (swelling), and sensation (pain), as well as a loss of function (*Color Plates 1, 19,* and *21*). Normal healing has minimal clinical manifestations of these attributes. When seen as usually described, these clinical manifestations should be regarded as clinical signs of

Table 2–2 Terminology Associated with Wound Healing Physiology

Terms	*Definitions (Reference)*
Angiogenesis	Development of new blood vessels in injured tissues. Function of endothelial cells.
Basement membrane	Thin layer of extracellular material that is found between the layers of the epithelia or between the epithelia and connective tissue. Also called *basal lamina*. (7)
Chemoattractants	Cause cell migration.
Chemotaxis	Attraction of a cell in response to a chemical signal.
Chronic wound	Wound that has "failed to proceed through an orderly and timely process to produce anatomic and functional integrity, or proceeded through the repair process without establishing a sustained anatomic and functional result." (4)
Collagenases	Enzymes that cleave (break) the bonds of the polypeptide chains in collagen at specific sites, aiding in its resorption during periods of connective tissue growth or repair. (7)
Complement system	11 proteins found in plasma with specific purpose to combat bacterial contamination. Also chemotactic for phagocytes; substances most responsible for acute inflammation. (2)
Extracellular matrix (ECM)	Intricate system of glycosaminoglycans (GAGs) and proteins secreted by cells; provides the framework for tissues. (7)
Free radicals	Highly reactive molecular species that have a least one unpaired electron in the outer shell. Attempt to react with other molecules to achieve an electrically more stable state in which the electron is paired with another. Important for normal cell functions, including metabolism and defense against infection. (25)
Galvanotaxis	Attraction of a cell in response to an electrical signal.
Glysoaminoglycans (GAGs)	Polysaccharides that contain amino acids, sugars, and glycoprotein. Termed *proteoglycans*. (60)
Growth factors (GFs)	Extracellular polypeptides—proteins able to affect cell reproduction, movement, and function. Term encompasses items c,d,e, below. Regulators of the wound healing cascade. May be deficient in chronic wounds. (7)
a. Autocrine stimulation	GF produced by a cell acting on itself.
b. Paracrine stimulation	GF produced by one cell type acting on another in the local area.
c. Endocrine stimulation	GF produced by a one cell type acting on distant cells.
d. Cytokines	Term for GF used by cell biologists. (15)
e Interleukins (ILs)	Term for GF used by immunologists. (15)
f. Colony-stimulating factor	Term for GF used by hematologists. (15)
Hemostasis	Coagulation to stop bleeding and initiate the wound healing process.
Hydroxyproline (HoPro)	A polypeptide chain of insoluble collagen.
Metalloproteinases (MMP)	Proteolytic enzymes that degrade proteins and ECM macromolecules.
Mitogens	Cause cell growth.
Mitogenic	Causing mitosis or cellular proliferation.
Neovascularization	Development of new blood vessels; another term for angeogenesis.
Phagocytosis	Ingestion, destruction, and digestion of cellular particulate matter. (7)
Proteases	Proteolytic enzymes that degrade proteins. (7)
Substrates	Substances acted upon by an enzyme, such as substances necessary for new tissue growth: protein, vitamin C, zinc.
Tensile strength	The most longitudinal stress that a substance can withstand without tearing apart.

excessive inflammation and are characteristic of impending infection.[7] The inflammation response is sometimes referred to as a "flare" because of the suddenness of the response, the color, and the associated temperature changes that are reminiscent of the flaring up of a fire. Inflammation is the body's immune system reaction and is essential for healing. The physiology of inflammation is well regulated in the normal acute healing wound. The process lasts 3–7 days. Acute inflammation begins at the moment of injury, setting into motion a biologic cascade of events. The major goals of the inflammatory phase of healing are to provide for hemostasis and to produce a clean wound site for tissue restoration. Signal sources within the wound attract responder cells and regulate the repair process.

Figure 2–2[8] shows the orderly progression through a distinct but overlapping series of processes, leading to scar formation and normal wound healing. This section will describe the key processes and cells of the inflammatory phase,

Table 2–3 Summary of Factors and Effects during Each Phase of Wound Healing in Chronic Wounds

Chronic Inflammatory Phase	Chronic Epithelialization Phase	Chronic Proliferative Phase	Chronic Remodeling Phase
Different stimulus of repair: a. From within b. Gradual c. Slowed	Diminished keratinocyte migration due to: a. Lack of moist environment b. Lack of oxygen c. Lack of nutritious tissue base d. Lack of stimulation by appropriate cytokine	Different composition of fibronectin: a. Partially degraded into fragments b. Fragments may perpetuate activity of matrix proteases c. Inhibit healing	Imbalance of collagen synthesis and lysis: a. Impaired scar tensile strength b. Overproduction of collagen: hypertrophic scarring
Inadequate perfusion and oxygenation: a. Muted phase process b. Ischemic tissue barrier to angeogenesis	Keratinocyte migration obstructed by wound edges that are: a. Rolled b. Thickened c. Nonproductive	Excess activity of proteases causes: a. Accelerated rate of connective tissue breakdown b. Destruction of polypeptide-signaling molecules c. Production of metalloproteinases that do not lyse collagen	Hyperoxygenation: a. Hypertrophy of granulation tissue b. Impediment to epidermal cell migration
Free radicals and oxygen reperfusion injury: a. Large production of free radicals b. Disruption in normal defense against free radicals c. Capillary plugging by neutrophils	Keratinocyte migration slowed due to: a. Large gap b. Slow filling of "dead space"	Chronic wound fluid inhibition of: a. Cellular proliferation: endothelial cells, keratinocytes, fibroblasts b. Cell adhesion Repeated trauma and infection: a. Increases the presence of proinflammatory cytokines b. Increases the presence of tissue inhibitors (metalloproteinases) c. Lowers the level of growth factors Impediments to wound healing: a. Elevated levels of matrix metalloproteinases b. Imbalance between levels of matrix metalloproteinases and their inhibitors Large tissue defect: a. Prolongs proliferation of tissue to fill the space Substrates relationship to stalling or plateauing: a. Inadequate substrates b. Bacterial competition for substrates necessary for tissue repair c. Continued lysis of new growth faster than synthesis of new material Long-term wound hypoxia effects: a. Negative effect on collagen production b. Decreased fibroblast proliferation c. Decreased tissue growth Impaired wound contraction: a. Wound remains large b. Delayed reepithelialization	Impairment of scar tensile strength: a. Wound breakdown b. Dehiscence

Source: Adapted with permission from Barbara Bates-Jensen, *A Quantitative Analysis of Wound Characteristics as Early Predictors of Healing in Pressure Sores.* © 1999. Barbara Bates-Jensen.

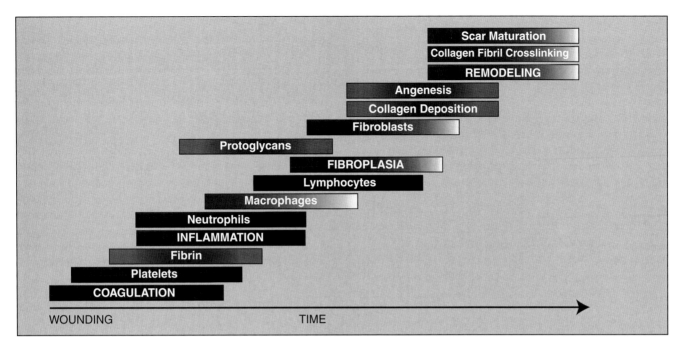

Figure 2–2 The normal wound healing response is characterized by an orderly progression through a series of distinct, but overlapping, rocesses. *Source:* Reprinted with permission from B.A. Mast, The Skin, *Wound Healing Biochemical & Clinical Aspects.* L.K. Cohen, R.F. Diegelmann, and W.J. Lindblad, eds. pp. 344–355 © 1992. W.B. Saunders Company.

beginning with the coagulation cascade to achieve platelet activation, hemostasis, the mitogenesis and chemotaxis of growth factors, hypoxia and the regulatory function of the oxygen tension gradient, complement system activation to control infection, neutrophil, macrophage, mast and fibroblast cell functions, the role of perfusion, and the "current of injury" stimulus for the repair process, followed by the attributes and processes that may be responsible for chronic wound healing during the inflammatory phase.

Coagulation Cascade or Hemostasis

Clotting and vasoconstriction, or hemostasis, occur immediately to reduce blood loss at the site of injury. Hemostasis is a major function of the platelets. Platelets, which are normally present in the intravascular space, are activated by collagen or microfibrils from the subendothelial layers exposed when injury occurs. The process known as *platelet activation* induces changes in platelet structure and function that are necessary for coagulation to occur, including thrombin, fibrin, and clot production, and, ultimately, hemostasis.[7] The fibrin clot becomes the primary foundation for collagen deposition and the pathway for the influx of monocytes and fibroblasts to the wound site.[9] Hypothermia, often associated with surgery, inhibits platelet activation and increases bleeding time. Unless corrected, the coagulation cascade may not proceed normally, and there is increased risk of blood loss and infection. Rewarming of the blood will restore both platelet function and normal clotting time.[10,11] Hypothermia is often undetected.

A second, equally important function of the platelet is the secretion of cytokines with multiple activities, including recruitment of leukocytes and fibroblasts to the injury.[12] Activated platelets release biologically active substances, or signal sources, known as *platelet-derived growth factor* (PDGF), *epidermal growth factor* (EGF), *transforming growth factor-β* (TGF-β), *heparin-binding epidermal growth factor* (HB-EGF), and *insulin-like growth factor-1* (IGF-1), all of which facilitate cell migration of neutrophils and macrophages to the area of injury.[7,12] The released growth factors are helpful in all phases of healing because they stimulate chemotaxis, mitogenesis, and collagen synthesis.[13]

Research Wisdom

1. Anticoagulation drugs (ie, heparin, wafarin, aspirin, and nonsteroidal antiinflammatory drugs) interfere with the coagulation cascade.
2. Core body temperature should be monitored for hypothermia. Even 0.2°C lowering of core body temperature will trigger peripheral vasoconstriction and tissue hypoxia.[14] This can be easily done by tempanic membrane thermometer.

Growth Factors

Growth factors are naturally occurring proteins (polypeptides) that are an integral part of wound healing. Growth factors can act on distant cells (endocrine stimulation), on adjacent cells (paracrine stimulation), and on themselves (autocrine stimulation).[7] Some growth factors cause cell growth (mitogenesis), others cause cell migration (chemoattractants), and some perform regulatory functions. The term *growth factor* includes all peptides that have growth-promoting activities and are referred to as *cytokines* by cell biologists, *interleukins* by immunologists, and *colony-stimulating factors* by hematologists.[15] Each growth factor is involved in specific pathways. Much research on the activities of growth factors since the early 1990s has demonstrated that growth factors have an integral part in the wound healing process. The platelets and the macrophages are the primary cells that produce and release growth factors, and, as such, they are critical to the wound healing process.

Growth factors are a built-in check-and-balance system within the body to ensure that overproliferation does not occur. For example, extended exposure to some growth factors (at least 4 hours) is required before cell division may occur.[7]

Wound Space Hypoxia

Following vasoconstriction, the wound space becomes hypoxic. The process of hemostasis curtails blood flow directly to the site of injury to stop bleeding by creation of fibrin clots in the local vessels. Lack of blood flow quickly depletes oxygen delivery to the wound space, producing an environmental change to a state of hypoxia. Hypoxia in the wound space is a key signal that controls wound healing. Too much oxygen in the wound space will *impede* wound healing. Hypoxia serves as a stimulus to tissue repair but also puts the tissues at risk for infection because it impairs the function of the neutrophils, lymphocytes, macrophages, and fibroblasts. Hypoxia is a signal that recruits endothelial responder cells and serves as a stimulant for angiogenesis, or the process of new blood vessel growth by the endothelial cells, which occurs during the proliferation phase. Local hypoxia also causes a shift to anaerobic glycolysis with increased lactate production that also is involved in activation of both angiogenesis and collagen synthesis. Lactate accumulation from white blood cells at the site contributes to the acidotic environment.[16] Thus, the hypoxic wound space becomes hyperlactic and acidotic.[5,17]

Infection and Oxygen

An oxygen tension gradient develops across the wound that is used for regulatory purposes. If the normal gradient of oxygen is eliminated or a macrophage-free tissue space is created, the process of angiogenesis may be temporarily or permanently inhibited.[18] Oxygen is essential to prevent infection and to meet the metabolic demands of the tissues, as well as the hydroxylation of proline necessary for useful collagen production in the remodeled wound. Neutrophils and macrophages require oxygen to kill bacteria and do not function efficiently in a hypoxic environment, where microorganisms may proliferate at a faster rate than neutrophils can phagocytose them, leading to infection.[19] Oxygen has been demonstrated to function equivalently to an "antibiotic" for prevention of wound infections.[20–22] Fibroblasts are aerobic cells and require oxygen for cell function, including division and collagen synthesis.[18] Signs of local hypoxia often go undetected. One example is the case of perioperative hypothermia-induced vasoconstriction and tissue hypoxia. Perioperative hypothermia and hypoxia have been directly related to the tripling of the incidence of perioperative surgical wound infection.[14]

Research Wisdom

Facilitate delivery of oxygen to the wound tissues by keeping the patient warm and well hydrated.[18,23] Improve tissue oxygen levels by administering oxygen by nasal cannula at 5 L/minute.[20]

The Complement System

A noncellular (ie, humoral) group of substances precedes the arrival of neutrophils to the wound space. This system, the complement system, consists of approximately 11 proteins that normally reside in the plasma. Components of the complement system are the substances responsible for acute inflammation through their ability to cause both humoral (ie, protein) and cellular (ie, phagocytic) defense mechanisms to move from the intravascular to the extravascular space, where bacteria accumulate. The primary function of the complement system is to facilitate bacterial destruction. Complement activation occurs by several specific substances, most often bacteria. The complement system acts either through the classical pathway of lysing bacterial cell walls, thereby destroying the infecting organism, or by the alternate pathway of opsonizing the invader (ie, coating the antigen with antibody), which makes the invader more appealing and recognizable to the phagocytic cells. In addition, complement acts as a chemotactic agent for attracting phagocytic cells, neutrophils, and macrophages to the site of infection and enhances their mechanism for oxidative killing.[2]

Two antibodies, IgG and IgM, serve as direct activators of the classical pathway of the complement system and are produced by the β-lymphocytes located in the spleen, lymph nodes, and submucosa of the gastrointestinal, respiratory, and genital tracts. They produce specific antibodies in response to specific antigens. These antibodies can neutralize viruses and lyse gram-negative bacteria and, as such, are potent inhibitors of antigens.[2]

Neutrophils

Neutrophils (polymorphonuclear neutrophilic leukocytes) migrate into the wound space, usually within the first 24 hours after wounding, and remain from 6 hours to several days.[2] Neutrophils are granulocytic leukocytes that function as phagocytic cells to clean the site of debris and bacteria. Initially, neutrophils are the most prevalent white blood cell at the injury site. They are able to use a special enzyme system to produce and use free radicals to attack invading bacteria.[24] Neutrophils proliferate in the hypoxic, acidotic environment and produce superoxide to fight bacteria and enhance effectiveness of antibiotics. Length of stay of the neutrophils is minimal if the bacterial count is low or declines. High bacterial counts prolong neutrophil activation and inflammation.[25] The neutrophil is considered to be a primary cell responsible for cleansing the wound of microorganisms, and lack of adequate numbers of neutrophils will retard healing in infected wounds. When bacterial counts in the wound exceed 10,[5] infection becomes apparent in the wound site. The wound produces pus, which is the accumulation of dead neutrophils that have phagocytized debris in the wound. The neutrophil has a short life span because it is unable to regenerate spent lysosomal and other enzymes used in the destruction of foreign substances. In addition to pus formation, the neutrophil produces numerous toxic byproducts that, if there is excessive neutrophil activity due to high bacterial counts, will negatively affect the wound tissue and even healthy tissue.[2]

When the wound is predominantly clean, neutrophil accumulation resolves. Whether or not neutrophil accumulation resolves or is prolonged (as may be the case in chronic wound healing), the monocyte becomes the primary white blood cell in the wounded tissues.[26] Once in the wounded area, monocytes are transformed into macrophages.

Macrophages

The macrophage is essential for transition from the inflammatory phase to the proliferative phase of healing because macrophage activities during the inflammatory phase permit initiation of angiogenesis and granulation tissue formation.[27] Growth factors transforming growth factor-β (TGF-β) and platelet derived growth factor (PDGF) are specific chemoattractants for macrophages.[7] Both neutrophils and macrophages function in a low-oxygen, high-acidotic environment. Macrophages perform several important functions during the inflammatory phase:

1. Phagocytosis of debris and control of infection by ingestion of microorganisms and excretion of ascorbic acid, hydrogen peroxide, and lactic acid. The body interprets the buildup of these excreted byproducts as a signal to send more macrophages, and the result of the increased macrophage population is a prolonged, more intense inflammatory response.
2. Autolytic debridement through synthesis and secretion of collagenases in preparation for the laying down of the new collagen matrix during the inflammatory phase and collagen degradation during the remodeling phase.[7]

The macrophage secretes a number of growth factors including angiogenic growth factors (AGFs), TGF-β, tumor necrosis factor-β (TNF-β), interleuken-1 (IL-1), and basic fibroblast growth factor (bFGF).[7] AGFs are signal sources that stimulate the budding of the endothelial cells from the damaged blood vessels and subsequent angiogenesis. Reestablishment of the blood supply is essential to deliver nutrients to the newly forming tissue. The growth factors released induce fibroblast proliferation, chemotaxis, and collagen deposition. Macrophage activity increases during the late phases of inflammation. The life span of the macrophage is thought to be months to years and is a component of wound fluid for a long period of time, transcending all phases of healing.[2]

Mast Cells

Mast cells are specialized secretory cells that, in the resting state, contain granules that are largely a heparin–protein complex in which the protein carboxyl groups serve as histamine-binding sites. There are a number of biologically active substances in mast cell granules, including neutrophil chemotactic factor.[28] Mast cells promote fibroblast proliferation through release of TNF-α, a weak mitogen for fibroblasts. Mitogens cause cell mitosis and cellular proliferation.[7] Histamine, a vasoactive amine, is initially released from the mast cells after injury and plays an important role in vascular dilation and permeability, inducing temporary mild edema. In low doses, histamine may stimulate collagen formation and healing.[28,29] Once the body has produced enough platelet and prothrombin reaction, the mast cell will produce heparin. Heparin stimulates the migration of endothelial cells. Other substances in the mast cells, eosinophil and neutrophil chemotactic factors, attract the leukocytic cells that, in turn, act as chemical signals for the recruitment of macrophages, leading to a modulation of the inflammatory phase. Macrophages promote later phases in the repair process through recruitment of fibroblasts.[28,30] The effect of the heparin is to accelerate the activity of the leukocytes (neutrophils and eosinophils) in the phagocytosis of the hematoma that occurs in the wound following damage to the blood vessels at the time of wounding.[31]

Perfusion

Circulatory activities that follow wounding are manifested as temperature changes in the wound and the surrounding tissues. Humoral and neurogenic factors, such as bradykinin, histamine, and prostaglandins, are responsible for causing vasodilation of the surrounding tissues. Increased perfusion increases local tissue temperature. The response is called *hyperemia*. This is not an inflammatory reaction. Pain, as a consequence of the surgical trauma to the tissues, irritates nerve endings and reflexively produces reflex hyperemia.[32] The vasodilation aids in movement of inflammatory cells from the vasculature into the site of injury. Vasodilatation of adjacent vessels follows vasoconstriction at the wound site and is accompanied by perfusion, increased capillary pressure, and permeability of small blood and lymphatic vessels, which permits the plasma protein molecules to migrate into the surrounding tissues with consequent edema, erythema, and stimulation of the pain afferents. Fibrin plugs seal off the lymphatic flow to prevent spreading of infection. Increased perfusion or blood flow brings needed nutrients to meet the increased metabolic demands of the tissues. High metabolic activities and the increased blood flow raises wound and surrounding tissue temperatures. Higher vascularity results in higher tissue temperatures. A regular temperature pattern of healing can be obtained by taking daily measurements of local skin temperatures following surgery. The temperature pattern can be obtained using liquid-crystal-bearing strips (see Chapter 4, Assessment of the Skin and Wound). If the zone of warmth does not decrease in width by the fourth postoperative day, it predicts the possibility of wound infection and disturbed healing.[32] This cascade of events is the physiologic basis for the familiar classic signs and symptoms of inflammation: a reddening of the surrounding tissues or, in individuals with darkly pigmented skin, a purple or violaceous discoloration; pain; heat; and edema. The rise in tissue temperature provides an environment favorable for cell mitosis and enhanced cellular activities.[33,34]

Current of Injury

Another component of healing is endogenous biologic electrical currents. All body cells, bone, skin, muscle, and nerves possess their own injury currents. Becker,[35] in the 1960s, demonstrated the existence of a direct-current electrical system that controls tissue healing. He called this the *cur-rent of injury*. The human body has an average charge on the skin surface of −23 mV.[36] Multiple experiments demonstrate that a negative charge exists on the surface of the skin with respect to the deeper skin layers. This results in weak electrical potentials across the skin, creating a "skin battery" effect. The battery is driven by a sodium ion pump, initiated by the sodium ions passing through the cells of the epithelium via specific channels in the outer membrane. Once in the cell, they diffuse to other cells of the epithelium; then they can be actively transported from these cells via electrogenic "pumps" located in all of the plasma membranes of the epithelium except the outer membrane. The result is a transport of NA^+ from the water bathing the epithelium to the internal body fluids and generation of a potential on the order of 50 mV across the epithelium.[37] If there is a break in the integrity of the skin, there will be a net flow of ionic current through the low-resistance pathway of the injured cells and fluid exudate that line the wound; if the wound space becomes dry, the voltage gradient will be eliminated.[22] Use of moist wound healing methods is clinical application of this theory.[38]

The ionic current flowing between the normal and injured tissue is a stimulus for the repair process. During the repair process, there is a distinct pattern of current flow and polarity switching, and when healing is complete, the current ceases. The bioelectric repair process is polarity-regulated, and cells of repair are attracted by the positive or negative pole. This is called *galvanotaxis*. The macrophages and neutrophils are attracted to the positive pole.[39,40] Weiss et al[41] found reduced mast cell representation in wounds after positive polarity stimulation seemingly inhibited by the positive pole, and suggested that as a mechanism for reduced fibrotic scarring. When the wound is inflamed or infected, neutrophils are attracted to the negative pole.[42] The negative pole attracts fibroblasts,[43] which stimulates protein and DNA synthesis, and increases CA^{2+} uptake, fibroblast proliferation, and collagen synthesis.[44–46] Negative polarity facilitates migration of epidermal cells.[47] Negative polarity is also associated with suppression of bacterial growth.[48–51] In chronic wound healing, it is proposed that the current of injury fails to occur. One rationale for the use of exogenous electrical stimulation for wound healing initially is based on the theory that electrical stimulation mimics the current of injury and will restart or accelerate the repair process. Clearly, there are significant research data to support the concept that electrical current plays an important role in the cell physiology of wound healing. The use of electrical stimulation for wound healing is explained in Chapter 21, Electrical Stimulation for Wound Healing.

Fibroblasts

Fibroblasts respond to the chemotactic signals from growth factors released by platelets, macrophages, granulocytes, and keratinocytes. These growth factors stimulate fibroblast proliferation. Alignment of the fibroblast cells within the wound site during the inflammatory phase is an early indication of the strength that will eventually be imparted to the wound. Alignment of the fibroblasts along the wound axis and creation of cell-to-cell linkages aid in the contraction of the wound and the strength of the final scar tissue.[2] During the inflammatory phase, the fibroblasts differentiate into a specialized cell called the *myofibroblast*.

INFLAMMATORY PHASE OF WOUND HEALING IN CHRONIC WOUNDS[52]

Defining critical attributes for chronic wound healing in the inflammatory phase of healing is difficult because the differences between the normal acute wound healing process and what is seen in chronic wound healing are only just being recognized. Three factors have been identified as causing an interruption in the inflammatory phase of repair, including the stimulus for repair, inadequate perfusion and ischemia, and free radicals and oxygen reperfusion injury.

Stimulus for Repair

One of the primary differences is the stimulus for repair. In acute wounds, there is vascular disruption from the outside of the body to the inside of the body, initiating the hemostasis system and, thus, the wound healing cascade. In chronic wounds, the injury or stimulus for repair may come from within and may be gradual in onset. Suh and Hunt[19] used burn injuries as an example. After burn injury, the depth of the injury increases for 3–4 days as injured microvessels thrombose, slowing the sequence of repair and inflammation. Suh and Hunt[19] suggest that the same mechanism may be responsible for the slower healing time in pressure wounds, where the tissue dies back to where the blood flow is barely adequate to sustain life of the tissue. They go on to explain that the vascular requirement for sustaining life may not be adequate for tissue healing.

Inadequate Perfusion and Ischemia

If the injury is initiated by trauma, as with acute wounds, the condition and poor perfusion of the tissues in which the wounding occurs results in a slow and laborious course of healing.[16,53] Usually, chronic wounds are the result of underlying pathologic vascular insufficiency of some type and, because hemostasis is the stimulus for the wound healing cascade, the process is muted. Chronic wounds heal slowly, and as the angiogenic stimuli become more and more removed from the initial wound edge, new blood vessels coalesce or drop out, resulting in a predominantly ischemic wound site.[16,53] In some instances, the ischemic tissue itself becomes an obstacle to healing because it is a barrier to angiogenesis.[16]

Free Radicals and Oxygen Reperfusion Injury

Oxygen-free radicals take part in many metabolic processes and act as part of the defense mechanism against infection. Free-radical species are generated during the process of oxidative phosphorylation and the electron transfer chain within the mitochondria. Normally, the free-radical species generated during these processes are used in a well-controlled manner, serve useful function in the cell metabolic processes, and do not escape to a significant degree from the mitochondria to other parts of the cell. Free radicals are chemically very reactive and may cause severe damage to many chemical compounds that are part of the cell, especially the lipids that make up the cell membrane. Enzymes within the cells usually catalyze the safe breakdown of oxygen-free radicals and, thus, protect the cell from these compounds. In addition, tocopherol (a vitamin E component) in the lipid membrane and ascorbic acid (vitamin C), acting as free-radical scavengers, are capable of breaking free radicals down safely.[24]

Tissue ischemia creates a series of events that includes the production of inflammatory mediators, mechanical capillary plugging by leukocytes, and oxygen metabolite formation that leads to further tissue damage.[24,54] The wound healing process may begin with white blood cell entry into the damaged tissues from blood vessel disruption. However, even this process may be slowed. Once the injury is present, the leukocytes attempt to initiate the inflammatory stage of healing, but they are unable to enter the wound tissue by passing through the capillary walls, due to increased rigidity of vessels and capillary plugging.[24] The leukocytes that do enter have difficulty with bactericidal activities, due to the decreased oxygen content in the wound bed from the underlying tissue ischemia.[19,54] The mechanism for capillary plugging by neutrophils and delayed entry into the wounded tissues is related to oxygen-free radical formation and reperfusion injury.

When blood flow is reestablished to the ischemic tissue, further damage to the tissues occurs from the disruption in the normal mechanisms of defense against injury from oxygen-free radicals. This is referred to as *reperfusion injury*. The mechanisms of reperfusion injury begin with ischemia and the conversion of the enzyme xanthine dehydrogenase to xanthine oxidase, setting the scene for the generation of free radicals. When blood flow is resumed to the ischemic site, the new availability of oxygen permits production of large amounts of free radicals derived from the xanthine oxidase.[24] These free radicals cause damage to the endothelium by lipid peroxidation. This overwhelms the normal free-radical defense mechanisms and leads to extensive injury of the endothelium, with ultimate destruction of the microcirculation. The consequence of these events is cell death. In addition, an already difficult situation may be complicated by the escape of more free radicals from the mitochondria.[24] Additional free radicals are released by neutrophils in response to activation from compounds released by endothelial cells during reperfusion. Both neutrophil activation and availability of xanthine oxidase increase free radicals at the wound site and result in increased endothelial damage.[24] When activated to produce free radicals, neutrophils lose their ability to deform to enter capillaries and adhere more easily to the endothelium, occluding capillaries.[24] The capillary occlusion, in combination with the neutrophil's inability to deform, may be the cause of decreased levels of functioning neutrophils and macrophages present in chronic wounds.[24] Research is now focused on prevention of the worst features of ischemia and the resulting reperfusion injury. Clinicians need to be aware of the implications of new treatments that may be developed as a consequence of this research.

EPITHELIALIZATION PHASE

Epithelialization commences immediately after trauma as a priority for the body to protect itself from invasion by outside organisms and occurs concurrently with the other phases. The signals for epithelialization begin during the inflammatory phase from growth factors released by the macrophages, neutrophils, and the current of injury to stimulate the response of the epithelial cells to migrate from the wound edges and dermal appendages. The majority of epithelial cells are keratinocytes because they accumulate keratin as they migrate to the surface of the skin. The skin is composed of multiple layers. At the deepest layer of the epidermis, the keratinocytes are connected to the basement membrane, which attaches the keratinocytes to the underlying dermis. Both the epidermis and the basement membrane must be reestablished in order to maintain an impermeable barrier during wound repair.[7] The epithelialization phase involves resurfacing of the wound, which is the function of the keratinocytes. The goal of epithelialization phase of healing is wound closure.

Keratinocytes

Keratinocytes make up the layers of the dermis and epidermis, as well as lining various body organs and dermal appendages (eg, sebaceous glands, sweat glands, and hair follicles). Kerotinocytes respond to signals from the macrophages, neutrophils, and current of injury within hours after injury. Responding kerotinocytes advance in a sheet to resurface the open space. The leading edges of the advancing keratinocytes become phagocytic and clean the debris, including clotted material, from their path. Cell sheets continue to migrate until the wound is covered and a new basement membrane is generated. Multilayered epithelial cells appear to migrate either as a moving sheet or in a complex "leapfrog" manner (also called *epiboly*).[7] A moist wound environment will speed the migration of keratinocytes toward

one another from the edges of the wound and from the dermal appendages. Full-thickness skin loss injuries suffer loss of the dermal appendages, an important source of new keratinocytes. As a consequence, epithelial cells can migrate only from the wound edges. The advancing front of epidermal cells cannot cover a cavity, so they dive down and curl under at the edges. For example, full-thickness pressure wounds develop a buildup of the epithelial cells at the wound edges, forming an epidermal ridge that curls under the edges and slows closure. It is as though the epithelial cells get tired of waiting for granulation tissue to fill in the wound defect, so they prematurely proliferate and migrate over the edge (see *Color Plate 3*). The migration of the epithelial cells is also oxygen dependent. When there are low levels of oxygen, epithelial migration cannot debride the wound.

In surgical wounds that are sutured, epidermal migration begins within the first 24 hours and is usually complete, in healthy adults, within 48–72 hours postoperatively. In other wounds, trauma to skin results in tissue degeneration, with broad, indistinct areas and where any edge is difficult to see. This forms a shallow lesion, with more distinct, thin, separate edges. As tissue trauma progresses, the reaction intensifies, with a thickening and rolling inward of the epidermis. The edge is well defined and sharply outlines the ulcer, with little or no evidence of new tissue growth. Repeated trauma and attempts at repair to the wound edges result in fibrosis and scarring. The edges of the wound become indurated and firm,[55] which results in possible impairment of the migratory ability of the keratinocytes.[56]

Elasticity of the replaced epidermal layers will affect the function of the skin as it overrides bony prominences and moving muscles or tendons. Once the wound has been resurfaced by epithelial cells, the cells begin the process of differentiating and maturing into type I collagen. The tensile strength of the remodeled skin will not exceed 70–80% of the original. The quality of the scar tissue is an indication of the final outcome. The fact that closure had been achieved by epithelialization does not mean that the wound is fully healed. The new skin at this time has a tensile strength of only roughly 15% of normal. The new skin must be treated carefully to avoid trauma, which can cause edema and infection, and can lead to reinflammation. Chronic inflammation will cause a thickening of the skin and less-elastic remodeled tissue.[57]

EPITHELIALIZATION PHASE OF WOUND HEALING IN CHRONIC WOUNDS[52]

Like interruption of the inflammatory phase, if the epithelialization process becomes interrupted or arrested, the result is a chronic wound. Causative factors are discussed that may arrest the epithelialization process by diminishing keratinocyte migration.

Diminished Keratinocyte Migration

Reepithelialization may be delayed in chronic wounds due to diminished keratinocyte migration from lack of a moist, oxygen-rich, nutritious tissue base, as is the case with debris-filled chronic wounds.[27] Decreased keratinocyte migration may also be due to a lack of stimulation from failure of the appropriate cytokine to be released during the initial processes of the inflammatory phase of healing.[27,58]

Keratinocyte migration may be difficult in chronic wounds because of the rolled, thickened, nonproductive wound edge. Additionally, reepithelialization may be delayed until the wound has filled sufficiently with granulation tissue to provide a moist environment for keratinocyte migration. In wounds with significant tissue loss, epithelialization is slowed by virtue of the larger area requiring resurfacing. If wound contraction is impaired such that the wound remains large, epithelialization will also be affected because of the continued large area to resurface. Research related to chronic wound healing in the epithelialization phase may provide more insight into the process of chronic epithelialization.

PROLIFERATIVE PHASE

The proliferative phase of wound healing overlaps with and follows the inflammatory phase, beginning 3–5 days postinjury and continuing for 3 weeks in wounds healing by primary intention.[26] The goals of this phase of healing are to fill in the wound defect with new tissue and to restore the integrity of the skin. The processes involved in the proliferative phase are angiogenesis, collagen synthesis, and contraction. The initial injury impairs tissue oxygenation, resulting in a hypoxic wound bed. Hypoxia, in conjunction with lactate produced through anaerobic metabolism and white blood cells, stimulates the release of AGFs by macrophages to attract fibroblasts to the wound site.[26,27] Fibroblasts and endothelial cells are responsible for the activities of the proliferative phase. Several differences exist for the chronic wound in the proliferative phase. These differences include:

- Fibronection composition
- Chronic wound fluid-inhibiting factors
- "Dead space" inhibition and prolongation of healing, stalling, or plateauing of healing associated with several factors
- Delayed reepithelialization, due to size of the "wound gap" or nonproductive wound edges
- Protracted inflammatory and proliferative responses

Each of these processes and differences will be described.

Angiogenesis

Restoration of vascular integrity is a function of the proliferative phase. During this phase, angiogenesis, also known as *neovascularization*, takes place. Growth factors, primarily basic and acidic FGF, TNF-β, EGF, and wound angiogenesis factor, play a major role in regulating angiogenesis.[7] Angiogenesis occurs as new capillary buds extend into the wound bed. New capillary buds arise from intact vessels adjacent to the wound. As endothelial cells proliferate and grow into the wound space, creating capillaries, they connect to prepare a new network of vessels filling the tissue defect. In the early stages of vessel growth, the vessels have loose junctions and gaps in the endothelial lining.[27] As a result, the initial capillaries are fragile and permeable, allowing passage of fluids from the intravascular space to the extravascular space; thus, new tissue is often edematous in appearance.[27] The thick capillary bed, which fills the matrix, supplies the nutrients and oxygen necessary for the wound to heal. The capillary loops have the appearance to the naked eye of small granules and lend the name *granulation* to both the tissue and the phase (*see Color Plates 2, 4,* and *8*).[7] The granulation tissue is first seen as pale pink buds, which, as they fill with new blood vessels, become bright, beefy, red tissue, as seen in *Color Plate 7.* Notice how the granulation starts at one side of the wound, then "marches" across the wound bed, as shown in *Color Plates 8* and *9.* At this time, the granulation tissue is very fragile and unable to withstand any trauma. Trauma to the new granulation tissue will cause bleeding that may reinitiate the inflammatory process and cause the laying down of excessive collagen, resulting in poor elasticity and a less desirable scar. Protection of the new granulation tissue is very important. This tissue is structurally and functionally different from the tissues it replaces and will not differentiate into the nerves, muscles, tendons, and other tissue that it replaces.[2]

Clinical Wisdom: *Granulation Tissue Complications*

Change from beefy, red granulation tissue to a dusky pink is an evaluation point. Wound fluid may also change in color, quantity, or both at the same time. This is often a sign of infection.

Fibroblasts

All connective tissue is composed of two major constituents—cells and extracellular material. The most important function of the fibroblasts is synthesis and deposition of the extracellular matrix (ECM) components—fibrous elements and ground substance. Fibrous connective tissue elements that give strength to the ECM include collagen, elastin, and reticulin. The nonfibrous portion includes ground substance that is primarily water, salts, and glysosaminogly-cans (GAGs). GAGs are polysaccharides that contain amino acids, sugars, and glycoprotein and are termed *proteogly-*

cans. Types of GAGs found in skin include chondroitin sulfate, hyaluronic acid, and dermatan sulfate.[59] GAGs are hydrophilic substances, a factor that causes them to attract large amounts of water and sodium. The turgor normally associated with connective tissue is a manifestation of the accumulation of fluid by the GAGs. Ground substance has semiliquid gel properties.[2]

Extracellular fibrous materials produced by fibroblasts include tropocollagen, a precursor of collagen. Tropocollagen is a soluble substance and needs to be transformed into insoluble collagen. The process is called *hydroxylation of proline* and results in the polypeptide chain hydroxyproline (HoPro). The measurement of HoPro is used, for research purposes, to assess collagen deposition, with collagen estimated as seven times the value of HoPro.[60] In vitro and in vivo studies show that collagen hydroxylation, cross-linking, and deposition are proportional to the arterial partial pressure of oxygen.[18] Hydroxyproline deposition is proportional to wound tensile strength in rats.[18] To achieve this transformation, ferrous iron, a reducing agent (eg, ascorbic acid), alpha ketoglutarate, and oxygen are required. Tropocollagen, thus transformed, is then combined with ground substance to form the scaffolding of repair.[2,59]

Elastin derives its name from its elastic properties. It is found in skin, lungs, blood vessels, and the bladder, and functions to maintain tissue shape.[2] A third fibrous connective tissue component is structural glycoprotein. Laminin and fibronectin are two of these fiber-forming molecules. Together, these connective tissues provide structural and metabolic support to other tissues.[2]

Matrix Formation

Granulation tissue fibroblasts coat with a layer of fibronectin matrix and produce the matrix, or scaffolding, for collagen deposition that will support blood vessel growth by the endothelial cells.[18] The endothelial cells migrate and proliferate along the scaffolding, building new capillaries as they go that are capable of providing oxygen and nourishment for the new collagen.[27,61] The optimal wound conditions to support fibroblast production of collagen and ground substances include the presence of cytokines (specifically, TGF-β) produced by the macrophage and by the fibroblast itself, and an acidic, low-oxygen-content wound bed. Fibroblasts secrete collagen until the wound is filled, then collagen production ceases as the fibroblast is downregulated. The process is called *fibroplasia*. Wound healing by fibroplasia requires a wound to be shaped like a boat or bowl to ensure that the granulation tissue fills the base before the epithelial edges of the wound meet. Wounds that are not of this shape are at risk for premature surface healing, leaving a cavity under the skin, which will subsequently break down.[62]

Cross-Linking of Collagen

Fibroblasts synthesize three polypeptide chains that coil to form a right-handed triple helix.[63] One of the polypeptide chains is HoPro. Now called *procollagen*, these spiraled chains are then extruded from the fibroblast out into the extracellular space. The next step is cleavage of the triple-helical molecule at specific terminal sites. Now the helix is referred to as *tropocollagen molecule*. Tropocollagens then amass and convolve with other tropocollagen molecules to form a collagen fibril. Once the collagen fibrils are formed, they are very disorganized. The amount of collagen filaments is not what gives the collagen matrix durability or tensile strength. Tensile strength is dependent on the microscopic welding, or bonding, of one filament to another. The sites where these bonds occur are called *cross-links*. Intermolecular bonds are the major force holding the tropocollagen molecules together. The greater the number of these bonds, the more the strength of the collagen filament will be enhanced. In an anoxic wound, cross-linking is inhibited.

Tropocollagen polymerizes (joins with many small particles to create a large molecule) and forms various types of collagen.[2] Types I and III collagen are found in the dermis and are involved with wound healing. New tissue growth in the wound follows a pattern of fibronectin secretion, type III collagen production, and, lastly, type I collagen.[27,61] The early immature type III collagen is gradually replaced with the normal adult type I collagen throughout the proliferation phase of healing, continuing through the remodeling phase of healing.

Type III collagen fibrils are smaller (40–60 nm), whereas type I collagen fibrils have a larger diameter (100–500 nm). The larger-diameter fibers have less elasticity than do the smaller. Approximately 80% of dermal collagen is type I, and these fibers provide the tensile strength to the tissue. The type III collagen fibers help the tissue to withstand a load over time. This is referred to as *creep resistance*. The proportion of large to small fibrils changes over the life span, with type III gradually replaced by type I. The proportion of large- to small-diameter fibrils is determinant of the dermal tensile strength.[59]

Normally, collagen fibers are organized and arranged in parallel lines along mechanical stress points, giving tissue strength.[27] Type I collagen is the major component of normal adult dermis but the predominant type of collagen synthesized in the wound is type III collagen.[61] Type III collagen is poorly cross-linked and not aligned in the same manner as type I collagen and, as such, provides minimal tensile strength to the new tissue.[27]

At this point, about 3 weeks after wounding, the greatest mass of collagen assembled by the tensile strength is roughly only 15% of normal. This new scar will not tolerate mobilization or rough handling, either of which will ultimately lead to creation of a new wound and further scarring.[63] Wound dehiscense and evisceration have been documented as occurring most frequently during this phase.[2]

Myofibroblasts and Contraction

The myofibroblasts contain an actin and myosin contractile system similar to what is found in smooth muscle cells.[18] Thus, they are able to contract and extend. The myofibroblast connects itself to the wound skin margins and pulls the epidermal layer inward. The myofibroblast ring forms what has been described as a "picture frame" beneath the skin of the contracting wound. The contracting forces start out equal in all wounds, but the shape of the "picture frame" predicts the resultant speed of contraction. Linear wounds contract rapidly, square or rectangular wounds contract at a moderate pace, and circular wounds contract slowly. One characteristic of pressure ulcers is that they take on a circular shape, and this is an indicator that they will contract slowly.[57] Wound contraction is seen as the change in wound shape and reduction in the open area of the wound and occurs at the final stage of wound repair. Myofibroblast function is mediated by growth factors. Wounds that heal by primary intention or partial-thickness wounds heal with very little wound contraction but, in full-thickness wounds, contraction may account for up to a 40% decrease in the size of the wound.[27,58] For successful healing, contraction needs to be maintained in balance. A diminished level of contraction leads to delayed healing, with possible excess bleeding and infection. Conversely, excess contraction can lead to loss of function, due to tissue contractures.[27]

Wound contraction pulls the wound edges together for the purpose of closing the wound. In effect, this will reduce the open area and, if successful, will result in a smaller wound, with less need for repair by scar formation. Wound contraction can be very beneficial in the closure of wounds in areas such as the buttocks or trochanter but can be very harmful in areas such as the hand or around the neck and face, where it can cause disfigurement and excessive scarring. Rapid, uncontrolled wound contraction in these areas must be avoided. Drawing together too tightly causes deformity of the repaired scar and impairment of tissue function. Skin grafting is used to reduce contraction in undesirable locations. The thickness of the skin graft influences the degree of contraction suppression. Pressure garments are another method of controlling wound contraction (see Chapter 13).

Oxygen and nutrition demand remains very high to support the cells of repair, fibroblasts, myofibroblasts, endothelial cells, and epidermal cells, which are reproducing at a rapid rate to create the collagen matrix. Nutrients, including zinc, iron, copper, vitamin C, and oxygen, are essential for fibroblast synthesis of the collagen matrix. The macrophages and neutrophils work to control infection as long as the wound remains open. The combination of activities raises tissue temperatures. The wound needs warmth at this time to promote cellular division and management of infection.

Research Wisdom: *Best Time To Apply Skin Grafts*

Split-thickness skin grafts suppress contraction by 31%, and full-thickness skin grafts diminish contraction by 55%. The best time for application of skin grafts is during the inflammatory phase, before contraction begins.[57]

PROLIFERATIVE PHASE OF WOUND HEALING IN CHRONIC WOUNDS[52]

Several differences exist for the chronic wound proceeding through the proliferative phase of healing. These include differences in the composition of fibronectin, chronic wound fluid, and a large tissue defect. Each causative factor will be discussed. Wysocki demonstrated differences in the composition of fibronectin (critical to the laying down of collagen) in chronic wounds, as compared with acute wounds.[64] The fibronectin in chronic wounds was partially degraded, whereas, in acute wounds, the fibronectin remained intact. The small fibronectin fragments seen in chronic wounds may perpetuate the activity of matrix proteases and inhibit healing.[65] Indeed, excess activity of proteases that break down connective tissue faster than it is formed and destroy important polypeptide-signaling molecules that coordinate healing may play a role in persistent nonhealing wounds.[66] Parks[67] has shown that chronic wounds exhibit production of two stromelysins (metalloproteinases that do not lyse collagen), which may represent unregulated production of proteinase that contributes to the inability of some chronic wounds to heal.

Chronic Wound Fluid

Interest in the wound environment has led researchers to look at the wound fluid as a reflection of the microenvironment of the wound from which it was collected. Human studies of wound fluids are complicated by inability to control carefully the variables related to the wound or the patient and the particular condition under which the wound fluids are collected, leading to varied results. It is fairly well accepted that wound fluid from acute wounds is mitogenic for wound-associated cells and that fluid collected from chronic wounds are inhibitory to these cells of regeneration.[68,69] However, the effect of wound fluid content on chronic wound outcomes has not been studied. Therefore, the clinician needs to be careful when interpreting the results of wound fluid studies and place the experiments in the context of the experimental design and methods.[68] What is presented here is a glimpse of some of the research findings. At some time in the future, wound fluid may provide important insight into the healing of chronic wounds and lead to new treatment strategies.

Chronic wound fluid has been shown to inhibit proliferation of endothelial cells, keratinocytes, fibroblasts, and cell adhesion.[70,71] These studies imply that the chronic wound environment may be missing elements critical for repair.[13] Bennett and Schultz[72] suggested that, in chronic wounds, repeated trauma and infection increase the presence of proinflammatory cytokines and tissue inhibitors or metalloproteinases, and lower the level of growth factors. Others[73,74] showed lower levels of PDGF, bFGF, EGF, and TGF-β in chronic pressure sores, compared with acute wounds. Yager et al[75] reported elevated levels of matrix metalloproteinases and imbalance between levels of matrix metalloproteinases and their inhibitors in the fluids of pressure ulcers, which may impede the healing of these wounds. Inhibitory effect of chronic wound fluid on fibroblasts was abolished by heating the wound fluid to 100° C, whereas heating it to 38° C had a significant effect.[69]

Large Tissue Defect

Full-thickness pressure ulcers often present with a "dead space" or a tissue gap, which prolongs proliferation because of the larger tissue defect to fill with new connective tissue and blood vessels.[19] Prolongation of the proliferative phase of healing can be observed in many chronic wounds. The wound will progress to a certain point of new tissue growth, then "stall," or plateau, with no further evidence of proliferation. The cessation of proliferation may be related to inadequate substrates necessary for new tissue growth, such as protein, vitamin C, and zinc.[16] Inadequate substrate availability may be due to increased levels of bacteria in the wound environment or to continued lysis of new growth faster than new material can be synthesized. The increased bacteria levels may compete with healthy cells for the necessary substrates for healing and prevent further tissue growth.[19] Siddiqui and colleagues[76] have suggested an alternate cause of decreased tissue proliferation. Using an in vitro system, the Siddiqui study demonstrated decreased collagen production and fibroblast proliferation in a chronically hypoxic wound environment, suggesting that long-term wound hypoxia exerts a negative influence on tissue proliferation.

REMODELING PHASE

The final phase of wound healing is the remodeling phase, which begins as granulation tissue is formed in the wound site during the proliferative phase and continues for 1–2 years postinjury[27,77] until it reaches maturation. During the remodeling phase of wound healing, scar tissue is rebuilt to provide for increased tensile strength. The tensile strength increases from the 15–20% strength associated with the initial scar tissue up to 80% of the original preinjury tissues by the end of the remodeling phase.[58,63] Remodeling is a delicate equilibrium between collagen synthesis and lysis.

The remodeling phase shows most clearly the overlapping of all the phases of secondary intention healing. Typically, it is described as the end of the proliferative phase, which is about 3 weeks postinjury. Actually, collagen matrix formation and remodeling begins concurrently with the formation of the granulation tissue. Unlike the other phases, no cell is predominant in this phase.[2] Regulation of the remodeling process is the function of growth factors, primarily TGF-β, PDGF, and FGF, that are stimulated during tissue injury and repair and by specific enzymes called *collagenases*. Collagenases are metalloproteinases (MMPs), which are proteolytic enzymes that degrade proteins and ECM macromolecules (ie, GAGs).[7]

Matrix Remodeling

The ECM and collagen deposition is continuously and gradually changing from the time it is initially produced in the wound bed, and this process continues even after the tissue integrity is restored.[27] Type III collagen, originally produced by the fibroblast, is gradually lysed by tissue collagenases, and type I collagen is produced to replace the lost tissues. The lysis of old collagen and production of new collagen leads to a change in the orientation of the scar tissue. The new type I collagen fibrils are laid down parallel to lines of tension in the wound and in a more organized fashion, with strong crosslinking and bundle construction.[27] During this phase, the highly vascular and cellular granulation scar tissue is gradually replaced with less vascular and less cellular tissues.[19] Fibronectin and hyaluronic acid (part of the ECM ground substance), along with type III collagen, are reduced, and proteoglycans are deposited with the new type I collagen, increasing the wound's resilience to deformation.[27] Lysis of old collagen is accomplished by the action of bacterial collagenase, lysosomal proteases, and tissue collagenase synthesized by macrophages, epidermal cells, and fibroblasts.[27,58]

Collagen Lysis

Collagenase and other proteolytic enzymes are produced during the inflammatory phase and throughout the proliferative phase as regulators of fibroplasia. Proteolytic enzymes are proteases that degrade proteins (ie, collagen). Collagenase has the capability of cleaving or breaking the cross-linkage of the tropocollagen molecules, aiding in its reabsorption during periods of connective tissue growth or repair.[7] In the healthy wound, collagenase is a regulator of the balance between synthesis and lysis of collagen. It is this ability to break down collagen that makes collagenase useful as a debriding agent. Breaking of the cross-linkage has the effect of making the tropocollagen molecule soluble so that it can be excreted from the body. The balance between collagen synthesis and collagen lysis is fine-tuned, with a goal that one process should not exceed the other. However, as the wound matures during remodeling, collagen lysis increases. The organization of the collagen fibers as they are laid down by the fibroblasts is part of this regulatory process. Better organization produces a better functional outcome of more elastic, smoother, and stronger fibers for the repaired scar tissues.

Collagen synthesis is oxygen dependent, but collagen lysis is not. Too much oxygen is believed to cause hypertrophy of the granulation tissues, called *hypergranulation*. Hypergranulation creates a humping of the tissue that inhibits the epidermal cell movements against gravity to cover and resurface the wound (see *Color Plate 23*). This is usually the result of an imbalance of collagen synthesis to collagen lysis. Some individuals have a genetic inhibition of lysis, meaning that the balance between collagen synthesis and collagen lysis is not balanced, and hypertrophic and keloid scars form. Chapters 4 and 11 discuss ways to control hypergranulation tissue.

Scar Formation

Clinical manifestations of the remodeling phase of healing are evidenced by changes in the appearance of the scar tissue. As collagen synthesis and degradation proceed, the vascularity and cellularity of the scar tissue diminish, with loss in scar tissue mass and obvious changes in the visual appearance of the wound site. The scar changes from bright red or pink to a silvery gray or white color, and the site becomes less bulky, flattening over time[19,77] until a normotrophic scar is achieved. Additionally, as the scar tissue matures, it becomes more flexible.[19]

As long as the scar exhibits a rosier appearance than normal, remodeling or maturation of the immature scar is under way.[57] The purpose of this process is an attempt by the scar to blend in, both cosmetically and functionally. An example is the surgical scar on the incision line that initially is bright red, then over time blanches and conforms to the body contours. The entire process of remodeling of wounds until maturation is described as taking from 3 weeks to 2 years postinjury.[57] Chapter 13 explains normal scar formation processes, explains complications, and discusses ways to manage scar formation for the most cosmetic and functional outcomes.

REMODELING PHASE OF WOUND HEALING IN CHRONIC WOUNDS[52]

In the chronic wound, an imbalance in collagen synthesis and lysis may be present, the causative factor that interrupts the remodeling phase. If collagen synthesis and lysis are not kept in balance, impairments in remodeling are evident. If collagen synthesis is impeded, the tensile strength of the wound is impaired and the wound may break down or dehisce (reopen) after integrity has been restored. If collagen lysis is impaired, collagen is allowed to proliferate with no checks, and hypertrophy or keloid formation may result.[78,79] Evidence indicates that MMP8, a collagenase produced by neutrophils, has high activity during this phase, and that may account for chronicity of the wound.[7] The reasons for these differences are not well understood.

Understanding the wound healing process and the physiologic events associated with wound healing, as well as potential differences in chronic wound healing, is the first step in evaluating healing. Assessment of the physiologic events of healing provides a method of measuring healing attributes in a wound at any given time.

FETAL WOUND HEALING

Researchers are looking to see what can be learned from fetal wound healing. It has been known for some time that there is a lack of scar formation in fetuses having fetal surgery in utero.[80–82] One feature of fetal wounds is that they are continually bathed in amniotic fluid, which has a rich content of hyaluronic acid (HA) and fibronectin, as well as growth factors crucial to fetal development. HA is a key structural and functional component of the ECM and fosters an environment that promotes cell proliferation and tissue regeneration and repair.[83] HA is laid down in the matrix of both fetal and adult wounds, but the sustained deposition of HA is unique to fetal wounds. An example of the effects of HA and amniotic fluid on healing of surgical wounds was reported by Byl et al in two studies.[84,85] Amniotic fluid, HA, and normal saline were applied to controlled incisional wounds. The surgeons were blinded to the fluids applied. Both the amniotic fluid- and HA-treated incisions healed faster than did the saline-treated wounds. In fact, the wounds treated with the amniotic fluid and HA appeared to close within minutes of the application. The healing was quicker and the quality of the scar was better in the HA and amniotic fluid groups than in the saline-treated incisions. The tensile strengths of the amniotic fluid- and HA-treated wounds were slightly weaker than those of the saline-treated group at the end of 1 week, but after 2 weeks, all groups had equal tensile strength.

There remain many questions to be answered about fetal wound healing. There are many differences between fetal development and adult repair and regeneration. For example, the transplacental circulation provides a partial pressure of oxygen of 20 mm Hg, which is markedly lower than that in adults, signifying that the fetus lives in a hypoxic environment.[86] This is in marked contrast to the adult environment, where oxygen is a critical factor in prevention of infection and in the repair process. Other factors are the differences in the fetal and adult immune systems, the histology of fetal skin during development, the function of adult versus fetal fibroblasts in collagen synthesis, and the absence of myofibroblasts.[87,88]

Research Wisdom

Hyaluronic acid (HA) is a gel that is degraded in vivo and breaks down rapidly when applied to wounds. A wound dressing, Hyaff (ConvaTec, a Bristol Myers Squibb company, Princenton, NJ), has just been produced from HA. This dressing, when applied to the wound, creates an HA-rich tissue interface and a moist wound environment conducive to granulation and healing (see Chapter 11).[89]

FACTORS AFFECTING WOUND HEALING

A chronic wound is defined as one that deviates from the expected sequence of repair in terms of time, appearance, and response to aggressive and appropriate treatment.[90] When the response to wounding does not conform to the described cycle of wound recovery after a period of 2–4 weeks, the wound may become stuck and unable to progress through the phases of healing without intervention. The typical way to diagnose chronic wounds is to use the pathophysiology leading to the ulcer. For example, there are ischemic arterial ulcers, diabetic ulcers (both vascular and neuropathic), pressure ulcers, vasculitic ulcers, venous ulcers, and rheumatoid ulcers, all of which are considered chronic wounds (Exhibit 2–1). Skin integrity and wound healing physiology are disrupted by the underlying pathology (intrinsic factors), by environmental influences (extrinsic factors), and by inappropriate management, (iatrogenic factors) that influence whether the wound will go on to heal or will become chronic or refractory. The following sections describe factors in each of these categories (Table 2–4). Chapter 12 discusses refractory wounds.

The nurse and the physical therapist have to manage the patient with a wound and to evaluate the intrinsic, extrinsic,

---

Exhibit 2–1 Examples of Chronic Wounds

- Ischemic arterial ulcers
- Diabetic vascular and neuropathic ulcers
- Venous ulcers
- Vasculitic ulcers
- Rheumatoid ulcers
- Pressure ulcers

---

and iatrogenic factors that may contribute to impaired wound healing. Early identification of wound healing factors that contribute to impaired wound healing will help the clinician to triage cases, reduce variability in cost and care, and improve the prognosis and outcomes for planned interventions.

Intrinsic Factors

Intrinsic factors are those that are related to medical status or physiologic properties within the patient that may affect skin integrity and/or healing. Intrinsic factors, including age, chronic disease, perfusion and oxygenation, immunosuppression, and neurologically impaired skin, are explained.

Age

Inflammation, cell migration, proliferation, and maturation responses are slowed with aging.[91,92] Skin changes that occur with aging include thinning of the epidermis, with increased risk of injury from shearing and friction, resulting in ulceration and skin tears. The skin also loses its impenetrability to substances in the environment. Irritants and certain drugs are more readily absorbed. The reproductive function of epidermal cells diminishes with age, and replacement is slowed. Elastin fibers are lost, and the skin becomes less elastic. The dermis atrophies, which slows wound contraction and increases risk of wound dehiscence.[93] Wound dehiscence is two to three times higher in patients over age 60, yet, as Eaglstein[92] notes, the causative factors may be infection, inadequate protein intake, or other medical complications—not solely age. There is diminished vascularity of the dermis.[93] Aging and chronic disease states often go together, and both delay repair processes, due to delayed cellular response to the stimulus of injury, delayed collagen deposition, and decreased tensile strength in the remodeled tissue. The regeneration process may be diminished as a result of impaired circulatory function. Aging alone is not a major factor in chronic wound healing. Research now demonstrates that, in elderly persons without chronic disease states, healing is only slightly retarded, compared with that of a young population.[94] Patient age did not significantly affect healing times for leg ulcers associated with venous insufficiency[95] or for neuropathic foot ulcers using total contact casting.[96] However, it appears to affect risk for skin breakdown with those persons who are older than 85 years, demonstrating a 30% risk of developing pressure ulcers.[97] Because chronic conditions are more common in older adults, age is at least a marker for conditions that predispose to chronic wounds and so is typically identified as a cofactor in impaired healing.[98]

Chronic Disease

Chronic diseases of all kinds—renal, pulmonary, and other systemic diseases—affect the cardiopulmonary system

Table 2–4 Factors Affecting Wound Healing

Intrinsic: *Related to Medical Status*	*Extrinsic:* *Related to Environment*	*Iatrogenic:* *Related to Wound Management*
Age	Medications	Local ischemia
Chronic Disease	Nutrition	Inappropriate wound care
Perfusion and Oxygenation	Irradiation and chemotherapy	Trauma
Immunosuppression	Psychophysiologic stress	Wound extent and duration
Neuorologically impaired skin	Wound burden and infection	

and the oxygen transport pathway that delivers oxygen from the lungs to the tissues and removes carbon dioxide. The cardiopulmonary system is affected by conditions that are hematologic, neuromuscular, musculoskeletal, endocrine, and immunologic.[99] For example, depending on the location or level of a neuromuscular lesion, breathing functions will be affected. This may contribute to reduced respiratory muscle function, which will affect lung volumes, flow rates, inspiratory and expiratory lung functions, and the delivery of oxygen to and removal of carbon dioxide from the tissues that are required for healing. Impaired cardiopulmonary function will affect mobility and must be considered as a risk for skin ulceration. In this case, the nurse and physical therapist must be aware of how to optimize the positioning and mobility of the patient to compensate for the effects of chronic disease on the body.

Patients with diabetes are at risk for poor healing, due to the effects of high blood glucose levels on leukocyte function, with increased risk of infection.[100] The microvascular and neuropathic components associated with diabetes also place the individual at increased susceptibility for impaired healing.[101] In body systems suffering immune suppression, such as is common in those who have diabetes, cancer, human immunodeficiency virus (HIV) infection, and acquired immune deficiency syndrome or who are undergoing immunosuppressive therapy, the body lacks the ability to produce an inflammation phase, which is the body's immune response to injury. As described, the inflammatory response sets off the cascade of repair. Absence or impairment of inflammation at the onset of trauma will impair the healing cascade through all phases of healing.[102]

Perfusion and Oxygenation

All phases of wound healing require adequate oxygen. Oxygen is carried in the blood and dissolved in the plasma by the red blood cells bound to the hemoglobin. In anemia, there is reduced hemoglobin and reduced oxygen-carrying capacity of the blood. However, research data suggest that anemia does not impair wound healing when there is adequate *perfusion* and *blood volume*.[103] Hypovolemia, the lack of adequate intravascular volume, has been shown to

impair healing because of insufficient volume to transport the oxygen and nutrients to the tissues and remove waste products.[103] Prolonged hypovolemia impairs collagen production and diminishes leukocyte activities.[94] External signs of mild hypovolemia are not evident. Diagnosis of hypovolemia is made by measurement of transcutaneous partial pressure of oxygen in the blood. Hypovolemia should be considered in situations that are common to the chronic wound population, such as use of diuretics, renal dialysis, or blood loss. Fluid administration can be used to correct for hypovolemia, but care must be taken to maximize intravascular volume without causing fluid overload.[94] Hartmann and colleagues[104] reported that fluid replacement, according to measurements of subcutaneous oxygen tension, improved accumulation of collagen in healing wounds by day seven in 29 patients after major abdominal surgery ($p < .05$).[104] Fluid replacement improves tissue perfusion,[105] although overhydration can also lead to perfusion difficulties related to the resulting edema. Thus, wounded patients with fluid volume imbalance may be at risk for impaired healing.

Theories and research abound in looking at reasons why there is a failure to respond to the signals of injury. One theory of the etiology of venous ulcer chronicity attributes the problem to a dysfunctional fibrinolytic system.[106] According to this theory, lipodermatosclerosis is part of the pathogenesis of venous ulcers that impairs the progression of the inflammatory phase, progressing to the proliferative phase. Other theories that have been proposed to explain the effects of venous disease on wound healing include the trapping of cytokines in the tissues,[13] the anticirculatory effects of fibrin cuff formation at dermal vessels,[107] and free radicals.[24] Free radicals are also implicated in the development of leg ulcers. The protective mechanisms become deranged during ischemia and are overwhelmed after reperfusion by the extent of free-radical production.[24]

Chronic venous hypertension leads to leukocyte accumulation in the skin and other tissues of the leg. There is good evidence that neutrophils and monocytes initiate the damage that eventually leads to skin ulceration.[24] In addition to free radicals, these cells replace proteolytic enzymes and inflammatory cytokines that lead to skin breakdown.[24] Oxygen-free-radical activity is elevated in individuals with diabetes mellitus and has been implicated in the etiology of vascular complications.[24] Arterial ulcers result from severe ischemia and the mechanisms of ischemia reperfusion injury. Diabetes also leads to increased susceptibility to peripheral arterial atheroma, leading to stenosis and occlusion that may lead to ischemia and ulceration.[24]

Immunosuppression

Wound healing is also delayed in patients with HIV or cancer and in those undergoing immunosuppressive therapy or the severely malnourished.[108] Immunosuppression retards the inflammatory response, is responsible for failure to mount any inflammatory response, and affects all phases of wound recovery.[102]

Neurologically Impaired Skin

Peripheral neuropathy is a common complication of chronic diabetes and alcoholism. Three types of neuropathy are found in individuals with neuropathy: sensory, motor, and autonomic. Neuropathy affects autonomic nervous system function of the sweat and sebaceous glands located in the skin, resulting in their impairment. When sweat and sebaceous gland function in the feet is impaired, the skin becomes dry and cracked, providing a portal of entry for infection. The skin acidity is also changed, resulting in impairment of the skin's ability to control surface bacteria normally controlled by the skin acidity. Patients with diabetes also have an impairment of the body's immune system, which is simply unable to generate an inflammatory phase of repair and, subsequently, unable to overcome infection. Combining all of these functional impairments results in a chronically infected wound in a patient with a comorbidity of diabetes. Chapter 18 describes the examinations to test for trineuropathy, including photos of the consequences of the three types of impairment.

Central nervous system neuropathy associated with spinal cord injury (SCI) also results in alteration of the functions of the autonomic nervous, motor, and sensory systems. If the lesion is above the sixth thoracic level, in the early stages postinjury, autonomic nervous system function is impaired, and the individual is often unable to maintain constant body temperature. This is because of a loss of the ability to dissipate or retain heat from the interior of the body to the periphery via vasomotor responses to heating. Reflex sweating is also lost with injury at these levels and places the SCI individual at risk for overheating.[109] Another complication of SCI is loss of vasomotor tone, leading to dilation of the veins of the lower extremity, with resultant peripheral edema and frequent deep vein thrombosis.[110] Neurologically impaired skin undergoes metabolic changes that take 3–5 years to stabilize following injury.[109] Changes that occur include:

1. An immediate, significant, and rapid increase in rate of collagen catabolism.
2. Decreased enzyme activity related to defective collagen biosynthesis in the skin below the level of injury. The increased rate of catabolism of collagen, coupled with defective collagen biosynthesis, produces fragile skin, which is more subject to skin breakdown.
3. Decrease in proportion of type I to type III collagen in the skin below level of injury. Properties of type III collagen include thinner, weaker, more widely spaced fibrils that contribute to the fragility of the neurologically impaired skin.
4. Decrease in density of adrenergic receptors in skin below level of injury could be the cause of abnormal vascular reactions.
5. Large increase in GAGs excreted in the urine, which robs the skin of the necessary elasticity to adapt to mechanical insults.

Mechanical factors also affect skin integrity for the SCI group. Muscle atrophy caused by paralysis reduces muscle bulk over bony prominences and exposes the skin covering them to mechanical forces; insensate skin cannot provide signals of impending damage. The combination of the biochemical and mechanical changes increases the vulnerability of the skin to ulceration[109] and will also negatively affect healing of those ulcers.

Extrinsic Factors

Extrinsic factors are those that come from sources in the environment that affect the body or the wound, such as medications, nutrition, irradiation and chemotherapy, psychophysiologic stress, and wound bioburden and infection.

Medications

Medications are often prescribed to control inflammatory responses in the body, including anticoagulants, immunosuppressive agents, antiprostaglandins, and antineoplastics. Steroids are immunosuppression medications that may be applied topically or systemically. Steroids are prescribed for diverse disorders, ranging from asthma to polymyalgia rheumatica. Steroids delay all phases of wound repair. They inhibit macrophage levels, reduce immunocompetent lymphocytes, decrease antibody production, and diminish antigen processing.[98,111] Applications of topical vitamin A and systemic vitamin A supplementation are effective in counteracting the effects of steroid medication.[112] Nonsteroidal antiinflammatory agents, phenylbutazone, and vitamin E also disrupt normal healing.[98] Data suggest that local anesthetics have some cellular impairment to healing but pain relief is achieved with no clinically significant impairment in the rate of healing.[98]

Nutrition

A few investigators have examined the role of nutritional support and intervention on chronic wound healing outcomes, with variable results. Myers et al[113] failed to demonstrate that nutritional support with consistent wound care was more beneficial to wound healing, as compared with consistent wound care alone. In contrast, Gorse and Messner[114] reported improved pressure sore healing in patients with adequate dietary intake. They studied the effect of topical dressings on 52 patients with stages II, III, and IV pressure sores and determined that those patients with adequate dietary intake demonstrated statistically improved healing, regardless of whether treated with hydrocolloid dressings ($p = .002$) or wet to dry saline dressings ($p = .02$).[114] Adequate dietary intake was defined as a diet order that met calculated requirements for protein and calories, as well as a nursing assessment that indicated generally good diet consumption. The 52 patients with pressure sores also demonstrated lower serum albumin levels, as compared with an age- and gender-matched group of 104 patients without pressure sores.[114]

Allman and colleagues[115] examined the use of air fluidized versus regular beds on wound healing in 65 hospitalized patients with pressure sores and included baseline nutritional status as part of the overall study. Wound healing was better ($p = .01$) among those patients on the air-fluidized therapy, with ulcers improving in 38 patients and no improvement in 27 patients. The baseline characteristic most associated with improved healing was dietary protein intake, with those who had improved healing consuming close to twice as much protein as those without improved healing (51.6 versus 27.1 g).[115] Most investigators will agree that nutritional impairment can lead to impaired healing. Certainly, what is less clear is whether providing adequate or increased levels of nutrition improves wound healing.

Malnutrition of protein and insufficient calories is a comorbidity related to chronic wound healing. Multiple studies cite malnutrition as a risk factor for wound healing.[116–118] A nutritional assessment should be considered for all patients with chronic wounds and is required for those individuals who are unable to take food by mouth or who experience weight loss. The Agency for Health Care Research and Quality (AHRQ), formerly known as the Agency for Health Care Policy and Research (AHCPR), published an algorithm for nutritional assessment and support as a guide for clinicians to manage nutritional needs of persons with pressure ulcers (see Chapter 3).[119] A serum albumin level below 3.5 mg/dL is a clinical indicator of a diagnosis of significant malnutrition if accompanied by total lymphocyte count less than 1,800 mm^3 or if body weight has decreased more than 15%.[119] Inadequate absorption may be a part of the problem.

Oral problems associated with eating and chewing have been identified as a component in pressure ulcer risk.[120] Dietary restriction, such as renal diets, will affect the protein available for wound repair. Vitamin C and zinc supplementation have been encouraged for wound healing. Hydration should also be considered as part of the nutritional assessment. Patients with fluid orders had a 35% reduced risk of developing pressure ulcers.[97] Malnutrition, which has long been recognized as a problem for pressure ulcer patients, is now being considered a problem for the patient with venous ulcer disease.[94] Chapter 3 discusses nutrition assessment, effects of nutrition on the physiology of healing, and interventions to prevent skin breakdown and promote healing.

Irradiation and Chemotherapy

The purpose of radiation therapy is to disrupt cell mitosis, and it has ongoing effects for the individual's life.[98] The damage may not be visible on the surface and may have a latent appearance. Injuries to the cells of repair, fibroblasts and endothelial cells, and to the vasculare of the area make tissues that have been irradiated at risk for breakdown and poor healing. The extent, dosage, frequency, and location of irradiation in relation to the wound site will determine the effect on wound healing. The effects of irradiation on tissue are not easily reversed.[93] Recovery depends on the dose of radiation and the half-life of the various cells.[98]

Chemotherapy affects cell division. Chemotherapy is accomplished with anticancer drugs that damage DNA or prevent DNA repair. The primary effects of chemotherapy occur during the treatment period and immediately following.[98] However, some drugs such as methotrexate may be used for other medical reasons on a long-term basis, and may interfere with tissue repair.

Psychophysiologic Stress

Understanding the role of psychophysiologic stress is another area of chronic wound research. It is estimated that 50–80% of illnesses have some components of stress, which is recognized as a risk factor in addictions, obesity, high blood pressure, peptic ulcers, colitis, asthma, insomnia, migraine headaches, and lower back pain, and may be a factor in some psychologic disorders. The role of stress in development of cancer is unknown but some believe there is a link.[121] Stress may be positive or negative. Positive stress allows us to perform all of our daily functions. Negative stress may weaken the immune system and needs to be managed.

Psychologic factors may play a role in impaired healing, as evidenced by Anderson and Andberg's[122] early work with persons with SCI, their life satisfaction, and incidence of pressure sores. Paraplegics who were college students were found to have more skin breakdown during final examination periods than at other times of the school year.[123] Caregivers of chronically ill patients who experienced wounds were found to take longer to heal than persons not living in such stressful situations. The chronically ill patient with multiple comorbidities has psychophysiologic stress from multiple disease processes.

Satisfaction with life activities has been inversely related to incidence of pressure ulcer development.[122] Several other investigators have examined the role of stress in relation to wound healing.[124–126] North[127] reviewed the effect of sleep on wound healing and concluded that sleep and relaxation may affect the physiological processes involved with wound healing. Holden-Lund[125] examined the use of guided imagery for relaxation and wound healing and demonstrated that stress (as measured by cortisol levels) and inflammation were reduced when using guided imagery. This work parallels the subsequent findings by Braden[124] that persons with lower cortisol levels did not develop pressure sores. West[126] also examined the role of stress but looked at the effect of perioperative stress on the repair process and concluded that perioperative stress decreases tissue and wound oxygen tension via vasoconstriction related to high levels of circulating catecholamines.

Noise, as a stressor, has also been explored in relation to wound healing. McCarthy and colleagues[128] reviewed the potential impact of noise on wound healing. Using an animal model, this group demonstrated impairment in leukocyte function in rats exposed to noise stress, as compared with rats not exposed to noise stress. Wysocki[129] more recently demonstrated decreased healing in rats when they were exposed to intermittent noise.

Sympathetic nervous system stimulation and subsequent release of adrenalin, noradrenalin, and cortisol may be the mechanism of the impact of stress on wound healing. Increased cortisol levels suppress migration of neutrophils, inhibiting synthesis of proinflammatory mediators, with resultant interference in the early inflammatory response in wounds. Additionally, increased cortisol levels block the proliferation of fibroblasts, leading to effects on the duration and strength of wound healing. Like much on stress and wound healing, the interaction between stress and the growth hormone-somatomedin system is not entirely understood. Lee and Stotts[130] reviewed the response of the growth hormone-somatomedin system on healing, as well as the negative effects of sleep changes and stress on the growth hormone-somatomedin system. They also describe the importance of the anabolic function of growth hormone on tissue repair and make recommendations for interventions targeted to healthy functioning of the growth hormone-somatomedin system. Suggestions include promoting adequate time for uninterrupted sleep and encouraging exercise as a mild stressor to promote secretion. Most of these exploratory studies and reviews have focused on the individual with an acute wound. Few data are known about the stress effect on chronic wounds.

Byl has pointed out that there may be some learned element in nonhealing. Studies demonstrate the existence of physical and chemical links between the mind and the immune system. The connection and the effect one has on the other is sometimes called *psychoneuroimmunology*—the interface of the brain and nervous system with the immune system. Perhaps the abnormal processes of healing can be learned. Many patients have their minds filled with unhappy thoughts that invite disease. Neuroplasticity research confirms the effects of negative learning on degradation of the representation of the hand on the somatosensory cortex. Negative thinking may have adverse effects on the cells of repair, the maintenance of inflammation, inadequate protein synthesis, or impaired circulation. Conversely, the patient may be able to reverse the adverse effects through a process of mental imagery, visualizing the process of healing (eg, increasing blood flow to the affected area by imagining the phagocytic cells gobbling up bacteria and debris, etc.) and by positive self-talk about healing. There is an increasing amount of research about the effects of visualization and meditation on healing and overcoming cancer and improving immune system function, even when medical science cannot explain the results.[131]

Bioburden and Infection

Excessive bioburden from necrotic tissue and infection have been associated with development of a chronic wound. For example, epidermal cells normally march forward as a sheet and lyse the necrotic debris from the wound edges, but they are impaired in this process of phagocytosis if obstructed by a large quantity of devitalized material. Devitalized tissue and foreign matter debris contribute to the proliferation of bacteria in the wound, which, in turn, will overwhelm the body with infection, possibly leading to sepsis. In such situations, the body will not be able to cleanse the wound without intervention. It is imperative to clean the wound down to healthy bleeding tissue to restart the inflammatory phase and the biologic cascade of healing. Bleeding creates a new acute battle zone and signal source for the responder cells. However, the response may fail to occur or be inadequate to initiate a new inflammation response if there is inadequate circulation.

Iatrogenic Factors in Chronic Wound Healing

Iatrogenic factors are those factors related to the specific way that the wound is managed. These include local ischemia, inappropriate wound care, trauma, and wound extent and duration.[93,94]

Local Ischemia

Local ischemia occurs in different ways, such as from pressure over a bony prominence or an inappropriate application of compression to a limb with mixed venous and arterial disease. Individuals who are smokers experience nicotine-induced vasoconstriction and tissue ischemia. Persons with a history of tobacco use are 76% more likely to develop a pressure ulcer than are nonsmokers.[120]

Inappropriate Wound Care

Inappropriate wound management, including a misuse of topical agents (eg, antiseptics) or poor technique in application of dressings and tapes that results in tears and blisters on surrounding skin or wound bed, has been implicated as a factor in development of a chronic wound.[93,94] Wound desiccation from lack of a dressing or inappropriate dressing choice is not uncommon. Drying out of the wound interferes with the "current of injury" function,[132] as well as with the mitotic and migratory function of cells. Dressing changes and wound cleansing disrupt the wound environment, causing chilling of the wound and surrounding tissues. Lock[133] and Myers[134] found that it takes up to 40 minutes for the tissues to regain their usual temperature and chilling impairs cell mitosis for up to 3 hours following. Chilling also disrupts leukocytic activity and oxyhemoglobin dissociation severely.[135]

Trauma

Trauma to wound tissue occurs frequently, impeding wound repair and influencing local wound infection.[136] Trauma retards the rate of healing, alters the tensions of respiratory gases in a wound remote from the injury site, and causes increased susceptibility to wound infection, probably due to decreased nutritive blood flow.[136] Trauma can be attributed to many different causes, including the following:

- High-pressure irrigation, such as in the whirlpool or with a Water Pik
- Sharp or mechanical debridement
- Improper pressure to new granulation tissue, traumatizing the fragile tissue and initiating a new inflammatory response, which retards healing and causes abnormal scarring
- Improper handling during removal of dressings, compression wraps, or stockings, frequently results in trauma to venous ulcers whose surrounding skin is often extremely fragile

---

Clinical Wisdom: *Avoiding Adverse Treatment Effects*

Careful evaluation of each treatment and technique, based on wound assessment, can avoid adverse treatment effects and change the course of the wound.

Wound Extent and Duration

There is evidence to support the role of wound surface area and wound depth as a factor in time to healing.[114,137–139]

There is intuitive logic in the belief that large-surface-area injuries (and multiple wounds, which also increase surface area to be repaired) increase the need for oxygen, nutrients, and adaptive resources required for healing because there is more damaged tissue to repair. Multiple sizable wounds present the host with a larger total surface area to repair.

Researchers looking at factors that can be used to predict wound healing have identified duration and size as two factors that are predictive of healing outcomes. Percentage of healing and ulcer area at week 3 were good predictors of 100% healing. Patients with venous ulcers that have a large initial size or who have moderate arterial insufficiency (ankle brachial index 0.5–0.8) have associated delayed healing times.[95] Shorter duration of ulceration and smaller size were predictive of time to heal.[140] Ulcers that are large, longstanding, and slow to heal after 3 weeks of optimal therapy are unlikely to change their course.[141] It is now possible to identify and diagnose correctly those leg ulcers that have a poor prognosis to respond to standard care, and consideration should be given to move them on to alternative therapies.[141]

CONCLUSION

The process of wound healing described occurs in the same way in all wounds, both open and closed, but is less observable in closed wounds. The processes that occur throughout wound healing are complex and sensitive to internal and external environmental forces. The goals of wound healing are to provide interventions that will mitigate the negative forces and to provide interventions that progress wounds through the sequence of repair or regeneration in an orderly and timely manner. In order for the nurse and physical therapist to have successful wound healing outcomes, it is important to understand and be able to recognize the key sequence of events. The ability to recognize the benchmarks of wound phase change is critical to monitoring the effects of treatment interventions and recognizing when the intervention is successful or not successful. Early identification that the wound has become "stuck" and unable to progress should trigger an appropriate response. Chronicity can happen during any phase of healing. A wound can also have an absence of a phase of repair. This occurs when the body simply fails to initiate the phase (eg, when there is inadequate circulation). These concepts are expanded in Chapter 4, Assessment of the Skin and Wound.

REVIEW QUESTIONS

1. Partial thickness wounds involving only the epidermis heal by which of the following processes?
   a. contraction and granulation
   b. epithelialization or epidermal resurfacing

c. epithelialization and granulation
d. inflammation remodeling

2. The clinician is assessing F.T.'s abdomen 3 days post abdominal-perineal resection surgery and notes erythema, slight edema, and slight increase in temperature at the incisional site. These findings are most consistent with which of the following?
   a. These are normal signs of the inflammatory phase of wound healing.
   b. The wound is exhibiting early signs of impending infection.
   c. The wound is in the proliferative phase of wound healing.
   d. The wound is exhibiting signs of abscess formation.

3. Which of the following statements is MOST accurate about fibroblasts?
   a. They are responsible for phagocytosis of bacteria and wound cleanup.
   b. They are responsible for wound contraction and scar hypertrophy.
   c. They are responsible for collagen lysis in the remodeling phase of healing.
   d. They are responsible for angiogenesis and collagen synthesis.

4. Which following statement regarding the inflammatory phase of wound healing is correct?
   a. Inflammation is detrimental to wound healing.
   b. The overall effect of inflammation is a wound area free of debris because leukocytes break down necrotic tissue and phagocytose bacteria.
   c. Inflammation occurs only in dirty, infected wounds and indicates the need for antibiotics.
   d. Steroids enhance wound healing by blocking the inflammatory response.

5. Vitamin A may facilitate healing in some clients because:
   a. It is essential for cellular repair.
   b. It significantly affects blood and tissue oxygen levels.
   c. It can partially correct the effects of steroids on wound healing.
   d. It potentiates antibiotic therapy, thus reducing inflammation.

6. Which of the following appear to be principal mediators for full-thickness wound repair?
   a. Endothelial cells and fibroblasts
   b. Neutrophils and platelets
   c. Fibroblasts and neutrophils
   d. Platelets and macrophages

7. Contraction plays an important role in wound healing for:
   a. wounds healing by primary intention
   b. wounds healing by secondary intention
   c. superficial abrasions
   d. all wounds

REFERENCES

1. Hunt TK, Hussain M. Can wound healing be a paradigm for tissue repair? *Med Sci Sports Exerc.* 1994;26:755–758.

2. Cooper D. The physiology of wound healing: An overview. In: Krassner D, ed. *Chronic Wound Care.* King of Prussia, PA: Health Management Publication; 1990:1–11.

3. Winter GD. Epidermal regeneration studied in the domestic pig. In: Hunt TK, Dunphy JE, eds. *Fundamentals of Wound Management.* New York: Appleton-Century-Crofts; 1979:71–111.

4. Lazarus GS, Cooper DM, Knighton DM, et al. Definitions and guidelines for assessment of wounds and evaluation of healing. *Arch Dermatol.* 1994;130:489–493.

5. Hunt TK, Heppenstall RB, Pines E, Rovee D, eds. *Soft and Hard Tissue Repair: Biological and Clinical Aspects.* New York: Praegar Publishers; 1984.

6. Hunt TK, Van Winkle W. *Fundamentals of Wound Management in Surgery, Wound Healing: Normal Repair.* South Plainfield, NJ: Chirurgecom; 1976:1e.

7. Kerstein MD, Bensing KA, Brill LR, et al. *The Physiology of Wound Healing.* The Oxford Institute for Continuing Education and Allegheny University of Health Sciences: Philadelphia; 1998.

8. Mast B. The skin. In: Cohen I, Diegelmann RF, Lindblad WJ, eds. *Wound Healing Biochemical and Clinical Aspects.* Philadelphia: W.B. Saunders Company; 1992:344–355.

9. Grinnell F, Billingham R, Burgess L. Distribution of fibronectin during wound healing in vivo. *J Invest Dermatol.* 1981;76(3):181–189.

10. Michaelson AD, et al. Reversible inhibition of human platelet activation by hypothermia in vivo and in vitro. *Thromb Haemost.* 1994;71(5):633–640.

11. Valeri CR, Khabbaz K, Khuri SF, et al. Effect of skin temperature on platelet function in patients undergoing extracorporeal bypass. *J Thoracic Cardiovasc Surg.* 1992;104(1):108–116.

12. Doherty D, et al. Human monocyte adherence: A primary effect of chemotactic factors on the monocyte to stimulate adherence to human endothelium. *J Immunol.* 1987;138(6):1762–1771.

13. Falanga VE, Eaglstein WH. The "trap" hypothesis of venous ulceration. *Lancet.* 1993;341(8851):1006–1008.

14. Sessler DI. Mild perioperative hypothermia. *N Engl J Med.* 1997; 336(24):1730–1736.

15. Fylling CP. Growth factors: A new era in wound healing. In: Krasner, DK, Kane D, eds. *Chronic Wound Care: A Sourcebook for Healthcare Professionals.* 2nd ed. Wayne, PA: Health Management Publications; 1997:344–346.

16. Hunt T, Hopf H. Wound healing and wound infection: What surgeons and anesthesiologists can do. *Surg Clin North Am.* 1997;77(3):587–606.

17. Knighton DR, Silver IA, Hunt TK. Regulation of wound-angiogenesis: Effect of oxygen gradients and inspired oxygen concentration. *Surgery.* 1981;90:262.

18. Byl N. Electrical stimulation for tissue repair: Basic information. In: Nelson R, Hayes KW, Currier DP, eds. *Clinical Electrotherapy.* 3rd ed. Stamford, CT: Appleton & Lange; 1999.

19. Suh D, Hunt T. Time line of wound healing. *Clin Podiatr Med Surg.* 1998;15(1):1–9.

20. Knighton DR, Halliday B, Hunt TK, et al. Oxygen as an antibiotic: The effect of inspired oxygen on infection. *Arch Surg.* 1984;119:199–204.

21. Hohn DC, et al. Effect of O_2 tension on microbicidal function of leukocytes in wounds and in vitro. *Surg Forum.* 1976;27:18–20.

22. Goodson WH, Andrews WS, Thakral KK, Hunt TK. Wound oxygen tension of large vs. small wounds in man. *Surg Forum.* 1979;30:92–95.

23. Jonsson K, Jensen J, Goodson WD, et al. Tissue oxygenation, anemia, and perfusion in relation to wound healing in surgical patients. *Ann Surg.* 1991;214(5):605–613.

24. Coleridge-Smith PD. Oxygen, oxygen free radicals and reperfusion injury. In: Krasner D, Kane D, eds. *Chronic Wound Care: A Clinical Source Book for Healthcare Professionals.* 2nd ed. Wayne, PA: Health Management Publications; 1997:348–353.

25. Knighton DR, Hunt TK. The defenses of the wound. In: Howard RJ, Simmons RI, eds. *Surgical Infectious Diseases.* 2nd ed. Stamford, CT: Appleton & Lange; 1988:188–193.

26. Clark R. Wound repair: Overview and general considerations. In: Clark R, ed. *The Molecular and Cellular Biology of Wound Repair.* New York: Plenum Publishing; 1996:3–50.

27. Calvin M. Cutaneous wound repair. *Wounds.* 1998;10(1):12–32.

28. Dyson M, Luke D. Induction of mast cell degranulation in skin by ultrasound. *IEEE Trans Ultrasonics, Ferroelectronics, Frequency Control.* 1986;33:194–201.

29. Dabrowski R, Masinski C, Olczak A. The role of histamine in wound healing: The effect of high doses of histamine on collagen and glycos-aminoglycan in wounds. *Agents Actions.* 1997;7:219–224.

30. Dexter TM, Stoddart RW, Quazzaz STA. What are mast cells for? *Nature.* 1981;291:110–111.

31. Ross J. *Utilization of Pulsed High Peak Power Electromagnetic Energy (Diapulse Therapy) To Accelerate Healing Processes.* Presented at the Digest International Symposium, Antennas and Propagation Society, Stanford, CA; Stanford University; June 20–22, 1977:146–149.

32. Horzic M, Bunoza D, Maric K. Contact thermography in a study of primary healing of surgical wounds. *Ostomy/Wound Manage.* 1996;42(1):36–42.

33. Lock PM. The effect of temperature on mitotic activity at the edge of experimental wounds. In: Sandell B, ed. *Symposium on Wound Healing: Plastic, Surgical and Dermatologic Aspects.* Sweden: Molndal; 1979:103–107.

34. Myers JA. Wound healing and the use of modern surgical dressing. *Pharm J.* 1982;229:103–104.

35. Becker RO. The significance of bioelectric potentials. *Med Times.* 1967;95:657–659.

36. Foulds IS, Barker AT. Human skin battery potentials and their possible role in wound healing. *Br J Dermatol.* 1983;109:515–522.

37. Vanable J Jr. Natural and applied voltages in vertebrate regeneration and healing. In: *Integumentary Potentials and Wound Healing.* New York: Alan R. Liss; 1989.

38. Jaffe LP, Vanable JW. Electric field and wound healing. *Clin Dermatol.* 1984;3:233–234.

39. Orinda N, Feldman JD. Directional protrusive pseudopodial activity and motility in macrophages induced by extracellular electric fields. *Cell Motil.* 1982;2:243–255.

40. Fukushima K, Senda N, Inui H, et al. Studies of galvanotaxis of leukocytes. *Med J Osaka Univ.* 1953;4:195–208.

41. Weiss DS, et al. Pulsed electrical stimulation decreases scar thickness at split-thickness graft donor sites. *J Invest Dermatol.* 1989;92:539.

42. Kloth LC. Electrical stimulation in tissue repair. In: McColloch JM, Kloth LC, Feeder JA, eds. *Wound Healing Alternatives in Management.* 2nd ed. Philadelphia: F.A. Davis; 1995:292.

43. Erickson CA, Nuccitelli R. Embryonic fibroblast motility and orientation can be influenced by physiological electric fields. *Cell Biol.* 1981;98:296–307.

44. Bourguignon GJ, Bourguignon LYW. Electric stimulation of protein and DNA synthesis in human fibroblasts. *FASEB J.* 1987;1:398.

45. Bourguignon GJ, Jy W, Bourguignon LYW. Electric stimulation of human fibroblasts causes an increase in Ca^{2+} influx and the exposure of additional insulin receptors. *J Cell Physiol.* 1989;140:379–385.

46. Bourguignon LYW, Jy W, Majercik MH, et al. Lymphocyte activation and capping of hormone receptors. *J Cell Biochem.* 1988;37:131–150.

47. Cooper MS, Schliwa M. Electrical and ionic controls of tissue cell locomotion in DC electric fields. *J Neurosci Res.* 1985;13:223–244.

48. Rowley BA, McKenna J, Chase G. The influence of electrical current on an infecting microorganism in wounds. *Ann NY Acad Sci.* 1974;238:543–551.

49. Barranco S, Spadaro J, Berger TJ, Becker RO. In vitro effect of weak direct current on staphylococcus aureus. *Clin Orthop.* 1974;100:250–255.

50. Kincaid C, Lavoie K. Inhibition of bacterial growth in vitro following stimulation with high voltage, monophasic, pulsed current. *Phys Ther.* 1989;69:29–33.

51. Szuminsksky NJ, Albers AC, Unger P, Eddy JG. Effect of narrow, pulsed high voltages on bacterial viability. *Phys Ther.* 1994;74:660–667.

52. Bates-Jensen B. A quantitative analysis of wound characteristics as early predictors of healing in pressure sores. *Dissertation Abstracts International. Vol. 59, No. 11.* Los Angeles: University of California; 1999.

53. Eaglstein W, Falanga V. Chronic wounds. *Surg Clin North Am.* 1997;77(3):689.

54. Wipke-Tevis D, Stotts N. Leukocytes, ischemia, and wound healing: A critical interaction. *Wound.* 1991;3(6):227–238.

55. Shea JD. Pressure sores: Classification and management. *Clin Orthop.* 1975;112:89–100.

56. Seiler WD, Stahelin HB. Implications for research. *Wound.* 1994;6: 101–106.

57. Hardy M. The physiology of scar formation. *Phys Ther.* 1989;69(22): 1014–1023, 1032.

58. Kirsner R, Eaglstein W. The wound healing process. *Dermatol Clin.* 1993;11:629–640.

59. Weiss EL. Connective tissue in wound healing. In: McCulloch JM, Kloth LC, Feedar JA, eds. *Wound Healing: Alternatives in Management.* 2nd ed. Philadelphia: F.A. Davis; 1995:16–29.

60. Byl N, McKenzie AL, West JM, et al. Low-dose ultrasound effects on wound healing: A controlled study with Yucatan pigs. *Arch Phys Med Rehabil.* 1992;73(July 1992):656–663.

61. Witte M, Barbul A. General principles of wound healing. *Surg Clin North Am.* 1997;77(3):509–528.

62. Harding KG, Bale S. Wound care: Putting theory into practice in the United Kingdom. In: Krasner D, Kane D, eds. *Chronic Wound Care: A Clinical Source Book for Healthcare Professionals.* Wayne, PA: Health Management Publications; 1997:115–123.

63. Hardy MA. The biology of scar formation. *Phys Ther.* 1989;69(12):1014–1023.

64. Wysocki AB. Fibronectin in acute and chronic wounds. *J ET Nurs.* 1992;19(5):35–39.

65. Hynes R. Molecular biology of fibronectin. *Annu Rev Cell Biol.* 1985;1:67–90.

66. Grinnell F, Zhu M. Identification of neutrophil elastase as the proteinase in burn wound fluid responsible for degradation of fibronectin. *J Invest Dermatol.* 1994;103(2):155–161.

67. Parks W. The production, role, and regulation of matrix metalloproteinases in the healing epidermis. *Wound.* 1995;7(5 Suppl A):23A–37A.

68. Staiano-Coico L, Higgins P, Schwartz S, et al. Wound fluids: A reflection of the state of healing. *Ostomy/Wound Manage.* 2000;46(1A):85S–93S.

69. Park H-Y, Shon K, Phillips T. The effect of heat on inhibitory effects of chronic wound fluid on fibroblasts in vitro. *Wound.* 1998;10(6):189–192.

70. Bucalo B, Eaglstein W, Falanga V. Inhibition of cell proliferation by chronic wound fluid. *Wound Repair Regeneration.* 1989;1(3):181–186.

71. Grinnell F, Ho C, Wysocki A. Degradation of fibronectin and vitronectin in chronic wound fluid: Analysis by cell blotting, immunoblotting, and cell adhesion assays. *J Invest Dermatol.* 1992;98(4):410–416.

72. Bennett NT, Schultz GS. Growth factors and wound healing. II. Role in normal and chronic wound healing. *Am J Surg.* 1993;166(1):74–81.

73. Cooper D, Yu EZ, Hennesey P, Ko F, et al. Determination of endogenous cytokines in chronic wounds. *Ann Surg.* 1994;219(6):688–691.

74. Pierce G, Tarpley J, Tseng J, et al. Detection of platelet-derived growth factor (PDGF)-AA in actively healing human wounds treated with recombinant PDGF-BB and absence of PDGF in chronic non-healing wounds. *J Clin Invest.* 1995;96(3):1336–1350.

75. Yager D, Zhang L, Liang H, et al. Wound fluids in human pressure ulcers contain elevated matrix metaloproteinase levels and activity compared to surgical wound fluids. *J Invest Dermatol.* 1996;107(5):743–748.

76. Siddiqui A, Galiano R, Connors D, et al. Differential effects of oxygen on human dermal fibroblasts: Acute versus chronic hypoxia. *Wound Repair Regeneration.* 1996;4(2):211–218.

77. Gogia P. Physiology of wound healing. In: Gogia P, ed. *Clinical Wound Management.* Thorofare, NJ: Slack; 1995:1–12.

78. Murray J. Scars and keloids. *Dermatol Clin.* 1993;11(4):697–708.

79. Stotts N. Impaired wound healing In: Carrieri-Kohlman V, Lindsay A, West C, eds. *Pathophysiological Phenomenon in Nursing.* Philadelphia: W.B. Saunders Company; 1993:343–366.

80. Adzick NS, Harrison MR, Glick PI, et al. Comparison of fetal, newborn and adult wound healing by histologic, enzyme-histochemical and hydroxyproline determination. *J Pediatr Surg.* 1985;20:315.

81. Harrison MR, Langer JC, Adzick, NS, et al. Correction of congenital diaphragmatic hernia in utero. V: Initial clinical experience. *J Pediatr Surg.* 1990;25:47.

82. Harrison MR, Adzick NS, Longaker MT, et al. Successful repair in utero of a fetal diaphragmatic hernia after removal of herniated viscera from the left thorax. *N Engl J Med.* 1990;322:1582.

83. Harris MC, Mennuti MT, Kline JA, et al. Amniotic fluid fibronectin concentrations with advancing gestational age. *Obstet Gynecol.* 1988;72:593.

84. Byl N, McKenzie A, Stern R, et al. Amniotic fluid modulates wound healing. *Eur J Rehab Med.* 1993;2:184–190.

85. Byl N, McKenzie A, West, JM, et al. Pulsed micro amperage stimulation: A controlled study of healing of surgically induced wounds in Yucatan pigs. *Phys Ther.* 1994;74:201–218.

86. Hock RJ. The physiology of high altitude. *Aci Amer.* 1987;22:52.

87. Chang B, Longaker MT, Tuchler RE, et al. *Do Human Fetal Wounds Contract?* Presented at the 35th Annual Meeting of the Plastic Surgery Research Council, Washington, DC; April 1990.

88. Longaker MT, Adzick, NS, Hall JL, et al. Studies in fetal wound healing. VII: Fetal wound healing may be modulated by elevated hyaluronic acid stimulating activity in amniotic fluid. *J Pediatr Surg.* 1990;25:430.

89. Edmonds M. Hyaluronic acid in recalcitrant ulcers. *Evidence Based Outcomes in Wound Management.* Symposium. Dallas, TX: ConvaTec; 2000.

90. Mulder GD, Jeter KF, Fairchild PA, eds. *Clinician's Pocket Guide to Chronic Wound Repair.* Spartanburg, SC: Wound Healing Publications; 1991.

91. Jones P, Millman A. Wound healing and the aged patient. *Nurs Clin North Am.* 1990;25(1):263–277.

92. Eaglstein W. Wound healing and aging. *Clin Geriatr Med.* 1989;5(1):183–188.

93. Mulder G, Brazinsky BA, Seeley J. Factors complicating wound repair. In: McCulloch JM, Kloth LC, Feeder JA, eds. *Wound Healing Alternatives in Management.* 2nd ed. Philadelphia: F. Davis; 1995:47–59.

94. Stotts NA, Wipke-Tevis D. Co-factors in impaired wound healing. *Ostomy/Wound Manage.* March 1996;42:44–56.

95. Marston W, Carlin R, Passman M, et al. Healing rates and cost efficacy of outpatient compression treatment for leg ulcers associated with venous insufficiency. *J Vasc Surg.* 1999;30(3):491–498.

96. Sinacore DR, Mueller MJ. Pedal ulcers in older adults with diabetes mellitus. *Top Geriatr Rehabil.* 2000;16(2):11–23.

97. Voss AC, Bender S, Cook AS, et al. *Pressure Ulcer Prevention in LTC: Implementation of the National Pressure Ulcer Long-Term Care Study (NPULS) Prevention Program.* Symposium for Advanced Wound Care, Dallas, TX: HMP Communications; 2000.

98. Stotts N, Wipke-Tevis D. Co-factors in Impaired Wound Healing. In: Krasner D, Kane D, eds. *Chronic Wound Care: A Clinical Sourcebook for Health Care Professionals.* 2nd ed. Wayne, PA: Health Management Publications; 1997:64–71.

99. Dean E. Oxygen transport deficits in systemic disease and implications for physical therapy. *Phys Ther.* 1997;77:187–202.

100. Yue D, McLennan S, Marsh M, et al. Effects of experimental diabetes, uremia, and malnutrition on wound healing. *Diabetes.* 1987;36(3):295–299.

101. Rosenberg C. Wound healing in the patient with diabetes mellitus. *Nurs Clin North Am.* 1990;25(1):247–261.

102. Norris S, Provo B, Stotts N. Physiology of wound healing and risk factors that impede the healing process. *AACN Clin Issues.* 1990;1:545–552.

103. Hunt TK, Rabkin J, von Smitten K. Effects of edema and anemia on wound healing and infection. *Curr Stud Hematol Blood Transf.* 1986;53:101–111.

104. Hartmann M, Jonsson K, Zederfeldt B. Effect of tissue perfusion and oxygenation on accumulation of collagen in healing wounds. Randomized study in patients after major abdominal operations. *Eur J Surg.* 1992;158(10):521–526.

105. Jonsson K, Jensen J, Goodson WD, et al. Assessment of perfusion in postoperative patients using tissue oxygen measurements. *Br J Surg.* 1987;74(4):263–267.

106. McCulloch JM. Treatment of wounds caused by vascular insufficiency. In: McCulloch JM, Kloth LC, Feeder JA, eds. *Wound Healing Alternatives in Management.* 2nd ed. Philadelphia: F. Davis; 1995: 216–217.

107. Burnand K, Whimster I, Naidoo A, et al. Pericapillary fibrin in the ulcer-bearing skin of the leg: The cause of lipodermatosclerosis and venous ulceration. *Br Med J Clin Res Educ.* 1982;285(6348):1071–1072.

108. Mosiello G, Tufaro A, Kerstein M. Wound healing and complications in the immunosuppressed patient. *Wounds.* 1994;6(3):883–887.

109. Garber SL, Biddle AK, Click CN, et al. *Pressure Ulcer Prevention and Treatment Following Spinal Cord Injury: A Clinical Practice Guideline for Health-Care Professionals.* Jackson Heights, NY: Paralyzed Veterans of America; 2000:12–14.

110. Twist D. Acrocyanosis in a spinal cord injured patient—effect of computer-controlled neuromuscular electrical stimulation: A case report. *Phys Ther.* 1990;70:45–49.

111. Leiebowitch SJ, Ross R. The role of the macrophage in wound repair. *Am J Pathol.* 1975;78:71–91.

112. Hunt TK. Vitamin A and wound healing. *J Am Acad Dermatol.* 1986;15:817.

113. Myers S, Takiguchi S, Slavish S, et al. Consistent wound care and nutritional support in treatment. *Decubitus.* 1990;3(3):16–28.

114. Gorse G, Messner R. Improved pressure sore healing with hydrocolloid dressings. *Arch Dermatol.* 1987;123:766–771.

115. Allman R, Walker J, Hart M, et al. Air-fluidized beds or conventional therapy for pressure sores: A randomized trial. *Ann Intern Med.* 1987;107:641–648.

116. Allman RM, Laprade CA, Noel LB, et al. Pressure sores among hospitalized patients. *Ann Intern Med.* 1987;105:337–342.

117. Bergstrom N, Braden B. A prospective study of pressure sore risk among institutionalized elderly. *J Am Geriatr Soc.* 1992;40:747–758.

118. Breslow RA, Hallfrisch J, Goldberg AP. Malnutrition in tubefed nursing home patients with pressure sores. *J Parenter Enteral Nutr.* 1991;15:663–668.

119. Bergstrom N, Bennett MA, Carlson C, et al. Treatment of pressure ulcers. *Clinical Practice Guideline,* No. 15. Rockville, MD: US Dept of Health and Human Services (DHHS), AHRQ Publication No. 95-0652, December 1994.

120. Ross PD. *Executive Summary—Phase I Prevention Results: The National Pressure Ulcer Long-Term Care Study.* Columbus, OH: Ross; 1999:1–6.

121. Dollinger L. Relaxation and cancer recovery. In: Dollinger M, Rosenbaum EH, Cable G, eds. *Everyone's Guide to Cancer Therapy: How Cancer Is Diagnosed, Treated, and Managed Day to Day.* Kansas City, MO: Andrews McMeel Publishing; 1997:197–200.

122. Anderson T, Andberg M. Psychosocial factors associated with pressure sores. *Arch Phys Med Rehabil.* 1979;60(8):341–346.

123. Crenshaw R, Vistnes L. A decade of pressure sore research. *J Rehab Res Dev.* 1989;26:63–74.

124. Braden B. The relationship between stress and pressure sore formation. *Ostomy/Wound Manage.* 1998;44(3A Suppl):26S–36S.

125. Holden-Lund C. The effects of relaxation with guided imagery on surgical stress and wound healing. *Res Nurs Health.* 1988;11(4):235–244.

126. West J. Wound healing in the surgical patient: Influence of the perioperative stress response on perfusion. *AACN Clin Issues.* 1990;1(3):595–601.

127. North A. The effect of sleep on wound healing. *Ostomy/Wound Manage.* 1990;27:56–58.

128. McCarthy D, Ouimet M, Daun J. Shades of Florence Nightingale: Potential impact of noise stress on wound healing. *Holistic Nurs Pract.* 1991;5(4):39–48.

129. Wysocki AB. The effect of intermittent noise exposure on wound healing. *Advances in Wound Care.* 1996a;9(1):35–39.

130. Lee K, Stotts N. Support of the growth hormone-somatomedin system to facilitate healing. *Heart Lung J Crit Care.* 1990;19(2):157–164.

131. Byl N. *The Doctor Within: The Inner Aspects of Healing.* American Physical Therapy Scientific Meeting, San Diego, CA: American Physical Therapy Association; 1997.

132. Illingsworth, C, Barker A. Measurement of electrical currents emerging during the regeneration of amputated finger tips in children. *Clin Phys Physiol Meas.* 1980;1;87.

133. Lock P. The effect of temperature on mitosis at the edge of experimental wounds. In: Lundgren A, Sover A, eds. *Symposia on Wound Healing: Plastic, Surgical and Dermatologic Aspects.* Sweden: Molndal; 1980.

134. Myers J. Wound healing and use of modern surgical dressing. *Pharm J.* 1982;229:103–104.

135. Thomas S. *Management and Dressings.* Pharmaceutical Press; 1990.

136. Conolly WB, Hunt T, Sonne M, et al. Influence of distant trauma on local wound infection. *Surg Gynecol Obstet.* 1969;128(4):713–717.

137. Ferrell B, Osterweil D, Christenson P. A randomized trial of low-air-loss beds for treatment of pressure ulcers. *JAMA.* 1993;269:494–497.

138. Gentzkow G, Pollack SV, Kloth LC, Stubbs, HA. Improved healing of pressure ulcers using dermapulse, a new electrical stimulation device. *Wounds.* 1991;3(5):158–169.

139. vanRijswijk L. Full-thickness pressure ulcers: patient and wound healing characteristics. *Decubitus.* 1993;6(1):16–21.

140. Skene A, Smith J, Dore C, et al. Venous leg ulcers: A prognostic index to predict time to healing. *Br Med J.* 1992;305(6862):1119–1121.

141. Phillips T, Machado F, Trout R, et al. Prognostic indicators in venous ulcers. *J Am Acad Dermatol.* 2000;43(4):627–630.

CHAPTER 3

Nutritional Assessment and Treatment

Mary Ellen Posthauer

CHAPTER OBJECTIVES

At the completion of this chapter, the reader will be able to:

1. Identify the guidelines for completing a nutritional screening and assessment.
2. Describe the role of proper nutrition in the process of wound healing.
3. Identify nutrients of particular importance to wound healing.
4. Screen patients at risk for nutrition deficiency, using a nutritional screening.
5. Use a nutritional assessment for clients with wounds.

INTRODUCTION

The role of nutrition is often the forgotten factor in wound healing. The identification of nutritional status of a client begins with a nutritional screening, followed by an assessment. A plan of care is developed, based on the data derived from the assessment process.

As defined by the American Dietetic Association (ADA), *medical nutrition therapy* involves the assessment of the nutritional status of patients with a condition, illness, or injury that puts them at risk. This includes review and analysis of medical and diet history, laboratory values, and anthropometric measurements. Based on the assessment, nutrition modalities most appropriate to manage the condition or treat the illness or injury are chosen and include the following:

Source: Adapted with permission from Kathleen Niedert and Mary Ellen Posthauer, *The Role of Nutrition in Wound Healing,* © 1994, 1996, 1998, 2001, Mead Johnson and Company, Evansville, Indiana.

- *Diet modification and counseling,* leading to the development of a personal diet plan to achieve nutritional goals and desired health outcomes.
- *Specialized nutrition therapies,* including supplementation with medical foods for those unable to obtain adequate nutrients through food intake only; enteral nutrition delivered via tube feeding into the gastrointestinal tract for those unable to ingest or digest food; and parenteral nutrition delivered via intravenous infusion for those unable to absorb nutrients.[1]
- *Nutritional screening,* the process of identifying characteristics known to be associated with nutrition problems. Its purpose is to pinpoint persons who are malnourished or at nutritional risk. Intervention takes place after screening occurs. The nutritional screening can be done by a health care team member.[1]

NUTRITIONAL SCREENING

Nutritional screening is the process of identifying characteristics known to be associated with nutritional problems. Its purpose is to pinpoint individuals who are malnourished or at nutritional risk. Intervention takes place after screening occurs. A screening can be completed by a member of the health care team, such as the dietitian, dietetic technician, nurse, physician, or other qualified health care professional. The Braden Scale for Predicting Pressure Sore Risk (see Chapter 15) includes nutritional screening information.[2] A nutritional screening algorithm (Figure 3–1) shows the methodology of nutritional screening. A sample screening form accompanies the case studies presented later in this chapter. A nutrition intervention to prevent wounds is included in Appendix 3–A at the end of this chapter.

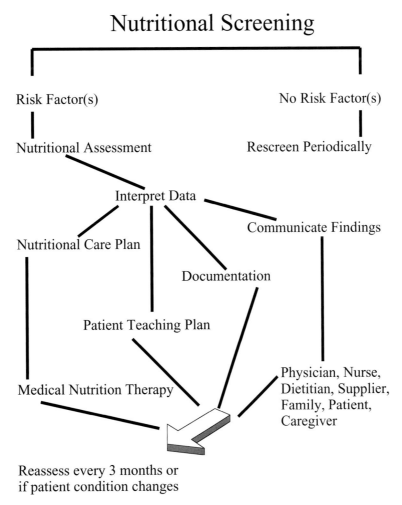

Figure 3–1 Nutritional screening algorithm. *Source:* Reprinted with permission from G. Turnbull, *The Role of Nutrition in Wound Healing, Mead Johnson Nutritional Publication No. MB183,* © 1998, Mead Johnson.

The elderly client often has multiple factors placing him or her at risk for pressure ulcer formation. Skin fragility, along with numerous medical conditions that occur with the elderly, increases risk and healing time.

Functional limitation, such as chewing or swallowing difficulties, affects the ability of the client to ingest adequate calories and fluids. Immobility affects a client's ability to either prepare meals or travel to a dining room for meals. Poor hearing and vision compromise the client's communication skills, often resulting in poor intake at meals. The saying "We eat with our eyes" is evident when poor vision hampers eating. Altered mental status often limits clients' abilities to feed themselves or to comprehend the importance of consuming a balanced diet. Advanced dementia often results in weight loss, dysphagia, malnutrition, and pressure ulcers. When clients become incapable of responding to caregivers' assistance to nourish them, the probability of developing pressure ulcers increases.

Medical condition and/or diagnosis often increase the risk of pressure ulcer development. For example, diabetes with chronic hyperglycemia may both cause and affect poor wound healing. High levels of glucose compete with transport of ascorbic acid into the cells, which is necessary for deposition of collagen. Hip fractures or spinal cord injuries that restrict mobility often result in increased pain and interfere with eating.

Drug therapy can often cause side effects such as nausea and gastric disturbances, which limit food and fluid intake. Corticosteroids increase the risk of wound complications such as infection and inhibit protein synthesis. Corticosteroids cause depletion of vitamin A from the liver, plasma, adrenals, and enzymes, and interfere with collagen synthesis and resistance to infection.[3]

Clients with pressure ulcers or those identified at risk for developing pressure ulcers should be monitored at appropriate intervals. Many long-term care facilities have wound care teams that make weekly rounds to assess the condition of the pressure ulcer and the implementation of the care plan. The nutritional status is monitored at a minimum of every 3 months for those at low nutritional risk and monthly for those identified to be at high risk or malnourished.

We are constantly debating quality of life issues. Prevention and treatment of pressure ulcers are key aspects of meeting the regulation concerning Quality of Life in the Omnibus Budget Reconciliation Act (OBRA) of 1987 (Public Law No. 101-239), which focuses on providing care that enables nursing home clients to live a dignified existence and to maintain the highest degree of physical, mental, and psychosocial well-being.[4] Effective prevention and treatment of pressure ulcers are key factors in reducing these costs and improving the quality of life for those at risk. Pressure ulcers are important quality indicators because, in long-term care, they may occur frequently; are preventable; can affect health, survival, and quality of life; and impact significantly on the cost of care and resource utilization.

The Health Care Financing Administration (HCFA), which regulates long-term care facilities, has targeted pressure ulcers, inadequate nutrition, and inadequate hydration as key survey issues. The development of a pressure ulcer for a person who was a low risk is automatically considered a sentinel event. HCFA has established a definition for high risk (see Exhibit 3–1).

Surveyors at both the federal and state level utilize an Investigative Pressure Ulcer Protocol to determine whether pressure ulcers are avoidable or unavoidable. The protocol investigates the facility's pressure ulcer treatment, prevention intervention, assessment (including nutrition), as well as the plan of care and ongoing evaluation. New federal enforcement provision, including Civil Money Penalty for each instance of a deficiency can result in fines ranging from $1,000 to $10,000.

Often, reimbursement rates do not cover the cost of care. Liquid oral supplements or fortified foods are not reimbursable under state or federal regulations but fall under the daily rate of care.

Legal consequences of malnutrition and pressure ulcers result in median monetary recovery of $250,000 and recovering in favor of the plaintiff in 68% of cases.[5]

The Agency for Health Care Research and Quality (AHRQ), formerly known as the Agency for Health Care Policy and Research (AHCPR), was established in 1989 under OBRA to enhance the quality, appropriateness, and effectiveness of health care services and access to these services. AHCPR published a series of clinical practice guidelines related to pressure ulcers, including *Pressure Ulcer in Adults: Prediction and Prevention*[6] in 1992 and *Treatment of Pressure Ulcers*,[7] released in 1994. The guidelines assist the dietetic professional in assessment and development of action plans for the nutritional care of clients with pressure ulcers.

Clinical Wisdom:
Ensuring Optimal Nutrition in Long-term Care

Maintaining or improving the nutritional status of the elderly individual who progresses from one care setting to another presents a challenge for the health care team. Identification of risk factors that contribute to undernutrition or malnutrition in nursing home facilities is essential. Federal regulations mandate that nursing facilities provide care that maximizes the resident's quality of life. Protein energy undernutrition has been associated with the development of ulcers, cognitive problems, infections, and increased mortality. Optimizing nutrition screening and interventions helps to achieve positive outcomes for the resident.

Source: Reprinted with permission from C. Russell and M.E. Posthauer, Ensuring Optimal Nutrition in Long-Term Care, *Nutrition in Clinical Practice*, Vol.12, No. 6, pp. 247–255, © 1997, American Society for Parenteral and Enteral Nutrition.

Exhibit 3–1 Definition of High Risk for Pressure Ulcer Development

- Impaired mobility or transfer
- End-stage renal disease
- Malnutrition
- Comatose

Source: Reprinted from *HCFA Quality Indicators for Minimum Data Set*, Health Care Financing Administration.

NUTRITIONAL ASSESSMENT

Nutritional assessment is a comprehensive approach completed by a registered dietitian that defines nutritional status using medical, nutritional, and medication histories; physical examination; anthropometric measurements; and laboratory data. It includes the "organization and evaluation of information to declare a professional judgement."[8(pp838,839)] Nutritional assessment includes interpretation of data from the screening process. The assessment process includes a review of data from other disciplines (ie, physical therapy and occupational therapy) that may affect the assessment process. Nutritional assessment precedes a care plan, intervention, and evaluation. The Nutritional Assessment and

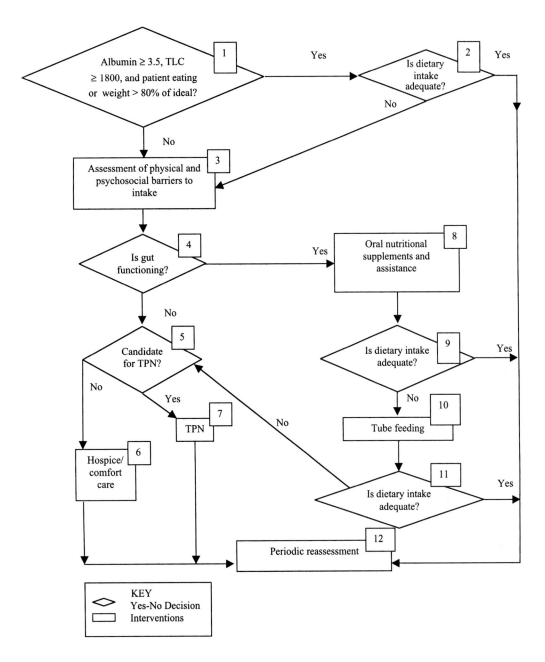

Note: TLC = total lymphocyte count; TPN = total parenteral nutrition.

Figure 3–2 Nutritional Assessment and Support decision tree. *Source:* Reprinted with permission from Bergstrom et al. (1994), *Treatment of Pressure Ulcers, Clinical Practice Guideline, No. 15*, U.S. Department of Health and Human Services: Public Health Service Agency for Health Care Policy and Research, AHCPR Publication No. 95-0652, December 1994.

Support decision tree (Figure 3–2), along with assessment recommendations made in Exhibit 3–2, can be used for guidelines in performing a nutritional assessment. A sample assessment form accompanies the case studies presented later in this chapter.

The dietitian reviews the screens and assessments from the various therapies to determine a nutritional care plan.

The speech therapist defines the diet texture, including the need for special feeding techniques, which are implemented by the dietary department. As an example, clients may require thickened liquids to prevent dehydration or aspiration. The occupational therapist often determines the need for self-help feeding devices, which promote eating independence. The dietitian is responsible for making certain that

Exhibit 3–2 Assessment Recommendations for Determining Proper Weight, Caloric Levels, and Degree of Nutritional Depletion

Recommended Weight for Height
Female: 100 lbs. per 5 ft. + 5 lbs. per inch > 5 ft.
Males: 106 lbs. per 5 ft. + 6 lbs. per inch > 5 ft.

Basal Energy Expenditure (BEE)
Female: $655 + (9.6 \times \text{wt. in kg}) + (1.8 \times \text{ht. in cm}) - (4.7 \times \text{age in years})$
Male: $66 + 13.7 \times \text{wt. in kg}) + (5.0 \times \text{ht. in cm}) - (6.8 \times \text{age in years})$

Estimated daily calorie levels are determined by multiplying the BEE and the appropriate injury and/or activity factor.

Injury Factors:

1.00 – 1.05	Postoperative (no complications)
1.05 – 1.25	Peritonitis
1.10 – 1.45	Cancer
1.15 - 1.30	Long bone fracture
1.20 – 1.60	Wound healing
1.25 – 1.50	Blunt trauma
1.30 – 1.55	Severe infection / multiple trauma
1.50 – 1.70	Multiple trauma with client on ventilator
1.60 – 1.70	Trauma with steroids
1.75 – 1.85	Sepsis

Burns (% total body surface):

1.00–1.50	0% - 20%
1.50–1.85	20% - 40%
1.85–2.05	40% - 100%

Activity Factors:

1.2	for clients confined to bed
1.3	for ambulatory clients
1.5 – 1.75	for most normally active persons
2.0	for extremely active persons

Protein Needs for Adults

Condition:	Albumin Level:	Protein Requirement:
Normal nutrition	3.5 g/dL	0.8 g/kg/day
Mild depletion	2.8 – 3.5 g/dL	1.0 – 1.2 g/kg/day
Moderate depletion	2.1 – 2.7 g/dL	1.2 – 1.5 g/kg/day
Severe depletion	2.1 g/dL	1.5 – 2.0 g/kg/day
COPD		100 – 125 g protein/day total

Exceptions:
Renal failure

Nondialyzed	0.5 – 0.6 g/kg/day	Hepatic failure	0.25 – 0.5 g/kg/day
Hemo-dialyzed	1.0 – 1.2 g/kg/day	Pulmonary compromised	1.2 – 1.9 g/kg/day (maintenance)
Peritoneal-dialyzed	1.2 – 1.5 g/kg/day		1.6 – 2.5 g/kg/day (repletion)

Another method to calculate protein needs—ratio of grams nitrogen to nonprotein calories (6.25 g protein – 1 g N.)

Patient Conditions:	Ratio of Nonprotein kcal: 1 g N
Adult medical	125 – 150:1
Minor catabolic	125 – 180:1
Severe catabolic	150 – 250:1
Hepatic or renal failure	250 – 400:1

Source: Reprinted with permission from Consultant Dietitians in Health Care Facilities, Practice Group of The American Dietetic Association, *Pocket Resource for Nutrition Assessment*, p. 30, © 1997.

Fluid Status
- Congestive heart failure / edema = 25 cc/kg of body weight
- Normal fluid status = 25 – 30 cc/kg of body weight
- 1 mL/kcal
- 100 mL/kg for first 10 kg body weight + 50 mL/kg for second 10 kg body weight + 15 mL/kg for remaining kg body weight
- OR shortcut to this method: (kg body weight – 20) x 15 + 1500 Ml

Source: J.C. Chidester and A.A. Spangler, Fluid Intake in the Institutionalized Elderly. Copyright The American Dietetic Association. Reprinted by permission from *JOURNAL OF THE AMERICAN DIETETIC ASSOCIATION*, Vol. 97, pp. 23–28, © 1997.

this special equipment is provided at meal time. Physical therapy sessions often result in the need for both increased calories and fluid, for which the dietitian will calculate and arrange provision at appropriate times.

Physical Conditions

Observe the client's skin condition, including signs of dehydration, edema, and/or ascites. These signs may be indicative of protein deficiency, renal disease, or hepatic disease. All have potential nutritional significance. Loose skin may be evidence of weight loss, and the interviewer should question the client about his or her usual weight. Make a visual scan for dry, flaky skin, skin that "tents" (which can relate to dehydration), or for nonhealing wounds, purpurae, or bruises.[9]

The older adult is particularly prone to pressure ulcers as a result of decreased mobility, multiple contributing diagnoses, poor nutrition, and loss of muscle mass, resulting in increased exposure to pressure and ulceration. Often, the physiologic effects of aging also affect nutrition in the older client (Table 3–1). The loss of skin elasticity and moisture, coupled with reduced feeling in susceptible areas, place the older client at risk for impaired skin integrity. Nutritional factors that contribute to skin breakdown include: protein deficiency, creating a negative nitrogen balance; anemia, inhibiting the formation of red blood cells; and dehydration, causing dry, fragile skin. Dehydration can also result in an increase in the blood glucose level and slow the healing process.[10] With advancing age comes decreased skin response to temperature, pain, and pressure. This affects the skin's elasticity and the healing process.[11] Dramatic changes in the skin occur with aging. Sweat glands decrease in number. There is atrophy and thinning of both the epithelial and fatty layers of tissue. In older individuals, there is little subcutaneous fat on the legs or forearms. This may be the case even if abundant abdominal or hip fat is present. One result of the general loss of fat from the subcutaneous tissue is the relative prominence of the bony protuberances of the thorax, scapula, trochanters, and knees. The loss of this valuable padding contributes to pressure ulcer risk in the aged.

Malnutrition is a condition of faulty or inadequate nutrition. The registered dietitian and other health care professionals should examine the client for physical signs of malnutrition. Risk factors for malnutrition are presented in Exhibit 3–3. The term *malnutrition* is often used synonymously with the more descriptive and inclusive term *poor nutritional status*. Poor nutritional status has been defined by the Nutrition Screening Initiative to include "not only deficiency, dehydration, undernutrition, nutritional imbalances, and obesity, but other excesses such as alcohol abuse. In addition, inappropriate dietary intakes for conditions

---

Clinical Wisdom: *Pressure Ulcer*

WARNING SIGNS!

The following are some signs that a resident may be at risk for or suffer from pressure ulcers:

- Patient subject to incontinence
- Needs help:
  –moving arms, legs, or body
  –turning in bed
  –changing position when sitting
- Weight loss
- Eats less than half of meals/snacks served
- Dehydration
- Has discolored, torn, or swollen skin over bony areas

REPORT AND TAKE ACTION

Below are some ACTION STEPS to help residents who are at risk for or suffer from pressure ulcers:

- Report observations and warning signs to nurse and dietitian!
- Check and change linens as appropriate.
- Handle/move the client with care to avoid skin tears and scrapes.
- Reposition frequently and properly.
- Use "unintended weight loss action steps" so resident gets more calories and protein.
- Use "dehydration action steps" so resident gets more to drink.
- Record meal/snack intake.

This guide was adapted from the Nutrition Care Alerts developed by the Nutrition Screening Initiative, a project of the American Academy of Family Physicians, the American Dietetic Association, and the National Council on the Aging, and sponsored by Ross Products Division of Abbott Laboratories *Source:* Adapted and reprinted with permission by the Nutrition Screening Initiative, a project of the American Academy of Family Physicians, the American Dietetic Association and the National Council on the Aging, Inc., and funded in part by a grant from Ross Products Division, Abbott Laboratories Inc.

---

that have nutritional implications and the presence of an underlying physical or mental illness with treatable nutritional implications are included. Finally, it also encompasses evidence that nutritional status may be deteriorating over time. Such evidence may be derived from clear-cut objective clinical signs (Table 3–2); by nonspecific clinical evidence; by responses to direct, specific questions about diet and nutrition (even if complaints are not volunteered); and by

Table 3–1 Physiological Effects of Aging and Their Effect on Nutrition

Physiological Changes	Implications and Intervention
Decreased visual acuity and peripheral vision	May restrict activity (eg, difficulty driving, fear of operating kitchen appliances)
Decreased focus or ability to dilate pupil to light changes	Inability to read dials, recipes, labels, prices; increased difficulty in food procurement and preparation
	In an institution, provide well-lighted areas and prevent glare, which can aggravate poor vision; orange, red, and yellow colors are best recognized
Decreased ability to hear higher-pitched tones	May self-impose restrictions on social activity (eg, eating out, asking store clerks questions)
	Speak directly to the person; allow for lip reading; remove background noise as possible; speak in lower tones at high volume
Decreased touch sensitivity	Possible clumsy spills and accidents carrying food or during meals
	Use textured versus smooth glasses, utensils, etc., which are easier to handle
Decreased smell or taste sensation, decreased number of taste buds, increased sour and bitter, with decreased salt and sweet sensations	Foods may lose appeal, have less flavor, or be less appetizing; motivation to prepare food decreased; may attempt to use more salt or sugar to compensate for loss of taste; add to this decreased appetite related to illness and effects of medications/depression or "diet," and intake may grow worse
	Use alternative herbs and spices, food demonstrations, or special cooking sessions
Dentition—loss of/missing teeth, ill-fitting dentures, decreased salivation, periodontal disease	Decreased ability to chew or swallow; decreased food appeal; dry mouth; may restrict variety and choose softer, low-fiber, high-calorie choices
	Serve moist rather than dry foods, reeducate on improving taste/appearance of food while avoiding excess calories
Stomach—parietal cells produce less hydrochloric acid	Slight difficulty digesting food; possible bacterial contamination of gastric juice, known as *bacterial overgrowth*, requires antibiotic therapy; achlorhydria associated with lack of intrinsic factor may result in pernicious anemia
	Use smaller, frequent meals; assess for macrocytic megaloblastic anemia, which may require vitamin B_{12} injections or iron supplements
Intestine—decreased enzyme excretion, vascular insufficiency, lactose intolerance, decreased gastrointestinal motility	Potential for impaired absorption of calcium, iron, zinc, protein, fat, and fat-soluble vitamins; may have difficulties digesting dietary calcium or protein; longer transit time may be mistaken for constipation; may have a need for increased protein of 1 g/kg/day versus recommended daily allowance of 0.8 g/kg/day
	Ensure calcium sources via diet or supplement
	Encourage adequate fiber and fluids and avoidance of harsh laxatives
Decreased bone density, loss of calcium from bone in jaw and skeleton	Tooth loss causes difficulty chewing; bone fractures lead to decreased mobility, which hinders procurement and preparation of food
	Stress calcium in diet as protective, not curative; caution against excess vitamin D intake; encourage calcium-rich foods in meals; refer for shopping assistance
Reduced basal metabolic rate, lean body mass, and activity with increased body fat	Decreased calorie needs; vulnerability to obesity
	Decreased activity may also result from retirement or chronic illness
	Stress weight control, prevention of weight gain, and avoidance of empty calories
Insulin resistance with increased adiposity and decreased insulin response to dietary sugar	Decreased tolerance for concentrated sweets/calories; type II diabetes mellitus
	Offer small, more frequent meals; modify diet to avoid simple carbohydrates, limit fat and calories, and increase dietary fiber; help patient to understand and accept diet rationale and implementation
Increased resistance to blood flow in peripheral blood vessels	Diagnosis of hypertension, accompanied by sodium restriction and possibly medication
	Discuss diet modifications, sources of sodium in food and over-the-counter medications, and use of alternative seasonings
General increases in frailty; poor balance and muscle weakness	Difficulty purchasing and preparing food
	Discuss labor-saving techniques; refer to meal services and shopping assistance
Loss of short-term memory	Potential for increased kitchen accidents, food poisoning, and skipping meals
	Reinforce kitchen safety and proper food handling

Exhibit 3–3 Risk Factors for Malnutrition

The following risk factors/categories are a guide to help the practitioner determine a client's risk level.

- Pressure ulcers or altered skin integrity
- Excessive activity level
- Immobility; ie, dependence, disability, or impairment in ADL
- Cancer and its treatments
- AIDS or HIV
- GI complications (eg, malabsorption, diarrhea, digestion, bowel changes)
- Catabolic or hypermetabolic conditions (eg, burns, stress, trauma, sepsis)
- Physical signs (eg, alopecia)
- Food allergies
- Alterations in anthropometric measures, weight or body mass index, marked overweight or underweight for height and age, midarm muscle circumference/triceps skinfold as appropriate, amputation, limb length, height, and head circumference.
- Declining sensory function (eg, loss of smell, taste, vision)
- Fat or muscle wasting (including cachexia)
- Obesity/overweight
- Chronic renal or cardiac problems, diabetes and related complications, hypertension
- Osteoporosis or osteomalacia
- Fluid and/or electrolyte imbalance
- Neurologic impairment
- Visual impairment
- Other acute and chronic disorders
- Extreme in age (eg, over 80 years old)

Source: © 1998, American Dietetic Association. "*Nutrition Care of the Older Adult*." Used with permission.

reliable reports from third parties (family, friends, caregivers, aides, social workers)."[12(p2)]

Anthropometry

Anthropometry is the measurement of body size, weight, and proportions, and is used to evaluate a client's nutritional status. Low body weight, when associated with illness or injury, increases the risk of morbidity. Obesity is common among nonambulatory clients whose caloric expenditure is low. Loss of height, for example, is an early indicator of osteoporosis.[13]

Body Mass Index

Body mass index (BMI) is used as an indicator of body fatness and/or desirable body weight. BMI is a weight/height ratio composed of body weight (in kilograms) divided by the square of the height in meters, or weight/height (703 × weight in lbs/height in inches.) The BMI is highly correlated with body fat, but increased lean body mass or a large body frame can also increase the BMI. It is generally agreed that a normally hydrated person with a BMI of 30 would be obese and that a person with a BMI of more than 27 would be at major risk for obesity.[14] A BMI of ≤ 21 with involuntary weight loss places a client at risk for pressure ulcer development.

Stress as a result of injury, surgery, burns, fractures, or wounds results in depletion of nutrient stores required for healing. Protein stores are used as energy sources if adequate carbohydrate and fat are not provided (Figure 3–3).

Height and Weight

Weight and body composition change with age. Weight tends to peak in the sixth decade, with a gradual decrease beyond the seventh decade. Shifts in body composition are noted, and the proportion of body weight that is fat increases, averaging 30% of the total body weight in the older adult, as compared with 20% of the total body weight in younger people.

Weight Variances

Variances in weight have significant impact on nutritional health, and degree of weight change has positive correlations

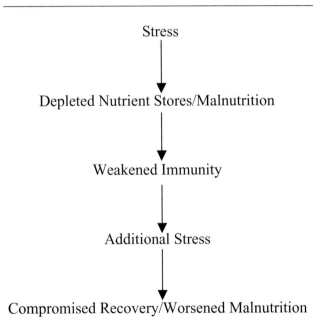

Stress

↓

Depleted Nutrient Stores/Malnutrition

↓

Weakened Immunity

↓

Additional Stress

↓

Compromised Recovery/Worsened Malnutrition

Figure 3–3 Stress resulting from injury or surgery. *Source:* From *Nutrition and Diet Therapy*, 5th edition, by C.B. Cataldo, L.K. DeBruyne, and E.N. Whitney © 1999. Reprinted with permission of Wadsworth, an imprint of the Wadsworth Group, a division of Thomson Learning. Fax 800 730-2215.

Table 3–2 Physical Signs of Malnutrition

Signs	Possible Causes
Hair	
Dull, dry, lack of natural shine	Protein-energy deficiency
Thin, sparse, loss of curl	Zinc deficiency
Color changes, depigmentation, easily plucked	Other nutrient deficiencies; manganese, copper
Eyes	
Small, yellowish lumps around eyes, white rings around both eyes	Hyperlipidemia
Pale eye membranes	Vitamin B12, folacin, or iron deficiency
Night blindness, dry membranes, dull or soft cornea	Vitamin A or zinc deficiency
Redness and fissures of eyelid corners	Niacin deficiency
Angular inflammation of eyelids	Riboflavin deficiency
Ring of fine blood vessels around cornea	Generally poor nutrition
Lips	
Redness and swelling	Niacin, riboflavin, iron, or pyridoxine deficiency
Gums	
Spongy, swollen, red; bleed easily	Vitamin C deficiency
Gingivitis	Vitamin A, niacin, or riboflavin deficiency
Mouth	
Cheilosis, angular scars	Riboflavin or folic acid deficiency
Tongue	
Swollen, scarlet, raw; sores	Folacin or niacin deficiency
Smooth with papillae (small projections)	Riboflavin, vitamin B12, or pyridoxine deficiency
Glossitis	Iron or zinc deficiency
Purplish	Riboflavin deficiency
Taste	
Diminished	Zinc deficiency
Teeth	
Gray-brown spots	Increased fluoride intake
Missing or erupting abnormally	Generally poor nutrition
Face	
Skin color loss, dark cheeks and eyes, enlarged parotid glands, scaling of skin around nostrils	Protein-energy deficiency, specifically niacin, riboflavin, or pyridoxine deficiency
Pallor	Iron, folacin, vitamin B12, or vitamin C deficiency
Hyperpigmentation	Niacin deficiency
Neck	
Thyroid enlargement	Iodine deficiency
Symptoms of hypothyroidism	

Source: © 1998, American Dietetic Association. "*Nutrition Care of the Older Adult.*" Used with permission.

with impact on health status. When evaluating the severity of weight variances (Exhibit 3–4), it is important to determine possible causes, such as recent surgery or the treatment initiated (eg, radiation or diuretic therapy), which can affect weight status.

The nutritional status of a client has a positive or negative effect on wound healing. Malnutrition or poor nutritional status impacts the healing. Malnutrition, dehydration, or unintentional weight loss (greater than 5% in 30 days, 7.5% in 90 days, or 10% in 180 days), whether secondary to poor appetite or other disease processes, places the client at risk for tissue breakdown and poor healing.

Therapeutic Diets

A diet order that imposes many restrictions can contribute significantly to reduced food intake and a marked decline in nutritional status. The denial of favorite foods and/or the

Exhibit 3–4 Severity of Weight Loss

Significant weight loss:[15]	Severe weight loss:
• 10% in 6 months	• > 10% in 6 months
• 7.5% in 3 months	• > 7.5% in 3 months
• 5% in 1 month	• > 5% in 1 month
• 2% in 1 week	• > 2% in 1 week

Source: © 1998, American Dietetic Association. *"Nutrition Care of the Older Adult."* Used with permission.

enforcement of a therapeutic diet may diminish the quality of life. Food is not nutritious unless eaten. Certain medical conditions may require diet modifications, but these can be met with simple adjustments and minimal restrictions.[16]

Treatments and Medications

Treatments and medications contributing to the risk for pressure ulcers include antidepressants and sleeping pills; drug-related immunosuppression; and steroid therapy. Many of the drugs designed to calm or reduce the agitation of clients may, in turn, reduce their mobility and activity levels, resulting in decreased intake of meals. Common side effects of some drugs, such as gastric disturbances, affect the nutritional intake of food and fluid. Radiation therapy, chemotherapy, and renal dialysis can result in increased nausea and vomiting, as well as decreased activity, placing the client at risk.

Exhibit 3–5 Lab Values Indicative of Increased Risk for Delayed Wound Healing

Serum Transferrin < 170 mg/dL
Prealbumin < 16 mg/dL
Serum Albumin < 3.5 mg/dL with normal hydration status
Hemoglobin < 12 g/dL
Hematocrit < 33%
Serum Cholesterol < 160 mg/dL
Total Lymphocyte Count < 1800/mm
Serum Osmolality > 295 mOsm/L
BUN/Creatinine > 10:1

Source: Reprinted from *Treatment of Pressure Ulcers: Clinical Practice Guidelines, No. 15,* AHCPR Publication No. 95-0652, Agency for Health Care Policy and Research, U.S. Department of Health and Human Services, Rockville, Maryland, December 1994.

Clinical Wisdom: *Unintended Weight Loss*

WARNING SIGNS!

- Needs help to eat or drink
- Eats less than half of meal/snack served
- Has mouth pain
- Has dentures that don't fit
- Has a hard time chewing or swallowing
- Coughs or chokes while eating
- Has sadness, crying spells, or withdrawal from others
- Is confused, wanders, or paces
- Has diabetes, chronic obstructive pulmonary disease (COPD), cancer, HIV, or other chronic disease

REPORT AND TAKE ACTION

Below are some ACTION STEPS to increase food intake, create a positive dining environment, and help residents get enough calories:

- Report observations and warning signs to nurse and dietitian!
- Encourage resident to eat.
- Honor food likes and dislikes.
- Offer many kinds of foods and beverages.
- Help residents who have trouble feeding themselves.
- Allow enough time to finish eating.
- Notify nursing staff if resident has trouble using utensils.
- Record meals/snack intake.
- Provide oral care before meals.
- Position resident correctly for feeding.
- If resident has had a loss of appetite and/or seems sad, ask what's wrong.

Source: Adapted and reprinted with permission by the Nutrition Screening Initiative, a project of the American Academy of Family Physicians, the American Dietetic Association, and the National Council on the Aging, Inc., and funded in part by a grant from Ross Products Division, Abbott Laboratories Inc.

Medication should be checked for possible side effects on nutritional intake, as well as the effect on the mental and physical status of the client. Constipation and diarrhea are both risk factors to address in a nutritional assessment. Laxative abuse can induce a state of malabsorption. Chronic diarrhea can lead to dehydration and weight loss, which increases the risk for malnutrition and pressure ulcers.

Lab Values

Laboratory indexes for nutritional assessment involve primarily tests related to protein metabolism. Protein status can be evaluated through a nitrogen-balance study, visceral protein blood levels, and gross tests of immune functions, such as total lymphocyte counts. It should also be noted that abnormal labs may be the result of poor appetite or other disease processes. Laboratory values indicating risk to wound healing are shown in Exhibit 3–5.

Laboratory values indicative of malnutrition include serum albumin below 3.5 g/dL, serum transferrin level (less than 180 mg/dL), or prealbumin (less than 17 mg/dL).[17] Serum albumin is a sensitive indicator of acute changes in clinical status from either infection, hydration, starvation, or a combination. Serum albumin has a long half-life of about 20 days, so concentration falls slowly during malnutrition. Deficit levels are classified as mild, moderate, or severe in Exhibit 3–6. A serum cholesterol (less than 160 mg/dL) with poor intake and weight loss places clients at risk for pressure ulcers. Hemoglobin (less than 12 mg/dL) and hematocrit (less than 33%) are important indicators of anemia. Deficits in hemoglobin and hematocrit have been correlated with the risk of developing pressure ulcers.

Exhibit 3–6 Serum Albumin Deficit Levels

Deficit levels of serum albumin can be classified as:
Mild, moderate, or severe

Mild	3.0–3.5 g/dL
Moderate	2.5–3.0 g/dL
Severe	< 2.5 g/dL

Source: Reprinted with permission from J. Maklebust and M. Sieggreen, *Pressure Ulcers: Guidelines for Prevention and Management*, 3rd Ed., p. 45, © 2001, Lippincott Williams & Wilkins.

Biochemical assessment data must be used with caution because it can be altered by hydration, medication, and changes in metabolism. Parameters for evaluating hydration status should include assessing urine output (I/O), weight, blood urea nitrogen (BUN)/creatinine ratio > 10:1, and skin turgor.

Chewing and swallowing problems resulting in poor oral intake can lead to malnutrition and pressure ulcers. Edentulous clients or those who have loose dentures as a result of weight loss often avoid foods high in protein that are difficult to chew, such as meat or meat alternates, and restrict their overall intake, thus increasing the chance for weight loss. If untreated, clients with swallowing problems or dysphagia become dehydrated, lose weight, and develop pressure ulcers. Loss of dexterity and/or the ability to self-feed is a risk factor because the result is often poor oral intake.

THE ROLE OF NUTRIENTS IN WOUND HEALING

A primary yet often overlooked component in wound healing is nutrition. With the spotlight on elaborate diagnostic tests, high-tech surgeries, and complex drug prescriptions, it is easy to lose sight of the basic concept of nutrition. More than just food, nutrition encompasses the many nutrients, calories, and fluids taken into the body, which are vital to the healing of wounds (Exhibit 3–7).

Carbohydrates

Carbohydrates are supplied by starch in the form of grains, cereals, legumes (peas and beans), pasta, bread, and natural sugars contained in fruits, vegetables, and milk. Added sugars also provide carbohydrates in the diet. Carbohydrates serve several functions (Exhibit 3–8).

Protein

All proteins consist of carbon, hydrogen, oxygen, and nitrogen atoms (it is the only nutrient containing nitrogen). Some proteins also contain phosphorus and sulfur. The body utilizes protein in numerous ways (Exhibit 3–9). These elements combine to form amino acids, which are the smallest molecular units of protein. Amino acids are components of collagen (the characteristic protein of connective tissue) and other structural proteins found in healing wounds. Food sources of protein include meat, milk products, and legumes.

Clinical Wisdom: *Adding Protein/Calories*

- Add dry milk to cream soups, mashed potatoes, casseroles, puddings, and milk-based desserts.
- Add 1/3 cup nonfat dry powdered milk to each cup of regular milk.
- Add cheese to vegetables, salads, potatoes, rice, noodles, and casseroles.
- Mix commercial supplements with ice cream or sherbet.
- Add yogurt to fruit and cereal.
- Add nuts, seeds, wheat germ to casseroles, breads, muffins, pancakes, and cookies.
- Sprinkle nuts, seeds, wheat germ on fruit, cereal, ice cream, and yogurt or use in place of bread crumbs.
- Add peanut butter to sandwiches, toast, crackers, muffins; use as a dip for vegetables or fruit; or add to milk and blend.
- Add dry beans to soups or casseroles.

Exhibit 3–7 Skin Integrity and Wound Healing: The Role of Nutrition

It has long been recognized but unappreciated that impaired nutritional status and inadequate dietary intake are risk factors for development of pressure ulcers. A well-balanced diet with adequate carbohydrate, protein, fat, water, vitamins, and minerals is necessary to maintain skin integrity.

Calories, protein, water, vitamin C, and zinc are often emphasized to promote wound healing. However, adequate intake of these nutrients or any nutrient alone does not facilitate healing. Sufficient calories plus all essential nutrients are required.

CALORIES

The body's first priority is for adequate energy. When the total amount of calories is too low, protein from both the diet and the patient's muscle stores will be used as an energy source; the patient will lose weight; and adipose tissue, as well as lean body mass, will be lost.

Every wound patient's calorie needs will be different. The caloric goal for patients with wounds is to prevent weight loss from occurring. In underweight patients, a slow, steady weight gain will increase the speed of wound healing. The three major nutrients—carbohydrate, protein, and fat—provide calories. Carbohydrates and fats are the preferred energy source for a healing wound.

PROTEIN

Dietary protein is needed for tissue maintenance and repair. Protein depletion impairs wound healing by preventing a desirable wound bed from forming. Repletion of calorie and protein status in undernourished patients is associated with shorter time to heal and improved wound strength. In general, a wound patient's daily dietary protein needs (expressed as grams of protein) can be estimated by dividing the patient's weight in half. For example, a patient who weighs 100 pounds would need approximately 50 g of protein daily to heal wounds. Too high a protein intake will increase fluid needs, and wound healing will be reduced if fluid needs are not met.

WATER

Water is an especially important nutrient for patients with wounds. Dehydration is a risk factor for development of wounds, and the water needs of patients with stages 3 and 4 pressure ulcers are very high. A good rule of thumb is to be sure that all patients receive a minimum of 1 mL of water for every kcal fed, or about 15 mL of water per pound of body weight per day. Wound patients need at least 200–2500 mL of water a day (2 quarts or more).

Water and other household beverages are adequate sources of water in most cases and can be given orally or by feeding tube. These fluids, however, are not adequate to replace the fluid and electrolyte losses that accompany vomiting, diarrhea, or other sources of gastrointestinal fluid losses. In these cases, a rehydration solution, such as Equalyte® (Ross Products Division of Abbott Laboratories), which is specifically designed to match and replace these losses, is needed.

VITAMIN C

Because nutritional deficiency has been associated with impaired wound healing, supplemental intake of vitamins and minerals is often thought to be important for wound healing. Although not appropriate for all patients, vitamin and mineral supplements are probably most beneficial for patients with a history of poor intake, who are, therefore, likely to have limited nutrient stores. A general one-a-day type vitamin and mineral supplement equal to 100% of the Reference Daily Intake (RDI) for vitamins and minerals is prudent for patients with wounds.

Vitamin C is essential in collagen synthesis. Collagen and fibroblasts compose the basis for the structure of a new healing wound bed. A deficiency of vitamin C prolongs healing time, decreases wound strength, and contributes to decreased resistance to infection. There is no evidence, however, that human wound healing is improved by providing doses of vitamin C many times greater than the RDI (60 mg/day). It is reasonable to increase vitamin C intake through consumption of fruits, vegetables, and juices for persons with extensive wounds who may rapidly exhaust their body reserves and for those with a history of poor intake.

ZINC

Zinc deficiency can occur through wound drainage or excessive gastrointestinal fluid losses or can be due to long-term low dietary intake. Chronic, severe zinc deficiency results in abnormal function of white blood cells and lymphocytes, increased susceptibility to infection, and delayed wound healing. Large amounts of dietary zinc, however, interfere with copper metabolism and are not advisable. The amount of zinc in a multiple vitamin/mineral supplement is generally adequate. It is much more preferable and safer to provide the RDI in zinc (12–15 mg/day) through a one-a-day type multiple vitamin and mineral supplement than to provide individual zinc supplementation at very high levels (such as zinc sulfate 200–300 mg daily or three times daily).

Courtesy of Charlette Gallagher-Allred, Ross Products Division, Abbott Laboratories, Columbus, Ohio.

Exhibit 3–8 Functions of Carbohydrates

Carbohydrates serve the following functions:

- Serve as the most readily available source of energy for the body
- Spare protein for its primary use; that of building and maintaining tissue
- Provide cellular components for regulating metabolism
- Provide flavor, color, and variety to the diet
- Provide 4 kcal/g energy

Clients on dialysis or with renal disease requiring limited protein are offered foods with high-quality protein, such as eggs, meat, fish, poultry, milk, and cheese. Proteins derived from animal sources are called high-quality or complete proteins because they contain all the amino acids essential in human nutrition in amounts adequate for use. The dietitian evaluates the appropriate quality and type of protein to meet the diet order for the client with renal disease. Clients who are obese or on low-cholesterol diets should select foods low in saturated fat, such as skim milk, lean fish, vegetable oils, and low-fat cheese.

Fats

Glycerides, composed of fatty acids and glycerol, are the most common fats in the diet and the body. Fat is provided largely from meat, dairy products (milk, butter, cream, and

Exhibit 3–9 Functions of Protein

Protein serves the following functions:

- Is involved in collagen synthesis, epidermal cell proliferation, skin integrity and resistance to infection, immune response, and gastrointestinal function
- Supplies structural and binding material of muscle, cartilage, ligaments, skin, hair, and fingernails
- Plays important roles as enzymes and hormones in chemical reactions and regulatory functions throughout the body and within cells
- Is a component of antibodies, immune system function
- Helps to maintain the fluid and mineral composition of various body fluids (fluid and electrolyte balance)
- Helps transport needed substances, such as lipids, minerals and oxygen, around the body
- Serves as building material for growth and repair of body tissues
- Provides 4 kcal/g

Exhibit 3–10 Functions of Fats

Fats serve several functions, including the following:

- Maintain normal cell membrane function
- Permit fat-soluble substances to move in and out of the cell
- Provide insulation under the skin from heat or cold
- Cushion the kidneys and other sensitive organs from shock and injury
- Provide flavor and aroma in food and carry the fat-soluble vitamins A, D, E, and K
- Serve as the most concentrated source of heat and energy, supplying 9 kcal/g
- Provide energy during long periods of food deprivation

eggs), fish and vegetable oils, nuts, and some fruits such as olives and avocados. Functions of fats in the body and diet are shown in Exhibit 3–10.

Vitamins

A vitamin is an organic compound that the body requires in small amounts for proper functioning. The body cannot produce vitamins. Thus, all vitamins must be obtained from food and beverages or from synthetic supplements. Vitamins facilitate various chemical reactions in the body, with different vitamins performing different functions. Vitamins play a key role in normal cell functioning and in the cell's ability to use energy. Vitamins also participate in protein synthesis and cell replication. The functions of specific vitamins are best known by the results of their deficiencies.

Vitamin supplements are recommended if the client's diet is poor or limited in calories, or if a vitamin deficiency is suspected. The pharmacist or physician can determine the appropriate time to take a vitamin supplement in relationship to other medications. A daily high-potency multiple vitamin/mineral supplement is given if vitamin and mineral deficiencies are confirmed or suspected. Supplements should be not greater than 10 times the Recommended Dietary Allowance (RDA). Vitamins and their therapeutic properties are given in Exhibit 3–11. Vitamins are classified into two groups, according to whether they are soluble in fat or water.

Fat-Soluble Vitamins

Vitamin A, D, E, and K are derived from the fat and oily parts of certain foods. They remain in the liver and fat tissue of the body until they are used. Because the body does not excrete excess fat-soluble vitamins, there is some risk of toxicity from overdose (resulting from overaccumulation).

Deficiencies of vitamin A have been associated with retarded epithelialization and decreased collagen synthesis.

Clinical Wisdom: *Pressure Ulcer Protocol*

Stage I

- 4 oz of vitamin C-fortified juice b.i.d. with meals
- 8 oz of milk t.i.d. with meals
- If weight is below target level, whole milk will be served

Stage II

- 4 oz of vitamin C-fortified juice t.i.d. with meals
- 8 oz of milk t.i.d. with meals
- 6 oz of high-calorie supplement at bedtime
- If weight is below target level, whole milk will be served

Stage III

- 4 oz of vitamin C-fortified juice b.i.d. with meals
- 8 oz of whole milk t.i.d. with meals unless overweight
- Increase protein at noon and supper to 3 oz
- 6 oz of high-calorie supplement at H.S.
- Request vitamin C and/or vitamin B complex be approved by doctor
- 50–100 mg zinc daily (× 60 days)
- 1000–2000 mg vitamin C daily (× 60 days) OR
- A multivitamin with zinc

Stage IV

- 4 oz of vitamin C-fortified juice t.i.d. with meals
- 8 oz whole milk t.i.d. with meals unless overweight
- Increase protein at noon and supper to 3 oz
- 6 oz of high-calorie supplement at H.S.
- 50–100 mg zinc daily (× 60 days)
- 1000–2000 mg Vitamin C daily (× 60 days) OR
- A multivitamin with zinc

Exhibit 3-11 Vitamins and their Therapeutic Property

Vitamin A	Required for inflammatory response, although excessive amounts of this vitamin may exacerbate the inflammatory response
Vitamin B	Required for cross-linking of collagen fibers in rebuilding tissue
Vitamin C	May increase the activation of leukocytes and macrophages to the wound site

Because vitamin A is a fat-soluble vitamin and not excreted from the body, deficiencies are rare.

Water-Soluble Vitamins

These include the vitamin B family and vitamin C, and are derived from the water components of foods. They are distributed throughout the water compartments of the body and, for the most part, are carried in the bloodstream. Unlike fat-soluble vitamins, they are not stored but are excreted in the urine when their concentration in the blood becomes too high.

Vitamin C (ascorbic acid) deficiency is associated with impaired fibroblastic function and decreased collagen synthesis, resulting in delayed healing, capillary fragility, and breakdown of old wounds. An age-associated decrease in ascorbic acid levels may increase the fragility of vessels and connective tissue, and lower the threshold for pressure-induced injury (Table 3–3).[18] Vitamin C deficiency also is associated with impaired immune function, decreasing the individual's ability to resist infection.[12] Because vitamin C is a water-soluble vitamin and cannot be stored in the body, deficiencies can develop quickly if adequate intake is not maintained. Vitamin C supplement is often recommended for patients with healing wounds.

Water

Water, which constitutes about 60% of the adult body weight, may be the most important nutrient of all. It is distributed in the body in three fluid compartments (intracellular, interstitial, and intravascular). Water serves many vital functions in the body (Exhibit 3–12).

Fluid requirements are met with 30 mL/kg of body weight or 1 mL/kcal, or a minimum of 1,500 mL/day (1.5 L) unless medically contraindicated. Additional fluids are needed for clients with draining wounds, emesis, diarrhea, elevated temperature, or increased perspiration. Clients on air-fluidized beds require 500 mL of additional fluids daily.

Exhibit 3–12 Functions of Water

Water serves many functions, including the following:

- Aids in hydration of wound site and oxygen perfusion
- Acts as a solvent for minerals, vitamins, amino acids, glucose, and other small molecules and enables them to diffuse in and out of cells
- Transports vital materials to cells and waste away from cells
- Serves as a lubricant around joints
- Helps to maintain body temperature

Table 3–3 Key Nutrients in Wound Healing

Key Nutrients	Function	Recommendation	Food Sources
Folic acid	Needed for production of red blood cells.	100% RDA	Liver, kidney, lean meats, eggs, dark green vegetables, whole-grain cereals.
Vitamin B_6	Needed for protein/hemoglobin synthesis.	0.4 mg	Meat, poultry, fish, whole-grain breads and cereals.
Vitamin B_{12}	Prevents anemia.	2.0 mg	Meat, poultry, fish, eggs, milk.
Thiamin	Necessary to obtain energy from food eaten. Promotes good appetite.	2.0 μ	Whole-grain and enriched breads and cereals, meats (especially pork), poultry, fish, eggs.
Zinc	Needed for wound healing, improved taste perception.	1.5 mg	Meat, liver, eggs, seafood.
Vitamin C	Aids in collagen formation and absorption of iron.	100% RDA	Citrus fruits, strawberries, cantaloupe, tomatoes, potatoes, green and red peppers, broccoli.
Iron	Necessary for formation of red blood cells. Transports oxygen to healing tissue.	100% RDA	Liver, meat, eggs, fortified cereal products.
Copper	Aids in collagen formation. Helps in formation of red blood cells and works with vitamin C to form elastin.	1.5–3 mg	Nuts, dried fruit, organ meat, dried beans, whole-grain cereal.
Vitamin A	Maintains healthy skin and mucous membranes.	100% RDA	Dark green and yellow vegetables, cantaloupe, liver, fortified milk, eggs.
Vitamin K	Regulates blood clotting.	100% RDA	Green leafy vegetables.
Fat	Contributes to cellular energy. Adds to meal satisfaction.	30% + total daily calories	Oils, margarine, butter, hydrogenated fats for cooking, fat in meat, high-fat dairy products, such as cream, cream cheese, ice cream.
Protein	Builds/repairs tissue. Helps fight infection.	1.25–1.5 g/kg of body weight for Stage III and IV Example: 70 kg person; 70 × 1.5 = 105 g of protein	Meat, poultry, fish, eggs, milk and milk products, cheese, dried beans and peas, tofu, nuts, peanut butter.
Carbohydrate	Supplies energy for healing so protein can be used for building cells and healing.	50% of total calories	Grain products as breads, cereals, pasta, pastries, cookies, rice. Starchy vegetables, such as potatoes, corn, lima beans, dried beans and peas. Fruits, sugars, honey, jam and jellies, sweetened beverages.
Water	Replaces fluid lost with draining wounds. Meets increased hydration needs for increased protein requirement.	30 ml/kg of body weight (unless cardiac or renal concerns) Example: 110 lb ÷ 2.2 kg = 50 kg × 30 mL = 1,500 ml fluid; 240 mL fluid = 1 cup fluid 1,500 mL = 6–8 glasses of water	

RDA = Recommended Daily Allowance

Source: Reprinted with permission from M.G. Ritter and S. Emerson, *Nutrition Healing, Continuing Care,* Vol. 8, No. 1, © 1989, Stevens Publishing Corporation.

Clinical Wisdom: *Dehydration*

WATCH FOR WARNING SIGNS!

The following are some signs that a resident may be at risk for or suffer from dehydration:
- Drinks less than 6 cups of liquid daily
- Has one or more of the following:
  - dry mouth
  - cracked lips
  - sunken eyes
  - dark urine
- Needs help drinking from a cup or glass
- Has trouble swallowing liquids
- Frequent vomiting, diarrhea, or fever
- Is easily confused/tired

REPORT AND TAKE ACTION

Most residents need at least 6 cups of liquid to stay hydrated. Below are some ACTION STEPS to help clients get enough to drink:
- Report observations and warning signs to nurse and dietitian!
- Encourage resident to drink every time you see the client.
- Offer 2–4 oz of water or liquids frequently.
- Be sure to record fluid intake and output.
- Offer ice chips frequently (unless the resident has a swallowing problem).
- Check swallowing precautions; then, if appropriate, offer sips of liquid between bites of food at meals and snacks.
- Drink fluids with the resident, if allowed.
- Make sure pitcher and cup are near enough and light enough for the client to lift.
- Offer the appropriate assistance, as needed, if resident cannot drink without help.

Source: Adapted and reprinted with permission by the Nutrition Screening Initiative, a project of the American Academy of Family Physicians, the American Dietetic Association and the National Council on the Aging, Inc., and funded in part by a grant from Ross Products Division, Abbott Laboratories Inc.

Exhibit 3–13 Signs and Symptoms of Dehydration

- If the client/resident is able to drink independently, keep water or other beverages at bedside so that they are easily accessible and in a container that can be handled easily.
- If client/resident doesn't initiate drinking, a suggested plan is to offer water each time the client/resident is turned (every 2 hours).

Look for:

1. Dry skin
2. Cracked lips
3. Thirst (may be diminished in the elderly)
4. Poor skin turgor (The pinch test for skin turgor may be an unreliable indicator for dehydration in the elderly. If the test is used, use only the skin on the forehead or sternum. Pinch gently. If well hydrated, the skin goes back into place in 2 seconds.)
5. Fever
6. Loss of appetite
7. Nausea
8. Dizziness
9. Increased confusion
10. Laboratory values may indicate dehydration. Serum creatinine hematocrit, BUN, K^+, CL^-, osmolarity would be increased. Sodium can be increased, normal, or low, depending on the underlying cause of the dehydration.
11. Decrease in blood pressure
12. Increase in pulse
13. Constipation (recent diarrhea can offer an explanation for the dehydrated state, and constipation is a common occurrence when dehydration exists)
14. Concentrated urine

Courtesy of Mary Ellen Posthauer, RD, CD, President of M.E.P. Healthcare Dietary Services, Inc., Evansville, Indiana.

tients who are at risk of dehydration must be monitored carefully. Signs and symptoms of dehydration are listed in Exhibit 3–13. Daily body weight can indicate large fluid losses or gains. For example, a weight loss of 2 kg in 48 hours indicates a corresponding loss of 2 L of fluid. Elderly clients declining in their sense of thirst should prompt the health care provider to offer hydration more frequently.

Minerals

Minerals are inorganic elements that are needed by the cells to build body structures, maintain fluid balance, and activate enzyme systems. Once ingested, mineral salts usually dissolve in body fluids and form ions. The skeletal

Clients with end-stage disease or severe congestive heart failure may have fluids calculated at 20–25 mL/kg body weight.

The dehydrated patient has weight loss (2%, mild; 5%, moderate; 8%, severe), dry skin and mucous membranes, rapid pulse, decreased venous pressure, subnormal body temperature, low blood pressure, and altered sensation. Pa-system depends on the minerals calcium, magnesium, and phosphorus for its structural rigidity.

Clinical Wisdom: *Tips to Increase Fluids*

- Hydration carts—offer fluids, such as juices, flavored water, or lemonade, three times a day
- Popsicles
- Jello cubes
- Soups
- Sorbet/sherbet
- Ice cream
- Milk/milkshakes
- Ice chips
- Offer 4 oz of water between meals

Microelements. Microelements are trace minerals needed in very small amounts and include iron, iodine, and zinc. Various minerals, such as iron, copper (Exhibit 3–14), manganese, and magnesium, play a role in wound healing, but the nature of their influence is unclear.[19] Zinc deficiencies have been associated with delayed healing and appear to act by reducing the rate of epithelialization and fibroblast proliferation. Deficiencies require replacement, but there is no indication that supplemental zinc is useful if a deficiency does not exist.[19]

Some clients are able to maintain their nutritional status by oral intake of a balanced diet, supplemented with multiple vitamins and minerals. Having performed a nutritional assessment, the dietetic professional can devise an appropriate individualized nutrition plan for these clients, which involves collaboration between the dietetics professional and other health care professionals. The Food Guide Pyramid (Appendix 3–B) is the basis for developing a plan of care for the client. The Modified Food Pyramid for 70+ Adults (Appendix 3–E) is the basis for developing a plan of care for the elderly client.

NUTRITION BASED ON WOUND ETIOLOGY

Surgical Wounds

The acute surgical wound is acquired as the result of an operative procedure and progresses in a timely fashion along the healing trajectory, with at least external manifestations of healing apparent early in the postoperative period. Key factors influencing healing include the systemic state of the client; nutritional status; presence of underlying medical conditions or malignancies; management of postoperative therapies, such as wound care; and skin prep/type of suture material used.

Burns

Major burns result in severe trauma. Energy requirements can increase as much as 100% above resting energy expenditure, depending on the extent and depth of the injury. This hypermetabolism is accompanied by exaggerated protein catabolism (eg, breaking down of amino acids for energy) and increased urinary nitrogen excretion. Clients suffering from trauma such as burns are in negative nitrogen balance because they are forcing their bodies to use protein for energy (Exhibit 3–15).

Protein is also lost through the burn wound exudate. Wound management depends on the depth and extent of the burn. The current trend is toward early excision and grafting. Metabolic needs are reduced slightly by the practice of covering wounds as early as possible to reduce evaporative and nitrogen losses and prevent infection.

Skin Tears

Lacerations occurring from falls, bumping, or shearing forces, due to poor lifting technique, are often found in the frail elderly. Skin becomes less elastic, has limited subcutaneous fat stores, is more susceptible to medication reactions, and is prone to tearing away. A skin tear that shows limited improvement in 7–14 days requires the initiation of more aggressive nutrition therapy, such as the addition of protein, calories, and fluid.

Exhibit 3–14 Functions of Zinc and Copper

Zinc is an essential cofactor for formation of collagen and protein synthesis.

Copper is required for cross-linking of collagen fibers in rebuilding tissue.

Exhibit 3–15 Nitrogen Balance

- Amount of nitrogen (N) consumed, as compared with the amount excreted
- Nitrogen equilibrium: N in = N out
- Positive nitrogen balance: N in > N out
- Negative nitrogen balance: N in < N out

Source: Reprinted with permission from Nitrogen Balance: Cataldo C, Debruyne, L., Whitney, E. *Nutrition and Diet Therapy*, p. 85, © 1999, Wadsworth Publishing.

Leg Ulcers

Many chronic, nonhealing ulcers occur on the lower legs and feet, particularly those of vascular origin. Management of lower-extremity ulcers is complex and resource intensive.

It is essential that a multidisciplinary team manage clients with lower-extremity ulcers because many pathologic conditions are typically associated with ulcerations on the lower extremities. It is extremely important to diagnose the cause of the wound, improve tissue perfusion via surgery if warranted, provide compression if needed, manage concurrent diseases, and provide support for possible alterations in life styles (ie, weight loss, proper diet, smoking cessation, etc.).

Dermatitis

The yeastlike fungus *Candida albicans* lives with the normal flora of the mouth, vaginal tract, and gut. Pregnancy, oral contraceptives, antibiotic therapy, diabetes, skin maceration, typical steroid therapy, certain endocrinopathies, and factors related to depression of cell-mediated immunity may allow the yeast to grow, resulting in candidiasis.

In the adult, oral candidiasis occurs for several reasons. It may occur in diabetic clients with depressed cell-mediated immunity, the elderly, and those with cancer, especially leukemia. Prolonged corticosteroid, immunosuppressive, or broad-spectrum antibiotic therapy and inhalant steroids may also cause infection.

NUTRITIONAL SUPPORT

Nutritional support describes a variety of techniques available for use when a client is unable to meet the nutrient needs by normal ingestion of food. Nutritional support ranges from providing the addition of a liquid nutritional supplement or various snack foods to the client's oral diet to feeding via tube placed into the gastrointestinal tract or, even more invasive, to administering nutrients into the venous system (total parenteral nutrition) when the gastrointestinal tract is not functional.

Enteral and Parenteral Feeding

Nutritional support is used to place the client into positive nitrogen balance (eg, the body maintains the same amount of protein in its tissues from day to day), according to the goals of care and whether it is compatible with the client's and family's wishes. Levels of nutritional intervention are presented in Exhibit 3–16. Enteral feeding (tube feeding) may be initiated when the ability to chew, swallow, and absorb nutrients through normal gastrointestinal route is compromised by conditions such as stroke, Parkinson's

Exhibit 3–16 Staging Nutritional Intervention

Level I

1. Estimate nutritional needs.
2. Monitor ability to self-feed; consider use of finger foods, adaptive utensils, refeeding programs, increased time, or feeding assistance.
3. Pay attention to food preferences and tolerances; optimize the eating environment by individualizing meal times and patterns as much as possible; ensure good food quality and variety.
4. Monitor food and fluid intake.
5. Consider an interdisciplinary assessment of chewing and swallowing ability.
6. Add medical nutritional products to supplement intake.
7. Limit use of unsupplemented liquid diets or other restrictive diets.
8. Routinely reassess nutritional status and response to nutritional intervention.
9. Document and reevaluate the plan of care.

Level II

1. Institute tube feedings to meet nutritional needs if this is compatible with overall goals of care.
2. Take precautions to prevent pulmonary aspiration and other complications.
3. Monitor nutritional intake through counting calories.
4. Routinely reassess nutritional status and response to nutritional intervention.

Document and reevaluate the plan of care.

Source: Adapted with permission from S.M. Campbell, *Pressure Ulcer Prevention and Intervention: A Role for Nutrition*, May 1994, pp. 14–15, © Ross Products Division, Abbott Laboratories, Columbus, Ohio.

---

disease, cancer, and dysphagia or when clients cannot meet their nutritional needs orally. Most enteral tube feeding formulas are nutritionally complete and are designed for a specific purpose. Parenteral nutrition (delivery of nutrient solutions directly into a vein, bypassing the intestine) is necessary in clients when enteral tube feeding is contraindicated, is insufficient to maintain nutritional status, or has led to serious complications. The Nutritional Assessment and Support decision tree (Figure 3–2) is used to determine when enteral and parenteral feeding should be considered.

DOCUMENTATION IN MEDICAL RECORD

Medical Nutrition Therapy documentation in the medical record should include:

- Amount of food consumed in both quantity and quality or type of food related to amount needed
- Average fluid consumed daily (mL), related to amount required
- Ability to eat: assisted, supervised, or independent, etc.
- Acceptance or refusal of diet, meals, and/or supplements
- Current weight and % gained or lost
- New conditions affecting nutritional status, such as introduction of thickened liquids or new diagnosis
- New medications affecting nutritional status
- Current labs (past 3 months)
- Condition and/or stage of wounds
- Current calorie, protein, or fluid requirements
- Recommendation for plan of care

Documentation requirements are the drivers for eligibility for reimbursement. In order for supplies and services to be covered and reimbursed, they must be "medically necessary" and supported by physician's orders, and they must include documentation that illustrates medical need. A sample Minimum Data Set (MDS) progress note and a tube feeding progress note for the dietetics professional to provide quality documentation are found in Appendixes 3–F and 3–G at the end of this chapter. Most payers require that changes in a client's treatment plans are well documented and that such changes be based on nationally accepted practice guidelines, such as AHCPR clinical practice guidelines.

Adequate documentation by the health care team should reflect the care required to prevent and treat pressure ulcers. Documented evidence of appropriate care includes:

- regular assessment/reassessment of pressure ulcer risk factors
- regular positioning schedule
- pressure-reducing support surfaces—bed and chair
- adequate nutritional intake—food/fluid intake
- routine skin assessment and care
- incontinence management
- local wound care, including management of necrotic tissue, adequate cleansing and dressing that support moist wound healing, monitoring of improvement or deterioration of each pressure ulcer
- evaluation (reevaluation of the plan of care if pressure ulcer is not improving over time)
- change in clinical outcomes (ie, lab values, weight status)

Documentation in the medical record must be consistent with the care that is actually provided.

Case Study 1: *CVA with Hemiplegia, Stage IV Pressure Ulcer, Dysphagia*

Name: George Smith
Age: 80
Sex: Male
Diagnosis: CVA with hemiplegia; stage IV pressure ulcer; dysphagia

History

Mr. Smith had a stroke with hemiplegia about 6 weeks ago. He resides in the Merry Long-Term Care Facility. The staff reports that Mr. Smith coughs when he is fed. The speech pathologist ordered a barium swallow, which was performed yesterday, and aspiration was noted. Mr. Smith has lost 10 lbs since his stroke.

Wound Care

Mr. Smith has developed a stage IV pressure ulcer on his left trochanter since his stroke. The wound measures 5 cm by 2.5 cm, with a depth of 2 cm. The wound has less than 25% necrotic tissue and does not display gross clinical signs of wound infection but has a large amount of serosanguineous drainage. The wound has not improved in 3 weeks, and the protocols were altered this week.

Nutritional Screening

Mr. Smith has which risk factors? (Please refer to the nutritional screening form [Exhibit 3–17].)

Nutritional Assessment

Anthropometric Measures.
Height: 6′3″ or 75″ × 2.5 = 187.5 cm
Weight: Actual = 180 ÷ 2.2 = 81.8 kg; Usual = 200 ÷ 2.2 = 90.90 kg (prior to stroke); Ideal = _____ ÷ 2.2 = _____ kg
How would you characterize Mr. Smith's weight measures over the last several weeks? What does this indicate with regard to his nutritional status?

24-Hour Dietary Recall.
Food intake: The patient's difficulty with swallowing has made it hard to "get anything down him," and he has only eaten a "few bites" of the meal offered him. He has had

continues

Case Study 1 continued

such severe coughing episodes that he now seems to be afraid to take anything by mouth.

Estimate the patient's food intake: Calories:_____;
Protein:_____

Fluid Intake: He has taken only a few "sips" of water since yesterday morning, but water and juices seem to make him cough even more.

Estimate the patient's fluid intake:_____ oz × 30 = _____ mL

Calculate Estimated Daily Requirements.

Calories: (AHCPR) 35 calories × _____kg = _____calories per day

Compare 24-hour recall to AHCPR requirement:
_____ calories– _____calories = _____ calories per day

Does this represent a deficit or a surplus?

_____

Protein: (AHCPR) 1.5 g × _____kg = 130 g per day
Compare 24-hour recall to AHCPR requirement:
_____g– _____g = _____g/day
Does this represent a deficit or a surplus?

_____

Fluid: 30 mL × _____kg = _____ + 200 mL (estimated wound exudate) = _____mL/day
Compare with 24-hour recall:
_____mL–_____mL = _____mL per day
Does this represent a deficit or a surplus?

_____

Lab Results.

Serum albumin = 3.3
Total lymphocyte count = 1,600
Finding:

_____

Recommendations

What would you recommend in this case? Is the patient an appropriate candidate for nutrition therapy? If so, what type and why? What other interventions might be appropriate in this case?

ANALYSIS

Case Study 1

Name: George Smith
Age: 80
Sex: Male
Diagnosis: CVA with hemiplegia; stage IV pressure ulcer; dysphagia

Nutritional Screening

Mr. Smith presents the following risk factors:

- Elderly
- Chronic wound: pressure ulcer
- Poor response to current wound treatment after 3 weeks
- Recent unintentional weight loss
- Functional limitations: chewing and swallowing difficulties (dysphagia), mobility, dexterity

Nutritional Assessment

Anthropometric Measures

Height: 6′3″ or 75″ × 2.5 = 187.5 cm
Weight: Actual = 180 ÷ 2.2 = 81.8 kg; Usual = 200 ÷ 2.2 = 90.90 kg; Ideal 196 ÷ 2.2 = 89.09 kg
Finding: Unintentional weight loss of 8% over last 4 weeks

24-Hour Dietary Recall

Food intake: Staff state that the patient's difficulty with swallowing has made it hard to "get anything down him" and that he has eaten only a "few bites" of the meal offered him. He has had such severe coughing episodes that he now seems to be afraid to take anything by mouth.

Estimated food intake: = 5 g protein, < 100 calories

Fluid intake: Staff states he has only had a few "sips" of water since yesterday morning but that water and juices seem to make him cough even more.

Estimated fluid intake = 6 oz × 30 = 180 mL

Calculated Estimated Daily Requirements

Calories: (AHCPR) 35 calories × 81.81 kg = 2,863 calories per day
Compared 24-hour recall to AHCPR requirement:
2,863 calories − 100 calories = 2,763 calories per day (deficit)
Protein: (AHCPR) 1.5 g × 81.81 kg = 123 g per day
Compared 24-hour recall to AHCPR requirement:
130 g − 5 g = 125 g/day (deficit)
Fluid: 30 mL × 81.81 kg = 2,454 + 200 mL (estimated wound exudate) = 2,654 mL/day
Compared with 24-hour recall:
2,654 mL − 180 mL = 2,474 mL per day (deficit)

Lab Results

Serum albumin = 3.3
Total lymphocyte count = 1,600
Finding: Malnutrition

continues

Case Study 1 continued

Recommendations

- Notify physician of nutritional assessment findings, lab results, and slow wound healing
- Because of the patient's dysphagia and the risk of aspiration, enteral nutrition therapy is recommended: category I (semisynthetic isotonic) medical nutrition therapy via percutaneous endoscopic gastrostomy

(PEG) tube
- Goal: 2,500 calories per day
- Goal rate = 200 mL/hr × 12.5 hours or 104 mL/hr continuous; flush 250 mL each shift
- Continue wound treatment protocol and routine wound assessments
- Recommend multivitamin with zinc

Case Study 2: *Dementia, Sigmoid Diverticulitis, Temporary Colostomy, Dysphagia, Stage III PU or Coccyx, Wound Infection*

Name: Susan Anderson
Age: 82
Sex: Female
Diagnosis: Dementia, sigmoid diverticulitis, temporary colostomy, dysphagia, stage III PU or coccyx, wound infection

History

Mrs. Anderson is bedbound, recuperating after surgery for sigmoid diverticulitis that resulted in the creation of a temporary colostomy. She also has dementia. Since the surgery, Mrs. Anderson is more agitated than usual. When the staff try to feed her, Mrs. Anderson appears to have to swallow many times with each mouthful and has a "wet-sounding" voice after eating. More recently, she has begun to refuse 50% of the meal and has become incontinent of urine. A speech pathologist has been contacted to evaluate her swallowing problems.

Nutritional Screen

Mrs. Anderson has which risk factors? (Please refer to the nutritional screening form [Exhibit 3–17].)

Nutritional Assessment

Anthropometric Measures

Height: 5′6″ or 66″ × 2.5 = 165 cm
Weight: Actual = 108 ÷ 2.2 = 49.09kg; Usual = 115 ÷ 2.2 = 52.27 kg

How would you characterize Mrs. Anderson's weight measures over the last several weeks? What does this indicate with regard to her nutritional status?

24-Hour Dietary Recall

Food intake: The resident has eaten only bites of food for the past 24 hours.
Estimate the patient's food intake:
Calories:_____
Protein:_____

Fluid Intake: The resident has had only a few sips of water and orange juice in the last 24 hours and "she just refuses everything."
Estimate the patient's fluid intake:_____ oz × 30 = _____ mL

Calculate Estimated Daily Requirements

Calories: (AHCPR) 35 calories × _____ kg = _____ calories per day
Compare 24-hour recall to AHCPR requirement:
_____ calories– _____ calories = _____ calories per day
Does this represent a deficit or a surplus?

_____

Protein: (AHCPR) 1.5 g × _____kg = 130 g per day
Compare 24-hour recall to AHCPR requirement:
_____ g– _____ g = _____ g/day
Does this represent a deficit or a surplus?

_____

Fluid: 30 mL × _____ kg = _____ + 250 mL (estimated wound exudate) = _____ mL/day
Compare with 24-hour recall:
_____ mL – mL = _____ mL per day
Does this represent a deficit or a surplus?_____

Lab Results

Serum albumin = 2.8
Total lymphocyte count = 1500
Finding:

_____

Recommendations

What would you recommend in this case? Is the patient an appropriate candidate for nutrition therapy? If so, what type and why? What other interventions might be appropriate in this case?

continues

Case Study 2 continued

ANALYSIS

Name: Susan Anderson
Age: 82
Sex: Female
Diagnosis: Dementia, sigmoid diverticulitis, temporary colostomy, dysphagia, stage III PU or coccyx, wound infection

Nutritional Screening

Mrs. Anderson has the following risk factors:

- Elderly
- Infection: wound
- Stage III ulcer or coccyx
- Functional limitations: chewing/swallowing, mobility, altered mental state
- Medical conditions: incontinence, gastrointestinal disorder

Nutritional Assessment

Anthropometric Measures

Height: 5'6" or 66" × 2.5 = 165 cm
Weight: Actual = 108 ÷ 2.2 = 49.09kg; Usual = 115 ÷ 2.2 = 52.27 kg
Finding: Unintentional weight loss over last 4 weeks; patient is 22 lb under ideal weight

24-Hour Dietary Recall

Food intake: Staff states that the resident has eaten "practically nothing" for the past 24 hours.
Estimated food intake: 0 protein; scant calories
Fluid intake: Staff states that resident has had only a few sips of water and orange juice in the last 24 hours and "she just refuses everything."
Estimated fluid intake: 6 oz × 30 = 180 mL

Estimated Daily Requirements

Calories: (AHCPR) 35 calories × 49.09 kg = 1,718 calories per day
Compared 24-hour recall to AHCPR requirement:
1,718 calories – scant calories = 1,718 calories per day (deficit)
Protein: (AHCPR) 1.5 g × 49.09 kg = 74 g per day
Compared 24-hour recall to AHCPR requirement:
74 g – 0 g = 74 g/day (deficit)
Fluid: 30 mL × 49.09 kg = 1473 + 250 mL (estimated wound exudate) = 1,723 mL/day
Compared with 24-hour recall:
1,723 mL – 180 mL = 1,543 mL per day (deficit)

Lab Results

Serum albumin = 2.8
Total lymphocyte count = 1,500
Finding: Malnutrition

Recommendations

- Notify physician and registered dietitian of nutritional assessment findings, lab results, slow wound healing, dysphagia
- Notify speech pathologist for speech/swallowing evaluation
- Because of functional limitations, including dysphagia and the risk of aspiration, recommend puree diet with nectar liquids
- Offer supplements at bedtime of 240 calories
- Offer supplements or nutrient-dense food if meals are refused
- Request that speech pathologist to instruct family and staff on appropriate swallowing techniques for assistance at meals, using nectarlike liquids per recommendation
- Have a goal of 1,700 calories per day
- Continue wound treatment protocol and routine wound assessments
- Recommend multivitamin with zinc

CASE STUDIES

Use Case Studies 1 and 2 (adapted from Mead Johnson Nutritionals, The Role of Nutrition in Wound Healing, MJ Publication No. MB183, Evansville, IN, December 1998) and information provided in this study guide to practice nutritional screening and nutritional assessment. Although the screening and assessment forms are essential tools, the dietetic professionals rely on their own professional judgment while implementing nutritional support.

Two residents with wounds are presented. In assessing these cases, please refer to Exhibit 3–17 (Nutritional Screening for Patients with Wounds) and Exhibit 3–18 (*Medical Nutritional Assessment for Patients with Wounds*).

Exhibit 3–17 Nutritional Screening for Patients with Wounds

Name: _____ Patient Number: _____ ❏ Male ❏ Female

DOB: _____ Age: _____ Diagnosis: _____

_____

_____

Physician: Diet Order:

Check all that apply

❏   Elderly (age 65 or older)

❏   Score of < 18 on Braden Scale

❏   Acute/surgical wound: ❏ Type: closed   ❏ open/dehisced

❏   Poor response to current wound treatment for past 2–4 weeks

❏   Recent unintentional weight loss/gain (5% or more over 1 month; 10% or more over 3 months)

❏   Functional limitations
           Types: ❏ altered mental state   ❏ hearing/speech
                    ❏ chewing/swallowing difficulties ❏ mobility
                    ❏ dexterity   ❏ vision

❏   Medical condition or diagnosis
           Types: ❏ arterial insufficiency   ❏ immunosuppression
                    ❏ cancer   ❏ incontinence (urinary and/or fecal)
                    ❏ cardiovascular disease   ❏ infections
                    ❏ COPD/pulmonary disease   ❏ kidney disease (chronic or end-stage)
                    ❏ diabetes   ❏ liver disease (chronic or end-stage)
                    ❏ dysphagia   ❏ malnutrition
                    ❏ gastrointestinal disorder   ❏ sepsis
                    ❏ hip fracture   ❏ spinal cord injury

❏   Drug Therapy   Type: ❏ antikinetics   ❏ immunosuppressants
                                         ❏ chemotherapy   ❏ radiation
                                         ❏ corticosteroids   ❏ renal dialysis

Action: ❏ Nutritional Assessment   ❏ Rescreen every 3 months

Screen completed by: _____   Date: _____

Evaluate the patient for the presence of any of the criteria above. If any are present, a Nutritional Assessment should be conducted. Information can be obtained from the patient's medical record or referral form.

Exhibit 3–18 Medical Nutritional Assessment for Patients with Wounds

Name: _____ Patient Number: _____ ❑ Male ❑ Female

DOB: _____ Age: _____ Diagnosis: _____

_____

_____

Physician: _____ Diet Order: _____

1. **Anthropometric measures:**
   Height: _____ ft _____ in
   Actual Weight: _____ lb ÷ 2.2 = _____ kg
   Usual Body Weight: _____ lb
   Target or Desirable Body Weight Range: _____ + _____ = _____ ÷ 2 + _____
   To Calculate Adjusted Body Weight for Obese Patients
   Actual body weight—ideal body weight × 0.25. Add this number back to the ideal body weight. Use this sum to calculate daily requirements rather than actual weight.

Weight loss/gain of 5% over last month?	❑ no	❑ yes ⇒ at risk
Weight loss/gain of 10% over 3 months?	❑ no	❑ yes ⇒ at risk

2. **24-Hour Dietary Recall** (list foods as reported by patient/caregiver)

   _____

   _____

   _____

   Estimated calorie intake _____   Estimated protein intake _____ g
   Estimated fluid intake _____ mL

3. **Estimated Daily Requirements for Patients with Wounds *** (use actual weight)
   Calories: 30–35 calories × _____ kg body weight = _____ calories per day
   Protein: 1.25 – 1.50 g × _____ kg body weight = _____ g protein per day
   Fluids: 30 mL × _____ kg body weight = _____ mL★ + _____ mL = _____ mL per day
   ★Resulting from : ❑ diaphoresis ❑ diarrhea ❑ vomiting ❑ wound drainage ❑ fever ❑ constipation ❑ fistula
   (Compare estimated requirements with findings from 24-Hour Dietary Recall)

4. **Lab Results**   serum albumin _____   total lymphocyte count _____
   (3.5 = normal, < 3.5 = malnutrition)   (1800 = competent immunity, < 1800 = impaired
                                              immunity/malnutrition)

5. **Recommendations**
   ❑ Diet prescription (ie, high calorie, high protein)
   ❑ Medical nutrition therapy
       ❑ oral supplement _____
       ❑ enteral nutrition _____
       ❑ parenteral nutrition _____

6. **Patient teaching plan**

   _____

   Assessment conducted by: _____ Date: _____

   * Agency for Health Care Policy and Research, US Department of Health and Human Services. *Treatment of Pressure Ulcers: Clinical Practice Guidelines.* No. 15. AHCPR Publication No. 95-0652. Rockville, MD: December 1994.

   Courtesy of Mead Johnson, Evansville, Indiana.

CONCLUSION

Malnutrition impedes healing for both chronic and acute wounds.[20] Poor nutritional status has been shown to influence healing time negatively in clients with deep pressure ulcers.[17,21] Indeed, the development of a pressure ulcer or failure of any type of wound to heal can be a grave indicator of malnutrition. In fact, malnutrition is one of the major risk factors for developing a pressure ulcer. The fact that aging is associated with both impaired healing[19] and reduced nutrient intake[22] sets the stage for the development and delayed healing of chronic wounds and slow to poor healing of acute wounds in the elderly.

Medical nutrition therapy can provide the means to meet these challenges. A diet that allows the client to enjoy favorite food using oral nutrition supplements (if needed) or enteral and parenteral nutrition support can effect optimal nutrition, thus having a positive impact on wound healing.

REFERENCES:

1. American Dietetic Association (ADA) Council on Practice Quality Management Committee. ADA's definitions for nutrition screening and nutrition assessment. *J Am Diet Assoc.* 1994;94:838–839.

2. Niedert K. *Nutrition Care of the Older Adult.* Chicago, IL: ADA; 1998:168–169.

3. Maklebust J, Sieggreen, M. *Pressure Ulcers: Guidelines for Prevention and Management.* 3rd ed. Springhouse, PA: Springhouse Corporation; 2001:356.

4. Omnibus Budget Reconciliation Act of 1987. Nursing Home Reform Legislation, 1987. Interpretive Guidelines: Transmittal #274, *State Operations Manual*, June 1995.

5. Bennett RG, O'Sullivan J, DeVito EM, Remsburg R. The increasing medical malpractice risk related to pressure ulcers in the United States. *J Am Geriatr Soc.* 2000;48:73–81.

6. Bergstrom N, Bennett MA, Carlson CE, et al. The Agency for Health Care Research and Quality (AHRQ), formerly known as the Agency for Health Care Policy and Research (AHCPR), Department of Health and Human Services (DHHS). *Pressure Ulcers in Adults: Prediction and Prevention: Clinical Practice Guideline.* AHRQ Publication No. 92-0047. Rockville, MD: AHRQ; May 1992.

7. Bergstrom N, Bennett MA, Carlson CE, et al. AHRQ, DHHS. *Treatment of Pressure Ulcers: Clinical Practice Guideline.* No. 15. AHRQ Publication No. 95-0652. Rockville, MD: AHRQ; December 1994.

8. Posthauer ME, Dorse B, Foiles RA, et al. ADA's definitions for nutrition screening and nutrition assessment. *J Am Dietetic Assoc.* 1994;8:838–839.

9. Niedert K. *Nutrition Care of the Older Adult.* Chicago, IL: ADA; 1998:192.

10. Maklebust J, Sieggreen M. *Pressure Ulcers: Guidelines for Prevention and Nursing Management.* 3rd ed. Springhouse, PA: Springhouse Corporation; 2001:37.

11. Lewis T, Grant R. Observations upon reactive hyperemia in man. *Heart (London).* 1925;12:73–120.

12. Nutrition Screening Initiative, a project of the American Academy of Family Physicians, ADA, and the National Council on the Aging, and funded in part by a grant from Ross Products Division, Abbott Laboratories, Inc. Washington, DC: Nutrition Screening Initiative; 1993:2.

13. Dwyer JT. *Screening Older Americans' Nutritional Health: Current Practices and Future Possibilities.* Washington, DC: Nutrition Screening Initiative; 1991.

14. Niedert K. *Nutrition Care of the Older Adult.* Chicago, IL: ADA; 1998:196.

15. Blackburn GL, Bristrain BF, Maini BS, et al. Nutritional and metabolic assessment of the hospitalized patient. *JPEN.* 1977;1:11–22.

16. Womack P, Breeding C. Liberalized diets for older adults in long-term care. *J Am Diet Assoc.* 1998;98:201–204.

17. vanRikwsijk L, Polansky M. Predictors of time to healing deep pressure ulcers. *Wounds.* 1994;6:159–165.

18. Bergstrom N, Bennett MA, Carlson CE, et al. AHRQ, DHHS. *Treatment of Pressure Ulcers: Clinical Practice Guideline.* No. 15. AHRQ Publication No. 95-0652. Rockville, MD: AHRQ; December 1994:29.

19. Bergstrom N, Bennett MA, Carlson CE, et al. AHRQ, DHHS. Treatment of Pressure Ulcers: Clinical Practice Guideline. No. 15. AHRQ Publication No. 95-0652, Rockville, MD: AHRQ; December 1994:30.

20. Maklebust J, Sieggreen M. *Pressure Ulcers: Guidelines for Prevention and Nursing Management.* 3rd ed. Springhouse, PA: Springhouse Corporation; 2001:39.

21. Brylinksy C. Nutrition and wound healing: An overview. *Ostomy/Wound Manage.* 1995;41:14–24.

22. Stotts N, Wipke-Tevis D. Co-factors in impaired wound healing. In: Krasner, D, Kane, D, eds. *Chronic Wound Care: A Clinical Source Book for Healthcare Professionals.* 2nd ed. Wayne, PA: Health Management Publications; 1997:63–72.

SUGGESTED READING

Niedert K. *Nutrition Care of the Older Adult.* Chicago, IL: ADA; 1998:196.

Sussman C. *Wound Care: Patient Education Resource Manual.* Gaithersburg, MD: Aspen Publishers; 1999.

Appendix 3–A: Nutrition Intervention To Prevent Wounds

The first goal in preventing pressure ulcers is to identify at-risk individuals needing prevention and the specific factors placing them at risk. Analysis of data from the National Pressure Ulcer Long-Term Care Study (NPULS) has identified patients who are most likely to develop a pressure ulcer. The nutrition characteristics of nursing home residents and the nutrition processes of care that are highly associated with the development of new pressure ulcers include:

- weight loss
- dependence in eating
- diabetes mellitus
- poor meal intake
- dehydration
- oral problems associated with eating
- missing diet order

Analysis of the NPULS data has also identified patients who are *less* likely to develop a pressure ulcer. These characteristics and processes of care are:

- mechanical diet
- fluid orders
- oral commercial medical nutritional products (such as Ensure®, Ensure Plus®, Promote®)
- enteral tube feeding (high-calorie and high-protein products, such as TwoCal® HN, and Ensure Plus® HN; and disease-specific products, such as Perative®)

In patients at risk for developing pressure ulcers or for worsening of ulcers, intensive therapy must be aimed at reducing risk factors. The following two levels of intervention and accompanying procedures will help health care providers to prevent and treat patients with wounds.

LEVEL I INTERVENTION—ORAL DIET

Immediately:

- Remove restrictive diets.
- Limit use of unsupplemented liquid diets.
- Refer to a registered dietitian.
- Order weekly weights.
- Begin a 24-hour assessment of food and fluid intake.
- Evaluate the patient's ability to self-feed (consider use of finger foods, adaptive utensils, refeeding programs, increased time, or feeding assistance).
- Identify food preferences and intolerances.
- Optimize eating environment.
- Individualize meal times and patterns.
- Use medical nutritional products.
- Begin a med pass program.

Within 7 days:

- Receive dietitian consultation or assessment that
  –estimates nutritional needs
  –evaluates weekly weight
  –evaluates 24-hour intake for food and liquid.
- Ensure good food quality and variety.
- Consider interdisciplinary assessment.
- Plan weekly reassessment of nutrition status and response to nutrition intervention.
- Document and reevaluate the plan of care.

Within 14 days, reassess goals of care:

- Advance to Level II intervention and begin tube feeding if nutrient needs are not met or weight loss continues.
- Begin palliative supportive care if aggressive nutritional therapy is not desired by patient, family, and health care professionals.

LEVEL II—TUBE OR PARENTERAL FEEDING

For those patients who cannot maintain adequate dietary intake with Level I interventions and should not be allowed to decline:

- Begin tube feeding.
- Prevent tube feeding complications, such as pulmonary aspiration and glucose/electrolyte abnormalities.
- Reassess nutritional status.
- Reassess response to nutritional interventions.
- Document and reevaluate plan of care weekly.

SUMMARY

Prevention, early intervention, and treatment programs are critical in caring for persons with wounds. Aggressive nutritional management as part of a comprehensive plan of care contributes to reduced cost of care and decreased patient pain and suffering. The nutritional intervention strategies advocated in this exhibit will help the health care provider to provide care consistent with the following nutrition therapy goals and interventions identified by the Agency for Health Care Policy and Research:

1. Ensure adequate dietary intake.
2. Perform nutritional assessment.
3. Encourage dietary intake with oral supplements.
4. Tube feed if oral intake is inadequate.
5. Ensure adequate vitamin and mineral intake.

Courtesy of Charlotte Gallagher-Allred, Ross Products Division, Abbott Laboratories, Columbus, Ohio.

Appendix 3–B: Food Guide Pyramid: A Guide to Daily Food Choices

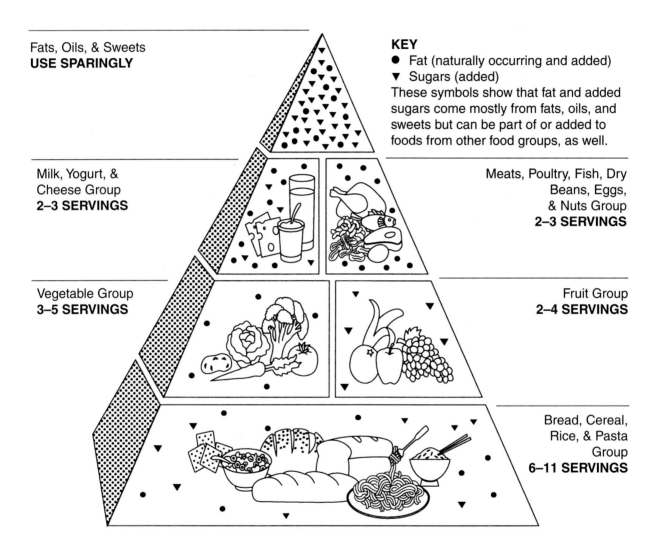

KEY
- ● Fat (naturally occurring and added)
- ▼ Sugars (added)

These symbols show that fat and added sugars come mostly from fats, oils, and sweets but can be part of or added to foods from other food groups, as well.

Fats, Oils, & Sweets
USE SPARINGLY

Milk, Yogurt, & Cheese Group
2–3 SERVINGS

Meats, Poultry, Fish, Dry Beans, Eggs, & Nuts Group
2–3 SERVINGS

Vegetable Group
3–5 SERVINGS

Fruit Group
2–4 SERVINGS

Bread, Cereal, Rice, & Pasta Group
6–11 SERVINGS

Use the Food Guide Pyramid to help you eat better every day—the Dietary Guidelines Way. Start with plenty of breads, cereals, rice, and pasta; vegetables; and fruits. Add two to three servings from the milk group and two to three servings from the meat group.

Each of these food groups provides some, but not all, of the nutrients you need. No one food group is more important than another—for good health, you need them all. Go easy on fats, oils, and sweets—the foods in the small tip of the pyramid.

Source: Reprinted from U.S. Department of Agriculture, Hunman Nutrition Information Service, Leaflet No. 572, August 1992.

Appendix 3–C: How To Use the Daily Food Guide

WHAT COUNTS AS ONE SERVING?

The amount you eat may be more than one serving. For example, a dinner portion of spaghetti would count as two or three servings of pasta.

Breads, Cereals, Rice, and Pasta

1 slice of bread
½ cup of cooked rice or pasta
½ cup of cooked cereal
1 ounce of ready-to-eat cereal

Vegetables

½ cup of chopped raw or cooked vegetables
1 cup of leafy raw vegetables

Fruits

1 piece of fruit or melon wedge
¼ cup of juice
½ cup of canned fruit
¼ cup of dried fruit

Milk, Yogurt, and Cheese

1 cup of milk or yogurt
1½ to 2 ounces of cheese

Meat, Poultry, Fish, Dry Beans, Eggs, and Nuts

2½–3 ounces of cooked lean meat, poultry, or fish
Count ½ cup of cooked beans, or 1 egg, or 2 tablespoons of peanut butter as 1 ounce of lean meat (about ⅓ serving)

Fats, Oils, and Sweets

Limit calories from these, especially if you need to lose weight.

Source: Reprinted from U.S. Department of Agriculture, Human Nutrition Information Service, *Leaflet No. 572*, August 1992.

Appendix 3–D: How Many Servings Do You Need Each Day?

	Women & some older adults	Children, teen girls, active women, most men	Teen boys & active men
Calorie level*	about 1,600	about 2,200	about 2,800
Bread group	6	9	11
Vegetable group	3	4	5
Fruit group	2	3	4
Milk group	**2–3	**2–3	**2–3
Meat group	2, for a total of 5 ounces	2, for a total of 6 ounces	3, for a total of 7 ounces

*These are the calorie levels if you choose low-fat, lean foods from the five major food groups and use foods from the fats, oils, and sweets group sparingly.

**Women who are pregnant or breastfeeding, teenagers, and young adults to age 24 need 3 servings.

A CLOSER LOOK AT FAT AND ADDED SUGARS

The small tip of the pyramid shows fats, oils, and sweets. These are foods such as salad dressings, cream, butter, margarine, sugars, soft drinks, candies, and sweet desserts. Alcoholic beverages are also part of this group. These foods provide calories but few vitamins and minerals. Most people should go easy on foods from this group.

Some fat or sugar symbols are shown in the other food groups. That's to remind you that some foods in these groups can also be high in fat and added sugars, such as cheese or ice cream from the milk group or french fries from the vegetable group. When choosing foods for a healthful diet, consider the fat and added sugars in your choices from all the food groups—not just fats, oils, and sweets from the pyramid tip.

Source: Reprinted from U.S. Department of Agriculture, Human Nutrition Information Service, *Leaflet No. 572*, August 1992.

Appendix 3–E: Modified Food Pyramid for 70+ Adults

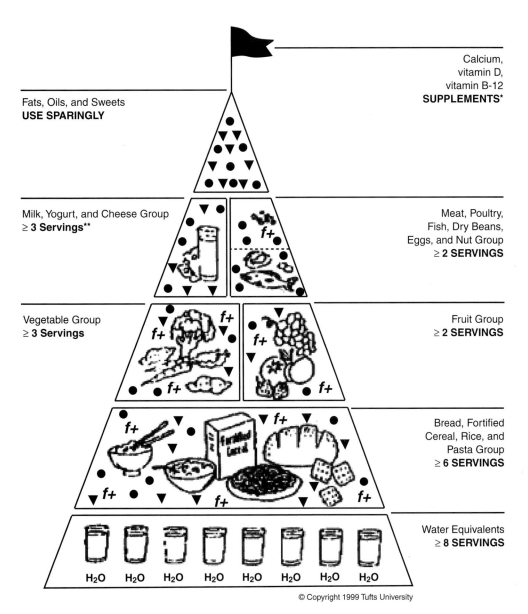

Calcium,
vitamin D,
vitamin B-12
SUPPLEMENTS*

Fats, Oils, and Sweets
USE SPARINGLY

Milk, Yogurt, and Cheese Group
≥ 3 Servings**

Meat, Poultry,
Fish, Dry Beans,
Eggs, and Nut Group
≥ 2 SERVINGS

Vegetable Group
≥ 3 Servings

Fruit Group
≥ 2 SERVINGS

Bread, Fortified
Cereal, Rice, and
Pasta Group
≥ 6 SERVINGS

Water Equivalents
≥ 8 SERVINGS

H₂O   H₂O   H₂O   H₂O   H₂O   H₂O   H₂O   H₂O

© Copyright 1999 Tufts University

KEY

●   **Fat** (naturally occurring and added)

▼   **Sugars** (added)

f+   **Fiber** (should be present)

These symbols show fat, added sugars, and fiber in foods
*Not all individuals need supplements; consult your health care provider
**≥ Greater than or equal to

Courtesy of Tufts University, © 1999 Tufts University, Medford, Massachusetts.

Appendix 3–F:
Medical Nutrition Therapy Quarterly/MDS Progress Note

NAME:_____		GENDER: ☐ M ☐ F	
TARGET WEIGHT _____ lbs HEIGHT:_____		AGE:_____ years	

1ST QUARTER		**2ND QUARTER**	**3RD QUARTER**
DIET ORDER:		Changed ☐ Y ☐ N	Changed ☐ Y ☐ N
SUPPLEMENT:		Changed ☐ Y ☐ N	Changed ☐ Y ☐ N
FORTIFIED FOODS:		Changed ☐ Y ☐ N	Changed ☐ Y ☐ N
TUBE FEEDING FLUSH		Changed ☐ Y ☐ N	Changed ☐ Y ☐ N
FOOD/FLUIDS % Intake	_____ B _____ HS _____ L _____ Fluids _____ S _____ Supplement	_____ B _____ HS _____ L _____ Fluids _____ S _____ Supplement	_____ B _____ HS _____ L _____ Fluids _____ S _____ Supplement
FEEDING ABILITY	☐ Dependent ☐ Independent ☐ Limited Assist ☐ Other ☐ Self-Help Devices	Changed ☐ Y ☐ N	Changed ☐ Y ☐ N
ORAL STATUS	☐ Chewing Prob ☐ Mouth Pain ☐ Swallowing Prob ☐ Dentures ☐ Edentulous ☐ Other	Changed ☐ Y ☐ N	Changed ☐ Y ☐ N
MEAL LOCATION	☐ DR ☐ Room/Day Room ☐ Restorative ☐ Other_____	Changed ☐ Y ☐ N	Changed ☐ Y ☐ N
COGNITIVE STATUS	☐ Alert/Oriented ☐ Depressed ☐ Cog. Impaired ☐ Disoriented/Confused ☐ Combative ☐ Wanders ☐ Comatose ☐ Other _____	Changed ☐ Y ☐ N	Changed ☐ Y ☐ N
CURRENT WEIGHT: _____ LBS _____% change ☐ 30 days ☐ 60 days ☐ 180 days		_____Wt _____% change ☐ 30 ☐ 60 ☐ 180	_____Wt _____% change ☐ 30 ☐ 60 ☐ 180
PLANNED WEIGHT CHANGE: ☐ Yes ☐ No		☐ YES ☐ NO	☐ YES ☐ NO
CALORIC/ HYDRATION REQUIREMENT:	_____ Calories _____ Protein _____ Fluid	Changed ☐ Y ☐ N	Changed ☐ Y ☐ N
SKIN CONDITION	☐ Intake ☐ Burns 2nd/3rd degree ☐ Edema ☐ Reddened Areas ☐ Surgical Wounds ☐ Other: _____ ☐ Open Lesion/Infections _____	☐ Intact ☐ Burns 2nd/3rd degree ☐ Edema ☐ Reddened Areas ☐ Surgical Wounds ☐ Open Lesion/Infections ☐ Other:_____	☐ Intact ☐ Burns 2nd/3rd degree ☐ Edema ☐ Reddened Areas ☐ Surgical Wounds ☐ Open Lesion/Infections ☐ Other:_____
PRESSURE ULCER(S)	☐ YES ☐ NO STAGE: 1 2 3 4 LOCATION:_____ SIZE:_____	☐ YES ☐ NO STAGE: 1 2 3 4 LOCATION:_____ SIZE:_____	☐ YES ☐ NO STAGE: 1 2 3 4 LOCATION:_____ SIZE:_____

continues

1ST QUARTER	2ND QUARTER	3RD QUARTER
LAB VALUES: 　　　　Date:_____ _____Albumin　　N　Hi　Lo _____BUN　　　　N　Hi　Lo _____Cholesterol　N　Hi　Lo _____Creatinine　N　Hi　Lo _____Folic Acid　N　Hi　Lo _____Glucose　　N　Hi　Lo _____Hematocrit　N　Hi　Lo _____Hemoglobin　N　Hi　Lo _____Hgb A1C　　N　Hi　Lo _____Potassium　N　Hi　Lo _____Sodium　　N　Hi　Lo _____Total Protein　N　Hi　Lo	LAB VALUES: 　　　　Date:_____ _____Albumin　　N　Hi　Lo _____BUN　　　　N　Hi　Lo _____Cholesterol　N　Hi　Lo _____Creatinine　N　Hi　Lo _____Folic Acid　N　Hi　Lo _____Glucose　　N　Hi　Lo _____Hematocrit　N　Hi　Lo _____Hemoglobin　N　Hi　Lo _____Hgb A1C　　N　Hi　Lo _____Potassium　N　Hi　Lo _____Sodium　　N　Hi　Lo _____Total Protein　N　Hi　Lo	LAB VALUES: 　　　　Date:_____ _____Albumin　　N　Hi　Lo _____BUN　　　　N　Hi　Lo _____Cholesterol　N　Hi　Lo _____Creatinine　N　Hi　Lo _____Folic Acid　N　Hi　Lo _____Glucose　　N　Hi　Lo _____Hematocrit　N　Hi　Lo _____Hemoglobin　N　Hi　Lo _____Hgb A1C　　N　Hi　Lo _____Potassium　N　Hi　Lo _____Sodium　　N　Hi　Lo _____Total Protein　N　Hi　Lo
PROGRESS:		
INTERVENTION:		
Signature:		
DATE:		

Appendix 3–G:
Monthly Medical Nutrition Therapy Tube Feeding Progress Note

F-74 (11/00)

NAME:_____ GENDER: ❏ M ❏ F

TARGET WEIGHT:_____ LBS HEIGHT: _____ AGE:_____years

Date:	Date:	Date:
TUBE FEEDING ORDER:	Changed Yes/No	Changed Yes/No
FLUSH:	Changed Yes/No	Changed Yes/No
FORMULA PROVIDES: Calories: _____ Free H$_2$O:_____ Protein:_____ Flush:_____ Total Water:_____	Changed Yes/No	Changed Yes/No
DIET: _____ **PUMP:**_____ **NPO:**_____ **BOLUS:** _____	Changed Yes/No	Changed Yes/No
TOTAL CALORIES PER TUBE: ❏ 1%–25% ❏ 51%–75% ❏ 26%–50% ❏ 76%–100%	Changed Yes/No	Changed Yes/No
NUTRIENT NEEDS: BEE_____ Activity Factor_____ Injury Factor _____ Total Calories_____ Protein _____g/kg Total Protein _____g Fluid _____cc/kg Total Fluids _____mL	Changed Yes/No	Changed Yes/No
SIGNIFICANT LAB VALUES:	LABS	LABS

WEIGHT:
  CURRENT WEIGHT: _____
  % CHANGE:_____
	Weight:_____
	
	% Change:_____
		Weight:_____
		
		% Change:_____

SKIN CONDITION: ❏ Intact ❏ Open Lesion/Infections ❏ Edema _____ ❏ Reddened Areas ❏ Pressure Ulcer Stage:_____	❏ Intact ❏ Edema ❏ Red Areas ❏ Open Lesion/Infections ❏ PU Stage:_____	❏ Intact ❏ Edema ❏ Red Areas ❏ Open Lesion/Infections ❏ PU Stage:_____
RECOMMENDATIONS:		
RD SIGNATURE:_____	_____	_____

CHAPTER 4

Assessment of the Skin and Wound

Carrie Sussman

CHAPTER OBJECTIVES

At the completion of this chapter, the reader will be able to:

1. Apply classification systems used to diagnose wound severity
2. Perform the process of wound assessment status
3. Perform assessment of the periwound status and adjacent tissues
4. Understand and apply the concept of wound phase diagnosis, based on the status of the phase of wound healing

This chapter continues the methodology of the diagnostic process described in Chapter 1 with step II, the assessment and functional diagnosis of the wound. Assessment is a process of assigning numbers or grades to events systematically. Tests are the instruments or means by which events are assessed or measured. Examination is the process of determining the values of the tests. To evaluate something properly or accurately, skills of evaluation are necessary. That is, a background is required in selecting appropriate tests, understanding the significance of the tests and measurements, and knowing how to interpret them. Both the examination and the evaluation require specific skills and understanding of the condition, how the information will be used to recognize its importance and value, and how to collect it appropriately and in an organized manner.[1] Examination and performance of tests are within the scope of practice of both physical therapist assistants and licensed practical/vocational nurses; however, evaluation of the data is a skill that is the purview of licensed physical therapists and registered nurses who have some knowledge of wound management. Simple monitoring of tissue attributes can be performed by unskilled persons after instruction, then reported back to the professional. The purpose of this chapter is to instruct the clinician in the why, who, when, where, what, and how to assess wound attributes leading to a functional diagnosis. Accepted terminology and the significance of each tissue attribute to be assessed are described and illustrated with color plates located in this book. Chapter 5 describes techniques for measurement of size and extent of wounding. Chapter 6, Tools To Measure Wound Healing, teaches how to use two methods to assign numbers or grades to the attributes described in this chapter.

Assessment of the wound and surrounding tissues through examination of various attributes provides data leading to two diagnoses—wound severity and biologic phase of wound healing. Additional examinations that are related to the wound etiology or coimpairments are described in chapters related to specific problems, such as noninvasive vascular testing, management of exudate and infection, management of edema, and therapeutic positioning.

During the initial assessment, the clinician may find that data collected trigger concerns requiring another opinion or a different level of care. For example, the initial assessment may indicate that the patient is not a candidate for sharp debridement because of concerns about circulatory or medical status. The nurse or physical therapist communicates these findings to the referring physician. The term for this is *prospective management*, and physical therapists and nurses are clinicians who have the ability to do prospective management of wound cases. Utilization management begins at baseline and is really prospective management because it is management of services to be delivered to the patient ahead of the actual delivery. Utilization management continues with every follow-up reassessment. At the end of this chapter, referral criteria are discussed. Why list referral criteria in a chapter on assessment? Utilization management mandates that, at the earliest possible time, the patient be diagnosed, appropriate medically necessary services be identified, and proper referral be made. Prospective, appropriate utilization management of health care services is critical under prospective payment and capitated delivery systems.

THE ASSESSMENT PROCESS

Purpose and Frequency

Wound assessment data are collected for four purposes: (1) to examine the severity (stage) of the lesion, (2) to determine the phase of wound healing, (3) to establish a baseline for the wound, and (4) to report observed changes in the wound over time. Assessment data enable clinicians to communicate clearly about a patient's wound, provide for continuity in the plan of care, and allow for evaluation of treatment modalities. Baseline assessment, monitoring, and reassessment are the keys to establishing the plan of care and evaluating achievement of target outcomes and progress toward goals. Valid, significant tests and measurements should be selected for the assessment process. Use the tests selected initially and for each retest throughout the course of care to evaluate progress toward target outcomes and to revise the treatment plan as required.

Attributes are assessed at the initial or baseline examination and at regular intervals, including dressing changes and more completely weekly or, at most, biweekly to measure progress or deterioration of the ulcer. Reassessment is done to measure change in either the status of the ulcer or in risk factors.[2] One study of stage III and stage IV pressure ulcers found that the percentage reduction in the ulcer area after 2 weeks of treatment was predictive of time to heal.[2] Expect improved status in 2–4 weeks.[3] If the reassessment indicates that the wound has deteriorated or has failed to improve with appropriate treatment after 2–4 weeks, the plan of care should be changed and adjunctive treatment considered.

Monitoring is a means of checking the wound frequently for signs and symptoms that may trigger a full reassessment, such as increased wound exudate or bruising of the adjacent or periwound skin. Monitoring includes gross evaluation for signs and symptoms of wound complications, such as erythema (change in color) of periwound skin and pus secondary to infection, and progress toward wound healing, such as granulation tissue growth (red color) and reepithelialization (new skin). Less skill is required for monitoring than for assessment and may be performed by unskilled caregivers, such as the patient's family or a nurse attendant. Monitoring takes place at dressing changes or other treatment application times.

Different care settings will have different requirements and will designate specific individuals to perform the assessment function. For example, in the home setting, the nurse or physical therapist may function as professional wound "case manager," who assesses the findings but may instruct a nonprofessional caregiver in wound attributes to be monitored. The caregiver would gather the data at dressing changes and predetermined intervals and report changes to the professional wound case manager, who would evaluate the results of the treatment plan. The professional wound case manager may see the patient's wound only intermittently for a complete reassessment. In a skilled nursing facility, there are usually requirements by federal licensing agencies that prescribe intervals for reassessment. If the patient is in an acute or subacute setting where there are very short lengths of stay, there may be only a single assessment.

Clinical Wisdom: *Monitoring Wound Progress*

Teach family and other caregivers to *monitor* the wound at each dressing change, looking for signs of wound infection, such as large amounts of purulent exudate (pus), periwound erythema (reddish, purplish), warmth, increased tenderness or pain at the site or elevated temperature, and signs of healing characteristics (bright red color and new skin, small amount of clear drainage).

Attributes to Assess

Evaluation of the severity of the wound by observation of the depth of tissue destruction, tissue response to injury, and signs of wound healing phase are presented. These components are used to provide a wound severity diagnosis and wound healing phase diagnosis. Assessment of the wound is separate from the assessment of the etiology of the wound, although the examinations chosen for the assessment may relate to or provide clues to the etiology. Management of wound etiologies is presented in Part III. For example, wounds with an etiology of venous insufficiency will have characteristics of the adjacent and periwound skin that are different from those of a pressure ulcer. A patient with a diagnosis of diabetic ulcer and insensitivity will have distinctive adjacent skin and tissue characteristics. Therefore, soft tissues adjacent to the area of wounding should be assessed for attributes of sensation, circulation, texture, and color. Findings of the adjacent soft tissues will be useful in determining medical necessity, establishing a treatment plan, and predicting outcomes of care for the wound. *Adjacent* refers to tissues extending away from the periwound. Therefore, it is a good clinical practice to include examination of the adjacent skin characteristics, as well as periwound skin characteristics.

Assessment encompasses a composite of characteristics. A single characteristic cannot provide the data necessary to determine the treatment plan, nor will it allow for monitoring progress or degradation of the wound. The indexes for wound assessment include all of the following: location, age of wound, size of the wound, stage or depth of tissue involvement, presence of undermining or tunneling, presence or absence of tissue attributes not good for healing (such as necrotic tissue in the wound and erythema of the periwound tissue), and attributes good for wound healing, such as condition of the wound edges, granulation tissue, and epithelialization. For many clinicians, the wound exudate characteristics are also essential indexes.

There are two schools of thought regarding tissue assessment. One looks only at the wound tissue. The second examines both the wound tissue and periwound skin and the soft tissue structures. Because the periwound skin is intimately involved in the circulatory response to wounding, as well as the risk for infection, it is prudent to evaluate both areas. The examination of the wound and periwound skin provides the data related to the wound healing phase diagnosis described later in this chapter. Exhibit 4–1 lists the common indexes for wound assessment.

Wound severity attributes to assess include determination of the tissue layers involved in the wound. Wounds that penetrate through more tissue layers are more severe than those that are less deep. This is the wound severity diagnosis. Depth of tissue involvement indicates the wound severity and has an impact on further wound assessment strategies, determination of an appropriate treatment plan, and predicted time to heal. For example, a partial-thickness wound would not be assessed for tunneling or undermining. It also has impact on prediction of risk for nonhealing and on reimbursement. For example, third-party payers know that a stage IV pressure ulcer requires more care and a longer length of stay than does a stage II pressure ulcer and that the risk of

complications is greater. The most commonly used method of diagnosing wound severity is with classification systems.

Wound Classification Systems

At the present time, a variety of wound classification systems is used to describe wound severity for different wound etiology. Although the classification systems were designed and researched with one specific wound type, they are often (sometimes inappropriately) used for any wound type. Although there are many wound classification systems, such as methods of classifying surgical wounds and severity scoring of lower leg ulcers, four wound classification systems are presented in this chapter. The National Pressure Ulcer Advisory Panel (NPUAP) pressure ulcer staging criteria developed for use with pressure ulcers, the Wagner staging system for grading severity of dysvascular ulcers, partial-thickness/full-thickness skin loss criteria, and Marion Laboratories red/yellow/black color system are described and discussed.[5,6] The NPUAP pressure ulcer staging system and the Wagner staging system are classifications based on tissue layers and depth of tissue destruction. The partial-thickness and full-thickness skin loss classifications are tissue layer descriptions of skin loss that are also commonly used. The final method discusses wounds based on color of the tissue. Marion Laboratories in Europe has developed a system that classifies the wound based on the color of the wound surface—red, yellow, or black. The International Consensus Committee on Chronic Venous Disease classification system is presented in Chapter 17, Exhibit 17–3. None of these wound classification systems should be used in reverse as a method of measuring wound healing.

NPUAP Pressure Ulcer Staging System

Classification by stages is used to describe the anatomic depth of soft tissue damage observed after the pathology has declared itself.[5] The pressure ulcer staging system is probably one of the most widely known wound classification systems. The staging system is most often applied to pressure ulcers, but it is used (sometimes inappropriately) to classify other types of wounds, as well. It is best used for wounds with a pressure or tissue perfusion etiologic factor, such as with arterial/ischemic wounds or diabetic neuropathic ulcers. The NPUAP and the Agency for Health Care Research and Quality (AHRQ), formerly known as the Agency for Health Care Policy and Research (AHCPR), used the initial pressure ulcer staging system proposed by Shea[7] as a basis for recommending a universal four-stage system for describing pressure ulcers by anatomic depth and soft tissue layers involved. The pressure ulcer staging system does not describe the entire wound and is limited to a description of the anatomic tissue loss; it is a diagnosis of severity of tissue insult before healing starts. The AHRQ adopted the NPUAP staging system for use in two sets of clinical practice guide-

---

Exhibit 4–1 Indexes for Wound Assessment

- Anatomic location
- Size (length, width)
- Volume: depth (also stage if initial assessment; note if unable to stage)
- Undermining/tunneling
- Age of wound in weeks or months
- Attributes not good for healing: necrotic tissue (including eschar[4]), hemorrhage (purple), periwound erythema and edema, edges not connected
- Attributes good for healing: granulation tissue, new epithelium, attached wound edges
- Wound exudate: color, amount, odor, consistency
- Pain: to touch, anytime, or during treatment
- Temperature: excess warmth, cool, normal body temperature for the area

lines.[3,8] It is widely accepted and commonly used to communicate wound severity, to organize treatment protocols, and as criteria for selection and reimbursement of treatment products for pressure ulcers. Table 4–1 presents the staging criteria for pressure ulcers, including the 1998 revised NPUAP definition of a stage I pressure ulcer.[9]

Clinical Wisdom: *Reverse Staging or Back Staging of Pressure Ulcers*

Once the ulcer is staged, that remains the stage and wound severity diagnosis. Correct terminology is *healing stage II, III, or IV.*

The pressure ulcer staging system is not an ideal system. It has many problems. Staging systems measure only one characteristic of the wound and should not be viewed as a complete assessment that is independent of other indicators. Staging classification systems do not assess for criteria in the healing process and hinder tracking of progress because of the inability of the staging system to demonstrate change over time. The definition of a stage I pressure ulcer does not account for the severity of soft tissue trauma beneath the unbroken skin, such as is seen with purple stage I ulcers. Stage I lesions vary in presentation and pose validity concerns. Some stage I lesions may be the indicator of deep tissue damage just beginning to manifest on the skin, and others may indicate only superficial insult where damage is somewhat reversible and not indicative of underlying tissue death. There are problems with the reliability of assessment of stage I ulcers in dark-skinned patients. In fact, in 1997, the NPUAP new definition of stage I pressure ulcers was developed to reflect better the ethnic diversity of persons with pressure ulcers (see Table 4–1). Not all of the indicators need be present for a stage I diagnosis.[10] Identification and meaningful interpretation of skin color changes in darkly pigmented skin require special assessment strategies. These strategies are described in the section on assessment of the periwound and wound tissues. Also, in Chapter 24, Therapeutic and Diagnostic Ultrasound, an ultrasound scanner that can detect tissue damage and provide early identification of stage I pressure ulcers is described.

Stage II pressure ulcers are lesions that are not necessarily caused by pressure and are more likely due to shearing, friction, or incontinence. The latter should be distinguished and treated in a different manner than pressure ulcers. Theoretically, pressure ulcer trauma starts at the bony tissue interface and works outward, eventually manifesting damage at the skin. However, stage II lesions are usually caused by friction or shearing of the tissues, causing superficial and partial-thickness damage to the epidermis and dermis. Stage II lesions start at the epidermis or skin and may progress to deeper layers.

Staging of pressure ulcers covered by eschar and necrotic tissue cannot be accomplished until removal of necrotic tissue allows determination of the extent of depth of tissue involvement. Pressure ulcers with necrotic tissue filling the wound bed are full-thickness wounds or stage III or stage IV wounds. The clinician cannot determine the level of tissue insult until the necrotic debris is removed. Another difficulty with staging occurs with patients with supportive devices because of the difficulty in accurately assessing the wound without removal of the supportive device. Finally, accurate, meaningful communication is difficult, because clinicians may not have the experience necessary to recognize the various tissue layers that identify the stage or grade. In addition, clinicians may be defining stages differently. Staging requires practice and a certain amount of skill that develops with time spent examining wounds.

Table 4–1 Pressure Ulcer Staging Criteria

Stage	Definition
I*	A stage I pressure ulcer is an observable, pressure-related alteration of intact skin whose indicators as compared to the adjacent or opposite area on the body may include changes in one or more of the following: skin temperature (warmth or coolness), tissue consistency (firm or boggy feel), and/or sensation (pain, itching). The ulcer appears as a defined area of persistent redness in lightly pigmented skin, whereas, in darker tones, the ulcer may appear with persistent red, blue, or purple hues.
II	Partial-thickness skin loss involving epidermis and/or dermis. The ulcer is superficial and presents clinically as an abrasion, a blister, or a shallow crater.
III	Full-thickness skin loss involving damage or necrosis of subcutaneous tissue that may extend down to, but not through, underlying fascia. The ulcer presents clinically as a deep crater with or without undermining of adjacent tissue.
IV	Full-thickness skin loss with extensive destruction, tissue necrosis or damage to muscle, bone, or supporting structures (eg, tendon, joint capsule).

Source: Reprinted with permission from the NPUAP Statement on Reverse Staging of Pressure Ulcers, The Pressure Ulcer Staging System. *NPUAP Report*, Vol. 4, No. 2, September 1995. © National Pressure Ulcer Advisory Panel.

Unfortunately, the staging system has been misinterpreted and applied in clinical practice as a way to monitor healing. It was not designed to do this. Biologically, wounds do not heal in the manner suggested by reversing the staging system. For example, a stage IV pressure ulcer cannot "heal" and become a stage II pressure ulcer. Staging pressure ulcers is used to document the maximum anatomic depth of tissue involved after all necrotic tissue is removed. Staging of pressure ulcers is a diagnostic tool useful to determine the extent of tissue damage only. It is used to aid examination of the *wound severity,* not *wound healing.* Elimination of reverse staging has left a void in the system to report and document wound healing quickly and efficiently. The situation has been complicated because of a reporting system developed by the Health Care Financing Administration (HCFA), requiring that providers continue to reverse stage in order to stay in compliance with HCFA regulations. Specifically, the Minimum Data Set (MDS) developed by HCFA relies on the reverse staging of wounds, both pressure ulcers and venous ulcers, to demonstrate progress of a wound toward healing. This has created a dilemma for the conscientious practitioner. One pragmatic suggestion is to stage for the wound severity at baseline, then, on subsequent reassessment, report decreasing stages as the wound shows attributes of healing (eg, initial stage IV wound has bad-for-healing attributes of eschar, slough, and exposure of tendon, muscle, or bone indicators, progressing to a stage III wound with presence of some good-for-healing attributes—absence of necrosis and presence of granulation tissue—to a stage II reepithelialization beginning and to stage I, healed).[11] Although this is a misuse of the staging system, it does have some merit, and, until there is broad acceptance of a research-based tool to monitor healing and a change in the government reporting system, this may be the only route open to the thoughtful clinician. The MDS post acute care has incorporated the Pressure Ulcer Scale for Healing, monitoring wound healing attributes (see Chapter 6).

Wagner Ulcer Grade Classification

The Wagner Ulcer Grade Classification system is used to establish the presence of depth and infection in a wound. The Wagner grading system was developed for the diagnosis and treatment of the dysvascular foot.[6] It is commonly used as an assessment instrument in the evaluation of diabetic foot ulcers. It is useful for both neuropathic and arterial/ischemic ulcer classification. There are six grades, progressing from 0 to 5 in order of severity. Table 4–2 presents the Wagner grading criteria, and Figure 4–1 shows how the natural history of breakdown in the diabetic, neuropathic foot corresponds to the Wagner 0–5 classification. The 0 classification

Table 4–2 Wagner Ulcer Grade Classification

Grade	Characteristics
0	Preulcerative lesions; healed ulcers; presence of bony deformity
1	Superficial ulcer without subcutaneous tissue involvement
2	Penetration through the subcutaneous tissue; may expose bone, tendon, ligament, or joint capsule
3	Osteitis, abscess, or osteomyelitis
4	Gangrene of digit
5	Gangrene of the foot requiring disarticulation

Source: Reprinted with permission from F.E.W. Wagner, The Dysvascular Foot: A System for Diagnosis and Treatment. *Foot and Ankle,* 2:64–122, © 1981, American Orthopaedic Foot and Ankle Society.

evaluates for predisposing factors leading to breakdown and, along with grades 1–3, is used for risk management, as described in Chapter 20.

Classification by Thickness of Skin Loss

Classification by thickness of skin loss—partial- or full-thickness skin loss—is a classification system commonly used for wounds whose etiology is other than pressure ulcers or neuropathic ulcers, such as skin tears, donor sites, vascular ulcers (venous ulcers in particular), surgical wounds, and burns. Wound thickness refers to partial-thickness or full-thickness loss of the skin, with or without penetration into subcutaneous tissues and deeper structures. Partial-thickness wounds extend through the first layer of the skin or epidermis, and into but not through the second layer of the skin or dermis (1–4 mm). Full-thickness wounds extend through the epidermis, the dermis, and beyond. Wounds deeper than 4 mm are full-thickness wounds and may be further categorized according to depth of involvement by using the term *subcutaneous tissue wounds.* Subcutaneous tissue wounds extend into or through subcutaneous tissues and may extend into muscles, tendons, and possibly down to the bone. Depth of injury classification identifies the specific anatomic level of tissues involved but does not report their condition or color.

Anatomic depth of tissue loss is predictive of healing.[1,12] Partial-thickness wounds heal by epithelialization and heal faster than do full-thickness and subcutaneous wounds. Full-thickness and subcutaneous wounds heal by secondary intention, which is a combination of fibroplasia or granula-

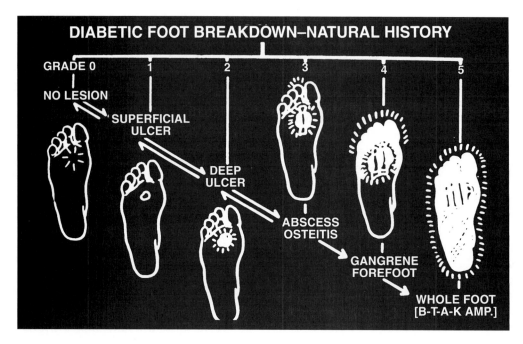

Figure 4–1 Diabetic neuropathic progression of foot breakdown. Courtesy of William Wagner, MD.

tion tissue formation and contraction. Table 4–3 provides the definitions of partial- and full-thickness skin loss.

Marion Laboratories Red, Yellow, Black Wound Classification

Classification by color is a popular system because of the simplicity of the concept and the ease of use of the system. A three-color concept—red, yellow, or black—is used for assessing the wound surface color.[13] The three-color system was originally conceived as a tool to direct treatment, with each color corresponding to specific therapy needs. The red

wound is clean, healing, and granulating. Yellow signals possible infection, need for cleaning or debridement, or the presence of necrotic tissue. Finally, the black wound is necrotic and needs cleaning and debridement. Red is considered most desired, yellow less desirable, and black least desirable. If all three types are present, select the least desirable as the basis for treatment. Table 4–4 shows the red, yellow, and black classification system with clinical manifestations.

The four wound classification systems discussed in this section and the types of wound most appropriate for use with each system are presented in Table 4–5.

Table 4–3 Partial-Thickness and Full-Thickness Skin Loss

Thickness of Skin Loss	Definition	Clinical Examples/Healing Process
Partial-thickness skin loss	Extends through the epidermis, into but not through the dermis	Skin tears, abrasions, tape damage, blisters, perineal dermatitis from incontinence; heal by epidermal resurfacing or epithelialization
Full-thickness skin loss	Extends through the epidermis and the dermis, extending into subcutaneous fat and deeper structures	Donor sites, venous ulcers, surgical wounds; heal by granulation tissue formation and contraction
Subcutaneous tissue wounds	Additional classification level for full-thickness wounds, extending into or beyond the subcutaneous tissue	Surgical wounds, arterial/ischemic wounds; heal by granulation tissue formation and contraction

Table 4–4 Red, Yellow, and Black Wound Classification System

Color	Indication
Red	Clean; healing; granulation
Yellow	Possible infection; needs cleaning; necrotic
Black	Needs cleaning; necrotic

Source: Data from J.Z. Cuzzell, The New RYB Color Code, *American Journal of Nursing*, Vol. 88, pp. 1342–1346, © 1988, American Nurses Association and N.A. Stotts, Seeing Red & Yellow & Black, The Three Color Concept of Wound Care, *Nursing*, Vol. 2, pp. 59–61, © 1990, Springhouse Corporation.

Wound Severity Diagnosis

Nurses use nursing diagnoses to classify skin and tissue impairments and to assist with developing care plans for wound care patients. Nursing diagnoses are expressed as specific diagnostic statements, which include the diagnostic category and the related-to-stem statement. *Impaired tissue integrity* is the broad diagnosis and would be correctly applied to stage III and stage IV pressure ulcers, for example. *Impaired skin integrity* is a subcategory and correctly applies to partial-thickness or full-thickness loss of skin. Impaired skin integrity should not be used for surgical incisions or deep tissue wounds. The diagnosis *risk for infection related to surgical incision* is more appropriate because of the disruption of the skin during surgery, making it more vulnerable to infection. The related-to-stem statements aid in communicating with other health care professionals and in planning care by targeting the defining characteristics for the diagnostic statement. For example, the diagnosis statement *impaired skin integrity* would be followed by a related-to-stem statement, such as *impaired skin integrity related to friction and moisture from urinary incontinence*. For nurses, the related-to-stem statement usually reflects etiologic factors in wound development and directs the plan of care and specific interventions.[14]

Physical therapists will also use a wound severity diagnosis that relates to depth of penetration of wounding. The wound diagnosis statement will have a stem statement *impaired integumentary integrity secondary to———*. The ending part of the statement will include the depth of skin involvement. End statements read *superficial skin involvement* or *partial-thickness skin involvement and scar formation*, *full-thickness skin involvement and scar formation*, or

Table 4–5 Wound Classification Systems and Wound Types

Wound Classification Systems	Pressure Ulcers	Venous Ulcers	Arterial, Ischemic Ulcers	Diabetic Ulcers (Neuropathic)	Other Wounds
NPUAP pressure ulcer stages	X		X (Those with pressure component)	X (Those with pressure component)	Stage II classification will be appropriate for skin tears and tape damage.
Wagner grades		X	X	X	
Depth of skin loss (partial-thickness to full-thickness skin loss)	X If the wound is full thickness, it requires examination of level of deep tissue involvement.	X If the wound is full thickness, it requires examination of level of deep tissue involvement.	X If the wound is full thickness, it requires examination of level of deep tissue involvement.	X If the wound is full thickness, it requires examination of level of deep tissue involvement.	Useful for skin tears, burns, and other skin wounds. If the wound is full thickness, it requires examination of level of deep tissue involvement.
Marion Laboratories red, yellow, and black system	X	X	X	X	Surgical wound is healing by secondary intention.

involvement extending into fascia, muscle, or *bone.* A total statement would read *impaired integumentary integrity secondary to partial-thickness skin involvement and scar formation.*[15] The statement refers to the functional impairment of the integument and different tissues, which has implications for functional impairment and disability. Physical therapists use the severity diagnosis to select examinations, plan treatment, and predict functional outcomes.

Diagnosis statements for both nurses and physical therapists are similar. Both use impairment diagnoses that affect function of the involved tissues.

ASSESSMENT OF WOUND STATUS

Data Collection and Documentation Forms

Information collection is easier, better organized, and more consistent when a form is used as a collection instrument. Forms may be paper-and-pencil instruments or templates on the computer screen. There are many forms being used, with the most common being the skin care flowsheet used by nurses. Methods of recording assessment data should allow for tracking of each assessment item over time, in objective and measurable terms that show changes in the wound status. Two tools, the Pressure Sore Status Tool (PSST) and the Sussman Wound Healing Tool (SWHT), can be used to record the findings and to measure each attribute objectively. Both are described, with forms and instruction provided, in Chapter 6. Useful forms for assessment of tissue will usually include the following items:

- periwound skin attributes
- wound tissue attributes
- wound exudate characteristics

Regardless of which instrument is used to collect findings, all attributes on the form should be considered. If the attribute is not applicable, the notation *N/A* should fill the blank. If an attribute is absent, record a zero. If present, a grade or check is required. Leaving a blank space on the form implies that the attribute was not considered or assessed.

If the patient's medical diagnosis suggests possible related impairments associated with the wound and periwound skin (eg, neuropathy or vascular disease), multiple forms may be required to report all the necessary elements that relate to the patient's condition. Chapter 7, Vascular Evaluation, and Chapter 18, Management of the Neuropathic Foot, have sample forms specific to recording data related to those problems.

Documentation requirements for wound assessment should be part of the facility policies and procedures. Documentation should be accurate and should clearly reflect the patient's condition, the examinations performed, the findings, the care rendered, and proper notification of the physician of significant findings. Documentation of similar findings by practitioners in the same department or facility should be consistent and reflect the facility policies.[16] Remember that someday, maybe 5 years from the time of initial assessment, the medical records may be subpoenaed into court. "Documentation can be either your shield against a potential malpractice lawsuit or the sword that strikes you down."[16(p40)]

Case Study: *Dangers of Differing Clinical Procedure and Facility Policy*

A physical therapist (PT) debrided a toenail on a patient with a medical history of neuropathy associated with diabetes. The toe went on to become infected, leading to below-the-knee amputation of the leg. The PT's action was called into question in a malpractice lawsuit. The debridement procedure followed by the PT was acceptable and documented, but it was the facility policy to have a patient with diabetic neuropathy evaluated in the vascular laboratory for transcutaneous oxygen levels before debridement. The PT did not document anything about evaluating the patient for circulatory status prior to performing the debridement procedure.

Observation and Palpation Techniques

Observation and palpation are classic components of physical diagnosis used to determine alteration in soft tissue characteristics, including the skin, subcutaneous fascia, and muscles leading to a soft tissue or structural diagnosis.[17] Proper lighting and positioning of the patient and tissue to be assessed will improve observation.

Begin the examination of tissues by evaluating for symmetry with the opposite side of the body and adjacent structures, by both observation and palpation. Look for consistency of symmetry of tissues in color, texture, contour, hardness/softness, and temperature that represent changes in the attributes of the skin, subcutaneous tissue, fascia, and muscle, compared with an area of normal skin and soft tissue.

Palpation requires the use of the hands as important sensitive diagnostic instruments. The hands should be clean and the fingernails of appropriate length. It is important for the clinician to develop a palpatory sense in the hands. For example, different parts of the hands are valuable for different tests. The back of the hand is more sensitive to temperature, the palms of the hands are best used to detect changes in tissue contours (induration, edema), and the finger pads are more sensitive to texture (fibrotic tissues) and fine discrimination. The thumbs are useful in applying pressure to check for hardness or softness at different tissue depths. Techniques of palpation include the use of slow, light movements. Avoid pressing too hard and trying to cover the area of examination too quickly. This will provide confusing messages to the sensory receptors of the examiner's hands.

Palpation skills require practice to refine the practitioner's palpatory sense. The first requirement is for the examiner to reduce other sensory inputs in the environment (noise, traffic, conversation), so as to concentrate and focus on the palpation examination. The next requirement is a common language to communicate the findings in easily understood terms. Paired descriptors, such as *superficial-deep, moist-dry, warm-cold, painful-nonpainful, rough-smooth, hard-soft*, and *thick-thin* are useful. The state of tissue changes can be reported as acute, subacute, chronic, or absent. They can also be graded on a scale of 0–3+ as a way of diagnosing the severity of the problem. A familiar example of this type of grading system is pitting edema; another is pulse strength. The use of this type of grading system is also helpful in reporting response to treatment intervention.

Clinical Wisdom: *Four Requirements for Palpatory Examination*

1. Concentration
2. Language to communicate findings
3. Light pressure
4. Slow movement

Assessment of Adjacent Tissues

The tissues adjacent to and surrounding a closed or open wound provide many clues that identify the health of the skin, the phase of wound healing, and the patient's overall health status. For clarity, the term *adjacent* is used to separate the tissues that may not show signs of wounding but that are predictive of healing from the tissues immediately surrounding the wounded tissue, referred to as *periwound skin*. First, it is important to review the anatomy of the skin (Figure 4–2). Skin or trophic changes are important predictors of the body's ability to respond to wounding. The attributes of the adjacent tissues that should be assessed are described in the following sections, including:

- Anatomy of the skin
- Skin texture (eg, dryness, thickness, turgor)
- Scar tissue
- Callus
- Maceration
- Edema
- Color

- Sensation (pain, thermal, touch, protective)
- Temperature
- Hair distribution
- Toenails
- Blisters

Anatomy of the Skin

The skin is composed of two primary layers: the epidermis, which is about 0.04 mm thick, and the dermis, which is about 0.5 mm thick (Figure 4–2). Each of the primary layers is stratified into several layers. The dermis is the true skin. It is tough, flexible, and elastic. The thickness of the skin varies from extremely thin over the eyelids to one-third of an inch thick over the palms of the hands and soles of the feet.

The epidermis is avascular, whereas the dermis is well vascularized and contains the lymphatics, epithelial cells, connective tissue, muscle, fat, and nerve tissue. The vascular supply of the dermis is responsible for nourishing the epidermis and regulating body temperature. The well-vascularized dermis will withstand pressure for longer periods of time than will subcutaneous tissue or muscle. The collagen in the dermis gives the skin its toughness. Hair follicles and sebaceous and sweat glands, located in the dermis, contribute epithelial cells for rapid reepithelialization of partial-thickness wounds. The sebaceous glands are responsible for secretions that lubricate the skin and keep it soft and flexible. They are most numerous in the face and sparse in the palms of the hands and soles of the feet. The sweat gland secretions control skin pH to prevent dermal infections. They are numerous in the soles of the feet and palms of the hands. The three together are referred to as *dermal appendages*. The sweat glands, dermal blood vessels, and small muscles in the skin (responsible for goose pimples) control temperature on the surface of the body. The nerve endings in the skin include receptors for pain, touch, heat, and cold. Loss of the nerve endings in the skin increases risk for skin breakdown by decreasing the tolerance of the tissues to external forces. Nails are also considered appendages of the skin. The deep or reticular layer of the dermis consists of fibroelastic connective tissue that is yellow and composed mainly of collagen. Fibroblasts are present in this tissue layer. The deep layer of the dermis merges with the subcutaneous fat and fascia and may be confused with yellow slough, but it should be evaluated for texture and vitality. A healthy reticular layer will be adhered and firm—not soft, mushy, or stringy, like slough. Often, granulation buds are seen protruding through the mesh of the reticular layer. *Color Plate 17* shows the reticular layer of the dermis, with the red granulation buds poking through the mesh layer in a partial-thickness wound.

Skin color varies greatly in humans, but the structure and the skin are very similar. Melanin produced from melanocytes accounts for the variation in pigmentation from very light to extremely dark. Numbers of melanocytes in dark and

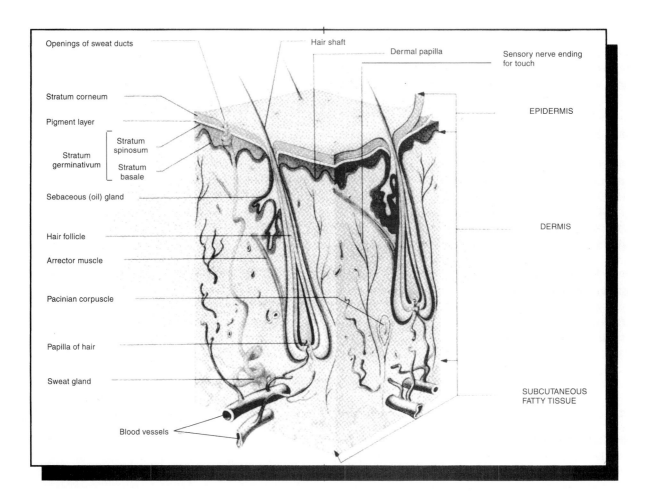

Figure 4–2 Anatomy of the skin. Courtesy of Knoll Pharmaceuticals, Mount Olive, New Jersey.

light skin are similar, but the size and activity of the melanocytes are greater in black skin than in light skin. The melanin pigmentation is concentrated in the stratum corneum layer, in a dark horny layer that can be wiped off when washing clean, black skin. Of course, this does not mean that all the color is removed, just the superficial layer. The thickness of the stratum corneum in both dark and light skin is the same, but the cells in dark skin are more compact, with more cell layers. For this reason, dark skin is more resistant to external irritants. Healthy dark skin is usually smooth and dry. Dry dark skin may have an ashen appearance.[18]

Clinical Wisdom: *Care of Darkly Pigmented Skin*

Care of darkly pigmented skin requires keeping the skin lubricated. Petrolatum, lanolin-based lotions, and sparing use of soaps are recommended.[18]

Skin Texture

Smooth, flexible skin has a feeling of fullness and resistance to tissue deformation that is called *turgor*. Turgor is a sign of skin health. Aging skin often shows signs of dryness due to atrophy and thinning of both the epithelial and fatty layers of tissue in the dermis. The feel of the skin reflects a loss of turgor. The areas most affected by loss of subcutaneous fat are the upper and lower extremities. This thinning of subcutaneous fat results in more prominent bony protuberances on the hips, knees, ankles, and bony areas of the feet, with a higher risk of pressure ulcer formation. Elderly skin also experiences a loss of elasticity due to shrinkage of both collagen and elastin. There is a weakening of the juncture between the epidermis and dermis, making the skin layers "slide" across each other and placing the person at risk for skin tears. Sebaceous glands and their secretions are diminished, resulting in skin that is dry, often itchy, and easily torn.[19] Impaired circulation also contributes to changes in the skin; it is usually associated with aging but may be due to a disease process, such as neuropathy associated with diabetes. Neuropathy impairs the secretion of sweat and sebaceous glands. Death of sweat and sebaceous glands contributes to slow resurfacing of partial-thickness dermal ulcers. Loss of sweat changes the pH of the skin, making it more susceptible to infection and bacterial penetration.

To assess skin texture, the clinician uses observation and palpation. Observe the skin, looking for evidence of dryness, such as flaking or scaling. To check skin turgor, gently pick up the tissues with thumb and forefinger, and observe how the tissues respond. For example, in older patients, loss of elasticity may be exhibited by the tissues' slow return to normal after pinching. In older patients it is best to check for general skin turgor on the forehead or sternal area. Palpate by gently rubbing your fingers across the patient's skin and feel for sliding of the epidermis away from the dermis.

Clinical Wisdom: *Skin Texture Assessment*

Observe skin for moisture content; look for evidence of dryness, such as flaking, scaling, and excoriations (linear scratches). Palpate the skin to assess turgor; gently grasp the tissues between thumb and forefinger, and observe for any delay in the tissues' return to normal position. Finally, rub your fingers across the patient's skin and feel the sliding of the epidermis from the dermis, due to weakened epidermal-dermal juncture.

Scar Tissue

Inspection of the adjacent skin should include checking for scar tissue. Check scar for smoothness, flexibility, thickness, and toughness. Scar tissue that is mature has greater density and toughness, and it is less resilient than surrounding skin. New scar tissue is thinner and more flexible than mature scar tissue and is less resilient to stress. Wounding in an area of scarring will have less tensile strength when healed than will a new wound and will be more likely to break down (see *Color Plate 39*).

New scar tissue will be bright pink. As the scar tissue matures, it will become nearly the same color as the periwound skin, except in persons with darkly pigmented skin. Hypopigmentation frequently follows injuries to dark skin. Loss of skin color may create more anxiety for the individual than the wound itself. If the wounding disruption is less than full-thickness loss of the epidermis, repigmentation will usually occur over time. However, new skin covering deeper lesions and new lesions will appear pink.[20] The area of scar may even turn white. Hypopigmented areas are more susceptible to sunburn than are normally pigmented areas. For some

individuals, burns and physical trauma may be followed by localized areas of hyperpigmentation. Like hypopigmentation, hyperpigmentation leads to anxiety for many individuals.

Observe for abnormal scarring characteristics. Hypertrophic scarring results from excessive collagen deposition, causing a very thick scar mass that remains within the area of the original wound. These scars are ugly and disfiguring, and may be bothered by itching or pain that may interfere with functional mobility (see *Color Plates 48*).

These scars are differentiated from keloid scars, which are also thickened scars but extend beyond the boundaries of the original wound (see *Color Plate 50*).[21] Although keloids are known in persons of all races, scarring is of special concern to African American persons and some Asians, as opposed to other dark-skinned individuals, because of frequency of keloid formation in this population, thus suggesting a genetic factor. Frequency of occurrence is equal among men and women. Keloids are like benign tumor growths. Keloids continue to grow long after the wound is closed and may reach large size. Any attempt to cut or use dermabrasion to buff away the keloid will result in even more scarring.[20] The mechanism of collagen deposition is totally out of control. Areas with keloids may be itchy and may be tender or painful.[18] New therapies are being used to control this phenomenon, but if a patient reports having had this problem or reports a familial tendency to form keloids, special attention should be made to address this problem at the time of initial assessment.

Hyperkerototic scarring is hypertrophy of the horny layer of the epidermis. It is commonly seen in diabetic patients and may be located in adjacent and periwound tissue (see *Color Plate 24* and Chapter 18). See Chapter 13, Management of Scar, for more information about scar tissue.

Callus

The most commonly encountered calluses occur on the plantar surface of the foot. They are usually found along the medial side of the great toe, over the metatarsal heads, and around the heel margin. Callus formation is a protective function of the skin to shearing forces of a prominent bone against an unyielding shoe surface. Neuropathy often leads to muscle imbalance and subsequent uneven weight distribution along the metatarsal heads, resulting in callus formation in those areas. The location of the callus is a clue to the underlying bony pathologic condition.[22] Untreated, the callus buildup will continue, creating additional shear forces between the bony prominence and soft tissues and resulting in breakdown of the interposing soft tissues. Hemorrhaging seen on a callus indicates probable ulceration beneath. Callus is an indicator of need for further assessment of the foot. Chapter 18 contains more information about callus management and pictures of callus.

Clinical Wisdom: *Observation and Palpation of Callus*

The callus will appear as a thickened area on the sole of the foot, and it will usually be lighter in color (often yellow), when compared with the adjacent areas. When palpated, the callus area will feel firm or hard to the touch. There may also be some scaling or flaking, roughness, or cracking of the callus. Cracked callus is a portal for infection. Further examination is recommended.

Maceration

Maceration is defined as "the softening of a tissue by soaking until the connective tissue fibers are so dissolved that the tissue components can be teased apart."[19(p198)] Macerated skin is drained of its pigment and has a white appearance and a very soft, sometimes soggy texture (see *Color Plate 15*). The skin is often described as being wrinkled like a prune. A familiar example is "dishpan hands." Softened tissue is easily traumatized by pressure and is a contributing factor in the development of pressure ulcers.[19] The source of moisture that soaks and macerates the skin may be perspiration, soaking in a tub, wound exudate, or incontinence, as well as wound dressing products. Macerated skin will be thinner than adjacent skin. Palpate very gently, so as to avoid trauma. Protect from pressure and shear.

Edema

Presence of edema may be associated with the inflammatory phase, the result of dependence of a limb, or an indication of circulatory impairment or congestive heart failure. *Edema* is defined as fluid excess in the tissues due to overload of interstitial or intracellular fluid, causing congestion. A consequence of trauma is increased extracellular fluids in the tissues that both block the lymphatic system and cause increased capillary permeability. The function of edema following injury is to block the spread of infection. The result is a swelling that is hard, and the application of pressure to the swollen area does not distort the tissues. The term *brawny edema* refers to this type of swelling and is associated with the inflammatory phase. Traumatic edema is usually accompanied by pain. Swelling resulting from lymphedema or from systemic causes is usually painless.[23]

There are two types of edema—nonpitting and pitting. Nonpitting edema is identified by skin that is stretched and shiny, with hardness of underlying tissues. Pitting edema is identified by firmly pressing a finger down into the tissues and waiting 5 seconds. When pressure is released, if tissues fail to resume the previous position and an indentation remains, there is pitting edema. Pitting edema is observed when there is tissue congestion associated with congestive heart failure, venous insufficiency, and lymphedema; or dependence of a limb. It is measured on a severity scale of 0–3+, where 0 = not present, 1+ = minimal, 2+ = moderate, and 3+ = severe.

Evaluate for body symmetry when examining for edema; also refer to the patient's medical history. Bilateral edema of the lower extremities can be a sign of a systemic problem, such as congestive heart failure, cirrhosis, malnutrition, or obesity, or it may be caused by dependence or use of certain drugs. Drug-induced edema is often pitting edema and may be caused by hormonal drugs, including corticosteroids, estrogens, progesterones, and testosterone. Other drugs to consider include nonsteroidal antinflammatory and antihypertensive drugs. Symptoms usually resolve if the drug is withdrawn.[23] Systemic edema may extend from the lower extremities up into the abdomen. Unilateral edema of the lower extremity of sudden onset may be due to acute deep vein thrombophlebitis and requires immediate referral to the physician. Other causes of unilateral edema are chronic venous insufficiency, lymphedema, cellulitis, abscess, osteomyelitis, Charcot's joint, popliteal aneurysm, dependence, and revascularization. Deep vein thrombophlebitis, chronic venous insufficiency, and lymphedema are the three most common causes.[23] If in doubt about the etiology of the edema, consult with the physician before planning further testing or an intervention. If edema is left in the tissue, the large protein molecules will clog the lymphatic channels and cause fibrosis. Chapter 10, Management of Edema, describes the management of edema with compression.

Measurement of Edema. Tissue volume increases when edema is present. Edema can be evaluated by palpation for change in contour of the tissues and by photographs. Two methods used for measurement of the extent of edema formation are girth and volume. Girth measurement of the limb is the most common method used in clinical practice because it is simple to perform. Although limbs are most easily measured, the torso can also be assessed for edema by taking girth measurements. Volumetric measurement is made by using water displacement. This is a quick and accurate measurement, using a volumometer filled with water. Volumometers are made of a heavy Lucite and come in different sizes for immersion of a foot and ankle, leg above the knee, or a hand (see Figure 4–3). They are strong and durable. Both methods work best when edema in a limb is being measured.

A simple form, such as Exhibit 4–2, either handwritten or preprinted, listing the measurements of both limbs side by side is a useful guide for consistency and completeness of the measurements and for making comparison between baseline and retest measurements quick and easy. Change in edema measurements is one way to assess the treatment outcomes.

3. Measure both limbs.
4. Record measurements (for both limbs) side by side. Repeat at next assessment. Compare.

The procedure for volume displacement measurements is as follows:

1. Fill volumometer with tepid water (about 95° F).
2. Immerse the affected extremity into water.
3. Catch overflow in a graduated cylinder to measure volume displaced.
4. Repeat with both limbs.
5. Record volume displacements to both limbs side by side on a form.

Target Outcomes for Edema Interventions. The edema will be absent, reduced, or controlled. Baseline girth or volume measurements were larger for the affected limb or area at baseline and are now equal to or closer to the measurements of the unaffected limbs.

If both limbs are affected, it will not be possible to do an opposite limb comparison. Measurements will be compared with the same limb or area. Palpation and observation, as well as decreased measurements, are used for evaluating change in edema. Change in severity of the pitting edema would be another measurement to report change in edema. Controlled edema means that, following an initial reduction, the edema has not returned to the prior level but remains in the tissues.

Edema Increased. Edema is increased when retested girth or volume measurements are *increased* in the affected

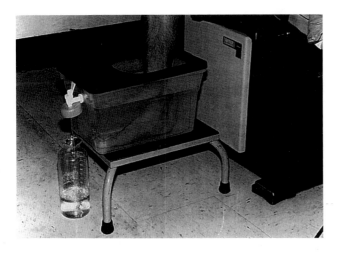

Figure 4–3 Volumetric edema measurement. *Source:* Reprinted with permission from G.M. Pennington, D.L. Danley, and M.H. Sumko. Pulsed, Non-Thermal, High-Frequency Electromagnetic Energy (DIAPULSE) in the Treatment of Grade I and Grade II Ankle Sprains. *Military Medicine: The Official Journal of AMSOS.* Vol. 158, No. 2, p. 102, © 1993, Association of Military Surgeons of the United States.

The procedure for girth measurements is as follows:

1. Mark and record the bony landmarks on the limb to guide the measurements, including the metatarsal heads, both malleoli, 3 cm above the lateral malleolus, 12 cm above the lateral malleolus, 18 cm above the lateral malleolus, and the lower edge of the patella.
2. Use a flexible tape measure to measure the circumference around these landmarks.

Exhibit 4–2 Lower Extremity Girth Measurements Form

Date						
	Right	Left	Right	Left	Right	Left
Locations: Metatarsal heads						
Both malleoli						
3 cm ↑ lateral malleolus						
12 cm ↑ lateral malleolus						
18 cm ↑ lateral malleolus						
Lower edge of patella						

limb, compared with the unaffected limb or area, when compared with baseline. Again, if both limbs are affected, it will not be possible to do an opposite limb comparison. Palpation and observation, as well as increased girth measurements, will need to be used for evaluating change in edema. The skin will be taut and the tissues hard and uncompressible. Increased edema could be an indication of change from absence of the inflammation phase to the acute inflammation phase. The increased edema would be accounted for by increased perfusion to the tissue. This edematous reaction may be more appropriately palpated than measured by instruments. The edema should be transitory and reduce as the inflammation phase passes.

Color

Assessment of adjacent skin color is a clue to skin circulation and disruptions in circulation associated with trauma or infection. Skin color tones reflect the condition of underlying blood vessels. In lightly pigmented skin, pressure closes capillaries and induces a blanching of the skin color that returns to normal color tones when pressure is released. If the color does not return to the color of the adjacent skin within 20 minutes after removal of pressure, this is called *unblanchable erythema*. Unblanchable erythema in lightly pigmented skin is redness that does not disappear when pressure is removed. Histology of unblanchable erythema shows erythrostasis in the capillaries and venules, followed by hemorrhage (see *Color Plates 14, 15, and 16* for unblanchable erythema).[24] The same indexes cannot be used in darkly pigmented skin.

Color Assessment for Darkly Pigmented Skin.
Identification of stage I pressure ulcers historically has relied heavily on color changes in the skin. Erythema may be seen in some situations in lighter-toned persons of color, but in darkly pigmented skin, the redness may not be seen.[20] *Darkly pigmented skin* is defined as skin tones that "remain unchanged (does not blanch) when pressure is applied over a bony prominence, irrespective of the patient's race or ethnicity."[25(p35)] Darkly pigmented skin is usually found in African Americans, Africans, Caribbeans, Hispanics, Asians, Pacific Islanders, Middle Easterners, Native Americans, and Eskimos. When assessment is made of darkly pigmented skin in patients with high risk for pressure ulcers, careful attention should be paid to color changes at sites located over bony prominences. Look for color changes that differ from the patient's usual skin color (as described by the patient or those who are familiar with the patient's usual skin color, or as observed in an area of healthy tissue).[25] Consider conditions that can cause changes in skin color, such as vasoconstriction (pallor) caused by lying on a cold surface or hyperemia (redness or deepening of skin tones) from lying on a bony prominence. Allow the area to be exposed to ambient room temperature for 5–10 minutes before examining. When darkly pigmented skin is inflamed, the site of inflammation becomes darker and appears bluish or purplish (eggplant-like color; see *Color Plates 19* and *21*). This is comparable to the erythema or redness seen in persons with lighter skin tones.[25] Change in color, as mentioned, is an indicator of hemorrhage of the microvasculature in the skin and may also be an indicator of deep tissue trauma that will later rupture and form a crater. When there is an extremely high melanin content, the color of the skin may be so dark that it is hard to assess changes in color at all.[19]

Another complicating factor in identifying erythema in darkly pigmented skin is differentiating inflammation from the darkening of the skin caused by hemosiderin staining. Hemosiderin staining usually occurs close to the wound edges, whereas injury-related color changes usually extend out a considerable distance and are accompanied by the other signs of inflammation. *Color Plate 10* shows hemosiderin staining at the margins of a wound in a dark-skinned person. Hemosiderin staining is a symptom of wound chronicity or repeated injury. The mechanism of hemosiderin staining is described later.

Color changes are apparent around acute (inflamed) and chronic open wounds (pigmentation). If color is not a reliable indicator, use other clinical indicators, such as sensation (pain), temperature (heat or coolness), or tissue tension (edema or induration and hardness) to confirm the diagnosis of inflammation in darkly pigmented skin.

Assessment of tissue circulatory status by use of color is also difficult in darkly pigmented skin. Consider the effects of gravity on vasomotor changes in the tissues of the extremities in elevated and dependent positions. Color changes will appear more subtle than those in light skin. Assess from a neutral position, then with the area elevated about 15° and dependent for about 5 minutes and compare.[26] Assessment of capillary refill time for persons with darkly pigmented skin should be tried at the tips of the second or third fingers.[13] Also consider examining the nail beds. If they are not pigmented, apply pressure to the second or third finger; if the skin under the nail blanches, it will give a color comparison for assessing pallor or cyanosis. The speed of color return following the slow release of pressure is an indicator of the quality of vasomotor function. The slower the return of color, the more diminished is the vasomotor function. Compare the speed of return with that in your own nail bed or that of another person with normal vascularity.[26]

Assessment should be made with good lighting. Avoid fluorescent light, which casts a blue color to the skin. Use natural or halogen lighting to assess skin tones. Flash photographs are recommended because the flash makes the demarcation between normal skin tones and those that are traumatized easier to see, and the picture provides a visual record of the patient's skin status.[25] Notice the demarcation between the normal skin tones and the traumatized area in *Color Plate 19*. The patient or family member who is familiar with the patient's natural skin tones should be the primary person to provide information relative to skin color changes.

Ecchymosis (Hemorrhage). Trauma to the skin and sub-cutaneous tissue causes rupture of the blood vessels and sub-cutaneous bleeding or hemorrhage, called *ecchymosis*. Ecchymosis is seen as a purple discoloration in white skin and a deepening to a purple color in darkly pigmented skin. In the literature, these have been described as "purple ulcers."[27] Purple ulcers cannot be classified according to the NPUAP staging system, and the significance of these ulcers is seldom recognized. The skin over the hemorrhagic area may be taut, shiny, and edematous (see *Color Plate 32*). It may be intact or rubbed off.[27] The purple ulcer has been described as the end stage of nonblanchable erythema, and it always signifies full-thickness skin loss. Biopsy specimens of the purple ulcer show hemorrhage and early gangrenous changes.[28] Hemorrhage and clotting occur as a consequence of an acute injury, such as trauma from pressure, a bump, or shearing, and includes trauma to new granulation tissue, as well as venous leakage from venous insufficiency (see *Color Plate 74*). Clotting cuts off oxygen to the tissues, with subsequent hypoxia and ischemia. If the blood is not reabsorbed into the tissues in a timely fashion, tissue necrosis will occur. It is not known exactly how long clotted blood can remain in the tissues before necrosis occurs. In most cases, these ulcers are not reversible. Witkowski[28] described a topical regimen using locally applied nitrates to cause vasodilation and de-creased adhesion and aggregation of cells, along with sys-temically administered hemorrheologic agents, to clinically reverse the process. Electrical stimulation, pulsed radio fre-quency stimulation, and ultrasound facilitate reabsorption of hemorrhagic materials, if started soon after injury (eg, 48–72 hours). Efficacy studies reported in the literature and pho-tographs that show the effects of these interventions are de-scribed in Chapters 21, 22, and 24. Case studies with color photos are shown in *Color Plates 74–79*.

Rupture of the vessels around a wound and seepage from venous hypertension cause deposition of blood in the subcu-taneous tissues. The blood stains the tissues by deposition of hemosiderin from lysed red blood cells and turns the skin a rust brown color that is called *hemosiderosis*. Hemosiderosis is seen as a ring around pressure ulcers (see *Color Plate 2*) or as the brown discoloration of the skin of the lower leg in patients with venous disease (see *Color Plates 55* and *56*). The discoloration may be permanent or it may gradually dis-appear.

Sensation

Sensory testing procedures and expected outcomes are de-scribed in this section. They include pain, protective sensa-tion, and thermal sensation.

Pain. New accreditation standards require that every pa-tient's pain be measured regularly and proper relief sup-plied[29]. Severe pain or tenderness, either within or around the wound, may indicate the presence of infection, deep tissue destruction, or vascular insufficiency. Use of a pin to test for pain sensation is considered outdated and is not rec-ommended. Absence of pain or insensitivity to touch and temperature may indicate neuropathy. Sometimes, pain-level reports are more a report of anxiety than pain. Observation of movements by the patient in the area of reported pain and reaction to gentle palpation are useful in distinguishing be-tween the two.

Ideally, the best and most reliable way to determine the intensity of pain is by report of the patient. Of course, this is not always possible. Several methods can be used to test and retest for pain. Retesting is very important if one of the ex-pected outcomes from treatment is pain reduced, eliminated, or controlled. Use the same testing measures before and after the use of an intervention. Commonly used tests for pain in-clude pain questionnaires that are either verbal or pictorial, visual analog scale, pain diary, or palpation and observation, for those who cannot communicate except by response to noxious stimuli.

Testing with a Pain Questionnaire. If the patient can communicate verbally, ask the patient to describe the pain. Guiding questions would include the following:

- Where is the pain?
- When do you have the pain? How long does it last?
- What type of pain do you have? Is it burning, throbbing, cramping, or prickling?
- Does the pain affect your sleep?
- Does it affect your mood?
- Do you take medication for the pain? What do you take?
- What are the effects of the medication?
- What positions or activities affect the pain?

For those who cannot communicate verbally but who can understand and respond, cue with questions such as, Can you show me where it hurts? Does it feel like it is burning?

In noncommunicating patients, observe during guided movement and palpation for facial grimacing, tenseness, and/or withdrawal response to noxious stimuli. For children and adults, use facial pictures to rate pain.

Testing with a Visual Analog Scale. A visual analog scale (Exhibit 4–3) is a line marked with 10 perpendicular lines and numbered 0–10, where 0 = no pain and 10 = the worst pain imaginable. Ask the patient to give a number on the line or point to a number to indicate pain severity. Record. This is a common procedure for assessing pain severity. It can be repeated to determine change in pain severity as a measure of treatment effect. Reliability may be questionable. Patients with either very high or very low pain thresholds may more accurately report pain level by another method.

Exhibit 4–3 Visual Analog Scale for Pain Measurement

0	1	2	3	4	5	6	7	8	9	10

Keeping a Pain Diary. The patient or caregiver can record the information on a pain diary form, such as Exhibit 4–4. This will be a valuable tool to measure change in pain over time and will provide feedback to the patient that pain is altered. If test results indicate that pain is present and is a problem, management of the pain with an intervention would be indicated, with a target outcome of pain free, pain reduced, or pain controlled. A change in pain status will be a functional outcome if there is a change in the patient's functional activities as a result of the change in pain status, such as the patient being able to tolerate active assistive range of motion to the wounded area and being able to sit up in a wheelchair.

Outcome measures to report after an intervention for pain management include the following:

- Pain free—the patient is pain free by observation or report of the patient or caregiver.
- Tension free—tissue tension reduction is tested by palpation or by checking for increased mobility of the area.
- Pain medication free—the patient may no longer require pain medication, or the amount or frequency may be reduced.
- Sleeping—the patient's pain is controlled and he or she has more hours of undisturbed sleep.
- Unreactive (to noxious stimuli)—the patient no longer responds to movement or palpation that previously produced pain.

Clinical Wisdom: *Premedication for Pain*

Response to the pain testing will guide the clinician about the need to premedicate the patient before performing a procedure. Sometimes, relaxation and anti-anxiety medication will be more appropriate than pain medication.

Protective Sensation. If neuropathy is suspected by medical history or observation, testing for sensation is indicated. A safe, accurate method for testing sensation has been developed using Semmes-Weinstein monofilaments. The monofilaments come in different force levels. Levels 4.17, 5.07, and 6.10 are used to check for protective sensation. Force levels increase as the numbers increase. The object of the test is to see whether the patient can detect pressure when the monofilament is placed against the skin and force applied that is sufficient to buckle the monofilament. Testing is usually performed on the sole of the foot. The procedure for measurement of sensation with Semmes-Weinstein monofilaments is as follows:

1. Start by applying to the sole of the foot.
2. Place the monofilament against skin.
3. Apply pressure until the filament buckles.
4. Ask the patient to identify where the monofilament was applied.

The patient should be able to detect the monofilament at the time it buckles.

The inability to detect the 5.07-level monofilament indicates a limited ability to use protective sensations. If the patient can distinguish this level of sensation at several points on the feet, the protective sensation is considered to be adequate to avoid risk of trauma.[30] A photograph of Semmes-Weinstein filaments and the appropriate interventions for patients with loss of protective sensation are given in Chapter 18.

Thermal Sensation. The test for thermal sensation is performed by using test tubes or small narrow bottles filled with warm and cold water. Be sure to test in a normal area before applying to possible insensate areas to avoid burns. Research reports that the lateral aspect of the foot is the area most sensitive to thermal sensation.[31] If the patient is unable to sense warmth, there will be a high risk of burns if heat is applied to

Exhibit 4–4 Pain Diary Form

Date	Time	Location	Activity	Pain intensity	Medication	Other symptoms

the skin. If the patient is unable to sense cold, there is a risk of injury from exposure to cold; the feet should be protected from frostbite if the patient is going to be exposed to very cold temperatures.

Research Wisdom

A patient may have unapparent mild core hypothermia that will affect wound healing and resistance to infection. Taking the tympanic membrane temperature is an accurate measure of core body temperature.[32]

Temperature

Adjacent Skin Temperature. Baseline skin temperature is one objective measurement of circulation that can be used to monitor circulatory response to treatment or to evaluate inflammation. Local body temperature can be tested by palpation or with a liquid crystal skin thermometer. Thermography using a liquid crystal skin thermometer is a semiquantitative method produces multicolor picture maps of the wound and adjacent tissues. These devices have good reliability and have been clinically tested for evaluation of primary wound healing status of surgical wounds. The method is quick, simple, reliable, and inexpensive to use.[32] Liquid crystal strips are available with different temperature ranges. Warm colors, such as brown and red, correspond to lower temperature and deep blue to highest temperatures. The color of the liquid crystal strip changes color in a few seconds after placing it on the tissue. It is easy to notice changes in the wound temperature during the first 8 postoperative days. During the first 3 postoperative days, the temperature of the wound and the adjacent tissues is the same, but by post operative day 4, there should be a discernible change, with the temperatures of the wound and surrounding tissues decreasing gradually. Zones of warmth around the wound become narrower, with sharply pronounced greater warmth over the incision than in the surrounding tissues. The heat measured in adjacent skin areas is not an inflammatory reaction but is reactive hyperemia. Hyperemia is the consequence of humoral substances released from cellular damage at the time of wounding—chiefly histamine—and pain that triggers neurogenic reactions, including vasodilatation.[32] Only a narrow zone adjacent to the wound represents inflammation. During the early postoperative period, the two areas are indistinguishable from one another. As the wound heals, the area of warmth narrows, decreases in temperature, and represents the area of true inflammation. Wound temperature depends on the degree of vascularity of the tissues: A higher grade of vascularity will result in a higher tissue tempera-

ture.[32] If the expected outcomes (that the wound and adjacent skin temperatures decrease by the fourth postoperative day) are not met, this indicates that the wound is not healing by primary intention and that secondary healing is imminent because of tissue necrosis or bacterial contamination.[32] If greater accuracy is required or temperature at a greater tissue depth is desired, there are several commercial instruments available. A thermistor is the least costly of the three commercial devices described here for measurement of skin surface temperature. A probe is placed against the skin and a reading taken. Another device is a radiometer, which determines temperature by measurement of surface reflection of infrared radiation. The thermistor and the infrared scanner, however, could be used in the clinic easily with minimal training. Use of the infrared scanner is described in Chapter 18.

Use of an inexpensive (about $2) liquid crystal skin fever thermometer strip that changes color with temperature change is a simple and useful way to assess the temperature of periwound skin. This is best done in areas that have adequate circulation, such as on the trunk. It is more sensitive to changes in temperature than the back of the hand, although not sensitive enough to record temperatures below 95° F (35° C), which are found in the distal parts of extremities. Skin fever thermometers usually have six thermochromic liquid crystal indicator lights in shades of brown, tan, green, and blue that respond to temperature shifts. To read the temperature, use the *highest* temperature window indicated by a color. Skin temperature is shown in 1° F intervals. The normal skin temperature in areas of good circulation is usually about 95° F. An increase in temperature of the surrounding skin measured on the fever thermometer, compared with adjacent area temperature, is an indication of an area of circulatory perfusion. This is the heat described as a classic sign of inflammation. Absence of an increase in periwound skin temperature from adjacent skin can be used as an indicator of wound chronicity. Skin temperature below 95° F (35° C) will not record on this type of thermometer. Other, more sensitive tests for temperature or blood flow should be considered.

Skin temperature is a useful measure for assessing many kinds of wounds, including surgical wounds, as described, and stage I pressure ulcers. An increase in skin temperature may indicate pressure ulcer formation over a bony prominence or the presence of infection, such as an abscess. It is a very useful tool for assessing inflammation and wounding in darkly pigmented individuals, in whom the margins of erythema are hard to see. Skin temperature can be taken at locations on the margins of discoloration and at the center over the bony prominence. The clock method, taking the temperature at the 12-, 3-, 6-, and 9-o'clock positions around the wounded tissue, is useful for recording this measurement when the wound is large. For small wounds, measure across the wound. The procedure for measuring skin temperature is as follows:

1. Make sure that the area of skin to be tested has been pressure free and exposed to ambient air temperature for at least 5–10 minutes before testing its temperature (a sheet can cover the patient for privacy).
2. Dry the skin of sweat before each measurement because moisture on the skin considerably modifies the image.[32]
3. Place a single layer of plastic against the skin as a hygienic barrier (this does not interfere with temperature accuracy).
4. Lay temperature strip flat on the plastic barrier.
5. Hold the strip in place at both ends lightly, so as not to compress capillaries, and wait for color of strip to change color. Allow at least 1 full minute for the color change to occur. In very inflamed tissues, it may occur immediately but may change further as it is held for the full minute.
6. Read the temperature while the strip is still against the skin.
7. For large wounds, measure at the wound edge at the 12- and the 6-o'clock positions and near the expected outer margin of the periwound erythema/discoloration. Repeat at the 3- and the 9-o'clock positions.
8. For small wounds, measure by placing the liquid crystal strip across the wound diameter.
9. Record temperature at each point.

Interventions are used to affect tissue perfusion and, thus, skin temperature. Skin temperature would be expected to increase if there is enhanced perfusion and vasodilation following superficial heating with whirlpool. Temperature changes in deeper tissues may occur following pulsed short-wave diathermy. However, the fever strip may not be sufficiently sensitive to measure any of these changes. If that is the case, the thermistor or infrared scanner thermometer is recommended. To measure the effects of an intervention, take a baseline measurement before treatment and repeat the measurement after treatment. Skin temperature should rise after treatment. If there is an expectation for hyperemia and mild inflammation, and the target outcome is to initiate the acute inflammation phase, measurement of tissue temperatures would help to verify the outcome.

Coolness also can be used as an assessment of circulation. Sometimes, there is an initial increase in skin temperature, followed by coolness after trauma. Like warmth, coolness without trauma may be an indicator of circulatory status. Some areas of the body naturally have less warmth, including the feet, toes, and fingers. The areas of the trunk or over well-perfused muscle tissues have greater warmth. If there is coolness in the digits or the feet, it is important to evaluate other signs and symptoms, such as hair growth, skin color, pulses, and skin texture for circulation. If those signs are also suggestive of circulatory impairment, they should trigger further circulatory examination, as described in Chapter 7. Coolness may also be an indicator of impaired tissue viability or tissue death following ischemia. A quantitative measure of tissue temperature as part of the assessment of wounds is not yet a standard of clinical practice. Articles appear in journals that describe temperature measurement as a useful method of assessment for inflammatory processes.[32–37] All of the procedures described are simple, noninvasive, and quick but, most importantly, have clinical significance and are more reliable than clinical observation alone.[32]

Hair Distribution

Normal body hair is distributed over all four extremities, extending down to the digits. Over time, body hair diminishes and is eventually lost. A diminished presence of hair is seen in aging skin or where there is impaired circulation. As circulation in a leg decreases, hair is lost distally. Hair distribution may be used as an indicator of the level of vascular impairment and an indication for vascular testing. Hair follicles are important to wound healing because they contribute epidermal cells for resurfacing partial-thickness wounds. Absence of hair should be considered a factor in the prognosis of wound healing if there is a partial-thickness wound in an area where hair is usually found, such as the lower leg.

Clinical Wisdom: *Assessment of Hair Distribution as an Indicator of Peripheral Circulation*

1. An easy checkpoint for adequate tissue perfusion to the lower extremities is examination of the great toe for hair growth. Hair growth on the great toes implies adequate circulation to support the hair follicles. When working with female patients, prior to examination, remember to ask whether they shave the hair on the great toe.
2. Move up the leg proximally from the ankle and assess the most distal point where hair distribution stops. Then palpate for skin temperature and pulses, and observe skin color in the area denuded of hair for circulatory changes.

Toenails

Part of a comprehensive examination of the feet includes not only the skin but also the toenails. Look at the color, thickness, shape, and any irregularities. Toenail pathology commonly seen includes hypertrophic, thick nails. Some toenails may look like a ram's horn. Ingrown toenails and fungal and pseudomonas infection, which give the toenail a green color, may be observed. Chapter 19, Management of the Skin and Nails, has a complete guide to assessment of the feet and nails. Findings of toenail abnormalities are referral criteria unless the clinician has knowledge and training in foot and nail care.[38]

Blisters

Trauma to the epidermis gives rise to a blister. The blister may be filled with clear fluid or, if the trauma is deeper than the epidermis and ruptures blood vessels, the blister fluid may be bloody or brown (see *Color Plate 77*). The blister roof is nature's best dressing, but it can hide deep tissue damage. Removal of the blister roof is controversial. If the blister fluid is clear, tissue damage may not extend into the dermis or deeper, and the wound will heal under the blister roof; the epidermis will eventually just fall off. It should not be disturbed and, in fact, may require protection. However, if the fluid is bloody, brown, or cloudy, as shown in *Color Plate 77*, deep tissue damage may be present, and unroofing the blister may be the only way to determine the extent of trauma, as shown in *Color Plate 78*. Ultrasound technology to identify depth of tissue edema and trauma, such as under a blister, is being tested with good outcomes. More on this technology is found in Chapter 24 and in *Color Plates 71–73*.

Assessment of the tissue under the blister without breaking the blister is helpful in evaluating when the blister needs to be unroofed. Gently press down with a fingertip on the tissue beneath the blister roof and compress it; release, and feel for the resiliency of the subcutaneous tissues. If there is good resilience, ie, it bounces back when the pressure is removed, the deep tissues may be mildly congested, but if the tissue feels soft, spongy, or boggy, there is high probability of tissue congestion and probable necrosis. Practice and careful concentration are needed to perform this palpation examination. One tip is to try pressing down on the skin on the opposite side of the body in the same location (eg, on the heel) and compare the resiliency when compressed.

ASSESSMENT OF THE PERIWOUND AND WOUND TISSUES

Assessment of the periwound and wound tissues is described in the following sections, according to clinical signs and symptoms that would be expected in each wound healing phase. There is a close relationship between assessment of the wound and periwound tissues and diagnosis of wound healing phase. Careful assessment of the wound and periwound tissue establishes the present, predominant wound healing phase. The *predominant* wound healing phase is the primary functional diagnosis for the wound at that time. There will also be a secondary functional diagnosis, signify-

ing transition to the next phase(s) or absence of subsequent phases(s). In this section, tissue assessment is presented by describing three aspects of healing: acute, chronic, or absent for each phase of wound healing (inflammation, proliferation, and epithelialization). Each aspect of each phase is a potential wound healing phase diagnosis. Table 4–6 lists the wound healing phases and the related wound healing phase diagnoses. An expected prognosis applies to each diagnosis and is also listed.

Acute Phase

As normal acute wounds heal, there is an orderly progression through the wound healing phases (inflammatory, proliferative, epithelialization, and remodeling). Chapter 2 describes the normal physiologic phases of wound repair.

Chronic Phase

Failure of the orderly progression of healing results in a chronic wound. The chronic wound may fail to initiate or stall in any phase of wound healing. When a wound stalls, plateaus, or simply gets stuck in one wound healing phase, the wound becomes chronic with respect to that phase. For example, a pressure ulcer often will become stuck in the inflammatory phase of wound healing, thus the term *chronic inflammation*. Another example is the wound that fills with granulation tissue but does not stop proliferating and goes on to form hypergranulation tissue *(Color Plate 23)*. This is termed *chronic proliferation*. A final example is the wound with impaired scarring, such as with hypertrophic scars or keloid formation. A wound in this condition does not stop laying down collagen. This is termed *chronic epithelialization*. Chapter 2 discusses the physiology that may be affecting wound phase chronicity.

Absent Phase

The wound that fails to pass through a wound healing phase is lacking attributes of that phase and is referred to as *absence of inflammatory phase, absence of proliferative phase,* or *absence of epithelialization phase*. Wounds that fail to progress through a wound healing phase differ from those that get stuck or exhibit characteristics of chronicity in one phase. Those wounds that are absent an inflammatory response, for example, will not demonstrate signs of inflammation, whereas wounds with chronic inflammation will show signs of a continued inflammatory response. Absence of the wound healing phase is a way of indicating that the wound has not initiated the phase, for whatever reasons. Absence of the wound healing phase signifies either the inability to heal or the need for help from an intervention to initiate the acute phase, leading to progression through phases,

Table 4–6 Wound Healing Phase Diagnosis and Prognosis

Wound Healing Phase	Acute Wound Healing Phase Diagnosis	Chronic Wound Healing Phase Diagnosis	Absence of Wound Healing Phase Diagnosis
Inflammatory	Acute inflammatory	Chronic inflammatory	Absence of inflammatory
Proliferative	Acute proliferative	Chronic proliferative	Absence of proliferative
Epithelialization	Acute epithelialization	Chronic epithelialization	Absence of epithelialization
Prognosis	Orderly, timely progression through phases of healing	Reinitiate acute phase, then progress through phases of healing. Reinitiate acute phase of healing and progress to a clean, stable wound.	Initiate healing phase, if able, and progress through phases. If able to initiate healing phase, progress to a clean, stable wound. If unable to initiate healing phase, refer.

eg, reperfusion through surgical intervention or enhanced blood flow from a physical agent.

WOUND HEALING PHASE DIAGNOSIS AND PROGNOSIS

When the periwound and wound tissue assessment is completed, the clinician will be able to review attributes present or absent, interpret the wound healing phase status observed, and create a care plan based on a diagnosis of wound healing phase. The wound healing phase diagnosis is used for the prognosis and to target treatment outcomes. Prognosis for a wound with a diagnosis of the acute healing phase (inflammatory, proliferative, or epithelialization) is progression through the phases of healing. A chronic wound healing phase diagnosis indicates a prognosis that the wound will progress through the phases of healing following reinitiation of the acute phase of healing that is impaired. Alternatively, the prognosis may be a clean, stable wound that may not heal or may need another intervention to achieve closure. If there is inability to initiate the absent phase and progress through the phases, the prognosis for the wound is nonhealing. Such a finding may suggest referral to another practitioner. More than one predominant wound healing phase can be apparent at the same time. For example, a wound with the chronic inflammatory phase is also in absence of the proliferative phase and in absence of the epithelialization phase. Chronic inflammatory would be the primary wound healing phase diagnosis, and absence of the proliferative phase and the epithelialization phase would be the secondary functional diagnosis, signifying that the wound is not progressing through the phases of healing. The wound healing phase diagnosis is

useful to demonstrate medical necessity for intervention by the nurse or physical therapist.

Inflammatory Phase

Assessment of the periwound and wound tissues during the inflammation phase includes attributes associated with the vascular response to wounding described in Chapter 2. The appearance of periwound and wound tissue will change as the wound progresses through the phases of healing. *Color Plates 1* and *2* show a wound that went from the chronic inflammatory phase to the acute inflammatory phase and subsequent progression to the proliferative phase. Four categories of wound characteristics are considered: periwound and adjacent tissue appearance (color, edema/induration, and temperature), wound tissue appearance (color and texture), wound edges, and exudate characteristics (odor, type, and quantity). The major attributes of adjacent and periwound tissue that are observed and palpated in the inflammatory phase include color, temperature, firmness/texture, sensation, and ecchymosis (hemorrhage)—bruising. In this section, the attributes of the wound and the periwound tissues are described during acute inflammation, chronic inflammation, and absence of inflammation.

Acute Inflammation

Signs of acute inflammation often extend well beyond the immediate wound and periwound tissues, and extend into adjacent tissues, as well; they indicate a healthy response and are a prerequisite to normal healing. Compare the characteristics seen during acute inflammation as a reference point for the evaluation of impaired responses.

Adjacent Tissues

Skin Color. *Erythema* is defined as redness of the skin and is one of the classic characteristics of the inflammatory phase. Initially, the adjacent skin may be erythematous due to reactive hyperemia, as mentioned. Erythema may not be evident in persons of color. Skin color attributes found in light and darkly pigmented skin are described in the section on assessment of adjacent tissue, discussed earlier. Reddened skin with streaks leading away from the area may indicate the presence of cellulitis. If assessed, check the patient's history for fever, chills, history of recurrent cellulitis, or medications being used to treat the condition. If no treatment has been initiated, these findings should be reported immediately to the physician.

Edema and Induration. The edema of acute inflammatory phase is a localized brawny edema that feels firm and distorts the swollen tissues, causing the skin to become taut, shiny, and raised from the contours of the surrounding tissues. This edema results from trauma (eg, pressure ulcers, burns, and surgical debridement) and is related to release of histamines. Histamines cause vasodilatation and increase vascular permeability, resulting in the movement of fluid in the interstitial spaces. It is usually accompanied by pain. Induration is abnormal hardening of the tissue at the wound margin by consolidation of edema in the tissues. A test for induration is to pinch the tissues gently; if induration is present, the tissues cannot be pinched. Induration follows reflex hyperemia or chronic venous congestion.[19]

Skin Temperature. Skin temperature should be palpated manually by using either the back of the hand or a liquid crystal skin fever thermometer, if the temperature is at least 95° F (35° C). More precise measurement can be made with an infrared scanner (see earlier description of measuring skin temperature). During acute inflammation, expect the temperature of the wound and adjacent tissues to be the same; then the temperature of the adjacent wound tissue will gradually decline, and the area of increased temperature will narrow as healing progresses.[32]

Pain. Spontaneous or induced pain in the adjacent tissues should be assessed either by palpation or by report, or both. Pain may indicate infection or subcutaneous tissue damage that is not visible, such as in pressure ulcers or vascular disease. Report of a sudden onset of pain accompanied by edema in a leg is a common indicator of a deep vein thrombosis. Unilateral edema accompanied by pain in the calf or palpation over a vein is an indicator of thrombophlebitis. Immediate referral for vascular assessment should follow these findings. More pain testing measures are described in the earlier section regarding assessment of sensation. Absence of pain in an obviously infected or inflamed wound should be investigated as an indication of neuropathy and need for further assessment of sensation.

Clinical Wisdom: *Acute Inflammation Signal*

Excessive signs of acute inflammation should be considered as a signal of impending wound infection.[39]

Differential Diagnosis of Inflammation and Infection

A differential diagnosis between inflammation and infection should be performed by the nurse or physical therapist during the tissue assessment. Inflammation with periwound characteristic symptoms of color change (red or purple), edema, pain, heat, and loss of function may progress to infection and necrosis. If the inflammatory process alone is present, there will be exquisite tenderness over the involved area. If, however, there is cellulitis or other infection, there will be streaks of redness extending away from the wound, and pain may become intense (see *Color Plate 53*). Wound exudate may be thick, yellow, tan, brown, or green with malodor. Amount may be moderate to large. Monitor for signs of systemic infection that can lead to sepsis, including fever of 101° F (39.4° C) or higher; chills; manifestation of shock, including restlessness, lethargy, confusion; and decreased systolic blood pressure.[13] Management and diagnosis of infection are discussed in Chapter 9.

Wound Tissue Assessment. A partial-thickness skin loss creates a shallow crater that looks red or pink or shows the yellow reticular layer—a thin, yellow, meshlike covering that is the deep layer of the dermis (see *Color Plate 17*). If it is bright and shiny, it is healthy and viable and should be left intact. *Color Plate 13* shows the anatomy of the tissues beneath the skin. If the wound penetrates through the dermis into the subcutaneous tissue, the wound will look as though it contains yellow fat, such as chicken fat, or white connective tissue called *fascia*. The fascia is a connective tissue that covers and wraps around all muscles, tendons, blood vessels, and nerves. Wounds that extend through the subcutaneous tissue into the muscle may have a pink or dark red appearance with a shiny layer of fascia on top.

Undermining/Tunneling. Excavation of the subcutaneous tissues during debridement creates a "cave" or undermining of the wound edges. Undermining can lead to separation of fascial planes (see *Color Plates 39 to 41*). Muscles lie together in bundles held together by fascia. Separation of the muscle bundles occurs when the fascia is cut. Separation of the fascial layers opens tunnels along the fascial planes between the muscles under the skin (see *Color Plates 39–41*). Tunnels may join together and form sinus tracts (see *Color Plate 38*). The tunnels are areas where infection can travel, leading to abscess. A wound in the acute inflammatory phase with undermining/tunneling will not have signs of infection or necrosis in those species. Differential diagnoses of inflammation and infection have been discussed previously. Muscle tissue is striated and jumps or twitches when palpated. Muscles are connected to bones by tendons. Tendons are covered with white fascia and look like ropes. The sheath of fascia covering the tendon is called *peritenon*. New granulation tissue will grow over intact peritenon.

Penetration of a wound into the joint may expose several anatomic structures, including ligaments that are white and striated, joint capsule that is white and shiny, and cartilage that is white, hard, and smooth, and is on the ends of bones. Bone is white, hard, and covered with a clear or white membrane called *periosteum*. The level of tissue exposed is used to stage or grade the wound severity, as described previously. Loss of peritenon or periosteum will compromise a skin graft.

Wound Edges. During acute inflammation, the wound edges are often indistinct or diffuse and change shape as wound contraction and epithelialization begins. Wound edges may be attached to the wound base or may be separated from it, forming walls with the base of the wound at a depth from the skin surface. Wound edges should be palpated for firmness and texture. Observe the margins for curling. See *Color Plates 33–36* to observe wound edges.

Wound Drainage. Wound drainage during the acute inflammatory phase is an indication of the status of the clotting mechanisms and of infection. Wound drainage that contains dead cells and debris is called *exudate*. Clear fluid drainage is called *transudate*. See Chapter 9 for more descriptions of exudate characteristics. During assessment, record the presence or absence, color, odor, quantity, and quality of the wound drainage.

Sanguineous Wounds. Initially, there will be bleeding into the wound space that is controlled by clotting. Wounds that have bloody exudate are called *sanguineous* and may have impaired clotting. This may be due to anticoagulant pharmacologic products that contain substances such as heparin or to disease processes, such as hemophilia. The amount of exudate will vary. Medical history, including a pharmacy history, and systems review should clarify the causes of the sanguineous drainage. Copious or persistent sanguineous drainage should be reported to the physician.

> **Clinical Wisdom:** *Reverse Staging or Back Staging of Pressure Ulcers*
>
> Once the ulcer is staged, that remains the stage and wound severity diagnosis. Correct terminology is *healing stage II, III, or IV.*

Serous Transudate. Serous transudate is clear fluid that exudes from the wound. It is usually yellow and odorless, and is seen in varying amounts during the inflammatory phase (see *Color Plates 43* and *46*).

Chronic Inflammation

Inflammation that persists for weeks and months is referred to as *chronic inflammation*. Chronic inflammation occurs when the macrophages and neutrophils fail to phagocytose necrotic matter, ingest foreign debris, and fight infection.[40] Therefore, necrotic matter or foreign debris is the type of material that would be expected to be found in the wound bed. Chronic inflammation is also related to the release of histamine from the mast cells and reflex hyperemia associated with vasodilatation of the surrounding vasculature. Repeated trauma to the wound will also develop into chronic inflammation.

Periwound Skin. Chronic inflammation is seen as a halo of erythema in lightly pigmented skin or a dark halo in darkly pigmented skin located in the periwound area. The latter may be easily mistaken because of its similar appearance with hemosiderin staining. There is minimal temperature change or cooling, compared with adjacent uninjured tissues. There may be some minimal firmness from edema in the periwound tissues. There is usually minimal pain response or there may be intense pain associated with arterial vascular disease or infection. Arterial ulcers over the malleolus and pressure ulcers are frequently seen with a halo of erythema but lack the blood flow to progress the wound (see *Color Plate 53*).

Wound Tissue. Wounds in the chronic inflammatory phase usually have necrotic tissue covering all or part of the wound surface. Necrotic tissue varies in color and may be black, yellow, tan, brown, or gray. Soft necrotic tissue, such as fibrin or slough, may be present in the wound bed. Fibrin forms on the wound surface and is associated with venous disease. Slough is necrotic fat and fascia adhering to the layer beneath it. See *Color Plates 26–32* for different appearances of necrotic tissues. Pale pink wounds may have chronic infection (see *Color Plate 11*). Chapter 8 describes the significance of the different qualities of necrotic tissue. Wounds that are chronically inflamed often have a portion of the wound surface that is in the proliferative phase with granulation tissue present, but the proliferation fails to progress. Not all pink tissue is granulation, however, because muscle tissue that is beneath newly removed necrotic tissue is pink or dark red (see *Color Plate 13*). During assessment, record the presence of necrotic tissue and the color. Wounds in the chronic inflammatory phase of healing often have a combination of several attributes present. For example, a wound can have black and yellow necrotic tissue, as well as pink granulation tissue or healthy muscle tissue (see *Color Plate 7*).

Clinical Wisdom: *Distinguishing Granulation Tissue from Muscle*

To distinguish granulation tissue from healthy muscle, palpate the tissue with a gloved finger. Granulation tissue is soft, spongy, and will not jump if pinched, but it may bleed. Muscle tissue is firm and resilient to pressure and will jump or twitch if pinched or probed.

Wound Drainage

Color and Odor. Wound drainage that is foul smelling and/or viscous yellow/gray or green exudate is often referred to as *pus*. The pus is a result of the demise of neutrophils after they have phagocytosed debris and excessive bacterial loads. When there is a high bacterial count (greater than 10^5), signs of active infection will be seen. Prolonged, chronic inflammation is the result when there is a bacteria-filled wound.[40]

Not all malodorous or yellow/gray exudate signifies infection. The odor and fluid may come from solubilization of necrotic tissue by enzymatic debriding agents or autolysis. Enzymatic and autolytic debridement are described in Chapter 8. Cleanse exudate from the wound to determine whether odor is transient or internal. If enzymatic or autolytic methods of debridement are used, the odor and debris should be removed by the cleansing. If odor remains or if exudate can be expressed from the wound or adjacent tissues that has color or odor, consider infection. Check for other symptoms of infection, such as heat, fever, and lethargy. Exudate color can suggest the type of infection. Normally, wound exudate is serous—a clear or light-yellow fluid. Green is usually associated with an anaerobic infection (see *Color Plates 42–47* and Chapter 9). Record color, texture, and odor on the assessment form.

Volume. Exudate volume is considered an indicator of wound outcome.[2] The amount of wound exudate volume should be estimated as scant/minimal, small, moderate, or large/copious. It is hard to record exudate quantity from a dressing or by expressing it from a wound, so these estimates are considered appropriate ways to record estimated quantity. Absence of exudate or dryness of the wound bed may indicate desiccation and the need for adding moisture. During assessment, record the presence or absence, color, odor, and quantity of exudate. The PSST has a Likert scale to rate each one of these aspects (Chapter 6).

Gelatinous Edema. Following a secondary trauma to the wound bed, such as sharp or enzymatic debridement, wound edema forms as a result of the leakage of plasma proteins from damaged or irritated capillaries, allowing moisture to accumulate and form an opaque, gelatinous mass in the base of the wound. The edematous mass contains many substances, all of which are contributory to sustaining a chronic inflammatory response. This mass is visible on examination.[41] Record if present (see *Color Plate 44*).

Absence of Inflammation

Absence of the inflammatory phase or inability of the body to present an immune response to wounding may be due to many causes, including an immune-suppression state (eg, human immunodeficiency virus infection/acquired immune deficiency syndrome, cancer, diabetes, drug or radiation therapy, overuse of antiseptics, or severe ischemia). Absence of an inflammatory response prevents the wound from progressing through the biologic phases of repair. It is different from chronic inflammation, with distinct signs and symptoms. In order for the wound to heal, interventions need to be considered to restart the inflammatory response. However, because of the coimpairments related to the problem, this may not be realistic. For example, a patient with an ischemic foot and an eschar over a wound on the heel has an absence of inflammation. This is nature's best protection from entry of infection. Protection of the eschar and the limb from trauma to prevent opening of the body to infection and new wounding would be the preferred treatment strategy (see *Color Plate 52*).[3]

Periwound Skin. Absence of an inflammatory phase is recognized by absence of a vascular response to wounding, including absence of color changes in the periwound skin and absence of tension or hardness; however, there may be a boggy feeling and minimal temperature difference or coolness, compared with adjacent tissue. Minimal pulses are palpable. Such findings would trigger further investigation of vascular status of the patient (see *Color Plate 52*).

Wound Bed Tissue. Wound bed tissue may be covered with hard, dry eschar to seal off debris and infection from the wound (see *Color Plate 52*).

Wound Drainage. Wound drainage may be scant or the tissues may be dry. Dryness may be due to sealing off of tissues or to improper treatment.

Summary of Three Inflammatory Phase Diagnoses and Prognoses

A diagnosis is the summary of data collected during the assessment process. Wound healing phase diagnosis is a diagnosis of the functional status of healing.[42] Table 4–7 summarizes the findings for each aspect of the inflammatory phase. The presence of edema, induration, erythema, elevated temperature, pain, or diffuse or indistinct wound edges is an indicator that the wound healing phase diagnosis is *acute inflammatory phase*. The *chronic inflammatory* wound healing phase diagnosis will be recognized by an inadequate circulatory response to the area of trauma. There will be a mild or limited erythema, minimal or absent edema and induration, and no elevation in tissue temperature. Often, the assessment findings include a wound with a large bioburden of necrotic tissue. There may be a copious and malodorous exudate, signifying an infection that the body cannot adequately suppress. *Absence of inflammatory* wound healing phase diagnosis is recognized by an absence of circulatory response to trauma. Sealing off the wound from the rest of the body by a hard, dry eschar gangrene is often nature's way of protecting the body from invasion. Absence of the inflammatory phase may also be due to scabbing over the wound surface or letting the deep wound tissues dry out.

Because the phases of healing overlap, the wound healing phase diagnosis if the wound is transitioning from one phase to the next is defined by the *primary* phase appearance. *Inflammatory* is the wound healing phase diagnosis if the attributes of inflammation are at least 50–75% of what would be expected in an acute inflammatory response (see *Color Plate 1*). If the wound attributes are chronic inflammatory for at least 50–75% of the symptoms associated with chronic inflammation, the diagnosis is *chronic inflammatory* phase (see *Color Plate 7*). When the wound attributes of acute inflammatory are less than 50% of what are expected and there is significant proliferation of granulation tissue in the wound bed, the primary wound phase diagnosis changes to proliferative phase (see *Color Plate 8*).

Proliferative Phase

Like the inflammatory phase, the proliferative phase is broken into three aspects: acute proliferative (the active biologic process of proliferation, including granulation tissue formation and contraction), chronic proliferative (the wound is stuck in the proliferative phase and not progressing to the

Table 4–7 Wound Healing Phase Diagnosis: Tissue Characteristics for Inflammatory Phase

Periwound Skin and Wound Tissue Characteristics	Acute Inflammatory Phase	Chronic Inflammatory Phase	Absence of Inflammatory Phase
Periwound skin color	• Unblanchable erythema in light-skinned patients • Discoloration or deepening of normal ethnic color in dark-skinned patients • Ecchymosis (purplish bruising) • Hemosiderosis (rust brown staining)	• Halo of erythema or darkening • Hemosiderin (rust brown) staining • Ecchymosis (purplish bruising)	• Pale or ashen skin color • Absence of erythema or darkening • Hemosiderin (rust brown) staining • Ecchymosis (purplish bruising)
Edema and induration	• Firmness • Taut, shiny skin • Localized swelling • Consolidation (hardness) between adjacent tissues • Gelatinous edema may be seen on wound tissue	• Minimal firmness • Absent • May feel boggy	

continues

Table 4–7 continued

Periwound Skin and Wound Tissue Characteristics	Acute Inflammatory Phase	Chronic Inflammatory Phase	Absence of Inflammatory Phase
Tissue temperature	• Elevated initially, decreases as inflammation progresses	• Minimal change or coolness	• Minimal change or coolness
Pain	• Present; wound is tender and painful unless neuropathy is present	• Minimal pain unless arterial etiology or infection, then may have intense pain	• Minimal or no pain unless arterial etiology, then may have intense pain
Wound tissue	• Blister with clear or bloody fluid • Shallow or deep crater with red to pink color • Red muscle • White shiny fascia • Yellow reticular layer of dermis with granulation buds	• Necrotic, varies in color from yellow to brown to black • Necrotic tissue covering full or partial surface area • Soft or hard necrotic tissue • Yellow fibrin or slough • Portion of wound may have granulation tissue • May also appear as clean, pale pink	• Covered with hard, dry eschar • Necrotic, varies in color from yellow to brown to black • Scab
Undermining/tunneling	• May be present in deep wounds • Has potential for infection and abscess	• May be present in deep wounds • Has potential for infection and abscess	• May be present in deep wounds • Has potential for infection and abscess
Wound edges	• Diffuse, indistinct, may still be demarcating from healthy tissues	• Distinct, edges may be rolled or thickened • Is not continuous with wound bed if deep wound cavity	• Has distinct well-defined wound edges • May be attached to necrotic tissue
Wound drainage	• Serous or serosanguineous	• Infection • Viscous • Malodor • Pus (yellow, tan, gray, or green) • Moderate to large amount	• Scant or dry
Color Plates	1, 14, 15, 17, 19	20, 25, 27, 36, 39, 42, 47	30, 52

next phase of epithelialization and remodeling), and absence of proliferative phase (the wound bed is clean but the wound is not proliferating or is not contracting). Each of the three aspect characteristics of proliferation is described.

Acute Proliferative Phase

Periwound Skin. Periwound skin during the proliferative phase regains color and contour symmetry with that of adjacent skin (edema resolved); if it is a recovering chronic wound, however, expect to see hemosiderin staining (pigmentation) around the wound margins (see *Color Plate 2*). Ecchymosis should be resolved. Skin turgor is normal and is not stretched or taut because the edema and induration are resolved (absent). Firmness is absent or minimal.

Periwound Skin Temperature. Periwound skin temperature, when palpated or measured on a skin thermometer, is the same as skin in adjacent areas or may be slightly elevated, due to enhanced perfusion of the tissues and higher metabolic activities associated with healing.

Pain. Minimal or no pain is experienced during this phase. It is an inappropriate indicator if there is neuropathy.

Undermining/Tunneling. The acute proliferative phase progresses after the wound has been debrided of necrotic tissue. Debridement of necrotic tissue creates a disruption of the tissue integrity of the skin and the underlying structures. The proliferative phase is concluding when the wound tissue integrity is reestablished. *Undermining* is defined as a closed passageway under the surface of the skin that is open only at the skin surface.[2] As previously described, wound undermining occurs following debridement of the skin and subcutaneous tissue and is erosion of the tissue, forming a cave under the wound edge (see *Color Plate 41*). Both undermining and tunneling are loss of tissue integrity. The loss of tissue integrity allows separation of the fascial planes between the bundles of muscles. Tunneling is like a subway progressing from the initial undermined excavation and occurs when there is debridement into the fascial and muscle layers. Tunneling may be unobservable from the surface and yet have a great extent, as shown in *Color Plates 37* and *38* of the same wound. Undermining and tunneling close as the tissues reestablish continuity during the laying down of the collagen matrix and granulation tissue in the proliferative phase. The extent of undermining is a measure of the total soft tissue involved in the wound. Reduction of the extent of undermining/tunneling is a measure of the progression of proliferation and reduced overall wound size. Note findings of undermining and tunneling as part of the tissue assessment. If the tunneling extends beyond about 15 cm, this is cause to notify the physician. Chapter 5 describes how to measure undermining/tunneling and calculate the extent of the overall wound.

Wound Tissue. Wounds that have a bowl-shaped cavity will fill with granulation tissue during the acute proliferative phase to create a surface across which epidermal cells may migrate. Tissue that develops during this phase has been given the term *granulation tissue* because the tissue has the appearance of granules piled upon one another. Biologically, this tissue is the collagen matrix. Granulation buds are clearly seen in *Color Plates 4* and *8*. Note how the cavity is filling in those photos to create a level surface with the adjacent skin. Acute proliferative phase starts when the wound bed tissue begins to show red or pink granulation buds and overlaps the late inflammatory phase. The collagen matrix is laid down and is infiltrated by and supports the growing capillary bed, giving it the red color. Reduced depth in a full-thickness wound is a measure of proliferation activity. The collagen matrix does not replace the structures or functions of the tissues that occupied the cavity prior to injury. This is scar tissue. The prevailing opinion is that this deep red color indicates a healthy healing wound. A contrary opinion is explained later, in the section entitled "Chronic Proliferative Phase."

Another feature that has been reported to appear during the acute proliferative phase of healing in a number of patients is the development of a yellow, fibrinous membrane on the surface of the granulation tissue. Removal of this membrane has been attempted, but it will recur in a few days. Wounds that develop this yellow membrane appear to be less susceptible to infection. These wounds continue to heal in a normal fashion. Recognizing this membrane during examination will prevent unnecessary disruption of the wound bed.[43]

Wound Edges. The wound edges are soft to firm and are flexible to touch. Edges will roll if the wound is full thickness, but when the wound tissue fills the cavity even with the edge of the wound, the edges will flatten and epithelialization and contraction will continue together (see *Color Plates 3–5* and *8–9*). At this point, the wound acquires a distinctive wound shape or "picture frame." The cells that control the movement of the picture frame, the myofibroblasts, are located beneath the wound edge. The cells are contractile and will move forward, drawing the wound together. During this process, the wound edges are drawn together like the drawing together of purse strings, shrinking the size of the open area measurably. The shape that the wound now assumes predicts the resulting speed of contraction. Linear wounds contract rapidly. Square or rectangular wounds contract at a moderate pace. Circular wounds contract slowly. Wound contraction is a major activity of the acute proliferative phase of healing. Contraction reduces the areas needing to close by epithelialization. Contraction in areas such as the gluteals and abdomen will be fine, but examples of locations where contracture is troublesome include the head, neck, and hand. Drawing together too tightly in those areas will cause a defect or contracture that will impair function and cosmesis. Wounds that would have a poor outcome if allowed to close by contraction would have a prognosis of need for surgical intervention at the start of the proliferative phase.[44]

Wound Drainage. During the acute proliferative phase, the wound drainage is serosanguineous and of moderate to minimal quantity and odor.

Chronic Proliferative Phase

Periwound Skin Color and Edema. Color of the skin at the wound edge may blanch or begin to draw together very tightly (see *Color Plate 36*). Gelatinous edema may be present, signifying an episode of trauma.

Periwound Skin Temperature and Pain. Compared with the temperature of the adjacent skin, periwound skin during the chronic proliferative phase may be cool or mildly elevated, and there may be some signs of intense pain. This could indicate that the wound has been traumatized and is having another episode of acute inflammation, or there may be presence of infection.

Undermining and Tunneling. Chronic proliferation develops when the tissue integrity is not reestablished. The tunneling can extend a long distance and presents an opportunity for infection to travel up the fascial plane. Tissues in the tunnel may be necrotic. Tunneling can become a sinus tract, which is defined as a cavity or channel underlying a wound that involves an area larger than the visible surface of the wound. An abscess may form in the tunnel or sinus tract.[2] When undermining/tunneling persists in a proliferating wound and the assessment findings include a black hole that has no reachable bottom, the wound needs urgent medical management.

Wound Tissue. A wound in the chronic proliferative phase may exhibit attributes of infection, poor vascular supply, desiccation, or hypergranulation. Poor vascular supply will appear as a pale pink, minimally granulating wound. A contrary opinion of some clinicians is that certain wounds that develop a livid red surface color may be infected and slow to heal (see *Color Plate 42*). Infection in granulating wounds is disruptive to healing. The features of infection that may be observed in granulating wounds are superficial bridging, friable tissue, bleeding on contact, pain in the wound, and a delay in healing. There are two stages in the proliferative phase when the granulation tissue may show these characteristics of infection—about 10 days postoperatively and at the end stage of healing, when the wound has progressed satisfactorily, then becomes indolent.[43] *Color Plates 10* and *11* show the same wound. In *Color Plate 10*, the wound was progressing through the proliferative phase. Seven days later, the wound had attributes of infection, the proliferation had ceased, and the wound was in the chronic proliferative phase. Trauma can also retard proliferation. Pale pink, blanched to dull, dusky red granulation tissue indicates poor vascular supply. Desiccated granulation tissue is dark, dull, garnet red. Hemorrhaging or bleeding of the granulation tissue vessels causes an acute inflammation to the area and promotes scarring. Hemorrhaging on the granulation tissue looks like a purple bruise on the surface. In *Color Plate 11*, note the small hemorrhagic area at the center of the wound, indicating rupture of blood vessels.

Chapter 2 explains how an imbalance of collagen synthesis and lysis can allow the collagen to proliferate unchecked, creating a hump of granulation tissue called "hypergranulation." Normally, the process of granulation decreases as the wound space decreases and the wound integrity is recovered. The granulation tissue fills the wound space to the surface; the epithelialization process then covers the wound. However, when the hypergranulation tissue overflows the wound bed, the epithelial cells cannot climb the hill of granulation tissue against gravity, and the result is that the epithelialization process is halted. See *Color Plate 23* for hypergranulation. If hypergranulation persists, the wound moves into a chronic proliferative phase. The "Clinical Wisdom" below describes some methods that are commonly used to control hypergranulation. There have been some suggestions about the use of dressings to control hypergranulation, but these methods are unproven and remain anecdotal.

Wound Edges. The chronic proliferative phase develops when the wound edges roll in and become hard and fibrotic, which inhibits further wound contraction. See *Color Plate 35* for an example of rolled fibrotic edges. Wounds of different pathogeneses develop this problem, including pressure ulcers and venous ulcers. This finding may trigger a referral to a surgeon to excise the rolled edge to restart the healing process.

Wound Drainage. Chronic proliferative exudate may be a yellow, gelatinous, viscous material on the wound granulation base that indicates the wound has been traumatized. This should not be confused with wound dressings such as amorphous hydrogels or treatments such as antimicrobial ointments. An infected wound in chronic proliferation may have a malodorous, viscous, reddish-brown, green, or gray exudate. *Color Plate 42* shows an apparently clean wound, but the wound dressing shows signs of moderate to large amounts of sanguineous and purulent, reddish-brown exudate. This wound is in the chronic proliferative phase and needs treatment to recover.

Clinical Wisdom: *Management of Hypergranulation*

Because hypergranulation will inhibit the reepithelialization of the wound surface, it must be prevented or controlled. Three methods used to achieve this purpose are as follows:

1. Cauterization by applying silver nitrate sticks to the surface will necrose the superficial granulation tissue, which can then be wiped off.
2. Excess hypergranulation tissue can be trimmed by rubbing with a gauze sponge or snipping with scissors.
3. Hypertonic saline is a nontoxic method to reduce hypergranulation (see Chapter 11).

Absence of Proliferative Phase

Periwound Skin: Color, Edema, Pain, and Temperature. The presence of hemosiderin staining or a halo of erythema will surround the wound, signifying a wound that is also in the chronic inflammatory phase. The skin may show signs of ecchymosis. Edema and pain will be minimal or absent. Temperature change is of minimal increase or coolness.

Wound Tissue. A wound in an absence of proliferative phase is either not producing granulation tissue or not contracting (see *Color Plate 33*). The wound tissue may look dry, dull red, and desiccated or may contain pale pink granulation tissue. There is lack of change in wound depth. Not much is written describing an absence of proliferative phase. The wound that is in the chronic inflammatory phase or absence of inflammatory phase also has absence of a proliferative phase. The wound is not progressing through the proliferative phase. Wounds in this situation often have a surface appearance of necrotic tissue and/or hemorrhage/ecchymosis. Any signs of ecchymosis would signify a restart of an inflammatory process within the wound. The chronic inflammatory phase and absence of the proliferative phase can both be used as functional diagnoses for the same wound. The prognosis would be for the wound to progress to the acute proliferative phase. The medical history and systems review should guide the clinician to investigate the impairments to the proliferation process.

Wound Edges. Wound edges may be rolled or jagged, and the shape is irregular. The wound does not change shape, signifying lack of wound contraction. Deep wounds may have absence of continuity of wound bed and edges. The wound is not reducing in size.

Wound Drainage. Wounds have absence of exudate or scant serous exudate. The wound in *Color Plate 45* is in the chronic inflammatory phase and has absence of a proliferative phase. Note the scant amount of serous exudate on the wound dressing. Treatment interventions should be reviewed to see why the wound lacks moisture.

Summary of Three Proliferative Phase Diagnoses and Prognoses

Table 4–8 summarizes the findings for each aspect of the proliferative phase. The presence of the following attributes signifies that the wound healing phase diagnosis is *acute proliferative phase*: beefy red granulation tissue in the wound bed (reduced depth); wound contraction (reduced surface open area, regular wound edges and shape); serous or serosanguineous exudate of moderate to minimal amount; and normalized peripheral skin temperature, turgor, and color. The prognosis is that reassessment will show reduction in depth and closing of the undermined/tunneled space, with measurable reduction in overall size estimate as the integrity of the tissue is reestablished.

Failure to progress as expected through the proliferative phase signifies a wound healing phase diagnosis of *chronic proliferative* or *absence of proliferative phase*. The evaluation of a halt to proliferation should be given careful consideration. For example, infection during the proliferative phase retards healing and causes a chronic proliferative phase. If superficial bridging, friable tissue, bleeding on contact, pain in the wound, and a delay in healing are observed, the evaluation would be positive for infection. Wounds with early signs of infection are treated with a regimen of oral antibiotics for 2–4 weeks, and those that have late healing signs of infection are treated with topical antibiotics.[43] The prognosis is that the wound will resume progression through the phases of healing following intervention with antibiotics. Failure to initiate an inflammatory phase will cause absence of a proliferative phase. Iatrogenic wound care may also cause the wound to have absence of a proliferative phase. The prognosis is that the inflammatory phase will be initiated (if body systems can support it) and will progress to the proliferative phase. Another possibility of prognosis is that the proliferative phase will be initiated following change in treatment.

Once again, the phases of healing overlap; the wound healing phase diagnosis if the wound is transitioning from one phase to the next is defined by the *primary* phase appearance. A wound healing phase diagnosis of *acute proliferative phase* means that most (50% or greater) of the wound surface appearance attributes—granulation tissue and contraction—are observed. If less than 50% of the proliferative phase attributes are identified, the wound is primarily in an

Table 4–8 Wound Healing Phase Diagnosis: Tissue Characteristics for Proliferative Phase

Periwound Skin and Wound Tissue Characteristics	Acute Proliferative Phase	Chronic Proliferative Phase	Absence of Proliferative Phase
Periwound skin color	• Continuity with adjacent skin • Hemosiderin staining if recovering chronic wound	• Continuity with adjacent skin • Paler than adjacent skin • Hemosiderin staining • Ecchymosis (purple bruising)	• Hemosiderin staining if chronic wound • Halo of erythema if in chronic inflammatory phase • Ecchymosis (purple bruising)
Edema and induration	• Absent	• Gelatinous edema may be present, signifying trauma	• Minimal edema present
Tissue temperature	• Temperature may be minimally elevated if wound is well perfused	• Minimal change or coolness	• Minimal change or coolness
Pain	• Pain free or minimal • Inappropriate indicator in presence of neuropathy	• Painful, may be indicator of local inflammation; if intense, consider infection	• Minimal or absent • Intense if infection present
Wound tissue	• Shiny, bright red to pink granulation • Sustained reduction in wound depth • Sustained wound contraction • Reduced size • Covering of yellow fibrinous membrane on granulation tissue • Livid red	• Hypergranulation • Desiccation (dark red color) • Poor vascularization (pale pink) • Ecchymosis (purple bruising) on granulation	• Necrotic tissue—stuck in chronic inflammatory phase • Ecchymosis (purple bruising) on granulation inflammation restarting • Dull red—desiccated granulation • Pale pink granulation • Lacking change in wound depth • Unsustained contraction—no reduction in size of surface area
Undermining/tunneling	• May be present in deep wounds • Closes as proliferation progresses	• May be present in deep wounds • Fails to close or may extend • Has potential for infection and abscess	• May be present in deep wounds • Fails to close or may extend • Has potential for infection and abscess
Wound edges	• Soft to firm • Flexible to touch • Rolled if full thickness • Change in wound shape from irregular to regular • Reduction in size of surface area • Drawing together • Adherence of wound edges by end of phase	• Tight drawing together to reduce size—contracture • Absence of continuity of wound bed and edges • Rolled • Fibrotic • Ecchymosis (purple bruising) on wound edge	• Unchanged size • Rolled or jagged irregular edges • Fibrotic • No change of shape—not drawing together • Absence of continuity of wound bed and edges

continues

Table 4–8 continued

Periwound Skin and Wound Tissue Characteristics	Acute Proliferative Phase	Chronic Proliferative Phase	Absence of Proliferative Phase
Wound drainage	• Serosanguineous or serous in moderate to minimal amount for wound size	• Yellow gelatinous following trauma • Infection: viscous malodorous, red/brown, green, purulent • Large amount	• Serous drainage scant to minimal amounts • Desiccated and dry
Color Plates	3 to 5, 8 to 10, 18	11, 23, 34, 35, 36, 42, 64	30, 31, 33, 39

inflammatory phase and has not yet reached the proliferative phase for diagnostic purposes. The diagnosis would be written *inflammatory phase/proliferative phase.*

A wound with infection of the granulation tissue has impaired healing and would carry a wound healing phase diagnosis of *chronic proliferative phase.* A clean wound that is not producing granulation tissue or contracting is in a wound healing phase of *absence of proliferative phase.*

Clinical Wisdom: *Describing a Wound in the Proliferative Phase*

Example of a narrative note describing a wound in the acute proliferative phase:
Evaluation: A wound on the right hip has beefy red granulation tissue. The wound edges are firm and soft. Wound is contracting into a rectangular shape.
Wound healing phase diagnosis: The wound healing phase diagnosis is proliferative phase.

Epithelialization Phase

Acute Epithelialization Phase

Periwound Skin. Because acute epithelialization begins at the time of wounding concurrently with the inflammation phase and overlaps the other phases, expect the signs of acute inflammation also to be observed in the periwound skin. As the acute inflammation process subsides, the periwound skin should return to the usual color for ethnicity and to the temperature of adjacent tissues, and should be firm but not hard, edematous, or fibrotic. Maceration of the periwound skin and new epidermis may occur from leakage of wound exudate or use of products that moisten the skin and saturate the cells. Maceration is especially damaging to new epithelium.

Macerated skin looks pale and wrinkled, and feels soft and thin to touch, making it very susceptible to trauma, such as from pressure.

Clinical Wisdom: *Protection of Skin from Maceration*

Skin barriers are products that can be used over the periwound skin and new scar tissue to protect them from maceration.

Wound Edges and Wound Bed Tissue. Epithelial cells start migrating toward the center from the wound edges to cover the defect with new skin within hours of wounding. Epithelialization occurs from several directions. The edges are a source of keratinocytes that cover the wound surface with epithelium. The wound edges must be adhered to the wound base for epithelial cell migration to cover the wound. The leading edge of the migrating cells is one cell thick. Gradually, the epithelium spreads across the wound bed, as shown in *Color Plates 5* and *6* of the same wound. The migrating tissue is connected to the adjacent skin and will pull it along to cover the opening.[44] The new skin will be bright pink, regardless of normal pigmentation, and may never regain the melanin factors that color skin (see *Color Plates 8* and *22*). New skin is formed as a very thin sheet, and it takes several weeks for the new skin to thicken. If the wound is less than full thickness, islands of pink epithelium may appear in the wound bed from migrating cells donated by the dermal appendages, the hair follicles, and the sweat glands. Cells from these islands and edges spread out and cover the open area. *Color Plate 64* shows a wound with an island of epithelium. *Color Plate 65* of the same wound shows the migration of the epithelium across the wound from the edges and from the island. Notice in *Color Plate 65* how the edges of the new epithelium are jagged. Full-thickness wounds lose these island contributors, and they never regenerate.[45] Full-thickness wounds begin to epithelialize when the edges are attached and even with the wound so that there are no sides or walls, and the epithelial cells can migrate from the edge across the wound surface. Edges are soft to firm and are flexible to touch, as shown in *Color Plate 18*. This wound went on to heal by epithelialization from the wound edges. The wound environment is critical to a successful epithelialization phase. The wound must be kept warm, moist, and free of trauma at all times.

Wounds may bypass this phase of repair if it is preferable to place a skin graft or muscle flap to close the wound. Large wounds and wounds in areas where contraction will be harmful or where it will simply take too long to cover the wound may benefit from surgical repair. The wound shown in *Color Plate 65* was closed at that time by a split-thickness skin graft to speed the repair process.

Clinical Wisdom: *Maintaining a Moist Wound Bed for Epithelialization*

Amorphous hydrogel dressings are useful wound moisturizers and, along with moisture-permeable films and sheet hydrogels, provide the warm, moist homeostatic environment critical for epithelialization.

Wound Drainage. A scant or small amount of serous or serosanguineous wound exudate is expected. The wound must be kept moist during this phase of healing because desiccation will destroy the epithelial cells.

Chronic Epithelialization Phase

Periwound Skin. The characteristics of the skin may be the same as chronic or absence of inflammatory phase. The periwound skin may show signs of ischemia, such as a pale or ashen color in the elevated position, which deepens to dark purple with dependence (rubor). Pain may be a constant, throbbing pain or intermittent claudication during walking, if it is associated with arterial occlusive disease. The appearance of the adjacent skin is usually dry, shiny, taut, and/or hairless. These are indicators of loss of hair follicles, sweat, and/or sebaceous glands. The wound shown in *Color Plate 81* is in the chronic epithelialization and chronic inflammatory phase. The appearance of adjacent and periwound skin changed as chronicity was altered and acute epithelialization and proliferative phases were initiated (*Color Plate 83*).

Wound Edges. Epithelialization of deep wounds occurs only at the edges and may involve thickening and rolling under of the edges. If the cells cannot continue to migrate across the wound, they will build up an epithelial ridge along the edge of the wound, as seen in *Color Plates 3* and *42*. Pressure ulcers typically develop a round shape when this occurs. Wounds in chronic epithelialization have cells piled on each until the rolled, thickened edges become fibrotic. The wound edges need to be modified and the wound bed filled before wound epithelialization will be reinitiated. Hyperkeratosis is another abnormality of the epithelialization phase. Hyperkeratosis is overgrowth of the horny layer of the skin. *Color Plate 24* shows a wound with hyperkeratosis and an irregular shape of a heel ulcer of a 100-year-old woman.

Scar Tissue. The majority of wound closure in humans is by granulation tissue formation, followed by epithelialization.[45] New epithelium of scar tissue is bright pink, regardless of the pigmentation of normal skin. In darkly pigmented skin, the scar tissue may never be repigmented. The bright pink color may fade over time to a lighter shade of pink as the vascular system is fully reestablished.

Wound Tissue. The wound bed tissue that is hypergranulating may develop a chronic epithelialization phase because the epithelial cells cannot migrate over the hump of granulation tissue against gravity (see *Color Plate 23*). The granulation tissue must be trimmed back to be level with the periwound skin for epithelialization to resume.

Wound Drainage. Wound drainage may be nonexistent and the wound dry. If no or scanty exudate is assessed, additional moisture may be needed to facilitate the migration of the epithelial cells. Epidermal cells migrate best in a warm, moist environment. Wound dryness can be due to improper dressing selection, loss of dressing, dehydration of the wound or patient, or other iatrogenic conditions. On the other hand, there may be heavy exudate from a partial-thickness ulcer that should be epithelializing, but the exudate washes out of the epidermal cells faster than they can migrate and attach to the wound surface. Excessive moisture associated with wound products may also cause this to occur. Management of the wound moisture would be required.

Absence of Epithelialization Phase

Absence of the epithelialization phase may be due to intrinsic, extrinsic, or iatrogenic causes that may be identified during the assessment.

Color. The color of the adjacent and periwound skin offers clues to the etiology of absence of the epithelialization phase. Absence of the epithelialization phase may be related to an intrinsic condition, such as arterial obstructive disease

(AOD). AOD limits blood supply and oxygen to the tissues and impairs the function of the skin to repair itself. Examination of adjacent skin will reveal absence of hair, dependent rubor, and pallor on elevation. The wound will have a punched-out appearance and a very limited ring of epidermal tissue around the wound that will not migrate across the wound, as shown in *Color Plate 54*. If no prior vascular testing is reported, these findings would indicate the need for further assessment of the vascular system. Chapter 7 should be consulted for testing suggestions.

Texture. Periwound skin that is dry and flaky, has an irregular texture, or is macerated provides limited epidermal cells to resurface the wound. The wound will lack epithelialization activity.

Skin Temperature. Skin temperature is a reflection of blood supply. Skin temperature cooler than 92–96° F on the torso and lower in the extremities (75–80° F) is an indicator that blood supply to the skin may be limited; warmer skin may be due to infection.

Edema. Chronic edema caused by tissue congestion such as lymphedema, congestive heart failure, or venous insufficiency stretches the skin and fills interstitial spaces with excess fluid, including large protein molecules. When the capacity of the tissue to hold fluid is exceeded, the fluid leaks through the skin. Because of the disease process, changes occur in the vascularity of the tissues, leading to loss of dermal appendages and dry stasis eczema. The changes are known as *lipodermatosclerosis*.[46] Skin changes associated with this disease process are shown in *Color Plates 59* and *60*. Patients with lipodermatosclerosis may show absence of epithelialization phase. More information on lipodermatosclerosis is presented in Chapter 17.

Wound Edges. Another example of an intrinsic factor that causes absence of epithelialization is decreased epidermal proliferation due to delayed cellular migration attributed to aging. There is slow or absence of new skin growth from edges or islands. Absence of epithelialization attributes include dry, flaky, hyperkeratotic skin at the wound edges. The dryness may be associated with a dry wound environment.

Wound Tissue. Hypogranulation results from an absence of the proliferative phase and failure to fill the wound bed and provide a surface for the epidermal cells to migrate across to cover the wound.

Summary of Three Epithelialization Phase Diagnoses and Prognoses

The *epithelialization phase* of healing begins with epithelial migration during the inflammatory phase of healing. Par-

tial-thickness wound epithelialization may progress from islands in the center of the wound, as well as from the wound edges. Full-thickness and deeper wound healing by epithelialization will be arrested if a large amount of wound debris interferes or if the wound edges fall off into a deep wound bed with steep walls or are nonadhered to the wound bed. Throughout the wound healing process, the phases overlap. It is not at all unusual for the epithelialization, inflammatory, and proliferative phases to overlap and attributes of each to be identified. Table 4–9 summarizes the findings during the epithelialization phase.

A wound phase diagnosis of *epithelialization phase* is based on findings that the wound is resurfacing. Partial-thickness wounds that are resurfacing from the middle or edges are in the *epithelialization phase*. Wounds that are greater than 50% attached at the edges and do not have steep walls that are epithelializing also are diagnosed as being in the *epithelialization phase*. Wounds in the acute epithelialization phase have an excellent prognosis for healing. Wounds in the chronic epithelialization phase need an intervention that will restart the healing process. The prognosis then would be that the wound will heal with intervention. For example, the surgeon may need to excise the fibrotic wound edges. An absent or chronic proliferative phase may need initiation before cells can migrate over the surface. Wounds that have absence of the epithelialization phase of healing have high risk for nonhealing unless intrinsic or iatrogenic conditions can be altered, eg, by reperfusion or application of moisture-retentive dressings.

Clinical Wisdom: *Describing a Wound in the Epithelialization Phase*

Example of narrative note describing a wound in the epithelialization phase:
Evaluation: A wound on the left medial ankle is adhered at 75% of the edges and epithelialization is progressing over 50% of the open area.
Wound healing phase diagnosis: The wound is in the epithelialization phase.

REFERRAL CRITERIA

Utilization management requires that the patient's problems be identified and triaged early to the medical care provider most appropriate to the patient's wound severity or wound healing phase diagnosis. Referral should be made when there are findings that require the attention of another discipline more skilled or more knowledgeable in management of the identified problem. Referral will depend on where the patient is to be seen, the available resources, and other very significant factors. For instance, skin lesions that

Table 4–9 Wound Healing Phase Diagnosis: Tissue Characteristics for Epithelialization Phase

Periwound Skin and Wound Tissue Characteristics	Acute Epithelialization Phase	Chronic Epithelialization Phase	Absence of Epithelialization Phase
Periwound skin	• Early phase has same characteristics as acute inflammatory phase • Returns to normal color for ethnicity as inflammation subsides • Hemosiderin stain if chronic wound	• May be same as chronic or absence of inflammatory phase • May be ischemic (pale) or ashen • May be purplish with dependency • Dry, flaky (hyperkeratotic—may be due to desiccation or aging skin) • Maceration: pale, wrinkled, soft, thin • Hemosiderin stain	• Scar tissue • Same as chronic or absence of inflammatory phase • Dry with hyperkeratosis or lipodermatosclerosis
Wound tissue	• Even with wound edges • Pink/red granulation • Reduction in wound surface area	• Not connected with wound edge • Hypergranulation	• Absence of resurfacing from edges or dermal appendages • Hypogranulation • Presence of scab or necrotic tissue
Undermining/tunneling	• Steep walls limit migration	• Steep walls limit migration	• Steep walls limit migration
Wound edges	• New skin moves out from wound edge and dermal appendages in irregular pattern • Bright pink color, regardless of usual skin pigmentation • Texture is soft to firm and flexible to touch, thin	• Epithelial ridge • Rolled under or thickened • Dry, flaky skin • Rounding off of wound shape	• Fibrotic wound edge • Rounding off of wound shape and edges • Macerated • Dry, flaky skin
Wound drainage	• Minimal to scant serous or serosanguineous	• Absent, dry; if hypergranulation, minimal/moderate	• Absent, dry
Scar tissue	• Thin layers of scar tissue • Thickens over time • Deep pink color initially; changes to bright pink color, regardless of usual skin pigmentation	• Hypertrophic scarring • Keloid scarring • Hyperkeratotic scarring	• Weak, friable epithelial tissue • Breaks or washes out
Color Plates	5, 22, 65	48–51	24, 33, 35, 48, 54, 58

Exhibit 4–5 Referral Sources

Physicians	Nursing	Allied Health
Dermatologist	Dermatology Nurse	Physical Therapist
Orthopaedic Surgeon	Enterostomal Nurse	Podiatrist
Plastic Surgeon	Geriatric Nurse Practitioner	Vascular Technician
Vascular Surgeon	Vascular Nurse	

have not been described in this chapter include scales associated with psoriasis; papules, such as warts and tumors; vesicles, such as chickenpox; and shingles, which are examples of skin conditions that may be seen on the adjacent skin and should be referred to a dermatologist. Wounds that have a history of nonhealing for long periods of time may be cancerous, and they should be referred to a dermatologist for biopsy evaluation. Deep wounds that can be probed to the bone should be considered positive for osteomyelitis and need evaluation by the orthopaedic surgeon. Wounds that are in the chronic inflammatory phase need enhanced perfusion to achieve conversion to an acute inflammatory phase. Vascular assessment would be a primary consideration, and the vascular technician may be the most qualified to provide the service. Reperfusion requires the expertise of the vascular surgeon. A wound with deep tunneling should be referred to the plastic surgeon. The physical therapist has skills in exercise, use of physical agents, and electrotherapeutic modalities, all of which enhance perfusion to tissues. Exhibit 4–5 is a list of possible referral sources.

CONCLUSION

Wound classification systems are used to identify the wound severity by the depth of tissue impairment, leading to a functional diagnosis of *impaired skin integrity* (if the dermis is not penetrated) or *impaired tissue integrity* (if the wound extends through the dermis and deeper). Wound healing assessment by physiologic wound healing phase includes three aspects for each physiologic phase: acute, chronic, or absent. Each phase describes the attributes of the acute, chronic, or absent state of the phase by symptoms found in the periwound skin and the wound tissues. The nurse or physical therapist needs to know where in the trajectory of healing the wound is at baseline assessment to plan treatment, make a diagnosis and prognosis of healing, select interventions, predict outcomes, and triage patients.

The assessment is usually completed by the same person, but this is not always the case. The evaluator may be a person more highly skilled and trained in interpretive skills than the collector. For example, examination and recording of the different wound characteristics may be done by a properly trained physical therapist assistant or a licensed practical nurse, and the evaluation of the findings, the wound healing diagnosis, and the prognosis may be completed by the physical therapist, the registered nurse, or the enterostomal nurse. Collection tools to grade, record, and monitor findings are described in Chapter 6. Documentation requirements for wound assessment should be part of the facility policies and procedures. Documentation should be accurate, should clearly reflect the patient's condition, and should be consistent with documentation by others in the same department or facility. If it is not documented, it did not happen.

REVIEW QUESTIONS

1. How do wound classification systems relate to the wound severity diagnosis?
2. What are the principal indexes for wound assessment?
3. What are the attributes of the adjacent tissues that should be assessed?
4. What tests and measures would be used to assess wound and adjacent tissue attributes?
5. How does assessment of darkly pigmented skin differ from that of lighter skin tones?
6. How would you apply the concept of wound healing phase diagnosis to the prognosis for the wound?

REFERENCES

1. van Rijswijk L. Frequency of reassessment of pressure ulcers, NPUAP Proceedings. *Adv Wound Care.* July/August 1995;8(Suppl 4):19–24.
2. van Rijswijk L, Polansky M. Predictors of time to healing deep pressure ulcers. *Ostomy/Wound Manage.* 1994;40(8):40–42.
3. Bergstrom N, Allman RM, Alvarez OM, et al. *Treatment of Pressure Ulcers.* Clinical Practice Guideline, No. 15. AHRQ Publication No. 95-0652. Rockville, MD: The Agency for Health Care Research and Quality (AHRQ), formerly known as the Agency for Health Care Policy and Research (AHCPR), U.S. Department of Health and Human Services (DHHS); December 1994.
4. Porter JM, Moneta GL. International Consensus Committee on Chronic Venous Disease. Reporting standards in venous disease: An update. *J Vasc Surg.* 1995:21;635:45.
5. National Pressure Ulcer Advisory Panel (NPUAP). Pressure ulcers: prevalence, cost and risk assessment: consensus development conference statement. *Decubitus.* 1989;2(2):24–28.

6. Wagner FW. The dysvascular foot: A system for diagnosis and treatment: *Foot Ankle.* 1981;3:64–122.

7. Shea JD. Pressure sore: Classification and management. *Clin Orthop.* 1975;112:89–100.

8. Bergstrom N, Allman RM, Carlson CE, et al. *Pressure Ulcers in Adults: Prediction and Prevention.* Rockville, MD: AHRQ, DHHS; May 1992.

9. National Pressure Ulcer Advisory Panel (NPUAP). *New Definition for Stage I Pressure Ulcers.* Buffalo, NY: NPUAP; 1998.

10. Henderson CT, Ayello EA, Sussman C, et al. Draft definition of stage I pressure ulcers: inclusion of persons with darkly pigmented skin. *Advances in Nursing Care.* 1997; 10(5):16–19.

11. Krasner D, Weir D. Recommendations for using reverse staging to complete the MDS-2. *Ostomy/Wound Manage.* 1997;43(3):14–17.

12. Ferrell BA, Osterweil D, Christenson P. A randomized clinical trial of low-air-loss beds for treatment of pressure ulcers. *JAMA.* 1993;269:494–497.

13. Cuzzell JZ. The new RYB color code. *AJN.* 1988;88(10):1342–1346.

14. Carpenito LJ. *Nursing Diagnosis, Application to Clinical Practice.* 6th ed. Philadelphia: JB Lippincott; 1995:701–713.

15. Integumentary Panel. Guide to physical therapist practice, II. *Phys Ther.* 1997;77:1163–1650.

16. Abeln S. Reporting risk check-up. *PT Magazine.* October 1997;5(10):38.

17. Greenman PE. Principles of structured diagnosis. In: *Principles of Manual Medicine.* 2nd ed. Baltimore: Williams & Wilkins; 1996:13–20.

18. Makelbust J, Sieggreen M. Glossary, pressure ulcers. In: *Guidelines for Prevention and Nursing Management.* 2nd ed. Springhouse, PA: Springhouse; 1996:8–9.

19. Makelbust J, Sieggreen M. Glossary, pressure ulcers. In: *Guidelines for Prevention and Nursing Management.* West Dundee, IL: S.N. Publications; 1991:14–15.

20. Throne N. The problem of the black skin. *Nursing Times.* August 1969;999–1001.

21. Weiss EL. Connective tissue in wound healing. In: McCulloch J, Kloth L, Feedar J, eds. *Wound Healing Alternatives in Management.* 2nd ed. Philadelphia: FA Davis; 1995:26–28.

22. Harkless LB, Dennis K. Role of the podiatrist. In: Levin ME, O'Neal LW, Bowker JH, eds. *The Diabetic Foot.* 5th ed. St. Louis, MO: Mosby-Year Book; 1993:516–517.

23. Ruschhaupt WF III. Vascular disease of diverse origin. In: Young JR, et al, eds. *Peripheral Vascular Diseases.* St. Louis, MO: Mosby-Year Book; 1991:639–650.

24. Parish CP, Witkowski JA. Decubitus ulcers: How to intervene effectively. *Drug Ther.* May 1983.

25. Bennett MA. Report of the task force on the implications for darkly pigmented intact skin in the prediction and prevention of pressure ulcers. *Adv Wound Care.* 1995;8(6):34–35.

26. Roach LB. Assessment: Color changes in dark skin. *Nursing 77.* January 1977:48–51.

27. Dailey C. Purple ulcers. Letters. *J ET Nursing.* 1992;19:106.

28. Witkowski JA. Purple ulcers. Letters. *J ET Nursing.* 1993;20:132.

29. Joint Commission on Accreditation of Healthcare Organizations (JCAHO). Pain management standards (standard RI 2–8 and PE 1.4). *Comprehensive Accreditation Manual for Hospitals.* JCAHO; 2001.

30. Cavanagh PR, Ulbricht JS. Biomechanics of the foot in diabetes mellitus. In: Levin ME, O'Neal LW, Bowker JH, eds. *The Diabetic Foot.* 5th ed. St. Louis, MO: Mosby-Year Book; 1993:225.

31. Levin ME. Pathogenesis and management of diabetic foot lesions. In: Levin ME, O'Neal LW, Bowker JH, eds. *The Diabetic Foot.* 5th ed. St. Louis, MO: Mosby-Year Book; 1993:43.

32. Horzic M, Bunoza D, Maric K. Contact thermography in a study of primary healing of surgical wounds. *Ostomy/Wound Manage.* 1996;42(1):36–42.

33. Pernet A, Villano JB. Thermography as a preoperative and followup method for surgery of the hand. *Int Surg.* 1984;69(2):171–173.

34. Hoffmann R, Largiader F, Brutsch. HP. Liquid crystal contact thermography—a new screening procedure in the diagnosis of deep venous thrombosis. *Helv Chir Acta.* 1989;56(1–2):45–48.

35. Chan AW, MacFarlane IA, Bowsher DR. Contact thermography of painful diabetic neuropathic foot. *Diabetes Care.* 1991;14(10):918–922.

36. Benbow SJ, Chan AW, Bowsher DR, et al. The prediction of diabetic neuropathic plantar foot ulceration by liquid-crystal contact thermography. *Diabetes Care.* 1994;17(8):835–839.

37. Kohler A, Hoffmann R, Platz A, Bino M. Diagnostic value of duplex ultrasound and liquid crystal contact thermography in preclinical detection of deep vein thrombosis after proximal femur fractures. *Arch Orthop Trauma Surg.* 1998;117(1–2):39–42.

38. Fishman T. *Foot and Nail Care.* Presented at the First Annual Wound Management Workshop, October 1995; Boca Raton, FL.

39. Kerstein M, Bensing KA, Brill LR, et al. *The Physiology of Wound Healing.* Allegheny University of Health Sciences and Oxford Institute of Continuing Education; 1998:11.

40. Cooper D. The physiology of wound healing: An overview. In: *Chronic Wound Care.* Wayne, PA: Health Management Publications; 1990:1–11.

41. Feedar J. Clinical management of chronic wounds. In: McCulloch J, Kloth L, Feedar J, eds. *Wound Healing Alternatives in Management.* 2nd ed. Philadelphia: FA Davis; 1995:140.

42. Sussman C. *Case Presentation: Patient with a Pressure Ulcer.* APTA Scientific Meeting, June 1996; Minneapolis, MN.

43. Harding KG. Wound care: Putting theory into clinical practice. In: Krasner D, ed. *Chronic Wound Care: A Clinical Source Book for Health Care Professionals.* 1st ed. Wayne, PA: Health Management Publications; 1990:24.

44. Hardy MA. The biology of scar formation. *Phys Ther.* 1989;69:1014–1024.

45. Knighton D, Fiegel VD, Doucette MM. Wound repair: The growth factor revolution. In: Krasner D, ed. *Chronic Wound Care: A Clinical Source Book for Health Care Professionals.* Wayne, PA: Health Management Publications; 1990:441–445.

46. Micheletti G. Ulcers of the lower extremities. In: Gogia PP, ed. *Clinical Wound Management.* Thorofare, NJ: Slack; 1995:100–101.

SUGGESTED READING

Sussman C. *Wound Care Patient Education and Resource Manual.* Gaithersburg, MD: Aspen Publishers; 1999.

CHAPTER 5

Wound Measurements

Carrie Sussman

CHAPTER OBJECTIVES

At the completion of this chapter, the reader will be able to:

1. Understand the three most commonly used methods of wound measurement: linear, tracing, and photography
2. Perform the methods for clinical wound measurement.
3. Use wound measurements to track rate of healing
4. Use rate of healing to evaluate outcome of treatment
5. Describe use of a validated tool that uses photography to measure wound healing

INTRODUCTION

Wound measurement accuracy and precision are critical to objective evaluation of wounds in clinical practice and for research. Many studies and suggestions regarding the best way to measure wounds to achieve a reliable result have been published. No method reported is completely reliable.[1] This presents a dilemma for the wound management clinician. If the measurements are not reliable, how can the clinician be sure that the wound is healing and that it is responding to the treatment interventions in a timely fashion? Common methods of wound measurement using linear ruler measurements and wound tracings with planimetry are simple and easy to use. Each has its advantages, disadvantages, and level of reliability, which will be discussed, as will more complex methods applying photography. Step-by-step procedures for performing measurements of wounds and the surrounding tissues, along with a sprinkling of user-friendly helpful hints and clinical wisdoms are provided. Wound volume measure-

ments present special challenges. Advanced technologies of the future may help to improve the reliability but, for a while, at least, will probably be too costly to implement in most wound care settings and will probably be used first for quantifying research results more accurately with standardized measurements. However, the clinician should be aware of the direction that wound measurement is taking in order to evaluate research reports. Two currently available advanced technologies will be explained.

Controlled clinical trials of many types of products on wound healing use reduction in ulcer surface area as the dependent variable, and results are reported as percentage of reduction in unit area per unit time (cm^2/mm^2 or %/day/week).[2] *Percentage of healing* refers to decrease of wound area from the baseline to the day of measurement for each reevaluation period. Method of calculation of this percentage is provided in this chapter. Percentage of healing reduction rates have been analyzed for different wound etiologies (pressure ulcers, venous ulcers, and diabetic ulcers) and are now becoming the standard way for predicting whether the wound will go on to heal, as well as for comparing the results and costs of different interventions.[3–8] Percentage of healing rates can be plotted on a graph (percentage of wound closure versus time of wound treatment) to show a trajectory of healing that will identify those patients whose wounds are on track to heal and those that are not, and the points on the trajectory can be used as end points to compare results, rather than complete healing.[9] Preparation of a trajectory plot is included in this chapter.

LOCATION

The anatomic name that clearly describes the wound location should be written. For example, *trochanter* is a clearer descriptor than is *hip* and signifies that the wound lies over the bony prominence (Figure 5–1). A circle over the anatomic site on the body diagram gives quick, easy identification of wound location on the completed wound measurement form.

The wound's anatomic location can be an indication of the wound etiology (Table 5–1). For example, wounds located over bony prominences are usually pressure wounds, wounds on the soles of the feet may be due to pressure and insensitivity (diabetic wounds), and wounds over the medial side of the ankle often are venous ulcers. Location provides important information about the expected wound healing. Wounds in areas of diminished blood flow, such as over the tibia, heal slowly.

If several wounds are clustered close together in a location, they should be noted by either different letters or by references such as *outer*, *inner*, *upper*, or *lower*. It is important to keep the same reference location ID for all the wounds by name throughout the course of care. If one of the wounds in the cluster heals, this should be noted in the documentation, and the same reference names for the remaining wounds should be retained for further documentation. If several wounds join together and become one, this should be recorded and a new ID name given to the revised wound site. Exhibit 5–1 shows an example of how to document wound location for multiple wounds.

BASELINE MEASUREMENT

Measurement done at the start of care establishes a baseline wound size. Measurements are performed at regular intervals. The rationale for measurement is to quantify and measure the progression of wound healing.[10] In the home care or long-term care settings, measurement is usually rec-

ommended, at least weekly. The professional case manager, nurse, or physical therapist may choose to select measurements that can be made easily. After training, an unskilled individual in the home can report to the skilled professional at a specified interval, such as weekly. Linear measurement of the size of the open surface area is an example of a type of measure that might be delegated. Significance would be interpreted by the professional case manager. For example, a number of studies have found that baseline wound size, when accompanied by other risk factors for healing, was a significant predictor of response to treatment and 100% healing.[5,8,11] Larger ulcers were less likely than smaller ones to heal rapidly, even with optimal therapy; the prognosis should be documented as needing longer time to heal or should trigger a referral.

Tests and measurements of wound size, their extent, and changes are important to providers, payers, and regulators, as well as the patient and the family. Well-documented wound measurements can be used as the best legal defense. They also provide positive feedback from the changes and progress toward recovery for the clinician, who can review the measurements and feel a sense of accomplishment. They may also be the alarm that all is not well. Because the information gathered is important to the interdisciplinary team, the language used requires uniform and consistent terminology to encourage good communication among the team members.

Overview of Monitoring Wound Healing Measurements

Table 5–2 provides an overview of the three different commonly used methods to monitor healing.[12] The table highlights purpose, requirements, and information derived from each method. Many measurement methods and suggestions are included in this chapter. Not all will be useful in all settings. Different skills and interests will determine the methods and measurements used. Table 5–3 is a guide for the common usage patterns for wound measurements. Measuring with sophisticated computer-assisted or technologic equipment has been omitted because these devices are usually research tools, rather than clinical practice approaches.

MEASUREMENT FORMS

Examination must be consistent, complete, and accurate. One way to manage uniformity, consistency, and completeness is with the use of forms. Forms guide the examiner in a logical sequence and assist in organizing the information gathered. Forms may be paper-and-pencil instruments or templates on the computer screen. They are real timesavers because one simply fills in the appropriate information on the preprinted form. Forms become a part of the documentation record. There are numerous forms in use for docu-

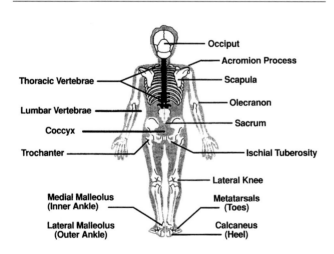

Figure 5–1 Common Locations for Chronic Wounds. Courtesy of Knoll Pharmaceutical Company, Mount Olive, NJ.

Table 5–1 Common Locations for Chronic Wounds by Etiology

Arterial Ulcers	Pressure Ulcers	Neuropathic Ulcers	Venous Ulcers
Lower leg dorsum	Bony prominences:	Plantar surface of foot	Above the ankle
Foot	Scull	Metatarsal heads	Medial lower leg
Malleolus	Ears	Heel	
Toe joints	Shoulder	Lateral border of foot	
Lateral border of foot	Scapulae		
	Sacrum		
	Coccyx		
	Trochanter		
	Ischial tuberosity		
	Knees—condyles, patella		
	Tibia/fibula		
	Malleolus		
	Heel		
	Metatarsal heads		
	Toes		

menting wound measurements. Exhibit 5–2 is a completed sample form for performing the wound measurement examination. The form fits into a 4 × 6-inch pocket notebook. A new form is used each week, and the forms are kept together in the notebook during the course of care for easy reference to prior week measurements. Having the measurements together in one place facilitates monitoring of the size changes on a weekly or biweekly basis. When the case is completed, the measurement sheets are put onto pages of note paper with tape and put into the permanent record. This notebook functions like the nurses' treatment or drug record books. When not in use, it can be kept in a specific location at the nurses' station or in the physical therapy department for reference. The form uses the clock method, described later, for moni-

toring wound depth and undermining. The sample wound form includes the following items:

- Wound anatomic location is noted, which on the form is called the *wound ID*.
- Size is given, including length by width open area, length by width area of erythema (color change), depth, undermining/tunneling, and overall wound size estimate (explained below).
- Period of the wound assessment is given: initial, interim observation week number (OB), and discharge (DC).
- The form also captures information about the wound healing phase. Initials are inserted next to *wound phase* to identify the current wound phase. The initials stand for the phase as follows: *I* for inflammatory phase, *P* for proliferative, and *E* for epithelialization, as described in Chapter 4.
- Discharge outcome status also should be checked as healed or not healed.

The sample form works well when used in conjunction with the Sussman Wound Healing Tool (SWHT),[13] described in Chapter 6. Data can be entered into a computer database and program outcomes monitored.

WOUND SIZE MEASUREMENT ACCURACY AND RELIABILITY

Accurate, complete, uniform, and consistent wound measurements are required to establish a wound diagnosis, plan treatment, and document results. Ways to maximize accuracy include the following:

- Take the measurement the same way each time, from a noted reference point on the body.

Exhibit 5–1 Documenting Wound Location

Documenting Wound Location with Narrative Note:

Example:

1. Single wound location: coccyx
2. Multiple wounds at a location:

Initial note: *Three wounds are located upper, middle, and outer side on the right trochanter.*
　The upper and middle wounds merge. Since they are upper to the outer wound, the same term upper is retained and the merger noted as in this example:
Follow-up note: The upper and middle wounds have merged and will in the future be referred to as the upper wound on the right trochanter.

Table 5–2 Monitoring Recovery of Chronic Wounds: Photo, Tracing, Measurements

Purpose	Photo	Tracing/Planimetry	Measurements
Objective	Establishes baseline wound status Wound size measurement Records change in recovery phase or wound stage	Records shape and size change at baseline and throughout recovery	Linear: estimates size Perimeter: estimates boundary Digitization: approximates surface area
Treatment planning	Validates overall treatment plan	Demonstrates short-term response to treatment plan	Demonstrates rate of recovery
Frequency	Baseline, weekly, or change in phase/condition, discharge	Baseline, weekly discharge	Baseline, weekly discharge
Time reference	Prospective	Prospective	Prospective Ongoing/interim

Requirements	Photo	Tracing	Measurements
Conditions	Correct light, body position, and device to indicate relative size	Use of standard anatomic landmarks and method to transfer tracing to medical record	Use of standard anatomic landmarks
Equipment	Camera and film	Tracing kit Graph paper	Measurement tool and recording notebook

Information	Photo	Tracing	Measurements
Type	Displays full color picture	Gives black and white picture of size and shape	Provides numeric information
Comparison	Provides color comparison of phase and size and tissue attributes	Represents topographic effects and size and change	Summarizes quantitative changes for use in a graph
Use	Clinical medical review, program management, referral source, reports, survey team, legal, patient compliance	Clinical medical review, program management, referral source, reports, survey team, legal, self care, patient compliance	Clinical medical review, program management, referral source, reports, survey team, legal, self care, patient compliance

- Use the same terminology and units of measure for each measurement.
- When possible, have the same person do repeat measurements.

Careful measurement records even small changes and shows the improved wound status or deterioration.

Recording the wound measurement is also an important part of accurate, consistent measurements. If it isn't recorded, it didn't happen.

- An assistant is helpful as a recorder of the measurements as they are taken. Use a prepared form, then fill in a measurement number at each space indicated on the form. This form can be preprinted or handwritten so nothing is forgotten. Record as soon as each parameter is measured. Memory is not accurate.
- Record a zero if a characteristic is assessed and found absent. This says that you observed the characteristic and assessed it. For example, partial-thickness wounds are superficial. By the depth measures spaces, a zero

Table 5–3 Common Usage Patterns for Recording Wound Measurements

Always	Often	Sometimes	Rarely	New
L × W area	Clock L × W area	Depth—greatest	Polaroid grid photo	Depth four points of clock
Tracing shape	Undermining—longest and "mapping"	Digital photography with computer technology	Stereophotography	Undermining four points of clock
	Instant photo with flash			Undermined estimate
	Point and shoot with flash			Area of erythema or discoloration in darkly pigmented skin
	Planimetry			Tracing "wound map"
				Tracing "wound map" with graph report

should be written. A blank space does not show that this characteristic was assessed.

WOUND SIZE MEASUREMENTS

Three types of wound measurements that track the change in the wound size over time are described in this section: surface area (SA) measurements (length by width), undermining or tunnels, and depth. The most common wound measurements are the SA length and SA width. The SA length and width of the wound are measured from wound edge to wound edge. The *greatest length and greatest width method* of measurement means that the wound is measured across the diameter of the greatest length and the greatest width. Then the length is multiplied by the width, which gives the estimated square area of the wound or SA. This measurement inflates the size area of the wound. The product results in a single number that can be easily monitored for change in size. These two dimensions are always measured and may be the only measurement recorded. Less frequently measured are undermining/tunnels and depth.

Another way to measure is called the *clock method*. The face of the clock is used to guide the measurement (see Figure 5–2). Select a 12:00 reference position on the wound. Twelve o'clock is usually toward the head of the body but, in situations such as severe contractures of the trunk and lower extremities, it may be more convenient and easier to reproduce the measurements if another convenient anatomic landmark is selected. For example, measurements in the foot may use the heel or the toes as the 12:00 reference point. In a fetally contracted person, a trochanteric pressure ulcer may be more easily tracked if the 12:00 reference point is toward the knee. Use a clock face and take the measurement from 12:00 to 6:00 and from 3:00 to 9:00.

Both wound measurement methods are acceptable. Choose a method that is comfortable and record which method is used, then use it *consistently*. Exhibit 5–3 lists some advantages and disadvantages of each.

Supplies Needed for Wound Measurement

Supplies assembled in advance help to improve efficiency and reduce examiner and patient fatigue (see "Helpful Hints for Measuring").

- Pen or pencil
- Disposable, plastic straight-edge ruler with linear measure ruled in centimeters
- Disposable gloves

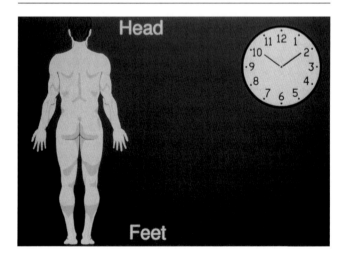

Figure 5–2 Orientation of 12:00–6:00 position of the body related to a clock face. Courtesy of Knoll Pharmaceutical Company, Mt. Olive, New Jersey.

Exhibit 5–2 Completed Wound Measurement Form

Wound Measurements

Initial	_x_
Discharge	____
OBWK#:	_0_
DC Status:	____

Date: _01/03/03_　　　　Patient Name: _G. Lucky_

Wound ID: _R Trochanter_　　　　　　　　　　　　Med Rec# _0397_

Wound Phase: _Chronic inflammation_

(all measurements in cm)

Linear Size:　　　　12:00–6:00　　(A) _4.4 cm_ × 3:00–9:00　(B) _3.3 cm_ = _14.52_ cm²
Erythema Size:　　　12:00–6:00　　(A) _6.5 cm_ × 3:00–9:00　(B) _4.5cm_ = _29.25_ cm²
Undermined:　　　　12:00 (A1) _0_　6:00 (A2) _0.5_　3:00 (B1) _1.5_　9:00 (B2) _0_
Depth:　　　　　　12:00 _0.3_　3:00 _0.3_　6:00 _0_　9:00 _0_
Overall Undermined Estimate:

$$A + A1 + A2 = (a)\ \underline{4.9}$$
$$B + B1 + B2 = (b)\ \underline{4.8}$$
$$(a)\ (b) = \underline{23.52}\ \ cm^2$$

Examiner: _B Sweet , PT_

(OB = the observation week # since start of care)

- Normal saline
- Disposable syringe with 18-gauge needle or angiocatheter (for cleaning)
- Gauze paper, form, or pocket-size notebook to record data (see Exhibit 5–2)

How To Measure

Before measuring, the wound should be cleaned and examined closely. Look carefully at the wound edges and see whether they are distinct so that you are measuring from wound edge to wound edge. Use the following steps:

1. Position patient.
2. Don gloves and remove wound dressing and packing.
3. Place in disposable infectious waste bag.
4. Clean wound with normal saline and syringe with 18-gauge needle or angiocatheter (see Chapter 9 for wound cleansing procedure).
5. Take measurements with disposable wound measurement ruler.
6. Measure the SA greatest length and greatest width from wound edge to wound edge.
7. Record each measurement *as it is taken.*

8. Dispose of wound dressing, measurement instrument, dressing, and gloves in infectious waste container after the procedure is completed.
9. Dispose of the syringe with 18-gauge needle in sharps container.
10. Apply fresh dressing.
11. Calculate wound surface area.
12. Repeat weekly or more frequently, if indicated.

The Clock Method To Measure Surface Area

Replace step 6 above with the following. Everything else remains the same.

6a. Establish the 12:00 position by choosing an anatomic landmark that will be easy to identify, and make a record for all following measurements. Example ✓ 12:00 toward head.
6b. Mark 12:00 with arrow on the skin. Repeat with marks at 6:00, 3:00, and 9:00.
6c. Measure from wound edge at 12:00 to wound edge at 6:00 position.
6d. Measure from wound edge at 3:00 to wound edge at 9:00 position.

Exhibit 5–3 Comparison of Two Wound Measurement Methods

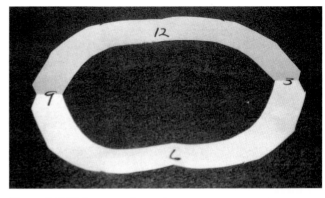

Figure 5–3 Using a template to improve measurement accuracy.

GREATEST LENGTH BY GREATEST WIDTH METHOD

Advantages

- Simple and easy to learn and use
- Most common method
- Reliable

Disadvantages

- Diameters change as size and shape change, so different diameters are measured each time
- Wound open area will be larger than in clock method

CLOCK METHOD

Advantages

- Simple and easy to learn and use
- Tracks same place on the wound over time
- More conservative measure of area

Disadvantages

- Requires more steps to perform
- More precision required to line up wound points along the clock "face"
- Less commonly used

Method 1

1. Map undermining around the *entire* wound perimeter by inserting a moist, cotton-tipped applicator into the length of the undermined/tunneled space and continuing around the perimeter. Dip the cotton tip into normal saline before insertion to make it slide in easier and be less likely to cause tissue trauma (see Figure 5–4).
2. At the end point, *do not force* further entry but gently push upward until there is a bulge in the skin. Mark the points on the skin with a pen and connect them. Measure two diameters as in the length by width. Calculate by multiplying length by width for *overall undermined estimate* (explained later).

Clinical Wisdom: *Using a Template To Improve Measurement Accuracy*

To improve accuracy and keep the measurements better aligned, cut a circle from paper folded in half twice and mark the four clock points at the four paper folds. Place over wound to use as a guide. Tape paper guide to the periwound skin to keep it from shifting.[14] Take all measurements with the template in place for uniformity of tracking the same wound locations for surface area, undermining, and depth (see Figure 5–3).

Measurement of Undermining/Tunneling

Measurement of undermining/tunneling shows the extent of wound damage into surrounding deep tissue. Three methods to measure undermining/tunneling are described. Choose one and use it consistently (see *Color Plates 39* and *40*).

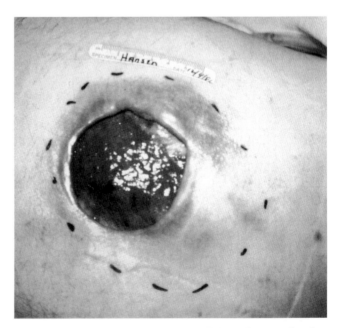

Figure 5–4 Mapping undermining around the entire wound perimeter. *Source:* Copyright © Evonne Fowler, MN, RN, CETN.

Method 2

1. The Sussman method for wound measurement applies the four points of the clock method to measurement of undermining/tunneling.[12] The four cardinal points of the clock—12, 3, 6, and 9—are used. Twelve o'clock will be toward the head unless otherwise noted (see section on clock method of measurement, above).

2. Wet the cotton-tipped applicator with normal saline and insert gently into tunnel. The place on the skin where the cotton tip causes a bulge can be marked, and the cotton-tipped applicator can be withdrawn.

3. The cotton-tipped applicator is gripped at the point where the skin and the wound edge meet and withdrawn. This is the length of the tunnel.

4. Next, place the length of the cotton-tipped applicator up to the withdrawal point against a centimeter ruler or measure from wound edge to mark on skin. Record length.

Method 3

1. Test the perimeter for undermining with a cotton-tipped applicator, then select the longest tunnel to record.

2. Use the clock to identify the location(s) on the wound perimeter where there is tunneling, then track the tunnel over time.

Research Wisdom: *Accuracy and Reliability of Wound Undermining Measurements*

Taylor[14] studied the variability of the measurements of wound undermining among physical therapists trained to use the Sussman wound undermining measurement method. Her findings show that the biggest variation occurred when 12:00 was chosen to coincide with the greatest length of the wound open surface area. This produced an inflation of the area measurements. Her results of reviewing measurements by 39 physical therapists over the 4-week study period demonstrated some interesting findings. For instance, there were three common errors: misreading the measuring device, errors in transferring the numbers, and calculation errors. As would be expected, there was more error in measurement when the wounds were smaller, compared with larger wounds. Overall, the coefficient of variation for open wound area measurements was 5% or less for intratester replication for 69% of the physical therapists and between 5% and 10% for the balance. The wound overall estimate had intertester variance of 10.5% or less for 100% of the study participants. Validation of the measuring technique was proven highly reliable and suggests that this measurement can be used to document progress in the healing of undermined wounds.[14]

☞ **Helpful Hint: Wound Stick Tunneler and Wound Stick Wand**

Two devices are available to aid in wound measurement: the Wound Stick Tunneler and the Wand. Both devices are long, thin rulers. The Tunneler is made of very thin, flat metal (see Figure 5–5). The Wand prototype resembles a fever thermometer and is made of smooth, unbreakable plastic. Both devices have centimeter ruling along the length of the device and can be gently inserted into the undermined space to the point of tissue resistance. Never force the instrument into the space. To use either device, insert the "1 cm" end into the length of the undermined space. The distance from the inside point of resistance to the edge of the wound is read on the ruler. Read the length from under the wound edge, not the visible number. Otherwise extent of undermining will be overstated. These devices can also be used to measure across the open area and from the wound bed to the skin surface for measurement of the depth as described. The depth is read directly from the ruler device. Both devices come in sterile packages and are for single-use application.[4] If the wound undermining/tunneling exceeds the length of the instrument, it would signify that a physician should be notified of possible sinus tract formation. Figure 5–6 shows how undermining is measured on a mock latex wound model. Extent can be read to nearest millimeter. See section on accuracy of measurements for more information.

Overall Undermined Estimated Size

Undermining/tunneling adds to the extent of tissue involved in the wound. The linear measurement of the extent of the wound undermining/tunneling at the same four points on the clock is added to the SA length and width. This is the overall length and overall width. Next, the overall length is multiplied by the overall width to derive an estimate of the *overall undermined estimated size* of the wound area (calculation is shown below).[12] The product is a single number that can be monitored and graphed to show the trajectory of healing over time in the manner shown in Figure 5–7. Figure 5–7 shows graphically how the overall undermined estimated size compares with the SA estimate.[12] If only the open surface area is monitored for change in size, the wound appears significantly smaller than it actually is, and incremental changes in size information are lost.

Extent of Wounding

Other information can be read from the trajectory graph, for example, large variations in the extent of the wound noted earlier between May and July. However, notice the linear reduction in wound extent from September to December. As the wound healed, undermined/tunneled spaces closed,

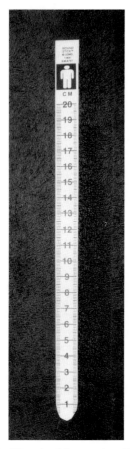

Figure 5–5 Florida Wound stick tunneler. Courtesy of USMS, Miami, Florida.

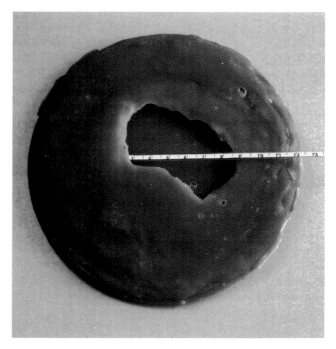

Figure 5–6 Using the wand to measure wound undermining on a latex wound model. Courtesy of Desmyrna R. Taylor, Loma Linda, California.

and tissue integrity was restored, the overall size reduced. Another finding observed from graphing is how the change in undermined estimate also parallels the change in wound phase. Note the abrupt jump in wound overall undermined estimate from 42.25 cm to 122.43 cm. This is frequently co-incident with the early proliferative phase. The expansion of the wound extent reflects the effects of wound debridement on loss of subcutaneous tissue integrity (the separation of fascial planes), producing tunneling. Loss of subcutaneous tissue integrity produces increased risk of infection. Subcutaneous tissue integrity is restored as the wound progresses through the proliferative phase to the remodeling phase.

Graphing the Trajectory of Healing

Graphs showing the wound healing trajectory, such as the one illustrated (Figure 5–7), are a very useful visual method to monitor healing over time. The graph can be generated as part of a database program or can be manually drawn on a piece of graph paper. Graphing to visualize the wound healing or deterioration status has been recommended for tracking the scores obtained using the Pressure Ulcer Scale for Healing (PUSH) tool (see Chapter 6, Tools To Measure Wound Healing). Recently, it has been suggested to use the wound healing

trajectory as a method to track significant points along the continuum of healing, rather than at a single end point, when determining the efficacy of treatment interventions.[9]

Calculating the Overall Estimate

1. Add the length of the SA from 12:00 to 6:00 to the undermined lengths at both 12:00 and 6:00. This is the overall length of the wound.
2. Add the width of the SA from 3:00 to 9:00 to the undermined lengths at both 3:00 and 9:00. This is the overall width of the wound.
3. Multiply the overall length by the overall width.
4. This equals the overall size estimate of the wound.

Example: Overall Size Estimate
12:00–6:00 length + 12:00 undermining + 6:00 undermining = overall length
3:00–9:00 width + 3:00 undermining + 9:00 undermining = overall width
Overall length × overall width = overall estimated area

Utility of Calculating Percentage of Change

Clinical assessment of wound size at baseline and at regular intervals, followed by determination of the percentage of change in wound size, along with other variables, may

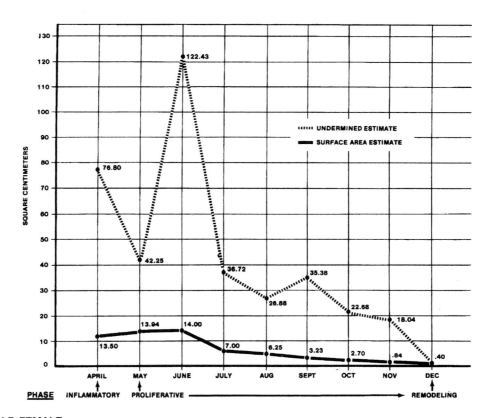

66-YEAR-OLD FEMALE
WOUND TYPE: PRESSURE WOUND
LOCATION: LEFT HIP

Figure 5–7 Wound healing trajectory: recovery of a pressure wound.

predict treatment outcomes for pressure ulcers and venous ulcers.[4] This is a compelling reason for regularly measuring wound SA and for performing the percentage of change calculation to quantify rate of change in size. Two clinical studies found that full-thickness pressure ulcers that decreased 47% and 39% in size during the first 2 weeks of treatment were much more likely to heal and were distinguishable from those that did not heal.[3,4] Other clinical studies looked at leg ulcers for predictors of healing and found that a > 30% reduction in ulcer area after 2 weeks of treatment was a significant predictor of healing.[11,15] Phillips et al[8] did a retrospective study of prognostic factors for venous ulcer healing. The findings were that ulcers that had at least 40% healing by week 3 predicted more than 70% of the outcomes correctly. Kantor and Margolis[7] concur that the percentage of change in area over the first 4 weeks of treatment represents a practical and predictive measure of complete wound healing.

The conclusion deduced from these studies is that both pressure ulcers and leg ulcers that do not reduce in size between 30% and 47% in a 2- to 3-week period are less likely to heal. The clinician can calculate the percentage of change of the wound, then use these numbers as a comparison with the research-reported findings to check whether the wound under care is on course for healing. Plotting the percentage of change on a graph will create a trajectory that will show whether the wound is following a course for healing or for nonhealing. Then an intervention to change the course can be initiated immediately if the wound is not on track. In Part IV, the percentage of change per week for most of the technologies considered in that section, based on the research evidence, is provided as a guide to expected outcomes with the therapy. Other criteria and clinical judgment will guide the decision of therapy choice.

It is clear that the precision of the wound measurement and the method of calculating the rate of change can influence research outcomes. It is less likely that the variations of concern to researchers described below will affect the clinician responsible for setting the goals of treatment and the ability to predict wounds that will go on to heal with standard care and those that should be triaged to adjunctive therapy. However, when reading the research, it is important to understand some of the nuances of the methodology of reporting the study data. Therefore, the information about the use of SA measurements in research is presented.

☞ Helpful Hints for Measuring

1. Wound Measurement Kit

If wound measurements are taken frequently, the job may be easier if you assemble a kit made up of the supplies in the supplies needed list for wound measurement that you keep with you in a small plastic carrier.

2. Use an Assistant

An assistant is helpful to:

- Position patient
- Comfort patient
- Act as recorder
- Control wound "sagging" (see below)
- Seek additional supplies or assistance

3. Patient Positioning

It is easier for everyone if both the patient and measurer are comfortable during the procedure. Some patients and some wounds are difficult to position for accurate measuring. Once a convenient and comfortable position to measure is found, record the position that works best. This will save time and effort and improve the uniformity of measures from time to time.
Example: coccyx wound—position: right sidelying; heel wound—position: left sidelying.

4. Order of Measuring

If measurements are always taken in the same order, the tracking of the wound will be more consistent. Suggestion is to take the length first, the width second. If the clock method is used, take 12:00, 6:00, 3:00, and 9:00—in that order—for improved consistency.

5. Controlling Sagging Wounds

Full-thickness wounds with undermining may sag because of lack of subcutaneous support and the pull of gravity. Tension on the tissue is hard to maintain. Try to keep sagging to a minimum and maintain uniform tension for accurate length and width measurements.

6. Wound Measurement Pocket Notebook (see Exhibits 5–1 and 5–2)

A 4 × 6-inch pocket notebook is useful for recording wound measurements. This can be a spiral notebook or a ring binder. If the information to be gathered is listed in the spiral notebook before doing the measurement, sort of like a handwritten form, it will help consistency, uniformity, and completeness. Another way is to use a preprinted form (see sample) with holes punched to fit a loose leaf notebook. An alphabetic index is also helpful in keeping the records separated by patient name. The small sheets can be taped to a large sheet and placed in the medical record in a cascading fashion. Then numbers do not have to be rewritten. They can also be entered into a computer.

Clinical Wisdom: *Remember the Goal*

When developing the patient's plan of care, it is important to remember the goal of assessing wound size to determine percentage of change from baseline.

Research Application of SA Measurements

Wound SA measurements are used by researchers to predict and track wound healing outcomes. Percentage of healing per unit of time (PHT), usually per week, is a valid way to identify healing and nonhealing. PHT now appears as a frequent variable in research reports, where it has been identified as a predictor of healing or nonhealing.[2–4,8,11,16,17] Clinicians need to be aware of this particular measurement, the method of calculation, and its application because of its newly identified importance. Methods of using PHT vary. Typically, the percentage of reduction in area from baseline calculation method presented here is the calculation method used to measure healing. This method tends to exaggerate the progress made by larger wounds relative to smaller ones, and the percentage of reduction in area minimizes the actual

---

Calculating Percentage Rate of Change in Wound Size

An interesting way to see how a wound is progressing is to look at the percentage rate of change. This is a way to measure and predict successful outcomes. It is a simple statistical calculation that uses the following formula:

1. Baseline (week 0) wound size (OA or overall OA size) measurement is used as the original size.
2. Subtract the next wound size OA or overall OA size measurement (interim) taken from the baseline.
3. Divide by baseline wound measurement and multiply by 100%.

Formula for computing rate of change in wound open area:

(Baseline open area (OA) – Interim open area (OA)/Baseline open area)   100%

Example:	Wound open area (OA) baseline week 0	$= 30 \text{ cm}^2$
	Wound open area (OA) week 1 (interim)	$= 28 \text{ cm}^2$
	OA baseline – OA week 1 (interim)	$= 30 - 28 = 2$
	Divide the remainder by the baseline OA	$= 2/30 = 0.066$
	To calculate percentage multiply $0.066 \times 100\%$	$= 6.6\% = $ Percentage rate of change

Note: A weekly percentage of change would use the prior week size measurement instead of baseline. Wounds often change drastically in size from one week to another in the early phases of healing and then the rate slows. Referring to the percentage of change measure on a weekly or biweekly basis is a good guide to how the wound is healing.

---

progress made by large wounds, relative to progress made in small wounds.[18] Wounds of different sizes or shapes present special problems. To compensate for these problems, Gilman[18] proposed a formula for measuring the wound perimeter change over time that would compensate for these problems (see Exhibit 5–4). The Gilman formula should be used if the population studied has a diversity of ulcer sizes.[17] Margolis and colleagues[17] found the Gilman method of measurement useful for reporting results of healing for venous ulcers and compared their results with those of other researchers looking at venous ulcers and diabetic leg ulcers. In all the studies, the results were nearly identical: Venous ulcers that healed in 4 weeks or more had an initial healing rate of 0.049–0.065 cm/week and diabetic ulcers a rate of 0.063cm/week, suggesting that there may be a fairly uniform rate of healing for chronic ulcers, regardless of etiology.[17] Because repairing wounds appear to heal at the same rate, there should be no correlation between initial ulcer size and the rate of healing. Margolis et al[17] suggested using the 0.062 cm/week rate of healing for all chronic ulcers and that a 4-week period seems to be enough time to establish a healing trend.

Before this can be used as a standard for all chronic wounds, consider the findings of Frantz and colleagues.[19] In an unpublished but reported study of pressure ulcers measured with stereophotogrammetry (SPG), they found that the trajectory for healing differed for partial- and full-thick-

Exhibit 5–4 Gilman Method of Measuring Wound Healing Using the Wound Perimeter

---

$\bar{d} = \Delta A / \bar{p}$

$\bar{d}$ = units of distance; $\bar{d}$ represents the average distance of advance of the wound margin over the study time *T*, in a direction toward the wound center,

ΔA = the difference in area of the wound before and after the study time *T*,

$\bar{p}$ = the average perimeter before and the wound perimeter after time *T*.

Source: Reprinted with permission from T.A. Gilman, Parameter for Measurement of Wound Closure, *Wounds: A Compendium of Research and Practice*, Vol. 2, No. 3, pp. 95–101. © Health Management Publications.

---

ness ulcers. Linear advance of the wound margin was 0.056 mm/day (0.0392 cm/week) for partial-thickness ulcers and 0.021 mm/day (0.0147 cm/week) for full-thickness ulcers. Median time to healing for the partial thickness ulcers was 28 days and 56 days for full-thickness ulcers. These findings suggest that norms for duration and rate of healing are specific to the level of tissue injury. More research on rate of healing of a large population sample with chronic wounds is needed to substantiate the trend before using these numbers as benchmarks for the rate of healing for all chronic wounds (see Exhibit 5–5).

Tallman et al[6] found that using the initial wound size as the baseline number for percentage of change in size calculation to determine the weekly healing rate gave healing rate instability from week to week, which decreased the ability to predict complete healing. They came up with another method to compare healing rates—taking the mean of all previous healing rates between each visit, which becomes the mean-adjusted healing rate, and using that rate as the baseline size to calculate the percentage of change. This method improved healing rate stability from week to week and allowed prediction of complete healing as early as 3 weeks from start of therapy ($p < .001$).[6] However, the sample in Tallman's study was small—15 elderly adults. Polansky and vanRijswijk[2] suggest using the *median* time of healing for study groups, rather than the *mean* time to plot healing time curves. Median time is the time when at least half of the patients have healed. The healing time curve provides a "moving picture" of healing and is developed using the Kaplan-Meir method called *survival analysis*. This methodology is particularly useful when there is a large study population and a significant number of patients that do not complete the entire study course; it may be useful also for prediction of healing of individual wounds.[9] These healing time curves provide more information about the healing than looking at the proportion healed at the end of a study. Healing trajectories are significantly different for healers and nonhealers with diabetic ulcers. Shifting of the wound healing trajectory from an impaired course to a more ideal course may be a way to evaluate the efficacy of the treatment plan.[9] The Polansky and vanRijswijk article describes the methodology involved in doing survival analysis for wound healing in a clear and relatively easy-to-understand way, and it is suggested reading for those considering a research project.[2]

Measurement of Wound Depth

Wound depth is defined as distance from the visible skin surface to the wound bed.[20] A method to track wound depth is desirable and needed because this measurement is an important indication of the proliferative phase of wound healing. Wound bed surfaces are irregular, and repair is not uniform. It is common practice to try to find the deepest site in the wound bed. This method is difficult to reproduce from measurement to measurement because the wound bed fills in irregularly, and what is the deepest spot one time may not be the same spot at the next measurement. Depth measurement accuracy is limited, regardless of how this measurement is made; however, the clock method sets repeated measurement sites that can be more closely reproduced at each measurement test than the use of a single "deepest" spot measurement. There is controversy, especially among researchers, about usefulness of the depth measures because of the inaccuracies recorded.[21]

The Clock Method for Measuring Wound Depth

1. Take depth measurements at the 12:00, 3:00, 6:00, and 9:00 positions.[12]
2. Insert a cotton-tipped applicator perpendicular to the wound edge.
3. Hold stick of applicator with fingers at wound skin surface edge.
4. Holding this position on the applicator stick, place applicator stick along a centimeter-ruled edge. Record for each position.
5. These depth measurements may or may *not* be at the deepest area.
6. A separate measurement may be taken and noted at the deepest area.

Partial-thickness wounds have a depth of less than 0.2 cm. Wounds with > 0.2 cm depth are difficult to measure and should be recorded as > 0.2 cm. Measure the depth of full-thickness wounds of greater than 0.2 cm depth. When a wound is undergoing debridement of nonviable tissue, the wound depth usually increases; but as the wound bed fills with granulation tissue, the depth decreases. Reduction in wound depth is a measurement of progression through the proliferative phase of healing.

Measurement of wound volume is difficult and is usually reserved for research. Two methods have been reported. One method involves filling the wound with a measured amount of normal saline from a syringe. This works best for wounds that can be positioned horizontally so that liquid doesn't spill out. Another method is the use of Jeltrate, an alginate hydrocolloid used by dentists. It has been reported that, by pour-

Exhibit 5–5 Factors Identified as Significantly Affecting Healing Outcomes

- Initial surface area size: Larger ulcers take longer to heal.[4,8]
- Duration: Ulcers of short duration are most likely to heal.[8]
- Healing rate: A 30–47% reduction in area size in the first 2–3 weeks predicts healing.[3,4,8]
- Circulation: Moderate arterial insufficiency (ankle/brachial index (0.5–0.8) increases risk of delayed healing.[5]
- Nutrition: Full-thickness pressure ulcers heal faster with good nutrition.[4]

ing the rapidly setting plastic into the wound, a mold of the wound can be made. Jeltrate is reported to be well tolerated by the wound tissue.[21] Regardless of which method of measuring wound volume is used, there will be significant inaccuracies. Is it necessary to measure wound volume? At this time, there is questionable value to the taking of volume measurements. Use of this parameter of measurement appears to be of most concern in the research arena and should not be of concern to the clinician.[21]

Measurement of Surrounding Skin Erythema

Erythema of the skin surrounding a wound may be a measure of the inflammation phase of healing or a sign of infection. Chronic wounds often show a halo of erythema but lack the other signs of inflammation. The periwound erythema can be identified as unblanchable redness or a darkening of the skin in darkly pigmented skin. See the "Clinical Wisdom" on page 135 regarding measurement of erythema in darkly pigmented skin. Streaking or significant signs of erythema projecting out a distance from the wound may be an indication of cellulitis, and medical measures are needed. Measurement can be taken using the greatest length and greatest width method, or the clock method can be used. The clock method is described.

The Clock Method To Measure Surrounding Skin Erythema

1. Measure across the wound surface area at the 12:00 to the 6:00 position to the outer margin of the periwound erythema.
2. Measure across the wound surface area at the 3:00 to the 9:00 position to the outer margin of the periwound erythema.
3. Compute the periwound area of erythema.

Estimated area of erythema:

12:00 to 6:00 length $\times$ 3:00 to 9:00 width = _____ cm^2

Example: 9:0 cm $\times$ 6.0 cm = 54 cm^2

Wound Tracings

Making a wound tracing, or the acetate method, is reported to be the most popular and practical method for measuring wound area. When the tracing is made on metric graph paper, it is called *planimetry*. It is most useful on wounds that are on flat surfaces, with limited usefulness for full-thickness wounds. Greater reliability using this method has been found for wounds whose edges begin to approximate over a bed of granulation tissue.[22] It is easy to learn, inexpensive, readily available, and requires minimal training.[23] Measuring the wound area from transparency tracings and placing it on graph paper to determine size by counting the centimeters has shown high intra- and intertester reliability (0.99). Compared with linear measurements with a ruler, there is less overestimation of the real wound area, although some error can be expected. Using the 1-cm graph paper to count squares has been reported to be quick and efficient.[22,24] Tracings can be made on acetate measuring sheets, such as those that are given out free by many companies for measuring wounds, or on household plastic wrap with a plastic transparency marking pen (the ink does not bead up). Tracings taped to a sheet of paper can be put in the patient record. However, because taped-on tracings can come loose or become ragged in a chart, the tracing and form can be photocopied and the copy placed in the chart. A tracing is a picture of the wound shape. Repeated tracings show change of size and shape over the course of recovery. Langemo and colleagues[22] compared the standard error of measurement for wounds of different shapes using four techniques: linear ruler length and width, planimetry, SPG length and width, and SPG area. Both length and width measurements best measured circular wounds, tracing worked best for pear-shaped wounds, and SPG had the lowest standard error of measurement for the L-shaped wound. SPG incorporates the use of enhanced digital photography with a computer system, using Wound Measurement System software (see Resources section at the end of this chapter)

Accuracy of measurement with tracing is dependent on how carefully the wound edges are followed as the tracing is drawn. Kloth and Feedar[25] documented measurements for patients in a research study. Sussman[26] suggested use of tracings applied to a graph form with a key for tissue assessment called *wound recovery form*[26] for clinical practice reporting wound healing progression. Following are suggested ways that tracings can be used:

- Tracings show change in the wound perimeter shape over time. Wound shape is a helpful indicator of the rate of healing. As described in Chapter 2, linear wounds contract rapidly, square or rectangular wounds contract at a moderate pace, and circular wounds contract slowly.[24]
- Tracings, when placed on a metric graph form (planimetry) show the wound size, as well as the shape of the healing wound (see Exhibit 5–6).
- A tracing can become a "wound map," showing features of the wound bed, such as necrotic tissue, and adjacent tissue characteristics, such as erythema (see Exhibit 5–6). Household plastic wrap is better for this because it is clear.

Exhibit 5–6 Wound Recovery Form with Tracing

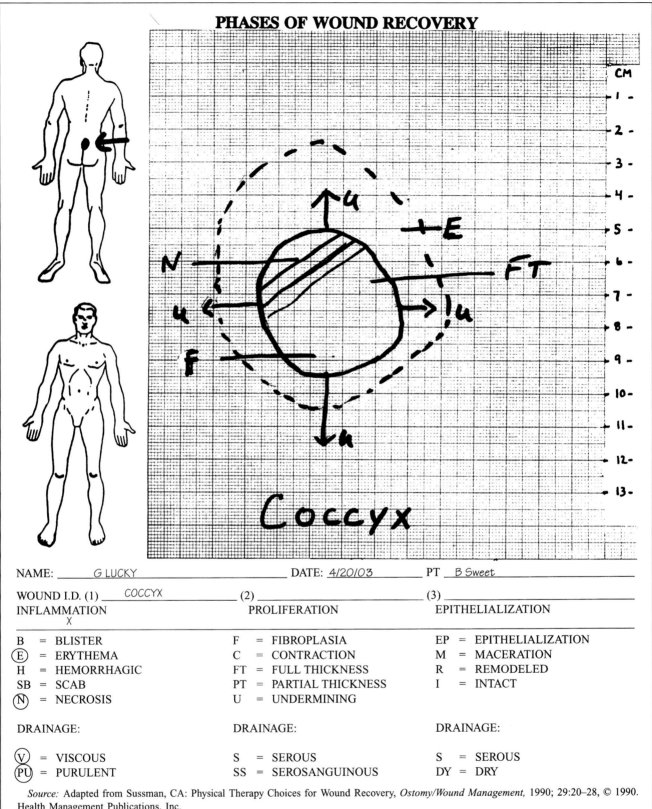

PHASES OF WOUND RECOVERY

NAME: _____G LUCKY_____ DATE: _4/20/03_____ PT __B Sweet_____

WOUND I.D. (1) ____COCCYX_____ (2) _____ (3) _____

INFLAMMATION	PROLIFERATION	EPITHELIALIZATION
X		

B	=	BLISTER	F	=	FIBROPLASIA	EP =	EPITHELIALIZATION
Ⓔ	=	ERYTHEMA	C	=	CONTRACTION	M =	MACERATION
H	=	HEMORRHAGIC	FT	=	FULL THICKNESS	R =	REMODELED
SB	=	SCAB	PT	=	PARTIAL THICKNESS	I =	INTACT
Ⓝ	=	NECROSIS	U	=	UNDERMINING		

DRAINAGE: DRAINAGE: DRAINAGE:

Ⓥ	=	VISCOUS	S	=	SEROUS	S =	SEROUS
ⓅⓊ	=	PURULENT	SS	=	SEROSANGUINOUS	DY =	DRY

Source: Adapted from Sussman, CA: Physical Therapy Choices for Wound Recovery, *Ostomy/Wound Management,* 1990; 29:20–28, © 1990. Health Management Publications, Inc.

- The wound map, if placed on the metric graph paper, can have features such as *actual* amount of undermining/tunneling around the wound perimeter drawn in, using the actual measurements and a ruler.
- The wound map tracing becomes the tissue attributes assessment documentation by the addition of information about the tissue. A key of tissue attributes with assigned letters for each attribute at the bottom of the graph form makes this an easy way to mark the tissue in the drawing. This is then a paper-and-pencil instrument to track wound healing over time. *Note:* The tissue attributes are the same as those represented in the SWHT described in Chapter 6.
- The wound tracing can be scanned into a computer, and a digitized measurement of the wound can be made, the area can be calculated, and the tracing can be stored on the computer.

Supplies Needed

Assemble all equipment needed:

- Two acetate measuring guides or one each plastic wrap over wound, topped by measuring guide
- Two pieces of plastic wrap, cut to approximately 6 × 8-inch pieces or larger, if wound plus periwound erythema is larger
- Fine-point transparent film-type marking pen so that ink won't bead up on the plastic (dark Pentel or Vis < Vis)
- Paper towel, folded in half lengthwise

- Paper or graph form
- Transparent tape

Make a Wound Tracing

1. Place two acetate measuring guides or two pieces of plastic wrap over wound so that the bottom piece is going across wound from 3:00 to 9:00 and the second piece is going from 12:00 to 6:00. This helps when separating the top layer from the bottom layer. Smooth each one to avoid wrinkles. Two layers are used to prevent contamination of the layer with the drawing. The layer that was in contact with the wound will be discarded with infectious waste after the tracing is completed.
2. Draw an arrow on the plastic wrap in the location and direction of the 12:00 position.
3. Trace the wound edges.

Optional Additions to Tracings

1. Draw any notable features within or around the wound surface area, such as outline of the necrotic tissue, exposed bone, etc. Label with a letter from wound assessment form key.[26]
2. Mark areas of erythema/darkened darkly pigmented skin with broken lines around the wound surface area.
3. Mark area of necrotic tissue or eschar with diagonal lines.
4. Mark other features with a circle and dots, and label.
5. Place the film with the drawing so the 12:00 arrow is in the conventional 12:00 position on the graph form. Tape the wound tracing onto the graph form. Make sure that the plastic is taut and free of wrinkles. See instructions for completing the wound assessment form that follows.
6. Copy wound tracing with copier for permanent record. Discard the graph with the plastic tracing.
7. Mark wound features with lines drawn at right angles to the feature and label.

Wound Assessment Form

The wound assessment form[26] is a paper-and-pencil instrument that consists of a centimeter graph sheet, a linear measure lined up with the graph coordinates to show size, and an anatomic figure front and back to mark location. The tissue characteristics are listed by phase: inflammatory, proliferative, and epithelialization. The key assists the clinician in the evaluation and the development of the wound phase healing diagnosis. The completed tracing is shown in Exhibit 5–6.

Supplies Needed

- Wound assessment form
- Wound tracing
- Transparent tape
- Fine-tip marking pen
- Copier (optional)

Use the Wound Assessment Graph Form

1. Prepare wound tracing (see above).
2. Place tracing on assessment form graph with arrow lined up with lines at 12:00 position.
3. Tape tracing in place unless it is adhesive backed.
4. Draw lines exactly the same length as length measurement taken from the undermining at clock points around wound perimeter, starting at wound edges and moving outward.
5. Draw lines from tissue characteristic out to the side of the graph and label with letter from key.
6. Print wound location at the bottom of the picture. Mark its location on anatomic figures.
7. This "wound map" is also a tissue assessment report.

Note: Tissue characteristics are described in Chapter 4.

Clinical Wisdom: *Using the Wound Tracing for Compliance*

The wound tracing is used as an incentive for compliance in diabetic patients. Two wound tracings are made on acetate film or plastic wrap. A date is placed on the tracing next to the wound edge. One copy is placed in the patient records, and the other is given to the patient. The next assessment day, the patient brings in his or her copy, and the copy from the chart is also presented. The wound is redrawn on both pieces of film and dated. The size change is then visually compared. Patients receive positive reinforcement for their compliance by seeing their wounds getting smaller (N. Elftman, *personal communication*, 1996).

☞ **Helpful Hints for Tracings**

1. A grid printed on an acetate film that peels off a plastic backing sheet can be used to make wound tracings. The sheet acts as a barrier to infection and is discarded. The tracing is then ready to place in the medical record.
2. The Polaroid Wound Photograph system has a grid available to be used when taking a wound photograph.

WOUND PHOTOGRAPHY

"A picture is worth a thousand words" used to be the best way to describe the value of wound photography. Now that old adage can be modified to say that "a picture of a wound is worth thousands of dollars."[1] Photo documentation is one way to prevent litigation in wound management. Wounds should be photographed if present on admission or when acquired and at discharge. The photograph serves as a permanent record of the wound at baseline and a record of its course during care. Unless consent for patient photography is part of the facility admission package, consent should be obtained before photography is used. In some facilities, the photographs of wounds are part of the patient's medical record; in others, it is kept separately. Wound photographs were reported to be part of the documentation procedures in 75% of the home health care agencies in the United States.[28]

Serial color photographs document wound tissue characteristics. The lighting will affect the color. Flash photography tends to give a blue tone to the photograph. Incandescent light gives a yellow tone. Photographs are used also to measure the wound size. The accuracy of wound measurement taken from a photograph is compromised by the problem caused by measuring wound area on curved surfaces.[23] Periodic photography is a method often used to validate the overall treatment outcome. Serial photos are great teaching tools for in-services, for referral sources, for reimbursement, and for patient encouragement. Photography can be done as simply as shooting an instant camera or by using more complex camera equipment. For example, an instant camera with a grid printed on the film is one method. See Figure 5–8 for an example of grid photography. The cost of digital camera equipment has dropped significantly but quality of resolution of the image using lower-priced digital cameras is still an issue, and this technology is not readily available to the average clinician. Another relatively new option is color print film, which can be shot with a standard 35-mm camera and is processed and returned in one or all three forms: photos, slides, and computer disk. The computer could be used to store the photographic records. Additional information can

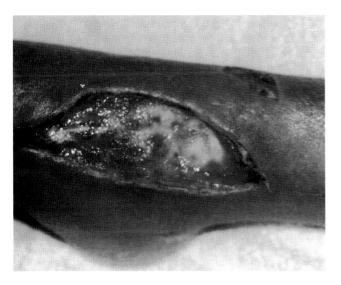

A

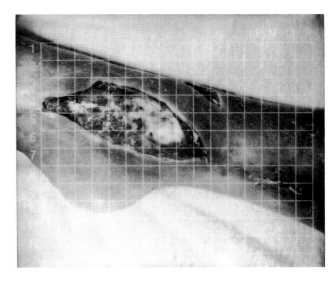

B

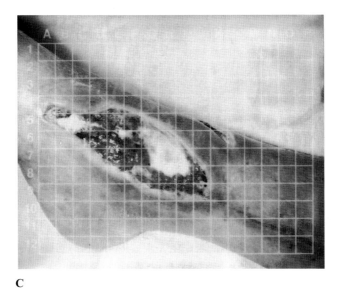

C

Figure 5–8 Grid photography (A–C). Shows change in wound size and attributes over time.

be added to each photo for recordkeeping. Scanning is yet another method for computer inputting of photographs that has become more widely available. Again, the quality of the scanner will influence the quality of the computer image. Enhanced digital or video photography with computer software designed to record, measure, document, track, and keep a database of wound information is available. Complex camera setups and computer systems are usually used by researchers but this is likely to change as the standards for recording and documenting wounds are revised and use of telemedicine expands. Regardless of which method is used, for good pictures, follow these tested suggestions:

- Use a good light source.
- Position patient and wound carefully, ensuring that the patient's private areas are screened from the camera.
- Position a linear measure (ruler) in the photo to show relative size.
- Use a string of known length to measure distance from the camera to the wound for more uniform recording.
- Use an identification sign with patient ID, wound location, and date in the photograph (unless dated by the camera).
- Select a camera with a close-up feature, if possible, to take the best close-up view of the wound.

- Use a ring flash attachment on a 35-mm close-up lens to eliminate shadows.
- Use an assistant to help maintain the position and perhaps to position the marker.
- Record wound and patient position for repeated photographing sessions, ie, right sidelying.

Helpful Hint: *Making an Identification Marker for Photographs*

1. Tape plastic measuring sheet to a 3 × 5-inch index card.
2. Put card into a plastic sandwich bag.
3. Put two strips of white tape on the plastic sandwich bag.
   –Write patient ID, wound location on first strip (example: W.J., coccyx).
   –Write date on second strip (example: 1/23/01).
4. Throw away the plastic bag.
5. Reuse the card.

PHOTOGRAPHIC WOUND ASSESSMENT TOOL

The Photographic Wound Assessment Tool (PWAT) is a modified version of the Pressure Sore Status Tool (PSST) (see Chapter 6, Tools To Monitor Wound Healing). It makes use of six domains of the PSST that can be determined from photographs alone and that do not require bedside assessment.[28] Each domain item of the PWAT is scored numerically, and a total score is calculated by summing the scores assigned to each of the six domains (see Exhibit 5–7). The range of possible total PWAT scores is between 0 and 24, with zero representing a healed ulcer.[28] The PWAT was applied and tested with pressure ulcers and leg ulcers and found to have high inter- and intrarater reliability among experienced wound clinicians, high concurrent validity, based on the degree of agreement between surface area calculation, obtained from the wound photograph (n = 46), and the surface area assessed, using wound tracings and linear measurements (the intraclass correlation coefficient [ICC] = 0.86 and 0.96, respectively). Serial photographs of 38 individuals were used to monitor the change of the wound over time. Researchers were able to divide the ulcers into "healers" and "nonhealers," based on the change in wound surface area, as measured by the PWAT. A comparison of PWAT scores revealed that there were almost statistically significant differences between the two groups ($p = 0.07$). Highest reliability was achieved when the PWAT was applied to pressure ulcers, compared with leg ulcers, probably reflecting its derivation from the PSST that was designed for assessment of pressure ulcers. Limitations to its use are the added costs associated with wound photography, the need for patient or decision maker approval before taking photographs, and how it affects the decision-making process by the clinician.[28] However, the PWAT may play an important role in the field of wound telemedicine. A tool that would help nurses and physicians have a reliable and easy-to-use method of quantifying the status of wounds from photographs could potentially improve the quality of outpatient wound care. Trials of telemedicine using digital photography show that wound evaluation on the basis of viewing digital images is comparable with standard wound examination and results in similar diagnosis, most of the time.[29]

REFERRAL CRITERIA

Why include referral criteria with the chapter on measurement? As wound measurements and remeasurements are performed, it may become immediately apparent that a prompt referral is necessary. The availability of expensive new technologies for treatment, such as growth factors and tissue-engineered products, has made it very important to recognize and understand the criteria for referral for these and other alternative or adjunctive treatments. To do that, the clinician must have a valid way of measuring the efficacy of standard care. Standard care for chronic wounds is well developed and includes pressure relief off loading or compression, debridement, moist wound healing, and good nutrition. Referral should be considered when the following four criteria are met.[30]

- Initial ulcer size and duration indicates that standard care is likely to fail (eg, large, deep ulcer of longer than 1 year duration)
- Rate of healing with standard care predicts failure (> 30% healing)
- Fails to heal in predicted time, based on guidelines of 30–47% reduction in size in 2–4 weeks

---

Exhibit 5–7 Six Domains of PWAT

---

1. Edges
2. Necrotic tissue type
3. Necrotic tissue amount
4. Skin color surrounding skin
5. Granulation tissue
6. Epithelialization

- Under special circumstances, such as unusual diagnosis or patient demand

Additional criteria to initiate referral at the time of wound measurement:

- Extent of wound involves bone and/or deep subcutaneous spaces—may indicate osteomyelitis or other infection
- Impending exposure of a named anatomic structure—wound extent should be evaluated medically
- Black holes or tunnels that cannot be measured—high-risk situation
- Wound tunneling may perforate the peritoneal cavity in either the abdomen or the rectum
- Wound size enlarging more than expected.

REFERRAL SOURCES

There are many health care practitioners who have experience in complex wound management. One or more of these professionals should be contacted for follow-up management if any of the referral criteria listed above are met. Some choices include the following:

Physicians	Nursing	Allied Health
Dermatologist	Dermatology nurse	Physical therapist
Orthopaedic surgeon	Enterostomal	Vascular technician
Plastic surgeon	Registered nurse	Podiatrist
Vascular surgeon	Geriatric nurse practitioner	
	Vascular nurse	

SELF-CARE TEACHING GUIDELINES

In today's health care environment, many levels of caregivers may be called on to measure and monitor the wound size parameters discussed in this chapter, then to report to the expert clinician their findings for interpretation. The most successful results occur when step-by-step instructions and return demonstration are given by the designated data collector. Prepare an instruction sheet for measuring and/or for tracing. Include a chart like the one in Exhibit 5–8 for recording the data. First, make an assessment of the person's abilities to follow the directions. If the patient or a lay caregiver is to do the measuring, limit the measurements to length and width. Teach the simple length by width multiplication so that only one number needs to be reported. Making a wound tracing is also within the ability of many caregivers. Tracing the wound will also help the caregiver to see that the wound is getting smaller as the report number decreases or to see the changes in drawing shape and size. This reinforces both

the caregiver's and the patient's compliance. If the wound is not getting smaller, it will be an attention-getter and encourage change in treatment planning. A form such as the one illustrated (see Exhibit 5–8) can be faxed to the wound case manager if visits cannot be made on a frequent basis, and the progress of the wound can be followed. If the person to monitor the wound is a paraprofessional, physical therapist assistant, or licensed practical nurse, other wound measurements can be taught and with a high level of expected reliability confidence.

Sample Instruction Sheet

Wound Measurements

Supplies Needed:
- Plastic measuring sheet
- Pen
- Plastic wrap
- Plastic sandwich bag (one or two)
- Hand-held pocket calculator

Wound measurements are taken once a week or biweekly.

1. Note the date.
2. Measure the longest diameter of the wound in each direction, head to toe (length) and side to side (width). Record the length and width in the appropriate boxes on the form as the measurements are taken.
3. Then multiply the two numbers together for a single total size measurement.

Instructions To Make a Wound Tracing at Home

1. Use either two pieces of plastic wrap or a plastic sandwich bag.
2. Place one layer of plastic against the clean wound. If the plastic becomes foggy, that is, like warm air condensing on eyeglasses, lift a corner of the plastic to

Exhibit 5–8 Wound Measurement Record

Name: _____ Medical Record # _____			
Date	Length	Width	Total
4/30/04	5 cm	3 cm	15 cm^2
5/15/04	4.5 cm	2.5 cm	11.25 cm^2
5/30/04	4.0 cm	1.75 cm	8.8 cm^2
6/15/04	2.5 cm	1.25 cm	3.13 cm^2

allow the heat and moisture to escape, and the fog will go away.

3. When you can see the edges of the wound, use a felt-tip marking pen and draw around the wound edges.
4. Mark the date of the drawing next to the edge of the wound. After the ink is dry (about 10 seconds), lift the top layer of plastic wrap or cut off the top layer of the plastic bag.
5. Save the wound tracing in another clean plastic lunch bag.
6. Discard the dirty plastic sheet.

CONCLUSION

This chapter described a number of different measurement strategies for monitoring wound extent and wound healing by tracking change in four different parameters of size: open SA, undermining/tunneling, depth, and overall wound estimate. Obviously, to perform all of the above measurements would be an overload for most people. All are used commonly. One method will appeal to one facility's practitioners and another to another facility's. This is an opportunity for collaboration. Have a team meeting and decide on the method that meets the needs of the majority of practitioners and conveys the desired information. There is enough similarity between methods that the information communicated through the continuum of care can and will be readily interpreted. The keys to successful measurements are consistency and accuracy. Once a method is selected, use it with rigor by all clinicians. Report on a regular, consistent basis.

REVIEW QUESTIONS

1. Describe two ways to take linear wound surface area and depth measurements.
2. Describe the benefits of each of the three types of wound measurements presented: linear, tracing with and without planimetry, and photography.
3. What is the benefit of performing the calculation of the percentage of change in SA at regular intervals?
4. How can an instrument to measure and score wound healing be useful in future health care systems?
5. What are the criteria for leaving standard care and referral for adjunctive therapy?

RESOURCES

- The Wound Stick Tunneler, USMS, Inc., 1172 S. Dixie Highway, Coral Gables, FL 33146
- The Wand and latex wound models: D. Taylor, Loma Linda University, School of Allied Health Professions, Loma Linda, CA
- Plastic/acetate measuring sheets are available from many wound care products companies listed in Appendix A.
- VeVMD Measurement Documentation: Vista Medical, Winnipeg, Manitoba, Canada, Web site http://www.vistamedical.org.
- Sussman C. *Wound Care Patient Education and resource Manual.* Gaithersburg, MD: Aspen Publishers; 1999.

REFERENCES

1. Salcido R. The future of wound measurement. *Adv Skin Wound Care.* 2000;13(2):54,56.
2. Polansky M, vanRijswijk L. Utilizing survival analysis techniques in chronic wound healing studies. *Wounds.* 1994;6(5):15–58.
3. vanRijswijk L. Full-thickness pressure ulcers: patient and wound healing characteristics. *Decubitus.* 1993;6(1):16–21.
4. vanRijswijk L, Polansky M. Predictors of time to healing deep pressure ulcers. *Ostomy/Wound Manage.* 1994;40(8):40–42, 44, 46–48.
5. Marston W, Carlin R, Passman M, Farber M, Keegy B. Healing rates and cost efficacy of outpatient compression treatment for leg ulcers associated with venous insufficiency. *J Vasc Surg.* 1999;30(3):491–498.
6. Tallman P, Muscare E, Carson P, Eaglstein W, Falanga V. Initial rate of healing predicts complete healing of venous ulcers. *Arch Dermatol.* 1997;133(10):1231–1234.
7. Kantor J, Margolis DJ. A multicenter study of percentage change in venous leg ulcer area as a prognostic index of healing at 24 weeks. *Br J Dermatol.* 2000;142(5):960–964.
8. Phillips T, Machando F, Trout R, Porter J, Olin J, Falanga V. Prognostic indicators in venous ulcers. *J Am Acad Dermatol.* 2000;43(4):627–630.
9. Robson MC, Hill D, Woodskein M, Steed D. Wound healing trajectories as predictors of effectiveness of therapeutic agents. *Arch Surg.* 2000;135(7):773–777.

10. vanRijswijk L. Frequency of reassessment of pressure ulcers: National Pressure Ulcer Advisory Panel Proceedings, 1995. *Adv Wound Care.* July/August 1995:19–24.

11. Arnold T, Stanley J, Fellows E, et al. Prospective, multicenter study of managing lower extremity venous ulcers. *Ann Vasc Surg.* 1994;8(4):356–362.

12. Sussman C, Swanson G. A uniform method to trace and measure chronic wounds. Presented at Symposium for Advanced Wound Care; April 1991; San Francisco, CA.

13. Sussman C, Swanson GH. The utility of Sussman wound healing tool in predicting wound healing outcomes in physical therapy. Presented at the National Pressure Ulcer Advisory Panel Fifth Biennial Conference; February 1997; Washington, DC.

14. Taylor DR. Reliability of the Sussman method of measuring wounds that contain undermining. Presented at American Physical Therapy Association Scientific Meeting; June 1997; San Diego, CA.

15. vanRijswijk L. Full-thickness leg ulcers: patient demographics and predictors of healing. Multi-center leg ulcer study group. *J Fam Pract.* 1993;36(6):625–632.

16. vanRijswijk L. Wound assessment and documentation. In: Diane K, Kane D, eds. *Chronic Wound Care: A Sourcebook for Healthcare Professionals.* Wayne, PA: Health Management Publications; 1997:16–27.

17. Margolis DJ, Gross EA, Wood CR, lazarus GS. Planimetric rate of healing in venous ulcers of the leg treated with pressure bandage and hydrocolloid dressing. *J Am Acad Dermatol.* 1993;28(3):418–421.

18. Gilman TH. Parameter for measurement of wound closure. *Wound.* 1990;2(3):95–101.

19. Frantz R, Bergquist S, Gardner S. *Measurements of Partial and Full Thickness Ulcers: Critical Parameters of Healing.* Washington, DC: American Nurses Association Council of Nursing Research; 1996.

20. Hess CT. *Nurse's Clinical Guide, Wound Care.* Springhouse, PA: Springhouse; 1995.

21. Gentzkow G. Methods for measuring size in pressure ulcers. National Pressure Ulcer Advisory Panel Proceedings, 1995. *Adv Wound Care.* July/August 1995:43–45.

22. Langemo DK, Melland H, Hanson D, Olson B, Haneter S, Henly SJ. Two-dimensional wound measurement: comparison of 4 techniques. *Adv Wound Care.* 1998;11(7):337–343.

23. Harding K. Methods for assessing change in ulcer status. *Adv Wound Care.* July/August 1995:37–42.

24. Majeske C. Reliability of wound surface area measurement. *Phys Ther.* 1992;72:138–141.

25. Kloth L, Feedar J. Acceleration of wound healing with high voltage, monophasic, pulsed current. *Phys Ther.* 1988;68:503–508.

26. Sussman C. Physical therapy choices for wound recovery. *Ostomy/Wound Manage.* July/August 1990; 29:20–28.

27. Bennett MA. Report of the task force on implications for darkly pigmented intact skin in the prediction and prevention of pressure ulcers. *Adv Wound Care.* November/December 1995:34–35.

28. Houghton PE, Kincaid CB, Campbell K, Woodbury MG. Photographic assessment of the appearance of chronic pressure and leg ulcers. *Ostomy/Wound Manage.* 2000;46(4):20–30.

29. Wirthlin D, Buradagunta S, Edwards R, et al. Telemedicine in vascular surgery: feasibility of digital imaging for remote management of wounds. *J Vasc Surg.* 1998;27(6):1089–1099.

30. Eaglstein W. What is standard care and where should we leave it? Presented at Evidence Based Outcomes in Wound Management Symposium; March 2000; Dallas, TX.

SUGGESTED READING

Gilman TH. Parameter for measurement of wound closure. *Wounds.* 1990;2(3):95–101.

Polansky M, vanRijswijk L. Utilizing survival analysis techniques in chronic wound healing studies. *Wounds.* 1994;6(5):15–58.

CHAPTER 6

Tools To Measure Wound Healing

Barbara M. Bates-Jensen and Carrie Sussman

CHAPTER OBJECTIVES

At the end of this chapter, the reader will be able to:
1. Explain validity, reliability, sensitivity, and specificity, as used for evaluating wound healing tools
2. Review the wound characteristics commonly included in wound healing tools
3. Describe the development and use of three wound healing tools:
   - Sussman Wound Healing Tool (SWHT)
   - Pressure Ulcer Scale for Healing (PUSH)
   - Pressure Sore Status Tool (PSST)

INTRODUCTION

Assessment of wound status to measuring healing should be performed at least weekly. Medicare requires a minimum of monthly reporting. How best to perform and document the wound assessment for the purpose of evaluating healing has not been agreed on, and several approaches have been proposed. Although there is general agreement that use of a systematic approach with evaluation of multiple wound attributes is helpful, there are no data available that demonstrate improved outcomes by using a standardized, research-based tool. However, it is prudent to use a systematic approach to increase communication among those involved in the wound care plan. Assessment of specific characteristics was covered in Chapter 4; the current chapter is devoted to tools that assess multiple characteristics in order for the clinician to evaluate whether healing has occurred. This chapter also includes information on instrument development and discusses tools used in evaluating wound healing.

There are several tools available that evaluate multiple wound characteristics to assess overall wound status and healing. Several instruments have been proposed to address the question of monitoring healing in pressure ulcers, including the Pressure Sore Status Tool (PSST),[1] the Sessing scale,[2] the National Pressure Ulcer Advisory Panel (NPUAP) Pressure Ulcer Scale for Healing (PUSH),[3] the Wound Healing Scale (WHS),[4] the Sussman Wound Healing Tool (SWHT),[5] the Photographic Wound Healing Tool (PWHT),[6] and the Assessment of Pressure Ulcer Healing Process (PUHP—Japanese).[7] Table 6–1 shows the wound characteristics and scoring systems used by each tool.

Measurements used to evaluate wound healing over time have included change in ulcer size or surface area, change in wound appearance, and stage of the wound. Use of a staging system has historically been very common as a method of evaluating healing. Although staging systems such as the NPUAP system[3] and the Wagner scale[8] (see Chapter 4) are appropriate for determining initial severity of tissue trauma, the systems have been misapplied as methods to measure healing by using the numerical classifications in reverse to down-stage the ulcer to signify healing. Use of a single wound characteristic has not been helpful in monitoring healing, determining treatment response, and prescribing therapy or predicting outcomes. Thus, there is a clear need for tools that include multiple wound characteristics as measures of healing in a more biologically accurate manner.

CRITERIA FOR EVALUATING WOUND HEALING TOOLS

Criteria to evaluate the appropriateness and utility of a tool include validity, sensitivity and specificity, reliability, responsiveness, and clinical practicality.

Table 6–1 Factors and Scoring Methods Used in Wound Healing Tools

Format	Pressure Sore Status Tool (PSST)	Pressure Ulcer Scale for Healing (PUSH)	Sessing Scale	Sussman Wound Healing Tool (SWHT)	Wound Healing Scale (WHS)*	Photographic Wound Healing Tool (PWHT)	Pressure Ulcer Healing Process (PUHP— Japanese)
Wound Characteristics Measured:							
Size	X	X		X		X	X
Depth or stage	X		X	X		X	X
Tissue characteristics							
Necrotic tissue	X	X	X	X	X	X	
Granulation tissue	X	X	X	X	X	X	X
Epithelial tissue	X	X	X	X	X	X	X
Surrounding tissue characteristics	X			X		X	
Exudate	X	X	X		X	X	X
Undermining and tunneling	X		X	X	X	X	X
Scoring Methods:							
Likert scale	X					X	X
Dichotomous scale							
Subscales with total score	X	X	X	X			X

*Method to measure changes in status over time unclear.

Validity

Validity is the accuracy with which an instrument or test measures what it purports to measure.[9] Validity is context-specific, meaning that a tool that is valid in one study may not be valid for another study. For instance, a tool that is valid for measuring healing in pressure ulcers may not be valid for measuring healing in lower extremity vascular ulcers. Validity, as it relates to tool development, is a cyclical process. When indicated, information from validity testing may be used to change a tool to increase validity, then the newly revised tool is retested.[10] Validity is not a static quality and changes over time. Validity is not an "all-or-nothing" quality; it is usually a matter of degree. There are three main qualities in validity: content, criterion, and construct.

Content Validity

Content validity is the degree to which a test or instrument measures an intended content area. The match between the objective to be measured and the items (content) on a tool relates to content validity. Content validity is typically evaluated during an instrument or tool's development. Content validity may be determined using an expert panel whose members (the number depends on the specific type of procedures used) rate in some manner the items on the tool and the total instrument as to ability to measure the objective. Guidelines are available for interpreting content validity but, in clinical practice, evaluation of how the tool was developed, who was involved, where knowledge of the tool's content was obtained, and the outcome of the expert panel is usually enough information. This is true because the ratings of the content specialists are only as good as their levels of expertise in the area measured.

Criterion Validity

Criterion validity evaluates the relationship between the instrument or tool and some other criterion. Criterion validity is concerned with the pragmatic issue: Is the tool a useful predictor? The functional usefulness of a tool is supported by criterion-related validity evidence.[10] There are two types of criterion available for evaluation—concurrent and predictive. Concurrent validity is testing the tool against present performance or status on a criterion. Predictive validity is testing the tool against future performance or status on a criterion. An example of concurrent validity for wound healing tools is the ability of a tool to separate partial- and full-thickness wounds, based on their scores on the tool. An example of predictive validity is the ability of a tool to predict healing or wound closure. Predictive validity is particularly important for wound healing instruments and bears further discussion. Predictive validity can be either positive or negative (for instance, a tool would be equally beneficial if it predicted those wounds that would not heal as it would in predicting those wounds that will heal).

Predictive validity of tools involves the evaluation of the tool's sensitivity and specificity. Sensitivity is the true positive rate for the instrument and is calculated by dividing the number of those with a condition and a positive test by the total number of those with the condition. Specificity is the true negative rate for the instrument and is calculated by dividing the number of those without a condition and a negative test by the total number of those without the condition. Sensitivity and specificity are inversely related. Predictive validity is important. Screening tools that have predictive validity are based on the assumption that, after detecting specific variables, an intervention can be applied that would affect the predicted outcome.

Sensitivity and Specificity. Sensitivity is the number of true positives obtained when using the tool. Sensitivity involves using the tool and determining those with the condition that were obtained by using the tool versus all of those with the condition. For example, a sensitive wound healing tool should be able to determine all of the wounds that have improved. Sensitivity involves precision and accuracy of the instrument. Can the tool accurately identify those wounds that have improved? Ideally, a tool should be able to pick up all or 100% of those with the condition being measured. However, most tools sacrifice some degree of sensitivity for specificity.

Specificity is the number of true negatives obtained when using the tool. Specificity involves using the tool and determining those without the condition that were obtained by using the tool versus all of those without the condition. In an ideal world, a tool should be 100% specific to the condition being measured.

Construct Validity

Construct validity is the third quality of validity and refers to evaluation of the attribute that the tool is attempting to measure. This form of validity is more concerned with the underlying attribute than with any scores produced by the tool. The major focus of construct validity is to establish support for the tool's ability to function, in accordance with the purpose for which it is being used. For instance, tools to measure wound healing should function by identifying wounds that are healing or nonhealing (the purpose for which the wound healing tool is being used).[10] Testing for this type of validity uses techniques such as known groups, where the researcher evaluates groups that are known to differ on the attribute being measured because of some characteristic. If the tool being tested demonstrates different scores for the two groups, this supports construct validity. Likewise, the tool can be evaluated for construct validity by using a similar instrument that measures the same attribute; if both tools come up with similar scores, this would support the construct validity of the new tool. The final aspect of validity is reliability. A tool cannot be valid if it is not reliable. A tool can be very reliable and still not meet the criteria for validity, but it is not possible to have a tool that is valid and not reliable.

Reliability

Reliability of a tool is its ability to be used with minimal random error. Reliability reflects the consistency of the measure obtained and is concerned with accuracy, dependability, consistency, and comparability of the tool. High reported reliability values on a tool do not guarantee that its reliability will be adequate in another sample or study.[9] As with validity, reliability estimates are specific to the population in the sample being tested. Reliability must be performed on each instrument used in a study. In clinical practice, this means that a wound healing tool that works for one organization may not work for another type of organization or another type of patient population. Each organization may have to test the tools to determine which work most reliably for them. There are several kinds of reliability tests for a tool.

Typically, three aspects of reliability are tested: stability, equivalence, and homogeneity. Stability reliability is also called *intrarater reliability* and evaluates the consistency of the tool with repeated measures. In this type of reliability, the same rater/observer uses the same tool on the same wound at different times. The goal is for the same rater to get the same score when observing the same phenomena repeatedly. This type of reliability may also be called *test-retest reliability*. Issues in wound healing tools with intrarater reliability relate to how much time should exist between measures. If the time period is long, the issue of concern is the possibility of different scores reflecting a true difference in the wound, and, if the time period is short, the concern exists regarding the possibility of the observer remembering a previous score.

Equivalence reliability may also be called *interrater reliability* and evaluates the multiple raters using the tool at the same time on the same wound. Interrater reliability is concerned with different raters getting the same score on the tool when evaluating the same wound. Adequate interrater reliability testing involves using at least 10 subjects or wounds and calculating the percentage of agreement between observers scores on the tool or computing a Cohen's Kappa, which is a statistical analysis of agreements that mathematically corrects the data for chance agreements. Both percentage of agreement and Cohen's Kappa statistics are reported in literature on wound healing tools.

The final aspect of reliability is homogeneity. Homogeneity is the similarity or "sameness" of items within an instrument. The calculations behind homogeneity reliability are complex but the thinking is simple. Homogeneity testing examines the extent to which all the items on the tool consistently measure the same objective.[9] This form of reliability evaluates the correlation of different items within the same tool or a measure of the similarity of the tool items. This is reported as a measure of internal consistency, typically, Cronbach's alpha coefficient. Other approaches to testing internal consistency are to use Cohen's Kappa statistic, which determines the reliability of each item with the probability of chance taken out; correlations of each item with the total tool score for the instrument; and correlating each item with each other item in the tool.[9] Factor analysis can also be used to evaluate an instrument's internal consistency. All forms of reliability may be reported for wound healing tools, so this basic discussion will help practitioners to understand better the use of an evidence-based instrument for wound assessment and healing.

Responsiveness

Responsiveness, or sensitivity to change, is another test criterion for a tool. An appropriate tool or method must be able to detect changes in the condition of the wound over time with repeated administrations. It is important for the instrument to be able to detect significant changes in the wound and to respond with a change in tool score. To some degree, sensitivity to change may be evaluated by assessing the tool's sensitivity and specificity. Responsiveness is the ability of the tool to respond quickly to changes in the wound status. One method of determining responsiveness of a tool is to evaluate change scores for reliability. Reliability of change scores is inversely dependent on the correlation between the initial score with the tool and the follow-up score.[10] If there is a strong correlation or relationship between the initial score and the follow-up score, the reliability of the change score will be lower. Likewise, if there is a weak relationship between the initial score and the follow-up score, the reliability of the change score will be much higher.

Clinical Practicality

Clinical practicality means that the tool must be simple, easy to learn, and easy to use, with clear instructions. It must be time-efficient and cost-effective. The tool must provide data that are meaningful enough to warrant the additional time and energy required to complete the assessment. Some aspects of clinical practicality can be evaluated during validity assessment, such as level of the language of the tool. The level of the language of the tool and the understandability of items should be reflective of the intended tool user. Similarly, scoring mechanisms and mathematical calculations must address the intended tool user.

WOUND CHARACTERISTICS

Most wound healing instruments include assessment of multiple wound attributes. This section provides a brief description of wound characteristics commonly included in instruments to measure healing. More comprehensive descriptions of wound characteristics are found in Chapter 4. The choice of which characteristics to include in a tool depends on the purpose of the instrument (prediction of healing, assessment of wound status, prescription of treatment, etc.) and, to some degree, the philosophy of the instrument developers.

Location

Assess the location of the wound by identifying where the lesion occurs on the patient's anatomy. Body diagrams are typically used to document wound location. Wound location has been shown to influence healing. However, which specific locations are beneficial or detrimental to healing are still to be determined.

Shape

As wounds heal, they often change shape and may begin to assume a more regular, circular/oval shape. The shape also helps to determine the overall size of the wound. Butterfly-shaped wounds occur in the sacrococcygeal area and are wounds with mirror images on each side of the coccyx. *Color Plates 3* and *4* show butterfly-shaped ulcers on the coccyx. The shape of the wound is determined by evaluating the perimeter of the wound. Shape of the wound is related to wound contraction. Wound contraction can be seen when the open surface area of the wound reduces and when the shape of the wound changes. Compare *Color Plate 3* with *Color Plates 4* and *5* to see the onset and progression of contraction and epithelialization. It is identified by a change in wound open area size and may be identified as a change in wound shape (eg, from irregular to symmetric, such as the circular or oval formation and rounding off of the edges of the wound seen in pressure ulcers; see *Color Plate 2*).

Size

Most tools include some measure of size. The most commonly used method in determining size is to measure (in cm) the longest and perpendicularly widest aspect of the wound surface that is visible. The surface area can be determined by multiplying the length by the width. It can be difficult to determine where to measure size on some wounds, because the edge of the wound may be hard to visualize or the edge may be irregular. This is a skill that takes practice. Use of the same reference points for determining size improves the reliability and meaningfulness of the measures. (Chapter 5, Wound Measurements, has step-by-step procedures for measuring size, depth, and undermining.)

Depth

Measure the depth of the wound using a cotton-tipped applicator. Insert the applicator in the deepest portion of the wound, mark the applicator with a pen, and measure the distance from the tip to the mark, using a metric measuring guide. Multiple measures of depth within the wound can increase reliability of depth evaluation. Some tools evaluate wound depth using descriptive terms instead of numeric measurements.

Edges

The edges of the wound reflect some of the most important characteristics of the wound. When assessing edges, look for how clear and distinct the wound outline appears. If the edges are indistinct and diffuse, there are areas where the normal tissues blend into the wound bed and the edges are not clearly visible. Edges that are even with the skin surface and the wound base are edges that are attached to the base of the wound. This means that the wound is flat, with no appreciable depth. Well-defined edges are clear and distinct and can easily be outlined on a transparent piece of plastic. Edges that are not attached to the base of the wound imply a wound with some depth of tissue involvement (*Color Plate 33*). The wound that is a crater or has a bowl/boat shape is a wound with edges that are not attached to the wound base (*Color Plate 41*). The wound has walls or sides. There is depth to the wound. As the wound ages, the edges become rolled under and thickened to palpation. The edge achieves a unique coloring. The pigment turns a grayish hue in both dark- and light-skinned persons (*Color Plate 35*). Wounds of long duration may continue to thicken, with scar tissue and fibrosis developing in the wound edge, causing the edge to feel hard, rigid, and indurated. Hyperkeratosis is the calluslike tissue that may form around the wound edges, especially with diabetic ulcers (see Chapter 18 and *Color Plate 24*). Evaluate the wound edges by visual inspection and palpation. *Color Plates 33–36* show wounds with different edges.

Undermining/Tunneling

Undermining and tunneling represent the loss of tissue underneath an intact skin surface. Undermining usually involves a greater percentage of the wound margins, with more

---

Clinical Wisdom:
Tips for Assessing Wound Edges

Definitions for help in assessing wound edges:

- Indistinct, diffuse—unable to clearly distinguish wound outline clearly
- Attached—even or flush with wound base, *no* sides or walls present, flat
- Not attached—sides or walls are present; floor or base of wound is deeper than edge
- Rolled under, thickened—soft to firm and flexible to touch
- Hyperkeratosis—calluslike tissue formation around wound and at edges

---

shallow length than tunneling. Undermining usually involves subcutaneous tissues and follows the fascial planes next to the wound. Undermining is defined as erosion under the edge of the wound, and tunneling is defined as separation of the fascial planes leading to sinus tracts. An undermined area can be likened to a cave, whereas a tunnel is more like a subway. Tunneling usually involves a small percentage of the wound margins; it is narrow and quite long, and it seems to have a destination.

Assess for undermining by inserting a cotton-tipped applicator under the wound edge and advancing it as far as it will go without using undue force. Raise the tip of the applicator so that it may be seen or felt on the surface of the skin and mark the surface with a pen. Measure the distance from the mark on the skin to the edge of the wound. Continue this process all around the wound. Then use a transparent metric measuring guide with concentric circles divided into four (25%) pie-shaped quadrants to help determine percentage of the wound involved (see *Color Plates 39–41*).

Necrotic Tissue Characteristics

Characteristics of necrotic tissue include *amount present, color, consistency,* and *adherence to the wound bed.* Choose the *predominant* characteristic present in the wound. Necrosis is defined as dead devitalized tissue. Color may be black, brown, gray, or yellow. Texture may be dry and leathery, soft, moist, or stringy. Odor may be present or absent. To determine whether the tissue being assessed is necrotic, see Chapter 8, Management of Necrotic Tissue, and *Color Plates 3, 26–31, 52,* and *53.* One common error in assessing necrotic tissue is to assess all yellow and white tissue as necrotic. Yellow tissue may be either healthy yellow fat, the reticular membrane of the dermis, or a tendon. White tissue may be connective tissue, fascia, or a ligament. *Color Plate 13* shows healthy yellow and white tissue. Healthy tissue usually has a gleam not seen in devitalized tissue. Note, however, that the topical treatment or exudate is not the source of the "gleam." Healthy tissue is not friable and has resilience when compressed. Dead tissue tears and does not spring back when compressed. Waiting 24 hours helps to see whether the tissue changes color to gray or brown, indicating loss of vitality.

Necrotic tissue type changes as it ages in the wound, as debridement occurs, and as further tissue trauma causes increased cellular death. There are two main types of necrotic tissue: slough and eschar. Slough generally indicates less severity than does eschar. Slough usually appears as a yellow to tan mucinous or stringy material that is nonadherent to loosely adherent to the healthy tissues of the wound bed (*Color Plates 3*, *28*, and *40*). Nonadherent material is defined as appearing scattered throughout the wound; it looks as though the tissue could be removed easily with a gauze sponge. Loosely adherent refers to tissue that is attached to the wound bed; it is thick and stringy and may appear as clumps of debris attached to wound tissue.

Eschar signifies deeper tissue damage. Eschar may be black, gray, or brown in color. Eschar is usually adherent or firmly adherent to the wound tissues and may be soggy and soft or hard and leathery in texture. A soft, soggy eschar is usually strongly attached to the base of the wound but may be lifting from and loose from the edges of the wound (*Color Plate 27*). Hard, crusty eschars are strongly attached to the base and the edges of the wound (*Color Plates 26, 30*, and *52*).

Clinical Wisdom: *Eschar Appearance*

Hard eschars are often mistaken for scabs. A scab is a collection of dried blood cells and serum on top of the skin surface, whereas an eschar is a collection of dead tissue and coagulated blood products within the wound.

Sometimes, nonviable tissue appears prior to a wound's appearance. This can be seen on the skin as a white or gray area on the surface of the skin. The area usually demarcates within a few days, and the wound appears and interrupts the skin surface.

The amount of necrotic tissue present in the wound is evaluated by one of two methods. One method involves using clinical judgment to estimate the percentage of the wound covered with necrosis. Place a transparent measuring guide with concentric circles divided into four (25%) pie-shaped quadrants over the wound. Look at each quadrant and judge how much necrosis is present. Add up the total percentage from judgments of each quadrant; this determines the percentage of the wound involved. A second method involves actual linear measurements of the necrosis. Measure the length and width of the necrosis and multiply to determine surface area.

Exudate

Evaluating exudate type can be tricky because of the moist wound healing dressings used on most wounds. Some dressings interact with wound drainage to produce a gel or fluid, and others may trap liquid and drainage at the wound site. Before assessing exudate type, gently cleanse the wound with normal saline or water and evaluate fresh exudate. Pick the exudate type that is *predominant* in the wound, according to color and consistency. Remember that a wound with necrotic tissue present will almost always have an odor. Amount can also be difficult to assess accurately for the same reasons that it is difficult to determine the type of exudate in the wound. Moist wound healing dressings interact with wound drainage to trap drainage at the wound site. Others may absorb varying amounts of exudate. To judge the amount of exudate in the wound, observe two areas: the wound itself and the dressing used on the wound. Observe the wound for the moisture present. Are the tissues dry and desiccated? Are they swimming in exudate? Is the drainage spread throughout the wound? Use clinical judgment to determine how wet the wound is. Evaluate the dressing used on the wound for how much it interacts with exudate. *Color Plates 42–47* show different exudate characteristics.

Surrounding Skin Characteristics

The tissues surrounding the wound are often the first indication of impending further tissue damage. The color of the surrounding skin may indicate further injury from pressure, friction, or shearing. *Erythema* is defined as reddening or darkening of the skin, compared with surrounding skin. Erythema following trauma is due to rupture of small venules and capillaries or may be caused by inflow of blood to start the inflammatory process, or both events. Distinguishing between the two is often difficult. Erythema is usually accompanied by heat, but it may be accompanied by cooling, indicating devitalization of tissue.[10] Distinguishing and assessing erythema in darkly pigmented skin is described in detail in Chapter 4 (see *Color Plate 19*). The ability to see the margins of the change in skin color is enhanced by lighting and may be seen more easily in a photograph than in the living tissues, especially in very dark skin tones. *Color Plates 6, 14*, and *15*, and *19* show erythema in both lightly and darkly pigmented skin. Dark-skinned persons show the colors "bright red" and "dark red" as a deepening of normal ethnic skin color or a purple or blacker hue (*Color Plates 19–21*). As healing occurs in dark-skinned persons, the new skin is pink and may never darken. In both light- and dark-skinned patients, new epithelium must be differentiated from tissues that are erythematous. To assess for blanchability, press firmly on the skin with a finger; lift the finger and look for blanching (sudden whitening of the tissues), followed by prompt return of color to the area. Nonblanchable erythema signals more severe tissue damage.

Clinical Wisdom: *Differentiation between Erythema and Reactive Hyperemia*

Erythema should be assessed after pressure has been relieved from the area for about 20 minutes, so as to eliminate effects of reactive hyperemia.

Edema

Edema in the surrounding tissues will delay wound healing in the pressure ulcer (*Color Plates 17–19*). It is difficult for neoangiogenesis, or the growth of new blood vessels into the wound, to occur in edematous tissues. Assess tissues within 4 cm of the wound edge. Nonpitting edema appears as skin that is shiny and taut, almost glistening. Identify pitting edema by firmly pressing a finger down into the tissues and waiting for 5 seconds; on release of pressure, tissues fail to resume normal position, and an indentation appears. Measure how far edema extends beyond the wound edges.

Induration

Induration is a sign of impending damage to the tissues. Along with skin color changes, induration is an omen of further pressure-induced tissue trauma. Assess tissues within 4 cm of the wound edge. Induration is an abnormal firmness of tissues with margins. Palpate where the induration starts and where it ends. Assess by gently pinching the tissues. Induration results in an inability to pinch the tissues. Palpate from healthy tissue, moving toward the wound margins. It is usual to feel slight firmness at the wound edge itself. Normal tissues feel soft and spongy; induration feels hard and firm to the touch.

Other Characteristics

Other characteristics that may be evaluated in the surrounding tissues include maceration and hemorrhage. *Maceration* is defined as a softening of connective tissue fibers by soaking until they are soft and friable. Macerated tissue loses its pigmentation, and even darkly pigmented skin looks blanched. This weakened tissue is highly susceptible to trauma, leading to breakdown of the macerated tissue and enlargement of the wound. *Hemorrhagic tissue* or *hematoma* is defined as a purple ecchymosis of wound tissue or surrounding skin (see *Color Plates 32, 71*, and *75*). The color plates show the deepening of tissue color or distinguishable purple ecchymosis that is an indicator of significant subcutaneous bleeding or hemorrhage. Wounds with hemorrhage have high probability of tissue death and, thus, enlargement of the wound. They are often referred to as "purple ulcers."

Clinical Wisdom: *Assessment of Hemorrhage or Hematoma Triggers Further Examination*

The presence of hemorrhage or hematoma would be a trigger for further examination, including temperature testing, as described in Chapter 4, to determine tissue vitality. Hemorrhage may trigger vascular consultation. The chapters in Part IV on electrical stimulation, pulsed electromagnetic fields, and ultrasound describe how these interventions promote absorption of hemorrhagic material.

Granulation Tissue

Granulation tissue is a marker of wound health. It signals the proliferative phase of wound healing and usually heralds the eventual closure of the wound. Granulation tissue is the growth of small blood vessels and connective tissue into the wound cavity. It is more observable in full-thickness wounds because of the tissue defect that occurs with full-thickness wounds. In partial-thickness wounds, granulation tissue may occur so quickly and in concert with epithelialization that it is unobservable in most cases. Granulation tissue is healthy when it is bright, beefy red, shiny, and granular with a velvety appearance. The tissue looks bumpy and may bleed easily. Well vascularized granulation tissue can be seen in *Color Plates 8, 9*, and *18*.

Clinical Wisdom: *Appearance of Unhealthy Granulation Tissue*

Unhealthy granulation tissue due to poor vascular supply appears as pale pink or blanched to dull, dusky red color (*see Color Plate 34*). Usually, the first layer of granulation tissue to be laid down in the wound is pale pink; as the granulation tissue deepens and thickens, the color becomes the bright, beefy red color, like *Color Plate 9*.

Try to judge what percentage of the wound has been filled with granulation tissue. This is much easier if there is history with the wound. If the same person follows the wound over multiple observations, it is simple to judge the amount of granulation tissue present in the wound. If the initial observation of the wound was done by a different observer or if the data are not available, simply use best judgment to determine the amount of tissue present.

Epithelialization

Epithelialization is the process of epidermal resurfacing and appears as pink or red skin. Visualizing the new epithelium takes practice. *Color Plates 5*, *6*, and *8* show the process of epidermal resurfacing. In partial-thickness wounds, the epithelial cells may migrate from islands on the wound surface or from the wound edges, or both. *Color Plates 64* and *65* show an example. In full-thickness wounds, epidermal resurfacing occurs from the edges only, usually after the wound has almost completely filled with granulation tissue. *Color Plates 5* and *6* show the same full-thickness wound as seen in *Color Plates 3* and *4*, with resurfacing evident from the wound edges. Epithelialization may first be noticed during the inflammation or proliferation phase of healing as a lightly pigmented pink tissue, even in individuals with darkly pigmented skin (*Color Plates 7–9*). Many people confuse new bright pink scar tissue or skin as erythema. *Color Plate 22* shows new pink scar tissue in a person with darkly pigmented skin. Use of a transparent measuring guide to help determine percentage of the wound involved in resurfacing and to measure the distance that the epithelial tissue extends into the wound from proliferative edges can be helpful.

Wound healing tools include a combination of these wound attributes to measure healing, according to the theory on which the tool is based and the framework behind the instrument.

TOOLS TO MONITOR WOUND HEALING

This chapter describes three tools to monitor wound healing, the SWHT, the PUSH, and the PSST. There are similarities in some aspects of the tools: All evaluate tissue attributes of the wound, and two evaluate surrounding skin. Methods of assessment, format, and scoring are different. Copies of the three tools and instructions for use are found in this chapter's appendixes. The PWHT, which is derived from the PSST, is described in Chapter 5.

Introduction and Development of the Sussman Wound Healing Tool

The SWHT was developed by Sussman and Swanson[5] as a physical therapy diagnostic tool to monitor and track the effectiveness of PT technologies used for pressure ulcer healing. The ability to predict pressure ulcer healing and treatment outcomes in PT has yet to be done reliably. The monitoring and tracking of healing and treatment outcomes are essential for clinical decision making and triage, and provide payers and providers improved utilization management.

The basis for the SWHT is the acute wound healing model (see Chapter 2) that describes the changes in tissue status and size over time, as the wound progresses through the biologic phases of wound healing. Some attributes of the wound that are observed during each phase are considered to be related to failure to heal or "not good for healing," and others are considered to be indicators of improvement or "good for healing." For example, a tissue attribute such as necrosis is thought to be negative or not good for healing, whereas wound attributes such as granulation tissue, which represents fibroplasia, and adherence of the wound edges are considered good for healing. The concept of the SWHT is to benchmark the wound attributes as it recovers and progresses throughout the healing phases. For example, the "not good" attribute, necrosis, should change over time from *present* to *absent*, thus moving from "not good for healing" to "good for healing." The "good for healing" attribute, fibroplasia—significant reduction in depth—should be granulation observed as the wound heals and changes from *absent* to *present*, indicating improved tissue status.

The initial design of the SWHT is a qualitative instrument, meaning that a wound would be described as having certain tissue attributes. It is composed of 10 wound attributes, combined with 9 descriptive attributes of size, extent of tissue damage plus location, and acute wound healing phase, which are not measurable. The 10 wound tissue attributes described were each assigned a score as *present* or *absent* and ranked as *not good* or *good* for healing. Five attributes ranked as *not good* include hemorrhage, maceration, erythema, undermining, and necrosis. Five attributes ranked as *good* include adherence at the wound edge, fibroplasia, appearance of contraction, sustained contraction, and epithelialization.

Sussman Wound Healing Tool Attribute Definitions

Part I: Tissue Attributes

The first five attributes, hemorrhage, maceration, undermining/tunneling, erythema, and necrosis are all classified as not good for healing. The location of undermining is defined as undermining at any location around the wound perimeter. The extent of undermining/tunneling is not recorded or included as part of the assessment; only the presence or absence of this attribute is evaluated. The second five attributes—adherence at wound edge, granulation tissue, contraction, sustained contraction, and epithelialization—are all classified as good for healing. Several of the good-for-healing items require a brief explanation.

Adherence at the wound edge means that there is continuity of the wound edge and the base of the wound at any location along the wound perimeter (*Color Plates 8*, *9*, *65*, and *81*). A partial-thickness wound will be adhered at the wound edge by definition. A full-thickness or deeper wound will have closed by either granulation or contraction to the point where some area of the wound edge will be even with the skin surface. Granulation tissue, or fibroplasia, is evaluated by measuring wound depth, with a significant reduction in depth indicating proliferation of granulation tissue formation. A significant reduction in depth is defined as at least 0.2 cm change in linear depth measurements since the prior assessment. *Color Plates 7–9* show a significant reduction in depth. Contraction is assessed as being present when the open surface area size of the wound reduces. This item is scored at subsequent assessments as the contraction continues or if it has stopped. If the wound enlarges, however, this item would change from present to absent, and a new appearance of contraction would be required to have a score of "present" again. Sustained contraction means there is a continued drawing together of the wound edges that is measured by a reduction in wound surface open area size. It is usually accompanied by a change in wound shape. *Color Plates 3–5* show the same wound as it goes through wound contraction. Sustained contraction is scored zero at the appearance of the contraction benchmark, then scored 1 at subsequent reassessment, following the appearance of contraction. Occasionally, something interferes with the wound contraction, and the wound does not reduce in size or increases. This attribute would be marked zero—absent—if the wound size does not reduce or enlarges after the appearance of contraction.

The not-good-for-healing attributes are all related to the inflammatory phase of healing. The attributes that are good for healing are related to the proliferative and epithelialization phases of healing. As the wound attributes change from not good to good, the wound is progressing through the phases corresponding to those of acute wound healing.

Part II: Size Location and Wound Healing Phase Measures

Wound depth and undermining indicate extent of wound. If a wound has a depth less than 0.2 cm, it is scored as zero at all four points and at general depth. Depth and undermining are two indicators of not good for healing.

11–15: Wound Depth. Five items on part II of the SWHT are related to presence of depth of at least 0.2 cm, both in general depth and at the four points of the clock—the 12-, 3-, 6-, and 9-o'clock positions. Depth is measured as described in Chapter 4, and if it is at least 0.2 cm, it is recorded as present. Extent of depth is not significant for this assessment as long as it is at least 0.2 cm. (See *Color Plates 2*, *7*, *10*, and *31* for full-thickness depth.)

16–19: Tunneling/Undermining. Undermining and tunneling are measured at all four points of the clock, like depth. However, the objective measure used to report this attribute

is also present or absent. With further testing and analysis, this attribute may prove to be redundant with part I. For the present time, it remains a part of the tool.

Additional Descriptive Attributes

Wound Location. Wound location is noted as the anatomic description most closely related to the wound site. Because lower torso and lower extremity wounds are most frequently seen, the locations have been broken down into the common sites for chronic wounds, and they have been clustered together for the upper body. Letters are also used to represent the wound location: *UB* for upper body, *C* for coccyx, *T* for trochanter, *I* for ischial, *H* for heel, and *F* for foot. Wounds in other locations can be added to the list if they are commonly seen in the practice setting by using letters on the form and adding a location descriptor to the key (eg, *K* = knee, *A* = abdomen, *Th* = thigh). One needs to be sure to include the side of the body where the wound is located—right or left—by putting an *R* or an *L* next to the location letter.

Wound Healing Phase. The wound healing phase refers to the four biologic phases of wound healing: inflammatory, proliferative, epithelialization, and remodeling. Letters are used to represent the current wound healing phase: *I* for inflammatory, *P* for proliferative, *E* for epithelialization, and *R* for remodeling. As described in Chapter 4, the wound healing phase may be chronic, acute, or absent. Letters can be placed before the phase, such as the letter *C* before the phase for chronic, no letter before acute, or the letter *L* for lacking or absent, as modifiers of the current phase. A change in phase over time is an expected outcome. Chronicity of a phase should change to an active state of the phase, followed by progression to the next phase in the trajectory. Absence of a phase indicates need for investigation as to why the phase has not been achieved. This item is listed but unscored.

Testing the SWHT

One of the first questions applied to the SWHT was whether a tool design based on the four-phase acute wound healing model could be applied to chronic wounds, such as pressure ulcers. The SWHT is in the process of being tested on a data set of 112 pressure ulcer cases. All of the patients who were included in the data set were long-term care residents with pressure ulcers. Many experts consider pressure ulcers to be chronic wounds from the time of onset. The analyses are as yet incomplete.

SWHT for Monitoring and Tracking Wound Healing

The utility of the SWHT in the clinical setting for monitoring and tracking healing is easy and practical. Each of the attributes of the SWHT is scored if tissue attributes of the wound or surrounding skin are present or absent. The total number of present not-good-for-healing attributes should diminish as the wound heals, and the total number of present good-for-healing attributes should increase in number. Change of score measures the change in healing and reduced severity of the wound. The scores are also useful for measuring the level of healing, indicating progress, lack of progress, or regression of healing. The SWHT has proven utility, both as a diagnostic tool that differentiates phases by assessment of healing attributes and as a tool for measurement of *change* in tissue status (eg, tissue attribute) and size (eg, change in depth and undermining) over time. Thus, the SWHT is designed to monitor and track healing, based on the acute wound healing model, and can be applied to acute or chronic wounds, such as pressure ulcers.

SWHT Reliability and Practicality

The SWHT has been clinically tested for reliability and clinical practicality by physical therapists (PTs) and PT assistants working in a long-term care facility during its 5 years of development and found to be very reliable for monitoring and tracking healing and nonhealing of pressure ulcers. It relies primarily on visual observation skills. No linear measurements, arithmetic calculations, or estimates of amount of tissue characteristic present are required. To health care professionals who treat wounds, the SWHT information communicates clearly wound progress or risk. Documentation is very simple, and outcomes are visual. For example, it takes the clinician about 5 minutes to complete the assessment. In a trial educational session to train new learners to use the SWHT, a group of 10 PTs and PT assistants who received 1 hour of training in the classroom using verbal description and photos to teach the method of assessment and definitions of the attributes, followed by 1 hour of clinical practice on pressure ulcer patients, learned to use it well.

Assessment of Treatment Outcomes

Assessment of treatment outcome was the initial reason for development of the SWHT. Most patients are referred to the PT by the nurse for treatment after conventional treatments fails to heal the wound. To qualify for an intervention by the PT, the patient and the wound often need to meet a criterion of no progress, regression, or a halt of healing. Therefore, it is critical for the PT and the nurse to be able to set target outcomes, then to assess the response to the treatment intervention. A wound assessed with the SWHT as not progressing after a course of conventional care by the nurse would meet the criterion for referral. Once referred, the SWHT is useful for reporting wound outcomes associated with the intervention prescribed by the PT, such as physical therapy technologies. Response to treatment with these interventions should demonstrate consistent change in tissue status that corresponds to the biologic model for acute wound healing. A change in tissue status benchmarks the healing process and becomes a target functional outcome for reporting purposes, such as the wound will be hemorrhage free, undermining free, necrosis free, and so forth. Reviewers can quickly determine a change in wound tissue status during the course of care because, as already described, the wound attributes should change from those that are not good for healing to those that are good for healing.

Using the SWHT

Two Parts of SWHT

Appendix 6–A shows the two parts of the long version of the SWHT and the procedure for using the SWHT. The SWHT is a paper-and-pencil instrument, comprising 19 attributes. Part I is the collection form of 10 tissue attributes. Part II is the list of 11 other attributes, including extent, location, and wound healing phase. All items on the SWHT are scored except location and the wound healing phase. Omission of a score indicates that the assessment was not completed. Scoring begins at baseline, week zero. The method of scoring for the tool is a number 1 for present and a zero for absent. This reporting format is readily compatible with computer technology and simplifies using the tool to build a database, such as the one described later. Completion of the form requires understanding of the definitions for each of the scored items. The assessment process is visual except for determining the presence of undermining/tunneling, which cannot be seen at the surface, and measurement of the open surface area of the wound.

SWHT Forms

Long Form

There are two forms of the SWHT, a long form (see Appendix 6–A) and a short form (see Exhibits 6–1A and B). Part I of the long form (Appendix 6–A) contains the 10 tissue attributes, listed in descending order of severity, next to definitions, followed by a column listing the rating option for the attribute as present or not present. The next column ranks the relationship to healing as not good or good. The last column is where the rating is listed as a score of present or absent. Part II lists measures and extent. The same scoring system of present or absent for 19 attributes of extent is applied. The attributes are the general depth of greater than 0.2 cm, the depth at the four clock points, and undermining at the four clock points. Date and week of care should be noted on the form. The benefit of the long form is having the definitions on the form. This would be helpful to a nurse or PT learning the system or for medical reviewers and surveyors looking for information about the rating system used for documentation.

Exhibit 6–1A SWHT Short Form Part I: Wound Tissue Attributes

Name: _____ Med Rec # _____ Examiner: _____

Week	0	1	2	3	4
1. Hemorrhage					
2. Maceration					
3. Undermining					
4. Erythema					
5. Necrosis					
6. Adherence					
7. Granulation (decreased deth)					
8. Appearance of contraction (reduced size)					
9. Sustained contraction (more reduced size)					
10. Epithelialization					

Key: Present = 1. Not present = 0.

	0	1	2	3	4
Total Not Good					
Total Good					

Source: Copyright © 1997, Sussman Physical Therapy, Inc.

Exhibit 6–1B SWHT Short Form Part II: Size, Location, Wound Healing Phase Measures, and Extent

Date	0	1	2	3	4
11. General Depth > 0.2 cm					
12. Depth @ 12:00 > 0.2 cm					
13. Depth @ 3:00 > 0.2 cm					
14. Depth @ 6:00 > 0.2 cm					
15. Depth @ 9:00 > 0.2 cm					
16. Underm @ 12:00 > 0.2 cm					
17. Underm @ 3:00 > 0.2 cm					
18. Underm @ 6:00 > 0.2 cm					
19. Underm @ 9:00 > 0.2 cm					
Location					
Wound healing phase					

Key: Present = 1. Not present = 0. Location choices: upper body (UB), coccyx (C), trochanter (T), ischial (I), heel (H), and foot (F); add right or left (R or L). Wound healing phase: absent (A), chronic (C), inflammation (I), proliferation (P), epithelialization (E), remodeling (R).

Source: Copyright © 1997, Sussman Physical Therapy, Inc.

Short Form

The short form (Exhibits 6–1A and B) of the SWHT is the same as the long form, except that the short form lacks the definitions printed on the form. The short form lists only the attributes and has columns to record data for multiple weeks. Part I can be printed on one side and part II on the other, and the paper can be cut to fit in a small, pocket-sized 4 × 6-inch loose-leaf notebook. Printing the forms as a pad punched with a hole pattern to match the notebook makes it easy and convenient to keep forms on hand. A printed set of the definitions and scoring can be printed on the same size paper, then kept in the notebook for reference. The notebook functions most smoothly if an alphabetic index the size of the notebook is used. The wound progress notebook can then be kept like a nursing treatment record book, with records alphabetically filed. The current patient wound healing records would then be readily available. The benefit of the notebook is that it will usually fit into a lab coat pocket and can be carried to the bedside or home. In a facility, like the treatment record book, it can be kept at the nurses' station, when not in use, for easy reference. An additional benefit of the short form is that it is easy to see a complete history of the change in tissue status over multiple weeks of assessment. Reading the report over time provides a quick and clear evaluation to monitor wound healing progress.

Exhibits 6–2A and B show a completed case record. At the time of discharge or monthly, the completed record of wound attributes is taped in tiling fashion, like telephone order prescription sheets, onto a sheet of paper and filed in the medical record.

Clinical Wisdom: *Use of Forms for Wound Measurement along with the SWHT*

Because wound measurement and tissue assessment or reassessment are usually done at the same time, it makes sense to record the information in the same record book. A wound measurement recording short form that fits in the same notebook as the SWHT meets this need. This form is used to record the size, depth, and undermining linear measurements. Each week, a new measurement form is added behind the SWHT form. By having the two forms together in the notebook, the examiner can check at a glance to see whether there is reduction in depth and open area. Chapter 5, Exhibit 5–2, shows a sample wound measurement form designed to fit this model.

Case Example Using the SWHT

Exhibits 6–2A and B show an example of a case where wound healing was monitored over a 5-week course of care,

as reported on the short form of the SWHT, parts I and II. A summary (Exhibit 6–3) of the case example shows how the SWHT can be used to document a change in wound tissue status from a predominance of not-good-for-healing to a predominance of good attributes. Exhibit 6–3 reflects the following:

- The patient had the presence at baseline, week zero, of hemorrhage, necrosis, and erythema, and absence of any attributes good for healing. The presence of these attributes at baseline is an indication that this wound will need aggressive intervention to improve.
- At week 2, there were multiple attributes that were indicators that this patient will be in the risk-for-not-healing group, including undermining and depth at all four clock points, further indicating the medical necessity for aggressive intervention to put the wound on a course of healing.
- Assuming that aggressive intervention was undertaken at week 2, the improvement in the wound tissue status from not good to good is significant by week 4.

Sussman Wound Healing Tool Database

Although the SWHT is a paper-and-pencil instrument, the SWHT wound database is maintained in a computer. The scoring system of using a 1 or a zero is computer-compatible for data management and data entry. The SWHT forms are printed on the computer as screens, and data are entered either prospectively or retrospectively. Data reports can be printed, and the captured data can be analyzed on an individual patient basis or by group. Further testing of the SWHT is planned at different sites.

Summary

Physical therapists and nurses can utilize the SWHT present/absent scoring system to assess healing, triage the case, guide treatment intervention, and report functional outcomes. The SWHT is a simple, easy-to-follow, and complete documentation system that provides payers and providers with improved utilization management.

Introduction and Development of the Pressure Ulcer Scale for Healing

In 1996, the NPUAP in the United States convened a task force to address the practice of reverse staging of pressure ulcers that was encouraged by Medicare documentation requirements using the Minimum Data Set (MDS) system in long-term care facilities. The objective was to develop a biologically accurate and easy-to-use instrument to replace reverse staging. The task force developed and tested a tool to measure pressure ulcer healing, and the PUSH tool was pre-

Exhibit 6–2A SWHT Part I: Wound Tissue Attributes

Week	0	1	2	3	4
Date: 2010	1/7	1/14	1/21	1/28	2/4
1. Hemorrhage	1	0	0	0	0
2. Maceration	0	0	0	0	0
3. Undermining	0	0	1	1	1
4. Erythema	1	1	1	0	0
5. Necrosis	1	1	1	0	0
6. Adherence	0	0	0	1	1
7. Granulation (decreased depth)	0	0	1	1	1
8. Appearance of contraction (reduced size)	0	0	1	1	1
9. Sustained contraction (more reduced size)	0	0	0	1	1
10. Epithelialization	0	0	0	1	1
Total "Not Good"	3	2	3	1	1
Total "Good"	0	0	2	5	5

Key: **Present = 1. Absent = 0.**

Source: Copyright © 1997, Sussman Physical Therapy, Inc.

Exhibit 6–2B SWHT Part II: Size, Location, Wound Healing Phase Measures, and Extent

Week	0	1	2	3	4
Date:	1/7	1/14	1/21	1/28	2/4
11. General depth > 0.2 cm	0	1	1	1	1
12. Depth @ 12:00 > 0.2 cm	0	1	1	1	1
13. Depth @ 3:00 > 0.2 cm	0	1	1	1	1
14. Depth @ 6:00 > 0.2 cm	0	1	1	1	1
15. Depth @ 9:00 > 0.2 cm	1	1	1	1	1
16. Underm @ 12:00 > 0.2 cm	0	0	1	1	0
17. Underm @ 3:00 > 0.2 cm	0	1	1	0	0
18. Underm @ 6:00 > 0.2 cm	0	1	1	1	0
19. Underm @ 9:00 > 0.2 cm	0	0	1	1	1
Location	RT	RT	RT	RT	RT
Wound healing phase	I	I	I	P	P

Key: Present = 1. Not present = 0. Location choices: upper body (UB), coccyx (C), trochanter (T), ischial (I), heel (H), and foot (F); add right or left (R or L). Wound healing phase: inflammation (I), proliferation (P), epithelialization (E), remodeling (R).

Source: Copyright © 1997, Sussman Physical Therapy, Inc.

Exhibit 6–3 Summary of Wound Attribute Change over a Five-Week Course of Care

WEEK 0	WEEK 2	WEEK 4
"NOT GOOD" for healing	*"NOT GOOD" for healing*	*"NOT GOOD" for healing*
Hemorrhage Undermining Erythema Necrosis Depth 9:00	Necrosis Undermining Erythema Depth 12, 3, 6, 9:00 Undermining 12, 3, 6, 9:00	Undermining Depth 12, 3, 6, 9:00 Undermining 9:00
"GOOD" for healing	*"GOOD" for healing*	*"GOOD" for healing*
None	Fibroplasia Appearance of contraction	Fibroplasia Appearance of contraction Sustained contraction Adherence Epithelialization
Wound healing phase	*Wound healing phase*	*Wound healing phase*
Inflammatory phase	Inflammatory phase	Proliferative phase

Source: Copyright © 1997, Sussman Physical Therapy, Inc.

sented in 1997 at the NPUAP biennial conference (see Appendix 6–B).

The PUSH tool incorporates three wound characteristics: surface area measurements, exudate amount, and surface appearance. These wound characteristics were chosen based on principal component analysis of 37 pressure ulcers followed every 2 weeks for a total of 8 weeks to define the best model of healing.[3] The three items identified in the model for the proposed tool (surface area, exudate amount, and surface appearance) were then tested on a new sample and performed similarly. The model of principal components explained 55–65% of the variance at weeks zero through week 8 for the study sample.[11] The results demonstrated good discrimination among the time points, particularly the earlier times, compared with the later times.

Validity

Two retrospective studies have validated the original findings. A multisite retrospective study evaluated 273 pressure ulcers using the PUSH tool over a time period of 10 weeks. Ulcers in the study included both partial-thickness stage II and full-thickness stage III and IV (58%) ulcers. Results demonstrated 58–74% of the variance over the 10 weeks was explained with the PUSH tool items. Inclusion of other variables did not contribute to the explanation of the variance. Pairwise comparisons showed evidence of sensitivity of the tool over time.[12]

The second retrospective study involved data from a sample of 2,490 nursing home residents, of whom 1,274 have a pressure ulcer at initial assessment.[13] However, only 269 ulcers met all criteria for study inclusion. All residents included in the study were participating in the National Pressure Ulcer Long-Term Care Study (NPULS).[14] The study demonstrated sensitivity of the tool over 12 weeks; however, only 40–57% of the total variance was explained by the PUSH tool items. Additional multiple regression techniques indicated that the tool explained 49% of the variance over the first 7 weeks. Beyond 7 weeks, the tool explained 29% of the variance. Based on findings from the second study, the PUSH tool was revised to increase the sensitivity of the tool to changes over time. The current version of the PUSH tool includes deciles for the categorical size item instead of the original quintiles, and the largest surface area on the size item was increased to 24 cm^2. The revised definitions were tested on the 269 cases from the NPULS data set, and the findings remained consistent with the original findings, with respect to variance and sensitivity to change. The authors suggest that content validity, correlational validity, prospective validity, and sensitivity to change can be met by the proposed tool. PUSH does allow a consistent, evidence-based methodology for reporting wound healing status among health care professionals. The PUSH is not a comprehensive assessment instrument for pressure ulcers, nor is it a research tool for measuring healing and should not be used for those purposes. Additional testing is needed to confirm the findings reported; however, in its present form, it is a clinically valid, practical alternative to reverse staging for reporting pressure ulcer healing.

Use of the tool involves measuring size, observation of exudate, and tissue type. The clinician measures the size of the wound, using length and width to calculate surface area (length × width) and chooses the appropriate size category on the tool (there are 10 size categories, from zero to 10). Exudate is evaluated as none (0), light (1), moderate (2), and heavy (3). Tissue type choices include closed (0), epithelial tissue (1), granulation tissue (2), slough (3), and necrotic tissue (4). Each of the three subscores are then summed for a total score. Exhibit 6–4 shows total scores plotted on a graph. Note the different trajectories of healing and nonhealing pressure ulcers.[15] The PUSH tool offers assessment of three wound characteristics and is best used as a method of quantitatively reporting the direction of healing over time. The PUSH tool does not include items that may be relevant to treatment decisions. Assessment of additional wound characteristics with other tools, such as the SWHT or PSST, could be used for baseline and more comprehensive assessment. The PUSH tool was designed for use as a trigger to identify when goals of treatment are being met and to identify patients who need to be reevaluated. Inappropriate reporting of healing indirectly compromises the quality of life of patients with pressure ulcers. A simple sensitive instrument to monitor the efficacy of treatment methods of pressure ulcer care would presumably improve the quality of life.[15]

The Health Care Financing Administration (HCFA) has pilot-tested the PUSH tool in skilled nursing facilities, and the tool is now incorporated in the Minimum Data Set for Post Acute Care (MDS-PAC) and in the Outcome and Assessment Information Set (OASIS) for home care. Incorporation of the PUSH tool in these data sets will standardize reporting of wound healing, and the PUSH tool will become the dominant wound healing tool for the future in the United States. It will be used by clinicians, surveyors, and payers to assess ulcer improvement or deterioration over time. This will have significant implications for the health care community.

The PUSH tool may be used with a pressure ulcer healing record form that allows for recording of subscores and total score on a periodic basis. The advantage of this form is the ability to note quickly any progress or degeneration of the wound. Another method of monitoring PUSH scores over time is available as a graph. The value of using graphs to track ulcer scores is the ability to spot trends in wound recovery quickly, as well as failure to progress. Exhibit 6–4 contains an example of a PUSH healing chart.[14]

Introduction and Development of the Pressure Sore Status Tool

The Pressure Sore Status Tool (PSST) is a pencil-and-paper instrument comprising 15 items (see Appendix 6–C). Two items that are not scored are location and shape. The remaining 13 items are scored and appear with descriptors of each item rated on a modified Likert scale (1 being the healthiest attribute of that characteristic and 5 being the worst attribute of the characteristic). The tool has a one-page sheet of instructions for use, in addition to the item descriptions (Appendix 6–C). The PSST was developed as an assessment tool for both clinical use and research. Over the years, PSST use has evolved to include measuring and predicting wound healing and is used in wounds beyond pressure ulcers. The PSST has provided a basis for many other wound assessment tools.

Validity

The items on the PSST were developed through the use of experts participating in a modified Delphi panel. The content validity of the tool was established with the use of a nine-member expert judge panel (mean overall content validity index = 0.91, $p = .05$). Content validity was established for each individual item on the tool and for the total tool with the judge panel. Concurrent validity was evaluated in a long-term care setting and involved comparing medical record documentation of pressure sore stage with the PSST depth item for a Pearson Product Moment correlation coefficient of $r = .91$ ($p = .001$).[16]

In a later study, the total PSST score was compared with recorded stage of the wound, and findings revealed a relatively strong positive relationship between the two scores (Pearson Product Moment correlation $r = .55$, $p = .001$). The study demonstrated little difference between the mean PSST scores of stage I versus stage II sores and for stage III versus stage IV sores, but significant difference between stage I and, II versus stage III and IV scores (stage I and II mean PSST score 23.35 versus stage III and IV mean PSST score 31.83; $p < .001$).[17]

Reliability

Reliability was demonstrated on adult patients in an acute care hospital with enterostomal therapy (ET) nurses or nurses with special training in wound management. The mean interrater reliability coefficient was 0.91.[1] Intrarater reliability

Exhibit 6–4 Example of PUSH Healing Chart

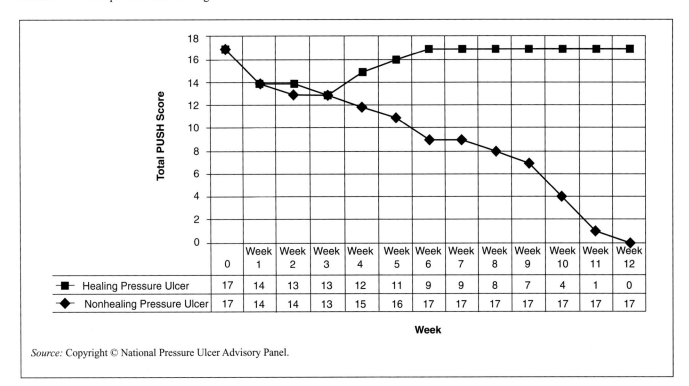

	0	Week 1	Week 2	Week 3	Week 4	Week 5	Week 6	Week 7	Week 8	Week 9	Week 10	Week 11	Week 12
■ Healing Pressure Ulcer	17	14	13	13	12	11	9	9	8	7	4	1	0
◆ Nonhealing Pressure Ulcer	17	14	14	13	15	16	17	17	17	17	17	17	17

Week

Source: Copyright © National Pressure Ulcer Advisory Panel.

estimates yielded a mean of 0.975. Although high reliability estimates had been established with expert nurses, a question remained as to the efficacy of the tool's use with practitioners who did not have extraordinary education or experience in wound assessment and management. Reliability of the PSST, when used by "regular" health care practitioners, was addressed in a long-term care facility. Fifteen practitioners with varied educational and experience backgrounds participated in the study. Two PTs, three licensed practical nurses, and 10 registered nurses participated in the study. Pairs independently assessed 16 wounds across a broad spectrum of severity on two occasions (2 hours apart). An expert nurse also independently assessed the same wounds as the practitioner pairs. Interrater reliability estimates were calculated between practitioners themselves and between practitioners and the expert rater. Intrarater reliability estimates were calculated in a similar manner, except that each rater's recordings were compared with a second assessment (taken within 2 hours of the first) for the same wound. Interrater reliability for the practitioners yielded a mean of 0.78. Reliability estimates for the practitioners versus the expert yielded a mean of 0.82. Intrarater reliability for the practitioners averaged 0.89.[16]

Because the PSST involves a Likert-type ordinal scale and the probability of chance agreements between two raters is 0.20 for any item, the data were also subjected to analyses using a polychotomous data stratagem. Resulting k statistics for each item on the scale yielded coefficients above 0.60.

Collectively, the results from the long-term care setting suggested that use of the PSST by general health care practitioners resulted in lower reliability than did its use by ET nurses but certainly within an acceptable range.

Sensitivity and Specificity

Predictive validity of the PSST was evaluated in a retrospective study of 143 pressure sores (51 partial-thickness wounds, 92 full-thickness wounds) over 6 weeks, with a minimum of three assessments per ulcer during the study period. The main outcome measure of the study was time to 50% healing, as measured by surface area. Data were analyzed with survival analysis techniques, with the main finding that surface area changes plus net PSST change at 1 week were most predictive of time to 50% healing. The positive predictive value of a net improvement in PSST score at 1 week was 65%, whereas the positive predictive value of a net deterioration in PSST score at 1 week was only 31%. Sensitivity in this sample was 61%, and specificity was 52%.[18]

The PSST is meant to be used once a pressure sore has developed; it is not a risk assessment tool. It is recommended that the pressure sore be scored initially for a baseline assessment and at regular intervals to evaluate therapy. Once a lesion has been assessed for each item on the PSST, the 13 item scores can be added to obtain a total score for the wound. The total score can then be plotted on the pressure sore continuum at the bottom of the tool to see regeneration or degeneration of the wound at a glance. Total scores range from 13 (skin intact but always at risk) to 65 (profound tissue degeneration).

PSST Scoring

The assessment and, ultimately, the quantification of clinical judgment forms the foundation for determining treatments and for evaluating effectiveness of therapy. After completing a full wound assessment using the PSST, the individual 13 items' scores can be summed to create the total PSST score. This total score can be monitored over time as an index to the status of the wound and to the effectiveness of the treatment. The total PSST score can be plotted on the continuum at the end of the tool, along with the date of assessment and, thus, can provide a visual aid to determining healing or nonhealing of the wound. A retrospective study[18] suggests that changes in the PSST score at 1 week plus changes in surface area measurements may have predictive value. A 1-week net decrease (improvement) in total PSST score plus a decrease in surface area was the best predictor of time to 50% wound closure in 143 partial- and full-thickness pressure sores within a 6-week study period. Thus, the total PSST score may provide a method of predicting outcomes. More research is needed in this area.

A PUSH score can be calculated from the PSST tool. The following guidelines will convert PSST subscale scores into PUSH subscale scores. Table 6–2 provides an example of conversion.

1. Wound Size: It is best to use actual surface area measurements, length × width, to determine which PUSH size category is appropriate. If actual measurements are not available, the following guide may be helpful:
   - If PSST size category = 1, then PUSH size category score = 0, 1, 2, 3, 4, 5, or 6
   - If PSST size category = 2, then PUSH size category score = either 7 or 8
   - If PSST size category = 3, then PUSH size category score = either 9 or 10
   - If PSST size category = 4 or 5, then PUSH size category score = 10
2. Exudate amount:
   - If PSST exudate amount score = 1, then PUSH exudate amount score = 0
   - If PSST exudate amount score = 2 or 3, then PUSH exudate amount score = 1
   - If PSST exudate amount score = 4, then PUSH exudate amount score = 2
   - If PSST exudate amount score = 5, then PUSH exudate amount score = 3
3. Tissue type:
   - If PSST Total Score = 13, then PUSH Type Score = 0 *OR* if Granulation = 1 *AND* Epithelialization = 1, then PUSH Type Score = 0
   - If Necrotic Tissue Type = 4 or 5, then PUSH Type Score = 4
   - If Necrotic Tissue Type = 2 or 3, then PUSH Type Score = 3
   - If Epithelialization < 5, then PUSH Type Score = 1
   - If Granulation < 5 *AND* Epithelialization = 5, then PUSH Type Score = 2

Assessment of Treatment Response

The PSST tool allows for temporal tracking of individual characteristics, as well as the total score. Each characteristic is assessed as described above and given a value from the Likert scale; thus, the scores can be monitored for improvement or deterioration in each characteristic. This quantifi-

Table 6–2 Example of PUSH Score Derivation from PSST Scores

PSST Items	PSST Scores	PUSH Items	PUSH Scores
1. Size	*4 (6.5 x 6.0 cm = 39 cm²)*	*1. Size* (724 cm²)	*10*
2. Depth	3		
3. Edges	2		
4. Undermining	1		
5. Necrotic Tissue Type	*3*		
6. Necrotic Tissue Amt.	4		
7. Exudate Type	4		
8. Exudate Amt.	*5*	*2. Exudate Amt.* (Heavy)	*3*
9. Skin Color	4		
10. Edema	1		
11. Induration	2		
12. Granulation	*3*	*Tissue Type** (Slough)	*3*
13. Epithelialization	4		
Total Score	**40**	Total Score	**16**

*Note that necrotic tissue is item 5 on PSST and 3 on PUSH, where slough is not classified as necrotic tissue if all necrotic tissue is absent.

Source: Copyright © National Pressure Ulcer Advisory Panel.

cation of observations allows for monitoring not only individual items and total score but also groups of characteristics. For example, the characteristics of necrotic tissue type and amount and exudate type and amount may be tracked to evaluate debridement or infection management.

Another benefit associated with the assignment of numeric values to items on the tool is the ability to set realistic goals. Clinical experience shows that not all pressure ulcers heal and certainly not always in the same setting. The PSST allows for more realistic goal setting as appropriate to the health care setting and the individual patient and pressure ulcer. For example, the patient with a large, necrotic, full-thickness ulcer in acute care will probably not be in the facility long enough for the wound to heal completely. However, the tool enables clinicians to set smaller goals, such as, "The wound will decrease in type and amount of necrotic tissue."

Clinical Wisdom: *Realistic Goal Setting*

In some instances, a pressure ulcer may never heal because of host factors or other contextual circumstances, so an example of a goal might be to maintain the total PSST score between 20 and 22.

Pressure sore severity, as well as overall health status of the patient, can also determine the appropriate management approach for ulcer healing. Severity states are a method of differentiating or stratification of various degrees of symptom intensity. In the case of the pressure ulcer, it refers to some measure of the degree of the tissue insult. The total PSST score can be used as a method of stratification to guide care planning. PSST scores can be divided into four suggested severity states, with total scores of 13–20 indicating minimal severity, 21–30 mild severity, 31–40 moderate severity, and 41–65 extreme severity. The goals of pressure sore management are to decrease the overall severity status of the wound and to make this decrease in a timely fashion. Figure 6–1 displays the suggested PSST severity state groups.

The severity status groups can be useful in designing general treatment algorithms. An example of a treatment algorithm for one wound in each severity state is presented below. These treatment algorithms are from the Wound and Skin Intelligence System (WSIS), a computer software program that incorporates the PSST instrument and provides treatment guidelines based on the PSST scores and the Agency for Health Care Research and Quality (AHRQ), formerly known as the Agency for Health Care Policy and Research (AHCPR), pressure sore treatment guidelines.[19]

PSST Minimal Severity Scores 13–20. Pressure sores with a PSST total score of 13–20 are generally stage I lesions, with intact skin at high risk for altered integrity, or

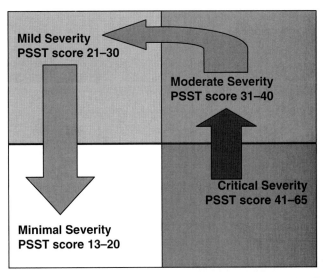

Figure 6–1 Severity states based on PSST scores. The goals of therapy are: (1) to decrease the overall severity state of the wound and, thus, the PSST score and (2) to make the decrease in a timely fashion. There is equal concern regarding severity of the wound and the duration of time that the wound spends in any severity state.

---

shallow stage II, partial-thickness pressure sores. Figure 6–2 presents a generic algorithm for treatment for wounds in this severity state. The main goals for wounds in this severity state are to prevent further damage and to provide a moist wound environment for healing.

PSST Mild Severity Scores 21–30. Pressure sores with mild severity include both partial-thickness and full-thickness wounds. Figure 6–3 presents a general treatment algorithm for partial-thickness wounds with mild severity scores, and Figure 6–4 presents general guidelines for full-thickness wounds with mild severity scores. The goals of care for partial-thickness wounds with mild severity scores are to absorb excess wound exudate, maintain a clean wound bed, and maintain a moist environment. Full-thickness wounds with mild severity scores offer more options for treatment because the wound can present as a clean, full-thickness wound or as a wound filled with necrotic debris.[20]

PSST Moderate Severity Scores 31–40. Figure 6–5 is a care plan for a full-thickness wound with necrotic tissue present. The goals of care for full-thickness wounds with moderate severity scores are to obtain/maintain a clean wound bed, provide a moist environment, absorb excess exudate, prevent premature closure, and reduce wound dead space. Wounds with moderate (and mild) severity scores have the most diverse presentations clinically, so choices regarding treatment are numerous.[20]

Figure 6–6 presents a general treatment algorithm for pressure sores with moderate PSST severity scores. Wounds

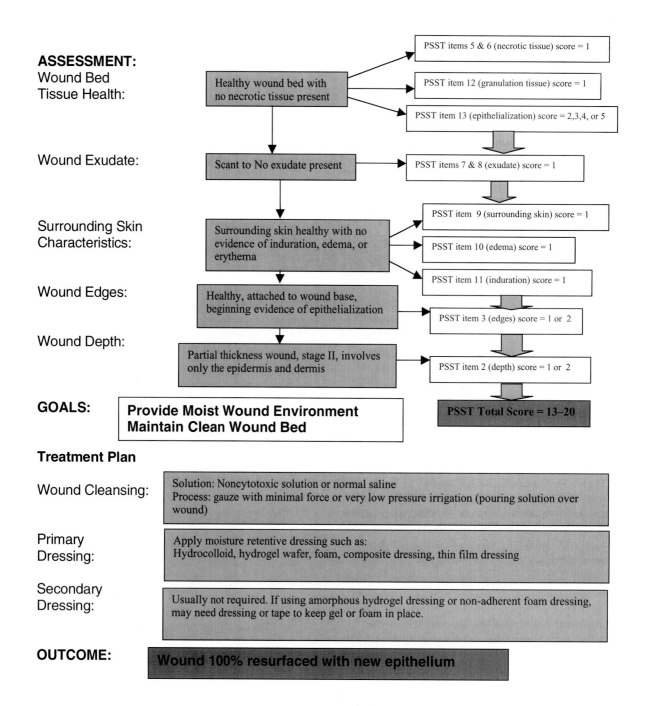

ASSESSMENT:

Wound Bed
Tissue Health:

Healthy wound bed with no necrotic tissue present	→ PSST items 5 & 6 (necrotic tissue) score = 1
	→ PSST item 12 (granulation tissue) score = 1
	→ PSST item 13 (epithelialization) score = 2,3,4, or 5

Wound Exudate:

Scant to No exudate present → PSST items 7 & 8 (exudate) score = 1

Surrounding Skin
Characteristics:

Surrounding skin healthy with no evidence of induration, edema, or erythema	→ PSST item 9 (surrounding skin) score = 1
	→ PSST item 10 (edema) score = 1
	→ PSST item 11 (induration) score = 1

Wound Edges:

Healthy, attached to wound base, beginning evidence of epithelialization → PSST item 3 (edges) score = 1 or 2

Wound Depth:

Partial thickness wound, stage II, involves only the epidermis and dermis → PSST item 2 (depth) score = 1 or 2

GOALS: Provide Moist Wound Environment
Maintain Clean Wound Bed

PSST Total Score = 13–20

Treatment Plan

Wound Cleansing:

Solution: Noncytotoxic solution or normal saline
Process: gauze with minimal force or very low pressure irrigation (pouring solution over wound)

Primary
Dressing:

Apply moisture retentive dressing such as:
Hydrocolloid, hydrogel wafer, foam, composite dressing, thin film dressing

Secondary
Dressing:

Usually not required. If using amorphous hydrogel dressing or non-adherent foam dressing, may need dressing or tape to keep gel or foam in place.

OUTCOME: Wound 100% resurfaced with new epithelium

Figure 6–2 Minimal PSST severity score treatment algorithm. *Source:* Adapted with permission from Wound and Skin Intelligence System™, *System Outputs Book*, ConvaTec, a division of Bristol-Myers Squibb, USA.

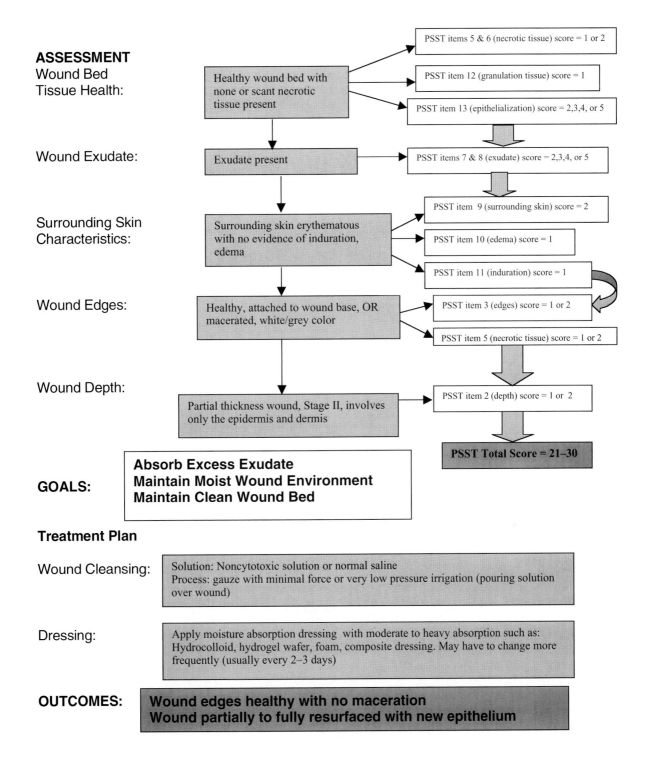

Figure 6–3 Mild partial-thickness PSST severity score treatment algorithm. *Source:* Adapted with permission from Wound and Skin Intelligence System™, *System Outputs Book*, ConvaTec, a division of Bristol-Myers Squibb, USA.

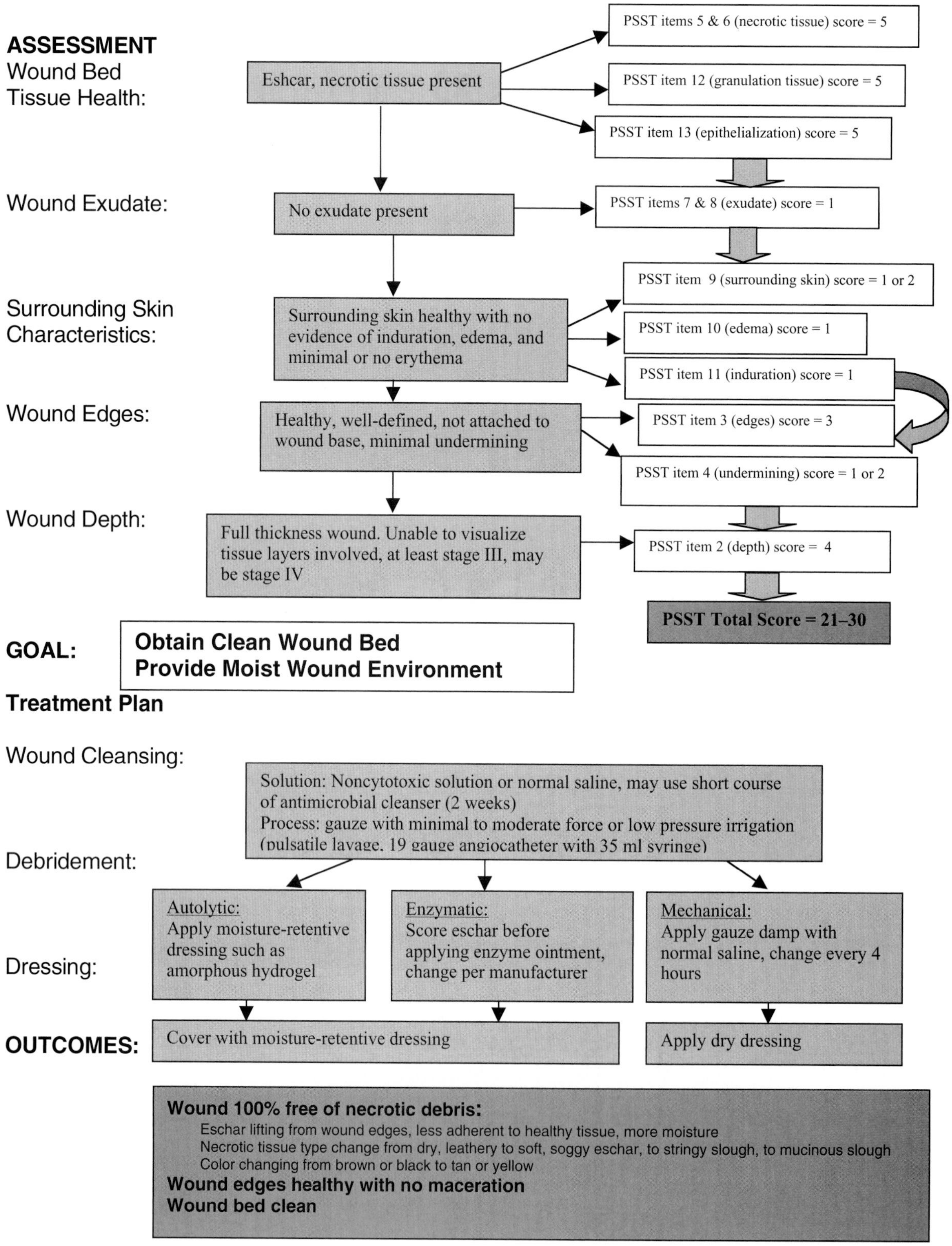

ASSESSMENT
Wound Bed
Tissue Health:

Eshcar, necrotic tissue present	→ PSST items 5 & 6 (necrotic tissue) score = 5
	→ PSST item 12 (granulation tissue) score = 5
	→ PSST item 13 (epithelialization) score = 5

Wound Exudate:

No exudate present → PSST items 7 & 8 (exudate) score = 1

Surrounding Skin
Characteristics:

Surrounding skin healthy with no evidence of induration, edema, and minimal or no erythema

→ PSST item 9 (surrounding skin) score = 1 or 2
→ PSST item 10 (edema) score = 1
→ PSST item 11 (induration) score = 1

Wound Edges:

Healthy, well-defined, not attached to wound base, minimal undermining

→ PSST item 3 (edges) score = 3
→ PSST item 4 (undermining) score = 1 or 2

Wound Depth:

Full thickness wound. Unable to visualize tissue layers involved, at least stage III, may be stage IV

→ PSST item 2 (depth) score = 4

PSST Total Score = 21–30

GOAL: **Obtain Clean Wound Bed**
Provide Moist Wound Environment

Treatment Plan

Wound Cleansing:

Solution: Noncytotoxic solution or normal saline, may use short course of antimicrobial cleanser (2 weeks)
Process: gauze with minimal to moderate force or low pressure irrigation (pulsatile lavage. 19 gauge angiocatheter with 35 ml syringe)

Debridement:

Autolytic: Apply moisture-retentive dressing such as amorphous hydrogel	Enzymatic: Score eschar before applying enzyme ointment, change per manufacturer	Mechanical: Apply gauze damp with normal saline, change every 4 hours

Dressing:

OUTCOMES: | Cover with moisture-retentive dressing | | Apply dry dressing |

Wound 100% free of necrotic debris:
Eschar lifting from wound edges, less adherent to healthy tissue, more moisture
Necrotic tissue type change from dry, leathery to soft, soggy eschar, to stringy slough, to mucinous slough
Color changing from brown or black to tan or yellow
Wound edges healthy with no maceration
Wound bed clean

Figure 6–4 Mild full-thickness PSST severity score treatment algorithm. *Source:* Adapted with permission from Wound and Skin Intelligence System™, *System Outputs Book*, ConvaTec, a division of Bristol-Myers Squibb, USA.

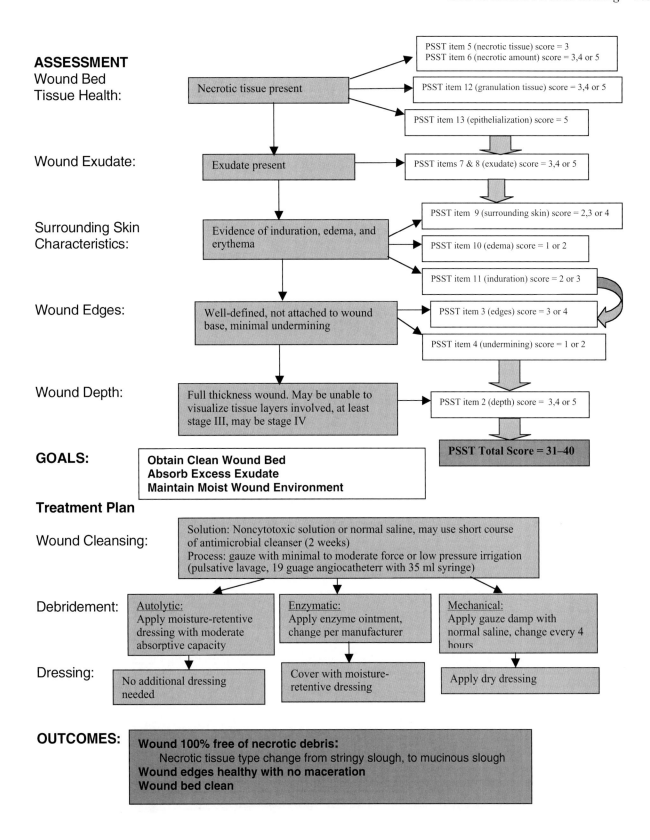

Figure 6–5 Moderate PSST severity score with slough treatment algorithm. *Source:* Adapted with permission from Wound and Skin Intelligence System™, *System Outputs Book*, ConvaTec, a division of Bristol-Myers Squibb, USA.

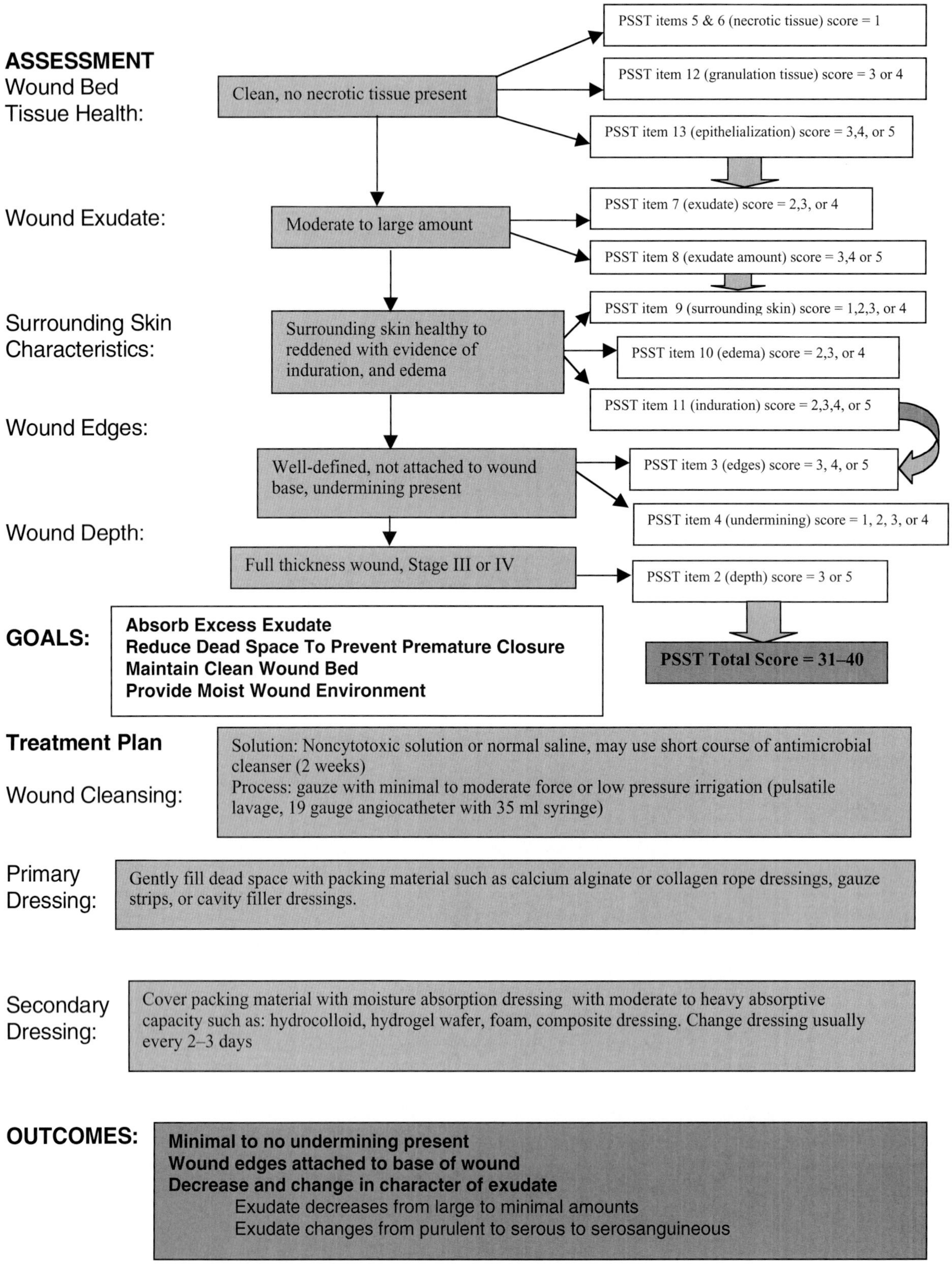

ASSESSMENT
Wound Bed
Tissue Health:

Clean, no necrotic tissue present

PSST items 5 & 6 (necrotic tissue) score = 1

PSST item 12 (granulation tissue) score = 3 or 4

PSST item 13 (epithelialization) score = 3,4, or 5

Wound Exudate:

Moderate to large amount

PSST item 7 (exudate) score = 2,3, or 4

PSST item 8 (exudate amount) score = 3,4 or 5

Surrounding Skin
Characteristics:

Surrounding skin healthy to reddened with evidence of induration, and edema

PSST item 9 (surrounding skin) score = 1,2,3, or 4

PSST item 10 (edema) score = 2,3, or 4

PSST item 11 (induration) score = 2,3,4, or 5

Wound Edges:

Well-defined, not attached to wound base, undermining present

PSST item 3 (edges) score = 3, 4, or 5

PSST item 4 (undermining) score = 1, 2, 3, or 4

Wound Depth:

Full thickness wound, Stage III or IV

PSST item 2 (depth) score = 3 or 5

GOALS:

Absorb Excess Exudate
Reduce Dead Space To Prevent Premature Closure
Maintain Clean Wound Bed
Provide Moist Wound Environment

PSST Total Score = 31–40

Treatment Plan

Wound Cleansing:

Solution: Noncytotoxic solution or normal saline, may use short course of antimicrobial cleanser (2 weeks)
Process: gauze with minimal to moderate force or low pressure irrigation (pulsatile lavage, 19 gauge angiocatheter with 35 ml syringe)

Primary
Dressing:

Gently fill dead space with packing material such as calcium alginate or collagen rope dressings, gauze strips, or cavity filler dressings.

Secondary
Dressing:

Cover packing material with moisture absorption dressing with moderate to heavy absorptive capacity such as: hydrocolloid, hydrogel wafer, foam, composite dressing. Change dressing usually every 2–3 days

OUTCOMES:

Minimal to no undermining present
Wound edges attached to base of wound
Decrease and change in character of exudate
        Exudate decreases from large to minimal amounts
        Exudate changes from purulent to serous to serosanguineous

Figure 6–6 Moderate PSST severity score with undermining or pocketing treatment algorithm. *Source:* Adapted with permission from *Wound and Skin Intelligence System™, System Outputs Book*, ConvaTec, a division of Bristol-Myers Squibb, USA.

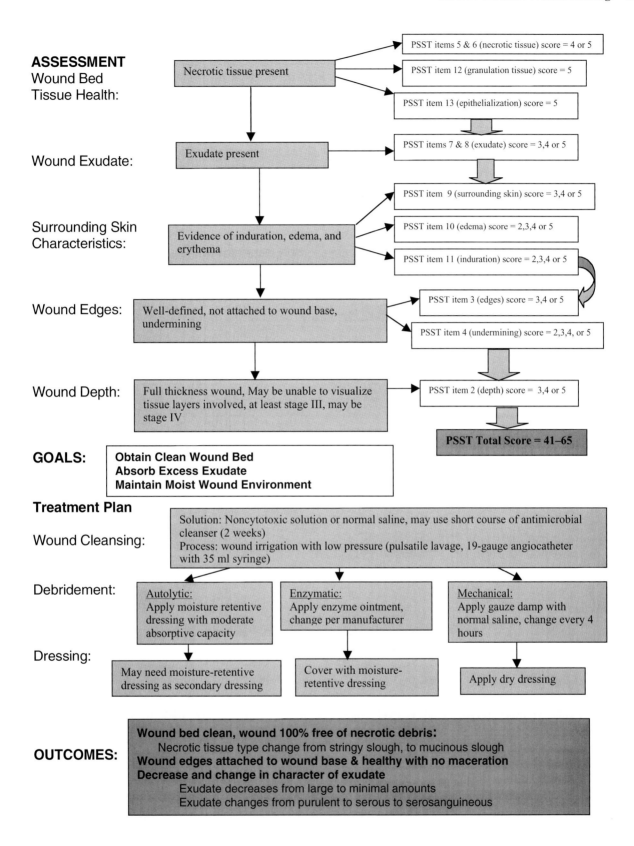

Figure 6–7 Critical PSST severity score with eschar treatment algorithm. *Source:* Adapted with permission from Wound and Skin Intelligence System™, *System Outputs Book*, ConvaTec, a division of Bristol-Myers Squibb, USA.

in this severity state are predominantly full-thickness stage III or IV pressure sores. Figure 6–6 presents the case of the full-thickness clean wound with dead space, and the treatment focus is on eliminating the dead space and prevention of premature wound closure. The goals of care for wounds in this severity state are to obtain/maintain a clean wound bed, absorb excess exudate, eliminate dead space to prevent premature wound closure, and provide a moist wound environment.

PSST Critical Severity Scores 41–65. Wounds with PSST total scores between 41 and 65 are generally stage III or IV full-thickness pressure sores with more critical clinical manifestations, including undermining and necrosis. The generic treatment plan for these wounds is some method of debridement. Figure 6–7 presents the algorithm for treatment for the typical wound in this severity state or the case of the wound with necrotic slough present. The algorithm provides the clinician with the choice of debridement options as the appropriate management method for wounds with necrosis. The goals of care for wounds in this severity state are to identify and treat infection, obtain/maintain a clean wound bed, absorb excess exudate, eliminate dead space to prevent premature wound closure, and provide a moist wound environment.[20]

The use of the PSST score for determining severity state and guiding treatment offers a new approach to managing pressure ulcers. This approach may be useful in designing broad generic treatment guidelines, but individualization of the care plan must still occur, based on the clinician's judgment. The treatment plans presented based on the PSST severity scores focus only on topical wound care, and the clinician must remember that attention to nutrition, adequate support surface use, and attention to the status of the whole patient is also part of the care plan.

Recently, the PSST has been revised for use with all chronic wound types. The new tool, the Bates-Jensen Wound Status Tool (BWST), is currently undergoing validity testing by an expert panel and will soon be available for use on wounds of all etiologies. Changes from the original tool are all based on evidence from users of the tool.

CLINICAL UTILITY OF WOUND HEALING TOOLS

Use of a wound healing tool should enhance communication between health care professionals involved in wound healing. By providing a framework for assessment and documentation with an attempt at quantification, the communication process becomes more meaningful. An objective method of assessing wound healing and monitoring changes over time allows for evaluation of the therapeutic plan of care and may be used to guide and direct therapy. This is particularly true in a managed care environment. For example, if a specific treatment modality is in use and the patient's wound status, as determined with the wound healing tool, has not changed in 2 weeks, reevaluation of the plan of care is warranted. Some studies have demonstrated that wounds with a 50% reduction in surface area within 2 weeks healed more expediently than did those without a 50% surface area reduction.[21,22] These data become an expectation for chronic wound healing. Use of wound healing tools may uncover other outcome criteria that will help to identify critical attributes during the course of healing.

Use of a research-based wound healing tool, such as those described in this chapter, can improve health care practitioner communication and the generalizability of research studies, allow discrimination in studies dealing with treatment modalities, and may help to improve understanding of wound healing. It can provide increased sensitivity, allowing greater precision and clarity in studies related to the treatment and development of pressure ulcers. An instrument that is sensitive to change in wound status will be helpful in the development of critical pathways for pressure ulcers and is useful as an outcome measure.

REVIEW QUESTIONS

1. Describe content validity, criterion validity, and predictive validity.
2. Stability reliability can be evaluated using which of the following methods?
   a. Test-retest techniques
   b. Interrater and intrarater measurements
   c. Internal consistency measurements
   d. Split-half techniques
3. List and describe five common wound characteristics used to evaluate wounds in healing instruments.
4. Explain the criteria you would use to select a wound healing tool for clinical reporting.
5. Describe how plotting the wound healing progression can be used.
6. Describe the validity and reliability of the SWHT, the PUSH, and the PSST.

REFERENCES

1. Bates-Jensen BM, Vredevoe DL, Brecht ML. Validity and reliability of the Pressure Sore Status Tool. *Decubitus.* 1992;5(6):20–28.

2. Ferrell BA, Artinian BM, Sessing D. The Sessing Scale for assessment of pressure ulcer healing. *J Am Geriatr Soc.* 1995;43:37–40.

3. Thomas DR, Rodeheaver GT, Bartolucci AA, et al. Pressure Ulcer Scale for Healing: Derivation and validation of the PUSH tool. *Adv Wound Care.* 1997;10(5):96–101.

4. Krasner D. Wound Healing Scale, version 1.0: A proposal. *Adv Wound Care.* 1997;10(5):82–85.

5. Sussman C, Swanson G. The utility of Sussman Wound Healing Tool in predicting wound healing outcomes in physical therapy. *Adv Wound Care.* 1997;10(5):74–77.

6. Houghton P. *Photographic Wound Healing Tool.* Oral abstract. Symposium for Advanced Wound Care; April, 2000.

7. Ohura T. *Assessment of Pressure Ulcer Healing Process.* Oral presentation. International Pressure Ulcer meeting, New York University, NY; June, 2000.

8. Wagner FW. The dysvascular foot: a system for diagnosis and treatment. *Foot Ankle.* 1981;64:122.

9. Burns N, Grove SK. The concepts of measurement. In: Burns N, Grove SK, eds. *The Practice of Nursing Research: Conduct, Critique & Utilization.* 4th ed. Philadelphia: WB Saunders; 2000:389–410.

10. Waltz CF, Strickland OL, Lenz ER. Reliability and validity of criterion-referenced measures. In: Waltz CF, Strickland OL, Lenz ER, eds. *Measurement in Nursing Research.* 2nd ed. Philadelphia: FA Davis; 1991:229–257.

11. Bartolucci AA, Thomas DR. Using principal component analysis to describe wound status. *Adv Wound Care.* 1997;10(5):93–95.

12. Stotts NA, Rodeheaver GT, Bartolucci AA, et al. *Testing the Pressure Ulcer Scale for Healing (PUSH) and Variations of PUSH.* Oral abstract. Proceedings from the Symposium for Advanced Wound Care and Medical Research Forum on Wound Repair, Miami Beach, FL; April 1998:D38–39.

13. Tohs AS, Rodeheaver GT, Bartolucci AA, et al. An instrument to measure healing in pressure ulcers: development and validation of the pressure ulcer scale for healing (PUSH). *J Gerontol.* 2001. In press.

14. Voss A, Benders C, Cook AS, et al. Pressure ulcer prevention in long-term care: implementation of the National Pressure Ulcer Long-term Care Study (NPULS) prevention program. Proceedings from the Symposium for Advanced Wound Care, Dallas; April 2000.

15. Sussman C, Cuddigan J, Ayello E, Lyder C, Langemo DK. Measuring pressure ulcer healing is critical to quality of life. Poster presented at Partnership for Health in the New Millenium: Launching Healthy People 2010, 2000; Washington, DC.

16. Bates-Jensen B, McNees P. Toward an intelligent wound assessment system. *Ostomy/Wound Manage.* 1995;41(Suppl 7A):80–88.

17. Bates-Jensen BM, McNees P. The wound intelligence system: early issues and findings from multi-site tests. *Ostomy/Wound Manage.* 1996;42(Suppl 7A):1–7.

18. Bates-Jensen BM. *A Quantitative Analysis of Wound Characteristics as Early Predictors of Healing in Pressure Sores.* Dissertation Abstracts International, Vol. 59, No. 11. Los Angeles: University of California; 1999.

19. Bergstrom N, Bennett MA, Carlson CE, et al. *Treatment of Pressure Ulcers. Clinical Practice Guidelines.* No. 15. Rockville, MD: U.S. Department of Health and Human Services. Public Health Service, Agency for Health Care Research and Quality (AHRQ), formerly known as the Agency for Health Care Policy and Research (AHCPR). AHRQ Publication No. 95-0652; December 1994.

20. Sanada H, Braden B, Bates-Jensen BM. Updating pressure ulcer care [Japanese]. Tokyo, Japan: Shorinsha Publishers; 1999.

21. Van Rijswijk L, Polansky M. Predictors of time to healing deep pressure ulcers. *Ostomy/Wound Manage.* 1994;40(8):40–50.

22. Van Rijswijk L. Full-thickness pressure ulcers: Patient and wound healing characteristics. *Decubitus.* 1993;6(1):16–30.

Appendix 6–A: Long Form SWHT and Procedures for Using the SWHT

Sussman Wound Healing Tool (SWHT)
WOUND ASSESSMENT FORM

NAME: _____

DATE: _____

EXAMINER: _____

MEDICAL RECORD NO.: _____

CIRCLE WEEK OF CARE: B 1 2 3 4 5 6 7 8 9 10 11 12

SWHT Vari-able	Tissue Attribute	Attribute Definition	Rating	Relationship to Healing	Score
1	Hemorrhage	Purple ecchymosis of wound tissue or surrounding skin	Present or absent	Not good	
2	Maceration	Softening of a tissue by soaking until the connective tissue fibers are soft and friable	Present or absent	Not good	
3	Undermining	Includes both undermining and tunneling	Present or absent	Not good	
4	Erythema	Reddening or darkening of the skin compared to surrounding skin; usually accompanied by heat	Present or absent	Not good	
5	Necrosis	All types of necrotic tissue, including eschar and slough	Present or absent	Not good	
6	Adherence at wound edge	Continuity of wound edge and the base of the wound	Present or absent	Good	
7	Granulation (Fibroplasia—significant reduction in depth)	Pink/red granulation tissue filling in the wound bed, reducing wound depth	Present or absent	Good	
8	Appearance of contraction (reduced size)	First measurement of the wound drawing together, resulting in reduction in wound open surface area	Present or absent	Good	
9	Sustained contraction (more reduced size)	Continued drawing together of wound edges, measured by reduced wound open surface area	Present or absent	Good	
10	Epithelialization	Appearance and continuation of resurfacing with new skin or scar at the wound edges or surface	Present or absent	Good	

MEASURES AND EXTENT (Depth and Undermining: Not Good)

	Depth/Location	SCORE		Undermining/Location	SCORE		Other	Letter
11	General depth >0.2 cm		16	Underm @ 12:00			Location	
12	General depth @ 12:00 >0.2 cm		17	Underm @ 3:00			Wound healing phase	
13	General depth @ 3:00 >0.2 cm		18	Underm @ 6:00			Total "Not Good"	
14	General depth @ 6:00 >0.2 cm		19	Underm @ 9:00			Total "Good"	
15	General depth @ 9:00 >0.2 cm							

Key: **Present = 1. Absent = 0.** Location choices: upper body (UB), coccyx (C), trochanter (T), ischial (I), heel (H), foot (F); add right or left (R or L). Wound healing phase: inflammation (I), proliferation (P), epithelialization (E), remodeling (R).

Source: Copyright © 1997, Sussman Physical Therapy Inc.

Location   _____

Wound healing phase   _____

Total "Not Good"   _____

Total "Good"   _____

Procedure for Using the SWHT

Completion of the SWHT is by observation and physical assessment, as follows:

1. Each wound of each patient needs its own SWHT attributes form.
2. The patient's name, medical record number, and date of assessment are written at the top of the form.
3. The examiner signs the document.
4. As the wound is assessed, the rater marks a 1 or a 0 to signify present or absent on the form next to each of the 19 attributes. The squares in the column must be marked with one of the two scores.
5. The wound location and the current wound healing phase are marked with the appropriate letter. Choose the appropriate letter to represent the anatomic location of the wound and place it in the square at the time of the initial assessment and subsequent reassessments. The location will not change.
6. Letters are also used to represent the current wound healing phase: mark an *I* for inflammatory, *P* for proliferative, *E* for epithelialization, and *R* for remodeling. In the appropriate box, the phase is noted initially and at each reassessment. The wound healing phase should change as the wound heals.
7. Undermining and depth require some physical assessment to determine presence or absence.
8. Open area measurements are made and listed on a separate form (see Chapter 5), then compared with subsequent measurements of these characteristics to determine contraction and sustained contraction, measured as reduction in linear size.
9. Scoring part I. Add the number of "not good for healing" attributes and the number of "good for healing" attributes listed. The score of "not good for healing" should diminish as the wound heals, and the score of "good for healing" attributes should increase.
10. A summary of the change is shown in Exhibit 6–4.

Appendix 6–B: Pressure Ulcer Scale for Healing and Instructions for Use

PUSH Tool 3.0

Patient Name:_____ Patient ID#:_____

Ulcer Location: _____ Date:_____

DIRECTIONS:
Observe and measure the pressure ulcer. Categorize the ulcer with respect to surface area, exudate, and type of wound tissue. Record a subscore for each of these ulcer characteristics. Add the subscores to obtain the total score. A comparison of total scores measured over time provides an indication of the improvement or deterioration in pressure ulcer healing.

Length	0	1	2	3	4	5	
	$0\ cm^2$	$< 0.3\ cm^2$	$0.3–0.6\ cm^2$	$0.7–1.0\ cm^2$	$1.1–2.0\ cm^2$	$2.1–3.0\ cm^2$	
x Width		**6**	**7**	**8**	**9**	**10**	**Subscore**
		$3.1–4.0\ cm^2$	$4.1–8.0\ cm^2$	$8.1–12.0\ cm^2$	$12.1–24.0\ cm^2$	$> 24\ cm^2$	
Exudate Amount	**0**	**1**	**2**	**3**			**Subscore**
	None	Light	Moderate	Heavy			
Tissue Type	**0**	**1**	**2**	**3**	**4**		**Subscore**
	Closed	Epithelial Tissue	Granulation Tissue	Slough	Necrotic Tissue		
							Total Score

Length × Width: Measure the greatest length (head to toe) and the greatest width (side to side) using a centimeter ruler. Multiply these two measurements (length × width) to obtain an estimate of surface area in square centimeters (cm^2). Caveat: Do not guess! Always use a centimeter ruler and always use the same method each time the ulcer is measured.

Exudate Amount: Estimate the amount of exudate (drainage) present after removal of the dressing and before applying any topical agent to the ulcer. Estimate the exudate (drainage) as none, light, moderate, or heavy.

Tissue Type: This refers to the types of tissue that are present in the wound (ulcer) bed. Score as a "4" if there is any necrotic tissue present. Score as a "3" if there is any amount of slough present and necrotic tissue is absent. Score as a "2" if the wound is clean and contains granulation tissue. A superficial wound that is reepithelializing is scored as a "1." When the wound is closed, score as a "0."

    4—Necrotic Tissue (Eschar): black, brown, or tan tissue that adheres firmly to the wound bed or ulcer edges and may be either firmer or softer than surrounding skin.
    3—Slough: yellow or white tissue that adheres to the ulcer bed in strings or thick clumps, or is mucinous.
    2—Granulation Tissue: pink or beefy red tissue with a shiny, moist, granular appearance.
    1—Epithelial Tissue: for superficial ulcers, new pink or shiny tissue (skin) that grows in from the edges or as islands on the ulcer surface.
    0—Closed/Resurfaced: the wound is completely covered with epithelium (new skin).

Version 3.0: 9/15/98
©National Pressure Ulcer Advisory Panel

PRESSURE ULCER HEALING CHART
(To Monitor Trends in PUSH Scores over Time)
(use a separate page for each pressure ulcer)

Patient Name:_____ Patient ID#:_____

Ulcer Location: _____ Date:_____

Directions: Observe and measure pressure ulcers at regular intervals using the PUSH Tool. Date and record PUSH Subscale and Total Scores on the Pressure Ulcer Healing Record below.

PRESSURE ULCER HEALING RECORD

DATE														
Length × Width														
Exudate Amount														
Tissue Type														
Total Score														

Graph the PUSH Total Score on the Pressure Ulcer Healing Graph below (see Exhibit 6–4)

PUSH Total Score	PRESSURE ULCER HEALING GRAPH													
17														
16														
15														
14														
13														
12														
11														
10														
9														
8														
7														
6														
5														
4														
3														
2														
1														
Healed 0														
DATE														

PUSH Tool Version 3.0: 9/15/98

Instructions for Using the PUSH Tool

To use the PUSH Tool, the pressure ulcer is assessed and scored on the three elements in the tool:

- Length × Width → scored from 0 to 10
- Exudate Amount → scored from 0 (none) to 3 (heavy)
- Tissue Type → scored from 0 (closed) to 4 (necrotic tissue)

Ensure consistency in applying the tool to monitor wound healing, definitions for each element are supplied at the bottom of the tool.

Step 1: Using the definition for length × width, a centimeter ruler measurement is made of the greatest head-to-toe diameter. A second measurement is made of the greatest width (left to right). Multiply these two measurements to get square centimeters, then select the corresponding category for size on the scale and record the score.

Step 2: Estimate the amount of exudate after removal of the dressing and before applying any topical agents. Select the corresponding category for amount and record the score.

Step 3: Identify the type of tissue. Note: if there is ANY necrotic tissue, it is scored a 4. If there is ANY slough, it is scored a 3, even though most of the wound is covered with granulation tissue.

Step 4: Sum the scores on the three elements of the tool to derive a total PUSH Score.

Step 5: Transfer the total score to the Pressure Ulcer Healing Graph. Changes in the score over time provide an indication of the changing status of the ulcer. If the score goes down, the wound is healing. If it gets larger, the wound is deteriorating.

Unmodified Version 3.0: 9/15/98
©National Pressure Ulcer Advisory Panel
Reprint Permission granted
Further reprint requests should be directed to:
NPUAP, 11250 Roger Bacon Drive, Suite 8
Reston, Virginia 20190-5202

Appendix 6–C: Pressure Sore Status Tool and Instructions for Use

PRESSURE SORE STATUS TOOL
Instructions for use

<u>General Guidelines:</u>

Fill out the attached rating sheet to assess a pressure sore's status after reading the definitions and methods of assessement described below. Evaluate once a week and whenever a change occurs in the wound. Rate according to each item by picking the response that best describes the wound and entering that score in the item score column for the appropriate date. When you have rated the pressure sore on all items, determine the total score by adding together the 13-item scores. The HIGHER the total score, the more severe the pressure sore status. Plot total score on the Pressure Sore Status Continuum to determine progress.

<u>Specific Instructions:</u>
1.   **Size**: Use ruler to measure the longest and widest aspect of the wound surface in centimeters; multiply length x width.

2.   **Depth**: Pick the depth, thickness, most appropriate to the wound, using these additional descriptions:
   1 =   tissues damaged but no break in skin surface.
   2 =   superficial, abrasion, blister or shallow crater. Even with and/or elevated above skin surface (eg, hyperplasia).
   3 =   deep crater with or without undermining of adjacent tissue.
   4 =   visualization of tissue layers not possible due to necrosis.
   5 =   supporting structures include tendon, joint capsule.

3.   **Edges**: Use this guide:
   Indistinct, diffuse   =   unable to clearly distinguish wound outline.
   Attached   =   even or flush with wound base, <u>no</u> sides or walls present; flat.
   Not attached   =   sides or walls <u>are</u> present; floor or base of wound is deeper than edge.

   Rolled under, thickened   =   soft to firm and flexible to touch.
   Hyperkeratosis   =   callous-like tissue formation around wound & at edges.
   Fibrotic, scarred   =   hard, rigid to touch.

4.   **Undermining**: Assess by inserting a cotton-tipped applicator under the wound edge; advance it as far as it will go without using undue force; raise the tip of the applicator so it may be seen or felt on the surface of the skin; mark the surface with a pen; measure the distance from the mark on the skin to the edge of the wound. Continue process around the wound. Then use a transparent metric measuring guide with concentric circles divided into 4 (25%) pie-shaped quadrants to help determine percent of wound involved.

5.   **Necrotic Tissue Type**: Pick the type of necrotic tissue that is <u>predominant</u> in the wound according to color, consistency, and adherence using this guide:
   White/gray non-viable tissue   =   may appear prior to wound opening; skin surface is white or gray.
   Non-adherent, yellow slough   =   thin, mucinous substance; scattered throughout wound bed; easily separated from wound tissue.
   Loosely adherent, yellow slough   =   thick, stringy, clumps of debris; attached to wound tissue.
   Adherent, soft, black eschar   =   soggy tissue; strongly attached to tissue in center or base of wound.
   Firmly adherent, hard/black eschar   =   firm, crusty tissue; strongly attached to wound base <u>and</u> edges (like a hard scab).

Source: Copyright © 1990 Barbara Bates-Jensen.

6. **Necrotic Tissue Amount**: Use a transparent metric measuring guide with concentric circles divided into four (25%) pie-shaped quadrants to help determine percentage of wound involved.

7. **Exudate Type**: Some dressings interact with wound drainage to produce a gel or trap liquid. Before assessing exudate type, gently cleanse wound with normal saline or water. Pick the exudate type that is <u>predominant</u> in the wound according to color and consistency, using this guide:

Bloody	=	thin, bright red
Serosanguineous	=	thin, watery pale red to pink
Serous	=	thin, watery, clear
Purulent	=	thin or thick, opaque tan to yellow
Foul purulent	=	thick, opaque yellow to green with offensive odor

8. **Exudate Amount**: Use a transparent metric measuring guide with concentric circles divided into four (25%) pie-shaped quadrants to determine percentage of dressing involved with exudate. Use this guide:

None	=	wound tissues dry.
Scant	=	wound tissues moist; no measurable exudate.
Small	=	wound tissues wet; moisture evenly distributed in wound; drainage involves $\leq 25\%$ dressing.
Moderate	=	wound tissues saturated; drainage may or may not be evenly distributed in wound; drainage involves $> 25\%$ to $\leq 75\%$ dressing.
Large	=	wound tissues bathed in fluid; drainage freely expressed; may or may not be evenly distributed in wound; drainage involves $> 75\%$ of dressing.

9. **Skin Color Surrounding Wound**: Assess tissues within 4 cm of wound edge. Dark-skinned persons show the colors "bright red" and "dark red" as a deepening of normal ethnic skin color or a purple hue. As healing occurs in dark-skinned persons, the new skin is pink and may never darken.

10. **Peripheral Tissue Edema**: Assess tissues within 4 cm of wound edge. Non-pitting edema appears as skin that is shiny and taut. Identify pitting edema by firmly pressing a finger down into the tissues and waiting for 5 seconds; on release of pressure, tissues fail to resume previous position and an indentation appears. Crepitus is accumulation of air or gas in tissues. Use a transparent metric measuring guide to determine how far edema extends beyond wound.

11. **Peripheral Tissue Induration**: Assess tissues within 4 cm of wound edge. Induration is abnormal firmness of tissues with margins. Assess by gently pinching the tissues. Induration results in an inability to pinch the tissues. Use a transparent metric measuring guide with concentric circles divided into four (25%) pie-shaped quadrants to determine percentage of wound and area involved.

12. **Granulation Tissue**: Granulation tissue is the growth of small blood vessels and connective tissue to fill in full-thickness wounds. Tissue is healthy when bright, beefy red, shiny, and granular with a velvety appearance. Poor vascular supply appears as pale pink or blanched to dull, dusky red color.

13. **Epithelialization**: Epithelialization is the process of epidermal resurfacing and appears as pink or red skin. In partial-thickness wounds it can occur throughout the wound bed, as well as from the wound edges. In full thickness wounds, it occurs from the edges only. Use a transparent metric measuring guide with concentric circles divided into four (25%) pie-shaped quadrants to help determine percentage of wound involved and to measure the distance that the epithelial tissue extends into the wound.

PRESSURE SORE STATUS TOOL   NAME

Complete the rating sheet to assess pressure sore status. Evaluate each item by picking the response that best describes the wound and entering the score in the item score column for the appropriate date.

Location: Anatomic site. Circle, identify right **(R)** or left **(L)** and use "**X**" to mark site on body diagrams:

____	Sacrum & coccyx	____	Lateral ankle
____	Trochanter	____	Medial ankle
____	Ischial tuberosity	____	Heel ____ Other Site

Shape: Overall wound pattern; assess by observing perimeter and depth.

Circle and <u>date</u> appropriate description:

____	Irregular	____	Linear or elongated
____	Round/oval	____	Bowl/boat
____	Square/rectangle ____		Butterfly ____ Other Shape

Item	Assessment	Date Score	Date Score	Date Score
1. Size	1 = Length × width < 4 sq cm 2 = Length × width 4–16 sq cm 3 = Length × width 16.1–36 sq cm 4 = Length × width 36.1–80 sq cm 5 = Length × width > 80 sq cm			
2. Depth	1 = Nonblanchable erythema on intact skin 2 = Partial-thickness skin loss involving epidermis and/or dermis 3 = Full-thickness skin loss involving damage or necrosis of subcutaneous tissue; may extend down to but not through underlying fascia; and/or mixed partial and full thickness and/or tissue layers obscured by granulation tissue 4 = Obscured by necrosis 5 = Full-thickness skin loss with extensive destruction, tissue necrosis or damage to muscle, bone or supporting structures			
3. Edges	1 = Indistinct, diffuse, none clearly visible 2 = Distinct, outline clearly visible, attached, even with wound base 3 = Well-defined, not attached to wound base 4 = Well-defined, not attached to base, rolled under, thickened 5 = Well-defined, fibrotic, scarred, or hyperkeratotic			
4. Under-mining	1 = Undermining < 2 cm in any area 2 = Undermining 2–4 cm involving < 50% wound margins 3 = Undermining 2–4 cm involving > 50% wound margins 4 = Undermining > 4 cm in any area 5 = Tunneling &/or sinus tract formation			
5. Necrotic Tissue Type	1 = None visible 2 = White/gray nonviable tissue &/or nonadherent yellow slough 3 = Loosely adherent yellow slough 4 = Adherent, soft, black eschar 5 = Firmly adherent, hard, black eschar			
6. Necrotic Tissue Amount	1 = None visible 2 = < 25% of wound bed covered 3 = 25% to 50% of wound covered 4 = > 50% and < 75% of wound covered 5 = 75% to 100% of wound covered			

Item	Assessment	Date Score	Date Score	Date Score
7. Exudate Type	1 = None or bloody 2 = Serosanguineous: thin, watery, pale red/pink 3 = Serous: thin, watery, clear 4 = Purulent: thin or thick, opaque, tan/yellow 5 = Foul purulent: thick, opaque, yellow/green with odor			
8. Exudate Amount	1 = None 2 = Scant 3 = Small 4 = Moderate 5 = Large			
9. Skin Color Surrounding Wound	1 = Pink or normal for ethnic group 2 = Bright red and/or blanches to touch 3 = White or gray pallor or hypopigmented 4 = Dark red or purple and/or nonblanchable 5 = Black or hyperpigmented			
10. Peripheral Tissue Edema	1 = Minimal swelling around wound 2 = Nonpitting edema extends < 4 cm around wound 3 = Nonpitting edema extends ≥ 4 cm around wound 4 = Pitting edema extends < 4 cm around wound 5 = Crepitus &/or pitting edema extends ≥ 4 cm			
11. Peripheral Tissue Induration	1 = Minimal firmness around wound 2 = Induration < 2 cm around wound 3 = Induration 2–4 cm extending < 50% around wound 4 = Induration 2–4 cm extending ≥ 50% around wound 5 = Induration > 4 cm in any area			
12. Granulation Tissue	1 = Skin intact or partial thickness wound 2 = Bright, beefy red; 75% to 100% of wound filled and/or tissue overgrowth 3 = Bright, beefy red; < 75% & > 25% of wound filled 4 = Pink, and/or dull, dusky red and/or fills ≤ 25% of wound 5 = No granulation tissue present			
13. Epithelialization	1 = 100% wound covered, surface intact 2 = 75% to < 100% wound covered and/or epithelial tissue extends > 0.5 cm into wound bed 3 = 50% to < 75% wound covered and/or epithelial tissue extends to < 0.5 cm into wound bed 4 = 25% to < 50% wound covered 5 = < 25% wound covered			
TOTAL SCORE				
SIGNATURE				

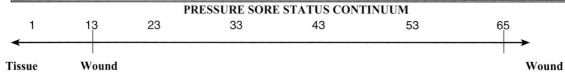

PRESSURE SORE STATUS CONTINUUM

1   13   23   33   43   53   65

Tissue Health   **Wound Regeneration**   **Wound Degeneration**

Plot the total score on the Pressure Sore Status Continuum by putting an "**X**" on the line and the date beneath the line. Plot multiple scores with their dates to see-at-a-glance regeneration or degeneration of the wound.

CHAPTER 7

Vascular Evaluation

Gregory K. Patterson

CHAPTER OBJECTIVES

At the completion of this chapter, the reader will be able to:

1. Describe two techniques for noninvasive vascular testing.
2. Compare and contrast vascular evaluation methods.
3. Describe the technique for obtaining an ankle brachial index.

INTRODUCTION

The initial evaluation of the wound care patient should always contain a thorough vascular assessment. Many of the patients referred to wound care specialists have wounds that are of vascular etiologies. These include arterial, venous, and diabetic wounds. Despite all of the modern wound care therapies, almost all of these wounds will not heal unless the underlying cause is assessed, treated, and confirmed to be not significant. If wounds do heal without treatment of their etiology, they most assuredly have a high rate of recidivism.

HISTORY AND PHYSICAL EXAMINATION

The evaluation of any patient, including the patient with wounds, begins with an adequate history. Exhibit 7–1 lists areas of medical history used to identify risk factors for vascular disease, both arterial and venous. It goes beyond the general medical history discussed in Chapter 1 and focuses on specific vascular-related events. The history and physical examination should include past medical and surgical histories, including the known presence of peripheral vascular disease (PVD), atherosclerotic cardiovascular disease, diabetes mellitus, renal disease, and history of elevated choles-

terol and triglycerides. Thorough surgical history includes all previous operations, especially vascular procedures, including peripheral arterial and venous procedures. Cardiac procedures should also be included, secondary to the fact that the greater saphenous vein is often utilized for bypass procedures. This can cause significant wounds, especially in the diabetic population, and can aggravate the patient with long-standing venous insufficiency. Medications are of importance, especially the use of steroids, rheologic agents, antihypertensive medications, anticoagulants, antiplatelet agents, and aspirin.

Critical evaluation of the patient's symptomatology can often distinguish the cause of the wound. In the discussion of symptoms with the patient with suspected arterial problems, attention should be given to the presence of pain. Typical *claudication* (Greek for "to limp") is pain in the calf only, with walking some distance. This pain should rapidly diminish after the activity is stopped. If this does not occur for long periods of time or if the pain is helped by positional changes, a neurologic cause, such as spinal stenosis or disk problems, should be entertained. This is the so-called pseudoclaudication or neuroclaudication. Rest pain is pain across the forefoot, mainly associated with positional elevation. Typical patients will state that, to relieve the pain at night, they will "hang" their feet over the side of the bed. With the venous patient, history of pain or "tiredness" should be discussed. With female vein patients, an obstetrical history should be elicited. This is to assess for presence of varicosities during pregnancy, secondary to the effect of high levels of estrogen on the vein walls.

The physical exam is extremely important and is aided by a thorough knowledge of the arterial and venous anatomy, including the lymphatic system (see Chapter 17). The examination should include inspection, palpation, and special diagnostic physical exam maneuvers. Inspection should

Exhibit 7–1 Past Medical History

Risk Factors for Peripheral Vascular Disease[1]

Cardiac history

- Heart disease (cardiac catheterization? results?)
- Heart attack (date of last event)
- Chest pain (note location of the pain, how is pain relieved? onset?)
- Stroke (date of event, note location of weakness or speech deficit)

Hypertension (severity, medications, age at onset, highest blood pressure reading)

Hyperlipidemia (last cholesterol level, medication, number of years)

Smoking history (number of packs per day × years smoked = number of pack-years) (For example: a patient smoking two packs per day for 20 years has a 40-pack-year smoking history.) (quit? year quit)

Diabetes (number of years, medications)

Concomitant illnesses (renal disease, collagen vascular disease, arthritis, pulmonary disease, malignancy [type of malignancy], back [spine] problems, etc)

Family history of arterial disease

Risk Factors for Venous Disease

Trauma (type, date)
Deep vein thrombosis (date, anticoagulants)
Prolonged inactivity
Pregnancies
Family history of venous disease
Obesity
Clotting disorders

Past Surgical History

Vascular surgery (date of procedure, indication)
Angiogram/venogram (dates, indication, intervention?)
General surgery (date of procedure, indication)

---

include the size and symmetry of the limb in question. It should be compared with the contralateral limb. Edema or swelling should be assessed. The color and texture of the skin, including the nail beds and capillary refill, should be checked. Texture should also be assessed for the presence or absence of hair, which is highly suggestive of arterial disease, as is muscle wasting. The overall venous pattern should be checked, and the presence of and location of all varicose veins should be documented. Scars, rashes, and pigmentation changes, such as hemosiderin deposits seen in chronic venous insufficiency, should be noted. See Table 7–1 for details concerning the differential between arterial disease and venous insufficiency.

> **Clinical Wisdom: *Trophic Changes***
>
> Trophic changes are skin changes that occur over time in patients with chronic arterial insufficiency. Trophic changes include absence of leg hair; shiny, dry, pale skin; and thickened toenails. These symptoms are due to the chronic lack of nutrition from a good blood supply to the extremity. Some of these changes occur naturally in elderly patients.

The next step of the physical exam should be palpation of all major pulse points and the assessment for any audible harsh sounds, called bruits. This can be done with a regular stethoscope. The major pulses checked should include the radial and brachial in the arm. The carotid artery in the neck and the femoral pulse in the groin are checked (see Figure 7–1). The popliteal pulse is often difficult to assess from the anterior approach (see Figure 7–2) but should be checked routinely, secondary to the rare but well-known problem of popliteal artery aneurysm. The popliteal can be assessed with the patient in the prone position, the so-called posterior approach (see Figure 7–3). The dorsalis pedis and posterior tibial arteries are assessed (see Figures 7–4 and 7–5). Wound assessment of all ulcers and wounds should be completed as with all wound patients.

> **Clinical Wisdom**
>
> The pulse exam includes locating and grading bilateral femoral, popliteal, dorsalis pedis, and posterior tibial artery pulses. The following system should be used to grade pulses:
>
> - 0 = No pulse
> - 1+ = Barely felt
> - 2+ = Diminished
> - 3+ = Normal pulse (easily felt)
> - 4+ = Bounding, aneurysmal ("pulse hits you in the face")

VASCULAR TESTING—INTRODUCTION

Beyond the standard history and physical, if further investigation of a patient's vascular status is needed, more objec-

Table 7–1 Comparison of Arterial and Venous Disease

	Arterial Insufficiency	Venous Insufficiency
Pain	Intermittent claudication, may progress to rest pain	Chronic, dull aching pain, progressive throughout the day
Color	Pale to dependent rubor, a dull to bright, reddish color, more common with advanced disease	Normal to cyanotic, more common with advanced disease
Skin Temperature	Piokilothermic, taking on the environmental temperature. Much cooler than normal body temperature	Usually no effect on temperature
Pulses	Diminished to absent without Doppler stethoscope	Usually normal, may be difficult to palpate, secondary to significant edema
Edema	Usually not present unless combined disease or can be related to cardiac disease and congestive heart failure	Present from mild to severe pitting edema. Can have weeping edema fluid from open wounds
Tissue Changes	Thin and shiny. Hair loss. Trophic changes of the nails. Muscle wasting.	Stasis dermatitis with flaky, dry, and scaling skin. Hemosiderin deposits—brownish discoloration. Fibrosis with narrowing of the lower legs, "bottle legs"
Wounds	Distal ulceration, especially on toes and in between in the web spaces. May develop gangrene and severe tissue loss.	Shallow ulcers in the gaiter distribution of the foot and ankle, usually the medial surface.

tive data in the form of vascular testing should be obtained. This testing can be in the form of noninvasive or invasive testing. Noninvasive testing, as the name implies, uses some form of imaging or method of measurement of the structure and physiologic function to determine information on some aspect of the vascular system. The most commonly used technique is that of ultrasound and its many derivatives. In the area of invasive testing, contrast injection and data acquisition, usually in the form of radiographs, are the most commonly employed. Familiarity with the various tests available and their limitations is essential to wound care professionals. This is important, especially if the wound care specialist is the person ordering and interpreting the tests.

CONTINOUS WAVE DOPPLER AND THE ANKLE BRACHIAL INDEX

In 1842, Christian Johann Doppler, a physicist, discovered the Doppler effect. This principle states that, when a sound source and a reflector are moving toward one another, the sound waves are spaced closer to one another. When the two are moving apart, the sound waves are farther apart. A modern example of this principle is that, as a train approaches, the whistle's pitch is higher, and as it passes, the pitch becomes lower. By using this principle today, we can determine the velocity and direction of blood flow. This is the basis of many of the modern noninvasive tests.

The most widely used noninvasive instrument is the continuous wave Doppler. This utilizes a piezoelectric crystal in a hand-held "pencil" probe. This crystal emits a sound wave that is reflected by the traveling red blood cells in the vessel of interest. This sound wave is reflected back to the probe and is transformed into an audible signal, which we can listen to subjectively or record on a graphic analyzer (see Figure 7–6).

The C.W. Doppler gives us a phasic flow pattern. The normal flow is triphasic. The first sound represents forward flow during systole; the second sound is a negative deflection. This represents a reversal of flow during diastole. The third and smallest sound represents a return of forward flow, caused by elastic recoil of the artery. As disease progresses, this triphasic flow diminishes to a biphasic flow. This is due initially to the loss of elastic recoil caused by "hardening" of the arteries. If the disease progresses further, the flow will decrease to a monophasic signal as the flow loses its pulsatile nature (see Figure 7–7).

The phasic flow patterns are mainly a subjective test. When we apply a blood pressure cuff and occlude the flow in

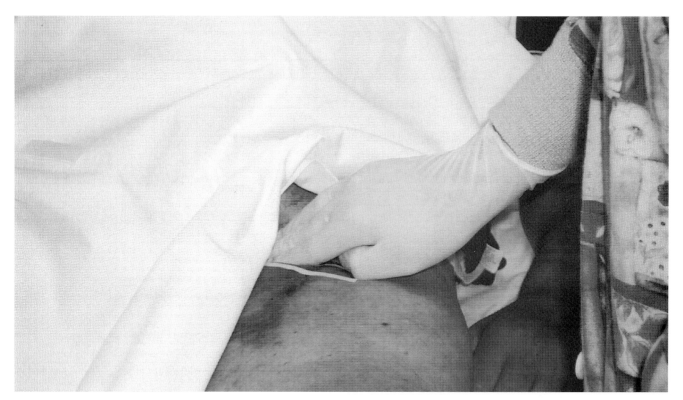

Figure 7–1 Palpation of femoral artery. Courtesy of Archbold Wound Care Center, Thomasville, Georgia.

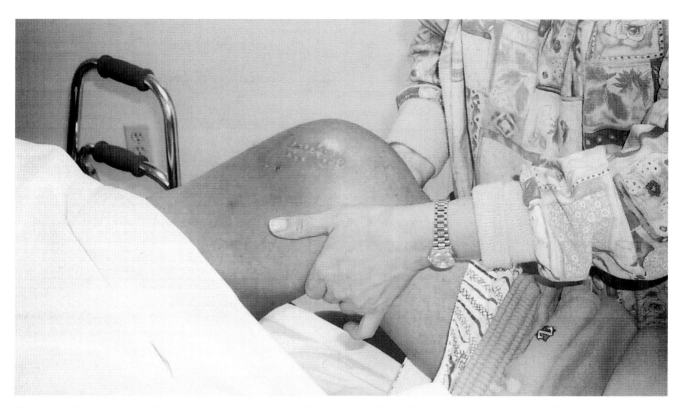

Figure 7–2 Palpation of popliteal artery (anterior approach). Courtesy of Archbold Wound Care Center, Thomasville, Georgia.

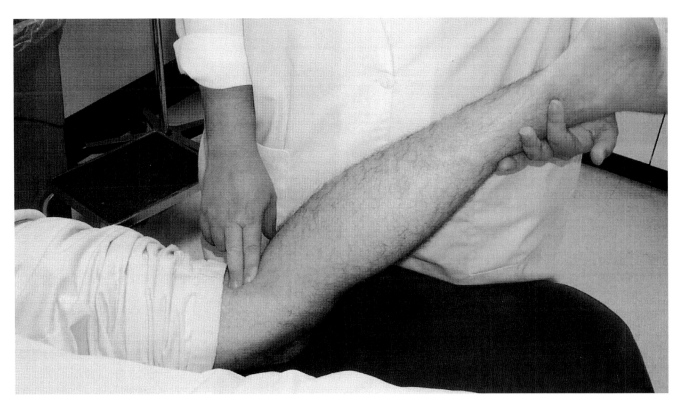

Figure 7–3 Palpation of popliteal artery (posterior approach). Courtesy of Archbold Wound Care Center, Thomasville, Georgia.

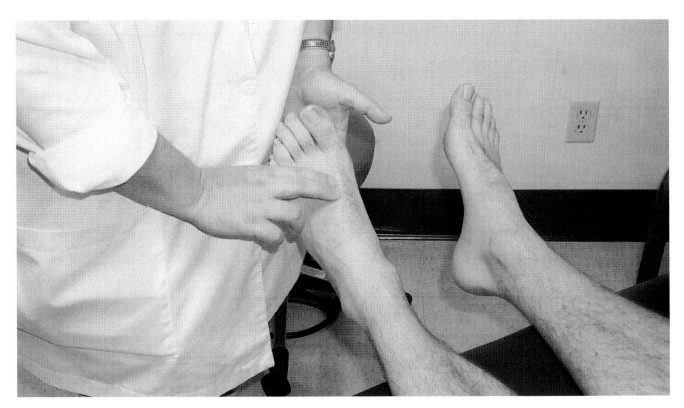

Figure 7–4 Palpation of doralis pedis artery. Courtesy of Archbold Wound Care Center, Thomasville, Georgia.

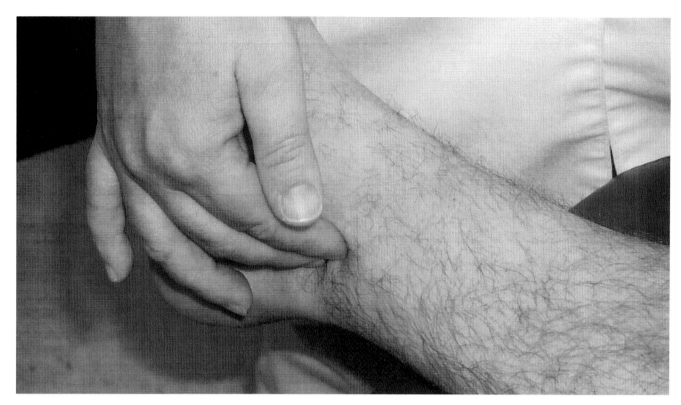

Figure 7–5 Palpation of posterior tibial artery. Courtesy of Archbold Wound Care Center, Thomasville, Georgia.

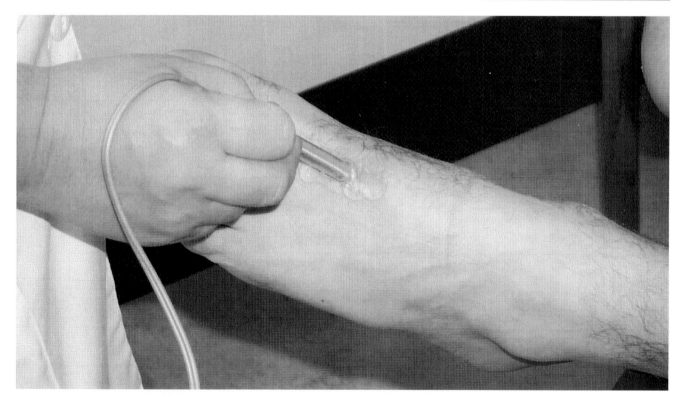

Figure 7–6 Continuous wave Doppler probe assessing dorsalis pedis artery. Courtesy of Archbold Wound Care Center, Thomasville, Georgia.

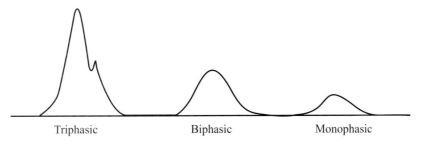

Triphasic   Biphasic   Monophasic

Figure 7–7 Phasic flow patterns.

the artery, then use the Doppler to access the return of flow as the pressure is decreased in the blood pressure cuff, we have obtained a Doppler blood pressure. The most common form of this is the ankle-brachial index (ABI). This compares or indexes the ankle pressure to the arm pressure. This value is obtained by first assessing the highest arm pressure, then placing the blood pressure cuff just above the ankle and obtaining the systolic number with the Doppler probe (see Figure 7–8). Both the posterior tibial artery and the dorsalis pedis artery values are observed. The ankle pressure is then divided by the arm pressure, giving a percentage value. In a normal patient, this value is greater than 1.0. There is some disease present when the number falls below 0.90–0.95. However, the patient usually becomes symptomatic with claudication pain at around 0.70. Rest pain usually occurs at 0.4–0.5. Tissue loss occurs at 0.3 and below. Table 7–2 presents ABI data on prediction of wound healing, and the ABI values and their significance are presented below.

One must remember that a patient describes claudication when walking. If a patient's symptoms are consistent with claudication and the ABIs are not, this may be because they were obtained at rest. Therefore, one can make a patient ex-

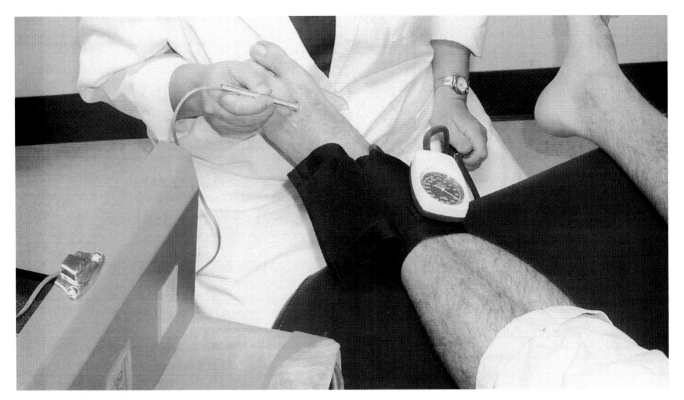

Figure 7–8 Obtaining ABI with C.W. Doppler probe. Courtesy of Archbold Wound Care Center, Thomasville, Georgia.

Table 7–2 Table of ABI Values

Dopplex® Ankle Pressure Index (API) Guide

Ankle Pressure (mmHg)

Brachial Pressure (mmHg)	30	35	40	45	50	55	60	65	70	75	80	85	90	95	100	105	110	115	120	125	130	135	140	145	150	155	160	165	170	175	180	185	190	195	200	
180	.16	.19	.22	.25	.27	.30	.33	.36	.38	.41	.44	.47	.50	.52	.55	.58	.61	.63	.66	.69	.72	.75	.77	.80	.83	.86	.89	.92	.94	.97	1.00					180
175	.17	.20	.22	.25	.28	.31	.34	.37	.40	.42	.45	.48	.51	.54	.57	.60	.62	.65	.68	.71	.74	.77	.80	.82	.85	.88	.92	.94	.97	1.00						175
170	.17	.20	.23	.26	.29	.32	.35	.38	.41	.44	.47	.50	.52	.55	.58	.61	.64	.67	.70	.73	.76	.79	.82	.85	.89	.91	.94	.97	1.00							170
165	.18	.21	.24	.27	.30	.33	.36	.39	.42	.45	.48	.51	.54	.57	.60	.63	.66	.69	.72	.75	.78	.81	.84	.87	.90	.93	.96	1.00								165
160	.18	.21	.25	.28	.31	.34	.37	.40	.43	.46	.50	.53	.56	.59	.62	.65	.68	.71	.75	.78	.81	.84	.87	.90	.93	.96	1.00									160
155	.19	.22	.25	.29	.32	.35	.38	.41	.45	.48	.51	.54	.58	.61	.64	.67	.70	.74	.76	.80	.83	.87	.90	.93	.96	1.00										155
150	.20	.23	.26	.30	.33	.36	.40	.43	.46	.50	.53	.56	.60	.63	.66	.70	.73	.76	.80	.83	.86	.90	.93	.96	1.00											150
145	.20	.24	.27	.31	.34	.37	.41	.44	.48	.51	.55	.58	.62	.65	.69	.72	.75	.79	.82	.86	.90	.93	.96	1.00												145
140	.21	.25	.28	.32	.35	.39	.42	.46	.50	.53	.57	.60	.64	.67	.71	.75	.78	.82	.85	.89	.92	.96	1.00													140
135	.22	.26	.29	.33	.37	.40	.44	.48	.51	.55	.59	.62	.66	.70	.74	.77	.81	.85	.88	.92	.96	1.00														135
130	.23	.27	.30	.34	.38	.42	.46	.50	.53	.57	.61	.65	.69	.73	.77	.80	.84	.88	.92	.96	1.00															130
125	.24	.28	.32	.36	.40	.44	.48	.52	.56	.60	.64	.68	.72	.76	.80	.84	.88	.92	.96	1.00																125
120	.25	.29	.33	.37	.40	.45	.50	.54	.58	.62	.66	.70	.75	.79	.83	.87	.91	.95	1.00																	120
115	.26	.30	.34	.39	.43	.48	.52	.56	.60	.65	.69	.74	.78	.82	.86	.91	.95	1.00																		115
110	.27	.31	.36	.40	.45	.50	.54	.59	.63	.68	.72	.77	.81	.86	.90	.95	1.00																			110
105	.28	.33	.38	.42	.47	.52	.57	.61	.66	.71	.76	.80	.85	.90	.95	1.00																				105
100	.30	.35	.40	.45	.50	.55	.60	.65	.70	.75	.80	.85	.90	.95	1.00																					100

GREATER THAN 1.00

Huntleigh Healthcare, a world leading manufacturer of pocket Dopplers, offers an extensive range of bi-directional pocket Dopplers with visual flow and rate display, together with a wide range of interchangeable probes for both vascular and obstetric applications.

WARNING: False high readings may be obtained in patients with calcified arteries because the sphygmomanometer cuff cannot fully compress the hardened arteries. Calcified arteries may be present in patients with history of Diabetes, Arteriosclerosis and Atherosclerosis.

Courtesy of Huntleigh Diagnostics Ltd., Cardiff, United Kingdom.

Significance of Ankle-Brachial Index Values

ABI ≤ 0.5 — Referral to vascular specialist (compression therapy contraindicated)

ABI = 0.5–0.8 — Referral to vascular specialist. Intermittent claudicant indicating peripheral arterial occlusive disease (compression therapy contraindicated)

ABI = 0.8–1.00 — Mild peripheral arterial occlusive disease (compression therapy with caution)

ABI = >1.00 — Referral to vascular specialist. Indicates calcified vessels if diabetic

ercise by walking, thus increasing vascular demand, decreasing vascular resistance, and decreasing overall relative blood flow. Utilizing this exercise testing will uncover some marginal patients. This is well described by Dr. S.T. Yao, in his classic 1970 article in the *British Journal of Surgery* 1970.[1] Some of the flaws in obtaining ABIs are operator error, plac-

ing the cuff too high on the lower leg, and dividing the arm pressure by the foot pressure, instead of vice versa.

Clinical Wisdom: *Diabetic Patients*

The ankle-brachial index can be falsely elevated in patients with diabetes. This is due to the calcification of the inner layer of the artery, ie, the cuff is unable to compress calcified distal vessel(s). This phenomenon is referred to as *noncompressible vessels*. Instead of ABI, proceed with transcutaneous oxygen testing, if available. Another option is to take toe pressures.

SEGMENTAL AND DIGITAL PLETHYSMOGRAPHY

An expansion of the standard ABI is the segmental plethysmography. This utilizes blood pressures along the entire leg in either a three- or four-cuff system. This obtains pressures from the high thigh, low thigh, below the knee, and above the ankle. All pressures are indexed again to the brachial artery or arm blood pressure. A significant decrease between two cuffs indicates an arterial lesion between these two locations, thus allowing for localization of arterial disease. This may be somewhat difficult to interpret if there is multifocal disease. Segmental plethysmography, or segmental pressures, as they are also known, are typically accompanied by pulse volume recordings (PVR). PVRs show the volume of change in the limb with each pulse beat. These are obtained with the same equipment, including the blood pressure cuffs, as with the segmental pressures. The cuffs are inflated to occlude arterial flow, then deflated to just below systolic pressure, so that only arterial flow is maintained in the limb. The readings are then obtained. These readings usually have a sharp upstroke, indicating systolic flow. They also have a corresponding dicrotic notch, indicating elastic recoil of the artery wall. With mild disease, there is loss of the dicrotic notch. With moderate to severe disease, there is decrease in the upstroke of the waveform. With severe disease, there is loss of the volume beneath the curve (see Figure 7–9).

Digital plethysmography, or "toe pressures," is the same as segmental pressures, except that a special, small-sized cuff is used and placed on the toe, usually the great halloo.

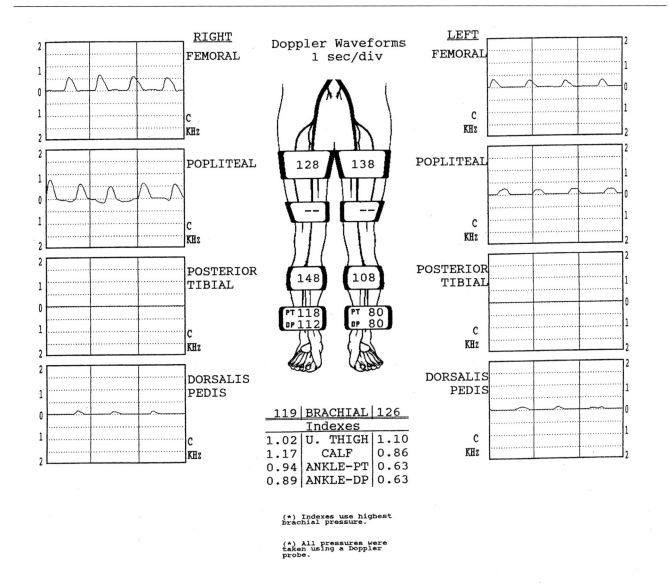

EVIDENCE FOR MILD OCCLUSIVE DISEASE ON RIGHT AT REST. SEVERE ON LEFT, PROBABLY SUPERFICIAL FEMORAL ARTERY IN NATURE. ABNORMAL TBI BILATERALLY.

continues

Figure 7–9 Segmental pressure study with pulse volume recordings.

Figure 7–9 continued

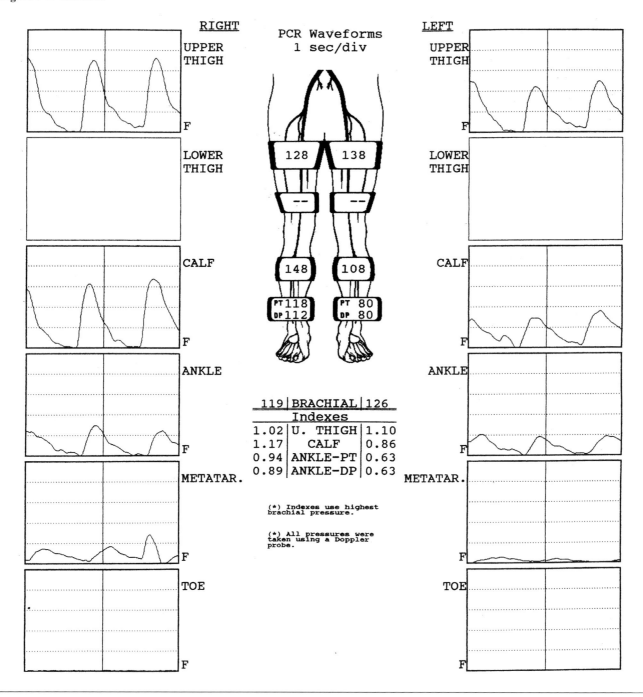

Because of the small-sized digital arteries and the increase in vascular resistance through these arteries, these pressures are reduced. When compared with or indexed to the brachial pressure as a toe brachial index, the normal value is greater than or equal to 0.7. ABIs are extremely useful with diabetic patients because of the process of medial calcific stenosis (MCS), which is a process where the media of the vessel wall is calcified. This causes a standard segmental pressure study to have values that are falsely elevated (greater than 1.0) be-

cause the vessel in question cannot be occluded to obtain a true systolic blood pressure. MCS does not affect digital arteries; therefore, they will be more indicative of arterial disease in diabetic patients.

ARTERIAL AND VENOUS DUPLEX

Duplex scanning is a combination of B-mode ultrasound scanning (gray scale ultrasound) and pulsed Doppler flow detector and spectral analyzer. B-mode ultrasound can show anatomic details with the assistance of color flow Doppler, which shows blood direction. When there is a blockage, there is reversal of flow with a mosaic color pattern. With the pulsed gated Doppler, the Doppler signal can be set to analyze inside the vessel only, so that the readings are not confused with other surrounding structures. In the case of arterial stenosis, the velocity or speed of the blood increases through the stenosis and is recorded in centimeters per second (cm/sec).[2–4] A good example of this is when you place your finger over the end of a water hose. The more of the opening you cover, the faster the water will come out.

In venous duplex scanning, B-mode scanning is used to detect any echogenic material, such as thrombus. The probe is pushed down on the vein to see whether it will collapse. Normally, a vein will compress easily, and an artery, because of its thick wall, will not. In the case of thrombosis, the vein will not compress easily. Color flow Doppler is used to assess for flow in the vein or around a thrombus. It is also used to assess for reflux, or backward flow due to chronic venous insufficiency.[5,6]

TRANSCUTANEOUS OXYGEN MEASUREMENTS

The end result of all vascular studies concerns the delivery of blood to the end tissues, but, in reality, the end result is the delivery of oxygen to the tissues. With this in mind, the actual measurement of oxygen at the skin level mirrors the delivery on the cellular level. Measurement of transcutaneous oxygen ($tcPO_2$) levels utilizes an airtight fixation ring affixed to the site in question. An electrode inside the ring is then heated above body temperature to 41° C. This allows diffusion of oxygen from the capillary level to the skin level and a measurement (in mm) of mercury is made. If the $tcPO_2$ is less than 20 mm Hg, the wound or ulcer will not heal. If the $tcPO_2$ is greater than 30 mm Hg, the wound or ulcer should heal without problems. This is also true of an ulcer that needs to be debrided. Safe debridement may be carried out if the $tcPO_2$ is greater than 30 mm Hg. In the case of amputation, less than 5 mm Hg indicates insufficient levels of oxygen for healing.[7]

> **Clinical Wisdom:** *Accuracy of tcPO$_2$ Measurements*
>
> Transcutaneous oxygen measurements are not reliable in patients with swelling or infection! Do not test these patients. The patient can be tested when the infection is clear and the swelling is gone.

Transcutaneous oxygen measurements have been shown to be predictive for healing of ulcers and amputation wounds,[8] and for determining the extent of chronic ischemia in limbs with and without wounds.[9,10] As mentioned earlier, the diabetic patient with PVD presents some difficulty in evaluating because of MCS. Toe pressure of digital plethysmography is the test of choice but, as is often the case, if the toes are involved, extensively calloused, or have been removed with minor amputation, $tcPO_2$ measurements are very useful. Transcutaneous oxygen measurements do have disadvantages. The reproducibility of the test and the fact that it takes approximately 30 minutes to perform at one level have prevented its widespread acceptance.

SKIN PERFUSION PRESSURES AND THE LASER DOPPLER

Often, the skin in many vascular patients seems to become the "first victim" of critical limb ischemia. With this in mind, the actual skin perfusion pressure (SPP) has been looked at for a prediction of critical ischemia. This is well published, mainly in the Scandinavian literature. There is a problem with the widespread use of this technique. Traditionally, SPP is performed using a Xenon radioisotope single-pass washout technique. This requires special equipment; the patient must keep the limb in question immobile for at least 20 minutes, and the procedure can be painful, necessitating analgesics.

New techniques of measuring SPP with a laser Doppler (see Figure 7–10) have been developed in the past several years. The laser Doppler uses a low-energy laser probe, secured in the bladder of a blood pressure cuff. These cuffs come in a variety of sizes, from large cuffs for thigh measures to tiny cuffs for toe digital SPP measurements (see Figure 7–11). The cuff is inflated to stop skin perfusion; after an adequate baseline is obtained, the cuff is slowly deflated. The skin perfusion is measured in volume percent units (LD1); the SPP is the reading that increases at least 40% over baseline (see Figure 7–12). The laser Doppler can also obtain pulse volume recordings of skin perfusion, thus allowing for further assessment of a patient's vascular status.

The laser Doppler has been shown to be 80% accurate at predicting critical limb ischemia.[11,12] It has also been shown to be a good predictor of healing of amputation wounds.[13] Castronuovo and colleagues' study of SPP in the diagnosis of critical limb ischemia used logistic regression analysis to predict the probability of healing versus the SPP (mm Hg). This revealed a sigmoid-shaped curve. Patients with an SPP greater than 45 mm Hg had a 100% healing rate. The 50% healing rate was for approximately 25 mm Hg.[11]

MAGNETIC RESONANCE ANGIOGRAPHY

The use of magnetic resonance imaging (MRI) has been applied to vascular studies in the form of magnetic resonance angiography (MRA). MRA has become a functional addition to invasive angiography.[14] MRA has advanced over the

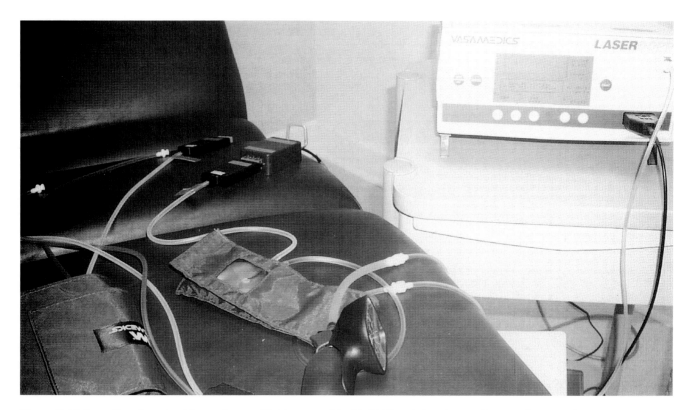

Figure 7–10 Laser Doppler unit with transducer cuffs. Courtesy of Archbold Wound Care Center, Thomasville, Georgia.

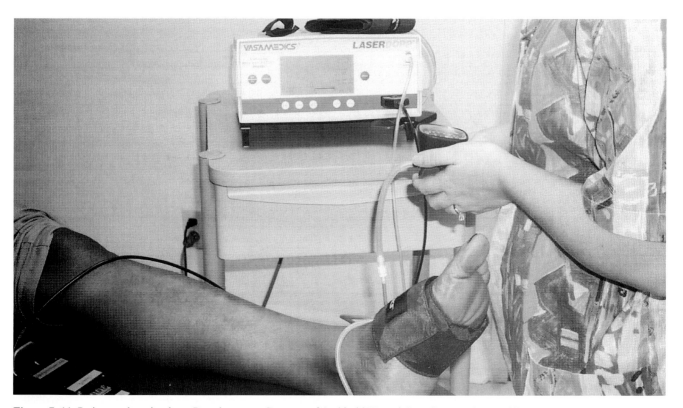

Figure 7–11 Patient undergoing laser Doppler exam. Courtesy of Archbold Wound Care Center, Thomasville, Georgia.

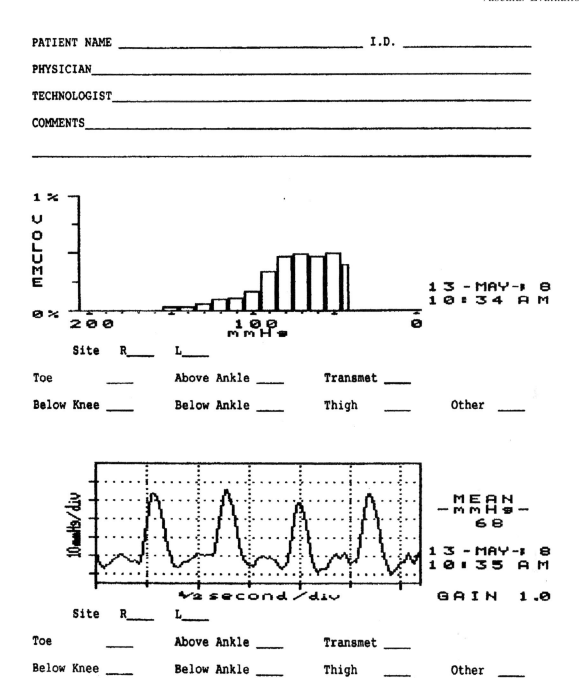

PATIENT NAME _____ I.D. _____

PHYSICIAN_____

TECHNOLOGIST_____

COMMENTS_____

_____

Site R____   L____

Toe _____   Above Ankle _____   Transmet _____

Below Knee _____   Below Ankle _____   Thigh _____   Other _____

Site R____   L____

Toe _____   Above Ankle _____   Transmet _____

Below Knee _____   Below Ankle _____   Thigh _____   Other _____

Figure 7–12 Normal laser Doppler exam with SPP = 90–100 mmHg and normal PVR wave forms.

last 15 years and now can visualize all of the same vessels and hemodynamically significant stenoses seen on contrast angiography. It has been very useful in imaging both the extracranial and intracranial cerebral circulation, as well as the heart and thoracic and abdominal aorta.[15]

MRA has several advantages over traditional contrast angiography. It is noninvasive for the most part. If contrast is used, it is a nonionic contrast, which does not cause any nephrotoxicity. It also has nonvisualization of cortical bone, which has been reduced in digital subtraction angiography but not completely eliminated. Probably the single greatest advantage is it can readily identify target recipient vessels not always identified on conventional contrast angiography.[16] This problem of visualizing occult distal vessels because of contrast washout may increase amputations before vascular reconstruction is attempted. MRA is also comparable in overall cost to contrast angiography.

MRA does have some disadvantages. It is experience-dependent by both radiologist and surgeons. This leads to "overreading" or overcalling the severity of the stenoses. It also needs the availability of a MRI unit, including specialized software and coils. Despite this, it is replacing angiography in some centers.

COMPUTED TOMOGRAPHY ANGIOGRAPHY

One of the newer applications of an existing radiologic test is that of computed tomography (CT) angiography. This test employs ultrafast helical CT scanners to obtain multiple serial images enhanced with contrast. These images are then reconstructed into a three-dimensional projected image. Many of the newer-generation CT scanners and the available software allow for some of the most "contrast-enhanced angiogram"-like pictures, when compared with true angiography. The acquisition of these images is relatively fast for the patient, but the problem lies in the reconstruction of these images. This process takes some highly sophisticated computer software and hardware and is currently very labor-intensive. Some of these CT angiograms can take 3–4 hours to reconstruct. This does not include time to scan the patient or to interpret the images. Currently, this imaging technique is mainly available in teaching institutions or very large medical centers. Future computer and reconstructive developments will undoubtedly determine CT angiography's future.

INVASIVE STUDIES AND CONTRAST ANGIOGRAPHY

Invasive vascular studies, as the name implies, require some invasive component beyond the standard intravenous aspect of the study. In the case of contrast enhanced angiography, this usually requires a femoral artery puncture or brachial artery cutdown. Catheters are then manipulated, which can cause plaques to break off and embolize or even to sustain inadvertent vessel wall damage. Serious complications can occur from the procedures, including heart failure, contrast-induced renal heart failure, and even death (0.05%).[17–19] Despite these complications, angiography remains the "gold standard" for vascular evaluation. If angiography is entertained, all patients should be in the care of a general or vascular surgeon. Angiography has definite advantages over other studies, which include anatomic landmarks for better localization of vessels in question, thus smaller incisions and directed approaches during revascularization. Intralamina intervention, such as angioplasty, is also a significant advantage beyond pure diagnostic tests, thus changing the role of angiography to a therapeutic modality.

One technically significant disadvantage of angiography is nonvisualization of distal runoff vessels. Several studies have shown that up to 70% of patients have failure to opacify the small distal runoff vessels during angiography.[14–21] This is due to a dilution effect of the contrast traversing multiple segments of stenoses. In some cases, there is not enough contrast to visualize the smaller vessels. Therefore, the vessels should be explored before amputation is considered or before patients undergo "on-table" intraoperative angiography and, in some cases, MRA.[20–23]

NEW TECHNOLOGIES

Each of the vascular study techniques presented shares a common starting point of being experimental at one time. Technology continues to bring us newer and improved methods of all aspects of medical care, vascular imaging and wound care included. One new technology recently introduced is that of orthogonal polarization spectral imaging (OPS) (see Figure 7–13). OPS provides real-time in vivo images of microcirculation (see Figure 7–14). It was originally developed by Dr. James W. Winkelton as a method to analyze blood noninvasively. One form can give diagnostic testing to produce a complete blood count, including white blood cell count, hemoglobin, and hematocrit without "sticking" the patient.

Orthogonal polarization spectral imaging's applications are just now being elucidated. OPS's ability to obtain high-contrast images using reflected light allows quantitative determination of capillary density, microvessel morphology, and luminal flow dynamics that have been inaccessible at various sites."[24–25] Direct correlation between improved microcirculatory blood flow in venous ulcers and rapid wound healing has been established.[26] It may be useful to assess wound microcirculation and could be used as a monitoring technique to assess efficacy of treatment before visual changes in chronic wounds occur. This could eventually lead to more rapid clinical decision making, better treatments, and improved healing times.

CONCLUSION

Due to the high incidence of vascular etiologies for wounds, each wound care patient should undergo a thorough history and physical examination. Once a major etiology is considered, further investigation by noninvasive vascular testing should be entertained. Secondary to the myriad of noninvasive vascular testing available, each wound care specialist should familiarize himself or herself with the testing that is available at the institution, including the insti-

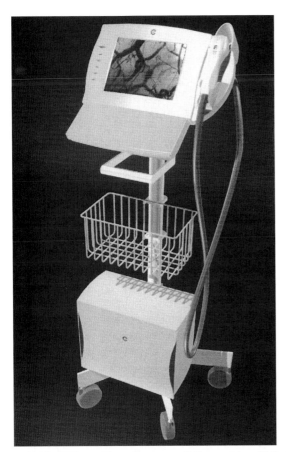

Figure 7–13 OPS machine. Courtesy of Cytometrics, Philadelphia, Pennsylvania.

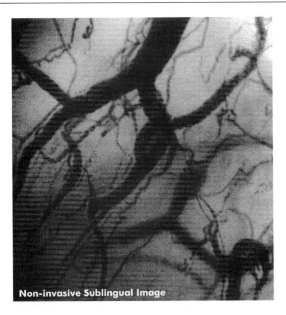

Non-invasive Sublingual Image

Figure 7–14 Image of the microcirculation under the tongue; note the individual RBCs that can be visualized. Courtesy of Cytometrics, Philadelphia, Pennsylvania.

tution's accuracy for this testing. Each wound care specialist should be familiar with and readily apply the ABI, and should include this as part of physical examination and assessment. If definitive diagnosis is reached with noninvasive testing or if invasive testing such as angiography is entertained, a directed consultation with a general or vascular surgeon is needed.

REFERRAL CRITERIA

The following indicators guide referral to a vascular surgeon or the vascular lab:

1. ABI greater than 1.0, $tcPO_2$ measurement greater than 30 mm Hg: semiurgent vascular appointment
2. Gangrene present: urgent vascular appointment
3. ABI
   a. Greater than 0.8: routine vascular appointment
   b. Between 0.5 and 0.8: semiurgent vascular appointment
   c. Below 0.5: urgent vascular appointment
4. Exposed bone or tendon at base of ulcer: urgent vascular appointment
5. Gross infection or cellulitis: urgent vascular appointment
6. ABI less than 1.0 with diminished or absent pulses: semiurgent vascular appointment
7. Nonhealing wounds despite 3+ pulses and good wound care: semiurgent vascular appointment

When in doubt, refer to vascular lab for further evaluation

SELF-CARE TEACHING GUIDELINES

The key to prevention of vascular diseases is patient education. Education is the key to preventing debilitating circulatory problems. Patients must learn the correct way to avoid added stress on their circulatory systems and when to notify their physician if there is a problem.

Self-Care Teaching Guidelines Specific to Arterial Insufficiency

1. Do not smoke! Even one cigarette a day can decrease circulation.
2. Follow physician's directions for controlling blood pressure, diabetes, and high cholesterol.
3. Inspect legs and feet daily, and report any signs of redness, pain, or ulceration immediately. Be sure to inspect between toes.
4. Wash and dry feet every day.
5. Lubricate skin to avoid cracks.

6. The first thing to go into the shoe in the morning should be a hand. Check to make sure there are no foreign objects that could injure the foot.

7. Cut toenails straight across. If possible, have a podiatrist cut the toenails.

8. Do not wear tight shoes.

9. Test bath water with a hand or thermometer ($< 98°$ F) to avoid burns.

10. Do not walk barefoot at any time, either inside or outside the home.

11. Wear comfortable, wide-toed shoes that cause no pressure (orthotics, if necessary).

12. Do not wear constricting clothes.

13. Wear clean cotton socks with smooth seams or without seams

Self-Care Teaching Guidelines Specific to Venous Insufficiency

1. Do not smoke!

2. Wear support stockings as prescribed.

3. Avoid crossing legs.

4. Elevate legs when sitting.

5. Inspect legs and feet daily, and report any increased swelling, new or larger ulcers, increased pain, redness, or infection.

6. Avoid trauma to legs, such as bumping or scratching.

7. Keep legs and feet clean.

8. Eat a well-balanced nutritional diet that is low in sodium.

REVIEW QUESTIONS

1. Taking segmental pressures is a noninvasive diagnostic test for arterial competence. In a comparison of lower extremity pressures with upper extremity pressures, which of the following is associated with a poor prognosis in terms of lower leg wound healing?
   a. Ankle/brachial index of 1.1
   b. Ankle/brachial index of 0.9
   c. Ankle/brachial index of 0.8
   d. Ankle/brachial index of 0.5

2. Which of the following descriptions is MOST characteristic of venous disease ulcers?
   a. Commonly occur on the tips of toes or over the malleolar head, with minimal exudate.
   b. Usually pale ulcer base, with necrotic tissue present.
   c. Wound edges are punched out and regular in appearance, and wound is usually painful.
   d. Commonly occur on the gaiter area, with irregular wound edges and moderate exudate.

3. Which of the following best reflects adequate tissue perfusion and oxygenation to support wound healing?
   a. Capillary refill time greater than 35 seconds
   b. Transcutaneous oxygen tension greater than 40 mm Hg
   c. Albumin levels greater than 2.5
   d. Palpable dorsalis pedis and posterior tibial pulses

REFERENCES

1. Yao ST. Haemodynamic studies in peripheral arterial disease. *Br J Surg.* 1970;57(10):761–766.

2. Kohler TR., Nance DR, Cramer NM, Vandenburghe N, Strandness DE Jr. Duplex scanning for diagnosis of aortoilliac and femoropopliteal disease: A prospective study. *Circulation.* 1987;76(5):1074–1080.

3. Edwards JM, Coldwell DM, Goldman ML, Strandness DE Jr. The role of duplex scanning in the selection of patients for transluminal angioplasty. *J Vasc Surg.* 1991;13(1):69–74.

4. Malone JM, Anderson GG, Lalka SG, et al. Prospective comparison of noninvasive techniques for amputation level selection. *Am J Surg.* 1987;154(2):179–184.

5. Heijborer H, Buller HR, Lensing AW, Turpie AG, Colly LP, Tencate JW. A comparison of real-time compression ultrasonography with impedance plethysmography for the diagnosis of deep-vein thrombosis in symptomatic outpatients. *N Engl J Med.* 1993;329(19):1365–1369.

6. Belcaro G, Labropoulos N, Christopoulos D, et al. Noninvasive tests in venous insufficiency. *J Cardiovasc Surg.* 1993;34(1):3–11.

7. Wagner WH, Keagy BA, Kotb MM, Burnham SJ, Johnson G Jr. Noninvasive determination of healing of major lower extremity amputation: The continued role of clinical judgment. *J Vasc Surg.* 1988;8:703–710.

8. Wyss CR, Matsen FA III, Simmons CW, Burgess EM. Transcutaneous oxygen tension measurements on limbs of diabetic and nondiabetic patients with peripheral vascular disease. *Surgery.* 1984;95(3):339–345.

9. Ballard JL, Eke CC, Bunt TJ, Killeen JD. A prospective evaluation of transcutaneous oxygen measurement of diabetic foot problems. *J Vasc Surg.* 1995;22:485–492.

10. Franzeck UK, Talke P, Bernstein EF, Goldbranson FL, Fronek A. Transcutaneous PO_2 measurements in health and peripheralarterial occlusive disease. *Surgery.* 1982;91(2):156–163.

11. Castronuovo JJ Jr, Adera HM, Smiell JM, Price RM. Measurement is valuable in the diagnosis of critical limb ischemia. *J Vasc Surg.* 1997;26(4):629–637.

12. Castronuovo JJ. Diagnosis of critical limb ischemia with skin perfusion pressure measurements. *J Vasc Technol.* 1997;21(3):175–179.

13. Adera HM, James K, Castronuovo JJ Jr, Byrne M, Deshmukh R, Lohr J. Prediction of amputation wound healing with skin perfusion pressure. *J Vasc Surg.* 1995;21(5):823–828.

14. Carpenter JP, Owen RS, Baum RA, et al. Magnetic resonance angiography of peripheral runoff vessels. *J Vasc Surg.* 1992;16(6):807–815.

15. Edelman RR, Mattle HP, Atkinson DJ, Hoogewoud HM. MR angiography. *AJR Am J Roentgenol.* 1990;154:937–946.

16. Owen RS, Carpenter JP, Baum RA, Perloff LJ, Cope C. Magnetic resonance angiography of angiographically occult runoff vessels in peripheral arterial occlusive disease. *N Engl J Med.* 1992;326:1577–1578.

17. Shehadi WH, Toniolo G. Adverse reactions to contrast media: A report from the Committee on Safety of Contrast Media of the International Society of Radiology. *Radiology.* 1980;137:299–302.

18. Hessel SJ, Adams DF, Abrams HL. Complications of angiography. *Radiology.* 1981;138:273–281.

19. Waugh JR, Sacharias N. Arteriographic complications in the DSA era. *Radiology.* 1992;182:243–246.

20. Patel KR, Semel L, Clauss RH. Extended reconstruction rate for limb salvage with intraoperative prereconstruction angiography. *J Vasc Surg.* 1988;7:531–537.

21. Ricco JB, Pearce WH, Yao JS, Flinn WR, Bergan JJ. The use of operative prebypass arteriography and Doppler ultrasound recordings to select patients for extended femoro-distal bypass. *Ann Surg.* 1983;198:646–653.

22. Scarpato R, Gembarowicz R, Farber S, et al. Intraoperative prereconstruction arteriography. *Arch Surg.* 1981;116:1053–1055.

23. Flanigan DP, Williams LR, Keifer T, Schuler JJ, Behrend AJ. Prebypass operative angiography. *Surgery.* 1982;92:627–633.

24. Groner W, Winkleman JW, Harris AG, et al. Orthogonal polarization spectral imaging: A new method for the study of microcirculation. *Nat Med.* 1999;5(10):1209–1212.

25. Harris AG, Langer S, Messmer K. The study of the microcirculation using orthogonal polarization spectral imaging. In: *Yearbook of Intensive Care and Emergency Medicine.* Berlin, Heidelburg, Germany: Springer Verlag; 2000:705–714.

26. Steins A, Junger M, Zuder D, Rassner G. Microcirculation in venous leg ulcers during healing: Prognostic impact. *Wounds* 1999;11(1):6–12.

SUGGESTED READING

Bates, Barbara. *A Guide to Physical Examination and History Taking.* 6th ed. Philadelphia: Lippincott Company; 1995.

Moore WS. *Vascular Surgery: A Comprehensive Review.* 4th ed. Phildelphia: Saunders; 1993.

Sussman C. Circulatory system disease and ulcers. *Wound Care Patient Education and Resource Manual.* Gaithersburg, MD: Aspen Publishers; 1999.

PART II

Management by Wound Characteristics

Barbara M. Bates-Jensen

The Bates-Jensen rules for wound therapy are as follows: *If the wound is dirty, clean it. If there's leakage, manage it. If there's a hole, fill it. If it's flat, protect it. If it's healed, prevent it.*

Understanding the impact of wound characteristics on treatment options provides a template for intervention. Often, the physical appearance of the wound is the driving force behind treatment options. Management of wound healing by examination of physical characteristics commonly observed in wounds is presented in Part II. The wound characteristics of necrotic tissue; exudate and infection; edema; the clean, proliferating wound; refractory wounds; and scar tissue require specific interventions by the clinician.

Part II begins with a chapter on management of necrotic tissue. A description of the significance and pathophysiology of necrotic debris in the wound bed opens the discussion. Specific necrotic tissue characteristics of consistency, color, adherence, and amount, as well as how necrotic tissue presents in wounds of different etiology are described. The characteristics of necrotic tissue in various wound types are described. The clinical presentation of slough and eschar is described.

Management of necrotic tissue involves wound debridement by one of four methods: mechanical, enzymatic, sharp, and autolytic. Each debridement method is presented, with indications for use, contraindications, advantages, and disadvantages of the method and procedures for implementation. Outcome measures based on the color and amount of necrotic tissue in the wound are presented as tools to measure the effectiveness of debridement interventions. The chapter concludes with self-care teaching guidelines for other health care workers, family caregivers, and patients.

Chapter 9 reviews management of exudate and infection. The significance and pathophysiology of wound exudate are

presented. Common wound exudate for various wound types is discussed. The definition and significance of wound infection are presented. Misdiagnosis of wound infection occurs frequently in clinical practice. Differentiation of infection and colonization of the wound is not a simple task for most clinicians. Comparing characteristics of the infected wound with the inflamed wound reveals significant similarities, as well as some key differences. One of the primary methods of differentiating between infection and inflammation is by wound culture. Bates-Jensen provides background and discussion on wound cultures with tissue biopsy, needle aspiration, and quantitative swab techniques. A procedure for each type of wound culture technique is included. The rising incidence of resistant organisms is presented with reference to methicillin-resistant *Staphylococcus aureus*.

One method of management of exudate and infection is wound cleansing. Wound cleansing and irrigation are discussed in relationship to use of antimicrobial cleansers, and specific cleansing procedures for various wounds are presented. The use of topical antimicrobials (antibacterials, antifungals, and antiseptics) is presented, with discussion on management of exudate with moist wound dressings completing the management interventions. Outcome measures for evaluating exudate management in terms of amount and type of exudate are presented. The chapter ends with self-care teaching guidelines for use with other health care workers, family caregivers, and patients.

Chapter 10 focuses on the management of edema. Wiersema-Bryant presents discussion of the etiologies associated with edema and strategies directed toward the management of edema. Management of edema includes a description of the procedures for managing edema and the parameters to measure in determining outcomes of interventions. Edema assessment and measurement of edema and edema control are presented as two primary categories of quantitative and qualitative findings. Quantitatively, leg circumference and leg volume can be measured to give a reference range of leg size, and, with care, pitting edema can also be measured and quantified. Procedures and guidelines for determining leg circumference, leg volume, and pitting edema are included. Qualitative assessment includes general appearance of the skin and leg, and patient statements about the edema.

Elimination and control of edema may be accomplished through leg elevation, exercise, and the use of compression therapy. Leg elevation facilitates the removal of fluid through utilization of gravity in assisting venous return. Compression therapy works with exercise to facilitate the movement of excess fluid from the lower extremity. Included as appropriate for edema management are leg elevation, elastic wraps, tubular bandages, paste bandages, graduated compression stockings, intermittent sequential compression devices, and exercise. A discussion of each method of edema management includes a definition of the method, the indications and contraindications for use, advantages and disadvantages of the method, and procedures for implementation of the method. Expected outcomes related to edema control with each method and helpful hints for using the method make these procedures very user-friendly. The chapter concludes with several case studies emphasizing the principles of edema management and, finally, self-care teaching guidelines, including a sample patient contract.

The next two chapters in Part II examine wound management of the clean wound and advanced wound therapy for the refractory wound. Geoffrey Sussman provides discussion on wound management of the clean wound with topical wound care products for moist wound healing. Discussion includes inert and passive products, such as gauze, lint and fiber products, and modern moist wound dressings. The features of an "ideal" wound dressing are presented. Generic wound product categories of film dressings, foams, hydrocolloids, hydrogels, alginates, hydroactive dressings, and combination/miscellaneous dressings are then presented. Each wound category includes a definition of the products, the composition and properties of the dressing, indications and contraindications for use, procedures for application and removal of the dressings, and expected outcomes for each category. Discussion of wound cleansing and use of topical antimicrobials is presented in relation to the clean wound. This chapter is supplemented with an appendix by Krasner on dressing categories for easy reference by the clinician.

Chapter 12 is a true collaboration, with multiple authors sharing their expertise on advanced wound therapies. The chapter begins with a definition of the refractory wound. Then each contributor provides background, indications, contraindications, and a case study using the advanced therapy. Negative pressure wound closure, wound temperature control, living skin equivalents, growth factors and the use of silver-impregnated dressings are all discussed. This chapter provides the clinician with a quick reference for determining appropriate use of advanced therapy for wound care.

The final chapter in this section, Chapter 13, focuses on the wound where skin integrity has been restored and management of scar tissue. Scott Ward provides a thought-provoking evaluation of methods to manage scar. The chapter begins with a review of scar tissue formation and dysfunctional scarring, such as keloid formation or hypertrophic scars. The interaction between scarring, contraction, and functional ability are discussed. Measurement and methods of scar assessment are presented, and the chapter then covers interventions for scars. Interventions for the management of scars include surgery (including realignment and use of tissue expanders), pharmaceutical agents, and use of physical agents to reduce pressure and skin tension on the scar site. Both molded splints and pressure garments are discussed as methods of pressure therapy. Use of noncustom pressure therapy, as with elasticized cotton tubular bandages, elastic wraps, or self-adherent stretch wraps, is discussed in relation to management of the scar. Exercise, silicone, massage, and other methods are also presented. The chapter includes self-care teaching guidelines and provides the clinician with an easy reference for management of scar tissue.

The chapters on wound management by wound characteristics in Part II all include tools, such as procedures for specific interventions, self-care teaching guidelines, and guidelines for measuring outcomes. The procedures and guidelines included in these chapters provide the clinician with a "toolbox" for daily practice in wound management. Each chapter focuses on simplifying the often-complex task of determining which interventions are appropriate for the patient with a wound. Each follows the simple rules for therapy stated at the beginning of this part introduction. If the wound is dirty, if necrotic debris and infection are present, clean the wound. Debride the devitalized tissue and identify and treat infection. If the wound is leaking excess exudate or if edema is present, manage the drainage. Control the edema and contain excess exudate. Provide for a moist wound environment, not a wet wound environment. If there is a hole, if significant tissue has been lost at the wound site, provide for tissue replacement with a wound dressing, or fill the hole. If the wound is flat, in the process of reepithelialization or presents with scarring, protect it from external trauma and complications related to scarring. Finally, if the wound is healed, prevention of future wounds is critical.

CHAPTER 8

Management of Necrotic Tissue

Barbara M. Bates-Jensen

CHAPTER OBJECTIVES

At the completion of this chapter, the reader will be able to:

1. Define the terms *eschar* and *slough*.
2. Describe two outcomes measures for management of necrotic tissue.
3. Identify indications for sharp debridement.
4. Describe two advantages and disadvantages for sharp, autolytic, enzymatic, and mechanical debridement.

SIGNIFICANCE OF NECROTIC TISSUE

As tissues die, they change in color, consistency, and adherence to the wound bed. As necrotic tissue increases in severity, the color progresses from white/gray to tan or yellow and, finally, to brown or black. Consistency of the necrotic tissue changes as the tissues desiccate or dry. Initially, consistency may be mucoid with a high water content. Later, the material becomes more clumpy and stringy in nature. Eventually, the tissues appear dry, leathery, and hard. Consistency of the necrotic debris is related to retaining moisture in the wound bed. As the wound is allowed exposure to air, the necrotic debris dehydrates, becoming leathery, dry, and hard. The level of tissue death and the wound etiology also influence the clinical appearance of the necrotic tissue. As subcutaneous fat tissues die, a collection of stringy, yellow slough is formed. As muscle tissues degenerate, the dead tissue may be more thick or tenacious. Histologic studies of human skin during pressure sore development demonstrate that, as the insult to the tissue progresses, the level of necrosis deepens.[1,2] Hard, black eschar represents full-thickness destruction, possibly occurring from prolonged ischemia and anoxemia or from a sudden large vessel disruption from shearing forces.[2] Fat and dermal necrosis and the formation of a slough may be compounded by infection from previous contamination by normal skin flora.[1,3,4] The debris may appear as yellow slough or a mucoid substance.[4,5] Prolonged ischemia may cause necrosis of underlying tissues and manifest as a gray area, blueness of the skin, or white devitalized tissue.[1,5,6] Tissue color varies as necrosis worsens, from white/gray nonviable tissue to yellow slough and, finally, black eschar.

Consistency refers to the cohesiveness of debris (ie, is it thin or thick? stringy or clumpy?). Consistency also varies on a continuum as necrosis deepens. The terms *slough* and *eschar* refer to different levels of necrosis and are described according to color and consistency.[1–3] Slough is described as yellow (or tan) and thin, mucinous, or stringy; eschar is described as brown or black, soft or hard, and representing full-thickness tissue destruction.[1,2] The more water content present in the necrotic debris, the less adherent the debris is to the wound bed. *Adherence* refers to the adhesiveness of the debris to the wound bed and the ease with which the two are separated. Necrotic tissue tends to become more adherent to the wound bed as the level of damage increases and as moisture in the wound decreases. Clinically, eschar is more firmly adherent than yellow slough. The boxed table below refers to color plates for necrotic tissue assessment. Plate captions give more information.

The amount of necrotic tissue retards wound healing because it is a medium for bacterial growth and a physical barrier to epidermal resurfacing, contraction, or granulation.[7–9] The more necrotic tissue present in the wound bed, the more severe is the insult to the tissue and the longer will be the time required to heal the wound.[1] In the process of treating the necrotic wound, the amount of necrotic tissue present leads to modification of treatment and debridement techniques. In addition, determining the severity of the tissue insult may be postponed if the amount of necrotic debris is sufficient to obscure visualization of the total wound. Necrotic tissue may be observed in chronic wounds with various etiologic factors.

Arterial/Ischemic Wounds

Necrotic debris in the ischemic wound may appear as dry gangrene. It may have a thick, dry, or desiccated, black/gray appearance. It is usually firmly adherent to the wound bed. It may be surrounded with an erythematous halo (see *Color Plates 47* and *53*).

Neurotrophic Wounds

Neurotrophic wounds usually do not present with necrosis but often have hyperkeratosis surrounding the wound. This hyperkeratosis looks like callus formation at the wound edges. The wound edges need to be decallused or saucerized frequently see Chapter 18, Figures 18–15B, 18–15C, and 18–21).

Venous Disease Wounds

Venous disease wounds may have either eschar or slough present. Often, venous wounds will appear with yellow fibrinous material covering the wound. Eschar may be attributed to desiccation of the wound and the necrotic debris (see *Color Plate 56*).

Pressure Sores

The necrotic debris that occurs in pressure sores relates to the amount of tissue destruction. In the early stage of pressure sore formation, the tissues may appear hard (indurated), with purple or black discoloration on intact skin. This is indicative of tissue death, and the necrosis appears as the wound demarcates. Exhibit 8–1 presents a critical thinking model, or guideline, for assessment of necrotic tissue and may be helpful in determining the best intervention choice.

Interventions

The therapeutic intervention for necrotic tissue presenting in the wound is debridement. Once the wound is predominantly clean and free of necrosis, debridement is no longer indicated. A variety of debridement choices are available to the clinician. Debridement choices often hinge on the wound appearance, the type of wound, and the type and amount of necrotic debris present in the wound. Some general guidelines may be helpful. Appendix 8–A presents debridement choices for a variety of wounds and necrotic tissue types. There are four main types of wound debridement: mechanical, enzymatic or chemical, sharp, and autolytic. Debridement strategies typically involve use of more than one form of debridement. Reimbursement for debridement is available for clinicians under several CPT (current procedural technology codes) and ICD-9 *diagnostic* codes. Coding varies according to health care professional status, and clinicians are advised to clarify codes specifically prior to billing for debridement services. In general, CPT codes 11040–11044 relate to full-thickness debridement as performed by physicians and physician extenders (nurse practitioners, clinical nurse specialists, or physician assistants). The CPT codes must be used in conjunction with ICD-9 *diagnostic* codes for Medicare billing. Code 86.22 is used when physicians perform the debridement procedure and code 86.28 should be used when the procedure is performed by nonphysicians. CPT codes 97601 and 97602 provide a mechanism for reporting interventions associated with active wound care as performed by occupational and physical therapists. Code 97601 refers to selective debridement technique without anesthesia, such as high-pressure waterjet, sharp selective debridement with scissors, scalpel or tweeezers, and topical applications including the enzymatic and autolytic agents. Code 97602 refers to nonselective debridement techniques without anesthesia, such as wet-to-moist gauze dressings or enzymatic agents. Reimbursement is a constantly changing

Assessment of Necrotic Tissue Types—*Color Plates*				
Color	Black/brown eschar	Tan/yellow slough	Yellow fibrinous	White/gray
Moisture content	Hard	Soft/soggy	Soft/stringy	Mucinous
Adherence	Firmly attached base and edges	Attached base only	Loosely attached	Clumps
Color Plate(s)	7, 20, 21, 26, 30, 52	1, 27, 31	3	28, 29, 31

Exhibit 8–1 Necrotic Tissue Assessment Guideline

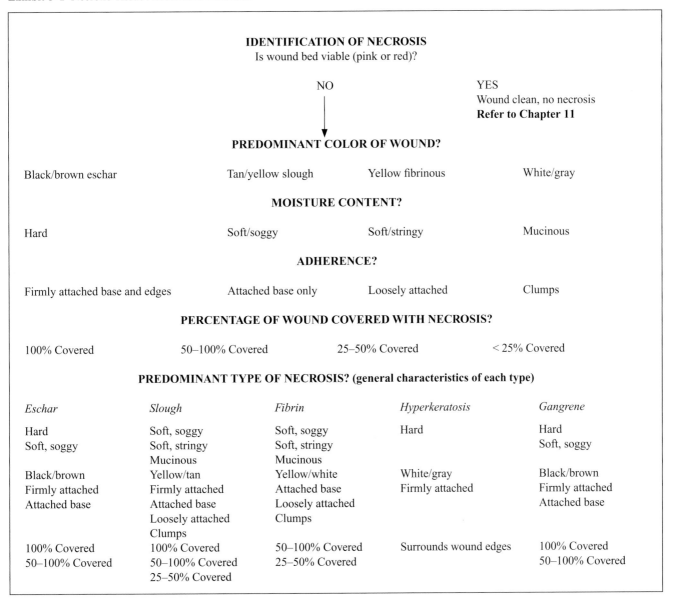

IDENTIFICATION OF NECROSIS
Is wound bed viable (pink or red)?

NO

YES
Wound clean, no necrosis
Refer to Chapter 11

PREDOMINANT COLOR OF WOUND?

Black/brown eschar	Tan/yellow slough	Yellow fibrinous	White/gray

MOISTURE CONTENT?

Hard	Soft/soggy	Soft/stringy	Mucinous

ADHERENCE?

Firmly attached base and edges	Attached base only	Loosely attached	Clumps

PERCENTAGE OF WOUND COVERED WITH NECROSIS?

100% Covered	50–100% Covered	25–50% Covered	< 25% Covered

PREDOMINANT TYPE OF NECROSIS? (general characteristics of each type)

Eschar	*Slough*	*Fibrin*	*Hyperkeratosis*	*Gangrene*
Hard	Soft, soggy	Soft, soggy	Hard	Hard
Soft, soggy	Soft, stringy	Soft, stringy		Soft, soggy
	Mucinous	Mucinous		
Black/brown	Yellow/tan	Yellow/white	White/gray	Black/brown
Firmly attached	Firmly attached	Attached base	Firmly attached	Firmly attached
Attached base	Attached base	Loosely attached		Attached base
	Loosely attached	Clumps		
	Clumps			
100% Covered	100% Covered	50–100% Covered	Surrounds wound edges	100% Covered
50–100% Covered	50–100% Covered	25–50% Covered		50–100% Covered
	25–50% Covered			

area and clinicians are advised to review current guidelines. Discussion of advantages and disadvantages of each debridement intervention follows.

Mechanical Debridement

Mechanical debridement involves the use of some outside force to remove the dead tissue. The most common types of mechanical debridement are wet-to-dry gauze dressings, wound irrigation (using syringe and needle), and whirlpool (see Chapter 25). The advantages of mechanical debridement include the following:

- Mechanical debridement uses treatment options that are familiar to most health care professionals.

- Wound irrigation can effectively decrease the bacterial burden on the wound, when done correctly, and it can be used in conjunction with other treatment options.

Whirlpool may soften necrotic debris for ease of removal by other methods.

The disadvantages of mechanical debridement relate primarily to use of wet-to-dry gauze dressings and outweigh potential benefits; they include the following:

- Wet-to-dry gauze dressings as a form of mechanical debridement are nonselective, removing healthy tissue in addition to dead tissue.
- Wet-to-dry gauze dressings are rarely applied correctly.

- Wet-to-dry gauze dressings may cause pain on removal.
- Wet-to-dry gauze dressings may be more costly in terms of labor and supplies.
- Wet-to-dry gauze dressings may cause maceration of the skin surrounding the wound.

Wet-to-dry gauze dressings continue to be the most commonly used debridement technique, despite the significant disadvantage of removing viable tissue, as well as nonviable tissue. The Agency for Health Research and Quality (AHRQ), formerly the Agency for Health Care Policy and Research (AHCPR), panel's expert opinion recommendation is to use this method cautiously, because it can traumatize new granulation tissue and epithelial tissue, and to administer adequate analgesia when this method is employed.[10]

Wound irrigation removes necrotic debris from the wound bed by using pressurized fluids. Pulsatile lavage (see Chapter 26) and high-pressure irrigation are two techniques for debridement. High-pressure irrigation involves the use of devices that deliver the irrigant solution to the wound at pressures between 8 and 12 pounds per square inch (psi). Use of a 35-mL syringe with a 19-gauge angiocatheter attached delivers fluids to the wound with high-pressure irrigation. This provides enough force to separate and remove necrotic tissue from viable tissue, yet not so much as to drive bacteria deeper into the wound tissues. The clinician performing high-pressure irrigation must use protective equipment to protect from potential bacterial contamination. Procedures for wet-to-dry gauze dressings and high-pressure irrigation are presented for reference and use.

Mechanical Debridement Procedures

Procedure: Wet-to-Dry Gauze Dressings.

Equipment Needed:
- Sterile normal saline
- Gauze (rolled or 4 × 4-inch squares)
- Cover/topper sponges
- Sterile gloves (one pair)
- Clean gloves (two pairs)
- Paper tape, trash bag

Frequency: Apply every 8 hours for wet-to-dry (see Chapter 11 for wet-to-moist gauze dressings).

Indications: Moist necrotic wounds (not effective on dry eschar).

Contraindications: Do not use on clean wounds because the healthy tissue will be "debrided."

Precaution: Patient may need premedication for pain at the time of dressing change.

Procedure:
1. Explain dressing and procedure to patient and caregiver.

2. Wash hands.
3. Prepare dressing supplies.
   a. Open gauze and moisten with normal saline.
   b. Open cover sponges.
   c. Tear tape.
4. Apply clean gloves (to protect from cross-contamination).
5. Remove dirty dressing and dispose in trash bag.
6. Remove gloves and dispose in trash bag (gloves have been contaminated with the dirty dressing).
7. Apply clean gloves (to protect from cross-contamination).
8. Evaluate wound (see Chapter 4 for more on wound evaluation).
9. Clean wound.
   a. Use 35-mL syringe and 19-gauge needle to apply wound cleanser directly into wound.
   b. Use normal saline or a nonionic surfactant wound cleanser.
   c. Antimicrobial solutions, such as povidine-iodine, destroy healthy wound tissues and should be used cautiously—*for short-term treatment, for appropriate bacterial flora only!* (See Chapter 9 for more on wound cleansers and infection.)
10. Remove gloves and apply sterile gloves (to prevent introduction of new bacteria into the wound). (When wound care is being carried out in the home or long-term care setting, the procedure may be performed using only clean gloves.)
11. Open the moistened gauze, fluff, and place in the wound loosely. Be sure to place some of the dressing in undermined or tunneled areas.
12. Cover the wound with the cover or topper sponges. Use one cover sponge for each gauze 4 × 4-inch square used in the wound or each 6–8 inches of roller gauze used in the wound.
13. Secure the dressing with paper tape, write the date and time, and initial the tape.
14. Dispose of the trash bag and wash hands.
15. Review procedure with patient and caregiver.

Procedure: Wound Irrigation.

Equipment Needed:
- Sterile normal saline
- Goggles, if splashing is anticipated
- Clean gloves (one pair)
- 35-mL syringe and 19-gauge needle or angiographic catheter
- Irrigation tray
- Trash bag
- Gauze sponges (4 × 4-inch squares or Kerlix super sponges) *or* cover/topper sponges

Frequency: Apply with each dressing change.

Indications: All wounds.

Contraindications: Use "gentle" irrigation on clean wounds and more vigorous irrigations on necrotic wounds (see Chapter 9).

Procedure:

1. Explain procedure to patient and caregiver.
2. Wash hands.
3. Prepare supplies.
    a. Open gauze or cover sponges.
    b. Fill syringe with irrigant.
        1) Use normal saline or a nonionic surfactant wound cleanser.
        2) Antimicrobial solutions, such as povidine-iodine, destroy healthy wound tissues and should be used cautiously—*for short-term treatment, for appropriate bacterial flora only!* (See Chapter 9 for more on wound cleansers and infection.)
4. Apply goggles and clean gloves (to protect from splashing and cross-contamination).
5. Remove dirty dressing and dispose in trash bag.
6. Remove gloves, dispose in trash bag, and apply clean gloves (to protect from cross-contamination).
7. Evaluate wound (see Chapter 4 for more on wound evaluation).
8. Flush wound with irrigant. Hold needle/catheter 1–2 inches from wound bed.
    a. Irrigate forcefully to debride loose, necrotic tissue mechanically.
    b. May attach a 14-French straight catheter to irrigate tunnels and large undermined areas.
    c. Irrigate gently if wound is clean or free of necrotic debris.
9. Dry surrounding skin with gauze or cover sponges.
10. Apply prescribed dressing, according to procedure for dressing.

Enzymatic or Chemical Debridement

Chemical or enzymatic debridement involves applying a concentrated, commercially prepared enzyme to the surface of the necrotic tissue, in the expectation that it will aggressively degrade necrosis by digesting devitalized tissue. A physician's order is required, and manufacturer's guidelines should be followed. Enzymatic ointments are not active in dry environments, and most are not intended for use on dry eschar without proper preparation of the eschar. Eschar must be cross-hatched with a scalpel and the wound surface kept moist for the preparations to be successful. Enzymes require a specific pH range for best results, and many are inactivated by heavy metals (such as those often found in wound cleansers, topical dressings, and antimicrobial solutions). Frequency of dressing changes depends on the type of enzyme used and range from once to three times daily.

Use of a secondary dressing is typically required, and most manufacturer guidelines recommend moist gauze dressings. Use of other moisture-retentive dressings may facilitate enzymatic debridement, but the choice of the dressing should match the expected dressing change frequency for the enzyme preparation. The surrounding skin must be monitored for potential maceration and the wound observed for potential infection. Enzymatic debridement is selective, only affecting the necrotic tissue and not damaging healthy wound tissues. However, once the wound is clean and free of necrotic debris, more appropriate dressings should be implemented because the enzyme preparations, although not harmful, are typically more costly.

Commercially available enzymes include collagenase, papain/urea, and fibrinolysin/deoxyribonuclease. The AHRQ guidelines used collagenase as an example of a topically applied enzyme and cited studies indicating that enzymatic debridement could result in a clean granulating wound bed in 3–30 days.[10] A review of the literature related to debridement suggested that, if the enzyme was ineffective, the observed debridement may be due to autolysis instead.[11] As mentioned above, use of moist wound healing topical dressings can facilitate debridement with enzyme preparations. Martin and colleagues[12] found that a hydrogel alone can obtain results to similar to that of an enzymatic agent, with less expense. In this study, 17 patients were evaluated in a randomized, controlled trial of enzymatic debridement for necrotic wounds.[12] Investigators found a mean time of 8 days to debride stage IV pressure ulcers for those treated with an amorphous hydrogel dressing, compared with a mean time of 12 days for those treated with an enzymatic preparation containing streptokinase/streptodornase. Although the times were not significantly different, they did indicate that an agent without enzyme activity could produce an effect similar to one with enzyme activity.

The advantages of chemical or enzymatic debridement are that it is selective, working only on necrotic tissue and that it is effective in combination with other debridement techniques, such as sequential sharp debridement and autolytic debridement. The disadvantages include the following:

- Often, enzymatic use is prolonged more than necessary, increasing costs of treatment.
- Enzymatic debridement can be slow to achieve success: It may take from 3 to 30 days to achieve a clean wound bed.

Choice of which enzyme preparation to use is unclear. Research with animal models on the effectiveness of papain/urea, fibrinolysin and deoxyribonuclease, and collagenase have been inconclusive in nature, with some demonstrating more effectiveness of collagenase[13] and others finding papain/urea more effective.[14]

Procedures for enzymatic debridement are included for reference and use.

Enzymatic Debridement Procedures

Procedure: Enzymatic Preparations.

Equipment Needed:
- Enzymatic preparation
- Gauze (4 × 4-inch squares) or cover/topper sponges
- Cleansing solution
- Sterile gloves (one pair)
- Clean gloves (one pair)
- Paper tape, trash bag

Frequency: Follow manufacturer's guidelines.

Indications: All necrotic wounds; moist necrotic wounds are best. If the wound has dry eschar, *cross-hatch* the eschar to improve healing. It is useful to match type of necrotic tissue to actions of enzyme activity, but not essential. For example, a venous disease ulcer will have more fibrin associated with the necrosis, and an enzyme that works on fibrin might be more effective.

Contraindications: Do not use on clean wounds, dry gangrene, or dry ischemic wounds, unless vascular consultation or ankle-brachial index (see Chapter 7) has been obtained and circulatory status determined.

Procedure:
1. Explain dressing and procedure to patient and caregiver.
2. Wash hands.
3. Prepare dressing supplies.
   a. Open gauze or cover/topper sponges and moisten with normal saline (most of the enzymatic ointments require a moist dressing for maximum effectiveness).
   b. Tear tape.
4. Apply clean gloves (to protect from cross-contamination).
5. Remove dirty dressing and dispose in trash bag.
6. Remove gloves and dispose in trash bag (gloves have been contaminated with the dirty dressing).
7. Apply clean gloves (to protect from cross-contamination).
8. Evaluate wound (see Chapter 4 for more on wound evaluation).
9. Clean wound (follow manufacturer's guidelines on use of cleaning solutions).
   a. Use 35-mL syringe and 19-gauge needle to apply wound cleanser directly into wound.
   b. Use normal saline or a nonionic surfactant wound cleanser.
   c. *Avoid* antimicrobial solutions, such as povidine-iodine, which destroy enzymatic activity in the enzyme preparations.
10. Remove gloves and apply sterile gloves (to prevent introduction of new bacteria into the wound). (May use a dressing other than gauze or cover/topper sponges as appropriate topical therapy as the secondary dressing for the wound. When wound care is being carried out in the home or long-term care setting, the procedure may be performed using only clean gloves.)
11. Apply the enzymatic ointment with a tongue blade or cotton-tipped applicator to wound bed. As an alternative, the enzymatic ointment may be applied directly to the gauze dressing to be applied to the wound surface.
12. Open the moistened gauze, fluff, and place in the wound loosely. Be sure to place some of the dressing in undermined or tunneled areas. (May use a dressing other than gauze or cover/topper sponges as appropriate topical therapy as the secondary dressing for the wound.)
13. Cover the wound with the cover or topper sponges. Use one cover sponge for each gauze 4 × 4-inch square used in the wound or each 6–8 inches of roller gauze used in the wound. (May use a dressing other than gauze or cover/topper sponges as appropriate topical therapy as the secondary dressing for the wound.)
14. Secure the dressing with paper tape, write the date and time, and initial the tape.
15. Dispose of the trash bag and wash hands.
16. Review procedure with patient and caregiver.

Sharp Debridement

Sharp or instrumental debridement may be performed as a one-time debridement or as sequential conservative instrumental debridement. One-time surgical debridement is rapid and effective, and may convert the chronic wound to an acute wound. Laser debridement may be considered as a form of surgical debridement and may be effective on those patients who are not candidates for the operating room. Sequential conservative debridement involves removal of loose avascular tissue with sterile instruments. Because sharp debridement involves use of a scalpel, scissors, or other sharp instrument to remove nonviable tissue, it is the most rapid form of debridement. Sharp debridement is indicated over other methods for removing thick, adherent, and/or large amounts of nonviable tissue and when advancing cellulitis or signs of sepsis are present. Both registered nurses and physical therapists (PTs) may perform sharp debridement for wounds in most states. Health care professionals who use sharp debridement must demonstrate their competence in sharp wound debridement skills and meet licensing requirements. Check state practice acts before proceeding.

One multicenter, randomized, controlled trial noted the following effects of sharp debridement on the healing rates of diabetic ulcers.[15] (The trial was designed to compare the effects of a topical growth factor versus placebo on wound healing in 118 patients.) All patients received sharp debridement as needed throughout the study period. Analysis subsequently demonstrated that, independent of treatment, centers that used sharp debridement relatively frequently experienced better healing rates than did those that used sharp debridement less frequently. The highest degree of healing (83%) occurred in the center that used sharp debridement most frequently. This finding suggests that a relationship exists between sharp debridement and wound healing.

Clinical Wisdom: *Licensing Issues*

Registered nurses and PTs may perform sharp debridement. Nurses must (and PTs should) complete an education course on wound debridement and competence validation of wound debridement skills. Competence validation involves performing debridement skills on a wound model, such as a pig's foot, and demonstration of debridement skills on patients, with a qualified mentor to document competence. Some states do not allow nurses or PTs to perform sharp debridement, so it is wise to check with the state board of registered nursing, the state nursing practice act, and the PT licensing agency for validation of practice requirements for performing wound debridement.

Of course, the main advantage of sharp debridement is the speed of converting a necrotic wound to a clean wound. When sharp debridement is performed as a one-time operative procedure, the chronic wound may convert to an acute wound, with resultant wound closure. Sharp debridement is a selective form of debridement when performed properly. Sequential conservative instrumental debridement is effective in combination with enzymatic, mechanical, and autolytic debridement and can speed the removal of necrotic debris when used in combination with other techniques. Conservative instrumental debridement can be performed in any health care setting by nonphysician clinicians and does not require transfer to an acute facility. The disadvantages of sharp debridement include the following:

- Sharp debridement requires a level of experience or skill and specific education.
- There is often questionable reimbursement when sharp debridement is performed by nonphysicians (nurses).

Reimbursement depends on individual state practice acts for nurses.

- Sharp debridement may be painful for the patient and, therefore, analgesia (topical or systemic) may need to be considered.
- There is a potential for blood loss and infection from the procedure.

There are special indications for sharp debridement in relationship to pressure ulcers. Sharp debridement should be performed when gross necrotic tissue, sepsis, or advancing cellulitis is present and should be done with physician collaboration and probable systemic antibiotic coverage. Ischemic wounds should not be debrided (by any means, but most certainly not with sharp debridement) unless the clinician is certain of collateral circulation by vascular studies or an adequate ankle-brachial index is present. Pressure ulcers on heels that present with black, hard eschar may be left intact, provided that they are inspected daily; if signs and symptoms of pathology develop (redness, sogginess, or mushy feel to the area or frank purulent drainage), they should be debrided immediately. Procedures for sharp debridement are presented for reference and use.

Clinical Wisdom: *Safe Sharp Debridement*

A key to successful, safe sharp debridement is knowledge of anatomy and assessment. The three-part *Sharp Debridement of Wounds* video series—*Introduction and Technique, Anatomy and Assessment of the Torso,* and *Anatomy and Assessment of the Lower Extremity*—is a training tool available to teach anatomy of common wound locations on the torso and lower extremities, assessment of necrotic tissue, instrument techniques, and procedures of sharp debridement.[16]

Sharp Debridement Procedure

Procedure: Sharp, Sequential Instrument Debridement.

Equipment Needed:
- Silver nitrate sticks, Gelfoam, or hemostatic dressing (optional)
- Sterile normal saline
- Gauze or cover/topper sponges
- Instrument set
- No. 10 and No. 15 scalpels and blades
- Wound dressing of choice
- Clamp (Kelly or mosquito)
- Suture removal set
- Sterile gloves (one pair)
- Clean gloves (one pair)
- Paper tape, trash bag

- Cotton-tipped applicators
- Scissors (small, fine, serrated, and large, with or without serrations)
- Forceps (Adson—with or without teeth—or Adson-Brown)

Frequency: Perform according to clinical judgment and physician's orders.

Indications: All necrotic wounds; moist necrotic wounds are best. If the wound has dry eschar, autolytic or enzymatic debridement may be used first to soften necrosis and facilitate sharp removal of debris.

Contraindications: Do not perform if you don't feel comfortable or don't know what you are cutting! Do not perform on clean wounds, dry gangrene, or dry ischemic wounds unless vascular consultation has been obtained and circulatory status determined.

Procedure:

1. Verify physician orders.
2. Explain procedure to patient and caregiver.
3. Premedicate patient for pain and relaxation.
   a. Topical: lidocaine (Xylocaine) spray or solution or benzocaine (Hurricaine) spray. Lidocaine spray can be used as a gauze compress directly to the wound site for 10 minutes for effective topical anesthesia or may be locally injected.
   b. Systemic: oral, intramuscular, or intravenous as a preoperative/predebridement regimen. Administer approximately 30 minutes prior to therapy to increase patient tolerance and compliance with procedure.
4. Assemble equipment.
5. Arrange for an assistant.
6. Provide adequate lighting.
7. Position patient.
8. Wash hands.
9. Prepare clean field and equipment.
10. Apply clean gloves (to protect from cross-contamination).
11. Remove dirty dressing and dispose in trash bag.
12. Clean wound (follow manufacturer's guidelines on use of cleaning solutions). Warm solution to 96° to 100° F for patient comfort, if possible.
    a. Use 35-mL syringe and 19-gauge needle to apply wound cleanser directly into wound.
    b. Use normal saline or a nonionic surfactant wound cleanser.
13. Evaluate wound (see Chapter 4 for more on wound evaluation).
14. Remove gloves and dispose in trash bag (gloves have been contaminated with the dirty dressing).
15. Apply sterile gloves (to prevent introduction of new bacteria into the wound). (When wound care is being carried out in the home or long-term care setting, the procedure may be performed using only clean gloves.)
16. Using the pickup forceps, lift the dead tissue or eschar that you are trying to debride and cut it with scalpel or scissors. Grasp dead tissue and hold it taut so that the line of demarcation is clearly visualized. Cut it with care and try to take it down in layers to prevent removal of healthy tissue. Pain and bleeding are signs of healthy tissue.
17. Remove as much nonviable tissue as possible, but limit procedure to 15–30 minutes.
    a. Request reevaluation when any of the following are present:
       1) Elevated temperature or patient is on downhill course
       2) No wound improvement over several weeks
       3) Cellulitis *or* gross purulence/infection
       4) Impending exposed bone or tendon
       5) Abscessed area
       6) Extensively undermined areas
    b. Aggressiveness of debridement should be guided by the following:
       1) The amount of necrotic tissue present
       2) Patient pain tolerance limits
       3) Time schedule and limits to avoid patient and provider fatigue (15–30 minutes)
18. Stop debriding when the following occur:
    a. There is impending bone or tendon.
    b. You are close to a fascial plane or other named structure.
    c. You get nervous.
19. Provide postdebridement care.
    a. Cleanse wound with normal saline.
    b. Apply wound therapy of choice.
    c. Document procedure.
20. Secure the wound therapy with paper tape, if necessary, write the date and time, and initial the tape.
21. Dispose of the trash bag and wash hands.
22. Review procedure with patient and caregiver. (See Exhibit 8–2 for more information on self-care teaching guidelines for wound care with necrotic tissue.)

Autolytic Debridement

Autolytic debridement is the process of using the body's own mechanisms to remove nonviable tissue. Autolysis may be accomplished by use of any moisture-retentive dressing. Maintaining a moist wound environment allows collection of fluid at the wound site, which promotes rehydration of the dead tissue and allows enzymes within the wound to digest necrotic tissue. Autolytic debridement typically involves adequate wound cleansing to wash out the partially degraded nonviable tissue. It is more effective than wet-to-dry gauze dressings because it selectively removes only the necrotic

Exhibit 8–2 Self-Care Teaching Guidelines

Self-Care Guidelines Specific to Necrotic Tissue	Instructions Given (Date/Initials)	Demonstration or Review of Material (Date/Initials)	Return Demonstration or Verbalizes Understanding (Date/Initials)
1. Type of wound and reason for necrotic tissue			
2. Significance of necrosis			
3. Topical therapy care routine:			
a. Clean wound.			
b. Apply enzymatic preparation (if appropriate).			
c. Apply autolytic dressing—transparent film, hydrocolloid, or hydrogel.			
d. Apply secondary dressing if using enzymatic preparation.			
4. Frequency of dressing changes			
5. Expected change in wound appearance during debridement			
6. When to notify the health care provider:			
a. Signs and symptoms of infection			
b. Failure to improve			
c. Evidence of undermining			
d. Impending bone or joint involvement			
7. Importance of follow-up with health care provider			

tissue and, therefore, protects healthy tissues. Mulder and colleagues[17] evaluated 16 patients in a randomized, controlled trial of a hypertonic hydrogel versus wet-to-dry gauze for wound debridement.[17] Their results suggested that the hydrogel could safely facilitate removal of dry adherent eschar from wounds. All of the wounds were chronic, with at least 75% necrotic tissue present. Other investigators have also found amorphous hydrogels to be effective in digesting and removing necrotic debris from wounds.[18–20] Autolysis is facilitated by cross-hatching if the wound is covered with dry eschar. The AHRQ panel recommends autolytic and enzymatic debridement approaches as being better for patients in long-term care or home care settings and for those who cannot tolerate other methods.[10]

Autolysis can be performed alone or in conjunction with other techniques, such as sequential conservative sharp debridement or enzymatic debridement. It is typically slower to achieve a clean wound bed, although progress should be seen within 6 days. It is essential to choose the appropriate dressing for autolysis. Dressing choice can be determined by the wound appearance. For instance, a wound that is covered with a dry eschar might be autolytically debrided using a thin film dressing, whereas a wound with obvious depth and moderate exudate would not be treated with a thin film dressing (an alginate dressing or one with more absorptive capacity would be the better choice).

Autolysis is usually performed using one of the following dressing choices (but any moisture-retentive dressing can achieve autolysis):

- Transparent film dressings (best for dry eschar; because they are nonabsorptive, they rapidly create a fluid environment)
- Hydrocolloids (best for moist wounds with necrosis because they provide some absorptive capacity while maintaining a moist wound environment)
- Hydrogels (promote autolysis by maintaining a moist wound environment)

The advantages of autolysis are that progress can be determined quickly (there should be observed progress within 6 days). Autolysis is selective, of relatively low cost, and effective in combination with other debridement techniques. Disadvantages include the caregiver education required to prepare for the wound appearance with autolysis; the odor and exudate under the dressing also may be disturbing. Procedures for autolysis using several dressings are presented for reference and use.

Autolytic Debridement Procedures

Procedure: Autolytic Debridement—Transparent Film Dressing.

Equipment Needed:
- Sterile normal saline
- Skin sealant
- Transparent film dressing

Frequency: Apply every 3–5 days. Always change dressing when drainage leaks out.

Indications: All necrotic wounds, but most beneficial for dry eschar; may cross-hatch eschar to facilitate autolysis.

Contraindications: Do not use for dry gangrene or dry ischemic wounds unless vascular consultation has been obtained and circulatory status determined.

Procedure:
1. Explain dressing and procedure to patient and caregiver.
2. Wash hands.
3. Prepare dressing supplies.
   a. Open transparent film dressing.
   b. Be sure that dressing size is at least 2 inches larger than wound area to be covered.
4. Position patient off of affected area.
5. Apply clean gloves (to protect from cross-contamination).
6. Remove dirty dressing and dispose in trash bag. (There is likely to be an odor, and the wound drainage may appear quite disturbing.)
7. Remove gloves and dispose in trash bag (gloves have been contaminated with the dirty dressing).
8. Apply clean gloves (to protect from cross-contamination).
9. Evaluate wound (see Chapter 4 for more on wound evaluation).
10. Clean wound (follow manufacturer's guidelines on use of cleaning solutions).
    a. Use 35-mL syringe and 19-gauge needle to apply wound cleanser directly into wound.
    b. Use normal saline or a nonionic surfactant wound cleanser.
    c. *Avoid* antimicrobial solutions, such as povidine-iodine, which destroy healthy wound tissues and should be used cautiously—*for short-term treatment, for appropriate bacterial flora only!* (See Chapter 9 for more on wound cleansers and infection.)

11. Remove gloves and apply sterile gloves (to prevent introduction of new bacteria into the wound). (When wound care is being carried out in the home or long-term care setting, the procedure may be performed using only clean gloves.)
12. Apply skin sealant to skin surrounding the wound and allow to dry until skin looks shiny (skin sealant protects the skin surrounding the wound from maceration and stripping during dressing removal).
13. Apply the transparent film dressing according to manufacturer's guidelines.
    a. When treating lesions in the sacral/coccygeal area, it is best to apply the dressing in a crisscross, overlapping fashion, using strips of the dressing.
    b. Avoid tension and wrinkling of the dressing.
14. Secure the dressing, write the date and time, and initial the dressing.
15. Dispose of the trash bag and wash hands.
16. Review procedure with patient and caregiver.

Procedure: Autolytic Debridement—Hydrocolloid or Hydrogel Wafer Dressings.

Equipment Needed:
- Sterile normal saline
- Hydrocolloid dressing or hydrogel wafer dressing
- Skin sealant (optional)
- Paper tape

Frequency: Apply every 3–5 days. Always change dressing when drainage leaks out.

Indications: All necrotic wounds. Dry eschar may benefit from cross-hatching to facilitate autolysis. This procedure is particularly effective in moist necrotic wounds with moderate amounts of exudate.

Contraindications: Do not use for cellulitis, documented wound infection, dry gangrene, or dry ischemic wounds unless vascular consultation has been obtained and circulatory status determined.

Procedure:
1. Explain dressing and procedure to patient and caregiver.
2. Wash hands.
3. Prepare dressing supplies.
   a. Open hydrocolloid/hydrogel dressing.
   b. Be sure that dressing size is at least 2 inches larger than wound area to be covered.
4. Position patient off of affected area.
5. Apply clean gloves (to protect from cross-contamination).
6. Remove dirty dressing and dispose in trash bag. (There is likely to be an odor, and the wound drainage may appear quite disturbing.)

7. Remove gloves and dispose in trash bag (gloves have been contaminated with the dirty dressing).
8. Apply clean gloves (to protect from cross-contamination).
9. Evaluate wound (see Chapter 4 for more on wound evaluation)
10. Clean wound (follow manufacturer's guidelines on use of cleaning solutions).
    a. Use 35-mL syringe and 19-gauge needle to apply wound cleanser directly into wound.
    b. Use normal saline or a nonionic surfactant wound cleanser.
    c. *Avoid* antimicrobial solutions, such as povidine-iodine, which destroy healthy wound tissues and should be used cautiously—*for short-term treatment, for appropriate bacterial flora only!* (See Chapter 9 for more on wound cleansers and infection.)
11. Remove gloves and apply sterile gloves (to prevent introduction of new bacteria into the wound). (When wound care is being carried out in the home or long-term care setting, the procedure may be performed using only clean gloves.)
12. Peel backing off the hydrocolloid or hydrogel wafer dressing and apply according to manufacturer's guidelines.
    a. Apply strips of tape to the wafer edges in a picture-frame manner; use of a skin sealant under the tape is advised to protect from stripping.
    b. Avoid use of skin sealants under hydrocolloid and hydrogel dressings.
13. Secure the dressing, write the date and time, and initial the dressing.
14. Dispose of the trash bag and wash hands.
15. Review procedure with patient and caregiver.

OUTCOME MEASURES

Three appropriate characteristics for evaluating the effectiveness of debridement are the type of necrotic tissue, the amount of necrotic tissue, and adherence of necrotic tissue to the wound. Outcome measures for necrotic tissue are specific to the type of debridement used during treatment. For example, outcome measures for sharp debridement are typically achieved faster than the same outcomes when other, less aggressive debridement techniques are used. Changes in necrotic tissue are intermediate outcomes; the final outcome measure is healing.

Amount of Necrotic Tissue

The amount of necrotic tissue should diminish progressively in the wound if therapy is appropriate. The amount of necrotic tissue can be measured by linear measurements (measuring the length and width of the necrotic debris), by determining the percentage of the wound bed covered, and by photography. To determine the percentage of the wound bed covered, use a transparent measuring device with concentric circles. Draw a horizontal and a vertical axis through the circles, creating four quadrants (each equal to 25% of the wound) and use the device to help judge the percentage of the wound involved. A rating scale similar to the following may be used to quantify amount of necrotic tissue or the actual percentage of wound coverage may be documented:

1 = None visible
2 = < 25% of wound bed covered
3 = 25–50% of wound covered
4 = > 50% and < 75% of wound covered
5 = 75–100% of wound covered

Type of Necrotic Tissue

The type of necrotic tissue should change as the wound improves and heals when conservative methods of debridement are used, including mechanical, autolytic, and enzymatic techniques. As the necrotic tissue is rehydrated, the appearance will change from a dry, desiccated eschar to a more soggy, soft slough and, finally, to a mucinous, easily dislodged tissue. The color usually changes as the necrosis is debrided. The black/brown eschar gives way to yellow or tan slough. Usually, eschar improves to slough material. Rating the type of necrotic tissue is best accomplished by the use of a scale similar to the following:

1 = None visible
2 = White/gray nonviable tissue and/or nonadherent yellow slough
3 = Loosely adherent yellow slough
4 = Adherent, soft black eschar
5 = Firmly adherent, hard black eschar

Adherence of Necrotic Tissue

Adherence of the necrosis should decrease as debridement proceeds. Initially, the necrotic tissue may be firmly attached to the wound base and all wound edges. As debridement proceeds, the necrosis begins lifting, loosens from the edges of the wound, and eventually disengages from the base of the wound, as well. Adherence is best evaluated using a rating scale similar to that for types of necrotic tissue.

General guidelines for length of time for debridement are presented in Table 8–1.

REFERRAL CRITERIA

Debridement in arterial/ischemic ulcers is contraindicated unless, and until, adequate circulatory status has been deter-

Table 8–1 Debridement Time Frames

Necrotic Tissue Type	Debridement Choice	Expected Outcomes	Time Frame Guide	Notes
Eschar	Autolysis	1. Eschar nonadherent to wound edges 2. Necrotic tissue lifting from wound edges 3. Necrotic tissue soft and soggy 4. Color change from black/brown to yellow/tan	14 Days	Depending on type of dressing used for autolysis, may proceed at more rapid rate.
Eschar	Enzymatic preparations	1. Eschar nonadherent to wound edges 2. Necrotic tissue lifting from wound edges 3. Necrotic tissue soft and soggy 4. Color change from black/brown to yellow/tan 5. Change from eschar to slough	14 Days	Requires compliance on dressing changes in order to be effective.
Eschar	Sharp	1. Removal/elimination of eschar, if done one time or significant change in amount and adherence, if sequential	Immediate if one time, 7 days if sequential	If sequential sharp debridement used in conjunction with enzymatic preparation or autolysis, may expect clean wound base in 7 days.
Slough or fibrin	Autolysis or enzymatic preparations	1. Necrotic tissue lifting from wound base 2. Necrotic tissue stringy or mucinous 3. Tissue color yellow or white 4. Change in amount of wound covered—gradual decrease to wound predominantly clean	14 Days	Will require moderate amount of exudate absorption and protection of surrounding tissues from maceration.
Slough or fibrin	Sharp	1. Removal/elimination of necrotic slough if done one time or significant change in amount and adherence, if sequential	Immediate if one time, 7 days if sequential	If sequential sharp debridement used in conjunction with enzymatic preparation or autolysis, may expect clean wound base in 7 days.

mined. If you don't feel comfortable or have limited or no experience in debridement, you may want to refer to a health care provider with more experience. The following patients may warrant referral to the physician or an advanced practice nurse:

- Patients with dry gangrene or dry ischemic wounds should be routinely referred for vascular consultation for circulatory status determination.
- Patients with elevated temperature or those on a downhill course should be evaluated further.
- Patients with no wound improvement over several weeks should be evaluated further. In this case, the nurse may want to consult other health care practitioners (PTs, dietitians, wound care nurses, enterostomal therapy (ET) nurses, and physicians).
- Patients with evidence of cellulitis *or* gross purulence/infection.
- Patients with impending exposed bone or tendon present in the wound.
- Patients showing evidence of an abscessed area or patients with extensively undermined areas present in the wound should be evaluated further.

SELF-CARE TEACHING GUIDELINES

Patient and caregiver instruction in self-care must be individualized to the topical therapy care routine, the individual patient's wound, the individual patient's learning style and coping mechanisms, and the ability of the patient/caregiver to perform procedures. These general self-care teaching guidelines must be individualized for each patient and caregiver. Exhibit 8–2 presents self-care teaching guidelines related to necrotic tissue management.

REVIEW QUESTIONS

1. Which of the following methods of debridement may be most useful with patients in long-term care facilities or in the home environment?
   a. sharp, enzymatic, and autolytic
   b. mechanical and autolytic
   c. sharp and mechanical
   d. autolytic and enzymatic

2. A client presents with a sacral wound that is 100% covered with thick, adherent black eschar. Which of the following debridement techniques is indicated?
   a. mechanical
   b. enzymatic
   c. autolytic
   d. sharp

3. Which of the following therapies could be classified as autolytic debridement?
   a. hydrogel dressings
   b. hydrocolloid dressings
   c. wet-to-dry gauze dressings
   d. thin film dressings
   e. a, b, c
   f. c and d
   g. a, b, d

4. The clinician notes the following upon assessment of a long-term care facility client's wound. The pressure ulcer is 75–100% filled with soft, yellow, stringy necrosis with a moderate amount of exudate. The necrotic debris is adherent to the base of the wound but is lifting from the edge of the wound. Which of the following represents the MOST appropriate treatment option for this wound?
   a. transparent film dressing
   b. gauze dressings for exudate management
   c. enzymatic ointment with secondary dressing for debridement
   d. whirlpool twice a week

5. The clinician is asked to see a client, age 81 years old, for pressure ulcer management. On evaluation, the clinician finds a large lesion (7.2 × 6.6 cm) on the trochanter covered with a thick, adherent, black eschar. The surrounding tissues are indurated, warm to touch, and erythemic. Systemically, the client's temperature is elevated, white blood cell count is elevated, and urine and sputum cultures were negative. Which of the following would be the best response by the clinician?
   a. application of a wet-to-moist gauze dressing
   b. use of enzymatic ointment and secondary gauze dressing
   c. request for physician surgical consult for sharp wound debridement
   d. use of transparent film dressings to soften eschar

REFERENCES

1. Shea D. Pressure sores: Classification and management. *Clin Orthop.* 1975;112:89–100.
2. Witkowski JA, Parish LC. Histopathology of the decubitus ulcer. *J Am Acad Dermatol.* 1982;6:1014–1021.
3. Enis JG, Sarmiento A. The pathophysiology and management of pressure sores. *Orthop Rev.* 1973;2:25–34.
4. Sather MR, Weber CE, George J. Pressure sores and the spinal cord injury patient. *Drug Intell Clin Pharm.* 1977;2:154–169.

5. Agris J, Spira M. Pressure ulcers: Prevention and treatment. *Clin Symp.* 1979;31:2–14.

6. Edberg EL, Cerny K, Stauffer ES. Prevention and treatment of pressure sores. *Phys Ther.* 1973;53:246–252.

7. Alterescu V, Alterescu K. Etiology and treatment of pressure ulcers. *Decubitus.* 1988;1:28–35.

8. Winter G. Epidermal regeneration studied in the domestic pig. In: Hung TK, Dunphy JE, eds. *Fundamentals of Wound Management.* New York: Appleton-Century-Crofts; 1979:71–111.

9. Sapico FL, Ginunas VJ, Thornhill-Hoynes M, et al. Quantitative microbiology of pressure sores in different stages of healing. *Diagn Biol Infect Dis.* 1986;5:31–38.

10. Bergstrom N, Bennett MA, Carlson CE, et al. *Treatment of Pressure Ulcers.* Clinical Practice Guidelines No. 15. Rockville, MD: U.S. Department of Health and Human Services (DHHS). Public Health Service, Agency for Health Care Research and Quality (AHRQ), formerly known as the Agency for Health Care Policy and Research (AHCPR) Publication No. 95-0652, December 1994.

11. Rodeheaver GT. Pressure ulcer debridement and cleansing: A review of current literature. *Ostomy/Wound Manage.* 1999;45(1A Suppl):80–86.

12. Martin SJ, Corrado OJ, Kay EA. Enzymatic debridement for necrotic wounds. *J Wound Care.* 1996;5(7):310–311.

13. Mekkes J, Zeegelaar J, Westerhof W. Quantitative and objective evaluation of wound debriding properties of collagenase and fibrinolysin/deoxyribonuclease in a necrotic ulcer animal model. *Arch Dermatol Res.* 1998;290:152

14. Hobson D, et al Development and use of a quantitative method to evaluate the action of enzymatic wound debriding agents in vitro. *Wounds.* 1998:10(4):105.

15. Steed DL, Donohoe D, Webster MW, Lindsley L. Diabetic Ulcer Study Group. Effect of extensive debridement and treatment on the healing of diabetic foot ulcers. *J Am Coll Surg.* 1996;183:61–64.

16. Sussman C, Fowler E, Wethe J. *Sharp Debridement of Wounds* (video series). Torrance, CA: Sussman Physical Therapy, Inc.; 1995.

17. Mulder GD, Romanko KP, Sealey J, Andrews K. Controlled randomized study of a hypertonic gel for the debridement of dry eschar in chronic wounds. *Wounds.* 1993;5(3):112–115.

18. Flanagan M. The efficacy of a hydrogel in the treatment of wounds with non-viable tissue. *J Wound Care.* 1995;4(6):264–267.

19. Bale S, Banks V, Haglestein S, Harding KG. A comparison of two amorphous hydrogels in the debridement of pressure sores. *J Wound Care.* 1998;7(2):65–68.

20. Colin D, Kurring PA, Quinlan D, Yvon C. Managing sloughy pressure ulcers. *J Wound Care.* 1996;5(10):444–446.

SUGGESTED READING

Black J, Black S. Surgical management of pressure ulcers. *Nurs Clin North Am.* 1987;22:429–438.

Bryant RA, ed. *Acute and Chronic Wounds: Nursing Management Second Edition.* St. Louis, MO: Mosby; 2000.

Davis JT. Enhancing wound-debridement skills through simulated practice. *Phys Ther.* 1986;66:1723–1724.

Fowler E. Instrument/sharp debridement of non-viable tissue in wounds. *Ostomy/Wound Manage.* 1992;38:26–33.

Gordon, B. Conservative sharp wound debridement. *J Wound Ostomy Continence Nurs.* 1996;23(3):137.

Haury B, Rodeheaver G. Debridement: An essential component of traumatic wound care. *Am J Surg.* 1978;135:238–242.

Krasner D, Kane D, eds. *Chronic Wound Care.* 2nd ed. Wayne, PA: Health Management Publications; 1997.

Knight DB, Scott H. Contracture and pressure necrosis. *Ostomy/Wound Manage.* 1990;26(1):60–67.

Mulder GD, Jeter KF, Fairchild PA. *Clinicians' Pocket Guide to Chronic Wound Repair.* Spartanburg, SC: Wound Healing Publications; 1992.

National Pressure Ulcer Advisory Panel. Pressure ulcers: Incidence, economics, risk assessment. In: *Consensus Development Conference Statement.* West Dundee, IL: S-N Publications; 1989:3–4.

Bergstrom N, Allman RM, Carlson CE, et al. Panel for the Prediction and Prevention of Pressure Ulcers in Adults. *Pressure Ulcers in Adult.* Prediction and Prevention Clinical Practice Guideline No. 3. AHCPR (www.AHRQ.gov) Publication No. 92-0047. Rockville, MD: DHHS, PHS, AHCPR; May 1992.

Rodeheaver G, Baharestani M, Brabec ME, et al. Wound healing and wound management: Focus on debridement. *Adv Wound Care.* 1994;7:22–38.

Thomaselli N. WOCN Position statement: Conservative sharp wound debridement for registered nurses. *J Wound Ostomy Continence Nurs.* 1995;22(1):32A.

Wound, Ostomy, Continence Nursing Society Standards Committee. *Standards of Care. Dermal Wounds: Pressure Sores.* Irvine, CA: Wound, Ostomy, and Continence Nursing Society; 1992.

Appendix 8–A Debridement Choices for Chronic Wounds

Wound Type	Tissue Type	Consistency	Adherence	Amount of Debris	Debridement Choices	Rationale and Notes
Pressure sores	Black/brown eschar	Hard	Firmly adherent, attached to all edges and base of wound	75–100% Wound covered	1. *Autolytic*—best choice is transparent film dressing. May use hydrocolloid or hydrogel; score eschar with scalpel for more rapid results. 2. *Enzymatic ointment with secondary dressing*—must score eschar with scalpel.	1. Transparent film dressings trap fluid at the wound surface with no absorptive capabilities, providing for more rapid hydration of the eschar and facilitating autolysis. Hydrocolloid/hydrogel dressings have an absorptive capacity and may require more time for autolysis. 2. Enzymatic ointments effective against collagen and protein may be most effective.
	Black/brown eschar or Yellow/tan slough	Soft, soggy Soft, stringy	Adherent, attached to wound base, may or may not be attached to wound edges	50–100% Wound covered	1. *Autolytic*—best choices are hydrocolloids and hydrogels; composite dressings may also be beneficial. 2. *Enzymatic ointment with secondary dressing.* 3. *Sharp, sequential, or one time*—may be used alone or in conjunction with any of the above methods.	1. Hydrocolloids and hydrogels provide for absorption of mild to moderate amounts of exudate while maintaining a moist wound environment to facilitate autolysis. 2. Enzymatic ointments effective against collagen and protein may be most effective. May need to protect intact skin from enzyme and excess exudate.
	Yellow/tan slough	Soft, stringy	Adherent, attached to wound base; may or may not be attached to wound edges or loosely adherent to wound base	Less than 50% wound covered	1. *Autolytic*—best choices are hydrocolloids and hydrogels. 2. *Enzymatic ointment with secondary dressing.* 3. *Sharp, sequential, or one time*—may be used alone or in conjunction with any of the above methods.	1. Hydrocolloids and hydrogels provide for absorption of mild to moderate amounts of exudate while maintaining a moist wound environment to facilitate autolysis.

Wound Type	Tissue Type	Consistency	Adherence	Amount of Debris	Debridement Choices	Rationale and Notes
Pressure sores (cont.)						2. Enzymatic ointments effective against collagen and protein may be most effective. May need to protect intact skin from enzyme and excess exudate.
	Yellow slough	Mucinous	Loosely adherent to wound base, clumps scattered throughout wound	50–100% Wound covered	1. *Autolytic*—best choices are hydrocolloids and hydrogels. 2. *Enzymatic ointment with secondary dressing.*	1. Hydrocolloids and hydrogels provide for absorption of mild to moderate amounts of exudate while maintaining a moist wound environment to facilitate autolysis. 2. Enzymatic ointments effective against collagen and protein may be most effective. May need to protect intact skin from enzyme and excess exudate. Should be discontinued when wound is predominantly clean.
Venous disease ulcers	Black/brown eschar	Hard	Firmly adherent, attached to all edges and base of wound	50–100% Wound covered	1. *Autolytic*—best choices are hydrocolloids and hydrogels. 2. *Enzymatic ointment with secondary dressing.*	1. Hydrocolloids and hydrogel dressings have absorptive capacity, which helps to prevent maceration of surrounding tissues and promotes autolysis. 2. Enzymatic ointments effective against fibrin may be most effective.

continues

Wound Type	Tissue Type	Consistency	Adherence	Amount of Debris	Debridement Choices	Rationale and Notes
Venous disease ulcers (cont.)	Yellow slough	Soft, soggy, or fibrinous	Firmly adherent, attached to all edges and base of wound	50–100% Wound covered	1. *Autolytic*—best choice are hydrocolloids and hydrogels. 2. *Enzymatic ointment with secondary dressing.* 3. *Sharp, sequential, or one time*—may be used alone or in conjunction with any of the above methods.	1. Hydrocolloids and hydrogel dressings have absorptive capacity, which helps to prevent maceration of surrounding tissues and promotes autolysis. 2. Enzymatic ointments effective against fibrin may be most effective. May need to protect intact skin from enzyme and excess exudate. Should be discontinued when wound is predominantly clean.
	Yellow slough	Fibrinous *or* Mucinous	Loosely adherent Clumps scattered throughout wound	Any amount of wound covered	1. *Autolytic*—best choices are hydrocolloids and hydrogels. 2. *Enzymatic ointment with secondary dressing.*	1. Hydrocolloids and hydrogel dressings have absorptive capacity, which helps to prevent maceration of surrounding tissues and promotes autolysis. 2. Enzymatic ointments effective against fibrin may be most effective. May need to protect intact skin from enzyme and excess exudate. Should be discontinued when wound is predominantly clean.

Wound Type	Tissue Type	Consistency	Adherence	Amount of Debris	Debridement Choices	Rationale and Notes
Arterial ischemic ulcers	Black/brown eschar	Hard	Firmly adherent, attached to all edges and base of wound	50–100% Wound covered	1. Autolytic—best choices are hydrogels. 2. Enzymatic ointment with secondary dressing.	Must be certain of circulatory status prior to initiating debridement. 1. Hydrogel dressings have absorptive capacity, which helps to prevent maceration of surrounding tissues and promotes autolysis. The amorphous hydrogels are nonadherent and require a secondary dressing. 2. Enzymatic ointments: may need to protect intact skin from enzyme and excess exudate. Should be discontinued when wound is predominantly clean.
		Soft, soggy	Adherent, attached to wound base; may or may not be attached to wound edges	50–100% Wound covered	1. Autolytic—best choices are hydrogels. 2. Enzymatic ointment with secondary dressing. 3. Sharp, sequential, or one time.	1. Hydrogel dressings have absorptive capacity, which helps to prevent maceration of surrounding tissues and promotes autolysis. The amorphous hydrogels are nonadherent and require a secondary dressing. 2. Enzymatic ointments effective against protein and collagen may be most effective. May need to protect intact skin from enzyme and excess exudate. Should be discontinued when wound is predominantly clean.

continues

Wound Type	Tissue Type	Consistency	Adherence	Amount of Debris	Debridement Choices	Rationale and Notes
Neurotrophic/ diabetic ulcers	White/gray	Hard	Hyperkeratosis, callus formation at wound edges	Involves all/partial wound edges	1. *Sharp, sequential, or one time*—saucerization or callus removal. 2. *Autolytic*—best choices are hydrocolloids and hydrogels.	1. Saucerization may be required at each dressing change. 2. Hydrocolloids and hydrogels soften the callus formation, and this may facilitate removal as the dressing is removed.

CHAPTER 9

Management of Exudate and Infection

Barbara M. Bates-Jensen

CHAPTER OBJECTIVES

At the completion of this chapter, the reader will be able to:

1. Describe the difference between wound colonization and wound infection.
2. Explain the effects of antimicrobial cleansing solutions on the wound environment.
3. Describe wound cleansing procedures.
4. Discuss issues related to obtaining wound cultures.
5. Describe methods of managing exudate.

Wound exudate (also known as *wound fluid* and *wound drainage*) is an important wound assessment feature because the characteristics of the exudate help the clinician to diagnose wound infection, evaluate effectiveness of topical therapy, and monitor wound healing. Wound infection retards wound healing and must be treated. Proper assessment of wound exudate is also important because it affirms the body's brief, normal, inflammatory response to tissue injury. Thus, accurate assessment of wound exudate and diagnosis of infection are critical components of effective wound management.

SIGNIFICANCE OF EXUDATE

The healthy wound normally has some evidence of moisture on its surface. Healthy wound fluid contains enzymes and growth factors, which may play a role in promoting reepithelialization of the wound and provide needed growth factors for all phases of wound repair.[1] The moist environment produced by wound exudate allows efficient migration of epidermal cells and prevents wound desiccation and further injury.[2,3]

In acute wounds healing by primary intention, exudate on the incision line is normal during the first 48–72 hours. After that time, the presence of exudate is a sign of impaired healing. Infection and seroma are the two most likely causes. In chronic wounds, increased exudate is a response to the inflammatory process or infection. Increased capillary permeability causes leakage of fluids and substrates into the injured tissue. When a wound is present, the tissue fluid leaks out of the open tissue. This fluid is serous or serosanguineous.

Evaluation of the wound type, the number and type of organisms present, and the condition of the patient are important in determining risk for infection. Evaluation of wound type includes assessment of acute versus chronic wounds and necrotic versus clean, nonhealing wounds. The number and type of organisms present in the wound are evaluated for burden on the wound, possible bacteria-produced toxins, and pathology of the organisms. Patient condition relates to immune function and local host defenses.

In the infected wound, the exudate may thicken, become purulent, and continue to be present in moderate to large amounts. An example of exudate character changes in infected wounds is the presence of *Pseudomonas* organisms, which produce a thick, malodorous, sweet-smelling, green drainage,[4] or *Proteus* infection, which may produce an ammonia odor. Wounds with foul-smelling drainage are generally infected or filled with necrotic debris, and healing time is prolonged as tissue destruction progresses.[5] Wounds with significant amounts of necrotic debris will often have a thick, tenacious, opaque, purulent, malodorous drainage in moderate to copious amounts. True wound exudate should be differentiated from necrotic tissue sloughing off of the wound, secondary to debridement efforts. Exudate from sloughing necrotic tissue is commonly attached to or connected with the necrotic debris. However, frequently, the only method of differentiation is adequate debridement of necrotic tissue from the wound. Necrotic tissue becomes more soluble most often as a result of enzymatic or autolytic debridement. Often, the removal of the necrotic tissue dramatically reduces the amount and changes the character of the exudate.

Wounds can become edematous when excessive amounts of plasma proteins leak from damaged capillaries and pervade the wound environment. The fluid of wound edema contains proteolytic enzymes, bacteria and bacterial toxins, prostaglandins, and necrotic debris, all of which contribute to prolonged chronic inflammation. Exudate also drains valuable and needed substrates, such as growth factors, from the wound bed and impairs the healing process. Excess exudate losses drain substrates and energy that could be used for wound healing processes.[4]

The character and amount of exudate change as pressure ulcers heal and has been found by some to be predictive of healing.[6,7] Xakellis and Chrischilles[6] examined 39 patients with pressure ulcers in a clinical trial and found that, when exudate was present at baseline, wounds healed more slowly, regardless of treatment.[5] The healing rate of wounds was reduced by two thirds when exudate was present at baseline. In contrast, others have not found exudate amount at baseline to be a significant predictor of healing.[8,9] However, most acknowledge the negative effects of large amounts of exudate on healing outcomes.

Assessment of Wound Exudate

Characteristics of exudate are color, consistency, adherence, distribution in the wound, presence of odor, and the amount present.[10] The color and consistency of wound exudate may vary, depending on the type of wound, degree of moisture in the wound, the wound recovery cycle, and the presence of organisms in the wound. Table 9–1 presents various types of wound exudate and associated characteristics. *Color Plates 42–47* (reading the dressing and wound exudate characteristics) will help the clinician to identify exudate types and make an appropriate assessment of significance.

Estimating the amount of exudate in the wound is difficult because of wound size variability and topical dressing types. Certain dressing types interact with or trap wound fluid to create or mimic certain characteristics of exudate, such as color and consistency of purulent drainage. For example, both hydrocolloid and alginate dressings mimic a purulent drainage upon removal of the dressing. Preparation of the wound site for appropriate exudate assessment involves removal of the wound dressing and cleansing to remove dressing debris in the wound bed. Then evaluate the wound for true exudate. Cooper[10] suggests estimating the percentage of exudate in the wound by clinical observation. This approach

works if the wound exudate is thick and can be observed in the wound bed. When wound exudate character is more serous in nature, clinical observation of the wound alone is insufficient to quantify the amount of drainage. For thinner wound exudate, the amount of drainage is estimated by noting the number of dressings saturated during a period of time. Although not part of exudate assessment, evaluation of the wound dressing provides the clinician with valuable data about the effectiveness of treatment. Evaluation of the percentage of the wound dressing involved with wound drainage during a specific time frame is helpful for clinical management that includes dressings beyond traditional gauze. In estimating the percentage of the dressing involved with the wound exudate, clinical judgment is quantified, because the clinician must put a number to visual assessment of the dressing. For example, the clinician might determine that 50% of the hydrocolloid dressing was involved with wound drainage over a 4-day wearing period. Based on the above data, the clinician might quantify judgment for this type of dressing, length of dressing wear time, and wound etiology as a "minimal" amount of exudate. Clinical judgment of amount of wound drainage requires some experience with expected wound exudate output in relation to phase of wound healing and type of wound, and knowledge of absorptive capacity and normal wear time of topical dressings. One problem with assessment of exudate amount is the size of the wound. What might be considered a large amount of drainage for the smaller wound may be considered a small amount for the larger wound, making clinically meaningful assessment of exudate more difficult to obtain.

Appropriate wound exudate assessment requires consideration of wound etiology. Independent of exudate differences related to etiology of the wound, certain characteristics of exudate indicate wound degeneration and infection. If signs of cellulitis (erythema or skin discoloration, edema, pain, induration, and purulent drainage) are present at the wound site, the exudate amount may be copious and seropurulent or purulent in character. The amount of exudate remains high or increases in amount, and character may change to frank purulence with further wound degeneration. Wound infection must be considered in these cases, regardless of etiology.

Arterial/Ischemic Wounds

Exudate in the ischemic wound may vary in amount and character. Arterial/ischemic wounds are often dry or have only a scant to small amount of serous exudate present.

Neuropathic Wounds

Neuropathic wounds may present with very little exudate present. One possible reason for decreased exudate is a limited inflammation response, due to concomitant vascular disease and immune status changes from diabetes. Generally,

Table 9–1 Wound Exudate Characteristics

Exudate Type	Color	Consistency	Significance
Sanguineous/bloody	Red	Thin, watery	Indicates new blood vessel growth or disruption of blood vessels
Serosanguineous	Light red to pink	Thin, watery	Normal during inflammatory and proliferative phases of healing
Serous	Clear, light color	Thin, watery	Normal during inflammatory and proliferative phases of healing
Seropurulent	Cloudy, yellow to tan	Thin, watery	May be first signal of impending wound infection
Purulent/pus	Yellow, tan, or green	Thick, opaque	Signals wound infection; may be associated with odor

the exudate is minimal and usually serous or serosanguineous in character.

Venous Disease Wounds

Venous disease wounds usually are highly exudative, both on initial presentation and throughout the course of healing. As the venous ulcer heals, edema is lessened, and the wound exudate increases. The excess fluid takes the path of least resistance, which in this case is the wound bed! Often, venous wounds will appear with yellow fibrinous material covering the wound, which must be differentiated from true exudate.

Pressure Sores

Pressure sores present with a variety of wound exudate characteristics and amounts. In partial-thickness pressure sores, the wound exudate is most likely to be serous or serosanguineous in nature and presents in minimal to moderate amounts. In clean full-thickness pressure sores, the wound exudate is similar, with minimal to moderate amounts of serous to serosanguineous exudate. As healing progresses in the clean, full-thickness pressure sore, the character of the exudate changes and may become bloody if the fragile capillary bed is disrupted and lessens in amount. For full-thickness pressure ulcers with necrotic debris, wound exudate is dependent on the presence or absence of infection and the type of therapy instituted. Exudate may appear moderate to large but, in fact, be related to the amount of necrotic tissue present and the liquefaction of the debris in the wound. Typically, the necrotic full-thickness pressure ulcer presents with serous to seropurulent wound exudate in moderate to large amounts (Figures 9–1A and 9–1B). With appropriate treatment, the wound exudate amount may also temporarily increase, although the character gradually assumes a serous nature.

SIGNIFICANCE OF INFECTION

Although bacteria colonize all chronic wounds, wound colonization by bacteria is not the same as infection. When host and wound conditions are favorable, infection can occur. Wound infection extends inflammatory response, delays collagen synthesis, retards epithelialization, and causes more injury to the tissues as the bacteria compete with fibroblasts and other cells for limited amounts of oxygen.[11]

Large acute wounds generally react to bacterial burden in a way different from that in small chronic ulcerative wounds. Acute wounds are more susceptible to bacterial invasion by skin flora, in particular, those with prolonged inflammatory responses.[8] Wounds with loss of large amounts of surface area (15% of body surface area or greater) are also at a higher risk for bacterial invasion. Sufficient numbers of skin flora organisms will cause acute wounds such as grafts and flaps to fail and, if untreated, lead to sepsis, whereas a chronic leg ulcer may remain unchanged for months or years, showing no signs of infection or sepsis, with the same or larger number of organisms present.[12] The same organisms that pose serious threat of infection and sepsis in some acute wounds present entirely different pictures in the small chronic wound, which may go on to heal, despite the presence of these organisms. Chronic wounds are often contaminated with skin flora, such as *Enterococcus*, *Staphylococcus*, *Bacillus*, or, occasionally, gram-negative organisms.[12]

Distinguishing between contamination and infection in wounds is often difficult. The process of differentiating between a contaminated wound and an infected wound is important to understand treatment choices better. Colonization is the process of a group of organisms living together, whereas infection is the invasion of tissues by microorganisms, resulting in a systemic reaction. Most clinicians will

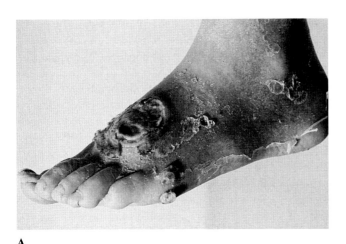

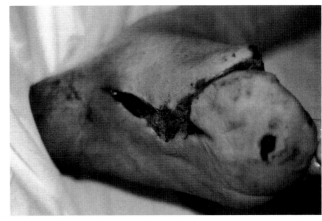

A   **B**

Figure 9–1A and B Obvious signs of infection.

agree that 10^4 to 10^5 organisms per gram of tissue indicate wound infection. Some laboratories use different references, so what may be considered colonization in one facility may be considered infection in another facility. In general, the overall condition of the patient also enters into the diagnosis process. Infection is signaled by a systemic reaction to the microorganisms, and contamination signals the presence of microorganisms in the wound.

High levels of bacteria are found in chronic wounds with necrotic debris. The number and density of aerobes and anaerobes are greater in necrotic wounds and those with undermining.[5] The presence of a foul odor is usually associated with anaerobic organisms. Sharp debridement of necrotic tissue virtually eliminates the anaerobic organisms (such as *Bacteroides*, *Streptococcus*, *Enterobacter*, and *Escherichia coli*) and decreases the aerobic organisms (such as *Staphylococcus aureus*) present in the wound.[5]

Methicillin-Resistant *Staphylococcus aureus*

Methicillin-resistant *S. aureus* (MRSA) presents special concerns for patients with wounds. *Staphylococcus aureus* is part of normal skin flora and is on the skin of approximately 20–50% of healthy adults and can persist in wounds.[13] Patients at highest risk for developing MRSA colonization and infection are those with a history of injection drug abuse, the presence of chronic disease, previous antimicrobial therapy, previous hospitalization, admission to an intensive care unit, or a prolonged stay in a health care institution.[14] All forms of *S. aureus*, including MRSA, can quickly invade and infect breaks in skin integrity, making wounds one of the most common sites of *S. aureus* infection and a site commonly colonized with *S. aureus* or MRSA.

In the early 1940s, penicillin was found to be effective against *S. aureus*; however, soon after its initial use, some

strains of *S. aureus* began to produce the enzyme penicillinase, which inactivates antimicrobials such as ampicillin, other penicillins, and cephalosporins. Methicillin was the first penicillinase-resistant semisynthetic penicillin and was (and is) used to treat *S. aureus* infections. The late 1960s and early 1970s saw the emergence of MRSA with the first reports of outbreaks in both acute and long-term care facilities.[13] Infections caused by MRSA raise concerns because resistance to methicillin is associated with resistance to other antimicrobials. A gene on the bacterial chromosome that codes for abnormal penicillin-binding protein (PBP) carries resistance to methicillin.[13] This abnormal PBP has a lower affinity for all penicillin, so very little methicillin binds to it. Therefore, all penicillins, which must bind to the PBP site in order to kill the bacteria, are ineffective. Some strains of MRSA mutate and become resistant to additional antimicrobials.

Of special concern is the recent finding of the potential for MRSA to acquire the gene-conferring vancomycin hydrochloride (Vancocin HCl) resistance from vancomycin-resistant enterococci (VRE), leading to vancomycin-resistant *S. aureus*.[13] Because vancomycin is the drug of choice for treating MRSA, resistance to vancomycin would present critical problems. Treatment of an MRSA wound infection involves antimicrobial therapy and prevention of cross-contamination. Topical antimicrobial therapy specific for MRSA-infected or -colonized wounds must be used cautiously for routine wound infections so that the antimicrobial will be available if the patient develops MRSA. Mupirocin (Bactroban) is specific for MRSA and can be used topically for wounds infected with the organism. Prevention of cross-contamination between patients requires significant education of caregivers—at all levels—and patients in use of universal standard precautions and good hand-washing procedures. Care must be taken to prevent not only contamination of multiple patients with the organisms, but also multiple body systems within the same patient. An alternative method to control MRSA is use of ultraviolet light (see Chapter 23).

Wound Contamination versus Infection

Clean wounds are contaminated with bacteria but usually progress through wound healing uneventfully. The clinician should suspect bacterial overburden if healing does not occur in clean wounds with appropriate topical therapy. Failure of the wound to progress may indicate a "silent" infection with colony counts above 100,000 organisms/mL but minimal outward signs of wound infection and superficial invasion of tissues.

Clinical Wisdom: *Bacterial Overburden*

The clinician should suspect high bioburden of bacteria in the clean wound if healing or improvement does not occur within a 2-week time frame and the patient is receiving appropriate topical therapy for the wound.

Wounds with continuing moderate to large amounts of seropurulent or purulent exudate and signs and symptoms of infection should be evaluated for infection. Local signs of wound infection include erythema or skin discoloration, edema, warmth, induration, increased pain, and purulent drainage, with or without a foul odor. Systemic signs of infection include elevated temperature and white blood cell count, and confusion in the older adult. Table 9–2 gives local and systemic characteristics of wound infection.

Assessment of Wound Infection

Assessment of wound infection involves assessment of the patient's overall condition, observation of the wound and surrounding tissues to differentiate wound inflammation versus the infected wound, and wound cultures to determine colony count. Clinical signs of inflammation are often mistaken for infection. Table 9–3 presents clinical manifestations of both inflammation and infection for comparison. Immunocompromised patients may fail to demonstrate any signs of infection or the signs may be significantly diminished. For example, in older adults, confusion or agitation may be the first indicator of infection, and elevated temperature occurs much later in the course of the illness. In some cases, the wound simply fails to progress without other obvious signs of infection. In the immunocompromised patient, identification of the organism may be critical to treatment, in that the responsible organism may be opportunistic in nature and not the typical culprit in wound infections.[15] Immunocompromised patients may also exhibit signs of infection when the bacterial burden is less than that required for producing infection in immunocompetent patients.

Clinical Wisdom: *Cellulitis and Wound Infection*

Advancing cellulitis indicates that the offending organism has invaded tissue surrounding the ulcer and is no longer localized. Advancing cellulitis begins as a small red or discolored area that is indurated, edematous, and warm to touch, and progresses to involve more extensive tissues. Left uncontrolled and untreated, cellulitis can result in sepsis.

The common method of confirming clinical infection is by colony count. The clinician diagnoses the infection based on clinical signs and symptoms and obtains a culture to aid in determining the appropriate antibiotic therapy. For example, in outpatient clinics, the usual sequence involves the clinician diagnosing the wound infection, based on signs and symptoms present, and obtaining a culture to confirm the correct selection of antibiotics for treatment. For inpatients diagnosed with infection, antibiotic therapy is generally initiated immediately, and the culture reports are used to adjust or modify the antibiotic regimen. Colony counts higher than 100,000 (10^5) are considered indicative of infection. A heavy bioburden (bacterial contamination in the wound) or compromised host resistance (for example, immunocompromised or diabetic patients) can both result in bacterial colony counts higher than 100,000 (10^5) organisms/mL, which is considered confirmation of clinical infection. Chronic wounds do not have to be sterile in order to heal. However, when the bacterial burden in the wound is over 10^5 organisms/g tissue, wound healing is impaired or delayed.[5,16] Wounds colonized with β-hemolytic streptococcus can exhibit impaired healing with colony counts less than 100,000/mL.[11] There are also wounds that heal uneventfully in the presence of bacterial colony counts of greater than 100,000/mL.

Table 9–2 Characteristics of Wound Infection

Local Signs of Infection	Systemic Signs of Infection
Erythema or skin discoloration	Elevated temperature
Edema	Elevated white blood cell count
Warmth	Confusion or agitation in older adults
Induration	Red streaks from wound
Increased pain	
Purulent wound exudate with or without foul odor	

Table 9–3 Comparison of Wound Characteristics in Inflamed and Infected Wounds

Wound Characteristic	Inflamed Wounds	Infected Wounds
Erythema	Usually presents with well-defined borders. Not as intense in color. May be seen as skin discoloration in dark-skinned persons, such as a purple or gray hue to the skin, or a deepening of normal ethnic color.	Edges of erythema or skin discoloration may be diffuse and indistinct. May present as very intense erythema or discoloration with well-demarcated and distinct borders. Red stripes or streaking up or down from the area indicates infection.
Elevated temperature	Usually noted as increase in temperature at wound site and surrounding tissues.	Systemic fever (may not be present in older adult populations).
Exudate: odor	Any odor present may be due to necrotic tissue in the wound, solubization of necrotic tissue, and the type of wound therapy in use, not necessarily infection.	Specific odors are related to some bacterial organisms, such as the sweet smell of *Pseudomonas* or the ammonia odor associated with *Proteus*.
Exudate: amount	Usually minimal; if injury is recent, should see gradual decrease in exudate amount over 3–5 days.	Usually moderate to large amounts; if injury is recent, will not see decrease in exudate amount—amount remains high or increases.
Exudate: character	Bleeding and serosanguineous to serous.	Serous and seropurulent to purulent.
Pain	Variable.	Pain is persistent and continues for an unusual amount of time. Must take wound etiology and subjective nature of pain into account when assessment is performed.
Edema and induration	May be slight swelling, firmness at wound edge.	May indicate infection if edema and induration are localized and accompanied by warmth.

Source: Adapted from J. Feedar, Wound Evaluation and Treatment Planning, *Topics in Geriatric Rehabilitation*, Vol. 9, No. 4, pp. 35–42, © 1994, Aspen Publishers, Inc.

It is clear that the determination of infection involves critical evaluation of the wound, the patient, and the pathogen. Evaluation of the pathogen occurs by colony count and provides the documentation of infection. Documentation of infection is based on the amount of the bacteria present in the wound tissue.

The level of bacteria in the wound tissue is determined to document the presence of a wound infection. As traditionally performed, swab cultures detect only surface contaminants and may not reflect the organism causing the tissue infection.[17] Quantitative wound culture is recommended for determination of infection. According to Stotts,[18] if a standardized technique is used, a quantitative swab technique can accurately document the bacterial burden in wounds. The technique for obtaining the culture specimen should mirror bacteria in the wound tissue, not simply bacteria on the wound surface.

Quantitative Wound Culture

Tissue biopsy, needle aspiration, and the quantitative swab technique are the most frequently used methods of quantitative wound culture. Each has an important place in clinical practice.

Tissue Biopsy

Tissue biopsy is removal of a piece of tissue with a scalpel or by punch biopsy. Before performing a tissue biopsy for wound culture, the area is cleansed with sterile solution that does not contain antiseptic. The area may be treated with topical anesthetic or injected with local anesthetic. The biopsy is performed and pressure applied to the area to control bleeding. The biopsy tissue is promptly transported to the laboratory, where it is weighed, flamed to kill surface contaminants, ground and homogenized, and plated in various media in varying dilutions. Findings are expressed in number of organisms per gram of tissue.[19,20]

Needle Aspiration

Needle aspiration involves insertion of a needle into the tissue to aspirate fluid that contains organisms.[21] Intact skin next to the wound is disinfected with a substance such as povidone-iodine and allowed to dry. Using a 10-mL disposable syringe and a 22-gauge needle with 0.5 mL of air in the syringe, the needle is inserted through intact skin; suction is achieved by briskly withdrawing the plunger to the 10-mL mark. The needle is moved backward and forward at different angles for two to four explorations. The plunger is gently returned to the 0.5-mL mark, the needle is withdrawn and capped, and the specimen is transported to the laboratory. In the laboratory, the fluid aspirated is diluted in broth and plated. Data are expressed in colony-forming units (CFU) per volume of fluid. If tissue is extracted by this technique, the weighing and grinding described for tissue biopsy processing also need to be done and, in this case, the data generated are in number of organisms per gram of tissue.

> **Clinical Wisdom:** *Performing Tissue Biopsy and Needle Aspiration*
>
> Physical therapists are not allowed by physical therapy practice acts to perform tissue biopsy or needle aspiration procedures. Physical therapists must work collaboratively with nursing to obtain these samples as required.

Quantitative Swab Technique

The swab technique often has been criticized as a method that produces information about colonization of the ulcer surface, rather than that in the tissue. One of the problems with the routine swab technique for culturing a wound is that it has been performed in a variety of ways and, therefore, cannot be relied on to address the issue of bioburden in the tissues. There is controversy on how to obtain a swab culture. Some recommend culturing the exudate in the wound prior to wound cleansing.[22,23] Others recommend that, after cleansing of the wound is complete, the culture is obtained using a Z technique (side to side across the wound from one edge to the other).[24,25] Others suggest irrigation of the wound with sterile water or saline and pressing the swab against the wound margin or ulcer base to elicit fresh exudate.[26]

The recommended method of quantitative swab culture involves cleansing the wound with a solution that contains no antiseptic solution. The end of a sterile, cotton-tipped applicator stick is rotated in a 1-cm² area of the open wound for 5 seconds.[26] Pressure is applied to the swab to cause tissue

fluid to be absorbed in the cotton tip of the swab. The swab tip is inserted into a sterile tube containing transport medium and transported to the laboratory. The end of the applicator that is not sterile is not inserted into the tube for culture. Serial dilutions of the organisms are made on agar plates. A swab moistened with normal saline without preservative provides more precise data than does the use of a dry swab.[27] Results are expressed as organisms per swab, CFU per swab, or in a semiquantitative manner, such as scant, small, moderate, and large (1+ to 4+) bacterial growths.

Tissue biopsy, needle inspiration, and the quantitative swab technique are used to evaluate the bacteria present in wound tissue, rather than on the surface of the wound, in the exudate, or in necrotic tissue. They are used to examine tissue for aerobic and anaerobic organisms. They also can be used to obtain a specimen for Gram's stain, a method recognized as a rapid diagnostic technique of infection.[27,28] For a Gram's stain, the tissue fluid is placed on a slide, treated with various stains, and viewed under the microscope. In wounds where swabs yielded less than 10^5 organisms, the Gram's stain is considered to show no bacteria.

Data show that the tissue biopsy, needle aspiration, and quantitative swab techniques are comparable in terms of sensitivity, specificity, and accuracy.[18] The following describes how the procedures are performed.

Procedures for Quantitative Wound Culture

Equipment Needed:
- Gloves (clean and sterile)
- Sterile saline (nonbacteriostatic)
- Container to transport specimen
- Lab requisition
- Appropriate dressing materials

Culture Technique-Specific Equipment Needed:
- Punch biopsy/scalpel
- Wound culture swab
- Anaerobic medium, if required
- 10-mL syringe with 22-gauge needle
- Cork

Procedure Preparation—For All Methods

1. Wash hands (reduces transmission of microorganisms).
2. Don clean gloves (gown, if necessary). (Maintains universal precautions.)
3. Remove soiled dressings and discard in plastic bag. Then remove and discard gloves (prevents contamination and spread of microorganisms).

4. Clean wound and surrounding skin with normal saline (cleaning removes contaminated debris).

Procedure: Swab Method

1. Don sterile gloves and remove swab from culturette tube, taking care not to touch swab or inside of tube (maintains universal precautions and aseptic technique).
2. Swab wound area 1 cm^2 with sufficient pressure to obtain wound fluid (ensures collection of a good specimen).
3. Use separate swabs if taking more than one specimen. Swab only a 1-cm^2 area of wound with each swab. (This ensures good culture specimen and prevents cross-contamination. Care must be taken to swab the wound instead of the wound edges to prevent contamination by skin flora and contaminated debris.)
4. Carefully place swab into culturette tube without touching swab or the inside, outside, or top of container (prevents contamination and keeps those areas free of pathogens that could be spread to others who handle the tube).
5. Crush ampule of medium in culturette and close securely, making sure swab is surrounded by medium (keeps specimen from drying out and provides supporting medium).

Procedure: Anaerobic Swab Culture Method

1. If collecting a specimen for anaerobic culture, take care to keep anaerobic transport culture tube in an upright position to prevent carbon monoxide from escaping. Close container securely after swab is placed in tube (maintains anaerobic environment).

Procedure: Syringe Method

1. Disinfect intact skin with antiseptic and allow skin to dry for 1 minute. (Anaerobic specimens are obtained from deep inside wounds.)
2. Place 0.5 mL of air in 10-mL disposable syringe with 22-gauge needle and insert needle into intact skin adjacent to wound. Withdraw plunger to achieve suction and move the needle back and forth at different angles (prevents contamination at needle withdrawal site).
3. Return the plunger gently to the 0.5-mL mark; do not insert drainage into the tissues. (This ensures good specimen and prevents contamination from skin flora. Syringe method is used when large amounts of pus or drainage are present or for collecting tissue.)
4. Cork needle to send syringe/needle to laboratory as one unit-containing specimen. Do not recap or attempt to disconnect needle from syringe. (This maintains universal precautions and prevents injury from needle stick and spread of microorganisms.)

Procedure: Tissue Biopsy

1. Don sterile gloves. Obtain a biopsy specimen using a 3- to 4-mm dermal punch or a scalpel. (This allows for determination of tissue level of microorganism contamination. Biopsy is usually performed by a physician or advanced practitioner.)
2. Place specimen in sterile container (prevents spread of microorganisms).

Procedure: Final Steps—All Methods

1. Remove and discard gloves in plastic bag (reduces transmission of microorganisms).
2. Wash hands.
3. Don sterile gloves and apply sterile dressing to the wound. (Dressing absorbs drainage and immobilizes and protects the wound.)
4. Label specimen container(s) with patient name, room number, date, time, and exact source of specimen. (This ensures proper identification of specimen. Proper source of specimen is important for laboratory to rule out normal flora from location.)
5. Place container in clean plastic bag, and have specimen transported to laboratory as soon as possible. (Plastic bag prevents spread of microorganisms. Immediate transport prevents overgrowth of microorganisms that can occur if specimen is left at room temperature for an extended length of time.)
6. Dispose of soiled equipment into appropriate receptacle (maintains universal precautions).
7. Wash hands (reduces transmission of microorganisms).

MANAGEMENT OF EXUDATE AND INFECTION

Management of exudate and infection includes wound cleansing; use of topical antimicrobials, antiseptics, and antifungals; and management of exudate with topical dressings.

Wound Cleansing

Effective wound cleansing removes debris that supports bacterial growth and delays wound healing. Wound cleansing delivers cleansing solution to the wound by mechanical force, aids with separation of necrotic tissue from healthy wound tissues, and removes bacteria and dressing residue from the wound surface. The process of wound cleansing involves selecting a cleansing solution and a method of delivering the solution to the wound. Exhibit 9–1 presents the Agency for Health Care Research and Quality (AHRQ, formerly known as the Agency for Health Care Policy and Research [AHCPR]) recommended guidelines for pressure ulcer cleansing.[16] Cleansing of all wounds can be performed using these principles.

Exhibit 9–1 AHCPR Recommended Guidelines for Pressure Ulcer Cleansing

1. Cleanse wounds initially and at each dressing change.
2. Use minimal mechanical force when cleansing ulcer with gauze, cloth, or sponges.
3. Do not clean wounds with skin cleansers or antiseptic agents (povidone-iodine, sodium hypochlorite solution, hydrogen peroxide, and acetic acid).
4. Use normal saline for cleansing most ulcers.
5. Use enough irrigation pressure to enhance wound cleansing without causing trauma to the wound bed. Safe and effective ulcer irrigation pressures range from 4 to 15 psi.
6. Consider whirlpool treatment for cleansing ulcers that contain thick exudate, slough, or necrotic tissue. Discontinue whirlpool when ulcer is clean.

Source: Reprinted from N. Bergstrom, M.A. Bennett, C.E. Carlson, et al., *Treatment of Pressure Ulcers,* Clinical Practice Guideline No. 15, December 1994, U.S. Department of Health and Human Services, Public Health Service, Agency for Health Care Policy and Research, AHCPR Publication No. 95-0652.

The cleansing solution chosen must be effective and safe to the wound. Isotonic normal saline is preferred as a solution because it is physiologic, nontoxic, and inexpensive. Saline does not contain preservatives and must be discarded 24–48 hours after opening.[29] Commercial wound cleansers are available to assist in wound cleansing for wounds requiring more cleansing capacity to remove adherent debris from the wound surface. These wound cleansers contain surfactants that act to lower surface tension and to loosen matter from the wound surface.[29] Nonionic surfactant wound cleansers are recommended as safe to the healing wound.

Clinical Wisdom: *Normal Saline for Wound Cleansing*

Two useful strategies for obtaining normal saline for wound care in the home setting:

1. Saline can be made at home by adding two teaspoons of table salt to 1 L of boiling water. Be sure to discard after 24 hours.
2. Another useful strategy is to use pressurized saline commonly used for contact lens wearers. This preserved saline may be used for a longer duration, and the pressure from the canister is not sufficient to cause wound trauma.

For healthy clean wounds, cleanse with normal saline and do not use antimicrobial solutions or skin cleansers. Clean wounds do not need to be cleansed with antimicrobial solu-

tions because the goal of care is to clear low levels of contaminants from the wound. In fact, they are harmful. Solutions such as povidone-iodine, acetic acid, hydrogen peroxide, and sodium hypochlorite (Dakin's fluid) are toxic to fibroblasts. Use of antimicrobial agents is contraindicated in the healthy proliferative wound because of the damage to the healthy tissues.[17,30,31] Contraindication of the use of antiseptic and antimicrobial solutions for cleansing clean pressure ulcers is based on laboratory studies of the toxicity of topical wound cleansers.[32,33] In general, most skin cleansers are not appropriate wound cleansers because they have been developed for use externally, not internally, as is the case with a wound. What is appropriate for cleansing the skin is not appropriate for open wounds because an open wound lacks the protection of intact epidermis and provides direct access to internal body structures. For healthy clean wounds, cleanse with normal saline. For healthy wounds, do not use antimicrobial solutions or skin cleansers.

For infected wounds, cleanse with normal saline or use a 10- to 14-day cleansing regimen with an antimicrobial solution. For infected wounds, do not use skin cleansers, and do not prolong the use of an antimicrobial solution. Antimicrobial agents may play a minor role in wound cleansing for infected wounds, wounds with large amounts of necrotic debris, or those with large amounts of exudate. Use of antimicrobial agents is best handled in a manner similar to that for antibiotic use, ie, for a short duration. Antimicrobial agents used as cleansing agents in the debris-filled wound should be used for 10–14 days and rinsed thoroughly from the wound with saline. Rinsing the wound with saline after cleansing with antimicrobial solutions decreases the cytotoxic effects in the wound. The antimicrobial cleanser should be discontinued after the course of therapy (10–14 days) or when the wound is clean and debris free.

Cleansing Method

There are several methods for cleansing the wound, including soaking, whirlpool, scrubbing, and irrigation. Soaking is a form of hydrotherapy (it includes a variety of types, from a bucket to a Hubbard tank) and may be useful for removal of gross contaminants and loosening necrotic tissue. The softening that occurs with the soaking helps to ease the separation of necrotic debris from healthy wound tissues. Wound soaking is appropriate only for wounds with large amounts of necrotic debris. Once a wound is clean and proliferating, whirlpool and wound soaking impede wound healing and, thus, are generally not appropriate.[17,29] Use of the new, battery-powered, disposable pulsatile irrigating devices that irrigate with solutions and simultaneously use suction to remove the irrigation fluid and the loosened wound debris has been shown to be more effective than whirlpool therapy in a study examining the rate of granulation tissue formation. This study found that those ulcers cleansed with pulsatile lavage had a rate of granulation tissue formation of 12.2% per week, compared with 4.8% per week for the whirlpool-treated group.[34]

Whirlpool may be useful for more than simply soaking and cleansing, as is the case with using whirlpool to increase perfusion to an area. (See Chapters 25 and 26 for information on pulsatile lavage and whirlpool.) Antimicrobial agents should not be used in the whirlpool or wound-soaking solution because of wound tissue toxicity.

Scrubbing the wound involves use of gauze or sponges in direct wound contact with mechanical force to enhance removal of debris and efficacy of cleansing solution used.[29] Scrubbing causes microabrasions in the wound, thus delaying healing. Use of a nonionic surfactant cleansing solution will limit the damage inflicted with scrubbing to the healing wound tissues. Use of nonabrasive sponges will also help to decrease the damage to the healing tissues. The more porous the sponge, the less damage inflicted on the wound surface.[29] Even use of nonionic surfactant cleansing solutions and nonabrasive porous sponges will injure the fragile wound tissue. Thus, no scrubbing is recommended.

Clinical Wisdom: *Shallow Wound Cleansing Procedure*

Cleanse from the center of the wound in a circular motion, working toward the edge of the wound and the surrounding tissues. Do not return to the center of the wound after cleansing at the edge of the wound or the surrounding tissues, because this will recontaminate the clean wound center.

Wound irrigation can be performed using a variety of instruments and equipment. Wound irrigation is particularly appropriate for cleansing deep wounds with undermining or tunneling present. Use a catch basin and towels to absorb and accumulate waste materials and irrigant runoff. Repeat the irrigation procedure at each dressing change. Protect eyes, face, and clothing of the clinician by using universal precautions. Some newer irrigation devices include a splashguard to help protect the clinician.

The amount of pressure used for irrigation is determined by the desire not to harm the healing wound tissues and to cleanse the wound effectively. The pressure of delivering the irrigant is commonly described as low or high pressure. Pressure force is described in pounds per square inch (psi). Pressure force under 4 psi is commonly referred to as low pressure and can be obtained by use of bulb syringes or just pouring solution over the wound bed.[29] Pressure force between 4 and 15 psi is considered high pressure and can be achieved by using commercial devices, a 35-mL syringe attached to a 19-gauge needle or angiocatheter, pulsatile lavage, or whirlpool therapy.

Clinical Wisdom: *Deep Wound Cleansing Procedure*

Use of a catheter or a syringe to irrigate wounds with undermining and tunneling will not injure the tissues and can effectively cleanse the tissues involved in the wound under the skin surface. Flush with copious amounts of irrigant solution, then gently massage the tissues above the tunneling to express the exudate accumulated in the tunnel. Repeat two or three times until the solution and fluids returned are clear (see Figure 9–2). After the wound cleansing, the undermined spaces are usually packed loosely with packing materials, such as roller gauze or alginate rope products, to prevent infection from traveling up the tunnel (see Figure 9–3).

High-pressure irrigation using any of these forms is a method of debridement—loosening and softening necrotic tissue for easy separation from healthy tissue. Pressurized irrigation removes bacteria and debris more effectively than do gravity or bulb syringe irrigation. As such, high-pressure irrigation is most effective, with an inflammatory process. Use of high-pressure irrigation is not the method of choice for the healthy, proliferating wound, because this can damage fragile blood vessels and new tissue growth.

A number of available irrigation devices deliver solutions with too much pressure, thus driving bacteria and irrigant solution deeper into wound tissues. Pressures over 15 psi can cause trauma to the wound bed, forcing bacteria deeper into wound tissues. For example, use of a Water Pik at the middle and high settings provides 42 psi and more than 50 psi, respectively, both of which are too high and will drive bacteria

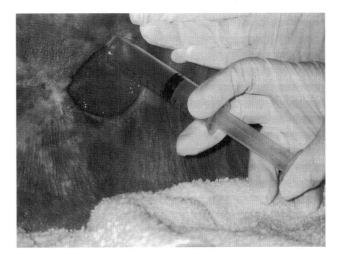

Figure 9–2 Irrigation of wound with syringe.

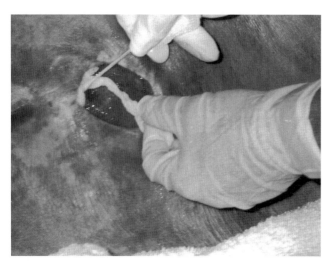

Figure 9–3 Packing wound with undermining.

farther into the wound tissues. Irrigation pressures between 4 and 15 psi are recommended.

The clinical outcomes from wound cleansing are determined by the purpose of the cleansing and the wound assessment. For predominantly clean wounds with new tissue growth, cleansing is used only to remove dressing residue, and if any additional cleansing is needed, a low-pressure irrigation system should be used (such as pouring the solution over the wound or using a bulb syringe or piston syringe to deliver the irrigant). The goals of therapy with low-pressure irrigation are to dislodge wound dressing residue, reduce wound surface contaminants, and protect fragile new tissue growth. For wounds with necrotic tissue or debris, a high-pressure irrigation system should be used. Whirlpool therapy and pulsatile lavage are not always available or appropriate for all patients, and other devices, such as the 35-mL syringe and 19-gauge needle or angiocatheter, may be the best choice. The goals of therapy are to loosen and soften the necrotic debris for easier separation from healthy tissues, to reduce the bacterial burden, to remove dressing remnants, and to prevent undue wound trauma.

Research Wisdom: *Wound Irrigation*

Use of a 35-mL syringe with a 19-gauge angiocatheter or needle attached delivers saline at 8 psi and provides more effective removal of bacteria and debris than does use of a bulb syringe.

Aseptic Technique

One of the continuing debates in wound management is what type of aseptic technique is necessary for wound care in various health care settings. Asepsis includes activities that prevent infection or break the chain of infection. It is generally divided into two types: surgical asepsis and medical asepsis. Surgical asepsis, or sterile technique, is the method used in surgery where all instruments and materials used are sterile and all health care providers involved wear sterile gloves, caps, masks, and gowns. Medical asepsis, or clean technique, involves procedures to reduce the number of pathogens and to decrease the transfer of pathogens. In surgical asepsis, the nurse prepares a sterile field, dons sterile gloves, and follows surgical aseptic techniques in caring for the wound. Sterile and clean techniques are compared in the following display.

There are various viewpoints on which approach is most suitable for wound care patients. Some general guidelines may help to clarify use of an aseptic technique. Sterile technique is most appropriate in acute care hospital settings, for patients at high risk for infection (advanced age, immunocompromised, diabetic) and for certain care procedures, such as sharp wound debridement. Clean technique is most appropriate for patients in long-term care settings, home care, and some clinic settings, and for patients not at high risk for infection and receiving routine wound care, such as dressing changes. Further research is needed to determine outcomes with use of clean technique. Table 9–4 compares general guidelines for clean versus sterile technique choices for wound care patients.

Hand Washing and Infection Control

What is clear about infection management and wound care is the importance of hand washing by the health care practitioner. Hand washing is the single most important means for preventing spread of infection. Use of universal standard precautions and hand washing by the wound care clinician promote health maintenance for patients and caregivers and, as such, are critically important to include when instructing others in wound care programs. Along with hand washing, caregivers must be instructed in appropriate disposal of infectious waste products, such as used wound dressings, gauze used for wound cleansing, and instruments used in wound care. In institutional settings, such as hospitals and long-term care facilities, there are procedures for disposal of contaminated materials in bags clearly identified as infectious waste (eg, double-bagging out of isolation rooms and use of red biohazard trash bags). In the home care arena, disposal of contaminated waste becomes more problematic, and the wound care clinician must address disposal based on the area served, local waste collection procedures, and agency protocols. In the home care setting, education of the caregiver regarding the procedures for waste disposal is essential for maintaining community health.

Sterile Technique	*Clean Technique*
Preparation of a sterile field	Preparation of clean field
Clean gloves	Clean gloves
Decontamination of the wound and surrounding skin	Cleansing of the wound and surrounding skin with an antimicrobial cleanser
Change gloves: Sterile gloves	Change gloves: Clean gloves
Use sterile forceps, scalpel, and scissors	Use sterile forceps, scalpel, and scissors
Allow only "sterile to sterile" contact of instruments and materials used for the procedure	Prevent direct contamination of materials and supplies, but no "sterile to sterile" rules apply
Apply sterile dressing	Apply clean dressing

Topical Antimicrobials*

The use of antimicrobials is confusing for clinicians. Systemic antimicrobial drugs (those agents given orally or intravenously) are often superior to topical agents (ointments, creams, or solutions put directly on the wound surface) because of the better penetration of systemic agents. However, topical antimicrobials are often effective in limiting surface colonization, so that tissue defenses can clean up without continual reinfection from superficial bacteria. Some superficial infections may respond better to topical agents and, in some cases, it is wise to use topical agents to avoid sensitizing the patient or creating resistant microorganisms. Some topical antimicrobials can damage healthy tissues, exacerbating tissue destruction or damaging tissue defenses. The

terms *antimicrobial, antibiotic, antibacterial,* and *antiseptic* are often used interchangeably; however, the definitions are slightly different, according to the Food and Drug Administration (FDA). Exhibit 9–2 presents definitions of these terms for easy reference.

The three main classes of antimicrobials used for wounds include antibacterials, antiseptics, and antifungals. Understanding how antimicrobials are prescribed is helpful for wound care clinicians. This is the process by which antimicrobials are ordered. The proper use of any antimicrobial requires determination of clinical infection in the wound, correct identification of the invading organism by culture and Gram's stain smears prior to beginning therapy, and consideration of pharmacology and toxicology when choosing the agent. If an agent must be chosen prior to receiving labora-

Table 9–4 Clean versus Sterile Technique General Guidelines

Factor	*Sterile Technique*	*Clean Technique*
Settings	Acute care hospitals Clinics in acute care facilities	Home care Long-term care facilities Community clinics Physicians' offices
Procedures	Invasive procedures Sharp debridement	Routine procedures Dressing changes
Patients	Immunocompromised Advanced age or very young age Diabetic	Patients NOT at high risk for infection

Exhibit 9–2 Definitions of Antimicrobial Terms

Term	Definition
Antimicrobial	An agent that inhibits or kills microorganisms
Antiseptic	A substance that prevents or arrests the *growth* by preventing multiplication (bacteriostatic) or *action* of microorganisms, either by inhibiting their activity or by destroying or killing them (bactericidal). Applies to substances used on living tissues (eg, povidone-iodine)
Antibiotic	An organic chemical substance produced by a microorganism that has the capacity in diluted solutions to destroy or inhibit the growth of bacteria and other microorganisms (eg, penicillin)
Antibacterial	An agent that destroys or stops bacterial growth (eg, bacitracin)
Antifungal	A wide variety of agents that inhibit or kill fungi (eg, nystatin)

Source: Adapted with permission from *Topical Agents for Open Wounds: Antibacterials, Antiseptics, Antifungals,* G. Gilman, ed., reviewed by G. Rodeheaver, J.W. Cooper, D.R. Nelson, and M. Meehan, © 1991, Hill-Rom International.

tory results, make the decision based on Gram's stain smears (either positive or negative), the most likely pathogens involved in the disease process (for example, *E. coli* for a fecally incontinent patient with a sacral pressure sore), and the efficacy of the agent in similar situations.

> **Clinical Wisdom:** *Factors Altering Response to Topical Antibacterials and Antiseptics*
>
> Patient response to antibacterial and antiseptic agents may be altered by age, disease processes (such as diabetes), malignancy, neurologic disorders, immune dysfunction, pregnancy, allergy, or concomitant drug therapy.

Multiple factors influence the transcutaneous penetration of antimicrobial agents, including physiochemical properties of the drug (polarity, stability, and solubility in base and lipids), nature of the pharmaceutical preparation (drug concentration, composition and properties of the base, and incompatible mixtures), method of application (inert delivery systems, time-released delivery systems, application in conjunction with occlusion, polar compounds to increase absorption, and substances that damage the stratum corneum to improve penetration), and nature of the skin (integrity of the epidermis, variability in skin thickness, and age). Problems associated with topical antimicrobial use in wound care are related to absorption of chemicals into the body tissues

*This information is adapted with permission from G. Gilson, ed. *Topical Agents for Open Wounds: Antibacterials, Antiseptics, Antifungals.* Reviewed by G. Rodeheaver, J.W. Cooper, D.R. Nelson, and M. Meehan. Charleston, SC: Hill-Rom International, Inc.; 1991.

through the wound bed. There are cases where absorption of certain chemicals contained in an antiseptic through the wound bed has caused systemic health problems. For example, iodine toxicity has occurred from use of povidone-iodine in open wounds.

Antibacterials

Antibacterial agents are chemicals that eliminate living organisms pathogenic to the host or patient. Some examples of antibacterials are bacitracin (Betadine, Cortisporin, Neosporin, Polysporin), gentamicin (Garamycin), metronidazole gel and cream (MetroGel, MetroCream, Noritate), mupirocin, and silver sulfadiazine (Silvadene, SSD). The use of antibacterials is common for most infections. In the elderly, the primary sites of infection, in order of frequency, are: urinary tract, pulmonary system, and wounds.[35,36] Broad-spectrum antibacterials are useful for mixed infections when there is more than one pathogen present and quick identification of the organism is difficult. Antibacterial topical administration occurs in smaller drug doses, compared with systemic antibacterials, due to direct contact with the affected area.[36] The same or better results may be achieved without the risk of toxicity. Systemic agents may be used in combination with topical agents, as in the treatment of impetigo. Topically administered drugs are in more direct contact with organisms so that problems of absorption, distribution, and availability to the infected site are reduced. Frequently, topical agents are used in conjunction with one another to give broader coverage, thereby increasing the rate of bactericidal action against a large spectrum of bacteria.[37]

Topical antibacterials may be used prophylactically. When used properly, they can be effective chemical barriers that may impede the entrance of pathogenic organisms and diminish the local or systemic morbidity associated with infected wounds. When using topical antibacterials prophylactically, there is always a danger of overgrowth of resistant organisms; therefore, use of antibacterials for prevention requires good clinical judgment for optimal effectiveness.[37]

Clinical Wisdom: *Wound Healing and Antimicrobials*

No antibacterial agent, whether bactericidal or bacteriostatic, will be curative when used in isolation. Attention to nutritional factors, management of underlying pathology, and relief of causative factors are also required.

Topical antibacterials used in a viscous vehicle provide a moist wound healing environment, facilitating epithelial migration.[38] The indications for topical antibacterials include significant bacterial infection diagnosed or suspected and an indication for prophylactic use, due to the patient's underlying disease and/or the patient's increased risk of infection resulting from surgical procedures, viral or metabolic diseases, chemotherapy or radiation therapy, and prolonged corticosteroid administration. Contraindications relate to the excessive use of antibacterials for minor infections and for nonbacterial pathogens.[37] Inappropriate use of antibacterials subjects the patient to risk of drug toxicity, risk of allergy, superinfection with resistant organisms, and unnecessary costs.[37,39]

Clinical Wisdom: *Routine Use of Topical Antibacterials*

Routine use of topical antibacterials is strongly discouraged because of the frequent development of resistant organisms. This is particularly true of mupirocin, because it is effective against MRSA and, if used inappropriately, will not be effective when most needed.

The base, or vehicle, is the form in which the antibacterial agent is available. In general, it is best to use a lotion or a paste for application to wet or weepy skin and wounds, and a greasy ointment for application to dry, cracked skin. Creams are convenient because, to some extent, they can be used for wet or dry surfaces and are easier to use. Many ointments contain lanolin or wood alcohols, and patients can readily develop contact sensitivity to these substances. Creams less often contain lanolin but usually contain a preservative or stabilizer, such as parabens or ethylenediamine dihydrochloride, both of which are known to be occasional sensitizers. Ointments may be confused with creams, particularly with the introduction of synthetic bases that claim to have the properties of both creams and ointments. Lotions are preferable to greasy applications for areas that rub against each other, eg, groin areas and in between the toes. Lotions are usually less occlusive than ointments. Appendix A contains an index of antibacterial agents. The index provides a listing of commonly used antibacterials and individual entries for each antibacterial. Individual antibacterials are presented with a description of the agent, the action, indications for use, precautions, directions, and packaging information.

Antiseptics

Antiseptics are a group of widely differing chemical compounds possessing bactericidal (kills bacteria) or bacteriostatic (prevents bacterial multiplication) properties. Some examples of antiseptics are povidone-iodine, acetic acid, hydrogen peroxide, and hypochlorites. They are employed in medical practice with the objective of preventing or combating bacterial infection of superficial tissues, as well as for sterilization of instruments and infected material. Chemically, antiseptics may be inorganic or organic. Oxidizing disinfectants liberate oxygen when in contact with pus or organic substances. Different bacteria are sensitive to different antiseptics. For example, acetic acid is commonly used against infections caused by *Pseudomonas aeruginosa*. Antiseptic agents are applied directly to tissue to destroy microorganisms or inhibit their reproduction or metabolic activity. By reducing organisms, it is believed that antiseptics may hasten wound healing and diminish local or systemic morbidity associated with wound infection.[40] However, many commonly used antiseptics are cytotoxic and actually inhibit wound healing; therefore, caution is recommended.[30] The major uses of antiseptics are as hand scrubs, cleansers, irrigants, and protective dressings. It is important to remember that the skin cannot be sterilized and that approximately 20% of the skin's normal resident flora are beyond the reach of antiseptics.[36] Excessive antiseptic use subjects the patient to risk of allergy, risk of drug toxicity, superinfection, and unnecessary costs, and pose significant public health concerns, due to ecologic pressure favoring selection of bacteria resistant to antiseptics.[40] Antiseptics, regardless of type, damage the healthy wound and impair wound healing.[31] Appendix A contains an index to antiseptics. The index provides a listing of commonly used antiseptics and individual entries for each antiseptic. Individual antiseptics are presented with a description of the agent, the action, indications for use, adverse reactions (with special attention to effects on wound healing), dosage, and packaging information.

Antifungals

Fungi comprise five widely differing classes of primitive flora. Thus, antifungal agents include a wide variety of chemical types of a rather narrow antifungal spectrum. Some examples of antifungals include nystatin (Mycostatin), keto-conazole (Nizoral), and miconazole nitrate (Monistat-Derm). Not all antifungal agents are fungicidal; many are only fungistatic, and certain of them may owe their efficiency to a keratolytic action.

Broad-spectrum antifungal agents, in general, are toxic irritants, as expected from their nonselectivity; however, many of these have limited absorption through the epidermis and so may be used in dermatologic preparations.[29] The indications for an antifungal are a significant fungal infection diagnosed or strongly suspected and an indication for prophylactic antifungal use, due to the patient's underlying disease, or the patient's increased risk of fungal infection, resulting from invasive procedures or environmental exposure (diarrhea, diaphoresis, poor hygiene, diabetes, etc). The major contraindication for antifungal use is known allergy to ingredients. Antifungals must be used for the prescribed time to eliminate the infection fully. Some areas are more difficult to treat, and some fungi are more difficult to eliminate because of the patient's underlying disease process. External factors may affect the antifungal agent's ability to penetrate the skin, including temperature, ambient water vapor pressure, and drying agents such as powders, which reduce the excess moisture in the skin folds and may aid in efficacy of antifungals. Nonsporing anaerobes are a significant pathogen in ulcers with a foul smell and exposure to fecal contamination.[36] Metronidazole topical gel (MetroGel) has been shown to be effective in eliminating or decreasing the odor associated with these wounds.[41–44] Appendix A contains an index of antifungal agents. The index provides a listing of commonly used antifungals and individual entries for each antifungal. Individual antifungals are presented with a description of the agent, the action, indications for use, precautions, available vehicle, dosage, and packaging information.

Research Wisdom: *Treatment of Malodorous Wounds*

Topical metronidazole has been shown to be effective in resolving odor in foul-smelling wounds. Use of a 1% solution or 0.75% gel applied twice daily reduced or eliminated odor in 80–\90% of wounds in 4–7 days. Odor was significantly decreased in 2 days.[41–44]

Topical Dressings for Management of Exudate

Effective management of exudate requires knowledge of absorptive capacity of dressing materials and attention to fragile wound margins. Excess exudate on the wound edges can lead to maceration and destruction of the critical wound edge. Use of petrolatum products or other hydrophobic ointments around the wound can provide some protection for the wound edges. Use of a topical dressing that adequately absorbs the wound fluid will also protect the wound edges.

Clinical Wisdom: *Caution about Petrolatum around Wound Edges*

If petrolatum products are being used and the patient is receiving physical therapy, nurses *must* notify the physical therapist. The therapist should be informed because petrolatum products interfere with physical therapy technologies and are hard to remove from the patient's skin prior to physical therapy interventions.

The choice of a dressing for a wound is, in many cases, dependent on the amount of drainage present in the wound and the expected drainage from the wound. For example, a wound that has been recently debrided of yellow necrotic tissue may have a history of moderate to large amounts of drainage; however, the amount of expected drainage postdebridement is less, usually minimal to moderate amounts. The topical dressing may also become not only the treatment but also the method of determining efficacy. For example, evaluation of the dressing upon removal from the wound allows the clinician to judge what percentage of the dressing material has interacted with wound drainage. Evaluation of the amount of dressing used by the wound exudate often determines whether treatment will continue with the same dressing or whether a new dressing will be applied. (See *Color Plates 42–47*, reading the dressing, for determining the effectiveness of topical dressings in management of wound exudate and how to distinguish exudate from the wound versus material from wound fluid and dressing interaction.) Table 9–5 presents the generic product categories with notes about the absorptive ability of each dressing type. This information may be useful in choosing dressings for the exudative wound. How to choose a wound dressing to manage exudate is explained in detail in Chapter 11, Management of the Wound Environment with Dressings and Topical Agents.

The type of wound under treatment also affects the choice of dressing for exudate management. An example is the venous disease ulcer under appropriate management with compression therapy and topical dressings. For the venous disease ulcer in the initial compression therapy stages, exudate amount will increase as edema in the extremities is being managed. Sometimes, exudate amount will remain copious for several weeks as the edema is brought under control. In general, the exudate amount can be expected to remain large for 2 weeks.

The presence of large amounts of exudate on the patient is significant. The skin surrounding the wound can become

Table 9–5 Topical Treatment—Wound Dressings

Wound Dressings: Generic Categories	Not Absorbent	Low to Minimal Absorption	Minimal to Moderate Absorption	Moderate to Large Absorption
Skin sealants	X			
Composite dressings		X	X	
Transparent film dressings	X			
Gauze—woven		X		
Gauze—nonwoven			X	
Gauze—impregnated	X			
Calcium alginates			X	X
Exudate absorbers—beads, pastes, powders, flakes			X	X
Hydrocolloids—regular, thin, pastes, granules		X	X	X (when used with other forms of dressings)
Hydrogels—sheets, wafers, amborphous		X	X	
Lubricating stimulating agents	X			
Foams		X	X	
Hydrocolloid-hydrogel combinations			X	X

macerated and, in some cases, a candidiasis or yeast infection may develop around the wound. The continual loss of proteins, fluids, and electrolytes in the wound exudate can cause fluid and electrolyte disturbances in severe cases; at a minimum, the loss of proteins and wound healing substrates can slow or impede the wound healing progress. Finally, the presence of a wound with large amounts of draining exudate takes a toll on the patient's daily quality of life, disrupting normal function.

OUTCOME MEASURES

Outcome measures are tools used to evaluate the results of therapy. Appropriate characteristics to assess in evaluating the results of exudate management are the amount of exudate in the wound, the type of exudate in the wound, and the involvement of the wound dressing with the exudate present in the wound. Measurement of exudate is an intermediate outcome measure; healing is the final outcome.

Amount of Exudate

The amount of exudate should diminish progressively in the wound if therapy is appropriate. The amount of exudate can be measured by using clinical judgment to evaluate the distribution of moisture in the wound and the interaction of exudate with the wound dressing. A rating scale similar to the following may be used to quantify amount of exudate:

1 = None = wound tissues dry
2 = Scant = wound tissues moist, no measurable exudate
3 = Small = wound tissues wet, moisture evenly distributed in wound, drainage involved ≤ 25% of wound dressing
4 = Moderate = wound tissues saturated, drainage may or may not be evenly distributed in wound, drainage involved > 25% to < 75% of wound dressing
5 = Large = wound tissues bathed in fluid, drainage freely expressed, may or may not be evenly distributed in wound, drainage involved > 75% of wound dressing

Type of Exudate

The type of exudate should change as the wound improves and heals. As the wound passes through the inflammatory phase of wound healing, serous drainage should become more serosanguineous, then sanguineous in nature. As infection or necrosis is resolved, the exudate type should also reflect improvement. Foul, purulent drainage should become merely purulent, then seropurulent, and finally serous and serosanguineous in character. Measurement of type of exudate is best accomplished by the use of a rating scale. A scale similar to the following may be helpful:

1 = Bloody = thin, bright red
2 = Serosanguineous = thin, watery, pale red to pink
3 = Serous = thin, watery, clear
4 = Purulent = thin or thick, opaque tan to yellow
5 = Foul purulent = thick, opaque yellow to green with offensive odor

REFERRAL CRITERIA

Determining whether a patient is a candidate for wound management requires adequate assessment of the patient, with attention to evaluation for possible referral. For example, the following patients would warrant referral to the physician and/or an advanced practice nurse for either a medical evaluation or immediate intervention or referral to another health care professional for consultation.

1. The person with a wound exudate that is copious, malodorous, and prolonged should be evaluated further for infection, cellulitis, abscess, or progressive degeneration. In this case, the advanced practice nurse may choose to manage the patient initially. If the condition worsens or the patient fails to improve over a 2-week time frame, the physician should be consulted.
2. Patients with an elevated temperature or those on a downhill course should be evaluated further. Intervene as in No. 1.
3. Patients with no wound improvement over several weeks should be evaluated further. In this case, the advanced practice nurse may want to consult other health care practitioners (physical therapists, dietitians, wound care nurses or enterostomal therapy (ET) nurses, and physicians).
4. Patients with evidence of cellulitis *or* gross purulence/ infection should be evaluated further. Intervene as in No. 1.
5. Patients with impending exposed bone or tendon present in the wound should be evaluated further. Intervene as in No. 3.
6. Patients with evidence of an abscessed area should be evaluated further. Intervene as in No. 3.
7. Patients with extensively undermined areas present in the wound should be evaluated further. Intervene as in No. 3.

SELF-CARE TEACHING GUIDELINES

Patient and caregiver instruction in self-care must be individualized to the topical therapy care routine, the individual patient's wound, the individual patient's and caregiver's learning style and coping mechanisms, and the ability of the patient/caregiver to perform procedures. The general self-care teaching guidelines in Exhibit 9–3 provide a model of information to teach and should be individualized for each patient and caregiver.

REVIEW QUESTIONS

1. Which of the following statements best describes wound colonization?
   a. Colonization can be confirmed by culture reports demonstrating 10^5 organisms/g of tissue.
   b. Colonization inhibits wound healing as microorganisms compete with fibroblasts for oxygen and nutrition.
   c. Colonization occurs only in wounds with significant amounts of necrotic tissue present.
   d. Colonization occurs in all wounds with normal bacterial flora and does not impede healing.
2. A client presents with a clean full-thickness wound. Which of the following solutions would be the best for use in cleansing?
   a. povidone-iodine
   b. normal saline
   c. sodium hypochlorite solution
   d. hydrogen peroxide
3. Cultures are indicated for which of the following pressure ulcers?
   a. all pressure ulcers involving loss of epidermis and dermis
   b. all full-thickness pressure ulcers
   c. pressure ulcers with signs and symptoms of localized/systemic infection or bone involvement
   d. pressure ulcers with necrotic tissue present and surrounding erythema
4. Which of the following provides a safe pressure for use in wound irrigation?
   a. Water Pik on a medium setting
   b. Water Pik on a high setting
   c. 35-mL syringe with 19-gauge angiocatheter attached
   d. Gauze soaked in solution
5. Which of the following reports typically indicates wound infection?
   a. Colony count of more than 1,000 organisms/mL
   b. Colony count of more than 5,000 organisms/mL
   c. Colony count of more than 10,000 organisms/mL
   d. Colony count of more than 100,000 organisms/mL

Exhibit 9–3 Self-Care Teaching Guidelines

Self-Care Guidelines Specific to Exudate and Infection Management	Instructions Given (Date/Initials)	Demonstration *or* Review of Material (Date/Initials)	Return Demonstration *or* Verbalizes Understanding (Date/Initials)
1. Type of wound and reasons for exudate			
2. Significance of exudate and infection			
3. Topical therapy care routine a. Clean wound.			
b. Apply absorptive dressing (note appearance of dressing when it interacts with wound drainage and on removal).			
c. Manage wound edges to prevent maceration.			
d. Apply secondary or topper dressing, as appropriate.			
4. Frequency of dressing changes			
5. Expected change in wound drainage during healing			
6. When to notify the health care provider a. Signs and symptoms of infection			
b. Failure to improve			
c. Presence of odor			
d. Pus or purulent drainage			
e. Copious amounts of drainage			
f. Elevated temperature or signs of confusion in the older patient			
7. Universal precautions a. Hand washing			
b. Use of gloves during care procedures			
c. Disposal of contaminated materials			
8. Antibiotic regimen a. Oral medication use			
b. Topical medication use			
c. Antimicrobial cleanser use			
9. Importance of follow-up with health care provider			

REFERENCES

1. Wysocki AB. Wound fluids and the pathogenesis of chronic wounds. *J Wound Ostomy Continence Nurs.* 1996;23:283–290.

2. Winter GD. Formation of the scab and the rate of reepithelialization of superficial wounds in the skin of the young domestic pig. *Nature.* 1965;193:293–294.

3. Kerstein MD. Moist wound healing: The clinical perspective. *Ostomy/ Wound Manage.* 1995;41(suppl 7A):37–45.

4. Stotts NA. Impaired wound healing. In: Carrieri-Kohlman VK, Lindsay AM, West CM, eds. *Pathophysiological Phenomenon in Nursing.* 2nd ed. Philadelphia, PA: WB Saunders Company; 1993:343–366.

5. Sapico FL, Ginunas VJ, Thornhill-Hyones M, et al. Quantitative microbiology of pressure sores in different stages of healing. *Diagn Biol Infect Dis.* 1986;5:31–38.

6. Xakellis GC, Chrischilles EA. Hydrocolloid versus saline-gauze dressings in treating pressure ulcers: A cost-effectiveness analysis. *Arch Phys Med Rehabil.* 1992;73(5):463–469.

7. Thomas DR, Rodeheaver GT, Bartolucci AA, et al. Pressure Ulcer Scale for Healing: Derivation and validation of the PUSH tool. *Adv Wound Care.* 1997;10(5):96–101.

8. Bates-Jensen BM. *A Quantitative Analysis of Wound Characteristics as Early Predictors of Healing in Pressure Sores.* Dissertation Abstracts International. Vol. 59, No. 11, University of California, Los Angeles; 1999.

9. Van Rijswijk L, Polansky M. Predictors of time to healing deep pressure ulcers. *Ostomy/Wound Manage.* 1994;40(8):40–50.

10. Cooper DM. The physiology of wound healing: An overview. In: Krasner D, Rodeheaver GT, Sibbald, RG, eds. *Chronic Wound Care: A Clinical Source Book for Healthcare Professionals.* Wayne, PA: HMP Communications; 2001.

11. Robson MC. Disturbances of wound healing. *Ann Emerg Med.* 1988;17:1274–1278

12. Thomson PD, Smith DJ. What is infection? *Am J Surg.* 1994;167(suppl 1A):7–11.

13. Pottinger JM. Methicillin-resistant *Staphylococcus aureus* in a sternal wound. In: Soule BM, Larson EL, Preston GA, eds. *Infect Nurs Pract.* St. Louis, MO: Mosby-Year Book; 1995:240–245.

14. Boyce JM. Methicillin-resistant *Staphylococcus aureus*: Detection, epidemiology, and control measures. *Infect Dis Clin North Am.* 1989;3:901–913.

15. Mosiello GC, Tufaro A, Kerstein MD. Wound healing and complications in the immunosuppressed patient. *Wounds.* 1994;6(3):83–87.

16. Daltrey DC, Rhodes B, Chattwood JG. Investigation into the microbial flora of healing and nonhealing decubitus ulcers. *J Clin Pathol.* 1981;34:701–705.

17. Bergstrom N, Bennett MA, Carlson CE, et al. *Treatment of Pressure Ulcers.* Clinical Practice Guideline No. 15. Agency for Health Research and Quality (AHRQ), formerly known as the Agency for Health Care Policy and Research (AHCPR) Publication No. 95-0652. Rockville, MD: AHRQ, U.S. Public Health Service, U.S. Department of Health and Human Services (DHHS); December 1994:15–22.

18. Stotts NA. Determination of bacterial burden in wounds. *Adv Wound Care.* 1995;8:28–52.

19. Robson MC, Heggars JP. Bacterial quantification of open wounds. *Milit Med.* 1969;134:19–24.

20. Wood GL, Gutierrez Y. *Diagnostic Pathology of Infectious Diseases.* Philadelphia, PA: Lea & Febiger; 1993.

21. Lee P, Turnidge J, McDonald PJ. Fine-needle aspiration biopsy in diagnosis of soft tissue infections. *J Clin Mibrobiol.* 1985;22:80–83.

22. Morrison MJ. *A Colour Guide to the Nursing Management of Wounds.* Oxford, England: Blackwell Scientific Publications; 1992.

23. Pagana KD, Pagana TJ. *Mosby's Diagnostic and Laboratory Test Reference.* St. Louis, MO: Mosby-Year Book; 1992.

24. Cuzzell JZ. The right way to culture a wound. *Am Nurs.* 1993;93:48–50.

25. Alvarez O, Rozint J, Meehan M. Principles of moist wound healing: Indications for chronic wounds. In: Krasner D, Rodeheaver GT, Sibbald RG, eds. *Chronic Wound Care: A Clinical Source Book for Healthcare Professionals.* 3rd ed. Wayne, PA: HMP Communications; 2001.

26. Levine NS, Lindberg RB, Mason AD, Pruitt BA. The quantitative swab culture and smear: A quick simple method for determining the number of viable aerobic bacteria on open wounds. *J Trauma.* 1976;16(2):89–94.

27. Georgiade NG, Lucas MC, O'Fallon WM, Osterhout S. A comparison of methods for the quantification of bacteria in burn wounds. *Am J Clin Pathol.* 1970;53:35–39.

28. Duke WF, Robson MC, Krizek TJ. Civilian wounds: Their bacterial flora and rate of infection. *Surg Forum.* 1972;23:518–520.

29. Barr JE. Principles of wound cleansing. *Ostomy/Wound Manage.* 1995;41(Suppl 7A):155–225.

30. Lineaweaver W. Cellular and bacterial toxicities of topical antimicrobials. *Plast Reconstr Surg.* 1985;75:394–396.

31. Rodeheaver G. Topical wound management. *Ostomy/Wound Manage.* 1988;20:59–68.

32. Foresman PA, Payne DS, Becker D, Lewis D, Rodeheaver GT. A relative toxicity index for wound cleansers. *Wounds.* 1993;5(5):226–231.

33. Hellewell TB, Major DA, Foresman PA, Rodeheaver GT. A cytotoxicity evaluation of antimicrobial and non-antimicrobial wound cleansers. *Wounds.* 1997;9(1):15–20.

34. Haynes, LJ, Brown, MH, Handley, BC, et al. Comparison of Pulsavac and sterile whirlpool regarding the promotion of tissue granulation. *Arch Phys Med Rehabil.* 1994;74(Suppl 5):54.

35. McConnell ES, Murphy AT. Nursing diagnoses related to physiological alterations: In: Matteson MA, McConnell ES, Linton AD, eds. *Gerontological Nursing: Concepts and Practice.* 2nd ed. Philadelphia, PA: WB Saunders; 1997.

36. Gilman G, ed. *Topical Agents for Open Wounds: Antibacterials, Antiseptics, Antifungals.* Reviewed by Rodeheaver G, Cooper JW, Nelson DR, Meehan M. Charleston, SC: Hill-Rom International; 1991.

37. Cooper BW. Antimicrobial chemotherapeutics. In: Soule BM, Larson EL, Preston GA, eds. *Infections and Nursing Practice: Prevention and Control.* St. Louis, MO: Mosby; 1995.

38. Speight TM. *Avery's Drug Treatment: Principles and Practice of Clinical Pharmacology and Therapeutics*, 3rd ed. Baltimore, MD: Williams & Wilkins; 1987.

39. Leaper DJ. Prophylactic and therapeutic role of antibiotics in wound care. *Am J Surg.* 1994;167(Suppl 1A):158S–159S.

40. Crow S, Planchock NY, Hedrick E. Antisepsis, disinfection and sterilization. In: Soule BM, Larson EL, Preston GA, eds. *Infections and Nursing Practice: Prevention and Control.* St. Louis, MO: Mosby; 1995.

41. Poteete V. Case study: Eliminating odors from wounds. *Decubitus.* 1993;6(4):43–46.

42. McMullen D. Topical metronidazole, part II. *Ostomy/Wound Manage.* 1992;38(3):42–48.

43. Jones P, Willis A, Ferguson I. Treatment of anaerobically infected pressure sores with topical metronidazole. *Lancet.* 1978;1:214.

44. Gomolin I, Brandt J. Topical therapy for pressure sores in geriatric patients. *J Am Geriatr Soc.* 1983;31:710–712.

CHAPTER 10

Management of Edema

Laurel A. Wiersema-Bryant and Bruce A. Kraemer

CHAPTER OBJECTIVES

At the completion of this chapter, the reader will be able to:

1. Identify etiologies contributing to edema formation.
2. Identify categories of medications that may be implicated in causing lower extremity edema.
3. Describe the four levels of compression and indications for use of each level.
4. Describe and compare five methods of compression for edema reduction.

INTRODUCTION

In this chapter, the reader will find a discussion of the etiologies associated with edema and strategies directed toward the management of edema. Management of edema includes a description of the procedures for managing edema and parameters to measure in determining outcome. Emphasis is placed on the steps the client needs to take to care for him- or herself because the management and control of edema requires an investment of time, energy, and dedication on the part of the client. At the end of the chapter, two case studies are discussed in an effort to apply the assessment, management plan, and outcome evaluation of the chapter content.

OVERVIEW OF THE PROBLEM

Venous disease with ulcers occurs in approximately 1% of the general population and 3.5% of persons over the age of 65 years. Edema in the client with venous disease occurs as a result of sustained increased venous pressure. This venous hypertension may occur primarily in the deep vein system

(femoral, popliteal, and tibial veins) or the superficial system (the greater and lesser saphenous veins or the perforator veins that join the deep and superficial system). These problems may occur in isolation or in combination. Respecting the underlying pathology is critical in the management of these clients. Increased venous pressure may be a result of chronic venous insufficiency (as described above), cardiac disease, pelvic tumors that place increased pressure on or occlude venous and lymphatic return, or morbid obesity, in which the weight of the abdomen may restrict venous and lymphatic return. In clients with edema secondary to cardiac disease, management of edema needs to be accomplished in concert with the cardiologist. A number of medications, especially the antihypertensive agents, may cause leg edema. These medications include calcium channel blockers, corticosteroids, estrogen and progesterone, testosterone, nonsteroidal antiinflammatory drugs, clonidine hydrochloride (Catapres, Clorpres, Combipres, Duraclon), minoxidil, guanethidine monosulfate, hydralazine hydrochloride (Hydra-Zide), rauwolfia derivatives, methyldopa (Aldoclor, Aldomet, Aldoril), and diazoxide (Hyperstat).[1,2] Managing a client with morbid obesity requires the assistance of the team in directing the client to appropriate exercise and weight management strategies. Fitting these clients with compression therapy is a challenge; in these individuals, we are asking for multiple lifestyle adjustments to be made to reduce the weight and manage the edema.

Increased interstitial volume is another reason for edema. These clients may suffer from a protein-losing enteropathy, liver cirrhosis, renal failure, and/or protein-calorie malnutrition. Care must be taken to manage the fragile skin, and edema management becomes a supportive therapy as the underlying medical problem is addressed. Another category of edema is that related to drug therapy with hormone replacement. Hormones in this category include corticosteroids, estrogen, testosterone, and progesterone. Clients experiencing edema secondary to hormone therapy generally respond well to leg elevation and exercise. If compression stockings are required, the low compression usually works well.

Clients with primary lymphedema require aggressive management and generally require compression at much higher levels than the individual with primary venous hypertension. Comprehensive management of lymphedema, including manual lymph drainage, is not addressed in this chapter. Readers interested in this topic are encouraged to obtain information from the National Lymphedema Network or other sources available to them.[3]

TESTS AND MEASUREMENT

Measurement of edema and edema control can be divided into two primary categories of quantitative and qualitative findings. Quantitatively, leg circumference and leg volume can be measured to give a reference range of leg size; with care, pitting edema can also be measured and quantified. Measuring leg circumference is an easy tool for clinical use; measuring leg volume is less "friendly" clinically, but it is a good measure of leg volume. Leg circumference can be measured with a disposable tape, obtaining measures of the calf 10 cm below the inferior rim of the patella at the visually largest portion of the calf (if different from the first measure) and 5 cm above the superior rim of the lateral malleolus. These measurements, plotted over time, provide a reference range for leg size and progress toward edema control. Leg volume measurement requires a large cylinder, which will hold the client's leg, and a basin to hold the water that is displaced. The cylinder or chamber is filled with water, and the client's lower leg is placed in the chamber, allowing the excess water to be displaced over the top and contained in the reservoir. The volume of water is then measured; the amount displaced will decrease as leg volume (edema) is decreased. Leg circumference is measured weekly or with each clinic/nursing visit. Measurement of pitting edema is often descriptive; however, edema can be quantified by using a simple grading scale, as outlined below:

0 to ¼-inch pitting = 1+ (mild)
¼ to ½-inch pitting = 2+ (moderate)
½ to 1-inch pitting = 3+ (severe)
>1-inch pitting = 4+ (very severe)

Qualitative measures to follow include the general appearance of the leg, the shininess of the skin, the amount of drainage from the ulcer(s), if present, and the client's sense of the heaviness or weight of the leg. It is also important to document the appearance of the leg when the wraps are removed, looking for areas of ridging and bulging between the layers

or above the level of the wrapping. Clients may also identify changes in how their clothing and shoes feel.

Clinical Wisdom: *Improper Bandaging of Edematous Foot*

The foot shown in Figure 10–1 displays pitting at the arch where the bandage was wrapped. This indicates that the bandaging was started up too far on the foot. The bandage should have been started at the toes.

MODES OF INTERVENTION AND PROCEDURES FOR INTERVENTION

Elimination and control of edema may be accomplished through leg elevation, exercise, and the use of compression therapy. It is often necessary to utilize a combination of these therapies to achieve the desired control of edema in the affected limb(s). Clients should be encouraged to elevate their legs as often as possible and, in general, to avoid any length of time with their legs in a dependent position. Exercise that results in working the calf muscle pump should be encouraged while using the appropriate compression garment or wrap. Clients may also find that elevation of the foot of the bed to facilitate leg elevation while sleeping is helpful; however, this is not useful for the client with heart disease, such as congestive heart failure. It is not unusual to find clients

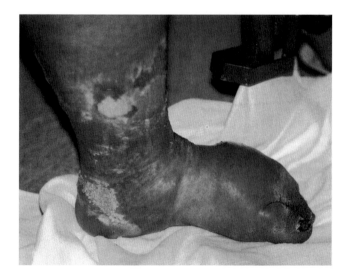

Figure 10–1 Pitting edema. *Source:* Reprinted with permission from R.B. Chambers and N. Elftman, Orthotic Management of the Neuropathic and Dysvascular Patient, in *Orthosis and Assistive Devices*, 3rd edition, B. Goldberg and J.D. Hsu, eds., p. 450, © 1997, Mosby-Year Book, Inc.

requesting a diuretic or water pill to facilitate the removal of the edema. The health care provider is encouraged to see this as an opportunity to provide client education as to the futility of diuretics as a primary treatment for edema. It is true that diuretics may be useful as an adjuvant therapy, especially if a sequential compression pump is to be utilized for the client with compromised cardiac function; however, diuretics are not the long-term solution to edema management. Appropriate for edema management are leg elevation, elastic wraps, tubular bandages, paste bandages, graduated compression stockings, intermittent sequential compression devices, and exercise. A discussion of each of these follows.

Leg Elevation

Leg elevation facilitates the removal of fluid through utilization of gravity in assisting venous return. For leg elevation to be successful, the legs must be elevated 18 cm above the heart.[4] Simply placing the feet on a stool is of no benefit. To facilitate leg elevation, the client may find it helpful to place one or two bricks under the foot end of the bed, which results in the legs being elevated higher than the heart during sleep. It is helpful to demonstrate this with the client by utilizing the exam table or bed to elevate the legs while reclining on the surface. The client should be encouraged to exercise the feet and ankles while elevating the legs. It is important to stress that leg elevation can be intermittent and that total bed rest is not recommended. Intermittent leg elevation during the day for 20–30 minutes at a time for a total of at least 2 hours a day is a reasonable goal.

Compression Therapy

Compression therapy works with exercise to facilitate the movement of excess fluid from the lower extremity. Several options are available for vascular support during compression therapy, depending on need (Table 10–1). The level of compression needed for edema secondary to venous disease, for example, is approximately 40 mm Hg at the ankle, ending with 12–17 mm Hg at the intrapatella notch.[4] It must be emphasized here that compression of 40 mm Hg is recommended for the client who is able to walk and work the calf muscles. A client with dependent edema who is unable to work the calf muscles will not tolerate this level of compression, and a lower level of compression—Class 1 or Class 2—should be considered. The four classes of compression used are as follows:

> Class 1: 14–18 mm Hg
> Class 2: 18–24 mm Hg
> Class 3: 25–35 mm Hg
> Class 4: 40–50 mm Hg

> **Research Wisdom:** *Guidelines for Safe Compression*
>
> Warning: *Do not* apply compression therapy to a limb with an ankle-brachial index (ABI) less than 0.8. Consult Chapter 7, "Noninvasive Vascular Testing," for ABI testing and significance. An ABI less than 1.0 suggests arterial vascular disease.

Elastic Bandages

Elastic bandages are relatively easy to apply, inexpensive, and easily removed. As with all compression garments/devices, it is best to apply the bandages within 20 minutes of waking and placing the feet below the level of the heart. Most compression wraps giving at least Class 2 compression are removed at night. Bandages do require practice to apply correctly, and the skill needs to be taught to the client and caregiver. Manufacturer's guidelines should always be followed when applying the elastic bandage. The most common application technique is the spiral; an alternative is the figure-of-eight. Figure 10–5 shows the four-layer bandage being applied in spiral fashion. Several types of bandages are now available with printed rectangles that, when stretched to squares, apply the correct level of compression. These bandages facilitate correct wrapping of an extremity (see Figure 10–2).

Tubular Bandages

Tubular bandages are also available to provide light compression (Figure 10–3). One should be careful to select bandages that are tapered at the ankle. Straight tubular bandages provide compression that is higher at the calf than at the ankle; these are not as useful for the client with edema.

Paste Bandages

Paste bandages, such as the Unna boot, are widely used in the treatment of leg ulcers (such as that shown in Figure 10–4A) and, as a result, in the control of edema. The boot was developed in the 1880s by a German physician, Paul Gerson Unna, and consists of a fine gauze impregnated with zinc oxide, gelatin, and glycerin (some varieties also include calamine). The gauze is applied without tension in a circular fashion from the foot to just below the knee (Figure 10–4B). Paste bandages do not provide compression; however, as the boot dries and stiffens, the leg cannot continue to swell. Application of a compression wrap over the boot (Figure 10–4C) will enhance compression and protect the client's clothing from the moist paste of the boot. A paste bandage is routinely changed every 4–7 days.

Table 10–1 Vascular Support Options

Level of Support	Examples	Recommendations for Use
Light support (8–14 mm Hg)	· Fashion hosiery · Jobst · Sigvarus	· Edema prevention for persons engaged in activities/work that require standing/sitting without much activity; examples: beautician, cashier, factory worker, some nursing positions
Antiembolism stockings (16–18 mm Hg)	· Anti-EM/GP (Jobst) · TED stockings	· Deep vein thrombosis prophylaxis · Nonambulatory clients with edema
Low compression (18–24 mm Hg)	· Relief (Jobst) · Elastic wraps · Paste bandage	· Nonambulatory clients with edema failing 16–18 mm Hg stockings · Clients with dependent edema
Low to moderate compression (25–35 mm Hg)	· Fast-Fit (Jobst) · Custom Fit · Double reverse elastic wrap · Four-layer bandage	· Edema secondary to venous insufficiency · Edema in client able to participate in exercise rehab
Moderate compression (30–40 mm Hg)	· Ultimate (Jobst) · Custom stocking (Jobst, Sigvarus) · Sequential pump · Four-layer bandage (Profore, Sure-Press)	· Edema with/without ulceration · Edema that persists in spite of lower-level compression options · Ulcer that failed to heal after 6 months
High compression (40–50 mm Hg)	· Vairox (Jobst) · Custom stockings (Jobst, Sigvarus) · Sequential pump	· Edema secondary to lymphedema

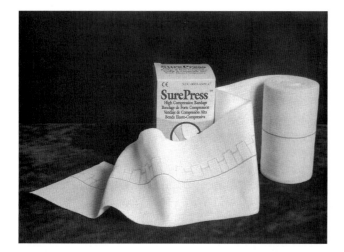

Figure 10–2 Short-stretch bandage. Courtesy of Convetec, Skillman, New Jersey.

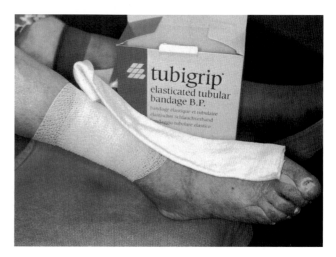

Figure 10–3 Short-stretch bandage. Courtesy of Convetec, Skillman, New Jersey.

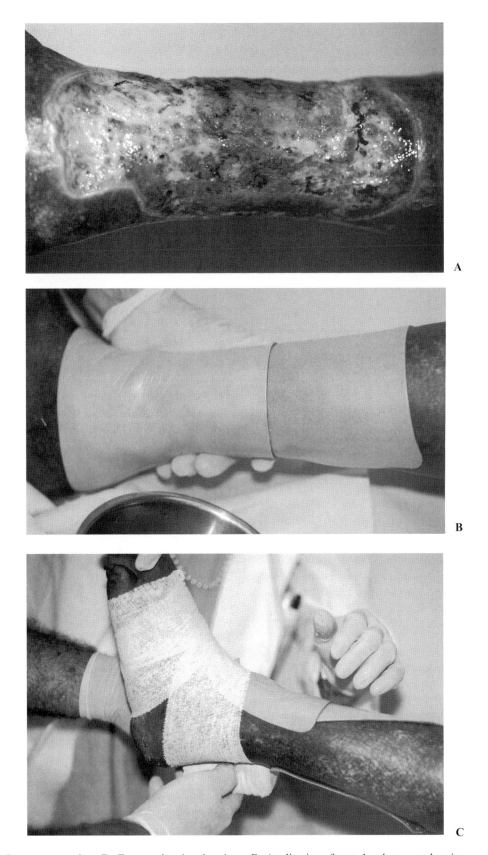

Figure 10–4 A, Large venous ulcer. **B,** Two overlapping dressings. **C,** Application of paste bandage over dressing.

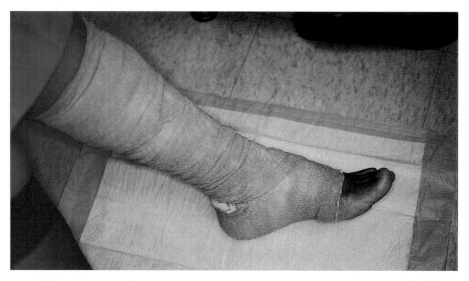

Figure 10–5 Four-layer bandage.

Four-Layer Bandage

An alternative to the paste bandage is the four-layer bandage developed at Charing Cross Hospital in London. The four-layer bandage provides graduated, sustained compression through the application of a series of layers, providing protection, padding, and compression (Figure 10–5). The dressing is removed weekly.

Graduated Compression Stockings

Graduated compression stockings assist venous return, thereby reducing edema (Figure 10–6). The client should be measured and fitted for compression stockings when the edema is absent or minimal. These stockings are then applied before the client has gotten out of bed or at least within 20 minutes of rising. Stockings may be difficult to get on, and devices are available to assist in donning. A nonambulatory client does not need moderate or high compression and will likely better tolerate a lower compression (18–24 mm Hg) stocking. Stockings do wear out and need to be replaced at the frequency recommended by the manufacturer. Many cli-

ents prefer to order two stockings (or two pairs) to prolong the life of the individual stocking and allow for laundering.

Compression Pump Therapy

Sequential compression therapy has gained popularity for the management of lower extremity edema. The leg sleeve (either knee-high or thigh-high) is divided into a 3-, 5-, or 10-chamber style, with peak pressures of 45–60 mm Hg at the ankle (Figure 10–7). The sleeve inflates first at the ankle, followed 2.5 seconds later at the calf chambers, and 3 seconds later at the thigh chambers. Each successive chamber inflates less, and the total inflation is sustained for approximately 5 seconds, followed by complete deflation. The cycle repeats every 7–8 seconds for the prescribed treatment period, which may range from 1 to 2 hours twice per day. Clients should be encouraged to follow treatment with application of either a fitted stocking or a compression bandage to maintain edema control. Use of compression therapy at night while sleeping is not recommended. Clients with congestive heart disease should be monitored closely for tolerance of the extra intravascular fluid burden with compression therapy.

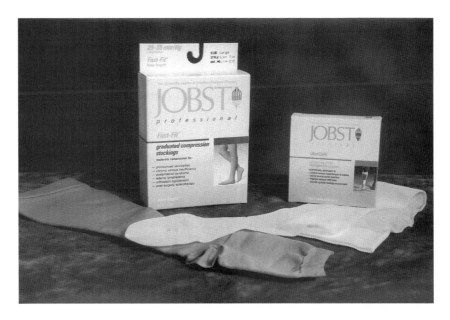

Figure 10–6 Compression stocking. Courtesy of Beiersdorf-Jobst, Inc., Charlotte, North Carolina.

Medicare Guidelines for Sequential Compression Therapy

The following are the Medicare guidelines at the time of this publication. Check with durable medical equipment suppliers to make sure that the guidelines are still as listed.

- Types of lymphedema pumps
  1. 3-Chamber
  2. 5-Chamber
  3. 10-Chamber
- Qualifying diagnosis: refractory lymphedema
  1. Lymph node removal/surgery
  2. Postirradiation fibrosis
  3. Malignant spread to lymph nodes with obstruction
  4. Scarring of lymphatic channels
  5. Milroy's disease
  6. Congenital anomalies
- General qualifying criteria
  1. Treatment for edema with custom-fabricated pressure stockings used without success
  2. Scarring of lymphatic channels
     a. Significant ulceration of lower extremities
     b. Several unsuccessful treatments with elastic wraps or pressure stockings unsuccessful
     c. Ulcers that have failed to heal after 6 months of continuous treatment

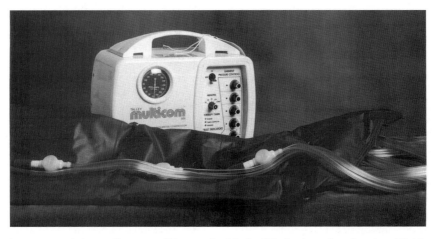

Figure 10–7 Compression pump and sleeve. Courtesy of Progressive Medical Technology, Inc., Lansing, Michigan.

- Authorization
  1. 3-Chamber: no ulcers
  2. 5-Chamber: ulcers present
  3. 10-Chamber: only after a 5-chamber has been used with minimal or no success, or if physician requests and documents condition accordingly

PROCEDURES FOR MANAGEMENT OF EDEMA

Leg Elevation and Exercise

Definition:
The legs are elevated higher than the level of the heart, with or without foot and ankle exercise, to allow gravity to assist in the removal of fluid from the legs.

Advantages:
- No costs associated with the procedure
- Effective when used regularly in combination with other form(s) of compression bandaging or stockings
- No special equipment required
- Involves client in active participation in edema reduction

Disadvantages:
- It requires consistent performance to be of benefit
- Some clients may be unable to elevate legs higher than the heart, such as those with morbid obesity, congestive heart failure, or orthopedic limitations
- The setting may not be conducive to reclining with legs elevated
- It may be ineffective in some forms of edema

Equipment Needed:
- A clean surface on which to recline
- A minute timer (optional)

Frequency:
Elevate legs for 20–30 minutes every 2–3 hours during the day for a total of approximately 2 or more hours per day.

Indications:
Edema of the lower extremities secondary to impaired venous return.

Contraindications:
- Morbid obesity
- Clients with arterial occlusive disease and ischemic pain with leg elevation
- Clients with congestive heart failure limiting ability to recline in a horizontal position
- Other medical conditions limiting client's ability to recline in a horizontal position

Procedure: Leg Elevation and Exercise
1. Recline horizontally on a clean, comfortable surface.
2. Elevate legs approximately 30° so that the feet are higher than the heart. Rest feet against the wall or footboard of the bed.
3. Set timer for 20–30 minutes (optional).
4. With one leg at a time, flex and extend foot against wall or footboard, then make circles (rotate) with the foot/ankle. Do 5–10 repetitions with each foot, then rest and repeat until the timer goes off.
5. Remove compression bandage and rewrap leg if compression bandage is being used.

Expected Outcome:
Edema and corresponding discomfort is relieved with leg elevation.

Clinical Wisdom: *Leg Exercise*

- Use of a kitchen-type minute timer is useful for ensuring an adequate amount of time.
- Encourage the client to work up to the 20–30 minutes if that is too much when starting out.
- Encourage the client to be creative at work in looking for opportunities to do the exercise.

Compression Wraps (Elastic Bandages)

Definition:
A compression wrap is a short-stretch elastic bandage that, when applied to the leg, exerts sufficient external compression to cause movement of excess fluid from the extremity.

Advantages:
- Wraps are inexpensive
- Wraps are readily available
- Wraps are easily removed
- Wraps involve clients in active participation of edema reduction

Disadvantages:
- Applying the bandage correctly requires practice.
- Care must be taken to avoid uneven tension when wrapping
- Wrap may telescope and fall down the leg with activity and will require reapplication
- Client may be unable to reach the toes comfortably in order to wrap from the foot to below the knee
- Client must be committed to application and wearing of the elastic bandage for it to work successfully

Equipment Needed:

- Short-stretch elastic bandage(s), of a width to accommodate foot and leg size (3- or 4-inch bandages are the most common sizes selected)
- Cotton padding or combination abdominal binder dressing (ABD)-type dressings (optional)

Frequency:

Apply wrap daily within 20 minutes of rising. Reapplication is required if wrap telescopes or slides down the leg.

Indications:

- Edema of the lower extremities secondary to impaired venous return
- Clients physically able to apply elastic bandages
- Clients who require edema reduction prior to fitting with compression stockings
- Clients who require low to moderate compression for the management of edema

Contraindications:

- ABI < 0.8
- Clients unable to wrap legs independently and have no caregiver able to assist
- Allergy to any component in the elastic bandage (for example, latex)

Procedure: Compression Wraps

1. Wash lower leg and foot and dry thoroughly.
2. Apply topical agent if ordered.
3. Apply wrap.
   a. Begin wrapping the bandage at the base of the toes, using two layers around the foot to anchor the bandage.
   b. Continue wrapping from toe to knee in a circular fashion by stretching the bandage approximately 50% of capacity or, if using imprinted bandages, until the rectangles become squares.
   c. If the leg is champagne-bottle-shaped, pad the ankle area with cotton padding or ABD-type dressing to minimize the shape disparity of the leg.
   d. With each turn around the leg, the wrap should overlap the previous layer by approximately 50%.
4. When the wrapping is complete, assess to make sure that wrap is not too tight by attempting to slide the index finger under one layer of the wrap. Assess skin under the anchoring clips (if used) to be certain the skin is not pinched.

Expected Outcome:

- Edema is decreased, as evidenced by a decrease in circumference of the calf and ankle
- Client/caregiver is able to provide a return demonstration correctly wrapping the leg
- Client arrives at follow-up visit(s) with leg(s) correctly wrapped

---

Clinical Wisdom: *Leg Bandaging*

- The index finger should be able to be slipped under the bandage if the dressing has been wrapped with the correct tension; if too tight, remove and rewrap.
- If the toes become numb and tingle, remove the bandage and rewrap.
- Encourage the client to walk for 30–60 minutes after wrapping, then remove and rewrap the bandage for correct compression.
- To maintain compression for a longer period, advise the client to walk after wrapping as above, then rewrap with a double-layer elastic bandage. Begin as above, holding the roll in the right hand, and wrap from toe to knee; then wrap again, beginning with the roll in the left hand, wrapping from toe to knee. Layering anchors the wrap, and it stays in place for a longer period of time.

Paste Bandage

Definition:

A paste bandage consists of a roll of gauze that has been impregnated with zinc oxide, gelatin, and glycerin (some have calamine added). The bandage is applied to the leg from the toe to the knee and left in place for 4–7 days. The bandage should be applied when the leg is without edema; as the bandage dries, it becomes resistant to additional swelling.

Advantages:

- It is useful for clients unable to comply with other modalities or contribute to self-care.
- It eliminates daily dressing changes.

Disadvantages:

- Client is unable to shower while bandage is in place.
- Client's ownership of the problem is transferred to the health care provider.
- Odor may be a factor when it is time to change the bandage.
- If the bandage is not wrapped correctly, new ulcerations may develop.

Equipment Needed:

- Prepackaged paste bandage (review manufacturer's guidelines that accompany the bandage)
- Gauze (3- or 4-inch wide roll)
- Compression wrap (Coban or elastic bandage)
- Gloves (clean)

- Scissors
- Receptacle to contain old dressing
- Soap and water to wash leg
- Wound care supplies, if indicated

Frequency:

Apply every 4–7 days; more frequent changes may be necessary if exudate is particularly heavy. Change immediately if the client experiences severe pain, excessive drainage, or foul odor.

Indications:

- Clients unable to comply with other modalities directed toward edema control
- Clients physically unable to wrap legs independently on a daily basis
- Clients who need interval assistance with edema control awaiting custom-fitted compression garments

Contraindications:

- Clients with poor personal hygiene
- Clients with significant arterial occlusive disease (ABI < 0.8)
- Clients with frail, friable skin
- Clients with active cellulitis
- Clients with infected ulcers

Procedure: Paste Bandage

1. Apply gloves. Remove old bandage by unwrapping or carefully cutting with bandage scissors as boot is lifted from the skin.
2. Wash foot and lower leg well. Use a soft brush to remove dry, scaly skin.
3. Dry foot and leg well (Figure 10–8A). A moisturizing cream may be applied.
4. Select paste bandage. Open all supplies.
5. Begin wrapping at the base of the toes (two revolutions) without applying tension (Figure 10–8B). Client should keep the foot and leg at a 90° angle.
6. Continue wrapping in a circular fashion around ankle and *enclosing* the heel (Figure 10–8C).
7. Overlap each turn by 50% as you continue to wrap up the leg to just below the knee (Figure 10–8D). A paste boot can and should be cut as often as necessary to avoid any folds, pleats, or wrinkles that may become pressure areas as the boot dries.
8. Strive for two to three layers of the bandage on the leg.
9. Smooth paste bandage and assess for wrinkles or folds, which should be removed.
10. Wrap from the toes to just below the knee with a single layer of gauze to facilitate drying and protection of clothing.
11. Remove gloves.

12. Apply an elastic bandage or short-stretch self-adherent wrap (Coban) from the base of the toes to the knee (Figures 10–8E and 10–8F). Overlap 50% with mild to moderate tension.

Expected Outcome:

- Wrap stays in place without complication for 7 days
- Leg edema is controlled, as evidenced by measures of circumference

---

Clinical Wisdom: *Paste Bandages*

- Client may wish to remove paste bandage immediately prior to clinic/nursing visit to allow time for showering. Leg must be elevated or an elastic bandage applied after showering if more than 20 minutes will elapse before new dressing can be applied.
- Some products recommend a figure-of-eight method of wrapping, whereas others recommend a circular overlap; check the package insert.
- Cast padding may be used to absorb heavy drainage.
- If boot feels too tight after client has been up and active for several hours, encourage client to elevate legs higher than the heart for at least 30 minutes.
- Paste boot can and should be cut frequently during application to avoid pleats, folds, or wrinkles that may cause damage to the skin as the boot dries.
- Assess client for allergies prior to application. Clients allergic to calamine should use a calamine-free bandage.
- A client with a narrow ankle and large calf (champagne bottle) may need to have the ankle padded with ABD-type dressings or cotton batting to avoid overpressurizing the calf.

Four-Layer Bandage

Definition:

The four-layer bandage consists of a wound contact layer and four bandages for sequential application to the leg. Correctly applied, the four-layer bandage system provides 40 mm Hg pressure at the ankle, decreasing to 17 mm Hg at the calf.

Advantages:

- It is useful for clients unable to comply with other modalities or to contribute to self-care
- It eliminates daily dressing changes

Disadvantages:

- Client is unable to shower while bandage is in place

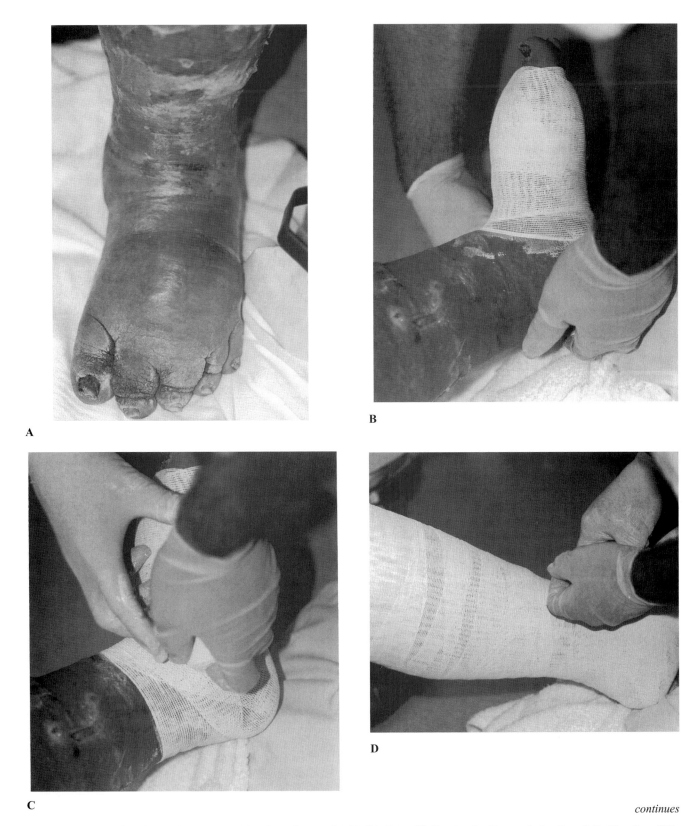

A

B

C

D

continues

Figure 10–8 Procedure for putting on a paste bandage. *Source:* for 10–8A, B, and F. Reprinted with permission from R.B. Chambers Elftman, Orthotic Management of the Neuropathic and Dysvascular Patient, in *Atlas of Orthosis and Assistive Devices*. 3rd edition, B. Goldberg and J.D. Hsu, eds., pp. 450, 451, © 1997, Mosby-Year Book, Inc.

Figure 10–8 continued

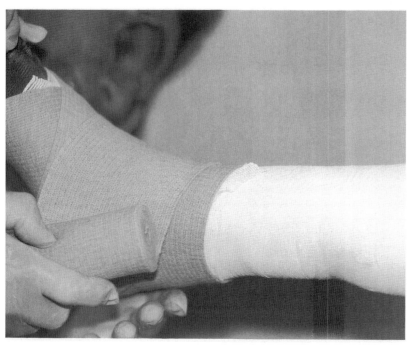

E

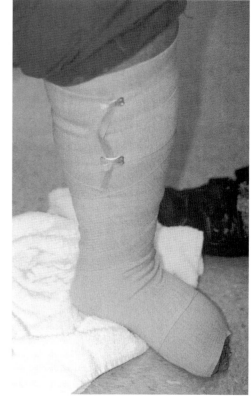

F

- Client's ownership of the problem is transferred to the health care provider
- Odor may be a factor when it is time to change the bandage
- If the bandage is not wrapped correctly, new ulcerations may develop

Equipment Needed:
- Four-layer bandage system (Profore)
- Gloves (clean)
- Scissors
- Receptacle to contain old dressing
- Soap and water to wash leg

Frequency:
Apply every 4–7 days; more frequent changes may be necessary if exudate is particularly heavy. Change immediately if the client experiences severe pain, excessive drainage, or foul odor.

Indications:
- Clients unable to comply with other modalities directed toward edema control
- Clients physically unable to wrap legs independently on a daily basis
- Clients who need interval assistance with edema control awaiting custom-fitted compression garments

Contraindications:
- Clients with poor personal hygiene
- Clients with significant arterial occlusive disease (ABI < 0.75)
- Clients with active cellulitis
- Clients with infected ulcers

Procedure: Four-Layer Bandage

1. Apply gloves. Remove old bandage by unwrapping or carefully cutting with bandage scissors as bandage is lifted from the skin.

2. Wash foot and lower leg well. Use a soft brush to remove dry, scaly skin.

3. Dry foot and leg well. A moisturizing cream may be applied.

4. Measure ankle and calf circumference.

5. Open four-layer bandage system and prepare supplies. Review package insert for directions if not familiar with the system.

6. Cover wound (if present) with contact dressing.

7. Wrap cotton padding layer without tension from the toes to just below the knee (Figures 10–9A and 10–9B).

8. Wrap a light, conformable bandage over the cotton padding layer, again without tension (Figure 10–9C).

9. Wrap a light compression bandage. Wrap from toe to knee (Figure 10–9D).

10. Wrapping in the direction of the first two layers, wrap the cohesive compression bandage with 50% stretch from the toes to just below the knee, using a figure-of-eight (Figures 10–9E and 10–9F).

11. Remove gloves and discard.

Expected Outcome:

- Wrap stays in place without complication for 7 days.
- Leg edema is controlled, as evidenced by measures of circumference.

Clinical Wisdom: *Four-Layer Bandages*

- Client may wish to remove bandage immediately prior to clinic/nursing visit to allow time for showering. Leg must be elevated or an elastic bandage applied after showering if more than 20 minutes will elapse before new dressing can be applied.
- If bandage feels too tight after client has been up and active for several hours, encourage client to elevate legs higher than the heart for at least 30 minutes.
- A client with a narrow ankle and large calf (champagne bottle) may need to have the ankle more heavily padded with the cotton padding to avoid overpressurizing the calf.

Compression Stockings

Definition:

Compression stockings are garments measured and fitted to the client that will provide external compression to the leg at a prescribed level. Stockings are available that will provide all levels of compression, from light support to high compression. Individual needs can be

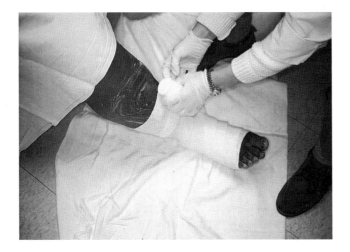

A

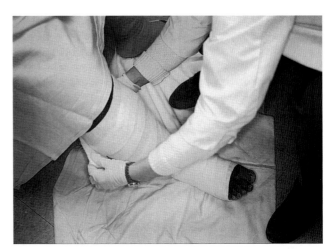

B

continues

Figure 10–9 A and **B**, Padding under four-layer bandage.

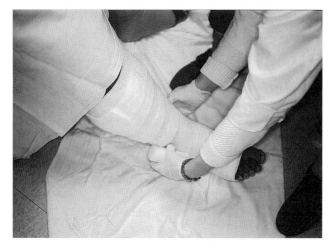

C

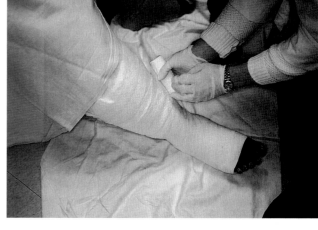

D

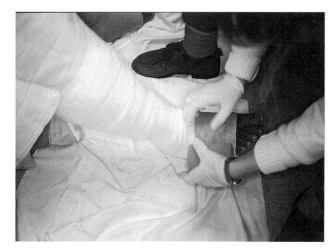

E

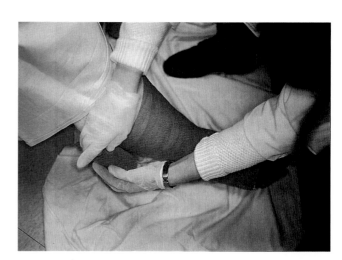

F

Figure 10–9 C, Light, comformable bandage covers padding without tension. **D,** The third layer is wrapped at 50% and in a figure-of-eight from the toes to just below the knee. **E** and **F,** The cohesive compression wrap is wrapped with moderate tension in direction of first layers; wrap is from toes to below the knee.

met through special order and a wide variety of ready-fit garments. Stockings are available knee-, thigh-, and waist-high.

Advantages:
- Stockings provide graded compression
- Stockings last from 4 to 9 months, depending on the manufacturer
- A variety of types is available, including custom made for the difficult-to-fit client
- Stockings are cosmetically acceptable

Disadvantages:
- Stockings may be difficult to get on clients who are disabled, have arthritis, or are elderly
- The cost of stockings is not universally covered by insurance providers
- The client must adopt a positive self-care attitude and be consistent with wearing the garment
- Stockings are not recommended for clients with extensive leg ulcers or circumferential wounds

Equipment Needed:
- Rubber gloves
- Stockings as ordered

Frequency:
Stockings should be applied before getting out of bed in the morning and removed just before going to bed at night.

Indications:
- Venous disease
- Lymphedema

Contraindications:
- Clients with arterial occlusive disease with ABI < 0.8 should use any stockings with caution
- Clients with allergy to latex should not use stockings made with latex

Procedure: Compression Stockings

1. Wash leg and foot and dry completely.
2. Measure ankle and calf circumference.
3. Apply lotion to the leg and foot, if needed; refer to manufacturer's guideline for type of lotion, because many products break down the fibers in the stocking, shortening the stocking wear life.
4. Turn stocking inside out, holding the heel portion, so that the stocking is pulled back over the foot portion (Figure 10–10A).
5. Place stocking over the foot and place heel in the heel portion of the stocking (Figure 10–10B).
6. Pull stocking back in place over the foot and to below the knee (Figure 10–10C). (Procedure is the same for thigh-high stockings. Waist-high pantyhose type must be applied without inverting the stocking.)
7. Smooth stocking to eliminate wrinkles (Figure 10–10D).

Expected Outcome:
- Client/caregiver is able to apply stocking with minimal difficulty
- Client arrives at office visits with stocking in place
- Edema in leg is kept under control, as evidenced by clinical improvement and a decrease in leg circumference

---

Clinical Wisdom: *Stockings*

- Clients should be measured for stockings when there is the least amount of edema in the leg—early morning or after using a sequential pump for 1–2 hours.
- Clients arriving for their appointment with stockings in a bag for you to put on do not understand the need for edema control.
- Review teaching.
- Inverting the stocking over the foot portion facilitates donning.
- Order two pairs at a time to allow one pair to be worn while the other is washed.
- Follow manufacturer's guidelines for washing.
- Stocking butlers are available as a device to assist a client in donning a stocking (see Figures 10–11A and 10–11B).
- Stockings are available in a variety of fabrics and colors. Cotton stockings are available from several manufacturers.

Clinical Wisdom: *Tubular Bandage as Alternative to Compression Stocking*

A tubular bandage may be used as an alternative to compression stockings (Figures 10–12A to 10–12C). For some patients, it is easier to don than compression stockings.

Sequential Compression Pump

Definition:
The sequential compression pump is a device that consists of a programmed pump and leg sleeves, which the client puts on. The pump is programmed to build and sustain compression from the lower leg/ankle to the thigh over a set period of time, then deflation occurs and, after a brief rest, the process starts all over again. Leg sleeves can be ordered for one or both legs.

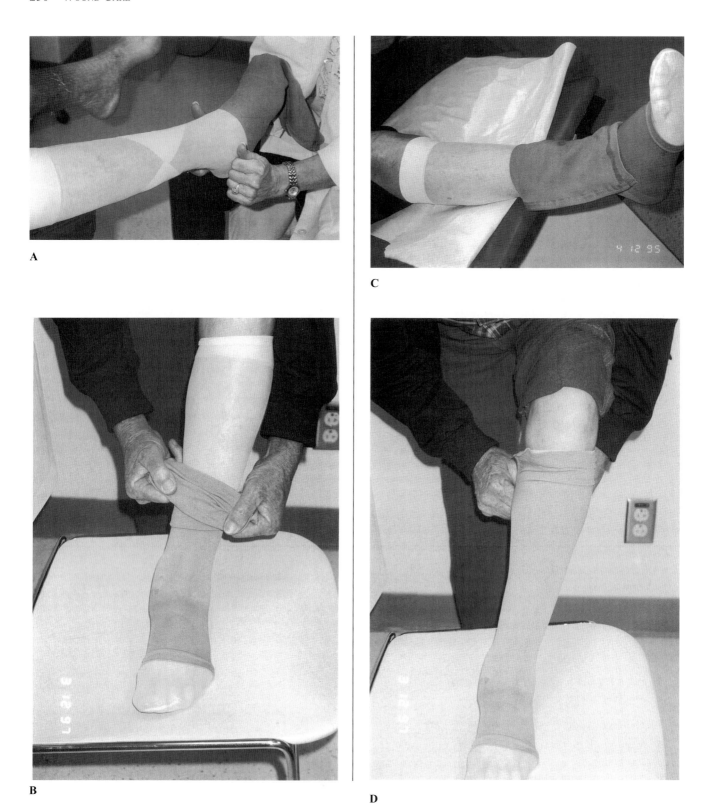

A

C

B

D

Figure 10–10 Applying compression stocking. **A,** Turn stocking inside out. A liner makes pulling on stocking easier. (Note dressing under the lining. The liner keeps the dressing positioned correctly.) **B,** Work stocking gradually up leg, smoothing out all wrinkles. (Stockings are available with or without toes.) **C,** Knee-high stockings halfway up showing zipper rear closure. **D,** Stocking extended to below the bend on the knee. Patient is positioing stocking. *Source:* Copyright © Evonne Fowler, MN, RN, CETN.

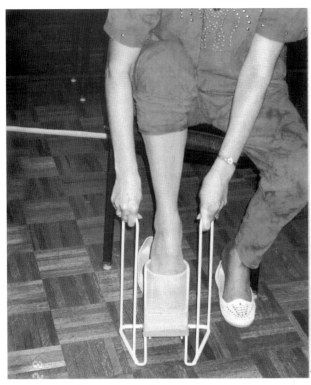

A

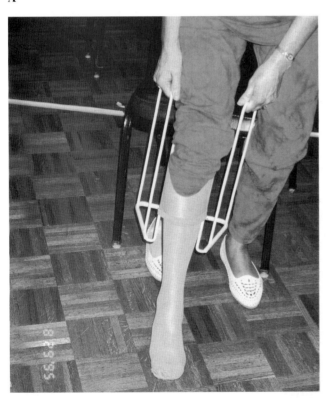

B

Figure 10–11 A and **B,** Using a stocking butler. *Source:* Copyright © Evonne Fowler, MN, RN, CETN

Advantages:

- The pump provides true graded compression that "milks" the edema from the leg
- The pump is used intermittently during the day
- Studies have shown the therapy to be effective in clients with venous disease and ulcerations
- The pump is easy to use

Disadvantages:

- During pumping, the client is restricted to a chair or bed
- Pumping may be too aggressive for clients with congestive heart failure
- The client will still need compression therapy of some type when not using the pump

Equipment Needed:

- Sequential compression pump, as ordered by physician
- Sleeves for one or both legs

Frequency:

Use for a 1- to 2-hour session twice during the day, preferably morning and late afternoon or evening.

Indications:

- 3-Chamber: edema, no ulcers
  1. Treated with custom pressure stockings without success
  2. Several treatments with elastic bandages without success
- 5-Chamber: edema, lower extremity ulcers
  1. Several treatments with elastic bandages without healing
  2. Treatment with custom pressure stockings unsuccessful
- 10-Chamber: only after 5-chamber used without success

Contraindications:

- Untreated congestive heart failure
- Inability to obtain sleeves that fit
- Cellulitis
- Active wound infection

Procedure: Sequential Compression Pump

1. Client should be in a comfortable reclining chair or in bed.
2. Pump should be plugged in with the controls (on/off) within easy reach of the client.
3. Remove stockings or elastic bandages (if possible).
4. Don and secure the sleeves.
5. Turn on pump. Most home units have an automatic "off" in 2 hours; if this feature is not on the pump, an alarm should be set for the prescribed time.

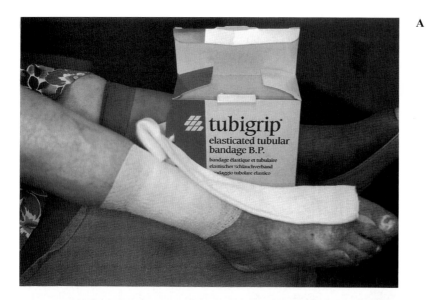

A

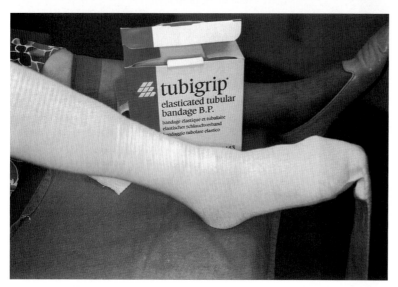

B

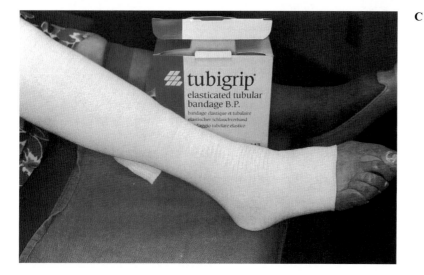

C

Figure 10–12 A to **C,** Using tubular bandage alternative. Courtesy of Convatec, Skillman, New Jersey.

6. Remove sleeves when prescribed time interval has passed; reapply compression wraps or stockings.
7. Clean sleeves periodically, according to manufacturer's recommendations.

Expected Outcome:

- Client tolerates procedure for 2 hours twice daily.
- Edema is relieved from extremity.

Clinical Wisdom: *Compression Pumping*

- If client is taking a diuretic, he or she should be advised to take it before pumping so that the peak effect will be realized as fluid is being pumped out of the leg(s).
- Clients who work may want to use the pump while at work. An extra pair of sleeves may be ordered so that only the pump travels back and forth, or a second pump may be obtained.

REFERRAL CRITERIA

When working with the client with peripheral edema, it is critical to know when to refer the client for additional evaluation and treatment. Knowing that there are many potential reasons for the edema and that many of these require a multifaceted approach to management, the practitioner needs to be aware of parameters that guide the making of referrals. The list below is to be considered as a guide only. In your practice, you may elect to accept, reject, or add additional parameters, depending on the type of client seen and referral opportunities available.

- Physical assessment reveals indicators of arterial occlusive disease, including pain and cramping of the calf with walking, absent peripheral pulses, localized lack of hair growth, thickening of toenails, and delayed capillary refill.
- The client has persistent edema for 1 month, despite compression wrapping, leg elevation, and exercise.
- The client develops new ulcerations or there is an increase in size of existing ulcer(s).
- The client has pain with leg elevation and exercise.

Where To Refer

Where and to whom the client should be referred needs to be established in conjunction with the medical director of the facility in which you practice. Some of the therapies require a physician's order (sequential compression pump) to receive reimbursement and, therefore, require that a physician see the client. Other circumstances are not quite so clear. It is also critical to take into consideration the client's insurance plan because it may, in fact, dictate a particular path for the referral process. Some of the potential referral directions include the following:

- Internal medicine physician for general medical problems, including hypertension, congestive heart failure, and other conditions
- Dermatologist for venous dermatitis, ulcer with uncertain pathology, nonhealing ulcer, and other conditions
- Vascular surgeon for indicators of arterial occlusive disease
- Wound healing clinic/center for nonhealing wound, refractory edema, comprehensive evaluation, etc.
- Rehab specialist for a client with need for exercise therapy and rehabilitation
- Lymphedema network for a client with lymphedema and need for specialized management and care
- Bariatric specialist for a client with obesity complicating management of the edema
- Home health care for assistance with and tolerance of application of compression devices

SELF-CARE TEACHING GUIDELINES

Teaching the client with edema the techniques for self-management is critical to the management of edema. In most cases, the edema does not represent a temporary, short-term problem. Therefore, management of edema requires that the client adopt lifestyle changes for a lifetime. It is important that the health care provider and the client respect that the problem of long-term edema management is owned by the client, not the practitioner. A client contract (Exhibit 10–1) may be of benefit in assisting the client to a position of ownership. For many clients, this may take some encouragement and effort because most clients come to the health care provider for a treatment and cure, not for the provider to instruct the client that he or she owns the problem and is key to its successful management.

In selecting a plan for managing the edema, ownership and responsibility need to be considered. Bandages/wraps that require the client to return for dressing changes, such as paste bandages and the four-layer system, may be a starting point for many. These systems, however, do not require active participation on the part of the client. Therefore, it is important to keep this in mind and move the client to an increasingly active role in his or her care as soon as possible. Several examples of edema management programs are illustrated by the two case studies that follow.

Exhibit 10–1 Sample Client Contract for Management of Venous Disease

Client name: _____

I.D. number: _____

Staff member: _____

Date of goal-setting interview: _____

Interval for reassessment:
___weekly   ___ monthly   ___ quarterly   ___ other

I, _____, understand that I have a problem with the veins in my leg(s). In order to take care of my leg(s), I understand that there are some things I must do. I agree to take care of my leg(s) as described below:

_____

_____

_____

_____

_____   _____
Client Signature/Date   Staff Member Signature/Date

Case Study 1: *A Case for Elastic Bandages*

R.A. is a 68-year-old man with a multiple-year history of swollen legs and ulcerations. The edema at the time of initial evaluation was severe, with pitting (3+) to just inferior to the knee. A large, irregular ulceration was present on the medial aspect of the left lower leg, with irregular borders and minimal periwound erythema. R.A. reported a heavy drainage from the leg, which prompted him to "try again" to get help for the problem. His past medical history was significant for a deep vein thrombosis (DVT) 15 years prior to this evaluation. Now retired, client had worked in a position that required long periods of standing with little walking. Medications were felt to be noncontributory. The client's legs initially were wrapped with elastic bandages in a circular fashion. He was found to have the bandages wrapped correctly when returning for appointments; however, after 3 weeks, little progress had been made. A 5-chamber sequential compression pump was added to the regimen, with significant progress in edema management over the next month. The client was felt at this time to have minimal edema and was fitted with 40 mm Hg compression stockings, and sequential pumping was to continue twice daily. At a 1-month follow-up, the client was found to have increased edema with deterioration of the ulcer. The client felt that he did better with the wraps. The stockings were discontinued, and R.A. resumed wrapping his legs with elastic bandages wrapped in a circular fashion, and a second layer counterclockwise to the first was added. He has continued to be followed every 3 months with this regimen and is doing well. R.A. wraps his legs daily and has decreased use of the pump to once per day. Edema has been kept under control with this combination, and the client is committed to the program.

Case Study 2: *Combination Therapy with Sequential Pump and Class 1 Stockings*

An 89-year-old woman presented to the clinic with more than an 18-year history of ulceration to the left lower extremity. Her history was significant for DVT in the left leg years earlier; the right leg was without significant change or edema. On assessment, the client's left leg was swollen, and the skin was shiny. There was a circumferential wound measuring 15 cm long anteriorly and 13 cm laterally; the drainage was clear yellow, and the wound edges were hypertrophic and scarred. The client is independent and refused home health nursing more frequently than twice per week. A sequential compression pump was ordered to be used for 1 hour twice daily, along with leg elevation every 2 hours. The client was able to do this herself and had been taking care of the wound without assistance. She had a family member raise the end of her bed with bricks. Wound care was directed toward keeping the area free of infection and the drainage contained. After 6 weeks of pumping, the leg was softer to the touch, but there was little change in the measurements. In collaboration with her internist, the client was given a diuretic, and the pump interval was increased to 1½ hours twice daily. With this regimen, the edema began to resolve. Subsequently, the client was recommended Class 1 stockings, which she was able to apply herself between intervals on the pump. At present, the wound has shown progress toward healing, with a decrease in length by 1.5 cm on the lateral side and 1.2 cm on the anterior surface. The skin of her leg is less tense and shiny; the circumference of her calf has decreased by 1.5 cm and the ankle by 2 cm. The mounded hyperkeratotic tissue has reduced in bulk, and the client feels that her leg "has lost some weight." The client is able to continue this program and to maintain her independence and church activities.

REVIEW QUESTIONS

1. At what level of leg elevation is the client likely to receive edema reduction?
   a. resting on a footstool while watching television
   b. horizontal when in bed (legs neutral to the heart)
   c. elevated 18 cm (7–8 inches) above the level of the heart
   d. watching television in a standard recliner chair
2. A new client has arrived and is determined to have dependent edema and is not ambulatory. What level of compression should you recommend?
   a. Class 4: 40–50 mm Hg
   b. Class 3: 25–35 mm Hg
   c. No level of compression will be tolerated and, therefore, none will be recommended
   d. Class 1 or 2
3. A client has been followed for 4 months and has persistent edema, despite a comprehensive program of leg elevation, exercise, and compression wraps. What is the next plan of action?
   a. Continue to compression wrap
   b. Review client medication profile
   c. Refer to appropriate provider
   d. Advise client that you are unable to help and that he or she will need to see someone else
   e. c, d
   f. a, b, c

REFERENCES

1. Ciocon JO, Fernandez BB, Ciocon DG. Leg edema: Clinical clues to the differential diagnosis. *Geriatrics.* 1993;48(5):34–45.
2. Terry M, O'Brien SP, Kerstein MD. Lower-extremity edema: Evaluation and diagnosis. *Wounds.* 1998;10(4):118–124.
3. National Lymphedema Network, 2211 Post Street, Suite 404, San Francisco, CA 94115. (415) 921-1306; Fax (415) 921-4284; hotline (800) 541-3259; http://www.lymphnet.org.
4. McGuckin M, Stineman MG, Goin JE, Williams SV. *Venous Leg Ulcer Guideline.* Philadelphia: University of Pennsylvania; 1997.

SUGGESTED READING

Airaksinen O, Partanen K, Kolari PJ, Soimakallio S. Intermittent pneumatic compression therapy in posttraumatic lower limb edema. *Arch Phys Med Rehabil.* 1991;72:667–670.

Ciocon JO, Fernandez BB, Galindo-Ciocon D. Leg edema in the elderly: A practical diagnostic approach. *Compr Ther.* 1994;20:586–592.

Ciocon JO, Galindo-Ciocon D, Galindo DJ. Raised leg exercises for leg edema in the elderly. *Angiology.* 1995;46:19–25.

Dealey C. *The Care of Wounds.* Oxford, England: Blackwell Scientific Publications; 1994.

Falanga V. Care of venous leg ulcers. *Ostomy/Wound Manage.* 1999;45(Suppl 1A):33S–43S.

Gutnik LM, Lovrien FC. An algorithm for evaluating swollen extremities in a community hospital: Recommendations and results. *South Dakota Med.* 1995;48(3):93–94.

Hess CT. Management of the patient with a venous ulcer. *Adv Skin Wound Care.* 2000;13:79–83.

Liehr P, Todd B, Rossi M, Culligan M. Effect of venous support on edema and leg pain in patients after coronary artery bypass graft surgery. *Heart Lung.* 1992;21:6–11.

Lippmann HI, Fishman LM, Farrar RH, Bernstein RK, et al. Edema control in the management of disabling chronic venous insufficiency. *Arch Phys Med Rehabil.* 1994;75:436–441.

Mayrovitz HN, Delgado M, Smith J. Compression bandaging effects on lov wer extremity peripheral and sum-bandage skin blood perfusion. *Ostomy/Wound Manage.* 1998:44(3):56–67.

Moffatt CJ, Franks PJ, Oldroyd M, Bosanquet N, et al. Community clinics for leg ulcers and impact on healing. *Br Med J.* 1992;305:1389–1391.

Struckmann J. The pathophysiology of venous ulceration. *Scope Phlebol Lymphol.* 1995;2(3):12–16.

Zink M, Rousseau P, Holloway GA. Lower extremity ulcers. In: Bryant RA, ed. *Acute and Chronic Wounds: Nursing Management.* St. Louis, MO: Mosby-Year Book; 1992:164–212.

CHAPTER 11

Management of the Wound Environment with Dressings and Topical Agents

Geoffrey Sussman

CHAPTER OBJECTIVES

At the completion of this chapter, the reader will be able to:

1. Have a clear understanding of the properties of ideal dressings
2. Be aware of the differences between inert dressings and interactive dressings
3. Understand the classification and use of the six main dressing product groups
4. Have knowledge of some of the newer products on the market
5. Understand more clearly the role of topical antiseptics in wound management

INTRODUCTION TO MOIST WOUND HEALING: THE BASIS FOR MODERN WOUND MANAGEMENT

Traditional theory has always indicated that

- wounds should be kept clean and dry so that a scab may form over the wound
- wounds should be exposed to the air and sunlight as much as possible
- where tissue loss is present, the wound should be packed to prevent surface closure before the cavity is filled
- wounds should be covered with dry dressing

The clear disadvantage of these principles is that the scab, which is made up of the dehydrated exudate and dead tissue, is a barrier to healing. This delay is caused by the epidermal cells that cannot move easily through the scab formed, which may lead to poor cosmetic results and scarring. Exposure to the air reduces the surface temperature of the wound, further delaying healing and possibly resulting in peripheral vasoconstriction, which affects the flow of blood to the wound, as well as the supply of oxygen, nutrition, and other factors. Exposure to the air will also increase the fluid loss and dry the surface. Where a wound is packed with dry gauze, the quality of healing is impaired due to adhesion of the material to the surface of the wound, causing it to dry out and risking trauma on removal.

Wounds managed in a moist environment covered by an occlusive dressing do not form a scab, so epidermal cells are able to move rapidly over the surface of the dermis through the exudate, that collects at the wound/dressing interface. The application of a totally occlusive or semi-permeable dressing to wound can also prevent secondary damage as a result of dehydration.

The initial work in understanding the functions of occlusive dressing began in 1948 with the publication by JP Bull[1] of a paper in *Lancet* entitled, "Experiments with a new plastic occlusive film dressings." Bull's work looked at the physical capabilities of a nylon derivative film. He concluded that the physical properties, in particular the water vapor permeability of nylon derivative film, made it suitable for wound dressings—the film being an effective barrier against microorganisms. He tested it on human skin to find whether the permeability of the film to water vapor would be sufficient to prevent the skin becoming sodden. He found that the bacterial flora of healthy skin under the occlusive dressing became modified, staph aureus disappeared, and a variety of organisms reduced.

Dr. RSF Schilling,[2] from the same group, specifically studied the use of the nylon derivative film in an industrial setting, as well as conducted a comparative trial with a waterproof dressing in common use at the time. The study concluded that the healing times of wounds treated with the nylon derivative film were significantly shorter when compared with similar wounds treated with a waterproof wound dressing, as commonly used in industry. Dr. George D. Winter[3], in his work, "Formation of the scab and the rate of epithelialization of superficial wounds in the skin of young domestic pigs," was able to demonstrate scientifically the difference between wounds of a similar nature when healing was open to the air, and when healing was under an occlusive dressing.

The experiment showed that wounds healing under moist conditions healed fifty percent faster than wounds open to the air healing under dry conditions. Winter's work has since formed the basis of the principles of modern moist wound management. The work was further extended in 1963 when Cameron D. Hinman[4] and others from the Division of Dermatology, University of California, published a study on the "Effects of air exposure and occlusion of experimental human skin wounds." In effect, Hinman repeated Winter's work, but this time with healthy adult male volunteers. He again used a sterile polyethylene film in artificially made wounds that were then either allowed to heal open to the air, or occluded. The results, once again, showed the same rate of success as the occluded wounds in Winter's work, thereby concurring with it.

Moist wound healing also simplifies debridement by assisting in the autolytic debridement of wounds. It facilitates wound cleaning, since the wound exudate is part of the healing cascade, and has been shown to carry a number of growth factors essential to the healing of wounds. It also protects granulating tissue and encourages epithelialization.

The aim of Wound Management is to provide the appropriate environment for healing by both direct and indirect methods, together with the prevention of skin breakdown. The history of the development and use of dressings has seen an evolution through many centuries—from inert and passive products, such as gauze, lint, and fiber products, to a dazzling range of modern moist wound dressings.

INERT WOUND DRESSINGS

In examining the continued use of passive products as described by Turner,[5,6] particularly gauze, it is clear that there are a number of negative aspects in the use of gauze. Gauze, being a fibrous material, tends to shed very readily and, as such, will contaminate the wound. Gauze is highly absorbent and, as a primary dressing, will tend to dry the surface of the wound rapidly. Gauze is permeable to bacteria, and moist gauze tends to be an environment for the growth of bacteria. This would risk penetration and ultimate contamination of the wound. Gauze is also adherent and will traumatize

the wound further on removal, risking damage to granulating tissue and pain.

In addition to gauze and lint, there are available other simple, modified absorbent pads covered with a perforated plastic film to prevent adherence to a wound, such as the trade name products Melolin and Telfa, which are used as both primary and secondary dressings. They are used in minor wounds and wounds with low exudation. Paraffin (petrolatum) gauze dressings, developed by Lumiere in World War I, were among the earliest modern dressings. Many variations have been developed over the years by changing the loading of paraffin in the base. These dressings, in general, produce a waterproof paraffin cover over the wound, which may lead to maceration because paraffin may not allow water vapor and exudate to pass through and may be trapped within the wound. These products are permeable to bacteria and are known to adhere to the wound, causing trauma on removal. Their use is limited to simple, clean, superficial wounds and minor burns. They are also used over skin grafts. They need to be changed frequently to avoid drying out and always require a secondary dressing.[7]

An alternative has been the development of equivalent dressing produced from synthetics fibers tightly meshed and impregnated with either an emulsified base or silicone. Examples are Adaptic and Aquaphor gauze.

IDEAL DRESSING

The properties of a good or ideal dressing have been described as follows:[5]

- Will remove excessive exudate from the wound but will not allow the wound to dry out, so as to maintain a moist environment
- Will allow gaseous exchange so that oxygen, water vapor, and carbon dioxide can pass into and out of the dressing
- Will be thermally insulating, so as to maintain the wound core temperature at approximately 37° C
- Will be impermeable to microorganisms to minimize contamination of the wound from outside the wound
- Will be free from either particulate or toxic contamination
- Will be nontraumatic and will not adhere to the wound, so that no damage is done to granulating tissue on removal

In addition, the following properties should be considered when selecting the appropriate dressing:

- Will provide the environment for healing
- Will be user-friendly (to ensure compliance)

- Will have ease of application and removal
- Will simplify treatment (minimal changes of dressing)
- Will be cost effective (ie, total management cost)
- Will be compatible with the wound
- Will have minimal need for secondary dressings
- May be suitable for combined use with compression therapy
- May be used in infected wounds
- Will remain in place

MODERN WOUND DRESSINGS

Film Dressings

Description and Effects

Film dressings are thin membranes coated with a layer of acrylic adhesive. They are moisture vapor- and oxygen-permeable; these properties vary from brand to brand, but not significantly. They are impermeable to microorganisms and moisture. Film dressings are flexible and allow easy assessment of the wound because they are transparent. They do not have the ability to absorb any exudate. The latest films being developed, however, have a very high moisture vapor permeability and, as such, will allow their use on more highly exuding wounds. Film dressings are elastic and extensible.[8,9]

The effects that make these dressings useful include the following:

- Providing a moist environment
- Enabling autolytic debridement
- Providing protection from chemicals, friction, shear, and microbes
- Transmittal of oxygen into and carbon dioxide and water vapor out of the dressing
- Functioning as a secondary dressing

Indications for Use

Film dressings are indicated in the management of minor burns and simple injuries (eg, scalds, abrasions, and lacerations) and as a postoperative dressing over suture lines. They are also used as a protective layer over intravenous catheters and for the prevention and treatment of superficial pressure areas.[10,11] A film dressing enables autolytic debridement and provides a moist wound healing environment.

Indications for Discontinuation

An increased level of exudation that causes pooling under the dressing may lead to maceration of both the wound and the surrounding skin. The dressing also should be discontinued if the wound becomes clinically infected.

Method of Application

An appropriately sized piece of film should be chosen to cover the wound and to provide an overlap of at least 4–5 cm from the edge of the wound. It is important to ensure that the skin around the wound is dry and free from oils or cream, because these may reduce the capacity of the product to adhere to the skin. The bottom backing paper is removed, and the film dressing is carefully applied over the wound, while maintaining light but firm stretching of the edges of the film to prevent it from sticking to itself. Once the dressing is in place, the upper cover is removed.

Film dressings are also used as a secondary dressing over hydrogels and alginates, and may be used as an alternative to tape for holding a dressing in place and to provide a waterproof covering. In addition to standard film dressings, there are island versions now available, comprising a simple absorbent pad covered by the film. These products are able to absorb small amounts of wound exudate and allow their use in wounds with low exudate. Simple, small versions of these dressings will also replace plastic first aid strips and have the advantage of not causing maceration common with plastic strips.

Removal

Film dressings may remain in place for up to 1 week or even longer. Changing of the dressing will depend on the position, type, and size of the wound. It is important to remove film dressings with care. The correct method is not to pull the dressing back across itself. This may cause a breakdown of intact skin, particularly in the elderly and in those with fine and dry skin. The film should be carefully pulled away from itself while applying light pressure to the center of the film dressing until it has been entirely removed.

Precautions and Contraindications

Care should be exercised in applying film dressings to damaged or frail skin because of the risks of further damage on removal. Film dressings are not recommended for use over deep cavity wounds, full-thickness burns, and wounds showing signs of clinical infection.

Outcomes Expected

Film dressings provide a transparent, flexible, waterproof, and breathing dressing that will protect simple wounds and encourage healing. They can be left in place for 1 week or more and are cost-effective, in that only one application of the dressing may be needed to manage the wound. When they are used postsurgery over sutures, they can remain in place until the sutures are removed.

The moisture vapor permeability test[9] is done under the conditions specified in the *British Pharmacopoeia 1980*. In

COMPARISON OF MOISTURE VAPOR PERMEABILITY OF DIFFERENT WOUND DRESSINGS

Dressing Brand	Cup Upright g/m²/24 hours	Cup Inverted g/m²/24 hours
Opsite™	839	862
Bioclusive™	547	605
Ensure™	436	436
Opraflex™	456	477
Dermafilm™	422	472
Tegaderm™	794	846

this test, the cup is either placed upright so that any loss of fluid is by evaporation or inverted so that the liquid comes in contact with the membrane. It should be noted that the loss of water vapor from intact skin is 240–1,920 g/m²/24 hours, and the water vapor loss from an open wound is about 4,800 g/m²/24 hours.

Combination Film Dressings

Ventex combines a vented film dressing and an outer absorbent pad. The vented film is applied directly over the wound, about 2–3 cm greater than the wound size; then the absorbent pad is stuck around the outer edge of the film. The pad remains in place until it is saturated with exudate. Then it is changed for a new pad without removing the vented film covering the wound. Viasorb also combines a vented film and absorbent pad, but they are not separate, so the entire dressing is changed. These dressings are indicated for use in exuding wound ulcers, pressure wounds, abrasions, and minor burns.

Foam Dressings

Description and Effects

Foam dressings are produced from polyurethane as soft, open cell sheets and may be single or multiple layers. They are also available impregnated with charcoal and with a waterproof backing.[8]

Foam dressings meet many of the standard requirements of the ideal dressings. They absorb exudate, protecting the surrounding skin from maceration and raise the core temperature of the wound, maintaining a moist environment. There are many polymer products with a similar appearance to foams; however, these are hydroactive dressings that adsorb moisture into their structure and swell up. They are absorbent dressings; however, they are not interchangeable with foam dressings in every situation. Foams are useful as both primary and secondary dressings. The effects of foam dressings include the following:

- Providing a moist environment
- Providing high absorbency
- Conforming to body shape
- Providing protection and cushioning
- Producing no residue
- Nonadhering to wound
- Providing thermal insulation
- Transmitting moisture vapor out of the dressing
- Requiring no secondary dressings

Indications for Use

Foams are indicated for a wide range of minor and major wounds, including exuding wounds (both superficial and cavity types), leg ulcers, decubitus ulcers, and sutured wounds. They can be used over skin grafts, donor sites, and minor burns. They may also be used as secondary dressings over amorphous hydrogels. Foams improve the functioning of amorphous hydrogels by removing excess exudate from the wound and raising the core temperature of the wound. This assists with autolysis. Foams may also be used around tracheostomy tubes and other drainage tubes and catheters.[12–14] The table below shows the form used by different manufacturers.

FOAM DRESSINGS

Dressing Brand	Main Constituent	Form
Allevyn™	Polyurethane	Three layers Film/hydrophilic foam/plastic net
Curafoam™	Polyurethane	Single uniform structure
Hydrasorb™	Polyurethane	Single uniform structure
Lyofoam™	Polyurethane	Two layers Hydrophobic foam/ hydrophilic contact layer
Lyofoam™ Extra	Polyurethane	Three layers Film/hydrophobic foam/hydrophilic contact layer

Indications for Discontinuation

Foam dressings should be discontinued when the level of exudation cannot be absorbed into the dressing in less than a 24-hour period.

Method of Application

The foam dressing is placed over the wound, allowing at least 3–4 cm greater than the size of the wound. The dressing should be kept in place with one of the following:

- In patients with fine or easily damaged skin:
  1. Lightweight cohesive bandage
  2. Tubular bandage
- In other patients:
  1. Adhesive tape (hypoallergenic)
  2. Tubular or lightweight cohesive bandage

The dressing can be used under compression bandaging and as a secondary dressing for amorphous hydrogels and alginates. In the case of a cavity device, select the appropriately sized device to fit comfortably into the cavity and insert it into the wound. It may remain in place for 1–4 days or until saturated with exudate. A sheet foam dressing can remain in place for up to 7 days or until the exudate has saturated to the edge of the dressing. Foam dressings may also be cut in shapes to allow better application to specific parts of the body. Foams can be cut in an L shape for application to fingers or toes. The method is to wind the shaft of the L shape around the finger or toe and secure with tape. The foot of the L is then folded over to complete the dressing and is also held in place with tape. A square piece of foam can also be cut diagonally to the center and folded within itself to form a cup that can be used over a healing wound.

Precautions

Foam dressings are of little value on dry wounds with a scab or eschar. Cavity dressings similarly should not be used alone in a dry cavity, but they may be used with an amorphous hydrogel.

Contraindications

There are no specific contraindications for the use of foam dressings. The author has clinically experienced a local reaction causing erythema, but this may have been due to an allergic reaction or to the increased blood flow caused by the thermal effect of the dressing.

Outcomes Expected

Foam dressings provide a satisfactory primary and secondary dressing for a wide range of wounds. They will aid in the removal of exudate, raise the core temperature of the wound, and protect the wound from external irritation. They will also protect the healthy skin around the wound from becoming macerated by the wound exudate.

Hydrogels

Description and Effects

Hydrogels are a group of complex organic polymers having a high water content—from 30% to 90%. These broad classes of polymers are swollen extensively in water, but they do not dissolve.

Hydrogels are three-dimensional, water-swollen, cross-linked structures formed from hydrophilic homopolymers or copolymers. Hydrogels are of two types. The first type is amorphous, being a nonfixed, three-dimensional macrostructure consisting of hydrophilic polymers or copolymers. The polymers absorb water, progressively decreasing viscosity. They are free-flowing and will easily fill a cavity space. These are amorphous gels. The second type is a fixed, three-dimensional macrostructure, usually presented as a thin flexible sheet. These gels swell, increasing in size until the gel is saturated; they do not change their physical form as they absorb fluid. Many also contain propylene glycol, and all contain a high proportion of water—up to 90%.[8] The table on the following page shows a comparison of water content of some amorphous hydrogel products.

Properties

Hydrogels are a moisture donor to a dry wound but are also able to absorb a certain amount of fluid. They have the following useful effects:

- Providing a moist environment
- Aiding in autolytic debridement
- Conforming to body shape
- Nonadhering to wound
- Providing both moisture donors and moisture absorbers

Indications for Use

Amorphous hydrogels, in general, are indicated for dry and sloughy wounds to rehydrate the eschar and enhance rapid debridement by autolysis. They are used on leg ulcers, pressure wounds, extravasation injuries, and necrotic wounds. They facilitate granulation and epithelialization by preventing the wound from drying out. They are used on simple and partial-thickness burns and on pressure wounds. Gels are used to prevent the drying out of such tissue as tendon. Gels are also a useful carrier of topical drugs to be applied to wounds, such as metronidazole and proteolytic enzymes. Hydrogels are suitable for use in infected wounds.

Water Content of Some Amorphous Hydrogel Products

Dressing Brand	Chemical Type	Water Content
Carrasyn Gel™	Triethanolamine, Carbomer 940, Acemannan	95%
DuoDerm Gel™	Sodium carboxymethyl-cellulose, Pectin, Propylene glycol	81.5%
Intrasite Gel™	Modified carboxymethyl-cellulose, Propylene glycol	78%
Purilon Gel™	Carboxymethyl-cellulose, Calcium Alginate	90%
Solugel™	Propylene Glycol Saline	75%
Saf-Gel™	Carbomer Propylene Glycol Sodium/Calcium Alginate	86%

Amorphous hydrogels are also used for management of the lesions of chickenpox and shingles.[10,15–18]

Indications for Discontinuation

Amorphous hydrogels should be discontinued if the exudate from the wound is excessive. It is generally considered that sheet hydrogels should be stopped if the wound is clinically infected.

Method of Application

Amorphous hydrogel should be applied to a wound to a minimum thickness of 5 mm and covered with a secondary dressing. The choice of secondary material will depend on the type and position of the wound, as well as availability and cost. The author has found that foams are the most satisfactory secondary dressings, by virtue of their properties of exudate absorption, thus maintaining the integrity of the gel for a longer time, protecting the surrounding skin from maceration, and raising the core temperature to aid in autolysis. Other products, such as film dressings, hydrocolloids, and simple nonadherent dressings, may be used. Gauze is also a suitable secondary dressing.

Hydrogels can remain in place with a clean wound for up to 3 days, then removed by irrigation with water or saline. When used for the lesions of chickenpox, they should be applied four or five times a day.

The sheet hydrogels are placed over the wound with at least 3- to 4-cm coverage greater than the wound. They are held in place with either tape or a light cohesive bandage, depending on the skin of the patient. In difficult areas, they should be held in place with a retention sheet, such as Hypafix, Fixomull, or Medipore. The sheet hydrogels do not cause maceration of the surrounding tissue. The sheets are left in place, depending on the wound type and the amount of exudation, but generally should be removed after 3–4 days. For some superficial burns, they may remain in place for up to 7 days. When removed, they cause no discomfort and leave no residue on the skin.

Precautions

Sheet hydrogels should not be applied to clinically infected wounds, due to their occlusive nature, without coverage with systemic antibiotics.

Contraindications

Amorphous hydrogels containing propylene glycol should not be used in patients known to be sensitive to propylene glycol. Sheet hydrogels should not be applied over small deep-cavity wounds or clinically infected wounds. They should also not be used in highly exuding wounds.

Outcomes Expected

Hydrogels will aid in the rapid removal of necrotic tissue and rehydrate dry wounds, assisting in granulation and reepithelialization. In burns, they reduce the heat and pain. The thicker sheet hydrogels, when used in the management of superficial pressure wounds, will also assist in the reduction of pressure by reducing friction and shear forces.

Hydrocolloids

Description and Effects

Hydrocolloids are a combination of gel-forming polymers with adhesives held in a fine suspension on a backing of film or foam. Hydrocolloid dressings are composed of a backing of either polyurethane foam or film and a mass, containing, in most cases, sodium carboxymethyl-cellulose and other gel-forming agents, such as pectin, gelatin, and elastomers. These form a self-adhesive mass.[8] These products are also available as granules, powder, and paste. When placed on a wound, the exudate combines with the polymers to form a soft gel mass in the wound. They were originally introduced as Stomahesive to protect good skin around ileostomies and colostomies. They vary from being occlusive to being semi-permeable. Hydrocolloids come in a wide range of shapes, sizes, and types. These include regular thickness, thin, bordered, padded, and in combination with alginates, as well as for cavity use as pastes, granules, and powder. When removed, the gel remaining is yellow and malodorous but not infected. The presence of bacteria under hydrocolloid dressings does not retard healing.

When applied to an exuding wound, the dressing absorbs exudate from the wound and forms a gel. This gel will vary in viscosity, depending on the brand of dressing. The dressing does not adhere to the wound itself, only to the intact skin around the wound. Hydrocolloids have the following effects:[19,20]

- Providing a moist environment
- Aiding in autolytic debridement of wounds
- Conforming to body shape
- Protecting from microbial contamination
- Providing a waterproof surface
- Requiring no secondary dressing

The table below shows a comparison of some hydrocolloid products.

Indications for Use

Hydrocolloids are indicated in the management of superficial leg ulcers, burns, donor sites (when hemostasis has been obtained), and pressure wounds. They may be used in small-cavity wounds, in combination with hydrocolloid paste, powder, or granules. Thin versions of these dressings are indicated as dressings over sutures in both minor and major surgery.[10,13,21–23]

Indications for Discontinuation

Hydrocolloids should be discontinued on surface granulation of the wound or if hypergranulation occurs.

Method of Application

Hydrocolloids on a superficial wound should be applied to the wound with at least 3–4 cm of product greater than the wound size. The skin should be dry to ensure good adhesion, and it is preferable to place one-third of the dressing above the wound and two-thirds below the wound; this will prolong the wear time of the dressing. The dressing may remain in place for 5–7 days or until strikethrough has occurred, ie, exudate has migrated to the outside edge of the dressing. The dressing should be carefully removed and the wound irrigated with warm saline before applying a new dressing.

In the case of small-cavity wounds, if relatively moist, the cavity should be filled with hydrocolloid paste, powder, or granules and covered with a sheet of hydrocolloid dressing. With a low to moderately exuding cavity, hydrocolloid paste should be inserted carefully and the wound again covered with a sheet of hydrocolloid dressing. The dressing should be changed after 3–4 days by irrigation of the cavity with warm saline and gentle removal of any remaining product before applying the new dressing.

Thin hydrocolloid dressings are applied after suturing of a surgical wound and, in most cases, can remain in place and be removed at the time of suture, clip, or Steristrip removal. These dressings have the advantages of being flexible and waterproof. They require no secondary dressing and help to appose wound edges by distribution of tension at the suture line across the surface area of the dressing.

Precautions and Contraindications

Care should be taken in using these dressings on patients with thin and fragile skin, because they may cause further damage on removal.

There are no absolute contraindications for use of hydrocolloids. Hydrocolloids are not indicated for use in very heavily exuding wounds or in clinically infected wounds. They also are not considered suitable for deep-cavity wounds.

Outcomes Expected

Hydrocolloids should help to remove necrotic tissue and slough from the wound and encourage angiogenesis and granulation of the wound. The presence of colonized bacteria in the wound does not contraindicate the use of these dressings.

Alginates

Description and Effects

Alginates are the calcium or calcium/sodium salts of alginic acid and are composed of polymannuronic and guluronic acids obtained from seaweed—mainly the genus *Laminaria*. When applied to a wound, the sodium ions present in the wound exchange for the calcium ions, producing a hydrophilic gel and providing calcium ions into the wound. This is part of the mechanism by which alginates act as a hemostat.

Alginates are gelling polysaccharides. They are presented as either calcium alginate, a mixture of sodium and calcium alginate in textile fiber sheets, or as a loose packing ribbon. Alginates combined with activated charcoal are also available. Alginates are combined with some hydrocolloid dressings to aid in the fluid-handling properties.

Sodium alginate has the empirical formula $C_6H_7O_6Na$, with a molecular weight in the range of 32,000–200,000.

Comparison of Hydrocolloid Dressing Products

Dressing Brand	Main Component	Backing	Forms
Comfeel™	Sodium carboxymethyl-cellulose	Polyurethane film	Standard, thin
Duoderm™	Carboxymethyl-cellulose	Polyurethane foam/film	Standard, thin
Tegasorb™	Polyisobutylene	Polyurethane film	Standard, thin
Restore™		Polyurethane film	Standard, thin

Sodium alginate has a complex structure, consisting essentially of two uronic acids, D-polymannuronic acid and L-guluronic acid. The ratio of these isomers will vary, depending on the species of seaweed from which the alginate is extracted and the method of production. Gels rich in polymannuronic acid form soft amorphous gels that partially dissolve or disperse in solutions containing sodium ions. Alginates rich in guluronic acid tend to swell in the presence of sodium ions, while retaining their basic structure.[8,24] Alginates have the following useful effects:

• Providing a moist environment
• Providing a high absorptive capacity
• Conforming to body shape
• Protecting from microbial contamination
• Providing hemostatis
• Nonadhering to wound

The table below shows a comparison of the chemical composition of different alginate products.

Indications for Use

Alginates are used in exuding wounds, such as leg ulcers, cavity wounds, and pressure wounds, and at donor sites (as a hemostat postsurgically) and other bleeding sites. They may be used in infected wounds.[10,14,25–28]

Indications for Discontinuation

Alginates should be discontinued if the level of exudation is insufficient to cause the fiber to gel. Alginates should not be premoistened with saline before application to a wound.

Method of Application

Sheet alginates should be placed in the wound to the shape of the wound and covered with a secondary dressing (such as a foam) or a nonadherent dressing and held in place with tape or a light cohesive bandage, depending on the condition of the patient's skin. If the wound is highly exudative, an additional covering with a simple absorbent pad is appropriate. In the case of a cavity wound, rope or packing alginate material should be placed gently in the cavity, taking care not to pack the material tightly into the space. When used on a donor site, the sheet alginate should be applied to the donor area after harvesting of skin and covered with a film dressing or foam. This will aid in rapid hemostasis and will provide the environment for reepithelialization of the skin. The dressing, in general, should remain in place in clean wounds for no longer than 7 days or when the gel loses its viscosity (this will vary, depending on the level of exudation from the wound). Wounds clinically infected should be changed daily. The alginate is removed by simple irrigation of the wound or cavity with warm saline. Freeze-dried alginates may be applied not only to the wound but also to cover the periwound skin because they gel only over the wound, thus protecting the periwound skin from maceration.

Precautions and Contraindications

Wounds clinically infected should be changed daily, with consideration given to the concurrent use of systemic antibiotics by the prescriber.

There are no known contraindications to the use of alginates. They are not suitable for use in dry wounds or wounds with thick, black eschar.

Outcomes Expected

Alginates will absorb exudate and provide the moist environment for granulation. They are suitable for use in infected wounds and are very effective in the management of bleeding, in particular, in postnasal surgery, postbiopsy, and when applied to donor sites. They will provide a comfortable dressing. Rapid healing of the skin is expected.

Combination Alginates

Manufacturers have combined alginates with other products to enhance the effects of each.

Calcium/Sodium Alginate Combination

CarboFlex is a combination of calcium and sodium alginate and Aquacel in a fiber sheet, bonded to a layer of activated charcoal and an outer layer of viscose. This product is a highly absorbent dressing with the ability to absorb odor. It

Comparison of Alginate Chemical Composition				
Name	Gulu-ronic Acid (%)	Mannu-ronic Acid (%)	Calcium Alginate (%)	Sodium Alginate (%)
Algoderm™	58	42	100	
Curosorb™	68	32	100	
Kaltostat™	66	34	80	20
Carboflex™	66	34	80	20
Sorbsan™	34	63	100	
Tegagen HG™			100	
Tegagen HI™			100	
Cutinova Alginate™	70	30	90	10
Calgicare™	65	35	80	20

is indicated in infected malodorous wounds, fungating neoplasms and ulcers, and superficial pressure wounds.

The sheet should be applied to the surface of the wound, ensuring that the alginate white layer is in contact with the wound and that the dark charcoal layer is on the outside. The product is covered with a secondary dressing and held in place with tape or a light cohesive bandage. The dressing should be changed every few days, depending on the level of exudate and the extent of infection. The use of systemic antibiotics in clinically infected wounds is indicated. The dressing is easily removed; removal may be assisted by irrigation with warm saline. This dressing, as with other alginates, is of no value in a dry wound with thick, dark eschar.

Alginate/Hydrocolloid Combination

Curaderm and Comfeel Plus. The combining of hydrocolloids and alginates in one dressing enhances the properties of the dressing and allows their use in more highly exuding wounds. They present in sheet form, similar in appearance to standard hydrocolloid sheets. They are used in a manner similar to that for hydrocolloids; however, they can remain in place for a longer time because of the better absorptive properties.

Hydroactive Dressings

Description and Effects

Hydroactive dressings have some similarities to hydrocolloids; however, they are not gel-forming products. They act by absorbing exudate into the structure of the dressing and swelling as the amount of exudate is absorbed. They maintain a moist environment at the interface of the wound.

Hydroactive dressings are multilayered dressings of highly absorbent polymer gel with an adhesive backing. These dressings are composed of an outer polyurethane film membrane, combined with a polyurethane gel and other absorbents (eg, sodium polyacrylate). They are semipermeable and are adhesive to the skin. They are available in a number of forms, including cavity fillers, foamlike, and thin types.[8] Hydroactive dressings have the following useful effects:

- Providing a moist environment
- Providing high absorbency
- Providing waterproof surface
- Regaining shape when stretched
- Aiding in autolysis
- Leaving no residue
- Semipermeability to moisture vapor

Indications for Use

Hydroactive dressings are indicated for use on exuding wounds, including leg ulcers, pressure wounds, minor burns, and exuding cavity wounds. They are of particular use over joints such as the elbow, knee, fingers, toes, and ankle because of their ability to expand and contract without causing constriction.[29–31]

There are foamlike forms of hydroactive dressings. These should not be confused with normal foam dressings because they react to exudate in a manner different than foams, by adsorbing the exudate into their structure. This can be observed by their change of shape. Hydroactive dressings absorb exudates rapidly, regardless of the level of exudation.

Indications for Discontinuation

Hydroactive dressings should be discontinued for the wound with little or no exudation or if the dressing is unable to absorb the level of exudate being produced by the wound.

Method of Application

The application of hydroactive dressings will vary, depending on the type of dressings used. Tielle is placed over the wound so that the central island of dressing completely covers the wound. Allow 2–3 cm greater than the wound size, then adhere to the surrounding skin. Cutinova is applied directly to the wound, allowing 3–4 cm of dressing greater than the wound size. It is preferable to warm the edges of the dressing slightly with the hand to aid in adhesion of the dressing. Cutinova Cavity, because of its ability to absorb exudate and expand, should be placed carefully into the cavity, not occupying more than 33% of the space. The outer wound should be covered with a suitable dressing, such as Cutinova Thin or Cutinova Hydro. These dressings may remain in place for up to 7 days, depending on the level of exudation. Care should be taken on removal in patients with thin or easily damaged skin. When removed, they will leave no residue from the dressing; however, it may still be necessary to irrigate the wound with warm saline if there is exudate present on the surface of the wound before redressing. Biotane and PolyMem are also hydroactive dressings and are presented as both a standard and an adhesive sheet. They are applied in a similar manner to the other hydroactive dressings.

Precautions and Contraindications

Hydroactive dressings are not considered suitable for use on clinically infected wounds or nonexuding wounds.

There are no known contraindications; however, care should be taken when using these products on fine and easily damaged skin.

Outcomes Expected

Hydroactive dressings will absorb exudate and provide a moist environment for granulation and epithelialization. They will provide a comfortable dressing that will remain in place and have a good wear time.

Miscellaneous Dressings

With constant research and development, new products have entered the market that do not fit into any of the standard groups mentioned. These products have properties resembling those of existing groups but are composed of different materials.

Exu-dry is a nonadherent absorbent pad composed of an outer layer of perforated polyethylene-laminated rayon and an inner layer of absorbent rayon/polypropylene blend, with a cellulose backing that wicks wound exudate and holds large quantities of fluid. It is indicated in highly exudative wounds—burns, in particular.[32]

Hydrofibers

Aquacel is a nonwoven, 100% sodium carboxymethyl-cellulose, spun into fibers and manufactured into sheets and ribbon dressing. This product mirrors the properties and actions of alginate dressings; however, it differs in that it rapidly absorbs exudate vertically and will not absorb laterally. It retains fluid within the structure of the fiber. The sodium carboxymethyl-cellulose fibers swell and convert into a gel sheet. This product is indicated in heavily exuding wounds, such as leg ulcers, pressure wounds, cavity wounds, minor burns, and donor sites.

The dressing is applied to the wound, allowing 2–3 cm greater than the wound size or wound cavity. The dressing will remain in place for 1–3 days, depending on the exudate level and when the product is saturated. Similar to freeze-dried alginates, hydrofibers may be applied to the periwound skin and the wound without the risk of maceration.

Combiderm is a multilayer absorbent pad combining a semipermeable hydrocolloid border with absorbent padding of hydrocolloid particles and a nonadherent cover against the wound. This product is highly absorbent and is able to hold the exudate within the dressing, preventing maceration to the surrounding skin. It maintains a moist environment. It is indicated on highly exuding wounds, pressure wounds, leg ulcers, and surgical wounds. It may be used as a secondary dressing over cavity wounds.

Cadexomer Iodine

Description and Effects

Cadexomer iodine is the combination of a polysaccharide polymer cadexomer and iodine at low strength. When this product is applied to a wound, the exudate is absorbed into the polymer structure, forming a gel and slowly releasing the iodine at about 0.1% continuously over 72 hours. The product will reduce the level of slough in the wound, absorb exudate, is antibacterial, and will also stimulate inflammatory growth factors. Iodosorb and Iodoflex are two presentations of this product.

Indications for Use

Cadexomer iodine is used on sloughy leg ulcers, pressure wounds, or other nonhealing wounds.

Indications for Discontinuation

Some patients experience pain on initial application of the product. In most cases, this subsides after 1 or 2 hours. There are a few patients who find it necessary to discontinue use of the product due to a low pain threshold.

Method of Application

Cadexomer iodine is applied directly to the wound as either powder, paste, or dressing. It is covered with a simple nonadherent dressing and left in place for up to 3 days. At dressing changes, the product, initially brown in color, becomes a white, pastelike gel that is washed away, and a fresh application of the product is applied to the wound.

Precautions and Contraindications

Should not be used on children under the age of 12 years or on patients with a known allergy to iodine. No more than 50 g as a single dose or 150 g in a week should be used.

Outcomes Expected

The wound should reduce odor, level of slough, and pain. The wound should show increased granulation and decrease in size.[33]

Charcoal

Charcoal is used in combination with a number of dressings, including foam and alginates. It is also available in specific dressings, eg, Actisorb Plus. The main function of charcoal dressings is the absorption of odor.

Collagen

Collagen is a vital structure in wound healing and is essential when cross-linked for the tensile strength in a wound. There are dressings composed of a collagen matrix, either bovine collagen or avian collagen. The role of the collagen is to stimulate fibroblast activity and to improve the healing cascade. There are many collagen products on the market. Their role clinically is still to be clarified.

Hyaluronic Acid Derivatives

Hyaluronan is a carbohydrate component of the extracellular matrix and plays an important role in the healing cascade. Forms of hyaluronic acid derivatives are in use clinically, and their role in wound healing also is not yet clear. Hyalofill is a hyaluronic acid derivative, Hyaff, and is being used in the management of nonhealing neuropathic ulcers and other chronic wounds. It is presented as a sheet or ribbon. Hyalofill should be applied to the entire surface of the wound, where it will absorb wound exudate and form a hyaluronic acid gel. The dressing is left in place for 3 days.[34]

Enzymes

The body produces a number of enzymes. Proteases are protein-splitting enzymes that have both positive and negative action on wounds. Proteolytic enzymes are applied topically to a wound to aid in the removal of slough and breakdown of nonviable tissue. This method of debridement has been used clinically for many years. The enzymes used in commercial products include papain in Accuzyme and Panafil, and collagenase in Santyl.

Hypertonic Saline

Description and Effects

When hypergranulation tissue is present in a wound, it is essential to reduce this tissue and to encourage new epithelium. One nontoxic method is to apply a dressing composed of an inert fabric impregnated with sodium chloride. The action of hypertonic saline is to draw fluid from surface cells by setting up an osmotic gradient between the highly concentrated solution in the dressing and the lower concentration of the cells. Examples of hypertonic saline are Mesalt and Curasalt.

Indications for Use

Hypertonic saline is used on hypergranulating and necrotic wounds.

Method of Application

The dressing should be applied only to the wound area and changed every 24 hours.

Indications for Discontinuation

The dressing should be discontinued if the patient experiences pain on application or if the wound is dry.

Outcomes Expected

Reduction in hypergranulation tissue is expected with use of this dressing.[35]

DRESSING CHOICE

Wounds are dynamic and, as such, the choice of dressing will vary and change as the wound changes. The product with which you may initially treat the wound will, in many cases, change as the wound itself changes. The choice should be based on the three major aspects of any wound: color, depth, and exudate (Table 11–1). The color will vary from pink (epithelializing), to red (granulating), to yellow (sloughy), to black (necrotic). The depth will include superficial, shallow, and deep cavity; the exudation will be none, minimal, moderate, or high.

Other aspects to consider are the presence of infection, the tissue surrounding the wound, the need to add graduated compression, the fragility of the skin, and any medical condition that may have an impact on the dressing choice.

SECONDARY DRESSINGS

The choice of secondary dressing will depend on the nature, position, and level of exudate. In general terms, film dressings and nonadherent dressings are suitable for lightly exuding wounds but not for high exudation. Foam dressings are useful over amorphous hydrogels and alginates (this does not apply to the foamlike hydroactive dressings). The use of gauze as a secondary dressing is limited, especially over hydrogels or alginates, because the gauze will reduce the ability of the dressing to function at its optimum level. The other consideration is the method of dressing retention. If the surrounding skin is good, the dressing may be held in place with high-quality tape. If the skin is poor, a tubular bandage or a lightweight cohesive bandage is suitable. See Appendix B, "A Quick Reference Guide to Wound Care Product Categories."

Table 11–1 Dressing Choice

Wound Type (Color/Exudate)	Aim	Wound Depth	
		Superficial	Cavity
Black/low exudate	Rehydrate and loosen eschar. Surgical debridement is the most effective method of removal of necrotic material. Dressings can enhance autolytic debridement of eschar.	Amorphous hydrogels Hydrocolloid sheets Proteolytic enzymes	
Yellow/high exudate	Remove slough and absorb exudate. Hydrocolloids, with or without paste or powder, for the deeper wounds. Hydrogels, alginates, and enzymes will aid in the removal of the slough and absorb the exudate.	Hydrocolloid Alginate Enzymes Hydroactive Cadexomer Iodine	Hydrocolloids with paste, granules, or powder Hydrogel Enzymes Alginates Hydroactive cavity Hydrocolloid/Alginate Foam cavity dressing Cadexomer Iodine
Yellow/low exudate	Remove slough, absorb exudate, and maintain a moist environment. Hydrogel, in particular, will rehydrate the slough. Hydrocolloids, films, and enzymes also will aid in autolysis.	Amorphous hydrogels Sheet hydrogels Hydrocolloids Film dressings Cadexomer Iodine	Amorphous hydrogels Hydrocolloids with paste Enzymes Hydrocolloid/alginate Cadexomer Iodine
Red/high exudate	Maintain moist environment, absorb exudate, and promote granulation and epithelialization. Foam dressings, alginates, and hydroactive dressings help to control exudate; use hydrocolloids with paste, powder, or granules for deeper areas.	Foam Alginates Hydroactive	Foam cavity dressing Alginates Hydrocolloid/Alginate Hydrocolloid with paste, powder or granules Hydroactive cavity
Red/low exudate	Maintain moist environment and promote granulation and epithelialization. Hydrocolloids, foams, sheet hydrogels, and film dressings will maintain the environment. It is possible to use a combination of amorphous hydrogels with a foam cavity dressing in deeper wounds.	Hydrocolloids Foams Sheet hydrogels Films In addition, the use of zinc paste bandages in superficial granulating venous ulcers is appropriate.	Hydrocolloids with paste, powder, or granules Amorphous hydrogels Foam cavity dressing

continues

Table 11–1 continued

Wound Type (Color/Exudate)		Wound Depth	
	Aim	Superficial	Cavity
Pink/low exudate	Maintain moist environment, protect, and insulate. Foams, thin hydrocolloids, thin hydroactives, film dressings, and simple nonadherent dressings will provide the necessary cover.	Foams Films Hydrocolloids (thin) Hydroactive (thin) Nonadherent dressing. In addition, zinc paste bandages may also be used.	
Red unbroken skin	To prevent skin breakdown. Hydrocolloids and film dressings provide the best protection.		

USE OF ANTISEPTICS IN WOUNDS

Antiseptics are an essential part of modern clinical practice. Their value as a hand-washing procedure prior to an aseptic procedure or for the preparation of the patient's skin prior to surgery is clearly documented. Studies have shown that the bacteria on the skin, whether resident or transient, are reduced by up to 95%. There is not, however, a considerable amount of research on the effects of antiseptics on open wounds. There will always be microorganisms present in a wound, to a greater or lesser extent. It has been argued that one of the most prolific researchers and publishers in the area of antiseptics and healing has said that antiseptics for this purpose may, in fact, be harmful, in that they damage healing tissue, thus allowing infection to gain a foothold.[36–40] It was Alexander Fleming in 1919 who said that it is essential in the estimation of the value of an antiseptic to study its effects on the tissues, rather than its effect on bacteria. Unfortunately, Fleming's wise counsel of so many years ago has tended to be ignored in modern practice. It is known that the surface of open wounds does not need to be sterile for healing to take place. Equally, there is no evidence to support that dressing changes performed once or twice a day with antiseptics guarantee protection from invasive infection.

The concern with antiseptics is their toxicity. A number of studies, particularly with the hypochlorites, have shown major problems. Brennan and Leaper,[37] in their study of the effects of antiseptics on healing wounds, used a devised rabbit ear chamber that was irrigated with a number of products. The effect on microcirculation was measured using laser Doppler. This study clearly showed the effects of various antiseptics on the microcirculation. In particular, Eusol was shown to occlude the microcirculation permanently after a 1-minute exposure, with no change in measured flow after 24 hours.[37]

Apart from the wound cell toxicity and the depression of collagen synthesis, hypochlorites may cause localized edema, hypernatremia, hyperthermia, and burns. It has also been reported that cases of renal failure associated with topical application of chlorinated solutions to pressure sores have occurred. This has been attributed to the release of a toxic lipid from bacteria, causing the bacteremia or endotoxic shock called *Schwartzman's reaction*.[41]

Hypochlorites as a chemical entity are chemically unstable, have a short shelf-life, are rapidly deactivated by organic material, and really are not cost-effective, requiring frequent changes of dressing. After all, sodium hypochlorite is a bleach. A further study by Brennan et al[39] showed that, in particular, hypochlorite retards the deposition of collagen, an essential element in the matrix for the healing of wounds by secondary intention.

The commonly used antiseptics fall into the diguanide group, one example being chlorhexidine, which is a bactericidal agent with Gram-positive and Gram-negative activity. It is ineffective against acid-fast bacteria, bacterial spores, fungi, or viruses. Skin sensitivity is reported, and chlorhexidine is incompatible with soap; the presence of blood and organic material also will decrease its activity. Antimicrobial activity is best at neutral or slightly alkaline pH. Chlorhexidine is used mostly as a hand or skin disinfectant.

The second antiseptic group contains the quaternary ammonium compounds, and there are a number of these—cetrimide being one example. Quaternary ammonium compounds are often used in combination with the chlorhexidine-type preparations, an example of which is Savlon.

These are also bactericidal against Gram-positive and Gram-negative organisms. They are relatively ineffective against bacterial spores, viruses, or fungi, and some strains of *Pseudomonas aeruginosa* and *Mycobacterium tuberculosis* are resistant. They can also cause hypersensitivity.

The third most commonly used antiseptic is povidone-iodine, an organic complex of iodine with polymers. It is a polyvinylpyrrolidine. It is bactericidal and sporicidal, and is active against fungi and viruses. Local irritation and sensitivity may occur, and it may cause burns if applied to denuded areas. It should not be used on patients with goiter. Its absorption may also interfere with thyroid function tests. It is incompatible with alkalis and is used as a skin preparation and as a disinfectant.

The topical application of an antiseptic will reduce the level of bacteria on the surface of the wound but will not penetrate into infected tissue.[42] If a wound is clinically infected, the use of systemic antibiotics should be considered as the most appropriate. Dr. Chris Lawrence considers that antiseptics and, to some extent, certain antibiotics, if used wisely, afford excellent antibacterial prophylaxis in a variety of skin wounds. However, unwise use of antibacterial agents—especially antibiotics—can create further problems. Dr. Lawrence, as do a number of other investigators, considers that convincing comparative clinical trials concerning the possible value of antiseptics are lacking. There is, however, sufficient in vitro evidence that would indicate that a problem exists with the prolonged use of antiseptics in chronic wounds.[43]

In general, the use of topical antiseptics in chronic wounds is considered to be of little benefit and may, in fact, be injurious to the tissue. The exceptions are patients with major arterial circulation deficiencies, such as diabetics and immunocompromised, neutropenic patients. A decision should be made for the individual patient, taking into account all of the positive benefits and risks. The use of low-strength povidone-iodine or nontoxic cadexomer iodine can be of benefit in some nonhealing chronic wounds.

ANTISEPTICS AND ACUTE WOUNDS

The use of topical antiseptics and antibiotics for acute wounds is entirely different from that for chronic wounds. In a traumatic wound, the risk of infection from contamination at the time of wounding is very high. Also, in the case of major burns, the presence of necrotic tissue is a focus for infection, and it is mandatory to use topical management. The aim of using antiseptics and antibiotics prophylactically is to reduce the level of bacteria in the wound and allow the body's own mechanisms to destroy the rest. The use of povidone-iodine, chlorhexidine, and chlorhexidine/cetrimide products is appropriate in the early management of acute traumatic wounds. The use of products such as silver sulfa-diazine cream (Silvadene, SSD) in burns is part of the early management of this type of wound.

ANTIBIOTICS

The use of topical antibiotics in chronic wounds should also be based on a general principle that topical use of antibiotics is not recommended because of the development of resistance and sensitization. However, in surface anaerobic contamination of some wounds, especially fungating wounds, the use of metronidazole gel (MetroGel) is appropriate, and there have been cases of methicillin-resistant *Staphylococcus aureus* where topical mupirocin (Bactroban) has been used. The other topical antibiotic used in clinical practice is silver sulfadiazine cream in some infected ulcers where *Pseudomonas* has been found to be present.[44–46] Appendix A has additional information on antiseptics and antibiotics.

WOUND CLEANSING

Cleansing of a wound at the time of dressing changes will depend on the nature of the wound. In general, if the wound is clean with little or no residue from the dressing, a simple irrigation with water or saline is the most appropriate. If there is dressing residue, slough, or dry or scaly tissue, then, in addition to water or saline, the use of a skin wash with surfactant properties will aid in the removal of the debris. The most important aspect is to minimize the direct contact with the granulating wound. It is considered best to use the cleansing materials at body temperature, because the application of a cold solution will reduce the temperature of the wound and may affect blood flow. The use of antiseptic cleansers is of little value in chronic wounds; however, they are of benefit in the initial cleaning of an acute wound.[47]

The other issue in relation to the use of any skin cleanser is the pH of the product. It is important to maintain an acid pH level of 5–6 in the wound and the periwound skin. It should be noted that most soaps are significantly alkaline in pH and will have a negative effect on the wound and the periwound skin.

REVIEW QUESTIONS

1. Name two negative aspects of the use of gauze as a primary dressing.
2. Modern dressings are divided into three functional groups. Give an example of each group:
   • Nonabsorbing
   • Absorbing
   • Moisture donating
3. Name two wound types where the use of topical antiseptics is indicated.

4. Name two dressings that can be used directly over a sutured wound.

5. Name two wound dressings suitable for exuding cavity wounds.

REFERENCES

1. Bull JP. Experiments with occlusive dressings of a new plastic. *Lancet.* 1948;213–215.

2. Schilling RSF. Clinical trial of occlusive plastic dressings. *Lancet.* 1950;293–296.

3. Winter GD. Formation of the scab and the rate of epithelization of superficial wounds in the skin of the young domestic pig. *Nature.* 1962;193:293–294.

4. Hinman CD. Effect of air exposure and occlusion on experimental human skin wounds. *Nature.* 1963; 200:377–378.

5. Turner TD. Products and their development in wound management. *Plast Surg Dermatol Aspects.* 1979;75–84.

6. Turner TD. Surgical dressings in the drug tariff. *Wound Manage.* 1991;1:4–6.

7. Thomas S. Pain and wound management: Community outlook. *Nurs Times.* 1989;85(Suppl):11–15.

8. Thomas S. *Handbook of Wound Dressings.* London: Macmillan; 1994.

9. Thomas S, Loveless P, Hay NP. Comparative review of the properties of six semipermeable film dressings. *Pharm J.* June 18, 1988;240:785–788.

10. Golledge CL. Advances in wound management. *Mod Med Aust.* May 1993;42–47.

11. Myers JA. Ease of use of two semi-permeable adhesive membranes compared. *Pharm J.* December 1, 1984;233:685–686.

12. Loiterman DA, Byers PH. Effects of a hydrocellular polyurethane dressing on chronic venous ulcer healing. *Wounds.* September/October 1991;3:178–181.

13. Myers JA. Lyofoam: A versatile polyurethane foam surgical dressing. *Pharm J.* August 31, 1985;235:270.

14. Foster AVM, Greenhill MT, Edmonds ME. Comparing two dressings in the treatment of diabetic foot ulcers. *J Wound Care.* July 1994;3:224–228.

15. Sussman GM. Hydrogels: A review. *Primary Intention.* February 1994;2:6–9.

16. Smith RA, Rusbourne J. The use of Solugel in the closure of wounds by secondary intention. *Primary Intention.* May 1994;2:14–17.

17. Thomas S, Jones H. Clinical experiences with a new hydrogel dressing. *J Wound Care.* March 1996;5:132–133.

18. Thomas S. Comparing two dressings for wound debridement. *J Wound Care.* September 1993;2:272–274.

19. Thomas S, Loveless P. A comparative study of the properties of six hydrocolloid dressings. *Pharm J.* November 16, 1991;247:672–675.

20. Rousseau P, Niecestro RM. Comparison of the physicochemical properties of various hydrocolloid dressings. *Wounds.* January/February 1991;3:43–45.

21. Marshall PJ, Eyers A. The use of a hydrocolloid dressing (Comfeel transparent) as a wound closure dressing following lower bowel surgery. *Primary Intention.* August 1994;2:39–40.

22. Banks V, Bale SE, Harding KG. Comparing two dressings for exuding pressure sores in community patients. *J Wound Care.* June 1994;3:175–178.

23. Thomas SS, Lawrence JC, Thomas A. Evaluation of hydrocolloids and topical medication in minor burns. *J Wound Care.* May 1995;4:218–220.

24. Thomas S. Observations on the fluid handling properties of alginate dressings. *Pharm J.* June 27, 1992;248:850–851.

25. Sussman GM. Alginates: A review. *Primary Intention.* February 1996;4:33–37.

26. Miller L, Jones V, Bale S. The use of alginate packing in the management of deep sinuses. *J Wound Care.* September 1993;2:262–263.

27. Thomas S. Use of a calcium alginate dressing. *Pharm J.* August 10, 1985;235:188–190.

28. Thomas S. Alginates: A guide to the properties and uses of the different alginate dressings available today. *J Wound Care.* May/June 1992;1:29–32.

29. Williams C. Treating a patient's venous ulcer with a foamed gel dressing. *J Wound Care.* September 1993;2:264–265.

30. Achterberg VB, Welling C, Meyer-Ingold W. Hydroactive dressings and serum protein: An in vitro study. *J Wound Care.* February 1996;5:79–82.

31. Collier J. A moist odour-free environment. *Prof Nurse.* September 1992;7(12):804–807.

32. Brown-Etris M, Smith JA, Pasceri P, Punchello M. Case studies: Considering dressing options. *Ostomy/Wound Manage.* June 1994;40:5: 46–52.

33. Sundberg JA. Retrospective review of the use of cadexomer iodine in the treatment of chronic wounds. *Wounds.* May/June 1997;3(9):68–86.

34. Foster AVM, Edmonds M. Hyalofill: A new product for chronic wound management. *Diabetic Foot.* Spring 2000;3(1):29–30.

35. Parsons L. Office management of minor burns. *Lippincott's Primary Care Pract.* March/April 1997;1(1):40–49.

36. Sleigh JW, Linter SPK. Hazards of hydrogen peroxide. *Br Med J.* 1985;291:1706.

37. Brennan SS, Leaper DJ. The effects of antiseptics on the healing wound: A study using the rabbit ear chamber. *Br J Surg.* 1985;72:780–782.

38. Lawrence CJ. Dressings and wound infection. *Am J Surg.* 1994; 167(Suppl):21S–24S.

39. Brennan SS, Foster ME, Leaper DJ. Antiseptic toxicity in wounds: Healed by secondary intention. *J Hosp Infect.* 1986;8:263–267.

40. Leaper DJ. Antiseptics and their effect on healing tissue. *Nurs Times.* May 1986;45–46.

41. Morgan DA. Chlorinated solutions: (E) useful or (e) useless. *Pharm J.* August 19, 1989;243:219–220.

42. Lawrence JC. The development of an in vitro wound model and its application to the use of topical antiseptics. In: *Proceedings of the First European Conference on Advances in Wound Management.* London: Macmillan; 1992:15–16.

43. Lawrence JC. Wound infection. *J Wound Care.* September 1993;2: 277–280.

44. Leaper DJ, Brennan SS, Simpson RA, Foster ME. Experimental infection and hydrogel dressings. *J Hosp Infect.* 1984;5:69–73.

45. Young JB, Dobrzanski S. Pressure sores: Epidemiology and current management concepts. *Drugs Aging.* 1992;2:42–57.

46. Brown CD, Zitelli JA. A review of topical agents for wounds and methods of wounding. *J Dermatol Surg Oncol.* 1993;19:732–737.

47. Dire JD, Welsh AP. A comparison of wound irrigation solution used in the emergency department. *Ann Emerg Med.* June 1990;704–707.

CHAPTER 12

Management of the Wound Environment with Advanced Therapies

Barbara M. Bates-Jensen, Joy Edvalson, Dayna E. Gary, Mark S. Granick, Elizabeth Hiltabidel, Nancy Tomaselli, Adela M. Valenzuela, with contributions by Paula Tashjian

CHAPTER OBJECTIVES

At the completion of this chapter, the reader will be able to:

1. Describe criteria for defining a refractory wound.
2. Identify six advanced wound therapies.
3. Compare and contrast advanced wound therapies.
4. Describe and explain indications for each advanced wound therapy.

INTRODUCTION
Barbara M. Bates-Jensen

Advanced wound therapy includes topical wound products and devices. Therapy in this category does not fall into other wound treatment categories and typically costs more than other wound therapies. Examples of advanced wound therapy include living skin equivalents, topical growth factors, devices that directly change the local wound environment, such as vacuum-assisted wound closure and temperature therapy, and silver-impregnated dressings and synthetic skin dressings. Each of these therapies is discussed under a separate section. There is some debate about when advanced wound therapies are appropriate to use. One suggestion is to use them only on wounds that fail to heal with standard wound treatment approaches. Another suggestion is to use them immediately on wounds identified as being potentially harder to heal. Both approaches depend on the ability of the clinician to define the appropriate wound candidate. Some of the wound therapies provide specific guidelines for appropriate use, and others provide more general indications. It has been suggested that use of advanced wound therapies would be particularly useful for the refractory wound.

Definition

Webster's dictionary defines *refractory* as "1. Resisting control or authority, stubborn or unmanageable, 2. Resistant to treatment or cure, 3. Unresponsive to stimulus, immune, insusceptible, 4. Difficult to fuse, corrode, or draw out."[1(p983)] The term *refractory* is typically used to define wounds that have not healed, despite appropriate treatment. It has come to be used to define difficult-to-heal wounds and wounds that do not progress toward healing. Wounds may be considered refractory when they present with certain wound characteristics, such as extensive necrosis, undermining, or tunneling. Some studies have found that undermining present on initial wound assessment was associated with poor wound healing outcomes.[2,3] Others did not find undermining at baseline assessment to be a significant predictor of healing.[4] The presence of necrotic tissue in wounds provides a physical impediment to healing, and, not surprisingly, several have found that healing outcomes in necrotic wounds is less than those without necrotic tissue.[5,6] These studies suggest that the presence of necrotic tissue is associated with slower healing times[6] and a decreased proportion of improving ulcers.[5]

Specific comorbidities that are known to compromise wound healing, such as immunosuppression,[7,8] diabetes mellitus,[9,10] vascular disease,[11] or hypovolemia,[12] may determine whether the wound is diagnosed as refractory. The patient may present with significant host burden that impairs healing, such as infection[13,14] wounds of prolonged duration, or extensive wounds.[5,15–18] Finally, a wound may be diagnosed as refractory when it fails to meet research-based temporal healing expectations. Clean full-thickness pressure ulcers should show signs of wound healing and improvement within 2–4 weeks[5,18] One retrospective study suggests that pressure ulcers that do not decrease in size and demonstrate overall improvement at 1 week may not progress to healing in a timely fashion.[4] Partial-thickness wounds should show improvement in one to two weeks.[19] Exhibit 12–1 presents a proposal for diagnostic criteria for the "refractory" wound. These criteria are simply guidelines for assisting clinicians in determining those wounds that may benefit from early use of advanced wound therapy.

GROWTH FACTORS
Nancy Tomaselli

There is a growing body of literature supporting the potential use of growth factors in wound healing. However, much of the research is still in its infancy, with most of the work continuing at the laboratory and animal model level. Several randomized controlled clinical trials have been done with recombinant platelet-derived growth factor-BB (rPDGF-BB).[20–22] Recombinant PDGF-BB was first reported in the treatment of pressure ulcers in a 1992 phase I/II prospective, controlled clinical trial of 20 patients.[20] Topically applied 100-µg/mL rPDGF-BB was applied to the wounds and produced an increase in the rate of wound closure, compared with other groups. In a follow-up multicenter study,[21] those wounds treated with rPDGF-BB showed a trend toward faster healing but the results were not statistically significant. Most recently, Rees and colleagues[22] reported statistically significant improvement in healing of pressure ulcers using a different preparation of rPDGF-BB than was previously tested. Basic fibroblast growth factor (bFGF) has also been evaluated in chronic wounds. Robson and colleagues[23] found bFGF to be safe and potentially effective in pressure ulcer healing. Other growth factors have been evaluated in pressure ulcers, including epidermal growth factor (EGF)[24] and interleukin 1-β (IL-1β).[25] The difficulty with growth factors and chronic wound healing is determining which growth factor should be used, at what adequate dose, and with what possible other growth factors. Studies using multiple growth factors are just beginning to surface.[26]

Exhibit 12–1 Proposed Refractory Wound Diagnostic Criteria

Wound Characteristics Present: undermining, tunneling, extensive necrotic tissue

Host Burden Present: extensive wounding, prolonged wound duration, infection

Healing Risk Factors Present: diabetes, vascular disease, immunocompromise, hypovolemia

Inadequate Temporal Outcome Expectations Present: full-thickness wounds failure to improve with appropriate treatment in 2–4 weeks, partial thickness wounds failure to improve in 1–2 weeks

The early use of exogenous growth factors to enhance wound healing focused on growth factors isolated from the patient's own tissue. Thrombin-induced platelet releasate (TIPR [Procuren]; Curative Health Services, Hauppauge, NY) is an autologous growth factor consisting of a clear, colorless, buffered solution containing naturally occurring growth factor proteins. The growth factors in TIPR include PDGF, transforming growth factor-β (TGF-β), EGF, and bFGF. These proteins have mitogenic and chemotactic properties necessary for wound healing. TIPR is obtained from a patient's own platelets with a single blood draw that usually provides an adequate supply for treating the wound. It is supplied in an aqueous buffered formulation and is applied to the wound bed on gauze for 12 hours, followed by 12 hours of aqueous saline gauze dressings.[27] This growth factor has been used for venous, diabetic, and pressure ulcers. An early phase I nonrandomized trial with chronic nonhealing cutaneous ulcers reported successful epithelialization in 93% of the chronic wounds, with an average time to complete reepithelialization of 7.5 weeks.[28] In a subsequent prospective, randomized, placebo-controlled, double-blind, crossover trial of 32 patients with wounds of mixed etiology, 81% treated in the positive arm achieved complete epithelialization in an average of 8.6 weeks of treatment. In the placebo arm, only 15% healed during the initial 8 weeks of placebo treatment, and, when those nonhealed ulcers were crossed over to the treatment arm, all 11 wounds resurfaced completely in an average of 7.1 weeks.[29] Analysis of 4 years of retrospective research demonstrates higher overall healing rates and lower amputation rates with platelet releasate and comprehensive wound care.[30] This multicenter, retrospective study evaluated wound healing and limb salvage outcomes over a 4-year period in over 3,000 patients treated in hospital-associated wound care centers. Those patients treated with comprehensive wound care plus platelet releasate demonstrated overall higher healing rates and lower amputation rates, compared with the group that received only comprehensive wound care.[30]

Later technology resulted in the production of single human growth factors by recombinant DNA technology. Recombinant human platelet-derived growth factor-BB (rhPDGF-BB, or becaplermin gel [Regranex Gel] (Ortho-McNeil Pharmaceutical, Inc., Raritan, NJ)) is the first recombinant growth factor to receive the United States Food and Drug Administration (FDA) approval. It was approved by the FDA in 1997 for the treatment of lower extremity diabetic neuropathic ulcers[31] and was first reported in the treatment of pressure ulcers in 1992.[20] In a phase I/II prospective, randomized, masked trail of 20 patients, 100 µg/mL topically applied PDGF-BB produced an increase in the rate of wound closure, compared with three other groups.[20,32] Mustoe et al[21] showed a trend toward healing acceleration, but the results did not reach statistical significance. Use of rhPDGF-BB (using becaplermin, a different formulation of PDGF-BB than in earlier studies) in pressure ulcers recently demonstrated improvement in wound healing than those wounds that did not use rhPDGF-BB.[22] Several prospective, double-blind, randomized, clinical trials have previously demonstrated that rhPDGF-BB as a topical application accelerates wound closure and actively helps to promote healing in diabetic neuropathic ulcers.[31]

Several other exogenous recombinant growth factors have been or are currently being investigated as wound healing agents. These include PDGF, bFGF, EGF, granulocytemacrophage colony-stimulating factor (GM-CSF), TGF-β, insulin-like growth factor I (IGF-I), and human growth hormone (HGH).[32] In addition, keratinocyte growth factor (KGF) and fibroblast growth factor (FGF) are currently being studied. Lastly, an autologous tissue coagulum graft prosthesis, AuTolo-Gel (Cytomedix, Inc., Deerfield, IL) is available. The product seals the wound with the patient's own blood products, initiates coagulation, and provides growth factors that accelerate the patient's own wound repair cascade. The inflammatory, proliferative, and maturation phases of wound repair are mediated by the autologous tissue coagulum. Blood is drawn from the patient for each treatment. The platelets and a small amount of plasma are added to proprietary activator products to form a gel that is applied topically by a physician and left in place for 5 days. The wound is then redressed with an alternative wound dressing for the next 7 days. The application of AuTolo-Gel, followed by an alternative dressing, is repeated, usually every 2 weeks until the wound heals. The product was designed to assist with healing in previously nonhealing, chronic wounds. To date, there are no randomized clinical trials for AuTolo-Gel.

Description and Effects

Regranex Gel is a topical gel that contains the active ingredient, becaplermin, formulated in an aqueous sodium carboxymethyl-cellulose-based (NaCMC) gel. Each gram of Regranex Gel contains 100 µg of becaplermin. The biological activity of becaplermin includes promoting recruitment (chemotaxis) and proliferation (mitosis) of cells involved in wound repair, and enhancing granulation tissue production (synthesis), which is similar to that of endogenous PDGF.

Indications for Use

Regranex Gel 0.01% is indicated for use in the treatment of diabetic neuropathic ulcers that extend into the subcutaneous tissue or beyond and have adequate blood supply.[31] When the product is used in conjunction with good wound care, it increases the incidence of complete wound healing. The cornerstones of good wound care include sharp debridement,[33] control of infection,[34] off-loading of pressure from the affected area,[35] and maintenance of a moist, clean wound

environment. The efficacy of becaplermin for the treatment of other types of wounds is currently being evaluated.[22]

Indications for Discontinuation

Becaplermin gel should be discontinued if the patient has extensive necrosis, untreated active infection, or ischemia. Once the ulcer is debrided, infection is treated, or the area is revascularized, the gel may be used. Continued treatment with becaplermin gel should be reassessed if the ulcer does not decrease in size by approximately 30% after 10 weeks of treatment or if complete healing has not occurred in 20 weeks.[31]

Method of Application

Regranex Gel is available in a 15-g multidose tube as a clear, colorless to straw-colored, topical gel. The dosage of gel to be applied will vary, depending on the size of the ulcer area. The formula to calculate the length of gel to be applied daily is length × width divided by 4.[31] For example, if the length of the ulcer measures 4.0 cm and the width measures 2.0 cm, multiply the length by the width and divide by 4 (4 × 2 = 8, divided by 4 = 2). A 2-cm length of gel should be used for this ulcer.

Clinical Wisdom

The amount of becaplermin gel to be applied to the wound should be recalculated by a wound care provider on a weekly or biweekly basis, depending on the rate of change in the surface area of the ulcer.

To apply the becaplermin gel, the calculated length of gel should be squeezed onto a clean surface, such as wax paper. The gel can then be transferred from the clean surface with an applicator, such as a cotton swab or tongue blade, and spread over the entire ulcer area at approximately 1/16 of an inch in thickness. The gel should be covered with a saline-moistened gauze dressing and left in place for approximately 12 hours. The dressing should then be removed and the ulcer rinsed with saline or water to remove the gel, then covered again with a second saline-moistened dressing without the gel for the next 12 hours. The gel should be applied once daily to the ulcer until complete healing occurs. If the ulcer does not decrease in size by approximately 30% after 10 weeks of treatment or if complete healing has not occurred in 20 weeks, continued treatment with the gel should be reassessed. Regranex Gel must be stored in the refrigerator. Do not freeze and do not use after the expiration date on the bottom of the tube.[31]

Precautions and Contraindications

Becaplermin gel is for external use only and is contraindicated in patients with known hypersensitivity to any component of the product or known neoplasms at the sites of application. Erythematous rashes occurred in 2% of patients treated with Regranex Gel. Wounds that close by primary intention should not be treated with Regranex Gel because it is a nonsterile, low-bioburden, preserved product. The effects of becaplermin on exposed joints, tendons, ligaments, and bone have not been established in humans. Carcinogenesis and reproductive toxicity studies have not been conducted. It is not known whether Regranex Gel can cause fetal harm when administered to a pregnant woman, can affect reproductive capacity, or is excreted in human milk. The safety and effectiveness in patients younger than 16 years old has not been established. It is also not known whether Regranex Gel interacts with other topical medications applied to the ulcer site.[31]

Expected Outcomes

When becaplermin gel is used in conjunction with good ulcer care, including initial sharp debridement, pressure relief, and infection control, the gel increases the incidence of complete healing of diabetic ulcers.[33]

Growth Factor Case Study

The patient is a 55-year-old Hispanic female with a 12-year history of type 2 diabetes; a 2-year history of Charcot deformity of the right foot; hypertension; peripheral neuropathy; nonhealing diabetic, neuropathic ulcer on the plantar surface of the right foot for 8 months; and tinea pedis of the toe webs. Figure 12–1 shows the ulcer predebridement, and Figure 12–2 is after debridement and initial application of becaplermin gel. The patient was using a walker and crutches to off-load pressure from the ulcer. Figure 12–3 shows improvement in the ulcer, with a decrease in size from 2.8 × 2.2 × 1.8 cm to 1.8 × 1.1 × 0.7 cm. Figure 12–4 shows further decrease in the ulcer size at 1.1 × 0.6 × 0.4 cm. Figure 12–5 shows complete wound closure, which took 14 weeks, once the ulcer was treated with becaplermin gel after weekly debridement. The patient is now in custom-molded shoes with no recurrence of the ulcer. (For basic information on growth factors and physiology of wound healing, see Chapter 2.)

LIVING SKIN EQUIVALENTS
Mark S. Granick

For over a century, skin grafting has been a valuable reconstructive tool. However, there are some problems and

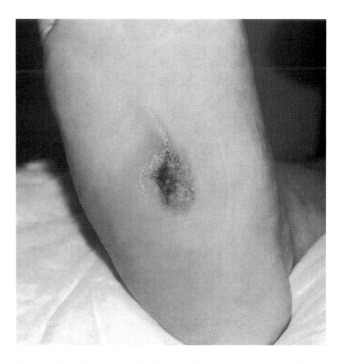

Figure 12–1 Ulcer pre-debridement. *Source:* Copyright © Nancy Tomaselli.

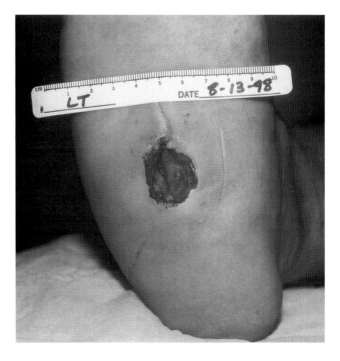

Figure 12–2 Ulcer post-debridement, Regranex growth factor treatment started. *Source:* Copyright © Nancy Tomaselli.

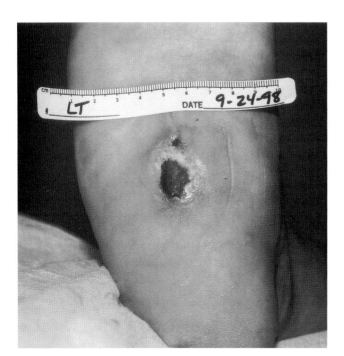

Figure 12–3 Ulcer after 6 weeks on Regranex growth factor treatment. *Source:* Copyright © Nancy Tomaselli.

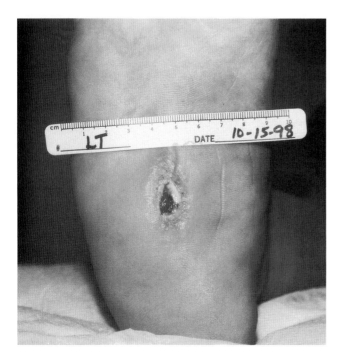

Figure 12–4 Ulcer 10 weeks after Regranex growth factor treatment started. *Source:* Copyright © Nancy Tomaselli.

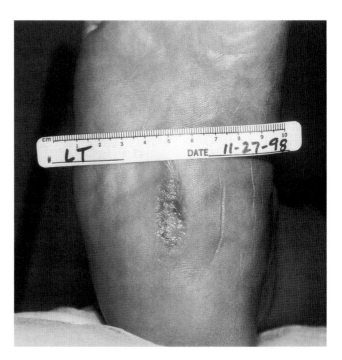

Figure 12–5 Complete wound closure. *Source:* Copyright © Nancy Tomaselli.

limitations with this technique. There is always a donor site, which can be painful or unsightly. The graft does not always take and heal the wound. In very large wounds or burns, the need for grafts can necessitate the use of reharvested donor sites, unusual donor sites, wide meshing of the grafts, and other creative strategies for obtaining wound coverage. There has clearly been a need for an off-the-shelf skin substitute that can promote healing, eliminate the donor site, be quickly and easily accessible, minimize contracture and scarring, and be immunologically compatible. There has been an evolution in product design that has led us to the living skin equivalents (LSEs).[36] Only one LSE is currently approved for use. The product is graftskin (Apligraf), and it is approved for the treatment of venous ulcers.

Dermagraft (Advanced Tissue Sciences, Inc., LaJolla, CA) is another product that failed to pass FDA approval until further clinical studies are completed. There are numerous other comparable constructs, either under development or in various phases of FDA testing. Because graftskin is the only commercially available LSE at this time, this section will primarily concentrate on that particular product. Our concept of what a living skin equivalent is, how it functions, and what it can accomplish revolves around the accumulating data concerning graftskin.

Description and Effects

Graftskin is a bilaminar construct consisting of a simulated dermal phase and a simulated epidermal layer.[37] The dermal component is a bovine collagen mesh, seeded with living neonatal fibroblasts. The fibroblasts are a pure fibroblast cell culture, derived from neonatal foreskin. The epidermal layer is a pure keratinocyte culture, similarly derived from neonatal foreskin. Histologically, it closely resembles normal skin without the rete ridges. The technical difficulties in creating pure cell cultures free of bacterial contamination and being able to deliver them to remote sites on demand for clinical use are incredible. At the moment, the FDA approval is for its use on venous leg ulcers, along with standard therapeutic compression.

Indications for Use

Although approved for use on venous ulcers,[38] the LSEs have been useful in obtaining healing in diabetic foot ulcers,[39] epidermolysis bullosa,[40] skin graft donor sites,[41] and burns.[36] Since graftskin has become commercially available, a wide variety of off-label uses have been employed and discussed, but few series have been published to date.

Indications for Discontinuation

There are few indications for discontinuation of the product. The presence of infection or allergic reaction would be strong indicators for discontinuing treatment with graftskin. Failure of the wound to improve significantly after two applications of the LSE would be another reason to cease further treatment with the product.

Method of Application

The product arrives in a thermally controlled box. It must be incubated until it is used, which needs to be soon after it is received. The graft is 7.5 cm in diameter. It is packaged on agarose media that is colored with a pH indicator in a Petri dish. The graft is gently lifted and placed on the wound with overlapping edges. A compression wrap is used to fix it in place.[42] It is indicated for use on wounds that are free of infection and necrotic debris. It may be necessary to pretreat the wound with mechanical debridement or topical antibiotics before applying the graft.

Clinical Wisdom

During graftskin use, all cytotoxic substances, such as Dakin's solution, chlorhexidine, or povidone-iodine, must be avoided.

Precautions and Contraindications

Graftskin is contraindicated in infected wounds or in people who are allergic to bovine collagen or the agarose shipping media.

Expected Outcomes

Initially, the LSE sticks to a clean wound and looks like a skin graft. After about a week, the material loses its appearance as a graft and takes on a gelatinous look. It is important not to disrupt the LSE during the first 2–3 weeks, due to these changes. It can easily be washed away. The LSE does not heal the way a skin graft does, despite its initial appearance. The LSE cells are rapidly replaced by the patient's own cells. The wound, which typically begins as a chronically indolent, inactive surface, becomes biologically more active. The wound healing cascade is stimulated. The LSE acts as a biologic growth factor factory, as well as providing a biologic occlusion at the surface. This increased activity continues for 6–8 weeks. If the wound achieves full healing, there is minimal contracture, and it achieves a remarkably normal appearance. In fact, the patient's own melanocytes repopulate the healing area to obtain a confluent color. If additional treatment is required, a new LSE can be applied.

Graftskin Case Study

The patient illustrated in Figures 12–6, 12–7, and 12–8 has chronic venous disease in her leg. She has been treated with chronic compression, with which she has been poorly compliant. Several years ago, she underwent a skin graft that healed an ulcer. She reappeared with a recurrence in the middle of her old skin graft. She was treated with graftskin. Initially, it looked like a healed skin graft. It then went through a gelatinous phase. The wound healed within 8 weeks and has remained healed for over 1 year.

ARTIFICIAL SKIN
Dayna E. Gary

There has long been a need for alternatives in the treatment of full-thickness or deep partial-thickness life-threatening burn injuries. These types of patients present unique wound challenges. The most common surgical treatment is the use of autografts and allografts, in the attempt to excise and close the wounds as soon as possible. The limitations of this conventional treatment are: the short supply of autograft, need for multiple surgeries, consequences of having large open wounds, and poor cosmetic and functional outcomes. Integra Artificial Skin (Johnson & Johnson Medical, Division of Ethicon Inc., Somerville, NJ) was initially developed in 1980 by Yannas and Burke[43] and is a dermal regeneration template that was developed to address these limitations.

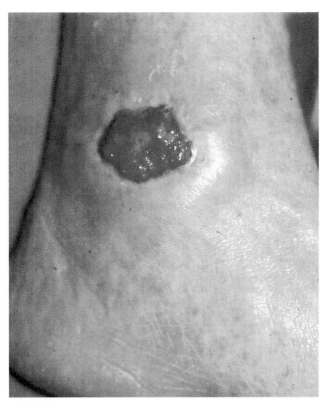

Figure 12–6 Recurrent venous ulcer. *Source:* Copyright © Mark S. Granick, MD, FACS.

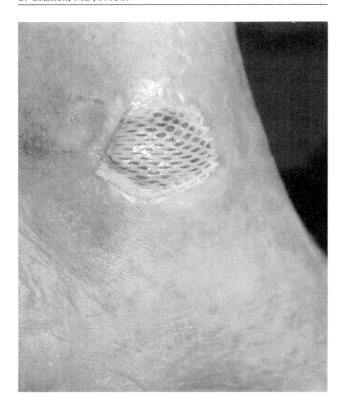

Figure 12–7 Apligraf living skin equivalent in place. *Source:* Copyright © Mark S. Granick, MD, FACS.

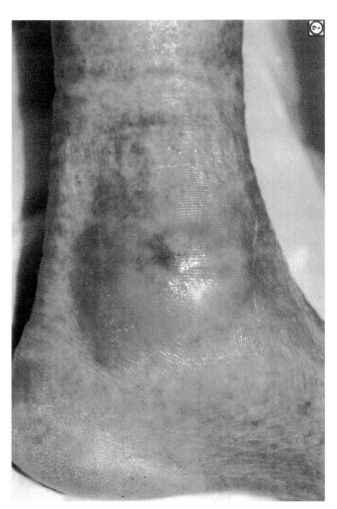

Figure 12–8 Complete wound closure within 8 weeks of therapy. The wound has remained healed for over one year. *Source:* Copyright © Mark S. Granick, MD, FACS.

Description

Integra Artificial Skin consists of two layers. The dermal replacement layer is made up of a porous matrix of fibers of cross-linked bovine tendon collagen and a glycosaminoglycan ([GAG] chondroitin-6-sulfate). The epidermal substitute layer is made of a thin polysiloxane (silicone) layer to control moisture loss from the wound.[44] The dermal replacement layer serves as a template for the infiltration of fibroblasts, macrophages, lymphocytes, and capillaries that form the neovascular network. The collagen deposition by the fibroblasts replaces the dermal replacement layer. Integra Artificial Skin has a prolonged shelf life and must be stored in a refrigerator at 2–8° C.[44] It is supplied in 4″ × 5″, 4″ × 10″, and 8″ × 10″ and can be bought by the sheet or by the box.

Indications

The FDA has approved the use of Integra Artificial Skin for the postexcisional treatment of life-threatening full-thickness or deep partial-thickness thermal injury where sufficient autograft is not available at the time of excision or not desirable due to the physiologic condition of the patient. It has been noted by many surgeons that this product has multiple off-label applications. It has been used successfully in the treatment of diabetic foot ulcers, venous stasis ulcers, and arterial ulcers. One advantage is that Integra Artificial Skin can be applied and the patient sent home. Weeks later, when the neodermis has formed, the patient can be brought in as an outpatient, and surgery for the epidermal graft can then be performed. Another advantage is that this product does not require perfect vascular supply to ensure success.

This product has been employed successfully for scar reconstruction, including scar resurfacing, keloids, treatment of donor sites, and treatment of chronic wounds.[2] It is beneficial in the treatment of necrotizing fasciitis by allowing for a height build-up via the layering of Integra Artificial Skin,[45] decreased wound contraction, and early wound closure. Two studies have indicated a good outcome with the use of cultured epithelial cells with Integra Artificial Skin. This technique allows for the early physiologic closure of large wounds with the Integra Artificial Skin and the epidermal grafting with cultured epithelial grafts to decrease donor site morbidity and/or deal with the challenge of little to no donor site availability.[46,47]

Contraindications

This product should not be used in those patients with a known hypersensitivity to bovine collagen or chondroitin materials. These are the components of the dermal replacement layer. Do not use Integra Artificial Skin in the presence of wound infection because the product will fail partially or completely. This product is more vulnerable than the typical skin graft.

Benefits

Integra Artificial Skin has many properties that make it advantageous. First and foremost, it allows for early excision of all burned tissue and coverage in one surgery that allows for physiologic closure.[48] This physiologic closure has been shown to reduce the nutritional requirements in patients who are typically very catabolic.[49] It requires thin epidermal donor sites that heal very quickly with less long-term scarring.[48,50] Histologic studies found that, at 7 days to 2 years after silicone removal/epidermal grafting, there was no scar formation, as well as no concentration of mast cells.[51] In a study looking at the outcomes over a 10-year span, areas grafted with Integra Artificial Skin were found to have effective wound healing after injury, near-normal cosmesis and mechanical behavior, normal antibacterial defense, and growth with patient growth.[44]

Disadvantages

Integra Artificial Skin requires two surgeries at least 2 weeks apart to allow for neodermis formation.[5] Usually for large burns, this is not a problem because they would be undergoing multiple surgeries if they were being treated by conventional methods. For smaller burns, this necessitates either a lengthened hospital stay or, if the patient is compliant, he or she can be sent home and must return for the second surgery. This product requires more heightened care operatively and postoperatively to ensure "take."[50] Postoperative technical problems include: hematoma formation, graft wrinkling with subsequent serous fluid collection, and separation of the silicone layer at the periphery.[44] There is also an increased risk of infection. Areas of infection must be drained or excised; otherwise, the infection rapidly spreads, causing partial or complete failure.

Instructions for Use

Preoperative and Operative Care. The standard burn center protocol for topical agents and antibiotics should be employed. Early and complete excision of burn eschar and necrotic and contaminated tissue should be performed, ensuring a viable graft bed, such as white dermis, pure yellow fat, or glistening fascia. Meticulous hemostasis must be achieved to prevent hematoma or seroma formation, and the graft bed should be smooth and flat to ensure good contact with the Integra Artificial Skin. If complete excision is not possible, a barrier must be in place to separate Integra Artificial Skin from unexcised skin, ie, excise and place allograft.

The FDA requires physicians to be trained prior to using Integra Artificial Skin, and physicians are the only team member allowed to apply this product.

In the operating room, the Integra Artificial Skin should be removed from the package and rinsed with sterile normal saline until the alcohol smell is gone. Integra Artificial Skin may be applied as a sheet or meshed at a 1:1 ratio. The meshed Integra Artificial Skin should not be expanded. The advantages of the meshed Integra Artificial Skin are that it decreases risk of fluid accumulation and hematoma formation, allows antimicrobials to penetrate wound bed, and improves conformability. The disadvantages of the meshed Integra Artificial Skin are that it does not allow for physiologic closure, is a possible pathway for bacteria to enter wound, and may encourage granulation tissue to form a mesh pattern.

Whether sheet or mesh, the Integra Artificial Skin is affixed with either staples or sutures.

Postoperative Care. The dressings consist of a stretch elastic net pulled tightly directly over the Integra Artificial

Skin. This promotes good contact of the Integra Artificial Skin with the wound bed, helps prevent dislodgement, and allows visibility. The antimicrobial dressings are placed directly over the elastic net. Options include: moistened Acticoat (Westaim Biomedical, Exeter, NH) or burn-roll soaked with 5% Sulfamylon solution. All solutions will need rewetting. Cover all the Integra Artificial Skin with antimicrobial dressing if it is meshed; cover seams if it is nonmeshed. Do not use Xeroform or any petrolatum products. Apply an outer dressing, such as Kerlix, and an Ace wrap for mild compression. Apply splints to immobilize joints for 3–5 days to prevent dislodgement. Occupational therapy and physical therapy may begin after 3–5 days. Special care must be taken not to sheer the Integra Artificial Skin or pull the edges apart. Use compressive wraps for ambulation.

Integra Artificial Skin should be monitored daily for infection, seromas, or hematomas. Such areas should be aspirated or removed immediately. The elastic net allows for observation of the Integra Artificial Skin and should remain intact during dressing changes if there are no complications. The outer dressings should be changed every 4–5 days. Do not allow immersion in water.

Expected Outcomes

The silicone layer is removed 14–21 days after application when the deposition of new dermal tissue and resorption of the collagen-GAG matrix has occurred. The neodermis has formed when it blanches under compression, there is separation/wrinkling of the silicone layer, and the color is a peachy/pink, yellow color. Do not remove the silicone layer until neodermis has formed completely. It should be easy to remove at this point. A thin epidermal graft of 0.003–0.007 inches is harvested. The grafts may be placed as a sheet or a mesh and should be attached per standard protocol.

Integra Artificial Skin is a dermal regeneration template that addresses the limitations of the conventional methods most commonly employed in the treatment of life-threatening full-thickness and deep partial-thickness burn injuries and has shown promising uses in off-label applications.

PROLONGED SILVER RELEASE DRESSINGS
Dayna E. Gary with Arglaes Case Study by Paula Tashjian

Silver has been used in the fight against infection since the late nineteenth century.[52] Silver kills microbes by poisoning respiratory enzymes and components of the microbial electron transport system, as well as impairing some DNA functions.[53,54] Until recently, there were only two choices in which to provide the beneficial properties of silver—silver sulfadiazine cream (Silvadene, Thermazene) and silver nitrate solution—both with significant limitations. Silver nitrate solution causes staining and must be applied in large quantities and multiple times per day to be effective.[55] Silver sulfadiazine cream must be cleansed and applied daily, often leaving a pseudo-eschar that must be removed. It has also been found to promote maceration and slow wound epithelialization.[56] Acticoat (Westaim Biomedical, Exeter, NH) and Arglaes (Medline Industries, Inc., Mundelein, IL) have been designed to overcome these limitations.

Acticoat and Arglaes are two dressings currently on the market that provide prolonged-release silver to fight infection and promote normal wound healing. These dressings provide a moist wound healing environment that decreases wound pain, prevents wound desiccation, and promotes the retention of exudate containing polymorphonuclear leukocytes and growth factors.[57] These dressings provide noncytotoxic antimicrobial control. In vitro cytotoxicity tests showed that Acticoat was significantly less cytotoxic than silver nitrate.[58] In vitro studies demonstrated the effectiveness of these dressings against Gram-negative, Gram-positive, and antibiotic-resistant bacteria, and against fungi.[59] These products eliminate the need for daily dressings, which decreases the chance of contaminating other wounds on the body, decreases risk of spread to others, decreases pain to the patient caused by daily dressings, is less disruptive to new epithelialization, decreases amount of dressing supplies needed, and decreases nursing care hours. Acticoat and Arglaes both offer these advantages; however, they are constructed differently and have some different characteristics that should be understood to make an appropriate dressing choice.

Acticoat

Acticoat is a made up of a rayon/polyester core that helps to manage moisture level and controls the release of silver surrounded by a silver-coated high-density polyethylene mesh that facilitates the passage of silver through the dressing. Acticoat is available in $4'' \times 4''$, $4'' \times 8''$, $4'' \times 48''$, $8'' \times 16''$, and $16'' \times 16''$. For heavily exudative wounds, the Acticoat is applied dry. The exudate causes the silver ions to be released. Otherwise, Acticoat needs to be moistened with sterile water approximately every 6 hours to ensure antimicrobial activity. The Acticoat moistening can be accomplished by placing holes into the top of the sterile water bottle and sprinkling the water onto the dressing or by the placement of small tubes with tiny holes in them applied on top of the dressing and flushed with sterile water. The goal is to keep the Acticoat moist, not wet, to prevent maceration. Do not moisten with saline. Acticoat should be changed every 3–5 days. If it has adhered, soak the dressing prior to removal to prevent damage. Figures 12–9, 12–10, and 12–11 show Acticoat dressing in place and the typical wound reaction with the dressing.

A multitude of studies have been performed on this dressing. Studies looking at the killing curve of this nanocrystal-

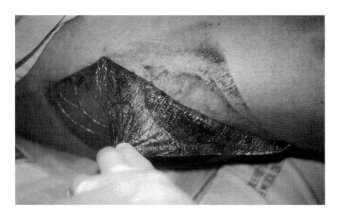

Figure 12–9 Acticoat dressing over posterior/lateral thigh donor site loosening from edges after standard self-shower/hydrotherapy. Mild staining usually resolves in 24–48 hours. *Source:* Copyright © Westaim Biomedical, Exeter, New Hampshire.

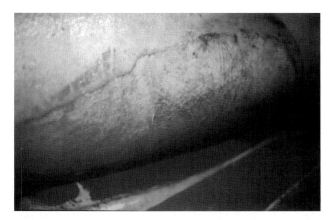

Figure 12–10 Benign exudate layer over posterior/lateral thigh donor site from Acticoat dressing. *Source:* Copyright © Westaim Biomedical, Exeter, New Hampshire.

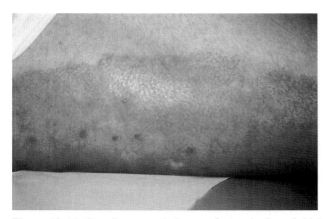

Figure 12–11 Complete wound closure of posterior/lateral thigh donor site. *Source:* Copyright © Westaim Biomedical, Exeter, New Hampshire.

line-coated dressing determined that bacterial survival was undetectable at 30 minutes. This fast kill rate is important because it shows that the dressing can be used as a barrier to bacterial penetration, as well as ensuring less opportunity to develop antimicrobial resistance.[60] A possible mechanism of wound contamination is bacterial translocation through the dressing. A rat model study indicated that the Acticoat had a significant impact on rat survival.[61] In vitro studies demonstrated the effectiveness of Acticoat against Gram-positive and Gram-negative pathogens. Zone of inhibition tests demonstrated the ability of Acticoat in inhibiting growth of bacteria for 9 days for Gram-positive and Gram-negative pathogens.[8] Bactericidal assays performed demonstrated the efficacy of Acticoat against antibiotic-resistant bacteria.[62] In vitro fungicidal efficacy of a variety of topical agents was performed, indicating that the Acticoat provided the fastest and broadest-spectrum fungicidal efficacy.[63]

Indications

Acticoat is indicated for a wide variety of acute and chronic wound types, including:

- Pressure ulcers
- Venous stasis ulcers
- Diabetic ulcers
- Surgical and traumatic wounds
- Partial-thickness burns
- Debrided full-thickness burns
- Grafts
- Donor sites

Contraindications

Acticoat would not be advantageous in healing, noninfected wounds. It is also not appropriate in wounds with eschar. The eschar must be debrided prior to application. Do not use oil-based cleansing agents or wound dressings. Do not moisten Acticoat with saline; use sterile water.

> **Clinical Wisdom**
>
> The Acticoat will need to be moistened at different intervals, depending on geography. In more humid areas, the Acticoat will need less wetting because it will stay moistened longer.

Arglaes

Arglaes literally means "silver glass." This "glass" is produced by heating the controlled-release polymers sodium phosphate and calcium phosphate. Arglaes is available as a film dressing and as an island dressing. The Arglaes barrier film dressing is a transparent film seeded with Arglaes in the polyurethane film and the adhesive. The Arglaes island dressing has the same controlled-release and antimicrobial properties as the film dressing, with the addition of a calcium alginate pad. The film dressing is available in 2-3/8″ × 3–1/8″, 4″ × 4–3/4″, and 6″ × 10″. The island dressing is available in 2-3/8″ × 3-1/8″, with the pad 1″ × 2″; 4″ × 4-3/4″, with the pad 2″ × 2″; and 6″ × 10″, with the pad 4″ × 6″. The application and removal of this product is similar to a transparent film. With the island dressing, it has been suggested that, to prevent a "drawing" sensation, the wound should be moistened with saline immediately before applying the dressing. Saline should also be used to remove any remaining gel after the removal of the island dressing.

Ovington[55] suggests that the current popular use for the film dressing is over the harvest sites of coronary artery bypass grafts, where it has been shown to decrease postoperative infections. It is also popular to use over central-line access sites to reduce the risk of infection. An in vitro study indicated the efficacy of this dressing against Gram-positive and -negative bacteria, and fungi, with a better efficacy toward Gram-negative pathogens.[59] Another study indicated that Arglaes appears to control bacteria in wounds and prevents bacterial contamination.[64] It was noted in one case study that Arglaes is effective against methicillin-resistant *Staphylococcus aureus* (MRSA).[65] Further studies indicating the role of Arglaes in wound care are needed. Arglaes is different from Acticoat, in that it does not require the moistening of the dressing with sterile water. It also provides a high moisture-vapor transmission rate (MVTR) that allows water vapor to evaporate from the patient's skin faster than standard film dressings, increasing wearing time and decreasing chance of maceration.

Indications

Arglaes is indicated for a wide variety of acute and chronic wounds, including:

- Intravenous line sites: central venous pressure lines (CVPs), peripheral intravenous central catheter (PICC)
- Surgical wounds
- Wide range of flat wounds
- Pressure ulcers
- Minor burns
- Moderately to heavily draining wounds (island dressing)

Contraindications

This dressing is not appropriate in well-healing, noninfected wounds. It should not be used in wounds with eschar. The eschar needs to be debrided prior to use. The island dressing should not be used on dry wounds to prevent further desiccation.

The use of silver to prevent and/or fight infection is well known. Until recently, the only choices available had multiple limitations. With the addition of Arglaes and Acticoat, there is now a choice of dressings that addresses these limitations.

VACUUM-ASSISTED CLOSURE
Elizabeth Hiltabidel and Adela M. Valenzuela

Definition

Vacuum-assisted closure (VAC) is a therapeutic product manufactured by Kinetic Concepts, Incorporated (KCI USA, Inc., San Antonio, TX) for the management of acute, subacute, and chronic wounds. The FDA approved the commercial marketing of the VAC in 1995. The VAC technique involves placing an open-cell foam dressing into the wound cavity and applying controlled subatmospheric pressure, typically 125 mm Hg below ambient pressure (Table 12–1). The therapy objective is to remove chronic edema, increase localized blood flow, and remove infectious material/fluid, with resultant enhanced formation of granulation tissue.[66]

Theory and Science of the Therapy

The application of negative pressure to the wound increases tension among adjacent cells, which is believed to alter the cells shape. This stimulates cell growth and division, drawing the edges of the wound to the center and promoting wound closure. The occlusive dressing provides a moist wound environment to promote more effective cellular activity and helps to prevent contamination of the wound site from outside bacteria.[67]

The production of granulation tissue in a wound depends on angiogenesis to provide a matrix to which collagen fibers support themselves. Negative pressure applied to a wound causes mechanical stress to the cells in close proximity to the open-cell foam and, thus, has been shown to increase the rate of cellular proliferation and neoangiogenesis. The application of negative pressure also removes excess interstitial fluid, which results in a decrease in the local interstitial pressure, thus restoring blood flow to those vessels compressed or collapsed by the excess pressure. Chronic wound fluid contains factors that, when applied to cells in culture, inhibit or suppress mitosis, protein synthesis, and fibroblast collagen synthesis. Active withdrawal of this fluid from nonhealing or slow-healing wounds decreases the inhibitory factors.[68]

An additional mechanism of action is the mechanical stimulation of cells by tensile forces placed on the surrounding tissue, due to collapse of the foam dressing. The concept that tissues respond to applied force has long been recog-

Arglaes Case Study

This case describes a 70-year-old African-American male, B.P., who presented with recurrent multiple full-thickness wounds on the right lower extremity. The area was extremely edematous, painful on elevation and rest, and heavily exudating. The wounds were covered with necrotic tissue, and there were tendons exposed on the foot. The patient's history was significant for non–insulin-dependent diabetes, peripheral vascular disease (PVD), recent myocardial infarction (MI), and pyoderma gangrenousum (PG). Previous wound biopsy showed inflammation, and a clinical diagnosis of PG was made. Past surgical history included a femoral-popliteal bypass 11/98, coronary angioplasty 10/84, and surgical wound sharp debridement 12/98. With current presentation, PG was initially suspected, because of the clinical history of PG; however, no biopsy was performed, and PG was eventually clinically ruled out. B.P. developed intermittent pseudomonas infections, which increased the pain and drainage from the wound sites, and systemic antibiotic therapy was utilized with each episode of infection. His wounds were treated with alginates or foam dressings and a 4-layer compression wrap for over 30 days, with little to no improvement. Surgical sharp debridement of the ulcers followed and still no progression to healing. Pain management was a challenge, and in-home, conservative sharp debridement could not be performed. His fasting blood

sugars at the time averaged 200–300, related to prednisone usage. Current medications included prednisone (40 mg), azathioprine (Imuran [50 mg]) and morphine sulfate controlled release (MS Contin [15 mg]) for pain, along with his routine cardiac and diabetic medication. A combination of a controlled-release silver film dressing (Arglaes) and compression were initiated on 1/26/99 after 2 months of unsuccessful treatment.

Even though a diagnosis was never confirmed, B.P.'s wounds responded very favorably to this combination of therapies. Several components, such as the bacterial burden in the wound bed and venous stasis disease, were the key to his wound care and treatment. Once the silver-impregnated film dressing and the nonelastic compression therapy were initiated, there was a dramatic improvement in the overall appearance of B.P.'s lower extremities. Within 30 days, the previously exposed tendons were covered with 100% granulation tissue, and the wounds had decreased in size. Less pain medication was required, and the patient tolerated in-home debridement on a prn basis. The pictures presented here demonstrate the progress of B.P.'s very challenging wounds. Figure 12–12 dated 1/26/99 was taken just before the silver film dressing and compression dressing were initiated. Figures 12–13, 12–14, and 12–15 were taken at 4-week intervals.

Table 12–1 Recommended Guidelines for Treating Wound Types

Wound Type	Cycle	Target Pressure (Black Foam)	Target Pressure (Soft Foam)	Dressing Change Interval
Acute/Traumatic	Continuous first 48 hrs	125 mm Hg	125–175 mm Hg; titrate up for more drainage	Every 48 hrs (every 12 hrs with infection)
Pressure Ulcers	Continuous first 48 hrs	125 mm Hg	125–175 mm Hg; titrate up for more drainage	Every 48 hrs (every 12 hrs with infection)
Surgical	Continuous first 48 hrs	125 mm Hg	125–175 mm Hg; titrate up for more drainage	Every 48 hrs (every 12 hrs with infection)
Meshed Grafts	Continuous for duration of therapy	75–125 mm Hg	125 mm Hg; titrate up for more drainage	None. Remove dressing after 3–5 days
Chronic Ulcers	Continuous for duration of therapy	50-75 mm Hg	125 mm Hg; titrate up for more drainage	Every 48 hrs (every 12 hrs with infection)
Fresh Flaps	Continuous for duration of therapy	125 mm Hg	125–175 mm Hg; titrate up for more drainage	Every 48 hrs (every 12 hrs with infection)
Compromised Flaps	Continuous for duration of therapy	125 mm Hg	125 mm Hg; titrate up for more drainage	Every 48 hrs (every 12 hrs with infection)

Source: The VAC® Physician & Caregiver Reference Manual,© 1999 KCI USA, Inc.

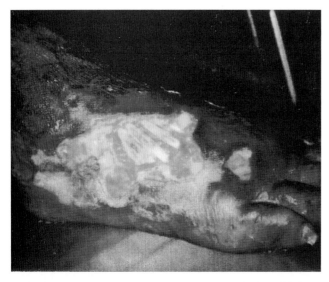

Figure 12–12 Full thickness right lower extremity ulcer with exposed tendons prior to beginning therapy with Arglaes silver impregnated film dressings and compression dressings. *Source:* Copyright © Paula Tashjian.

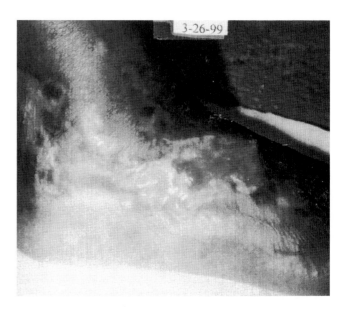

Figure 12–14 Lower extremity ulcer with granulation tissue now even with or flush with the skin surface, and evidence of wound contraction in smaller wound size. *Source:* Copyright © Paula Tashjian.

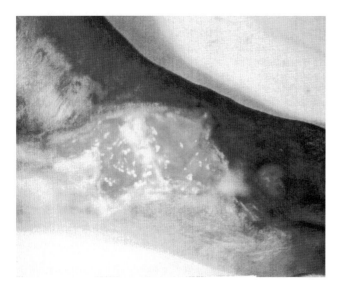

Figure 12–13 Lower extremity ulcer after 1 month of therapy with Arglaes silver impregnated film dressings and compression dressings. Previously exposed tendons are completely covered with granulation tissue. *Source:* Copyright © Paula Tashjian.

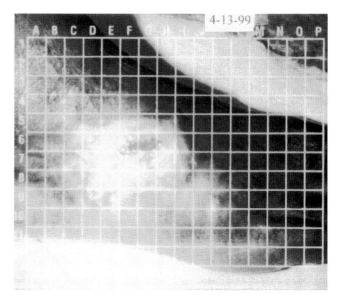

Figure 12–15 Lower extremity ulcer with new epithelial tissue and significant progress in healing. *Source:* Copyright © Paula Tashjian.

nized in relation to bone lengthening (Illazarov procedure) and to soft tissues (tissue expanders). The application and/or release of forces on tissues surrounding wounds results in deformation of cells anchored in the tissues. Cellular deformation results in release of secondary messengers, followed by changes in expression of immediate-early genes, with subsequent increases in cellular proliferation and protein synthesis.[69]

There are numerous clinical case studies that have been reported in the literature to show enhanced wound healing related to VAC therapy.[70–72] Joseph et al[66] did a blinded prospective randomized trial, looking at the healing rates of chronic nonhealing wounds using VAC versus wet to moist dressings. The study showed that, after 6 weeks of treatment, the percentages of change in wound volume were 78% reduction with VAC and 30% with wet to moist dressings. The most significant difference in volume was change in depth of 66% for VAC and 20% for wet to moist. Complete wound closure was not a realistic end point of the study because wounds were of variable sizes and anatomic location. Chronic wounds of large volume may require 16–20 weeks for complete closure, whereas 80–90% closure may occur in 3–6 weeks. Therefore, a 90% reduction in volume over time was used as the dependent variable in multivariate analysis. In cases where complete wound closure was not achieved, wounds treated with the VAC system showed a layer of granulation tissue. An adequate (100%) granulation bed was rarely seen in the wet to moist group.[66]

Indications for Therapy

VAC therapy is used to enhance healing and promote closure in a variety of open wounds. Chronic full-thickness wounds, such as stages III and IV pressure ulcers, along with venous, arterial, and neuropathic ulcers, have all been proven appropriate for negative-pressure wound therapy. Subacute and acute wounds, including burns, dehisced incisions, split-thickness meshed skin grafts, and muscle flaps, also have been shown to benefit from VAC therapy.[68,73] The authors have successfully used VAC conservatively on select wounds complicated by fistulae, as an off-label application, and wounds with exposed bone, tendon and/or orthopedic hardware (see Table 12–2 for choosing the specific type of polyurethane foam for use with VAC therapy).

Contraindications

Contraindications for treatment with VAC include necrotic tissue, untreated osteomyelitis, malignancy in the wound, and fistulas to organs or body cavities. Precautions to consider include active bleeding, anticoagulant use, and difficult wound hemostasis. The *VAC Recommended Guidelines for Use*[74] states that fistulae to organs or body cavities are contraindications for the therapy. KCI USA, Inc. has been doing extensive research on the use of VAC on wounds complicated with fistula and has applied to the FDA to remove fistulas from the list of contraindications and to list it as a precaution. These authors, under direct supervision of physicians, have been successful with placement of VAC on wounds complicated with multiple types of fistulae and over body organs. When vital organs are exposed, precautions, such as the placement of absorbable Vicryl mesh or its equivalent, should be considered.[68]

VAC is not a miracle cure. It enhances the body's natural capability to heal by accelerating the formation of granulation tissue, improving perfusion through removal of excess interstitial fluid (edema) and reducing bacterial colonization. It will not revascularize clogged veins or cure untreated infections.[68]

Cost Analysis

In a study by Philbeck et al,[75] records for 1,032 Medicare home care patients with 1,170 wounds that failed to respond to previous interventions—and subsequently treated with the VAC—were reviewed. Reductions in wound area were compared with rates reported by Ferrell et al[76] in 1993, and costs were analyzed. Ferrell reported trochanteric and trunk pressure ulcers averaging 4.3 cm^2, treated with a low-air-loss (LAL) surface and saline-soaked gauze closed at an average of 0.090 cm^2 per day. For comparison with Ferrell's outcomes, Philbeck et al analyzed their stages III and IV trochanteric and trunk wounds treated with LAL and the VAC Those averaged 22.2 cm^2 in area and closed at an average 0.23 cm^2 per day. The average 22.2 cm^2 wound in the Philbeck study, treated as described by Ferrell, would take 247 days to heal and cost $23,465. Using VAC, the wound would heal in 97 days and cost $14,546. The cost comparison took into account the costs of materials—including equipment rental—and home care nursing visits. Philbeck concluded that VAC therapy is an efficacious and economical treatment modality for a variety of chronic wounds.[75]

In an independent analysis of the same patient data used in Philbeck's study, the Weinberg group[77] considered only wounds that were over 30 days old and had failed previous interventions (n = 979). Once treated with VAC therapy, 77% of those wounds closed or were progressing toward closure after 60 days. Weinberg concluded that, on average, VAC therapy would successfully heal more chronic wounds than would standard therapies, and that VAC would cost $1,925 less per patient.[77]

Research and case studies have demonstrated that the use of VAC therapy can decrease hospital stays, office visits, and/or home visits. Costs for VAC equipment rental and dressing supplies will vary among institutions and geographic locations. Caregivers need to stay abreast of Medicare, state aid, and managed care contracts regarding the reimbursement of VAC therapy, because they are continuously being reviewed and revised.

Application Technique

The application of the VAC system is a simple technique, with equipment that is very user-friendly. The digital readout on the pump guides the user through different options, such as pressure settings and problem solving. Equipment that is unfamiliar to health care providers can be intimidating; therefore, the authors recommend that institutions de-

Table 12–2 Recommended Guidelines for Foam Use

Indications	VAC® Polyurethane (black foam)	VAC® Soft foam (white foam)	Both	Either
Deep, acute wounds with moderate granulation tissue growth	X			
Deep wounds with extremely rapid growth in granulation tissue			X	
Deep pressure ulcers	X			
Superficial wounds		X		
Venous stasis ulcers		X		
Postgraft therapy				X
Compromised flaps	X			
Fresh flaps	X			
Tunneling/sinus tracks/undermining		X		
Diabetic ulcers				X
Dry wounds	X			
Deep trauma wounds			X	
Superficial trauma wounds				X
Burns	X			

Source: The VAC® Physician & Caregiver Reference Manual,© 1999 KCI USA, Inc.

velop a technique for the use of the VAC system (see Figure 12–16). Users should be educated on the equipment, application, removal, and monitoring of the therapy in order to achieve positive patient outcomes. Once health care professionals are comfortable with the therapy, the cost benefits, including time savings and improved patient outcomes, will be realized.

WARM-UP WOUND THERAPY SYSTEM
Joy Edvalson

Most wounds are hypothermic—averaging 5.6° F cooler than core body temperature.[78] Hypothermia causes vasoconstriction, depresses neutrophil activity, reduces the ability of the cells to use oxygen-free radicals to kill bacteria, and lowers collagen deposition. Hypothermia not only impairs the normal function of the immune system, it also weakens host resistance to wound infection and delays wound healing.[79–81] With warming wound therapy, the skin and subcutaneous tissues are warmed toward core body temperature (normothermia), which increases blood flow to the wound by vasodilatation. Increased blood flow delivers more subcutaneous oxygen and growth factors to the wound, which improves cellular functions.[82] (See Chapter 25 for more information on thermal regulation with heat.)

The Warm-Up wound therapy system (Augustine Medical, Eden Prairie, MN) provides safe and precise warming technology to create a controlled, humidified, noncontact healing environment for wounds. The system is comprised of a temperature control unit that can be operated from an AC adapter or with a rechargeable battery pack; a sterile wound cover that is water-resistant, semiocclusive, disposable, and latex free; and a warming card that delivers radiant warmth to the wound bed area (see Figure 12–19). The wound cover is designed to surround the wound and provide a noncontact environment that will not disrupt new cell growth. The wound cover also insulates against heat loss in order to maintain an ideal environment for wound healing. The trans-

VACUUM ASSISTED CLOSURE (VAC®)
WOUND CLOSURE SYSTEM

PERSONNEL WHO TYPICALLY PERFORM TECHNIQUE: MD, RN, PA, NP, PT

EQUIPMENT NEEDED:
Gloves	VAC® pump
Scissors	VAC® cannister kit—includes cannister and tubing
Wound cleanser	VAC® dressing assembly—sponge, drape, and catheter

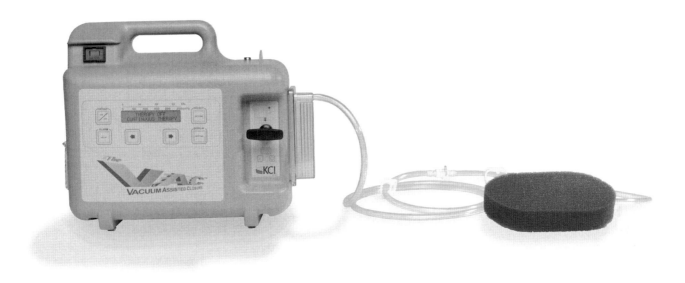

METHOD	KEY POINTS
PREPARING PATIENT	
1. Explain procedure to patient.	Position will depend on location of wound.
2. Assist patient into correct position.	
PROCEDURE	
1. Don gloves.	Follow Standard Precautions.
2. Remove old dressings and dispose of dirty dressings and gloves.	
3. Don gloves.	
4. Clean wound and remove gloves.	Use wound cleanser or normal saline.
5. Dry and prepare periwound.	Shave hair on border around wound, if applicable.
6. Open dressing assembly package, remove the catheter from inside the sponge, and set it aside for later use.	
7. Place the VAC® pump on a level surface or hang on the foot board, turn machine on, and set appropriate settings.	Use the green button on the far left-hand corner to turn machine on. Settings must be ordered by an MD.
8. Insert the cannister in the pump machine.	To assist with cannister placement, pull out on the black knob on the right side of the pump.
9. Cut sponge to fit within the wound.	Make sure the pattern cut is slightly smaller than the wound, fitting the size and shape of the wound, including tunnels and undermining areas.
10. Don gloves.	
11. Place the sponge to fit into the wound cavity.	Sponge should not lay over the wound edge.
12. Lay the vented catheter tip on top or inside of sponge, directing it away from pressure points.	
13. Remove drape backing, exposing the adherent side.	Located behind the green tab. Dressing should be cut to size, 4 inches beyond the wound edge before removing backing.
14. Place the transparent film over the sponge and catheter, pinching off the areas around the tubing.	For fragile periwound skin, use a skin prep prior to drape application or frame the wound with a hydrocolloid.

continues

Figure 12–16 continued

METHOD	KEY POINTS
15. Secure tubing with an additional piece of tape (pad underneath tubing) several cm away from the dressing.	
16. Connect the catheter snap end to the cannister tubing snap end and release clamps (2).	Clamps are to be used when disconnecting patients from suction.
17. Turn therapy on.	Therapy on/off button is located on the face of the machine.
18. Check for air leaks.	Pinch around the tubing to seal off air leaks. Apply a second piece of transparent film dressing. The sponge should appear like a raisin if suction has been established.

DOCUMENTATION

1. Date, time, procedure
2. Assessment of the wound
3. Patient tolerance of procedure
4. Settings of the KCI® VAC® system
5. Nurse's signature and initials

Figure 12–16 Sample VAC® technique. *Note:* The KCI® VAC® system (pump) must be rented, and disposables must be purchased from KCI®. The following are wound contraindications for use of the VAC® system: fistulae to organs or body cavities, presence of necrotic tissue, osteomyelitis (untreated), cancer in the wound margins. Closely monitor patients on anticoagulants. The pressure setting (mm Hg) and interval of dressing changes must be ordered by the physician. Protocols for dressing changes as described by KCI® should be followed. *Source: The VAC® Physician and Caregiver Reference Manual,* © 1999 KCI USA, INC.

VAC Case Study

This is a 71-year-old male, admitted to the hospital for left hip chronic wound with drainage. His status was postop, open reduction internal fixation (ORIF) for left hip fracture 1 month prior to admission. He had no known allergies and was on several routine medications. He wadadmitted for incision and drainage (I&D) of the hip wound. The surgery showed a large hematoma, with infection down to the hardware. Infection was cleaned up, and part of the fascia latta was debrided, due to infection. Eight days later, he developed another infection and was taken to the operating room again for a subsequent I&D. Previous wound care treatments had been wet to moist normal saline packing two to three times a day and pulsatile lavage.

Medical History: Insulin-dependent diabetic, pericardial calcification

Surgical History: Pericardial calcium resection, left below-the-knee amputation, back surgery

Wound Assessment: VAC therapy was initiated 4 days after surgery. The wound was anatomically vertical along the left lateral thigh. The wound bed was 80% beefy red granulation tissue, with 20% exposed tendon and hardware (Table 12–3). Drainage was clear serous fluid with no odor noted. Periwound was nonerythematic with wound edges attached. Measurements were 25cm × 7cm × 3cm, with a 5-cm depth at the 2:00–5:00 position. Client had been on a course of vancomycin hydrochloride (Vancocin) IVPB and is currently on rifampin (Rifadin) PO. Client complained of excruciating pain on palpation of wound and was medicated with hydromorphone hydrochloride (Dilaudid I.V. with dressing changes. There were no special support surfaces on the patient. Physical therapy (for strengthening) and nutritional services were following the patient at this time (see Figures 12–17 and 12–18).

Indications/Goals for VAC Therapy: Nonhealing wound. Closure of chronic wound and/or preparation for flap/skin graft.

Review of Clinical Course with VAC Therapy: After 3 weeks of therapy, there was significant progress in wound filling and contraction. The patient was discharged to home on VAC therapy, with the expectation of complete wound closure.

Table 12–3 Review of Left Hip Wound Clinical Course with VAC® Therapy

Date	Length	Width	Depth	Undermining	Color	Exposed Hardware	Odor
7/24/00	25 cm	7 cm	3 cm	5 cm between the 2:00 and 5:00 position	80% beefy red	20% hardware and tendon exposed	none
7/26/00	25 cm	5 cm	3 cm	6 cm @ the 4:00 position	95% beefy red, 5% yellow	minimal hardware exposed	none
7/28/00	24 cm	5.5 cm	1 cm	2 cm @ the 4:00 position	90% beefy red	10% exposed hardware	none
8/4/00							
8/9/00	24 cm	4 cm	0	2 cm @ the 3:00 position	95% beefy red	5% exposed hardware	none
8/16/00	24 cm	3 cm	0	1 cm @ the 3:00 position	97% beefy red	3% exposed hardware	none

8/19/00 Discharged to home on the VAC® therapy.

After 3 weeks of therapy, there was significant progress in wound filling and contraction. The patient was discharge home on VAC® therapy, with the expectation of complete wound closure.

parent film in the wound cover provides for wound observation and monitoring while the foam collar absorbs excess exudate. The infrared warming card slides into a sleeve in the top of the wound cover and warms to a temperature of 38° C (100.4° F). The Warm-Up wound therapy system provides a stand alone therapy that eliminates the need for additional dressings or wound-packing materials. Once applied, the wound cover can remain in place for 72 hours or as clinically indicated.

Indications for Use and Discontinuation

Warming therapy is indicated for a wide range of full-thickness and partial-thickness wounds. including pressure ulcers, surgical wounds, and lower extremity ulcers, such as venous, arterial, and diabetic/neuropathic ulcers. Case studies have shown that, with warming therapy, tunneling wounds do not require packing.[83–85] When traditional pack-

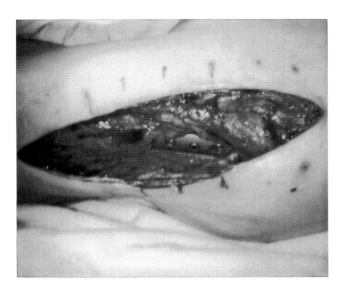

Figure 12–17 Left lateral thigh wound post incision and drainage, 25cm × 7cm × 3cm will be exposed hardware. *Source:* Copyright © KCI USA, Inc.

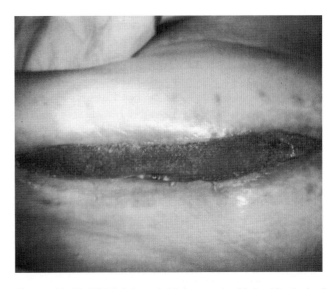

Figure 12–18 8/16 left lateral thigh wound with healthy bed of granulation tissue after VAC treatment. *Source:* Copyright © KCI USA, Inc.

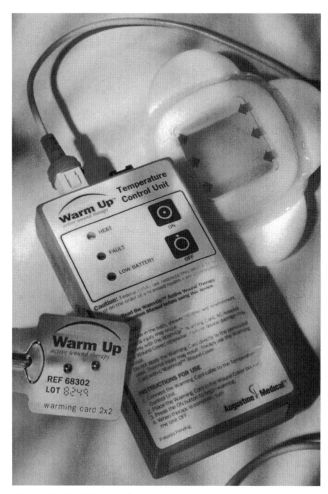

Figure 12–19 Warm-Up* therapy, temperature control unit, cover, and warming card.

* Warm-Up is a trademark of Augustine Medical, Inc., registered in the United States as well as other countries.

Source: Photo is reproduced herein with permission © 2000 Augustine Medical Inc. All rights reserved.

ing is not used, it removes the variable of who is packing, how much he or she is using, and whether or not the wound bed is being traumatized with the packing. In treating an undermining or tunneling wound, the clinician needs to select a wound cover that covers the entire area of the undermining and/or tunneling. Warming therapy can be used until the wound has completely resolved or until final epithelialization is inevitable and the clinician believes another treatment is appropriate, ie, when the wound is at surface level. If the patient develops an allergic response to the wound cover's adhesive, it should be removed.

Method of Application

Measure and cleanse the wound, then select the appropriately sized wound cover and corresponding warming card. Wound covers are currently available in six different sizes,

with two of these wound covers specifically designed for the sacral area. The wound cover is applied by removing the release paper covering the adhesive and applying the wound cover to the periwound area. The use of a skin protectant barrier is sometimes indicated if there is a known sensitivity to adhesives. Then the warming card cable is inserted into the temperature control unit port. The warming card slides into a pocket on the wound cover by directing the warming card between the arrows. Press the "ON" button on the temperature control unit to begin warming therapy. When the warming session is completed after 1 hour, the warming card is removed from the wound cover. Press the "OFF" button to turn off the temperature control unit. An AC adapter is provided and can be used either during warming sessions or when the temperature control unit needs recharging. The warming therapy is used for 1 hour, three times daily. The method of application is a simple procedure that can be done consistently by clinicians and caregivers.

Precautions

When using the Warm-Up wound therapy system, follow the manufacturer's instructions. Do not use the temperature control unit, AC adapter, or warming card in the bath, shower, or other wet environment, due to the risk of electrical injury. Do not apply the warming card directly to the wound or periwound area. When using the warming card, always use an appropriately sized Warm-Up therapy wound cover to obtain the best result.

As with other wound care products, active known infections, including osteomyelitis, should be treated concurrently. Warming therapy provides a moist environment and will encourage autolytic debridement; therefore, patients with dry, stable ischemic ulcers should be thoroughly assessed and informed before initiating this or any other moist therapy. Debridement of nonviable, necrotic tissue should be initiated for clinically indicated wounds, as appropriate, prior to beginning warming therapy.

Wounds resulting from third-degree burns are considered a contraindication for the use of warming therapy.

Outcomes Expected

Warming therapy is beneficial in the treatment of patients with chronic wounds by creating an optimal environment for healing. It is anticipated that wounds will have an increase in granulation tissue and will progress toward wound closure and, ultimately, proceed to wound resolution. Typically, clinicians should expect an increase in exudate during the first 7–10 days after Warming therapy is begun. This increased exudate is a normal response to Warming therapy moving the wound into the inflammatory phase.

In published, clinical studies, many patients with venous ulcers report a reduction in wound pain when treatment with Warming therapy begins.[86,87] It has also been shown in clinical studies to accelerate wound healing rates in pres-

Warm-Up Therapy Case Study

On October 7, 1998, a 41-year-old female with multiple sclerosis was referred to home care with a small but significantly undermined sacral surgical wound after removal of a baclofen pump. She received daily in-home nursing visits for traditional, moist wound care, consisting of wound cleansing and moist wound packing, followed by an absorbent cover dressing. Following 3 months of care, there was no change in the depth or other characteristics of the sacral wound.

On January 15, 1999, the wound measured 0.5 cm in circumference with a 7 cm tunnel that was lateral and obliquely angled. There was a mild wound odor with serosanguineous drainage. By February 26, the tunnel measured 6.2 cm deep. The wound continued to demonstrate progress, and the tunneling depth measured 2.5 cm by March 19. On March 26, the wound had regressed and now measured 6.5 cm in depth. Traditional moist wound treatment, which included packing the tunnel, had failed to resolve the wound.

On April 2, the sacral wound measured 5.9 cm in tunneling depth, and warming therapy was initiated (see Figure 12–20). Active warming therapy consisted of three 1-hour warming sessions per day with wound, cover changes every three days and as needed if wound leakage occurred. Following 33 days of active warming therapy, the tunnel had granulated to the surface, and the wound margins were epithelializing (see Figure 12–21). A moist hydrogel and protective dressing were placed on the wound, and 3 days later, the wound had resolved completely.

Cost Analysis

The cost of treatment prior to and following the intervention of warming wound therapy, including labor and wound care products:

October 7, 1998 through April 2, 1999, employing traditional moist wound therapy: $24,773.16. Wound unresolved with 5.9-cm tunnel.

April 2 through May 8, 1999, employing Warm-Up therapy: $8,534.08. Wound resolved.

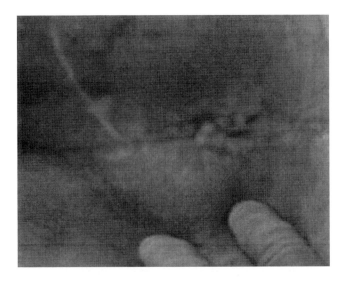

Figure 12–20 Sacral wound with 5.9 cm tunnel, Warm-Up therapy initiated. *Source:* Copyright © 2001, Joy Edvalson, RN, MSN, CWOCN.

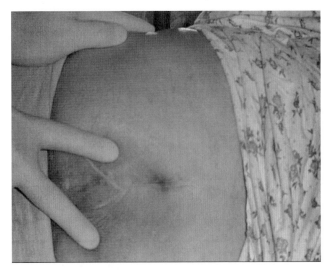

Figure 12–21 Sacral wound following 33 days of active warming therapy. The tunnel had granulated to the surface and the wound margins were epithelializing. *Source:* Copyright © 2001, Joy Edvalson, RN, MSN, CWOCN.

sure ulcers and venous ulcers, compared with standard treatment.[78,81,86,88] Using Warming therapy in the treatment of venous ulcers can be done in combination with compression. The compression used would need to facilitate access three times a day to the wound cover for placement of the warming card.

Because using warming therapy is relatively simple, family members are more willing to participate in providing wound care in the home with both cover changes and warming card insertions. This provides an overall reduction of cost, due to the decreased interval of skilled nursing visits in the home care environment. Instead, the skilled nursing visits are primarily for assessing wound progress. By empowering the patient and caregivers in their wound care, compliance does not seem to be an issue.

REVIEW QUESTIONS

1. Which of the following advanced wound therapies would be most appropriate to treat a dehisced sternal wound?
   a. Living skin equivalent
   b. Warming therapy
   c. VAC therapy
   d. Becaplermin topical growth factor
2. A refractory wound may present with all of the following EXCEPT:
   a. Healing progress with nonadvanced wound therapy
   b. Undermining, tunneling, and/or extensive necrotic tissue
   c. Host burden factor of 1 year duration of the wound
   d. Comorbidity of diabetes mellitus
3. List one indication and one contraindication for each of the following advanced wound therapies:
   a. Living skin equivalents
   b. Artificial skin
   c. Silver-impregnated dressings
   d. VAC dressings
   e. Warm-Up therapy
   f. Becaplermin growth factor

REFERENCES:

1. *Merriam-Webster's Collegiate Dictionary, 10th edition.* Springfield, MA: Merriam-Webster; 1993.

2. Allman RM, Walker JM, Hart MK, Laprade CA, Noel LB, Smith CR. Air-fluidized beds or conventional therapy for pressure sores: A randomized trial. *Ann Intern Med.* 1987;107:641–648.

3. Bates-Jensen BM. The Pressure Sore Status Tool a few thousand assessments later. *Adv Wound Care.* 1997;10(5):65–73.

4. Bates-Jensen BM. *A Quantitative Analysis of Wound Characteristics as Early Predictors of Healing in Pressure Sores.* Dissertation Abstracts International, Vol. 59, No. 11, University of California, Los Angeles; 1999.

5. Van Rijswijk, L. Full-thickness pressure ulcers: Patient and wound healing characteristics. *Decubitus.* 1993;6(1):16–30.

6. Xakellis GC, Chrischilles EA. Hydrocolloid versus saline-gauze dressings in treating pressure ulcers: A cost-effectiveness analysis. *Arch Phys Med Rehabil.* 1992;73(5):463–469.

7. Barbul A, Lazarou SA, Efron DT, Wasserkrug HL, Efron G. Arginine enhances wound healing and lymphocyte immune responses in humans. *Surgery.* 1990;108(2):331–336.

8. Mosiello GC, Tufaro A., Kerstein M. Wound healing and complications in the immunosuppressed patient. *Wounds.* 1994;6(3):83–87.

9. Bagdade JD, Root RK, Bulger RJ. Impaired leukocyte function in patients with poorly controlled diabetes. *Diabetes.* 1974;23(1):9–15.

10. Pecoraro RE, Ahroni JH, Boyko EJ, Stensel VL. Chronology and determinants of tissue repair in diabetic lower extremity ulcers. *Diabetes.* 1991;40:1305–1313.

11. Coleridge-Smith PD, Thomas P, Scurr JH, Dormandy JA. Causes of venous ulceration: A new hypothesis. *Br Med J Clin Res Educ.* 1998;296(6638):1726–1727.

12. Hartmann M, Jonsson K, Zederfeldt B. Effect of tissue perfusion and oxygenation on accumulation of collagen in healing wounds. Randomized study in patients after major abdominal operations. *Eur J Surg.* 1992;158(10):521–526.

13. Sapico FL, Ginunas VJ, Thornhill-Hoynes M, et al. Quantitative microbiology of pressure sores in different stages of healing. *Diagn Biol Infect Dis.* 1986;5(1):31–38.

14. Robson MC, Stenberg BD, Hegger JP. Wound healing alterations caused by infections. *Clin Plast Surg.* 1990;17(3):485–492.

15. Allman R M. Pressure ulcers among the elderly. *N Engl J Med.* 1989;320(13):850–853.

16. Gorse GJ, Messner RL. Improved pressure sore healing with hydrocolloid dressings. *Arch Dermatol.* 1987;123:766–771.

17. Gentzkow GD, Pollack SV, Kloth LC, Stubbs HA. Improved healing of pressure ulcers using dermapulse, a new electrical stimulation device. *Wounds.* 1991;3(5):158–169.

18. Van Rijswijk L, Polansky M. Predictors of time to healing deep pressure ulcers. *Ostomy/Wound Manage.* 1994;40(8):40–50.

19. Ferrell BA, Osterweil D, Christenson P. A randomized trial of low-air-loss beds for treatment of pressure ulcers. *JAMA.* 1993;269:494–497.

20. Robson MC, Phillips LG, Thomason A, et al. Recombinant human platelet-derived growth factor-BB in the treatment of pressure ulcers. *Ann Plast Surg.* 1992;29:193–201.

21. Mustoe TA, Cutler NR, Allman RM, et al. Phase II study to evaluate recombinant platelet-derived growth factor-BB in the treatment of pressure ulcers. *Arch Surg.* 1994;129:213–219.

22. Rees RS, Robson MC, Smiell SM, Perry BH. Becaplermin gel in the treatment of pressure ulcers: A randomized, double-blinded, placebo controlled study. *Wound Repair Regen.* 1998;6:A478.

23. Robson MC, Phillips LG, Lawrence WT, et al. The safety and effect of topically applied recombinant basic fibroblast growth factor on healing of chronic pressure sores. *Ann Surg.* 1992;216:401–408.

24. Brown GL, Curtsinger L, Jurkiewicz MJ, et al. Stimulation of healing of chronic wounds by epidermal growth factor. *Plast Reconstr Surg.* 1995;96:251–254.

25. Robson MC, Abdullah A, Burns BF, et al. Safety and effect of topical recombinant human interleukin-1B in the management of pressure sores. *Wound Repair Regen.* 1994;2:177–181.

26. Robson MC, Hill DP, Smith PD, et al. Sequential cytokine therapy for pressure ulcers: Clinical and mechanistic response. *Ann Surg.* 2000;231(4):600–611.

27. Finney JL, Jones H, Margolis DJ. Management of wounds: Wound repair, growth factors and engineered tissue. *Product Monograph.* Hauppauge, NY: Curative Health Services; 1999.

28. Knighton DR, Fiegel VD, Austin LL, Ciresi KF, Butler DL. Classification and treatment of chronic nonhealing wounds. *Ann Surg.* 1986;204:322–330.

29. Knighton DR, Ciresi K, Fiegel VD, Schumerth S, Butler E, Cerra F. Stimulation of repair in chronic, nonhealing, cutaneous ulcers using platelet-derived wound healing formula. *Surg Gynecol Obstet.* 1990;170:56–60.

30. Glover JL, Weingarten MS, Buchbinder DS, Poucher RL, Deitrick GA, Fylling CP. A four year outcome-based retrospective study of wound healing and limb salvage in patients with chronic wounds. *Adv Wound Care.* 1989;10(1):33–38.

31. Regranex (becaplermin) Gel 0.01% (product labeling), Raritan, NJ: Ortho-McNeil Pharmaceutical, Inc; 1998.

32. Robson MC. Exogenous growth factor application effect on human wound healing, *Prog Dermatol.* 1996;30:1–7.

33. Steed DL, Donohoe D, Webster MW, Lindsley L. The Diabetic Ulcer Group. Effect of extensive debridement and treatment on the healing of diabetic foot ulcers, *J Am Coll Surg.* 1996;183:61–64.

34. American Diabetes Association. Foot care in patients with diabetes mellitus. *Diabetes Care.* 1997;20(Suppl 1):S31–32.

35. Oxford Clinical Communications Inc. *A Brief History of Wound Healing.* Yardley, PA: Oxford Clinical Communications; 1998;1–49.

36. Hansbrough JF, Franco ES. Skin replacements. In: Granick MS, Long CD, eds. Wound healing: State of the art. *Clin Plast Surg.* 1998;25:407–423.

37. Falanga V, et al. Rapid healing of venous ulcers and lack of clinical rejection with an allogenic cultured human skin equivalent. *Arch Dermatol.* 1998;134:293–300.

38. Falanga V, Sabolinski M. A bilayered living skin construct (Apligraf™) accelerates complete closure of hard to heal venous ulcers. *Wound Rep Regen.* 1999;7:201–207.

39. Pham HT, et al. Evaluation of a human skin equivalent for the treatment of diabetic foot ulcers in a prospective, randomized, clinical trial. *Wounds.* 1999;11:79–86.

40. Falabella A, et al. The use of tissue-engineered skin (Apligraf) to treat a newborn with epidermolysis bullosa. *Arch Dermatol.* 1999;135:1219–1222.

41. Muhart M, et al. Behavior of tissue-engineered skin: A comparison of a living skin equivalent, autograft, and occlusive dressing in human donor sites. *Arch Dermatol.* 1999;135:913–918.

42. Falanga V. How to use Apligraf to treat venous ulcers. *Skin Aging.* 1999;Feb:30–36.

43. Yannas IV, Burke, JF. Design of an artificial skin I. Basic design principles. *Journal of Biomedical Materials Research.* 1980;14(1):65–81.

44. Sheridan RL, Hegarty M, Tompkins RG, Burke JF. Artificial skin in massive burns: Results to ten years. *Eur J Plast Surg.* 1994;17:91–93.

45. Orgill DP, Straus FH II, Lee RC. The use of collagen-GAG membranes in reconstructive surgery. *Ann N Y Acad Sci.* 1999;888:233–248.

46. Loss M, Wedker V, Kunzi W, Meuli-Simmen C, Meyer VE. Artificial skin, split-thickness autograft and cultured autologous keratinocytes combined to treat a severe burn injury of 93% of TBSA. *Burns.* 2000;26(7):644–652.

47. Boyce ST, Kagan RJ, Meyer NA, Yakuboff KP, Warden GD. The 1999 clinical research award. Cultured skin substitutes combined with Integra Artificial Skin to replace native skin autograft and allograft for the closure of excised full-thickness burns. *J Burn Care Rehabil.* 1999;20(6):453–461.

48. Clayton MC, Bishop JF. Perioperative and postoperative dressing techniques for Integra Artificial Skin: Views from two medical centers. *J Burn Care Rehabil.* 1998;19(4):358–363.

49. King P. Artificial skin reduces nutritional requirements in a severely burned child. *Burns.* 2000;26(5):501–503.

50. Heimbach D, Lutterman A, Burke J, et al. Artificial dermis for major burns. *Ann Surg.* 1988:208(30):313–319.

51. Stern R, McPherson M, Longaker MT. Histologic study of artificial skin used in the treatment of full-thickness thermal injury. *J Burn Care Rehabil.* 1990;11(1):7–13.

52. Russell AD, Hugo WB. Antimicrobial activity and action of silver. *Prog Med Chem.* 1994;31:351–370.

53. Cervantes C, Silver S. Metal resistance in *Pseudomonas*: Genes and mechanisms. In: Nakazawa T, Furukawa K, Haas D, Silver S, eds. *Molecular Biology of Pseudomonads.* Washington, DC: American Society for Microbiology; 1996.

54. Modak SM, Fox Jr CR. Binding of silver sulfadiazine to the cellular components of *Pseudomonas aeruginosa.* *Biochem Pharmacol.* 1973;22:2391–2404.

55. Ovington LG. The value of silver in wound management. *Podiatry Today.* 1999:;12:59–62.

56. Klein DG, Fritsch DE, Amin SG. Wound infection following trauma and burn injuries. *Crit Care Nurs Clin North Am.* 1995;7:627–642.

57. Field CK, Kerstein MD. Overview of wound healing in a moist environment. *Am J Surg.* 1994;167:2S–6S.

58. Burell RE. A preclinical trial safety evaluation of a new silver coated burn wound dressing. *Proceedings of the American Burn Association.* Chicago: American Burn Association; 1996.

59. Wright JB, Hansen DL, Burrell RE. The comparative efficacy of two antimicrobial barrier dressings: *In vitro* examination of two controlled release of silver dressings. *Wounds.* 1998;10(6):179–188.

60. Yin HQ, Langford R, Burrell RE. Comparative evaluation of the antimicrobial activity of Acticoat antimicrobial dressing. *J Burn Care Rehabil.* 1999;20(3):195–200.

61. Burrell RE, Heggers JP, Davis GD, Wright JB. Efficacy of silver-coated dressings as bacterial barriers in a rodent burn sepsis model. *Wounds.* 1999;11(4):64–71.

62. Wright JB, Lam K, Burrell RE. Wound management in an era of increasing bacterial antibiotic resistance: A role for topical silver treatment. *Am J Infect Control.* 1998;26:572–577.

63. Wright JB, Lam K, Hansen D, et al. Efficacy of topical silver against fungal burn-wound pathogens. *Am J Infect Control.* 1999;27:344–350.

64. Williams C. Arglaes controlled release dressing in the control of bacteria. *Br J Nurs.* 1997;6(2):114–115.

65. Falconio-West M, Sacramento L. *Silver Dressing Improves Healing in MRSA Wound.* Presented at the 31st Annual Wound, Ostomy and Continence Conference; June 1999, Minneapolis, MN.

66. Joseph E, Hamori CA, Bergman S, Roaf E, Swann NF, Anastasi GW. New therapeutic approaches in wound care: A perspective randomized trial of vacuum assisted closure versus standard therapy of chronic nonhealing wounds. *Wounds.* 2000;12(3):60–67.

67. Bates-Jensen BM, Sussman C, Bates-Jensen, BM, eds. *Wound Care: A Collaborative Practice Manual for Physical Therapists and Nurses.* Gaithersbug, MD: Aspen Publishers; 1998.

68. Mendez-Eastman S. Negative pressure wound therapy. *Plast Surg Nurs.* 1998;18(1):27–29,33–37.

69. Morykwas M, Argenta L, Shelton-Brown E, McGuirt W. Vacuum-assisted closure: A new method for wound control and treatment: Animal studies and basic foundation. *Ann Plast Surg.* 1997;38(6):553–561.

70. Hartnett JM. Use of vacuum-assisted wound closure in three chronic wounds. *J Wound Ostomy Continence Nurs.* 1998;25(6):281–290.

71. Meara JG, Guo L, Smith JD, Pribaz JJ, Breuing KH, Orgill DP. Vacuum-assisted closure in the treatment of degloving injuries. *Ann Plast Surg.* 1999;42(6):589–594.

72. Wu SH, Zecha PJ, Feitz R, Hovius SER. Vacuum therapy as an intermediate phase in wound closure: A clinical experience. *Eur J Plast Surg.* 2000;23:174–177.

73. Genecov DG, Schneider AM, Morykwas MJ, Parker D, White WWL, Argenta LC. A controlled sub-atmospheric pressure dressing increases the rate of skin graft donor site reepithelialization. *Ann Plast Surg.* 1998;40(3):219–225.

74. Kinetic Concepts Incorporated. VAC recommended guidelines for use, wound closure. *Physician & Caregiver Reference Manual.* San Antonio, TX: Kinetic Concepts; 1999.

75. Philbeck TE, Whittington KT, Millsap MH, Briones RB, Wight DG, Schroeder WJ. The clinical and cost effectiveness of externally applied negative pressure wound therapy in the treatment of wounds in home healthcare Medicare patients. *Ostomy/Wound Manage.* 1999;45(11):41–50.

76. Ferrell BA, Osterweil D, Christenson P. A randomized trial of low-air-loss beds for treatment of pressure ulcers. *JAMA.* 1993;269(4):494–497.

77. Weinberg Group. *Technology assessment of the VAC for in-home treatment of chronic wounds.* Washington, DC: The Weinberg Group; 1999.

78. Kloth L, Berman J, Dumit-Minkel S, Sutton C, Papanek P, Wurzel J. Effects of a normothermic dressing on pressure ulcer healing. *Adv Skin Wound Care.* March/April 2000;13(2):69–74.

79. Ikeda T, Tayefeh F, Sessler DI, et al. Local radiant heating increases subcutaneous oxygen tension. *Am J Surg.* 1998;175:33–37.

80. Xia Z, Sato A, Hughes M, Cherry G. Stimulation of fibroblast growth in vitro by intermittent radiant warming. *Wound Repair Regen.* 2000;8(2):138–144.

81. Santilli S, Valusek P, Robinson C. Use of a noncontact radiant heat bandage for the treatment of chronic venous stasis ulcers. *Adv Wound Care.* 1999; 12(2):89–93.

82. Rabkin TM, Hunt, TK. Local heat increases blood flow and oxygen tension in wounds. *Arch Surg.* 1987;122(187):221–225.

83. Cuttino C. *A Clinical and Cost Outcome Study: Healing of an Ischial Pressure Ulcer.* Eden Prairie, MN: Augustine Medical; 2000.

84. Edvalson J. *Resolution of a Tunneling Wound: Use of Warming Therapy Instead of Packing.* Augustine Medical; 1999.

85. Taylor B. *A Clinical and Cost Study: Management of an Abdominal Wound.* Augustine Medical; 2000.

86. Cherry G, Phil J, Wilson J. The treatment of ambulatory venous ulcer patients with warming therapy. *Ostomy/Wound Manage.* 1999;45(9):65–70.

87. Robinson C, Santilli S. Warm-Up active wound therapy: A novel approach to the management of chronic venous stasis ulcers. *J Vasc Nurs.* 1998;16(2):38–42.

88. Price P, Bale S, Cook H, Harding K. The effect of a radiant heat dressing on pressure ulcers. *J Wound Care.* April 2000;201–205.

CHAPTER 13

Management of Scar

R. Scott Ward

CHAPTER OBJECTIVES

At the completion of this chapter, the reader will be able to:

1. Discuss the process of scar formation.
2. Discuss impairments caused by scar formation.
3. Describe common examination techniques used to assess and document scar tissue.
4. Describe intervention strategies used to treat impairments related to scar formation.

INTRODUCTION

Scar tissue, as a component of wound healing, can lead to functional and cosmetic complications. The hypertrophy associated with keloid or hypertrophic scar formation is disfiguring and is particularly problematic when located at body sites commonly exposed to the public (ie, face, hands, arms, etc.). Contraction of the forming scar often leads to further disfigurement, as well as restriction of function. Functional deficits occur principally when the scar is situated over a joint surface, particularly over joints of the extremities. Scarring of the face may also compromise functions such as feeding or speech. Pruritis, some pain, or other annoying parathesias may also accompany scar formation.

The problems of scar formation have been described as early as the writings of Hippocrates as a torsion resulting from healed burns.[1] Early documentation of surgical correction of scar contractures is included in the writings of Camillo Ferrara (in 1570)[1] and Wilhelm Fabry of Hilden (1560–1634).[1] Fabry of Hilden also described the use of splinting apparatuses to help correct joint deformities secondary to scar contraction. Similar, but certainly more modern, methods of treatment are used today in laboring to control the problems created by active scar formation.

Contemporarily, scar tissue is managed operatively, pharmaceutically, or with conservative measures, including pressure therapy, silicone, exercise, splinting, positioning, and massage. Each of these treatments has demonstrated success that has been documented or is accepted anecdotally because of accounts of clinical success. Further, many of these treatments have been used in combination in an attempt to accentuate the expected outcomes of treatment that include improved function and appearance. Common to each of these treatments is that they effect a correction of some problem related to the progression of scarring, but it must be understood that none of these interventions cure or stop the process of scarring. Current scientific investigation is uncovering more information about the cause of scarring and may lead to new therapies, such as the use of growth factors, that would be aimed more directly at the actual development of scar.

FORMATION OF SCAR TISSUE

Inflammation occurs following any tissue trauma. Several cell lines are recruited during the inflammatory response to control local infection, debride damaged tissue, nourish surviving and regenerating cells, and release factors that stimulate repair. One cell line that is stimulated to proliferate is fibroblasts. The fibroblast is the cell of origin for scar tissue. Fibroblasts produce elastin and collagen. The secreted elastin becomes elastic fibers that provide normal dermis, or scar, with elasticity and flexibility; however, the ratio of elastic fibers to collagen is less in scar than in normal skin. Collagen secreted by the fibroblasts develops into collagen fibers that are arranged in parallel coils and mainly provide tissue with tensile strength but also afford some flexibility within the normal dermis. The collagen secreted by fibroblasts in scar tissue is laid down in an unorganized, whorllike pattern. Collagen in both keloid scar and hypertrophic scar is produced at a much greater rate than in normal skin. Ground substance, or extracellular matrix, is comprised of substances including, among others, proteoglycans and glycosaminoglycans. The ground substance provides normal dermis, as well as scar, some cushion, and it allows for the diffusion of oxygen and nutrients in the vicinity. Scar tissue is well vascularized and highly metabolic.

Although scar formation begins with the proliferation and stimulation of fibroblasts during inflammation, the process of scarring continues for weeks, if not months, in most individuals. The growth factors that contribute to the proliferation and activity of fibroblasts in the wound continue to be released through the proliferative and remodeling phases of wound healing. Examples of some of the growth factors that elicit chemotaxis and proliferation of fibroblasts and that are also involved in stimulation of fibroblasts to produce collagen include platelet-derived growth factor (PDGF), tumor necrosis growth factor-β (TGF-β), and insulin-like growth factor (IGF). The interaction of these growth factors with other substances in the scar is not understood well enough to explain the reason for aberrant scar formation.

Collagen is continually deposited in scar to strengthen the wound site and is also degraded in an attempt to remodel the wound. Some wounds demonstrate an imbalance between the rate of collagen deposition and degradation. If the rate of collagen production exceeds the rate of degradation, a scar that is raised and thick forms.[2,3] Scar may be referred to as *normotrophic*, *hypertrophic*, or *keloid*. A normotrophic scar is a visible scar that is not raised above the height of the normal skin (see *Color Plate 6*). A hypertrophic scar is raised but does not grow beyond the original wound boundaries (see *Color Plate 48*). A keloid scar is raised and does extend past the original boundaries of the wound (see *Color Plates 49 and 50*). As scar actively forms, it is red, raised, and lacks suppleness. During this "phase" of scarring, the scar is commonly referred to as *immature scar*. As the scar matures in due course, the redness fades, the scar levels out to some degree, and the scar tissue softens (see *Color Plate 51*). It commonly takes 6–18 months for a scar to "mature."[4]

There are several clinically observed and documented markers that allow for some prediction of scar formation. The depth of the wound is related to scar formation, in that the deeper the wound, the more likely it is that the wound will scar. The increased chance of scarring is likely due to extended healing time and the associated formation of granulation tissue.[5] In this same light, the length of time it takes for a wound to heal, thereby also implicating the chronicity of inflammation, will also influence scar formation. Skin

with more pigment has been described as being more susceptible to scarring.[3] Skin tension appears to be a contributor to scarring.[3] Microdamage to tissue caused by tension may lead to inflammation that stimulates fibroblasts to create collagen. Young people tend to scar more than the elderly people do. This might be due to the "tighter" skin and generally more active lifestyle (causing frequent skin tension) of younger individuals, compared with the "loose" skin and decreased elasticity of the skin in elderly people. It is generally thought that location of a wound may contribute to the amount of eventual scarring, even though scars have been described on all parts of the body. Keloids most commonly appear somewhere between the ears and the waist or from the elbow to the shoulder.[5] Hypertrophic scarring has been described to more likely occur at the shoulder, upper arm, upper back, dorsal feet, and buttocks.[6] Clinically, keloid scars or hypertrophic scars can form on any body surface. Further, there is probably some genetic predisposition to scar formation.[7]

Complications of Scar Formation

Cosmetic changes are considered to be a possible complication of scarring. The location of the scar might be thought to influence it initially, and this may be true to a degree. For example, a facial scar is likely to be more a consistent challenge than a scar that is commonly hidden on the body. However, it must also be considered that this does not hold true if the person swims daily or if the person lives in a warm climate that necessitates shorts or other light clothing. Generally, interactions with people beyond health care providers, family, and friends may be difficult and, therefore, a person may confine himself or herself socially.

Quality of life issues are a concern to patients with scarring, particularly following a trauma such as a burn, and this view also reflects a perceived low level of self-esteem.[8,9] Patients' perceived quality of life may be diminished secondary to the presence of scar because, as just mentioned, they may hesitate to participate in their normal activities or to commence social relations, thereby losing some of their sense of worth or contribution. Disfigurement can result in a deceased self-esteem for women and men.[10] Low self-esteem and quality of life can also be affected by other complications of scarring, such as scar contraction, changes in sensation, itching, and color variability in the scar.

Hypertrophic scar contracts while it is maturing.[11,12] Contraction of scar may intensify a cosmetic deformity but can also result in restriction of mobility and potential for chronic soft-tissue length changes. Any scar that is associated with or located over a joint surface has the potential to render fixed contracture. This particular problem is one of the major factors requiring long-term clinical care and follow-up of scars. The types of contracture can most often be predicted, based on the location of the scar. When a scar is forming over a joint or on a particular side of an extremity, the contraction will affect the related motion. For example, a scar located on the anterior surface of the elbow (the antecubital fossa) will be expected to contract the arm into flexion and could lead to limits of extension of the elbow. Scars on the dorsal surface of the toes will "pull" the toes into extension and limit toe flexion. If intervention is not provided and the scar contraction is allowed to progress, it can become a fixed scar contracture. The process of contracture formation also results in the shortening of allied soft tissue, such as muscle, ligament, and joint capsule. The combination of all of these shortened structures makes it an extremely difficult challenge to recover any functional mobility without invasive surgical revision. The regrettable part of the need for surgical revision of scar contracture is that the person is subjected to the possibility of the very same outcome because of the scarring that results following the revision.

Sensation is affected because of abnormal innervation of scar. Scar is typically less densely innervated than is normal skin. Patients will experience a "dulled" ability to recognize any of the protective sensations normally present in the skin, such as touch, pain, and temperature.[13] Because of these elevated sensory thresholds, a patient may be at risk for trauma to the scar and should be taught to inspect the scar regularly for scrapes, cuts, small burns, or other damage. Interestingly, even though there is a loss of cutaneous temperature sensation, some patients complain of their scar being very sensitive to "the cold." Patients may describe numbness, tingling, or shooting pain in the scar during cold weather.

Itching or pruritis is also common in maturing scar tissue. Itching may also persist as a chronic problem in some scars. The itching is probably a result of several contributing factors. A low level of inflammation may be present in forming scar, and substances released during inflammation, such as histamine and substance-P, can contribute to itch. The scar also lacks oil-producing glands. The deficiency of skin oils results in a dry surface that may cause itching. It should also be noted that the dry scar is less supple and, therefore, more prone to "cracking," which may lead to the development of sores. A patient should be instructed to apply lotion to the scar frequently. If the scar is allowed to stay dry, it may itch more. Patients should also avoid scratching the itch because of the risk of blistering or skin breakdown. Lotion may help to decrease itchiness and prevent the scar from "cracking." Lotions that are perfumed should be avoided because they might cause a rash or skin irritation.

Additional ingredients, such as vitamin E or aloe, are often included in lotions because they are purported to decrease or cure scar. Although neither of these additives will aggravate or worsen a scar, there is also no current evidence that they will improve the appearance of a scar or cure the scar.

Clinical Wisdom

If a patient is experiencing a rash or skin irritation, the soap currently being used for for hygiene and body washing should be discontinued and the patient should try a mild, nonperfumed lotion. If you are not sure whether it is the soap or lotion that is causing the irritation, have the patient change the soap first for a few days. If the rash has not gone away, try a nonperfumed lotion. If both the soap and lotion are changed to nonperfumed brands and the rash does not go away, a physician should be consulted.

A patient may also notice and report that a scar changes color from time to time. Color changes are probably between varying shades of red, purple, brown, and gray. Position often affects the color changes. Generally, the color intensifies if a limb is in a dependent position. Elevation of the same body part should help diminish the amount of color. Extreme ambient environmental temperatures, either hot or cold, might also increase the color of a scar. Color changes associated with position or temperature are not permanent. However, if a maturing scar is exposed to sunlight, there is a risk that the scar will become permanently hyperpigmented. The mechanism for this hyperpigmentation is not understood at this time. A maturing scar *must* be kept protected from sunlight.

Clinical Wisdom: *Sun Protection*

You should have your patient apply a waterproof sun block or a sunscreen that is at least a sun protection factor (SPF) 30 when planning any outdoor activity. It is also wise to wear light, sun-protective clothing and hats to guard against the rays of the sun. The extra clothing is recommended even when the patient is wearing compression garments. Remember, too, that the harmful rays are also present on cloudy days.

TESTS AND MEASUREMENT

Several characteristics and sequelae of scars can be examined to improve determination of appropriate intervention strategies. Assessment of the scar tissue itself is aimed at determining whether the scar is immature or mature. This is important because a scar that is immature is considered to be more likely to respond to treatment. Specific characteristics of the scar that help in determining maturity and outcome include pigmentation, pliability, height, and texture. Pigmentation may be documented by describing the color of the scar.

Generally, immature scars appear hypervascular and, therefore, may be red or violescent. The same scar may turn a deep purple if it is on a body part that is held in a dependent position or is exposed to cold for a period of time. This coloration begins to fade and should generally return to near-normal skin tone through the process of scar maturation. After the scar has matured, it may be either hypo- or hyperpigmented. Patients should understand that variations of the pigment of the scar are probably permanent if they are present following scar maturation.

Clinical Wisdom: *Cosmetics*

Patients with permanent discoloration of scar might benefit from the use of cosmetics. Cosmetics are most useful over areas of visible scarring, such as the hands and face. There are hypoallergenic forms of makeup that can be used to provide a covering for discoloration and minor deformity. Cosmetics with a sunscreen should be selected to protect the scar tissue from the sun.

Palpating the scar and appraising the stiffness of the tissue commonly assess pliability of the scar. Simply pinching the scar may be useful in determining pliability. A scar that is not pliable will be difficult to pinch up between the fingers because of the stiffness of the tissue. Normal pliable skin allows for very localized mobilization of the skin, without much spread to adjacent skin. Also, scar that is not pliable will often move as a "unit" when mobilized. Mature scars are generally, but not always, more pliable that maturing scars.

Documentation of height provides some indication for the level of hypertrophy of the scar. Height may be difficult to quantify; however, a description that the scar is raised above the plane of the normal adjacent skin demonstrates hypertrophy. The scar will not necessarily flatten as it matures, without some intervention. The texture of the scar may also indicate hypertrophy. As scar tissue is being actively deposited and becomes hypertrophied to any degree, the texture of the scar deviates from that of normal skin. Texture might be described with a variety of adjectives, such as *rough*, *uneven*, or *bumpy*. Although not necessarily scientific or certainly not quantitative, these terms do relay the presence of an atypical texture, compared with normal skin.

Sequelae of scar that need to be examined are impairments secondary to scar contraction. A decrease in range of motion and associated joint mobility is a major impairment caused by scar contraction. Assessment procedures for examining the loss of range of motion might include standard goniometry, for example. Assessment of functional limitation secondary to contraction, including activities of daily living and instrumental activities of daily living, should be completed.

Disfigurement is one of the possible problems associated with contraction. Written description and photography are two assessment methods that can be used to portray the present disfigurement. For example, scarring that occurs on the dorsum of the hand, involving the web spaces of the fingers, may described as "development of web space syndactyly."

Sensation is another impairment that follows scarring. Sensation testing may be performed to assess the degree of sensory ability over a scar. Decreases in sensation may then be documented and used as important information to include in patient education regarding skin protection.

Clinical measurement of scar tissue, including documentation of intervention treatments, has historically been provided simply by objective description of the scar. There are a few documented scar measurement tools that allow some objectification of observed scar traits; however, each of these scales involves observation and some judgment regarding the scar. In 1990, Sullivan and colleagues[14] published the Vancouver Scar Scale as a method for assessing burn-related scars. This scale uses the variables of pigmentation, vascularity, pliability, and height of the scar to describe the current status of the tissue. Scores are assigned based on variances of these variables from normal, with normal being zero. A higher score represents a worse scar. Table 13–1 provides a representation of the scale and the representative values used to score the scar.

Additional scar rating or appearance scales have been described, using photographs of the scar. One such scale uses scar characteristics, including smoothness of scar surface, a depressed scar border, scar thickness, and pigmentation of the scar, which are rated by rating color pictures of scars.[15] The quality of the photograph and the experience of the evaluator may affect the reliability of this tool; however, if it is used within a particular setting, it may provide useful ways not only of objectifying scar but of documenting it by photograph, as well. Exhibit 13–1 provides a representation of the scale used to assess scar using this method.

INTERVENTIONS FOR THE TREATMENT OF SCAR

Surgical

Surgery is considered in cases where conservative measures of scar control have not completely corrected or controlled scarring. Surgical intervention is indicated to improve specific cosmetic or functional deformities. Results of the surgery depend on the location of the scar, the timing of the surgery, the extent of the deformity, and the surgical technique.

Scar at most anatomic locations can be revised; however, areas such as the head and face, neck, and axillae respond more poorly to surgical modification than do other areas.[16]

Table 13–1 Ratings Used in the Vancouver Scar Scale to Measure Scar Formation

Pigmentation	Vascularity	Pliability	Height	Score
Normal—color that closely resembles the color over the rest of the body	Normal—color that closely resembles the color over the rest of the body	Normal	Normal—flat	0
Hypopigmentation	Pink	Supple: flexible with minimal resistance	Raised < 2 mm	1
Hyperpigmentation	Red	Yielding: giving way to pressure	Raised < 5 mm	2
	Purple	Firm: inflexible, not easily moved, resistant to manual pressure	Raised > 5 mm	3
		Banding: ropelike tissue that blanches with extension of the scar		4
		Contracture: permanent shortening of scar producing deformity or distortion		5

Note: The higher the score reported, the worse the scar.

Source: Reprinted with permission from T. Sullivan et al., Rating the Burn Scar, *Journal of Burn Care Rehabilitation*, Vol. 11, pp. 256-260, © 1990, Lippincott Williams & Wilkins.

Most scar revisions are performed after the scar tissue has matured. However, individual considerations and the extent of any deformity must be considered when decisions about reconstructive surgery for correction of scar are made. The larger the deformity or scar, the more extensive the surgery will be. A patient's particular needs, goals, and medical history are important matters for deliberation when finalizing any judgment regarding surgery.

Surgical techniques vary, and the type used for any scar revision will be influenced by the factors previously discussed. Small scars can simply be excised and the excision-site then primarily closed. Larger scars may be excised and a graft placed to cover the wound. The selection of the graft type is important and may lead to further scar for- mation. Generally, split-thickness meshed skin grafts will scar to some degree, whereas full-thickness skin grafts, skin flaps, or split-thickness sheet grafts are less likely to scar. Of course, there is a risk that a donor site for a skin graft might scar. There is clearly a risk for the donor site of a full-thickness skin graft or a skin flap to scar. Such donor sites will require further skin coverage, either with another split-thickness skin graft or, if the donor site is small enough, primary closure. Another technique used in revising larger scars is serial excision, or segmental scar reduction. This is achieved by excising a central portion of the scar and primarily closing the wound. This procedure is then replicated over a period of several months until the entire scar has been removed.

Exhibit 13–1 Ratings Used in a Photographic Scar Scale to Measure Scar Formation

1. Scar Surface

–1 ------------ 0 -------------- 1 -------------- 2 -------------- 3 -------------- 4
smooth   normal   rough   rough   rough   rough

2. Scar Border Height

–1 ------------ 0 -------------- 1 -------------- 2 -------------- 3 -------------- 4
  depressed   normal   raised   raised   raised   raised

3. Scar Thickness

–1 ------------ 0 -------------- 1 -------------- 2 -------------- 3 -------------- 4
  thinner   normal   thicker thicker   thicker   thicker

4. Color Differences (between scar and adjacent normal skin)

–1 ------------ 0 ------------- 1 -------------- 2 -------------- 3 -------------- 4
hypopigment   normal   hyperpigment hyperpigment hyperpigment hyperpigment

Note: The scale ranges from –1 to 4 for each characteristic. Generally, the higher the score reported, the worse the scar.

Source: Reprinted with permission from E.K. Yeong et al., Improved Burn Scar Assessment with Use of New Scar-rating Scale, Journal of Burn Care Rehabilitation, 18: 353-355, 1997, *Journal of Burn Care Rehabilitation*, Vol. 18, pp. 353-355, © 1997, Lippincott Williams & Wilkins.

Realignment of scar tissue may be considered when the scar forms causing abnormally high skin tension lines. This contributes to contracture formation. Z-plasty, Y-V plasty, and local advancement or rotational flaps are surgical techniques used to realign or replace scar and break up tension lines.

Tissue expanders, which are silicone balloons surgically implanted in the subcutaneous fat or under the muscle, are injected with saline and are used to increase the surface area of normal skin adjacent to the scar. This expanded area of skin can eventually be transferred as a flap to cover an excised area of scar. Tissue expansion allows for better matches of skin color, thickness, and texture than do techniques such as grafting.

In any case of scar revision, a patient must be informed that the scar may form again. This would then require continuing treatment to control the new scar.

Pharmaceutical

Some scar tissue responds to injection of cortisone-related medications. Such medications likely are effective be-

cause of their capability to increase activity of collagenase in breaking down the scar. Injections of this type are recommended only for small scars.

Pressure Therapy

Although previous publications of the effect of pressure on wound healing[17] and scar[18] existed, pressure therapy burgeoned in the 1970s, following the publication of the successful use in treating burn scars.[19] Actual pressures under a pressure garment will vary.[20] It appears, however, that these variable pressures still generally provide an adequate clinical response of controlling scar.[21]

Pressure therapy is typically recommended when a wound takes longer than 14 days to heal. The longer the healing time, the more likely it is that a wound will form scar tissue. It is by and large advised that pressure garments or devices be worn for an average of 23 hours a day while the scar is maturing. Companies manufacture choices of colors for the garments. Manufacturers also are generally willing to fabricate uncharacteristic garments for special circumstances, such as a hand with an amputated finger. The fit of the supports should be checked from time to time because the garments will stretch and wear out. Alterations to existing garments and the fitting of new garments should be carried out as often as necessary to promote the sought-after outcome.

Manufacturers of pressure garments offer garments that fit the face, neck, upper extremity, torso, hand, and lower extremity. Although the different manufacturers may have slightly different methods for measuring each body part for a pressure garment, generally, limb circumferences every 1 inch to 1-1/2 inches are required. Assuring a proper fit of the face, torso, and hands is a bit more complex than the limbs, and manufacturers' methods for taking measurements of these parts vary to some extent. Each company's specific directions for measurement techniques can be obtained by contacting the manufacturer directly. A listing of custom pressure garment suppliers can be found at the end of the chapter.

After a patient bathes or showers, he or she should be instructed to apply some lotion to the scar and to put on a clean pressure garment. The garment previously worn should be washed and dried. The pressure garment can be washed either by hand or on a delicate cycle in a washing machine with mild detergent and warm (not hot) water. If the garment is washed by hand, it should be rinsed thoroughly after washing. The pressure garment should be dried in the air (do not dry in the dryer or by placing the garment on a heater). The garment will dry faster if it is first rolled up in a towel and gently wrung in the towel to remove extra water. Pressure garments will not tolerate dry cleaning. Pressure garments should not be ironed. It is recommended that each patient have at least two of each type of garment worn so that a clean one can always be available.

Compliance with the wearing of pressure supports might be an issue with some patients. Commonly expressed concerns about wearing the garments include the appearance, the discomfort (tightness), getting the garment on and off, and how hot they make the patient. Compliance will increase as patients wear the garment for a longer period of time and if they are given a choice of colors of garment. Education about the benefits and care of the garments will also enhance compliance to treatment.[22]

There may be some difficulty in donning a pressure garment located on the same limb being treated with pressure therapy. Attempting to pull the pressure garment over dressings is difficult and commonly dislodges the dressings. This problem can generally be overcome by pulling on nylon hosiery over the dressed limb, then donning the pressure garment over the nylon hosiery.

Pressure to scar can also be applied through the use of elastic wraps, self-adherent stretch wraps, or elasticized cotton tubular bandages (see Figure 13–1). Manufacturers of custom pressure garments also produce noncustom, general fit supports. These less expensive, noncustom options can also be advantageous in treating lymphedema or postwound edema. Early pressure can decrease edema formation and facilitate wound healing. This may also have some effect on eventual scarring because, as mentioned previously, delayed wound healing has been linked to increased scar formation.

Certain areas of the body may be difficult to fit appropriately with a fabric pressure garment. For example, due to the contours of the central portion of the face, palm of the hand, interscapular region, and sternal region, the fabric generally bridges between bony prominences or over anatomic arches. Foam, thermoplastic splinting material, and rubberized compounds can be placed under a pressure garment to conform better to these areas (see Figure 13–2). These "inserts" can also be used to augment pressure provided by a well-fitting pressure garment in areas such as the web spaces of the hand (see Figure 13–3). Custom-fitted, rigid, transparent, plastic material has also been used successfully to control scarring of the face and could certainly be considered for other areas.[23,24]

Massage

Massage has been advocated as a treatment for scar, both to loosen adhesions formed between the scar and adjacent tissue and to prevent or decrease scarring. Evidence for the effectiveness of massage on scar is scarce. The use of some form of friction massage should be useful in mobilizing superficial tissues by loosening the adhesions of scar to the tissue, based on the mechanical effects of the massage. Massage does not appear to decrease scarring or to improve variables of scar formation, such as vascularity, pliability, and height.[25] Although massage does not appear to improve the scar itself, supplementary benefits of massage may include lubrication of the scar to prevent drying and cracking of the skin, a decrease in reported pruritis, and the psychologic benefits of touch. Aggressive massage of early forming scar tissue should be avoided because it may cause blisters or skin breakdown.

Silicone

A silicone polymer gel (the viscosity of silicone used for scar treatment) is produced in sheets or pads that are applied directly over a maturing scar. These manufactured gel pads are commonly offered in several shapes and sizes for application to scars on different areas of the body. Silicone gel has been used successfully in treating scar hypertrophy.[26,27] The mechanism of action behind the success of silicone gel treatment is not known. Silicone gel is most commonly used over small areas, as opposed to large surface areas. It is also used in areas where sufficient pressure cannot be applied to a scar. Reported complications associated with silicone gel application include local rash, skin breakdown, and a lack of

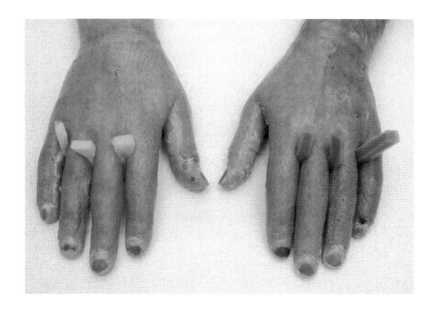

Figure 13–1 Self-adherent wrap and cotton elasticized pressure supports may be used to control edema and scarring. Coban™ self-adherent wrap was applied to the fingers in this figure. Tubigrip™ was used to cover the arm and hand in this figure. *Source:* Copyright © 2001, R. Scott Ward, PT, PhD.

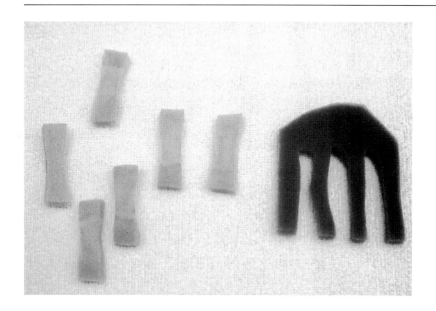

Figure 13–2 Examples of how foam was cut for placement in the wed spaces of the fingers under a pressure support glove. *Source:* Copyright © 2001, R. Scott Ward, PT, PhD.

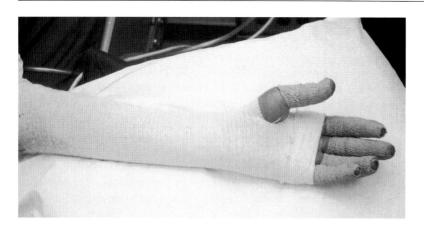

Figure 13–3 Application of the foam inserts placed in the web spaces of hands. A pressure support glove is then applied over these inserts. The foam inserts increase the pressure applied to web spaces of fingers and toes and can be used over other areas that may require additional pressure. *Source:* Copyright © 2001, R. Scott Ward, PT, PhD.

durability of some brands of silicone. If a rash develops, the use of the gel product should be temporarily suspended. In general, the rash clears up readily and, because the rash does not predictably reoccur at the same location, the gel may be reapplied, once the site is clear of the rash. Skin breakdown appears to occur in cases where a rash develops and the use of the gel sheet is not interrupted. No systemic complications related to the use of silicone have been reported.

Exercise

Exercise is vital in counteracting the contraction associated with active hypertrophic scar. Directed exercise to prevent deconditioning, functional limitation, and disability is also extremely important. When determining an exercise prescription for a patient with scar, several factors about the scar should be considered, including location of the scar, size of the scar (surface area of the scar), and status of the scar (phase of wound healing). For example, in some acute situations immediately following a grafting procedure or following tendon repair associated with a skin wound, any type of exercise may be delayed to allow for appropriate healing. Patient variables that also must be considered in the preparation of an exercise prescription include: the patient's medical history and current medical status, the patient's age, the patient's level of cognition, the patient's perceived or real level of cooperation, and the patient's goals for recovery.

A patient should always be encouraged to put as much stretch on the scar as is safely indicated by the therapist to prevent as much scar contraction as possible. Blanching of the scar is a reasonable clinical indication that the scar is being sufficiently stretched, and the stretch should not exceed the pain tolerance of the patient. Stretching of a scar should be done with a slow, sustained elongation of the tissue. Stretching and exercise will also help to prevent other associated soft tissues from shortening.

Types of Applicable Exercise

Active Exercise. Active exercise should be the preferred method of exercise in treating scar. This type of exercise allows a patient to control the extent and amount of stretch placed on a scar. Active exercise will also help to overcome any loss of strength or endurance associated with varying levels of muscle disuse sometimes associated with scar formation. An active exercise program should be prescribed and monitored by a therapist.

Active-Assisted Exercise. Active-assisted exercise allows a patient who cannot quite achieve full range of motion to be assisted by the therapist. Patients should be encouraged to complete as much of the motion as they can by themselves; then the therapist can apply additional stretch to maximize tissue elongation. Weights may be used to enhance a stretch.

The patient may also provide the assistance to active motion by using equipment such as reciprocal pulleys.

Passive Exercise. Passive exercise is effective but does not encourage patient independence. This form of stretching may be necessary if a patient is otherwise unable to stretch a scar because of such problems as weakness or paralysis, or when the patient is otherwise cognitively unable to participate in a prescribed active exercise program. Passive exercise, controlled by the therapist, may also be indicated when a wound is acute enough that a well-intentioned but overzealous patient might compromise healing. The therapist should be cautious not to overstretch the scar or exceed a patient's pain tolerance. Therapists should be aware that overly aggressive stretching might lead to heterotopic ossification.[28] Passive exercise should progress to active-assisted or active exercise as soon as possible.

Strength Exercise. There may be variable times of recovery from wounds. As previously mentioned, delayed wound healing also is associated with increased scar formation. Any reason for a decrease in normal use of a muscle (or muscle group) can lead to a decrease in strength of that muscle. Strength testing should be a part of any physical examination associated with scarring. If strength deficits are found, a prescribed series of resistance exercises should be provided to regain lost strength. Strengthening exercises will also assist with any decreases in endurance or conditioning.

Directed Functional Exercise. Scar contraction can also lead to an inability to strengthen a muscle through its normal range of motion. These scar contraction-related impairments of strength or range of motion can lead to functional limitations. Age-appropriate functional exercises should be instituted to improve motor skills, enhance confidence in daily activities, and allow the patient to resume his or her expected daily role in society.

Splinting

Splints are generally indicated for the positioning of a scar to avoid deformation or to maintain or increase the stretch on a scar. The therapist can fabricate splints or some effective prefabricated splints are also available. Thermoplastic material is the most common item used by therapists to fabricate custom splints. It is common that these splints, when used for scar, are fabricated as *conforming splints*. A conforming splint is one that is custom-fit to a patient and matches the patient's anatomic shape. A custom-fit, conforming splint decreases the likelihood of a poorly fitted splint and might also apply some pressure to the scar, therefore assisting in controlling scar formation.

Splints may also be referred to as *static splints*, *dynamic splints*, or *serial splints*. A static splint has a fixed shape and maintains a position through immobilization of the splinted part.[29] Static splints are commonly used in the early phases of scar formation. They are generally molded and applied following an exercise treatment to maintain the elongation of the scar achieved during the session. They may be left on for an extended period of time to preserve gains of range of motion. Dynamic splints apply a force, or a stretch, to a body part or allow resistance to movement for exercise.[29] This type of splint can be used to continue a gentle force to scar, thus providing an extended period of stretching. Serial splints are basically static splints that are remolded to a newly achieved position of a body part. Serial splints (or casts) might be used if a scar is particularly difficult to stretch. A maximal tissue stretch is completed, then the splint is reformed to the new stretched position. This procedure is followed "serially" until full range of motion is realized.

Splinting should be discontinued if there is any associated pain, sensory disturbance (numbness, tingling, etc.), or skin breakdown.

Positioning

Positioning may be used to sustain tissue elongation to counter scar contraction.[30] General positions of preference are listed in Table 13–2. Custom-made or prefabricated splints may be used as "positioning" devices. However, positioning devices need not be sophisticated or expensive. For example, pillows may be used to position the hips or shoulders, and high-top tennis shoes make a reasonable positioning device for the foot and ankle.

Physical Agents

Thermal agents are the common therapeutic modalities used to treat scar or the sequelae of scarring. Warming the scar, in particular, may have the most effect on the tissue because of the high concentration of collagen in scar. Gersten[31] demonstrated that collagen extensibility could be increased with therapeutic applications of ultrasound. The combined work of Gersten and others groups also provided the strong advocation that collagen tissue is most effectively stretched when a blend of heat and gentle stretch are provided.[32,33] Superficial forms of heat may also provide the most effective method of heating surface scar and allowing enhanced elongation of the tissue; however, very little research exists to support the efficacy of superficial heat on integumentary scarring.

Because scars are also normally hypesthetic, caution must be taken when applying thermal agents to the scar tissue. A sensory examination should be completed, and frequent inspections of the tissue should be done to ensure that no

Table 13–2 Preferred Anticontracture Positions for Major Joints.

Joint/ Joint Complex	Preferred Position
Neck	Hyperextension, no rotation
Shoulder	Abduction (90°), slight horizontal flexion
Elbow	Extension, supination
Wrist/hand	Slight wrist extension, slight MCP flexion, PIP/DIP extension, thumb abduction
Trunk	Straight postural alignment
Hip	Extension, abduction (20°), no rotation
Knee	Full extension
Ankle/foot	Neutral ankle (no plantar flexion), neutral toes

tissue damage is occurring secondary to the heat or coupling media.

Patient Education and Self-Care

Patients and their families or other caregivers should be trained to apply and assess scar control techniques. This includes care of the scar, pressure supports, silicon gel, exercise, splints, and positioning. Sufficient time for observation of the techniques, followed by opportunities to practice the techniques while supervised, will enhance the confidence of the patient/caregivers in their abilities. Providing written or pictorial supplemental materials can be useful additions to an education program. Having a patient/caregiver demonstrate the appropriate application of interventions is a logical discharge goal for patients with actively forming scar.

Patients/caregivers must be educated about the reasons for treatments being used and the goals of the interventions. An increased understanding will lead to more "buy-in" of the treatment. Patients are more likely to take some personal responsibility regarding their care if they truly "buy in" to the plan.[34] Reassurance that you will be willing to provide further assistance and advice, should it be needed, will also quell some concerns they might have about forgetting a component of the intervention or questions arising concerning the progression of the scar. The supplemental material provided might be sufficient for some, but a contact phone number with an invitation to call can also be reassuring.

Case Study

B.G. is a 34-year-old Caucasian female with healed full-thickness burns to the dorsum of her left hand and the dorsal surface of all left fingers. She is 3 weeks post–split-thickness autografting to the hand wound. Her burn injury included partial-thickness burns to her left arm that have fully healed. She is otherwise healthy, with no significant past medical history.

On examination, there is no evidence of scarring on the left arm over the site of the partial-thickness burns. The skin-grafted areas of the left hand are showing signs of scarring. The tissue is red, has a mildly decreased pliability, and is slightly raised and uneven. Range of motion measurements demonstrated the following limitations: the left wrist is 0–80° extension, 0–65° flexion; an average loss of 20° of motion in the left MCPs of the fingers; an average loss of 25° in the PIP joints of the fingers; an average loss of 15° in the DIP joints of the fingers; a loss of 20° in thumb abduction; and a 10° loss of the thumb MCP and IP flexion. The patient is also concerned about the appearance of the scar.

Therapy interventions for the problem at its current level include:

- Passive stretch of all joints affected by decreased range of motion. These stretches will be taught to the patient and should be performed six or more times daily.
- Active range of motion exercises, including encouraging full use of the hand in normal daily functional activities. The active motion exercises should be performed following each session of passive stretches. The hand should be used actively for all normal activities.
- Measurement and application of a custom-fit, anti-scar support glove. The patient will be educated on the application and care of the pressure garment. One to two additional gloves will be ordered.
- Application of moisturizer to the scar, as needed for itching and discomfort of the scar. The patient will be educated in the indication for application of moisturizer, including itching, discomfort of the scar, and "scaliness" of the scar.

All of these interventions will continue through to maturation of the scar, which may be 6–18 months. The frequency of the stretching and range of motion exercises may be decreased, depending on the level of ongoing limitation and impairment.

The discharge outcome for this patient would be a scar that closely matches normal skin pigment, is relatively pliable, is smooth, and that does not limit mobility and function of the hand.

DISCUSSION

When considering treatment for a scar, all aspects of the scarring process must be deliberated. This includes the appearance of the scar and the limitations that result from the contraction of the scar. It is important to remember that scarring is a process and that it commonly takes several months for a scar to mature. Therefore, much of what is done to treat scar cannot be employed on only a short-term basis. This requires high-quality patient education and follow-up to monitor the progression of the scarring properly in quest of the best possible clinical outcome.

REVIEW QUESTIONS

1. How is scar tissue formed and what are predictors for scar formation?
2. Describe the characteristics of scar and impairments related to scar contraction.
3. What interventions may be useful in treating the disfigurement of a scar that is immature and hypertrophic?
4. What interventions may be useful in treating range of motion impairment secondary to scar contraction?

RESOURCES

Custom Pressure Garment Manufacturers

Barton-Carey Medical Products
269 63 Eckel Road, Suite 303
Perrysburg, OH 43551
(800) 421-0444

Bio-Concepts, Inc.
2424 East University Drive
Phoenix, AZ 85034-6911
(800) 421-5647

Gottfried Medical, Inc
4105 West Alexis Road
Toledo, OH 43623
(800) 537-1968

Jobst Institute, Inc.
5825 Carnegie Blvd.
Charlotte, NC 28209-4633
Phone: (800) 537-1063

Medical Z
6800 Alamo Downs Parkway
San Antonio, TX 78238
Phone: (800) 368-7478

REFERENCES

1. Thomsen M. It all began with Aristotle—the history of the treatment of burns. *Burns Incl Therm Inj.* 1988;14(Suppl):S1–S8.

2. Ketchum LD. Hypertrophic scars and keloids. *Clin Plast Surg.* 1977;4:301–310.

3. Rockwell WB, Cohen IK, Erlich HP. Keloids and hypertrophic scars: A comprehensive review. *Plast Reconstr Surg.* 1989;84:827–837.

4. Hunt TK. Disorders of wound healing. *World J Surg.* 1980;4:289–295.

5. Cohen IK and McCoy BJ. The biology and control of surface overhealing. *World J Surg.* 1980;4:289–295.

6. Deitch EA, Wheelahan TM, Rose MP, et al. Hypertrophic burn scars: Analysis of variables. *J Trauma.* 1983;23:895–898.

7. Lewis WHP, Sun KKY. Hypertrophic scar: A genetic hypothesis. *Burns.* 1990;16:176–178.

8. Blumenfield M, Reddish PM. Identification of psychologic impairment in patients with mild-moderate thermal injury: Small burn, big problem. *Gen Hosp Psychiatry.* 1987;9:142–146.

9. Cobb N, Maxwell G, Silverstein P. Patient perception of quality of life after burn injury: Results of an eleven-year study. *J Burn Care Rehabil.* 1990;11:330–333.

10. Sheffield CG III, Irons GB, Mucha P Jr, et al. Physical and psychological outcome after burns. *J Burn Care Rehabil.* 1988;9:172–177.

11. Hunt TK. Disorders of wound healing. *World J Surg.* 1980;4:289–295.

12. Clark JA, Cheng JCY, Leung KS, Leung PC. Mechanical characterization of human postburn skin during compression therapy. *J Biomech.* 1987;20:397–406.

13. Ward RS, Tuckett RP. Quantitative threshold changes in cutaneous sensation of patients with burns. *J Burn Care Rehabil.* 1991;12:569–575.

14. Sullivan T, Smith J, Kermode J, McIver E, Courtemanche DJ. Rating the burn scar. *J Burn Care Rehabil.* 1990;11:256–260.

15. Yeong EK, Mann R, Engrav LH, et al. Improved burn scar assessment with use of new scar-rating scale. *J Burn Care Rehabil.* 1997;18:353–355.

16. Kraemer MD, Jones T, Deitch EA. Burn contractures: Incidence, predisposing factors, and results of surgical therapy. *J Burn Care Rehabil.* 1988;9:261–265.

17. Blair VP. The influence of mechanical pressure on wound healing. *Ill. Med J.* 1924;46:249–252.

18. Cronin TD. The use of a molded splint to prevent contracture after split skin grafting on the neck. *Plast Reconstr Surg.* 1961;27:7–18.

19. Larson DL, Abston S, Evans EB, Dobrkovsky M, Linares HA. Techniques for decreasing scar formation and contractures in the burned patient. *J Trauma.* 1971;11:807–823.

20. Mann R, Yeong EK, Moore M, Colescott D, Engrav LH. Do custom-fitted pressure garments provide adequate pressure? *J Burn Care Rehabil.* 1997;18:247–249.

21. Cheng JCY, Evans JH, Leung KS, Clark JA, Choy TTC, Leung PC. Pressure therapy in the treatment of post-burn hypertrophic scar: A critical look into its usefulness and fallacies by pressure monitoring. *Burns Incl Therm Inj.* 1984;10:154–163.

22. Rosser P. Adherence to pressure garment therapy of post traumatic burn injury. *J Burn Care Rehabil.* 2000;21(Part 2):S178.

23. Rivers E, Strate RG, Solem LD. The transparent face mask. *Am J Occup Ther.* 1979;33:100–113.

24. Shons AR, Rivers E, Solem LD. A rigid transparent face mask for control of scar hypertrophy. *Ann Plast Surg.* 1981;6:245–248.

25. Patino O, Novick C, Merlo A, Benaim F. Massage in hypertrophic scars. *J Burn Care Rehabil.* 1998;19:268–271.

26. Gold HM. A controlled clinical trial of topical silicone gel sheeting in the treatment of hypertrophic scars and keloids. *J Am Acad Dermatol.* 1994;30:506–507.

27. Sang TA, Monafo WW, Mustoe TA: Topical silicone gel: A new treatment for hypertrophic scars. *Surgery.* 1989;106:781–787.

28. Van Laeken N, Snelling CFT, Meek RN, Warren RJ, Foley B. Heterotopic bone formation in the patient with burn injuries: A retrospective assessment of contributing factors and methods of investigation. *J Burn Care Rehabil.* 1989;10:331–335.

29. Duncan RM. Basic principles of splinting the hand. *Phys Ther.* 1989;69(12):1104–1116.

30. Rudolf R. Construction and the control of contraction. *World J Surg.* 1980;4:279–287.

31. Gersten JW. Effect of ultrasound on tendon extensibility. *Am J Phys Med.* 1955;34:362–369.

32. LaBan MM. Collagen tissue: Implications of its response to stress in vitro. *Arch Phys Med Rehabil.* 1962;43:461.

33. Warren CG, Lehmann JF, Koblanski JN. Elongation of rat tail tendon: Effect of load and temperature *Arch Phys Med Rehabil.* 1976;57:122–126.

34. Peloquin SM: Linking purpose to procedure during interactions with patients. *Am J Occup Ther.* 1988;42:775–781.

PART III

Management by Wound Etiology

Barbara M. Bates-Jensen

Determining the cause or etiology of a wound is a critical element in creating a comprehensive treatment plan for patients with wounds. The chapters in Part III focus on management by wound etiology. Specific attention to acute surgical wounds, pressure ulcers, vascular ulcers, and neuropathic ulcers is presented in the chapters in Part III. Emphasis is placed on understanding the pathophysiology involved in the wound type, assessment methods, and prevention and management of specific wound types. Improving and expanding knowledge of wound etiology empowers clinicians to provide quality comprehensive care in clinical practice.

Chapter 14 presents management of the acute surgical wound. The chapter begins by defining acute versus chronic wounds. When does an acute wound become a chronic wound? Better understanding of acute wounds improves ability to monitor and treat all wounds. Types of surgical wound healing—primary intention, secondary intention, and tertiary intention—are presented. Extrinsic factors that affect wound healing during the preoperative, intraoperative, and postoperative time periods are described. Surgical wound classifications are presented and reviewed. Interventions for managing hypovolemia, thermoregulation strategies, and methods of optimizing tissue oxygen perfusion are described.

Intrinsic factors affecting healing of the acute surgical wound, such as age, concurrent conditions, nutritional status, and oxygenation and tissue perfusion are all discussed, with special attention to the patient with diabetes. Examination of the surgical incision includes evaluation of wound characteristics, such as incision location, length, presence of healing ridge, type and amount of exudate, type of wound closure materials, and approximation of wound edges. The incisional examination forms the basis of acute surgical wound assessment and is presented by phase of wound healing (inflammatory, proliferative, and remodeling).

Discussion includes types of dressings used for primary and secondary dressings. Wound healing in secondary intention and tertiary intention wounds is discussed and contrasted with primary intention incisions.

Outcome measures for evaluating healing in incisional wounds following the phases of wound healing are presented and described, with examples of appropriate documentation of the healing incision. The chapter concludes with a case study for review of material and self-care teaching guidelines for use with other health care providers, family caregivers, and patients.

Chapters 15 and 16 describe issues related to management of pressure ulcers. Chapter 15 is devoted to pathophysiology and prevention of pressure ulcers. It begins with a definition of pressure ulcers and an extensive review of the pathophysiology of pressure ulcer development. The relationship between time and pressure in the development of pressure ulcers is presented, as well as the clinical presentation of pressure ulceration and the most prevalent locations for pressure ulcer development. Specific information is included on assessment of the dark-skinned individual for risk of pressure ulceration.

The history of staging systems and the current system recommended by the Agency for Health Care Policy and Research and the National Pressure Ulcer Advisory Panel are described. The issues of pressure ulcer assessment and the use and misuse of staging classification systems are a subject of debate and controversy. Pressure ulcer development does not necessarily occur from one stage to the next, and there may be different etiologic factors for various stages. Chapter 15 reviews this issue.

Discussion of pressure ulcer pathophysiology and etiology would not be complete without mention of other interacting factors. Factors that contribute to pressure ulcer development by force over the bony prominence and those that affect the tolerance of the tissues to pressure are presented and described. Particular attention is given to immobility or severely restricted mobility because it is the most important risk factor for all populations and a necessary condition for the development of pressure ulcers. The most common risk assessment tools are presented and discussed.

Appropriate prevention interventions can be focused on eliminating specific risk factors. Thus, early intervention for pressure ulcers is risk factor-specific and prophylactic in nature. The prevention strategies are presented by risk factors, beginning with general information and ending with specific strategies for a particular risk factor. Chapter 15 includes specific information on the use of support surfaces, with definitions of pressure-reducing and pressure-relieving devices, pillow bridging, and passive repositioning. Extensive discussion on nutrition interventions and management of incontinence is included. Skin hygiene and maintenance interventions round out the prevention strategies. Chapter 15 concludes with outcome measures for evaluating the success of a pressure ulcer prevention program and extensive self-care teaching guidelines for other health care providers, family caregivers, and patients.

In Chapter 16, Rappl continues the discussion of support surfaces that began in Chapter 15. Rappl provides a look at therapeutic positioning for pressure ulcer prevention. Persons who become sitting dependent more than ambulatory and those who use the lying-down or the sitting position for the majority of their day are at high risk of skin breakdown. Also, for the patient with an existing pressure ulcer, proper positioning in the most active and functional position possible, both in sitting and in recumbent positions, improves the healing rate of the ulcer and minimizes the likelihood of developing new ulcers. Chapter 16 provides an overview of therapeutic positioning knowledge. The areas the clinician should examine to determine the need for intervention are presented and described. The basics of therapeutic positioning and a discussion of how therapeutic positioning affects body system impairments are presented. The chapter includes a table on functional diagnosis and relationship to prognosis, interventions, and outcomes related to therapeutic positioning. The ideal sitting position is described, and basic seating principles related to pelvic control, thigh control, seat depth, and footrest are discussed. Finally, specifics in positioning the patient with an existing ulcer, both in sitting and in lying down, are described. An extensive discussion of methods of determining appropriate wheelchairs and sitting position, as well as procedures for recumbent positioning for patients, is presented.

Donayre provides an in-depth analysis of the diagnosis and management of vascular ulcers in Chapter 17. The chapter begins with a review of general anatomy and physiology of the circulatory system and pathophysiology related to lower extremity ulcers. Thorough history and physical assessment are essential for the patient with a lower leg ulcer, and Donayre provides this information for each ulcer type; in addition, risk factors for arterial/ischemic, venous, and diabetic ulcers are discussed. Donayre describes presentation and assessment of common findings related to lower leg ulcers, such as intermittent claudication, rest pain, altered ankle-brachial index, edema, and tissue changes. Associated diagnostic tests for the lower leg are described. Differential diagnosis for leg ulcers is a key factor in determining appropriate treatment. Treatment that is appropriate for a venous ulcer may be contraindicated for an arterial/ischemic ulcer. The presenting clinical manifestations, diagnostic tests, and differential wound assessments are presented for each lower leg ulcer type. Medical and surgical management related to arterial/ischemic, venous disease, and diabetic ulcers is described. Special attention is given to diagnosing osteomyelitis in the diabetic and describing pathophysiology of edema related to venous disease, with indications for clinical management.

Chapter 18 opens with Elftman's discussion of the necessity of interdisciplinary collaboration in the management of neuropathic ulcers. The neuropathic patient often has dysvascular components that must be addressed by a medical team, rather than by one specialty. The trineuropathy assessment, with attention to sensory, motor, and autonomic neuropathy, is explained. Gradual and sudden-onset peripheral neuropathy are compared for easy differential diagnosis. Diabetic neuropathy is the major focal point of Chapter 18. Common infections and dermatologic changes are presented. The definitions of wet and dry gangrene are presented, and the two conditions are compared. Footwear assessment guidelines and interventions, based on the Wagner ulcer grade, are explained. Chapter 18 includes in-depth explanations of sensory, pressure, vibratory, and foot deformity evaluation. Charcot's deformity is explained and the method of assessment described. Management with orthotic devices is explained. Specific instructions for procedures, such as how to make a foam toe separator, are included. Interventions to decrease pressure, such as total-contact casting, use of splints and inserts, and neurowalkers, are all discussed. A chapter on care of the skin and nails of the neuropathic foot by Conlan contains practical detailed instructions. The chapter concludes with self-care teaching guidelines for use with patients and family caregivers and documentation requirements for neuropathic ulcers.

Chapter 19 continues the examination of lower extremities with a focus on the skin and nails of the foot. Kelechi provides vivid photographs to help clinicians with diagnosis of common foot problems in the older adult. The chapter presents the underlying pathology, differential diagnosis, treatment, and plan for evaluation for three common foot problems, including tinea pedis, onychomycosis, and plantar fasciitis. Tinea pedis is the most common form of dermatophytoses, or fungal infection of the feet. Tinea pedis, most commonly known as athlete's foot, is a disorder that can be classified into three categories: interdigital infections, scaling hyperkeratotic moccasin-type infections of the plantar surface, and highly inflammatory vesiculobullous eruptions. Diagnosis and treatment of each is presented and discussed.

Plantar fasciitis is the most common form of heel pain and is due to inflammation, microruptures, hemorrhages, and collagen degeneration of the plantar fascia. The major underlying factor is overuse injury to soft tissue involving repetitive, excessive loading impact on heel strike over time. Interventions address treatment of pain, restoring flexibility to the ankle and arch, strengthening the muscles in and around the foot, and gradual resumption of activities. Conservative approaches are presented. Onychomycosis (tinea unguium) is an infection of the toenails in which fungal organisms invade the nail unit via the nail bed or nail plate, causing insidious, progressive destruction of the nail plate, if left untreated. Treatment measures are presented and include measures for topical nail reduction using urea compound (20–40%) in petrolatum under thin film dressing and topical antifungal agents. This chapter concludes with a brief discussion of miscellaneous conditions of the foot.

The final chapter in this section, Chapter 20, presents management of malignant cutaneous wounds and fistulas. Palliative care and the role of the wound care clinician, when faced with wounds with little or no healing potential, plays a strong part in the material presented in this chapter. Malignant cutaneous wounds and fistulas are often complex, difficult-to-manage wounds. Clinicians must use creativity and sensitivity in dealing with patients who present with malignant cutaneous wounds or fistulas. Basic goals of therapy are presented with attention to symptom palliation. Techniques are described and discussed on pain management, odor control, management of bleeding, and pouching for output. Several techniques are illustrated, with step-by-step photographs to complement the text. This chapter provides a thoughtful, caring framework for the clinician dealing with malignant cutaneous wounds and fistulas.

Although similarities exist in the treatment of any wound, treatment approach varies depending on wound etiology. The chapters in Part III form a foundation on knowledge of wounds of various etiologies. This foundation should provide clinicians with a stronger and more individualized approach to the person with a wound.

CHAPTER 14

Acute Surgical Wound Management

Barbara M. Bates-Jensen and James D. Wethe

CHAPTER OBJECTIVES

At the completion of this chapter, the reader will be able to:

1. Define key characteristics of the acute surgical wound.
2. Describe assessment factors for the acute surgical wound.
3. Describe factors that affect wound healing in the acute surgical wound during the preoperative, intraoperative, and postoperative periods.
4. Explain the relationship between tissue perfusion and oxygenation, and wound healing.

ACUTE SURGICAL WOUND DEFINITION

Acute wounds are defined as disruptions in the integrity of the skin and underlying tissues that progress through the healing process in a timely and uneventful manner. The acute elective surgical wound is an example of a healthy wound in which healing can be maximized. However, not all surgical wounds are uncomplicated, with maximal healing potential or the possibility of uneventful healing. For example, acute surgical wounds can occur in unhealthy tissues, in a compromised host, or as a result of unexpected or significant trauma. Surgical wounds may be allowed to heal by one of three methods: primary intention, secondary intention, and tertiary intention (Table 14–1). Wounds healing by primary intention are wounds with edges approximated and closed. Secondary wounds are wounds left open after surgery. Secondary healing wounds heal with scar tissue replacement in the tissue defect. Tertiary wound healing, or delayed primary closure, involves aspects of both primary and secondary wound healing. In tertiary wound healing, the wound is left open initially and, after a short period of time, the edges are approximated and the wound is closed. Wound healing by secondary intention or dehisced wounds may not follow a timely and uneventful healing course and, thus, may be considered "chronic" wounds by some clinicians.[1]

When does an acute wound become a chronic wound? The easiest and perhaps the least controversial defining characteristic of the acute wound that becomes chronic is failure to follow the normal wound healing temporal sequence. In general, the acute surgical wound should complete the proliferative phase of wound healing in 4 weeks. For example, the wound should have filled with granulation tissue and be resurfaced with epithelial tissue. Acute surgical wounds that progress at a slower pace or fail to progress can be considered chronic.

The surgical incision healing by primary intention might be described as the ideal wound for healing. The wound is controlled with attention to tissue handling and proper use of surgical instruments by the surgeon, and the wound edges are apposed and aligned immediately to decrease the risk of infection. The acute surgical incision wound healing by primary intention is the focus of this chapter.

FACTORS AFFECTING HEALING IN ACUTE WOUNDS

Healing in acute surgical wounds involves the interaction of extrinsic and intrinsic factors. Extrinsic factors relate to those agents outside the person, whereas intrinsic factors are those influencing the person internally or systemically.

310

Table 14–1 Types of Surgical Wound Healing

Wound Healing Type	Definition
Primary intention	Wound edges approximated and closed at time of surgery
Secondary intention	Wound left open after surgery and allowed to heal with scar tissue replacing the tissue defect
Tertiary or delayed primary closure	After surgery, wound left open initially and after short period of time, wound edges are approximated and wound is closed

Extrinsic Factors

The physical environment before and during surgery, the surgical preparation, the technique of the surgeon, and types of sutures are all examples of extrinsic factors affecting acute wound healing. Thus, for the surgical wound, evaluation of the perioperative period is indicated, because it plays a role in the wound outcome. Wound infection is the major cause of surgical wounds failing to progress through the healing process in a timely and uneventful manner. Operating room protocols, attention to instrumentation, and appropriate surgical technique are all means of decreasing the risk of infection and ensuring optimal healing from the outset for the surgical wound.

Preoperative Period

The length of time the patient spends in the hospital prior to surgery influences the rate of surgical wound infection. As the length of hospital time increases prior to surgery, the risk of wound infection increases.[2] Preparation of the operative site also influences the risk of wound infection. Showering immediately prior to surgery, using a hexachlorophene soap, has been shown to result in a decrease in infection rate, compared with not showering.[2] Shaving the operative area and the method used to shave the area have also been implicated in surgical wound infection.[2]

> **Research Wisdom:** *Operative Site Preparation*
>
> Use of an electric razor, clipping hair, and not shaving the operative area are all associated with wound infection rates lower than those with use of a nonelectric razor to shave the operative area.[2] Despite the research, however, most preparations still include nonelectric shaving, most commonly performed in the operating room. The poor implementation of the research may be due to the absence of electric razors or clippers in the operating room.

Intraoperative Period

Limiting the infection rate intraoperatively is largely under the control of the surgeon. Sometimes, infection control is hard to obtain. For example, the surgeon has limited power over the nature of the problem for which the surgery is performed, the operative site, and the general condition of the patient; all are more complicated factors that are not easily controlled. The type of surgical procedure influences the risk of infection. Surgical procedures are classified according to the risk of infection.[3] Table 14–2 presents wound classifications for surgery. Clean wounds are those nontraumatic injuries in which no inflammation is encountered during the procedure and there is no break in sterile technique. Clean-contaminated wounds are procedures wherein the gastrointestinal (GI) or respiratory tract is entered without significant contamination. A contaminated wound is one in which a major break in sterile technique or gross spillage from the gastrointestinal tract occurs. Procedures in which acute bacterial inflammation or pus is encountered with devitalized tissue or contamination are classified as dirty or infected wounds.

Increased length of time for the operative procedure increases the risk for wound infection significantly. One study found that the infection rate doubled each hour that the surgical procedure continued.[2] Strict adherence by operating room personnel to a protocol has also resulted in decreased wound infection rates.[4]

The surgeon must be concerned with wound tension, vascular supply, and proper surgical technique. If the wound cannot be closed without a significant amount of tension or if the vascular supply is poor, there is increased risk of dehiscence and infection.[5] Suturing technique can assist with optimal wound healing outcomes. Use of buried sutures can improve primary wound healing by decreasing potential dead space underneath the incision, giving tensile support for 4–6 weeks while the wound is still weak, and decreasing tension on the apposed wound edges.[5] Surface sutures may provide additional concerns for optimal healing because they provide additional "wounds" to heal alongside the incision.

Table 14–2 Surgical Wound Classifications

Wound Classification	Surgical Label	Definition
I	Clean	• Nontraumatic injuries • No inflammation found during procedure • No break in sterile technique
II	Clean-contaminated	• Procedures involving GI or respiratory tract • No significant contamination
III	Contaminated	• Major break in sterile technique • Gross spillage from GI tract
IV	Dirty or infected	• Acute bacterial inflammation found • Pus encountered • Devitalized tissue encountered

Postoperative Period

The stress response associated with surgery has also been implicated as a cause of impaired wound healing. The stress of surgery is known to stimulate the sympathetic nervous system, with a resultant sympathetic nervous system-mediated vasoconstriction. The effect of high levels of circulating catecholamines in the immediate postoperative period causes the resulting vasoconstriction, with factors leading to the trigger of the sympathetic nervous system, including hypoxia, hypothermia, pain, and hypovolemia.[6] In the immediate postoperative period, measures of subcutaneous tissue/wound oxygenation are lower after major operations and correlate with extensive, more complex surgical procedures.[6] Attempts to restore tissue and wound oxygen deficits relate to minimizing the risks of hypothermia, pain, hypovolemia, and hypoxia simultaneously in the immediate postoperative period.

Clinical Wisdom: *Maximizing Wound Healing*

Critical measures to maximize wound healing in the immediate postoperative period include all of the following. Keep the patient:

• Warm
• Well hydrated, intravenously or orally
• Pain free by use of patient-controlled analgesia, if possible
• Well oxygenated by use of supplemental oxygen, if needed

Thermoregulatory responses are diminished in the surgical patient because of the prolonged exposure to the cold operating room environment. Patients treated with active rewarming by use of heated blankets during the recovery period respond with a faster return of normal tissue/wound oxygen levels than do those allowed to return to normothermia without rewarming interventions.[6] Routine use of measures to warm the patient actively during the surgical procedure, such as warming blankets and the use of warmed intravenous fluids, along with active monitoring during surgery, help to prevent thermoregulatory problems. It is easier to prevent thermoregulatory problems than to remedy them.

Correcting hypovolemia with adequate fluid infusion prevents continuing vasoconstriction caused by hypovolemia. Fluid replacement occurs simultaneously with rewarming efforts. Assessment and management of pain and tissue perfusion are also recommended to ensure optimal wound healing.[6]

Additional factors crucial to optimal surgical wound healing in the postoperative period are intrinsic factors that can be controlled, which are discussed in the following section.

Intrinsic Factors

Intrinsic factors affecting healing of the acute surgical wound are those that influence the person systemically. Intrinsic factors include age, concurrent conditions, nutritional status, and oxygenation and tissue perfusion.

Age

The physiologic changes that occur with aging place the older individual at higher risk for poor wound healing outcomes. Decreased elastin in the skin and differences in collagen replacement influence healing in older adults.[7] A decreased rate of replacement of cells affects the rate of wound healing and, in particular, reepithelialization of the skin.[7]

> **Clinical Wisdom:** *Risk of Delayed Wound Resurfacing in the Older Adult*
>
> The delay in wound resurfacing puts the older patient at risk for wound infection. Daily wound assessments and use of topical dressings for protection are required for a longer period of time than necessary for younger patients.

Immune system function declines with age, and this may account for increased risk of infection in older adults. The microorganisms proliferate in the wound before they can be removed, due to the diminished immune response. Older adults present with chronic diseases, circulatory changes, and nutritional problems, all of which increase the risk for poor or delayed wound healing. Decreased motor coordination and diminished sensory function increase the potential for injury, wound complications, and repeated wounding at the same site.

Concurrent Conditions

The presence of certain diseases, conditions, or treatments can influence wound healing outcomes. Diabetes mellitus is one condition that interferes with wound healing. Diabetes is associated with small vessel disease, neuropathy, and problems specific to glucose control—all of which predispose the person to impaired wound healing. Diabetic wound healing problems include increased risk of infection, delayed epithelialization, impaired or delayed collagen synthesis, and slowed wound contraction and closure.[8] Hyperglycemia can affect the cellular response to wounding. There may be a delayed response or impaired functioning of the leukocyte and fibroblast cells, both of which are essential for wound repair.[8]

The effect of surgery on the diabetic patient can be dramatic. The diabetic responds to the stress of surgery by releasing a series of hormones: epinephrine, glucagon, cortisol, and growth hormone. The stress hormones reduce the amount of circulating insulin while increasing circulating glucose. Elevated glucose levels can reduce the effectiveness of neutrophils' phagocytotic function and alter the deposition of collagen by fibroblasts, leading to a decrease in wound tensile strength.[8] Elevated glucose levels can also lead to cellular malnutrition, because insulin is the key for allowing nutrient use in cells. When glucose cannot be used as energy, proteins and fats are used as fuel, depleting necessary substrates for wound healing. The ability to control the glucose level in the postoperative period is probably advantageous for positive wound healing outcomes in the diabetic. Maintaining serum glucose levels below 200 mg/dL is recommended for patients with wounds.[3] In the immediate postoperative period, close monitoring of blood glucose and insulin supplements, as indicated, are required for adequate wound healing. Careful attention to blood glucose levels can assist significantly in positive outcomes and prevent an acute surgical wound from becoming a chronic wound.

> **Clinical Wisdom:** *Urine Glucose Levels*
>
> Urine glucose levels are not sensitive enough to provide good glucose control because of the high renal threshold for glucose (approximately 180 mg/dL). The use of blood glucose monitoring for more definitive management is a critical assessment strategy.

Other conditions also affect wound healing. Cardiovascular disease presents risks for wound healing because of the associated perfusion alterations, impaired blood flow, and vascular disease. Atherosclerosis is a common cause of inadequate perfusion of wounds.[9] Immunocompromised patients are an additional group at risk for poor healing outcomes. The immune system plays a significant role in wound healing, and any impairment (e.g., aging, malnutrition, and cancer) can have serious sequelae for the patient with a wound.

Treatments that affect wound healing include steroids, antiinflammatory drugs, antimitotic drugs, and radiation therapy. Steroids inhibit all phases of wound healing, affecting phagocytosis, collagen synthesis, and angiogenesis. The effects of steroids can be reversed with the use of topical vitamin A. The vitamin A is applied directly to the wound and acts as an inflammatory agent. Vitamin A is appropriate to apply to open wound beds. Wounds healing by primary intention, closed with edges well approximated, may not be appropriate candidates for topical vitamin A.

> **Clinical Wisdom:** *Vitamin A Use for Wounds*
>
> The usual dose of topical vitamin A is 1,000 U applied three times a day to the open wound bed for 7–10 days.

Other antiinflammatory drugs also inhibit wound healing, with effects seen predominantly in the inflammatory phase. Cancer therapies, antimitotic medications, and radiation therapy work by impeding the normal cell cycle in rapidly dividing cells. The antimitotic activity interferes with new tissue generation in the wound. In addition, radiation therapy has both acute effects on cellular function and long-term sequelae for healing. The long-term effects of radiation therapy on wound healing are caused by hypoperfusion of tissues in the irradiated field. Hypoperfusion induced by irradiation is due to damage, deterioration, and fibrosis of the vasculature.[3]

Nutritional Status

Adequate nutrition is essential for wound healing. In the healthy surgical patient, malnutrition may not be an issue. However, with the population aging and more procedures being performed on older adults, nutritional status is a concern for wound healing. Adequate amounts of calories, proteins, fats, carbohydrates, vitamins, and minerals are all required for wound repair. Inadequate amounts of any nutrients negatively influence wound healing.[10]

Proteins are needed for neovascularization, fibroblast proliferation, collagen synthesis, and wound remodeling. Amino acids are the structural components of proteins and are essential parts of deoxyribonucleic acid (DNA) and ribonucleic acid (RNA). DNA and RNA provide the pattern for cell mitosis and enzymes required for tissue generation. Protein malnutrition results in loss of body stores of amino acids and insufficient substrates for wound repair and new tissue growth.

Carbohydrates and fats provide necessary energy required for cellular function. When there are inadequate amounts of carbohydrates and fats (calorie malnutrition), the body uses catabolism to break down proteins in order to meet energy requirements. Glucose balance and available essential fatty acids are essential substrates for wound healing.

Vitamins and minerals play an important role in wound healing. Several vitamins and minerals have specific functions for wound healing. Vitamin A is a fat-soluble vitamin and is responsible for supporting epithelialization, angiogenesis, and collagen formation. It is also important for the inflammatory phase of wound healing. The water-soluble B vitamins are cofactors in enzymatic reactions. Vitamin C has been associated with wound healing. Vitamin C is essential for angiogenesis and collagen synthesis. Vitamin C also supports fibroblast function and is critical for leukocyte function. For patients with wounds, infection, or significant injury, supplemental vitamin C is often provided to assist in meeting the increased metabolic and wound healing needs. Consensus on specific guidelines for appropriate supplemental doses of vitamin C is not available; however, megadoses of vitamin C have not been proven beneficial. Vitamin C use and elimination increase with exercise, stress, injury, increases in metabolic rate, and smoking. Vitamin D is required for bone healing and absorption of calcium, which is important in enzyme systems. Vitamin K is necessary for coagulation and hemostasis. Vitamin E is used for fat metabolism; excess amounts are not beneficial to wound healing.

Minerals also play a role in wound healing. Usually, the minerals of concern are zinc and iron. Zinc plays an essential role in enzyme systems and immune system function and is

---

Clinical Wisdom: *Vitamin E and Wound Healing*

Many people think that vitamin E has healing properties. In fact, vitamin E delays healing and fibrosis.[10] It is the delay of fibrosis or scarring that may be responsible for decreased scar formation at the injury site.

---

a cofactor for collagen synthesis. Zinc deficiency contributes to disruption in granulation tissue formation, diminished tensile strength, dehiscence, and evisceration.[10] Low levels of zinc are found in older adults and low-income patients, with losses associated with diarrhea, renal failure, diuretic and laxative use, and parenteral and enteral nutrition.[11] Iron is a cofactor in collagen synthesis and acts to transport oxygen. Iron deficiency may be present in those with changes in eating habits, intestinal damage, or increased metabolic needs.

Oxygenation and Perfusion

Adequate wound oxygenation is essential for wound healing. The initial injury causes hypoxia, and the resultant growth factor release supports initial capillary budding. Oxygen is influential in angiogenesis, fibroblast function, epithelialization, and resistance to infection.[12–14] Tissue perfusion is intertwined with tissue oxygenation. Satisfactory tissue perfusion is essential for oxygenation. Ample circulating blood volume carries oxygen-rich hemoglobin to the tissues. Tissue perfusion alone, however, does not guarantee wound oxygenation. Problems related to tissue perfusion and oxygenation may be due to cardiovascular or pulmonary disease, as well as other conditions, such as hypovolemia. Thus, maintaining vascular volume is critical for ensuring adequate tissue perfusion. The clinician must balance fluid replacement to prevent both underhydration and overhydration. Excess hydration can lead to hypervolemia and edema, which may decrease tissue oxygenation. To optimize oxygenation in the presence of adequate tissue perfusion, use of pulmonary hygiene interventions, assessment and monitoring of tissue oxygen levels, and low-flow supplemental oxygen may be warranted.[15] Pulmonary hygiene, including incentive spirometry, deep breathing and coughing, and postural drainage, improves the pulmonary toilet and increases the likelihood of adequate oxygenation of the wound. Low-flow oxygen can saturate hemoglobin so that the supply to the tissue is ample. Promoting activity such as repositioning and early ambulation can also be beneficial for peripheral tissue perfusion and oxygenation.[15] Oxygenation and perfusion are vital to wound healing, and postoperative interventions to improve the circulatory and oxygen-carrying capacity of the tissues or blood (the oxygen saturation of tissues) can enhance wound healing.

ASSESSMENT OF THE ACUTE SURGICAL WOUND

Assessment of the acute surgical wound involves physical examination of the wound site and surrounding wound tissues in relation to the wound healing process (Figure 14–1). Physical examination of the wound and the surrounding tissues includes measurement of the incision; observation of the wound tissues, with attention to epithelial resurfacing, wound closure, wound exudate, and surrounding wound tissues; and palpation of the incision, with attention to collagen deposition and surrounding tissues. The linear measurement of the length of the incision and the anatomic location of the incision provide a baseline measure. Measure the length of the incision in centimeters.

Observation and palpation of the incision line provide insight to the healing process that occurs in the underlying tissues. Healing proceeds in the surgical incision as it does in other wounds with inflammation—proliferation of new tissues and remodeling. In the surgical incision, the wound healing processes are not always visible. Thus, the standard for assessment of healing may be best based on time since the surgical injury. It is important for clinicians to track the amount of time postsurgery, because the healing progress of the wound can be measured against the standard time expectations for acute wound repair. Knowledge of the wound healing process provides a critical foundation for assessment of the acute surgical incision. During the inflammatory process, assessment focuses on identification of signs and symptoms of inflammation, evaluation of wound closure materials and wound dressings, and appraisal of epithelial resurfacing. The central point during the proliferation phase of wound healing is evaluation of collagen deposition, wound exudate, and tissues surrounding the incision. Assessment during the remodeling phase is directed toward examination of collagen remodeling at the incision-site.

Incisional Assessment during the Inflammatory Phase

The major assessment finding in the first 4 days postoperatively is the identification of inflammation. The surgical incision may feel warm to the touch, and there may be surrounding erythema and edema at the incision-site. Signs of inflammation are expected and normal during the first 4 days postoperatively.

Clinical Wisdom: *Signs of Inflammation*

It is normal to observe signs of inflammation such as warmth, erythema or discoloration, pain, and edema at the incisional wound site during the first few days after surgery.

Patients with immune system compromise due to age, a disease process, or therapy (such as steroid treatments) may not be able to mount an effective inflammatory process; thus, the signs of inflammation at the incision are not visible. The lack of inflammation at the incision-site is an indication of immune system compromise. Thus, an incision with no indication of inflammation is an abnormal finding during the first 4 days after surgery. The process of epithelial resurfacing also occurs during the inflammatory phase of wound healing.

In the acute surgical incision, new epidermal tissues are generated quickly because of the presence of intact hair follicles and sebaceous and sweat glands, as well as the short distance the epithelial cells must travel to resurface the incision. The surgical incision is resurfaced with epithelium within 72 hours postsurgery. The new epidermis provides a barrier to bacterial organisms and, to a small degree, external trauma. The tensile strength of the incision is relatively weak, and the incision is not able to withstand force.

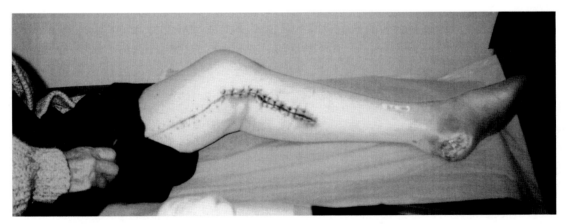

Figure 14–1 Surgical incision healing by primary intention. Note the lack of wound edge approximation and no healing ridge at the posterior half of the incision. Sutures remain present along the posterior incision. Courtesy of Evonne Fowler, MN, RN, CETN, Banning, California.

The astute clinician can observe changes in the new incision indicating the presence of new epithelial tissue. The incision is evaluated for the close approximation of the wound edges and color of the incision line. Wound edges should appear well aligned, with no tension observed.

Clinical Wisdom: *Incisional Color Changes*

As the new epithelial tissue migrates across the incision, the color of the incision may change from bright red to pink; although this is not observed in all patients, it is a useful clinical change that demonstrates maturing epithelial tissue.

A wound dressing is no longer necessary to prevent bacterial contamination of the incision, once epithelial resurfacing has occurred. However, the wound dressing has other benefits at this point. Some clinicians suggest that the presence of the dressing at this point may be a reminder of the wound's presence and the need to use care in the wound area. The dressing provides a physical barrier to rough edges of clothing to limit local irritation, and the dressing can help the patient to include the wound in a new body image by allowing gradual viewing of the wound.

Wound closure materials are assessed for the reaction of the surrounding incisional tissues. The use of sutures of any type to approximate the wound edges creates small wounds alongside the incision wound. The wounds from the sutures increase the inflammation at the wound site and can cause ischemia if the sutures are pulled taut with increased tension, either from poor technique or wound edema postoperatively. The continued presence of sutures or staples provides additional tensile strength for the wound, but the sutures can also cause increased risk of infection and the potential for wound ischemia. Use of Steristrip tapes for wound closure or early removal of sutures with Steristrip tape replacement can decrease the problems associated with sutures. Removal of the wound sutures or staples in a timely manner is a proactive healing intervention. Removal of sutures in healthy surgical patients in 7–10 days postoperatively can be used as a general guideline, depending on surgical site.

Incisional Assessment during the Proliferative Phase

Palpation of the surgical incision reveals the underlying process of collagen deposition. The new collagen tissues can be palpated as a firmness along the incision, extending 1 cm on either side of the incision.[4] This firmness to the tissues, caused by new collagen deposition in the wound area, is called the *healing ridge*. The healing ridge should be palpable along the entire length of the incision between day 5 and day 9 postoperatively.[4] If the healing ridge is not palpable within 5–9 days, the wound is at risk for dehiscence or infection.[4]

Evaluation of surgical incisional wound exudate requires knowledge of what wound exudate is expected in the course of healing. The character and the amount of the exudate changes as wound healing progresses. The wound exudate immediately after surgery is bloody. Within 48 hours, the wound drainage becomes serosanguineous in nature and, finally, the exudate is serous. The amount of the wound exudate should gradually decrease throughout the healing period. An increase in wound exudate usually indicates compromised wound healing caused by infection. New drainage from a previously healed incision heralds wound dehiscence, infection, and, in some cases, fistula formation.

The tissues immediately surrounding the incision should be observed and palpated for the presence of edema and induration, and for color changes. The presence of edema retards the wound healing process, because the excess fluids in the tissues provide an obstacle to angiogenesis and raise the potential for wound ischemia. Skin color changes may indicate the presence of bruising or hematoma formation caused by surgery. The skin color will appear dark red or purple. Skin color changes may also indicate impending infection. Signs of erythema, warmth, and edema, as well as increased pain at the incision wound are indicators of possible wound infection. Evaluation of the healing ridge, wound exudate, and surrounding incisional tissues provides information on the progress of the proliferative phase of wound healing.

Incisional Assessment during the Remodeling Phase

The remodeling phase of wound healing is best assessed in the surgical incision by evaluation of the color of the incision. As the scar tissue is remodeled and organized structurally, the color of the tissue changes. The remodeling phase of wound healing can last 1–2 years. The incision color changes throughout the first year, gradually changing from bright red or pink to a silvery gray or white. The tensile strength of the wound gradually increases over the first year, eventually achieving approximately 80% of the original strength of the tissues. The main focus of interventions at this stage is to limit force on the wound site. Interventions to limit force and tension at the wound site include teaching the patient to avoid heavy lifting, bending, or straining at the site.

MANAGEMENT OF THE ACUTE SURGICAL WOUND

Management of the surgical incision includes attention to factors that affect wound healing, as addressed earlier, as well as dressing care. The surgical dressing includes the primary and secondary dressing. The primary, or first, surgical dressing is the dressing in direct contact with the wound. The direct wound contact requires that the primary dressing be nontraumatic to the wound. The primary dressing provides absorption of drainage, maintains a sterile wound environment, and serves as a physical barrier to further wound trauma. The primary dressing should be nonadherent to the wound site. The traditional gauze dressing becomes adherent to the new incision and, upon removal, causes new tissue injury. Use of nonadherent, absorptive dressings can facilitate wound healing because the nonharmful nature of the dressings allows wound healing to proceed.

The primary dressing absorbs wound exudate and wicks it away from the wound site, allowing the exudate to be absorbed into the secondary dressing. Secondary wound dressings provide increased absorptive capacity or hold the primary dressing in place. Secondary wound dressings are applied on top of the primary dressing and may be composed of the same materials as the primary dressing. The secondary dressing plays an important role for wounds when increased amounts of wound exudate are anticipated. The secondary dressing absorbs drainage from the primary dressing and wicks the exudate away from the wound bed and into the absorbent material of the dressing.

Clinical Wisdom: *Surgical Incisional Dressings*

The vast majority of primary intention surgical wound dressings continue to be gauze. Conversion to moist wound healing in the immediate postoperative period may facilitate wound healing and provide for patient comfort when changing dressings. Education of the surgeon on "better" primary wound dressings is also helpful.

Securing the wound dressing is usually done with the use of tape. Premature and frequent dressing changes can damage the tissues surrounding the incisional wound and negatively affect wound healing. Use of Montgomery straps, skin sealants, or hydrocolloid frames around the wound and underneath the tape can eliminate skin stripping around the incisional wound from frequent dressing changes. Frequent dressing changes are more likely to be a problem with wounds healing by secondary intention, tertiary intention, or draining wounds. (See Chapter 11, Management of the Wound Environment with Dressings and Topical Agents, for more information about wound dressings.)

SECONDARY AND TERTIARY INTENTION WOUND HEALING

Surgical wounds left open to heal by secondary or tertiary intention have a reparative trajectory similar to that of chronic wounds. Secondary intention healing is allowing wounds to heal without surgical closure. Wounds healing by secondary intention must heal by scar tissue replacement. The tissue defect at the wound site must fill with new collagen tissue during the proliferative phase of wound heal-

ing. The inflammatory phase of wound healing may be prolonged because of the contaminated nature of the wound. (See Chapter 2, Wound Healing Physiology and Chronic Wound Healing.)

Tertiary intention is a combination of both primary and secondary intention wound healing. The wound is allowed to heal secondarily, then primarily closed for final healing.[5] Tertiary wound healing is designed for specialized wounds in which primary intention is preferred but not possible at the time of wounding. The delay in primary closure may be to clear infection, allow some wound contracture, or create a healthy granulation base for a graft.[5]

Most surgical wounds left to heal by secondary or tertiary intention are those in which the risk of infection is increased or the tissue loss is such that the wound edges cannot be approximated without unacceptable tension on the incision. Reversal of both conditions—infection and extensive tissue loss—can be maximized in the early weeks following surgery. The administration of systemic antibiotics, when appropriate, and careful wound observation and care can lessen infection risk. The process of wound contraction and proliferation of granulation tissue occurs as the healing response attempts to decrease the total surface area of the wound[5] and to decrease the tissue loss.

The primary wound dressing takes critical importance in the wound healing by secondary or tertiary intention. Nonadherent, absorptive dressings optimize wound healing for secondary and tertiary intention wounds. Assessment of the wound for signs and symptoms of infection includes evaluation of the character and amount of wound exudate and examination of the wound and surrounding tissues for erythema, edema, induration, heat, and pain. Wounds healing by secondary or tertiary intention should be evaluated using the same parameters used for chronic wounds. Evaluate the wound size and depth, the presence or absence of necrotic tissue, the characteristics and amount of exudate, the condition of the surrounding tissues, and the presence of the healing characteristics of granulation and epithelialization.

OUTCOME MEASURES

Outcome measures for acute surgical incisions relate to healing progress according to time since injury. The outcome measures for incisional wounds are presented according to the time frame since surgery.

Postoperative Day 1 through Day 4

The following signs and symptoms represent measures of positive outcomes for acute surgical incision wounds. The presence of an inflammatory response, including erythema or skin discoloration, edema, pain, and increased temperature at the incision-site during the first 4 days after surgery, is a normal healing response. The lack of inflammation at the new surgical incision is a negative outcome. Wound exudate should be bloody in character initially and, toward day 3 and day 4, should change to serosanguineous in nature. The amount of wound exudate should gradually decrease from a moderate amount to scant exudate by day 4. Many surgical wounds have no exudate past days 2 or 3, especially facial wounds. Failure of the wound exudate to decrease in amount and to change in character from bloody to serosanguineous is a negative indicator for healing. Epithelial resurfacing should be complete by day 4. The incision appears bright pink, as opposed to the initial red color of the incision. Lack of epithelial resurfacing of the surgical incision indicates delayed healing and less than optimal outcomes.

One negative outcome that can occur at any time during the postoperative course of the patient is the development of a hematoma (swelling or mass of blood, usually clotted, confined in the tissues and caused by a break in a blood vessel). External evidence of hematoma formation includes swelling or edema at the site; a soft or boggy feel to the tissues initially, which may be followed by induration at the site; and color change of the skin (similar to bruising).

Postoperative Day 5 through Day 9

The major healing outcome in the surgical incision on days 5 through 9 is the presence of the healing ridge along the entire length of the incision. The healing ridge indicates new collagen deposition in the wound site. Lack of development or incomplete development of the healing ridge may be prodromal to wound dehiscence and wound infection. A deficient or nonexistent healing ridge is a negative outcome measure for wound healing. Wound exudate character should change from serosanguineous to serous and gradually disappear over days 4–6. The exudate amount should diminish from a minimal amount to none present. Any increase in the amount of wound exudate during days 5–9 should be viewed as a negative outcome and heralds probable wound infection.

The suture materials should begin to be removed from the incisional site during days 5–9. Adhesive tape strips or Steristrips may be used to provide additional wound tensile strength. Failure to remove any of the wound suture materials during days 5–9 may indicate a negative outcome for the wound.

Continued signs of inflammation at the incision-site during days 5–9 are indicative of delayed wound healing. Signs of erythema or edema, extensive pain, or increased temperature at the incision wound during this time frame indicate that wound healing is not normal. Prolonged inflammation may occur as a result of underlying infection, immunocompromise, or continued trauma at the wound site. Documentation of all characteristics of the incision and healing are important for continuity of care throughout the wound recovery period

but especially during this time frame, because the patient will likely be changing health care settings. For example, the surgical patient is often discharged from the acute care hospital to the home setting very soon after surgery.

Postoperative Day 10 through Day 14

The major outcome measure for day 10 through day 14 is the removal of external incision suture materials. Internal or "buried" sutures remain in place. Failure to remove external suture materials during this time frame will prolong incision healing. Healing is delayed by increasing the risk of infection from the suture microwounds and the continued insult to the tissues by the presence of the foreign objects (the suture materials), prolonging the inflammatory response.

Postoperative Day 15 through 1–2 Years

During the end of the proliferative phase of wound healing and throughout the remodeling phase, attention is directed toward the changes in the incisional scar tissue. The collagen deposited alongside the incision is gradually realigned, restructured, and strengthened. The outcome measure for this time period is predominantly based on the changes in the incisional scar tissue color. The color of the incision changes from a bright pink after the initial epithelial resurfacing, gradually fading to pink and, eventually, turning a pearly

---

Case Study:
Lack of Inflammatory Response Postoperatively

M.J., a 71-year-old Caucasian woman, was admitted for bowel surgery with resection of the descending colon and low anterior anastomosis. M.J.'s history included long-term steroid therapy for rheumatoid arthritis. On postoperative day 1, her midline incision primary dressing showed evidence of bright red bleeding. The wound edges were well approximated, with staples as the closure material. Assessment of the incision on postoperative days 2 and 3 revealed no evidence of any edema, warmth, erythema, or discoloration at the incision-site. Exudate was moderate and serosanguineous to seropurulent in nature. By postoperative day 4, the incision was not fully resurfaced with new epithelial tissue; signs of inflammation, although now present, were diminished; and the exudate remained seropurulent and moderate in amount. She showed signs of confusion and agitation (signs of infection in older adults); lab tests confirmed the presence of wound infection. In this case, the absent signs of inflammation were early warning signs of impaired healing and wound infection.

gray or silvery white color. The noticeable induration and firmness associated with the healing ridge gradually softens during this time frame also. Negative outcomes include reinjury of the incisional line, such as herniation of the wound site, and complications associated with scarring, such as keloid formation or hypertrophic scarring. Functional ability with the scar tissue becomes a key outcome measure for many surgical incisional wounds during this time frame. A positive outcome measure at year 1 for the incisional wound includes lack of significant hypertrophic scarring or wound herniation, maximal functional ability with the new scar, and acceptable cosmetic results of healing, with a silvery white or gray scar line. Tables 14–3 and 14–4 present the positive and negative outcome measures for time frames from the point of surgery to the end of remodeling. Chapter 13 discusses the management of scar.

CONCLUSION

There are many strategies that clinicians use to optimize wound healing in the acute surgical incision. The astute and attentive clinician may diminish risk of complications, identify delayed or impaired healing, and provide for a supportive healing environment. The key to successful intervention for the patient with an acute surgical incision is knowledge of normal healing mechanisms and temporal expectations,

knowledge of factors that impair wound healing, and vigilant attention to both. The case study below helps to demonstrate the interaction between knowledge of normal healing and the time sequence associated with wound healing, and factors that interfere with normal healing.

REFERRAL CRITERIA

Watchful assessment of the patient with an acute surgical incision can influence prompt referral to the physician or advanced practice nurse for evaluation and intervention for complications of wound healing. The following criteria are helpful guidelines for referral of the patient to another level of health care and to other specialties for their expertise:

- The patient with markedly increased bloody drainage during the immediate postoperative period may be at risk of hemorrhage from undetected leaking blood vessels in the surgical field.
- Patients who exhibit a change in exudate characteristics, from bloody or serosanguineous to purulent, should be evaluated for wound infection or abscess formation and treated with appropriate antimicrobial therapy.
- Any increase in amount of exudate after postoperative day 4 is indicative of wound infection or abscess formation and, as above, requires primary care provider evaluation and appropriate antimicrobial therapy.
- The absence of a healing ridge along the entire length of the incision wound by postoperative day 9 indicates impaired healing and, often, abscess formation. Prompt referral to the primary care provider usually results in drainage of the abscess area, antimicrobial therapy, and a wound left to heal by secondary intention.
- The patient with the presence of signs and symptoms of wound infection, including erythema, edema, elevated temperature, and increased pain along the incision after day 4, *and/or* signs of systemic infection, including elevated temperature, elevated white blood cell count, or confusion in the older adult, requires evaluation. These signs and symptoms suggest a wound infection, and the primary care provider should evaluate and treat appropriately.
- The patient with a frank wound dehiscence or fistula formation requires evaluation by the primary care provider, usually the surgeon, and may need a referral to an enterostomal therapy (ET) nurse (a nurse specializing in management of draining wounds) for management.

SELF-CARE TEACHING GUIDELINES

The patient's and caregiver's instruction in self-care must be individualized to the type of surgical incision and the individual patient's wound, the specific incisional dressing management routine, the individual patient's learning style and

Case Study: *Incisional Wound Healing*

P.L., a 78-year-old African American man, was admitted for radical prostatectomy surgery for prostate cancer. P.L. has a history of diabetes mellitus, hypertension, obesity, and peripheral vascular disease. His diabetes is managed with oral hypoglycemic agents and an 1800-calorie diabetic diet (with which he is noncompliant). P.L. lives alone on a small pension and fixed income and is a smoker. He was admitted with a random blood sugar of 198 mg/dL.

Preoperatively

Assessment of P.L. revealed several risk factors for impaired healing: uncontrolled diabetes mellitus, obesity, advanced age, hypertension, and peripheral vascular disease. Control of blood sugar level was identified as a goal in the preoperative period, and P.L. was started on sliding-scale insulin therapy with blood glucose monitoring. P.L.'s history of hypertension and peripheral vascular disease put him at risk for poor tissue perfusion; thus, in the immediate postoperative period (days 1 and 2) he was put on supplemental oxygen per nasal cannula to optimize tissue oxygenation. Obesity is a risk factor for excess incision wound tension, which increases potential for poor perfusion of the incision wound, due to the presence of excess subcutaneous fat.

Postoperative Day 4

P.L.'s 15-cm midline abdominal incision showed evidence of inflammation with edema, skin discoloration, and warmth at the site. There was evidence of epithelial resurfacing, and the incision line was bright pink. There was a continued minimal amount of serous drainage and staples remained in place. The primary gauze dressing was changed daily. Blood sugars ranged from 110 to 132 mg/dL on insulin therapy. Oxygen was administered the first 2 days postoperatively at 2 L per nasal cannula.

Postoperative Day 9

P.L. was discharged from the hospital to his home with home health care nursing follow-up. Upon discharge from the hospital, P.L.'s incision was bright pink with no exudate present. The incision was completely resurfaced with new epithelial tissue present along the entire incision, and half of the staples had been removed. A healing ridge was palpable along the anterior 13 cm of the wound but not palpable at the posterior aspect of the wound.

Postoperative Day 10

The home health nurse evaluated P.L.'s incision and found surrounding skin discoloration, increased pain, and edema present at the posterior aspect of the wound. No healing ridge was palpable at the posterior aspect of the wound, although collagen deposition was evident along the anterior 13 cm of the wound. Half of the original staples were still present in the incision line. The physician was notified, and P.L. was referred to the physician's office for evaluation of the incision.

Postoperative Day 12

The physician removed the remaining staples, performed an incision and drainage (I and D) of the posterior aspect of the incision in the office, started P.L. on systemic antibiotics, and left the posterior aspect of the wound open to heal by secondary intention, using moist saline gauze dressings.

Postoperative Day 15

P.L.'s posterior incision is 75% filled with granulation tissue and there is minimal serous exudate present. The anterior aspect of the incision is well healed and pale pink. P.L.'s incision wound went on to heal uneventfully by secondary intention over the next 10 days.

coping mechanisms, and the ability of the patient/caregiver to perform procedures. The general self-care teaching guidelines in Exhibit 14–1 must be individualized for each patient and caregiver.

REVIEW QUESTIONS

1. Which of the following provides the best example of the acute surgical wound?
   a. Surgical wound healing by secondary intention
   b. Dehisced surgical wound
   c. Pressure ulcer
   d. Surgical incision

2. Which of the following statements best describes the effects of age as an intrinsic factor affecting wound healing?
   a. Aging decreases elastin in the skin; affects collagen replacement; decreases the rate of replacement of cells, delaying reepithelialization; and causes a decline in immune function.
   b. Aging decreases protein synthesis, causes lower levels of serum albumin, and causes a decline in immune function.
   c. Aging causes collagen weakness, leading to poor binding with ground substances, and causes a decrease in fibroblast function and poor white blood cell function.

Table 14–3 Positive Outcome Measures for Incisional Wound Healing

Outcome Measure	Days 1–4: Inflammation	Days 5–9: Proliferative	Days 10–14: Proliferative	Day 15–Years 1–2: Proliferative-Remodeling
Incision color	Red, edges approximated	Red, progressing to bright pink	Bright pink	Pale pink, progressing to white or silver in light-skinned patients; pale pink, progressing to darker than normal skin color in dark-skinned patients
Surrounding tissue inflammation	Edema, erythema, or skin discoloration; warmth, pain	None present	None present	None present
Exudate type	Bloody or sanguineous, progressing to serosanguineous and serous	None present	None present	None present
Exudate amount	Moderate to minimal	None present	None present	None present
Closure materials	Present, may be sutures or staples	Beginning to remove external sutures/staples	Sutures/staples removed, Steristrips or tape strips may be present	None present
Epithelial resurfacing	Present by day 4 along entire incision	Present along entire incision	Present	Present
Collagen deposition (healing ridge)	None present	Present by day 9 along entire incision Present along entire incision	Present	

d. Aging increases blood glucose levels, leading to poor leukocyte function and inadequate protein synthesis.

3. Factors affecting wound healing in the immediate postoperative period include which of the following?
   a. hydration, pain management, and protein intake
   b. tissue perfusion, pain management and temperature
   c. tissue perfusion, protein intake, age, and concurrent conditions
   d. volume status, pain management, tissue perfusion, and temperature

4. The clinician assessing a client's abdomen 3 days post abdominal-perineal resection surgery notes erythema, slight edema, and slight increase in temperature at the incision-site. These findings are most consistent with which of the following?
   a. These are normal signs of the inflammation phase of wound healing.
   b. The wound is exhibiting early signs of impending infection.
   c. The wound is in the proliferative phase of wound healing.
   d. The wound is exhibiting signs of abscess formation.

5. The clinician is evaluating a client status post abdominal surgery on postoperative day 8. In assessing the midline abdominal incision, the clinician should be aware of which of the following?
   a. Signs of inflammation, including redness, warmth, pain, and edema are expected signs of normal healing at this time.
   b. A moderate amount of serous to serosanguineous drainage is expected during this phase of healing.
   c. A healing ridge or collagen matrix deposition should be palpable along the incision line.
   d. The wound edges should begin to show signs of approximation by this time

Table 14–4 Negative Outcome Measures for Incisional Wound Healing

Outcome Measure	Days 1–4: Inflammation	Days 5–9: Proliferative	Days 10–14: Proliferative	Day 15–Years 1–2: Proliferative-Remodeling
Incision	Red, edges approximated but tension evident on incision line	Red, edges may not be well approximated; tension on incision line evident	May remain red, progressing to bright pink	Prolonged epithelial resurfacing, keloid or hypertrophic scar formation
Surrounding tissue inflammation	No signs of inflammation present: *no* edema, *no* erythema or skin discoloration, *no* warmth, and minimal pain at incision site; hematoma formation	Edema, erythema, or skin discoloration; warmth, pain at incision site; hematoma formation	Prolonged inflammatory response with edema, erythema, or skin discoloration; warmth and pain; hematoma formation	If healing by secondary intention, may be stalled at a plateau (chronic inflammation or proliferation), with no evidence of healing and continued signs of inflammation
Exudate type	Bloody or sanguineous, progressing to serosanguineous and serous	Serosanguineous and serous to seropurulent	Any type of exudate present	Any type of exudate present
Exudate amount	Moderate to minimal	Moderate to minimal	Any amount present	Any amount present
Closure materials	Present, may be sutures or staples	No removal of any external sutures/staples	Sutures/staples still present	For secondary intention healing, failure of wound contraction or edges not approximated
Epithelial resurfacing	Present by day 4 along entire incision	Not present along entire incision	Not present along entire incision, dehiscence evident	Not present or abnormal epithelialization, such as keloid or hypertrophic scarring
Collagen deposition (healing ridge)	None present	Not present along entire incision	Not present along entire incision, dehiscence evident	Abscess formation with wound left open to heal by secondary intention

Exhibit 14–1 Self-Care Teaching Guidelines

Self-Care Guidelines Specific to Acute Surgical Incisions	Instructions Given (Date/Initials)	Demonstration *or* Review of Material (Date/Initials)	Return Demonstration *or* States Understanding (Date/Initials)
1. Type of incisional wound and specific cautions required a. No heavy lifting and other measures to prevent hernia formation			
b. Showering or bathing area			
c. Importance of adequate nutrition for wound healing			
2. Significance of wound exudate, incision wound tissue color, surrounding tissue condition, and presence of healing ridge			
3. Wound dressing care routine a. Wash hands, then remove old dressing and discard			
b. Clean wound with normal saline			
c. Apply primary dressing to wound			
d. Apply secondary dressing if appropriate			
e. Secure dressing with tape			
f. Universal precautions and dressing disposal			
g. Frequency of dressing changes			
4. Expected change in wound appearance during healing process a. Scheduled removal of closure materials			
b. Incision color change as wound heals (bright red or pink to pale pink and finally to silvery white or gray)			
5. When to notify the health care provider a. Signs and symptoms of wound infection (erythema, edema, pain, elevated temperature, change in exudate character or amount, discoloration in tissues surrounding incision wound)			
b. Absent or incomplete healing ridge along incision after postoperative day 9			
6. Importance of follow-up with health care provider			

REFERENCES

1. Lazarus GS, Cooper DM, Knighton DR, et al. Definitions and guidelines for assessment of wounds and evaluation of healing. *Arch Dermatol.* 1994;130:489–493.

2. Cruse PJE, Foord F. The epidemiology of wound infection: A ten-year prospective study of 62,939 wounds. *Surg Clin North Am.* 1980;60:27–40.

3. Stotts NA. Impaired wound healing. In: Carrieri-Kohlman VK, Lindsay AM, West CM, eds. *Pathophysiological Phenomena in Nursing: Human Responses to Illness.* 2nd ed. Philadelphia: W.B. Saunders Company; 1993:443–469.

4. Cooper DM. Acute surgical wounds. In: Bryant RA, ed. *Acute and Chronic Wounds: Nursing Management.* St. Louis, MO: Mosby-Year Book; 1992:91–104.

5. Moy LS. Management of acute wounds. *Dermatol Clin.* 1993;11:759–766.

6. West JM. Wound healing in the surgical patient: Influence of the perioperative stress response on perfusion. *AACN Clin Issues.* 1990;1:595–601.

7. Gerstein AD, Phillips TJ, Rogers GS, Gilchrest BA. Wound healing and aging. *Dermatol Clin.* 1993;11:749–757.

8. Rosenberg CS. Wound healing in the patient with diabetes mellitus. *Nurs Clin North Am.* 1990;25:247–261.

9. Weingarten MS. Obstacles to wound healing. *Wounds.* 1993;5:238–244.

10. Stotts NA, Washington DF. Nutrition: A critical component of wound healing. *AACN Clin Issues.* 1990;1:585–594.

11. Wagner PA. Zinc nutriture in the elderly. *Geriatrics.* 1985;40(3):111–125.

12. Jonsson K, Jensen JA, Goodson WH, Hunt TK. Wound healing in subcutaneous tissue of surgical patients in relation to oxygen availability. *Surg Forum.* 1986;37:86–89.

13. Pai MP, Hunt TK. Effect of varying oxygen tensions on healing of open wounds. *Surg Gynecol Obstet.* 1972;135:756–758.

14. Knighton DR, Silver IA, Hunt TK. Regulation of wound-healing angiogenesis: Effect of oxygen gradients and inspired oxygen concentration. *Surgery.* 1981;90:262–269.

15. Whitney JD. The influence of tissue oxygen and perfusion on wound healing. *AACN Clin Issues.* 1990;1:578–584.

SUGGESTED READING

Bryant RA, ed. *Acute and Chronic Wounds: Nursing Management.* 2nd ed. St. Louis, MO: Mosby, 2000.

Krasner D, Kane D, eds. *Chronic Wound Care.* 2nd ed. Wayne, PA: Health Management Publications; 1997.

CHAPTER 15

Pressure Ulcers: Pathophysiology and Prevention

Barbara M. Bates-Jensen

CHAPTER OBJECTIVES

At the completion of this chapter, the reader will be able to:

1. Define each stage in the pressure ulcer classification system, according to the National Pressure Ulcer Advisory Panel.
2. Explain frequency of risk assessment for home care, long-term care, and acute care.
3. Describe the Braden Scale for predicting pressure sore risk.
4. Identify and explain three interventions for preventing pressure ulcers.
5. Define prevalence and incidence.

PRESSURE ULCER DEFINITION

Pressure ulcers are areas of local tissue trauma, usually developing where soft tissues are compressed between bony prominences and any external surface for prolonged time periods.[1,2] A pressure ulcer is a sign of local tissue necrosis and death. Pressure ulcers are most commonly found over bony prominences subject to external pressure. Pressure exerts the greatest force at the bony tissue interface; therefore, there may be significant muscle and subcutaneous fat tissue destruction underneath intact skin.

PRESSURE ULCER SIGNIFICANCE

The incidence and prevalence of pressure ulcers are sufficiently high to warrant concern. Pressure ulcers represent a significant health concern for those in long-term care facilities, rehabilitation systems, and for special populations.

Prevalence and incidence in long-term care facilities vary significantly from study to study. Prevalence rates range from 2.3% to 28%.[3,4] Incidence in long-term care is equally diverse, with reports as low as 3.1% in Veteran's Administration nursing homes[5] to a high of 73.5% in a study of a single nursing home.[6] To get a better understanding of whether or not there have been improvements in pressure ulcer care, Berlowitz and colleagues[7] examined the temporal trends in pressure ulcer development from 1991 to 1995 in a chain of 100 private, for-profit nursing homes. Pressure ulcers were measured using the Minimum Data Set, and risk-adjusted rates demonstrated a 25% decrease in pressure ulcer development over the 5-year period.

Rehabilitation facilities present special concerns related to pressure ulcer development because patients in rehabilitation facilities have conditions that limit mobility, such as spinal cord injury, traumatic brain injury, cerebral vascular accident, burns, multiple trauma, or a chronic neurologic disorder. Studies in this area are few. Prevalence rates are reported between 11–12%[8,9] and 25%.[10] Incidence rates over 2 months have been reported at 4%.[11] Individuals with spinal cord injury are at higher risk for pressure ulcer development, with incidence rates reported at 20% for those undergoing spinal surgery[12] to 31% over 1 year's time.[13] Prevalence rates are reported at 10%, based on physical examination during the first annual exam at Model Spinal Cord Injury Centers.[14] Among hospitalized patients of all ages, the prevalence of pressure ulcers has been estimated at 10–14% in two multisite studies.[15,16]

Although, in some cases, it appears that pressure ulcer care has improved, there are many problems with methodology in studies on pressure ulcer incidence and prevalence, including: database use versus clinical site data, sampling issues, and calculation issues. These areas of concern make it difficult to draw firm conclusions about the status of pressure ulcers and the significance of the problem. The reality is that pressure ulcers occur in all health care settings and cost health care systems in terms of actual dollars spent in care and time and labor spent in caregiving.

Pressure ulcers have become a quality issue for all areas of health care. Pressure ulcer incidence and severity are used as markers of quality care by regulators in long-term care facilities and in home care agencies and acute care hospitals. This emphasis on pressure ulcers across the spectrum of health care settings highlights the importance of the condition for clinicians. As a result of these potential risks for pressure ulcers, the Department of Health and Human Services' health goals for the nation, *Healthy People 2010*,[17] has identified a 50% decrease in the prevalence of pressure ulcers in nursing homes as a part of the nation's health agenda. Pressure ulcers have also received attention in the courtroom. Organizations have been prosecuted for negligence related to pressure ulcer care and development, and, in a landmark case, a care-home operator was found guilty of manslaughter for a resident's death related to improper care for her pressure ulcers.[18] Clearly, pressure ulcers are a significant problem for all clinicians.

PRESSURE ULCER PATHOPHYSIOLOGY

Pressure ulcers are the result of mechanical injury to the skin and underlying tissues. The primary forces involved are pressure and shear.[19-23] Pressure is the perpendicular force or load exerted on a specific area, causing ischemia and hypoxia of the tissues. High-pressure areas in the supine position are the occiput, sacrum, and heels. In the sitting position, the ischial tuberosities exert the highest pressure, and the trochanters are affected in the sidelying position.[20,24]

As the amount of soft tissue available for compression decreases, the pressure gradient increases. Likewise, as the tissue available for compression increases, the pressure gradient decreases; thus, most pressure ulcers occur over bony prominences where there is less tissue for compression and the pressure gradient within the vascular network is altered.[24] Figure 15–1 demonstrates this relationship.

The changes in the vascular network allow an increase in the interstitial fluid pressure, which exceeds the venous flow. This results in an additional increase in the pressure and impedes arteriolar circulation. The capillary vessels collapse, and thrombosis occurs. Increased capillary arteriole pressure leads to fluid loss through the capillaries, tissue edema, and subsequent autolysis. Lymphatic flow is decreased, allowing further tissue edema and contributing to the tissue necrosis.[21,23,25-27]

Pressure, over time, occludes blood and lymphatic circulation, causing deficient tissue nutrition and buildup of waste products, due to ischemia. If pressure is relieved before a critical time period is reached, a normal compensatory mechanism, reactive hyperemia, restores tissue nutrition and compensates for compromised circulation. If pressure is not relieved before the critical time period, the blood vessels collapse and thrombose. The tissues are deprived of oxygen, nutrients, and waste removal. In the absence of oxygen, cells use anaerobic pathways for metabolism and produce toxic byproducts. The toxic byproducts lead to tissue acidosis, increased cell membrane permeability, edema, and eventual cell death.[21,25]

Tissue damage may also be due to reperfusion and reoxygenation of the ischemic tissues or postischemic injury.[28,29] Oxygen is reintroduced into tissues during reperfusion following ischemia. This triggers oxygen-free radicals known as *superoxide anion*, hydroxyl radicals, and hydrogen peroxide, which induce endothelial damage and decrease microvascular integrity.

Time and Pressure

Ischemia and hypoxia of body tissues are produced when capillary blood flow is obstructed by localized pressure. How much pressure and what amount of time is necessary for ulceration to occur has been a subject of study for many years. In 1930, Landis,[30] using single-capillary microinjection techniques, determined normal hydrostatic pressure to be 32 mm Hg at the arteriole end and 15 mm Hg at the venule end. His work has been the criterion for measuring occlusion of capillary blood flow. Generally, a range from 25 to 32 mm Hg is considered normal capillary blood flow and is used as the marker for adequate relief of pressure on the tissues.

Pressure is the greatest at the bony prominence and soft tissue interface and gradually lessens in a cone-shaped gradient to the periphery.[20,31,32] Thus, although tissue damage apparent on the skin surface may be minimal, the damage to the deeper structures can be severe. In addition, subcutaneous fat and muscle are more sensitive than the skin to ischemia. Muscle and fat tissues are more metabolically active and, thus, more vulnerable to hypoxia with increased susceptibility to pressure damage. The vulnerability of muscle and fat tissues to pressure forces explains pressure ulcers where large areas of muscle and fat tissue are damaged with undermining due to necrosis, yet the skin opening is relatively small.[26]

Intensity and Duration of Pressure

There is a relationship between intensity and duration of pressure in pressure ulcer development. Low pressures over a long period of time are as capable of producing tissue damage as are high pressures for shorter periods of time.[20] Tissues can tolerate higher cyclic pressures versus constant pressure.[33] Pressures differ in various body positions. Pressures are highest (70 mm Hg) on the buttocks in the lying position, and in the sitting position can be as high as 300 mm

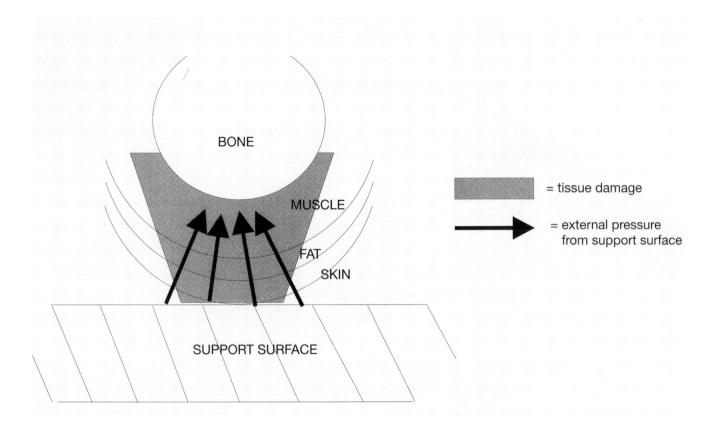

Figure 15–1 Pressure gradient at the bony prominence.

Hg over the ischial tuberosities.[20,24] These levels are well above the normal capillary closing pressure and are capable of causing tissue ischemia. When tissues have been compressed for prolonged periods of time, tissue damage continues to occur, even after the pressure is relieved.[31] This continued tissue damage relates to changes at the cellular level that lead to difficulties with restoration of perfusion.

Figure 15–2 shows the relationship between time, pressure, and tissue destruction.

Four levels of skin breakdown occur, depending on the amount of time exposed to unrelieved pressure.[34] Hyperemia can be observed within 30 minutes or less; it is manifested by redness of the skin and dissipates within 1 hour after pressure is relieved. Ischemia occurs after 2–6 hours of continuous pressure; the erythema is deeper in color and may take 36 hours or more to disappear after pressure is relieved. Necrosis is the third level and occurs after 6 hours of continuous pressure. The skin may take on a blue or gray color and become indurated. Damage that has progressed to this level disappears on an individual basis. Ulceration is the fourth and final level and may occur within 2 weeks after necrosis with potential infection; it resolves on an individual basis.

In dark-skinned patients, it is often difficult to discern redness or erythema of the skin. Redness and erythema may appear as a deepening of normal ethnic color or as a purple hue to the skin.[35,36] (See *Color Plate 21*.) Other manifestations in dark-skinned patients are local changes in skin temperature and skin texture. The immediate response of inflammation of the tissues can be seen by an increase in skin temperature. As the tissues become more disturbed, the temperature decreases, signaling underlying tissue damage. Skin texture may feel hard and indurated, and observation of the skin may reveal heightened skin features or an orange-peel appearance.[35,36] (See Chapter 4 for more information on assessment of the dark-skinned patient.)

CLINICAL PRESENTATION OF PRESSURE ULCERS

The clinical presentation of a pressure ulcer is a predictable cutaneous chain of events. The first clinical sign of pressure ulcer formation—blanchable erythema—presents as discoloration of a patch or flat, nonraised area of the skin larger than 1 cm. This discoloration presents as redness or erythema that varies in intensity from pink to bright red in light-skinned patients (see *Color Plates 14–15*). In dark-skinned patients, the discoloration appears as a deepening of normal ethnic color or as a purple hue to the skin (see *Color*

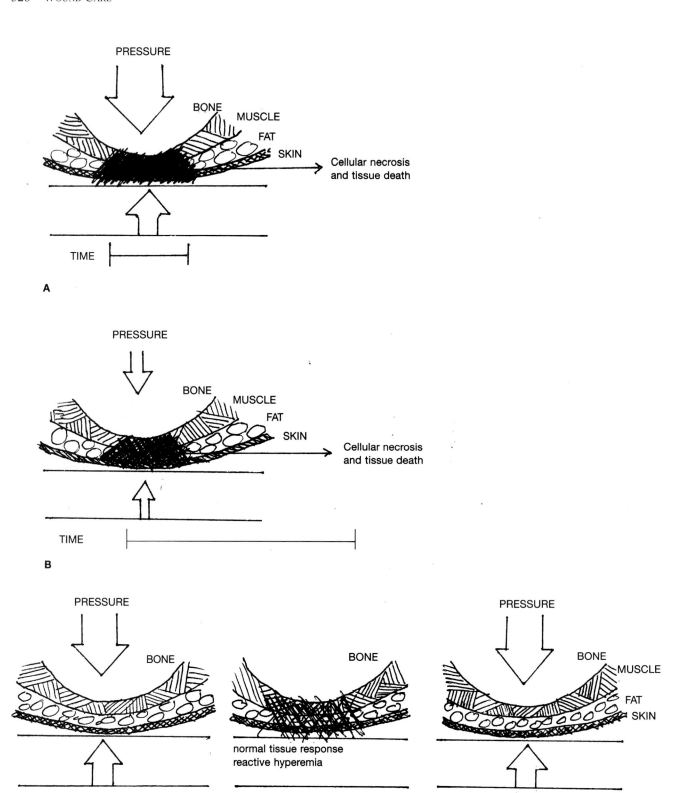

Figure 15–2 Relationship of time versus pressure. **A,** High pressure over a short period of time. **B,** Low pressure over a long period of time. **C,** Intermittent pressure.

Plate 19). Other characteristics include slight edema and increased temperature of the area. In light-skinned patients, the severity of the tissue insult can be evaluated by testing for blanchability of tissues. After finger pressure is applied to the area, complete blanching occurs, followed by quick return of redness, once the finger is removed. In dark-skinned patients, it is difficult to discern blanching. Use of temperature is a more valuable assessment of the severity of the tissue damage in the dark-skinned patient. Initial skin trauma and discoloration exhibit an elevated skin temperature, as compared with that of healthy tissues. The beginning clinical indicators of pressure ulceration all relate to the signs of inflammation in the tissues. At this beginning stage of damage, if the pressure is relieved, the skin can return to normal in 24 hours.[37] If pressure is not relieved, the damage progresses.

Nonblanchable erythema involves more severe damage and is commonly the first stage of pressure ulceration (see *Color Plate 15*). The color of the skin is more intense. It varies from dark red to purple or cyanotic in both light- and dark-skinned patients. Dark-skinned patients exhibit deepening of normal skin color, a purple or gray hue to the skin, and changes in skin texture, with induration and an orange-peel appearance.[35,36] Skin temperature is now cool, compared with healthy tissues, and the area may feel indurated. In light-skinned patients, nonblanchable erythema is detected by testing for blanching of tissues. The damage to tissues is more severe and is indicated by the inability of the tissues to blanch. This stage of tissue destruction is also reversible, although tissues may take 1–3 weeks to return to normal.[37]

The result of further deterioration in the tissues is evidenced as the epidermis is disrupted with subepidermal blisters, crusts, or scaling present. If properly treated, the situation may resolve in 2–4 weeks.[37] The early pressure ulcer reflects continued tissue insult and progressive injury. The early ulcer is superficial, with indistinct margins and a red, shiny base (see *Color Plate 14*). It is usually surrounded by nonblanchable erythema. If not dealt with aggressively, progression to a chronic, deep ulcer is inevitable. Superficial ulcers begin at the skin surface and progress to deeper layers. Deep ulcers do not originate at the skin surface; they begin at the bony prominence–soft tissue interface and spread to involve the skin structures (see *Color Plates 19–20*).

The chronic deep ulcer usually has a dusky red wound base and does not bleed easily (see *Color Plate 36*). It is surrounded by nonblanchable erythema or deepening of normal ethnic tone, induration, and warmth, and possibly is mottled. Undermining and tunneling may be present with a large necrotic cavity (see *Color Plates 28 and 30*). Eschar formation may be a result of larger vessel damage from shearing force and may be the result of large vessel damage below skin level.[37] Eschar is the formation of an acellular dehydrated compressed area of necrosis, usually surrounded by an outer rind of blanchable erythema. Eschar formation indicates a full-thickness loss of skin (see *Color Plates 20–21, 25, and 29*).

Location

More than 95% of all pressure ulcers develop over five classic locations: sacral/coccygeal area, greater trochanter, ischial tuberosity, heel, and lateral malleolus (see *Color Plates 3, 11, 24, 35, and 52–54*).[22] Common pressure ulcer sites occur over bony prominences and depend on the patient's position; areas with large amounts of soft tissue between bone and skin are least susceptible to breakdown.[34] Meehan,[38] in a prevalence survey of 148 hospitals, found the sacrum the most common location of pressure ulcers and the trochanter the location of the most severe ulcers. Correct anatomic terminology is important in identification of the true location of the pressure ulcer. For example, many clinicians often document pressure ulcers as being located on the patient's hip. The hip, or iliac crest, is actually an uncommon location for pressure ulceration. The iliac crest is located on the front of the patient's body and is rarely subject to pressure forces. The area that most clinicians are referring to is correctly termed the *greater trochanter*. The greater trochanter is the bony prominence located on the side of the body, just above the proximal, lateral aspect of the thigh or "saddle-bag" area. The majority of pressure ulcers occur on the lower half of the body. The location of the pressure ulcer may have an impact on clinical interventions. For example, the patient with a pressure ulcer on the sacral/coccygeal area with concomitant urinary incontinence will require treatments that address the incontinence problem (see *Color Plate 16*). Ulcers in the sacral/coccygeal area are also more at risk for friction and shearing damage, due to the location of the wound. Figure 15–3 presents the usual locations of pressure ulcer development with correct anatomic terminology.

Pressure ulcers commonly occur over bony prominences, but ulcers can develop at any site where tissues have been compressed, causing tissue ischemia and hypoxia. Patients with contractures are at special risk for pressure ulcer development because of the internal pressure of the bony prominence and the abnormal alignment of the body and its extremities. (Refer to Chapter 16 on therapeutic positioning.)

Clinical Wisdom: *Contractures and Pressure Ulcer Formation*

The compression of tissues may be greater in the presence of contractures, and the management of the contracture must be considered when assessing the patient for risk of pressure ulcer development.[39]

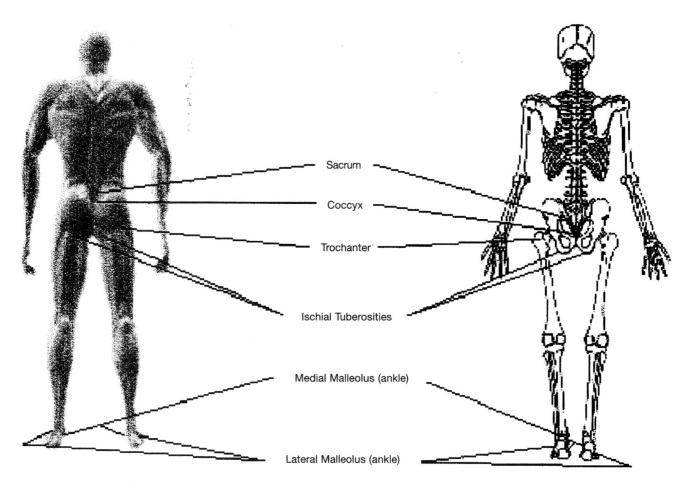

Figure 15–3 Anatomic locations. *Source:* Copyright © 1996, *Applied Health Science.*

PRESSURE ULCER STAGING

Pressure ulcers are commonly classified according to grading or staging systems based on the depth of tissue destruction. The stage is determined on initial assessment by noting the deepest layer of tissue involved. The ulcer is not restaged unless deeper layers of tissue become exposed.[40] Historically, one problem in assessment was the lack of a universal staging system for classifying the severity of pressure ulcers. Many of the staging systems available are based on Shea's initial 1975 article[41] describing a method of classifying pressure sores. Shea believed that a pathology-based classification system would simplify communication for health care professionals, provide a mechanism for identification of pressure ulcers, and suggest a broad guide for determining whether operative care was needed. Shea defined each grade of pressure ulceration by the anatomic limit of soft tissue damage that could be observed. His numeric classification system suggested an orderly evolution of pressure ulceration. The National Pressure Ulcer Advisory Panel (NPUAP)[2] and the Agency for Health Care Research and Quality (AHRQ), formerly known as the Agency for Health Care Policy and Research (AHCPR),[42] recommend use of a universal four-stage classification system to describe depth of tissue damage. The recommended system is similar to Shea's original system, with the major exception being that of defining stage I lesions. Exhibit 15–1 shows the staging system recommended by the NPUAP.

The issue of pressure ulcer assessment and the use and misuse of staging classification systems is a subject of debate and controversy. Pressure ulcer development does not necessarily occur from one stage to the next, and there may be different etiologic factors for various stages. Ulcers do not heal by reverse staging. Staging systems measure only one characteristic of the wound; should not be viewed as a complete assessment, independent of other indicators; and should not be the sole criterion in determining treatment plans (see Chapter 4 on wound assessment). Staging classification systems do not assess for criteria in the healing process and hinder tracking of progress because of inability to demon-

Exhibit 15–1 Pressure Ulcer Staging Criteria

Pressure Ulcer Stage	Definition
Stage I	An observable pressure-related alteration of intact skin whose indicators, as compared with the adjacent or opposite area on the body, may include changes in one or more of the following: skin temperature (warmth or coolness), tissue consistency (firm or boggy feel), and/or sensation (pain, itching). The ulcer appears as a defined area of persistent redness in lightly pigmented skin, whereas, in darker skin tones, the ulcer may appear with persistent red, blue, or purple hues. (See *Color Plates 14–15.*)
Stage II	Partial-thickness skin loss involving epidermis or dermis, or both. The ulcer is superficial and presents clinically as an abrasion, blister, or shallow crater. (See *Color Plate 17.*)
Stage III	Full-thickness skin loss involving damage or necrosis of subcutaneous tissue, which may extend down to but not through underlying fascia. The ulcer presents clinically as a deep crater, with or without undermining of adjacent tissue. (See *Color Plate 45.*)
Stage IV	Full-thickness skin loss with extensive destruction, tissue necrosis, or damage to muscle bone or supporting structures (such as tendon, joint capsule). (See *Color Plates 1, 3, 7, 37,* and *39.*)

strate change over time. The staging system does not allow for movement within and between stages.[43] Many clinicians use the staging system as a measure of healing, despite the inherent difficulties associated with back-staging or down-staging (use of the stages in reverse order, eg, a wound moving from stage IV to stage II). Determining the stage of the pressure ulcer is a diagnostic tool for evaluating the level of tissues exposed. Once the stage of destruction is determined, the stage should not change, even as the wound heals. In a full-thickness pressure ulcer (stage III or IV), the wound defect is filled with granulation tissue as the wound heals. The granulation tissue does not replace the structural layers of muscle, fat, and dermis that were present in the original tissues. Back-staging of pressure ulcers is inappropriate use of the staging criteria and does not reflect physiologic healing phenomena.[43]

The terms *partial thickness* and *full thickness* are commonly used to describe wounds of various skin depths that heal by either regeneration or scar formation. Partial-thickness wounds involve only the epidermis and dermis. Full-thickness wounds involve complete destruction of the epidermis and dermis, and extend into deeper tissues.

Superficial lesions involving the epidermis and dermis generally heal in days to weeks. Deeper lesions involving the subcutaneous tissues and muscle may require weeks to months to heal.[44] Tissue trauma extending to bone or joint structures may result in osteomyelitis and further prolong healing time. Ulcers involving the subcutaneous tissue layers may be obscured by necrosis or eschar and additionally may present as areas of both partial- and full-thickness tissue losses. Chapter 2 also discusses the anatomy of the skin.

PRESSURE ULCER PREDICTION: RISK FACTOR ASSESSMENT

Discussion of pressure ulcer pathophysiology and etiology would not be complete without mention of other interacting factors. Pressure ulcers are physical evidence of multiple causative influences. Factors that contribute to pressure ulcer development can be thought of as those that affect the pressure force over the bony prominence and those that affect the tolerance of the tissues to pressure. The conceptual schema of Braden and Bergstrom[45] divides factors into categories according to the role played in eventual pressure ulcer development. Figure 15–4 illustrates Braden and Bergstrom's conceptual framework for pressure ulcer development.

Mobility, sensory loss, and activity level are related to the concept of increasing pressure. Extrinsic factors (shear, friction, and moisture), as well as intrinsic factors (nutrition, age, and arteriolar pressure) relate to the concept of tissue tolerance. Several additional areas may influence pressure ulcer development: emotional stress, temperature, smoking, and interstitial fluid flow.[46]

Pressure Factors

Immobility, inactivity, and decreased sensory perception all affect the duration and intensity of the pressure over the bony prominence. Immobility or severely restricted mobility is the most important risk factor for all populations and a necessary condition for the development of pressure ulcers. Mobility is the state of being movable. Thus, the immobile

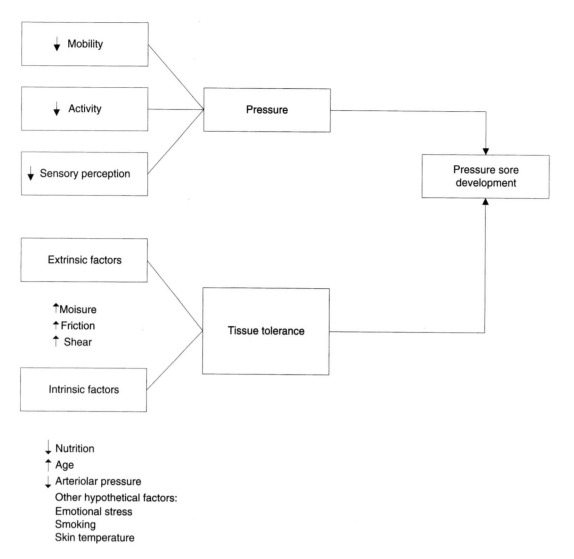

Figure 15–4 Factors contributing to the development of pressure ulcers. *Source:* Reprinted with permission from Barbara Braden, PhD, RN, FAAN. Reprinted from *Rehabilitation Nursing*, 12(1), 9, Association of Rehabilitation Nurses, 4700 W. Lake Avenue, Glenview, IL 60025-1485. Copyright © 1987. Association of Rehabilitation Nurses.

patient cannot move, and facility or ease of movement is impaired. Exton-Smith and Sherwin[47] demonstrated that 90% of individuals with 20 or fewer spontaneous nocturnal body movements developed a pressure ulcer, whereas none of the persons with greater than 50 movements per night developed a pressure ulcer. Closely related to immobility is limited activity levels.

Research Wisdom: *Immobility*

Immobility or severely restricted mobility is the most important risk factor for all populations and a necessary condition for the development of pressure ulcers.

Activity is the production of energy or motion and implies an action. Activity is often clinically described by the ability of the individual to ambulate and move about. Those persons who are bed or chair bound and, thus, inactive, are more at risk for pressure ulcer development.[42,48] A sudden change in activity level may signal significant change in health status and increased potential for pressure ulcer development. Sensory loss places patients at risk for compression of tissues and pressure ulcer development because the normal mechanism for translating pain messages from the tissues is dysfunctional.[40] Patients with intact nervous system pathways feel continuous local pressure, become uncomfortable, and change their position before tissue ischemia occurs. Patients with spinal cord injury have a higher incidence and prevalence of pressure ulcers.[49,50] Patients with paraplegia or quadriplegia are unable to sense increased pressure, and if their body weight is not shifted, pressure ulceration develops. Likewise, patients with changes in mental status functioning are at increased risk for pressure ulcer formation. They may not feel the discomfort from pressure, not be alert enough to move spontaneously, not remember to move, not be too confused to respond to commands to move, or be physically unable to move.[40]

Extrinsic Factors

Shear

Extrinsic risk factors are those forces that make the tissues less tolerant of pressure. Extrinsic forces include shear, friction, and moisture. Shear is a parallel force. Whereas pressure acts perpendicularly to cause ischemia, shear causes ischemia by displacing blood vessels laterally and, thus, impeding blood flow to tissues.[51–53] Figure 15–5 shows the effect of shearing on the tissues.

Shear is caused by the interplay of gravity and friction. Shear is a parallel force that acts to stretch and twist tissues and blood vessels at the bony tissue interface and, as such, shear affects the deep blood vessels and deeper tissue structures. The most common circumstance for shear occurs in the bed patient in a semi-Fowler's position (semisitting position with knees flexed and supported by pillows on the bed or by elevation of the head of the bed; Figure 15–6). The patient's skeleton slides down toward the foot of the bed, but the sacral skin stays in place (with the help of friction against the bed linen). This produces stretching, pinching, and occlusion of the underlying vessels, resulting in ulcers with large areas of internal tissue damage and less damage at the skin surface.

Clinical Wisdom: *Shear Injury*

Shear is the reason many pressure ulcers are much larger than the bony prominence over which they occur. In clinical practice, this explains, in part, pressure ulcers with large undermined areas.

Friction

Friction and moisture, although not direct factors in pressure ulcer development, have been identified as contributing to the problem by reducing tolerance of tissues to pressure.[53] Friction occurs when two surfaces move across one another (see Figure 15–5). Friction acts on the tissue tolerance to pressure by abrading and damaging the epidermal and upper dermal layers of the skin. Additionally, friction

acts with gravity to cause shear. Friction abrades the epidermis, which may lead to pressure ulcer development by increasing the skin's susceptibility to pressure injury. Pressure combined with friction produces ulcerations at lower pressures than does pressure alone.[53] Friction acts in conjunction with shear to contribute to development of sacral/coccygeal pressure ulcers on patients in the semi-Fowler's position.

Moisture

Moisture contributes to pressure ulcer development by removing oils on the skin, making it more friable, as well as interacting with body support surface friction. Constant moisture on the skin leads to maceration of the tissues. The waterlogged tissues lead to softening of the skin's connective tissues. Macerated tissues are more prone to erosion, and, once the epidermis is eroded, there is increased likelihood of further tissue breakdown.[54] Moisture alters the resiliency of the epidermis to external forces. Both shearing force and friction increase in the presence of mild to moderate moisture. Excess moisture may be due to wound drainage, diaphoresis, and fecal or urinary incontinence.

Urinary and fecal incontinence are common risk factors associated with pressure ulcer development. Incontinence contributes to pressure ulcer formation by creating excess moisture on the skin and by chemical damage to the skin. Fecal incontinence has an added detrimental effect: the presence of bacteria in the stool, which can contribute to infection, as well as to skin breakdown. Fecal incontinence is more significant as a risk factor for pressure ulceration because of the bacteria and enzymes in stool and the subsequent effects on the skin.[40,55] In the presence of both urinary and fecal incontinence, the pH in the perineal area is increased by the fecal enzymes' conversion of urea to ammonia. The elevated pH increases the activity of proteases and lipases found in stool, which, in turn, cause increased permeability of the skin, leading to irritation by other agents, such as bile salts.[56–58] Inadequately managed incontinence poses a significant risk factor for pressure ulcer development, and fecal incontinence is highly correlated with pressure ulcer development.[48,59]

Intrinsic Risk Factors

Nutrition

There is some disagreement on the major intrinsic risk factors affecting tissue tolerance to pressure. However, most studies identify nutritional status as playing a role in development. Hypoalbuminemia, weight loss, cachexia, and malnutrition are all commonly identified as risk factors predisposing patients to pressure ulcer development.[60–63] Malnutrition is associated with pressure ulcer development.[60,62] Individuals with low serum albumin levels are associated

Bony Prominence
without Pressure

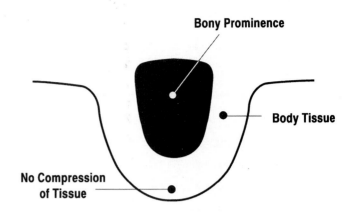

Bony Prominence
with Pressure

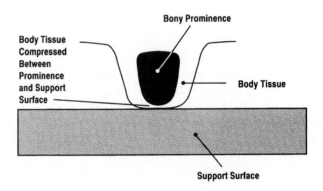

Bony Prominence
with Pressure plus Shear

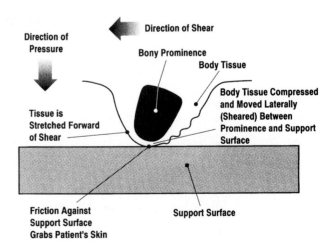

Figure 15–5 Effects of shearing and friction in conjunction with pressure on the skin. Courtesy of RIK Medical, Boulder, Colorado.

Shear Effect of Raising the Head of the Bed

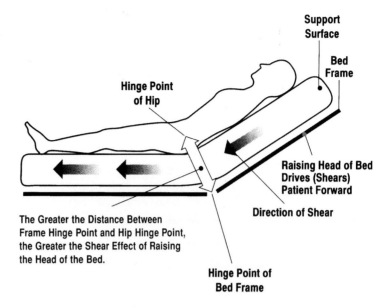

Bottoming Out

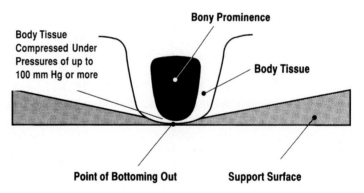

Figure 15–6 Semi-Fowler's position and shearing effect. Courtesy of RIK Medical, Boulder, Colorado.

with both having a pressure ulcer and developing a pressure ulcer.

Age

Age itself may be a risk factor for pressure ulcer development, with age-related changes in the skin and wound healing increasing the risk of pressure ulcer development.[64] The skin and support structures undergo changes in the aging process. There is a loss of muscle, a decrease in serum al-bumin levels, diminished inflammatory response, decreased elasticity, and reduced cohesion between the dermis and epidermis.[64,65] These changes combine with other changes related to aging to make the skin less tolerant of pressure forces, shear, and friction.[64]

Medical Conditions and Psychologic Factors

Certain medical conditions or disease states are also associated with pressure ulcer development. Orthopaedic injuries, altered mental status, and spinal cord injury are such conditions.[49,50,63,66,67] Others have examined psychologic factors that may affect risk for pressure ulcer development.[68,69] Self-concept, depression, and chronic emotional stress have been cited as factors in pressure ulcer development.

Risk Assessment Tools

For practitioners to intervene cost-effectively, a method of screening for risk factors is necessary. There are several risk assessment instruments available to clinicians. Screening tools assist in prevention by distinguishing those persons who are at risk for pressure ulcer development from those who are not. The only purpose in identifying patients at risk for pressure ulcer development is to allow for appropriate use of resources for prevention. The use of a risk assessment tool allows for targeting of interventions to specific risk factors for individual patients. Selection of which risk assessment instrument to use is determined by reliability of the tool for the intended raters, predictive validity of the tool for the population, sensitivity and specificity of the instrument under consideration, and ease of use and time required for completion. The most common risk assessment tools are Norton's Scale, Gosnell's Scale, and Braden's Scale for Predicting Pressure Sore Risk.

Norton's Scale

The Norton tool is the oldest risk assessment instrument. Developed in 1961, it consists of five subscales: physical condition, mental state, activity, mobility, and incontinence.[70] Each parameter is rated on a scale of 1–4, with the sum of the ratings for all five parameters yielding a total score, ranging from 5 to 20. Lower scores indicate increased risk, with a score of or below 16 indicating "onset of risk" and scores 12 and below indicating high risk for pressure ulcer formation.[71] Others, such as the Gosnell tool, have revised the Norton tool and developed additional tools for assessing risk.

Gosnell's Scale

Gosnell based her scale on further refinement of the Norton Scale. Gosnell kept the original categories on the Norton Scale, changed the general condition category to nutrition, and renamed the incontinence category to *continence*.[72,73] She added skin appearance, medication, diet and fluid balance, and intervention categories to the tool, along with detailed instructions for use. Gosnell reversed the numerical scaling so that the higher score would indicate the higher the risk of pressure ulcer development, so a Gosnell score of 5 is the lowest risk, and a score of 20 is the highest risk (see Exhibit 15–2).

Braden's Scale for Predicting Pressure Sore Risk

The Braden Scale was developed in 1987 and is composed of six subscales that conceptually reflect degrees of sensory perception, moisture, activity, mobility, nutrition, and friction and shear.[45,46] All subscales are rated from 1 to 4, except for friction and shear, which is rated from 1 to 3. The subscales may be summed for a total score, with a range from 6 to 23 (see Exhibit 15–3).

Lower scores indicate lower function and higher risk for developing a pressure ulcer. The cutoff score for hospitalized adults is considered to be 16, with scores of 16 and below indicating at-risk status.[46] In older patients, some have found cutoff scores of 17 or 18 to be better predictors of risk status.[62,74] Levels of risk are based on the predictive value of a positive test. Scores of 15–16 indicate mild risk, with a 50–60% chance of developing a stage I pressure ulcer; scores of 12–14 indicate moderate risk, with a 65–90% chance of developing a stage I or II lesion; and scores below 12 indicate high risk, with a 90–100% chance of developing a stage II or deeper pressure ulcer.[62,75] The Braden Scale has been tested in acute care and long-term care settings with several levels of nurse raters and demonstrates high interrater reliability with registered nurses. Validity has been established by expert opinion, and predictive validity has been studied in several acute care settings, with good sensitivity and specificity demonstrated.[46,62] The Braden Scale has a firm evidence base and solid research as a foundation for use.

> **Clinical Wisdom:** *Quick Risk Assessment Screening*
>
> The Braden Scale activity subscale can be used as a quick screening tool. Those patients who receive a score of 1 (indicating patients who are ambulatory) may be considered at low or no risk, and no further assessment is required. All other patients should receive the full Braden Scale assessment, and prevention interventions should be instituted specific to level of risk and individual risk factors present.

Regardless of the instrument chosen to evaluate risk status, the clinical relevance is threefold. First, assessment for risk status must occur at frequent intervals, which are determined by the level of care. All health care organizations should monitor assessment at admission to the health care organization (within 24 hours) and 48 hours later. The later assessment more accurately reflects true risk for the individual. The patient should also be assessed at predetermined intervals determined by patient acuity. In acute care hospital critical care units, the suggested interval is daily and, in general medical-surgical units, three times a week. In home care, weekly intervals are suggested because this correlates well

Exhibit 15–2 Gosnell's Tool

GOSNELL SCALE—PRESSURE SORE RISK ASSESSMENT

I.D. _____

Age _____ Sex _____

Height: _____ Weight: _____

Date of Admission _____

Date of Discharge _____

Medical Diagnosis:

  Primary _____

  Secondary _____

Nursing Diagnosis:

_____

Instructions: Complete all categories within 24 hours of admission and every other day thereafter. Refer to the accompanying guidelines for specific rating details.

DATE	Mental Status	Continence	Mobility	Activity	Nutrition	TOTAL SCORE
	1. Alert 2. Apathetic 3. Confused 4. Stuporous 5. Unconscious	1. Fully Controlled 2. Usually Controlled 3. Minimally Controlled 4. Absence of Control	1. Full 2. Slightly Limited 3. Very Limited 4. Immobile	1. Ambulatory 2. Walks with Assistance 3. Chairfast 4. Bedfast	1. Good 2. Fair 3. Poor	

Date	Vital Signs				Diet	24-Hour Fluid Balance		COLOR	GENERAL SKIN APPEARANCE			Interventions		
	T	P	R	BP		Intake	Output	1. Pallor 2. Mottled 3. Pink 4. Ashen 5. Ruddy 6. Cyanotic 7. Jaundice 8. Other	**Moisture** 1. Dry 2. Damp 3. Oily 4. Other	**Temperature** 1. Cold 2. Cool 3. Warm 4. Hot	**Texture** 1. Smooth 2. Rough 3. Thin/ Transp 4. Scaly 5. Crusty 6. Other	No	Yes	Describe

PRESSURE SORE RISK ASSESSMENT MEDICATION PROFILE

Medication	Dosage	Frequency	Route	Date Begun	Date Discon.

GOSNELL SCALE—GUIDELINES FOR NUMERICAL RATING OF THE DEFINED CATEGORIES

Rating	1	2	3	4	5
Mental Status: An assessment of one's level of response to his environment.	**Alert:** Oriented to time, place, and person. Responsive to all stimuli, and understands explanations.	**Apathetic:** Lethargic, forgetful, drowsy, passive, and dull. Sluggish, depressed. Able to obey simple commands. Possibly disoriented to time.	**Confused:** Partial and/or intermittent disorientation to TPP. Purposeless response to stimuli. Restless, aggressive, irritable, anxious, and may require tranquilizers or sedatives.	**Stuporous:** Total disorientation. Does not respond to name, simple commands, or verbal stimuli.	**Unconscious:** Non-responsive to painful stimuli.

continues

Exhibit 15–2 continued

Rating	1	2	3	4	5
Continence: The amount of bodily control of urination and defecation.	**Fully Controlled:** Total control of urine and feces.	**Usually Controlled:** Incontinent of urine and/or feces not more often than once q 48 hrs OR has Foley catheter and is incontinent of feces.	**Minimally Controlled:** Incontinent of urine or feces at least once q 24 hrs.	**Absence of Control:** Consistently incontinent of both urine and feces.	
Mobility: The amount and control of movement of one's body.	**Full:** Able to control and move all extremities at will. May require the use of a device but turns, lifts, pulls, balances, and attains sitting position at will.	**Slightly Limited:** Able to control and move all extremities but a degree of limitation is present. Requires assistance of another person to turn, pull, balance, and/or attain a sitting position at will but self-initiates movement or request for help to move.	**Very Limited:** Can assist another person who must initiate movement via turning, lifting, pulling, balancing, and/or attaining a sitting position (contractures, paralysis may be present).	**Immobile:** Does not assist self in any way to change position. Is unable to change position without assistance. Is completely dependent on others for movement.	
Activity: The ability of an individual to ambulate.	**Ambulatory:** Is able to walk unassisted. Rises from bed unassisted. With the use of a device such as cane or walker is able to ambulate without the assistance of another person.	**Walks with Help:** Able to ambulate with assistance of another person, braces, or crutches. May have limitation of stairs.	**Chairfast:** Ambulates only to a chair, requires assistance to do so OR is confined to a wheelchair.	**Bedfast:** Is confined to bed during entire 24 hours of the day.	
Nutrition: The process of food intake.	Eats some food from each basic food category every day and the majority of each meal served OR is on tube feeding.	Occasionally refuses a meal or frequently leaves at least half of a meal.	Seldom eats a complete meal and only a few bites of food at a meal.		

Vital signs:	The temperature, pulse, respiration, and blood pressure to be taken and recorded at the time of every assessment rating.
Skin appearance:	A description of observed skin characteristics: color, moisture, temperature, and texture.
Diet:	Record the specific diet order.
24-hour fluid balance:	The amount of fluid intake and output during the previous 24-hour period should be recorded.
Interventions:	List all devices, measures, and/or nursing care activity being used for the purpose of pressure sore prevention.
Medications:	List name, dosage, frequency, and route for all prescribed medications. If a PRN order, list the pattern for the period since last assessment.
Comments:	Use this space to add explanation or further detail regarding any of the previously recorded data, patient condition, etc. OR Describe anything which you believe to be of importance but not accounted for previously.

Source: Copyright © 1988, Davina Gosnell.

Exhibit 15–3 Braden Scale for Predicting Pressure Sore Risk

Patient's Name _____		Evaluator's Name _____		Date of Assessment	

SENSORY PERCEPTION ability to respond meaningfully to pressure-related discount	**1. Completely Limited:** Unresponsive (does not moan, flinch, or grasp) to painful stimuli, due to diminished level of consciousness or sedation. OR limited ability to feel pain over most of body surface.	**2. Very Limited:** Responds only to painful stimuli. Cannot communicate discomfort except by moaning or restlessness. OR has a sensory impairment which limits the ability to feel pain or discomfort over 1/2 of body.	**3. Slightly Limited:** Responds to verbal commands, but cannot always communicate discomfort or need to be turned. OR has some sensory impairment which limits ability to feel pain or discomfort in 1 or 2 extremities.	**4. No Impairment:** Responds to verbal commands. Has no sensory deficit which would limit ability to feel or voice pain or discomfort.	
MOISTURE degree to which skin is exposed to moisture	**1. Constantly Moist:** Skin is kept moist almost constantly by perspiration, urine, etc. Dampness is detected every time patient is moved or turned.	**2. Very Moist:** Skin is often, but not always moist. Linen must be changed at least once a shift.	**3. Occasionally Moist:** Skin is occasionally moist, requiring an extra linen change approximately once a day.	**4. Rarely Moist:** Skin is usually dry, linen only requires changing at routine intervals.	
ACTIVITY degree of physical activity	**1. Bedfast:** Confined to bed.	**2. Chairfast:** Ability to walk severely limited or nonexistent. Cannot bear own weight and/or must be assisted into chair or wheelchair.	**3. Walks Occasionally:** Walks occasionally during day, but for very short distances, with or without assistance. Spends majority of each shift in bed or chair.	**4. Walks Frequently:** Walks outside the room at least twice a day and inside room at least once every 2 hours during waking hours.	
MOBILITY ability to change and control body position	**1. Completely Immobile:** Does not make even slight changes in body or extremity position without assistance.	**2. Very Limited:** Makes occasional slight changes in body or extremity position but unable to make frequent or significant changes independently.	**3. Slightly Limited:** Makes frequent though slight changes in body or extremity position independently.	**4. No Limitations:** Makes major and frequent changes in position without assistance.	

continues

Exhibit 15–3 continued

NUTRITION *usual* food intake pattern	1. Very Poor: Never eats a complete meal. Rarely eats more than 1/3 of any food offered. Eats 2 servings or less of protein (meat or dairy products) per day. Takes fluids poorly. Does not take a liquid dietary supplement. OR is NPO and/or maintained on clear liquids or IVs for more than 5 days.	2. Probably Inadequate: Rarely eats a complete meal and generally eats only about 1/2 of any food offered. Protein intake includes only 3 servings of meat or dairy products per day. Occasionally will take a dietary supplement. OR receives less than optimum amount of liquid diet or tube feeding.	3. Adequate: Eats over half of most meals. Eats a total of 4 servings of protein (meat, dairy products) each day. Occasionally will refuse a meal, but will usually take a supplement if offered. OR is on a tube feeding or TPN regimen which probably meets most of nutritional needs.	4. Excellent: Eats most of every meal. Never refuses a meal. Usually eats a total of 4 or more servings of meat and dairy products. Occasionally eats between meals. Does not require supplementation.	
FRICTION AND SHEAR	1. Problem: Requires moderate to maximum assistance in moving. Complete lifting without sliding against sheets is impossible. Frequently slides down in bed or chair, requiring frequent repositioning with maximum assistance. Spasticity, contractures, or agitation leads to almost constant friction.	2. Potential Problem: Moves feebly or requires minimum assistance. During a move skin probably slides to some extent against sheets, chair, restraints, or other devices. Maintains relatively good position in chair or bed most of the time but occasionally slides down.	3. No Apparent Problem: Moves in bed and in chair independently and has sufficient muscle strength to lift up completely during move. Maintains good position in bed or chair at all times.		
				Total Score	_____

with registered nurse visit schedules. In long-term care, residents should be assessed once a week for the first 4 weeks then routinely, such as quarterly, with the Minimum Data Set. Of course, regardless of health care setting, risk assessment should be performed whenever a significant change occurs in the patient's general health and status. The registered nurse should perform risk assessment. However, in many instances, the registered nurse will need input from the direct care provider, such as a family member or a nursing attendant.

The second clinical implication is the targeting of specific prevention strategies to identified risk factors. The final clinical implication is for those patients in whom prevention is not successful. For patients with an actual pressure ulcer, the continued monitoring of risk status may prevent further tissue trauma at the wound site and development of additional wound sites. The prevention interventions presented are based on the Braden Scale Risk Assessment instrument items. Exhibit 15–4 presents a flow diagram for determining prevention strategies based on risk factor assessment.

Exhibit 15–4 Flow Diagram for Determining Prevention Strategies Based on Risk Factor Assessment

Presence of tissue trauma over bony prominence?
(usual locations: sacral/coccygeal, trochanter, ischial tuberosity, malleolus, heel)

NO   YES, provide for wound assessment and treatment plus prevention strategies

Patient NOT chair or bed bound and thus at no or low risk?
(patient scores a 1 or 2 on Braden Scale activity subscale)

NO, complete full risk assessment   YES, do not need further risk assessment

Pressure ulcer risk factors present?

Immobility	Inactivity	Decreased Sensory Perception	Nutrition	Friction and Shear	Moisture Urinary and Fecal Incontinence

Prevention interventions by risk factors:

Immobility, Inactivity, and Decreased Sensory Perception		Malnutrition	Friction and Shear	Moisture Incontinence
passive repositioning, pillow bridging, pressure-reducing/relieving support surfaces		provide nutrition supplement: protein, calorie, vitamin C, zinc, iron	cornstarch, lubricants, pad protectors, transparent film, thin hydrocolloid dressings, turning, and draw sheets	absorbent products, diagnosis of incontinence, general skin care

RISK STRATIFICATION AND RISK ADJUSTMENT

Risk stratification is arranging data related to quantifiable outcomes, resource utilization, or other phenomena associated with pressure ulcer prevention or treatment by level of risk to facilitate analysis and to reflect more accurately effect of case mix. For example, using the Braden Scale for Risk Assessment instrument, patients can be stratified or grouped according to their levels of risk, as follows:

- Mild Risk = 15–18 Braden Score
- Moderate Risk = 13–14 Braden Score
- High Risk = 10–12 Braden Score
- Very High Risk ≤ 9 Braden Score

Risk adjustment or stratification can give a more realistic picture of the progress in prevention as acuity levels wax and wane. Risk adjustment supplies a more realistic comparison between one institution's outcomes and those of other agencies/facilities. Risk stratification can also provide a tool to see where strengths and weaknesses in the program of prevention might exist.

Clinical Wisdom

Risk adjustment or stratification can also be used with pressure ulcer assessment data. For example, the Pressure Sore Status Tool (PSST) can be useful as an instrument to determine severity levels of pressure ulcers as follows:

- Minimal severity = 13–20 PSST Total Score
- Mild severity = 21–30 PSST Total Score
- Moderate severity = 31–40 PSST Total Score
- Critical severity = 41–65 PSST Total Score

PRESSURE ULCER PREVENTION: EARLY INTERVENTIONS

Prevention strategies are targeted at reducing risk factors present. Appropriate prevention interventions can be focused on eliminating specific risk factors. Thus, early intervention for pressure ulcers is risk factor-specific and prophylactic in nature. The prevention strategies are presented by risk factors, beginning with general information and ending with specific strategies for a particular risk factor. The Braden Scale is the basis for these prevention interventions. Prevention interventions should be instituted that are appropriate to the patient's level of risk and specific to individual risk factors.[42] For example, the risk factor of immobility is managed very differently for the comatose patient versus the spinal cord-injured patient. The comatose patient requires caregiver education and caregiver-dependent repositioning. The spinal cord-injured patient requires self-care education and may be able to perform self-repositioning. Thus, the intervention for the risk factor of immobility is very different for these two patients.

Immobility, Inactivity, and Sensory Loss

Patients with impaired ability to reposition and who cannot independently change body positions must have local pressure alleviated by any of the following interventions.[40,42,75]

- Passive repositioning by the caregiver
- Pillow bridging
- Use of pressure-relief or pressure-reduction support surfaces for chair and bed

In addition, measures to increase mobility and activity and to decrease friction and shear should be instituted. Overhead bed frames with trapeze bars are helpful for patients with paraplegia, stroke patients with upper body strength, and obese patients, and may increase mobility and independence with body repositioning. Wheelchair-bound patients with upper body strength can be taught and encouraged to do wheelchair pushups to relieve pressure and allow for reperfusion of the tissues in the ischial tuberosity region. For patients who are weak from prolonged inactivity, providing support and assistance for reconditioning and increasing strength and endurance will help to prevent future debility.[40] Mobility plans for each patient should be individualized, with the goal of attaining the highest level of mobility and activity individually possible. Mobility plans are the responsibility of nurses and physical therapists working together in all health care settings. It is essential that health care professionals train and observe home caregivers in the mobility plan and, in particular, passive repositioning techniques. Caregivers in the home are often left to fend for themselves for prevention interventions and may be frail and have health problems themselves. A return demonstration of a repositioning procedure can be very informative to the health care provider. The health care provider may need to coach, improvise, and think of creative strategies for caregivers to use in the home setting in order to meet the patient's need for movement and tissue reperfusion.

Passive Repositioning by Caregiver

Turning schedules and passive repositioning by caregivers is the normal response for patients with immobility risk factors. Typically, turning schedules are based on time or event. If time based, turning schedules are usually every 2 hours for full-body change of position and more often for small shifts in position. Event-based schedules relate to typical events during the day, eg, turning the patient after each meal. Full-body change of position involves turning the patient to a new lying position, eg, turning the patient from the right sidelying position to the left sidelying position or the supine position. When the sidelying position is used in bed, avoidance of direct pressure on the trochanter is essential. To avoid placing pressure on the trochanter, position the patient in a 30° laterally inclined position instead of the commonly used 90° sidelying position, which increases tissue compression over the trochanter.[76] The 30° laterally inclined position allows for distribution of pressure over a greater area (see Figure 15–7). Use of diagrams with clock faces and body position of patient are helpful in reminding staff when and how to position the patient[77] (see Figure 15–8).

Small shifts in position involve moving the patient but keeping the same lying position,[78] eg, changing the angle of the right sidelying position or changing the lower extremity position in the right sidelying position. Both strategies are

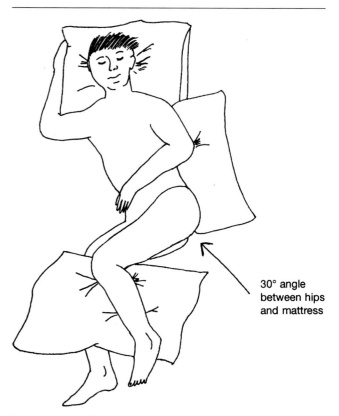

30° angle between hips and mattress

Figure 15–7 Thirty-degree laterally inclined position. *Source:* Copyright © Barbara M. Bates-Jensen and Lynette Merriman.

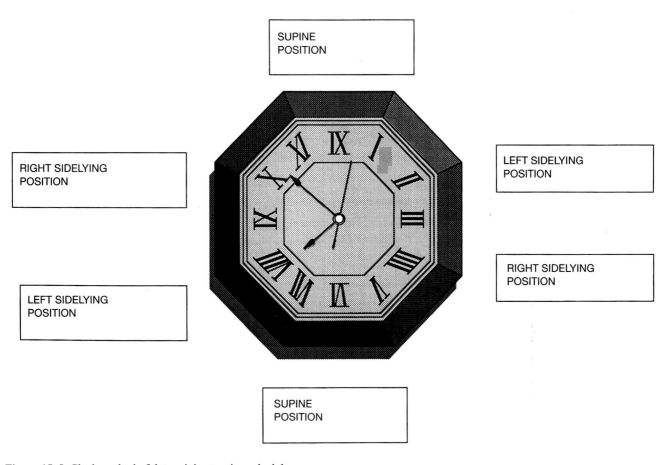

Figure 15–8 Clock method of determining turning schedule.

helpful in achieving reperfusion of compressed tissues, but *only full body change of position completely relieves pressure.*

There are techniques to make turning patients easier and less time-consuming. Turning sheets, draw sheets, and pillows are essential for passive movement of patients in bed. Turning sheets are useful in repositioning the patient to a sidelying position, and draw sheets are used for pulling the patient up in bed and help to prevent dragging the patient's skin over the bed surface. Two-person repositioning is a simple task with the turning sheet and can be accomplished in a very small amount of time with little risk of dragging the patient's skin across the bed linens:

1. Position one person on each side of the bed.
2. Bend the patient's knees and fold the patient's arms across the chest.
3. Roll up the draw sheet next to the patient's body and grasp firmly.
4. On a prearranged verbal cue, both persons lift the patient and move him or her up in bed.

5. Next, one person pulls on the turn sheet to roll the patient passively toward the side.
6. The person on the other side of the bed immediately places pillows behind the patient's back for support.
7. Additional pillows are then used for easing pressure on other bony prominences.

The recommended time interval for full change of position turning is every 2 hours, depending on the individual patient profile.

Similar approaches are useful for patients in chairs. Full-body change of position involves standing the patient and resitting him or her in the chair. Small shifts in position for those in chairs might be changing lower extremity position. For the chair-bound patient, it is also helpful to use a footstool to help reduce the pressure on the ischial tuberosities and to distribute the pressure over a wider surface. Attention to proper alignment and posture is essential. Individuals at risk for pressure ulcer development should avoid uninterrupted sitting in chairs and should be repositioned every hour. The rationale behind the shorter time frame is the extremely high pressure generated on the ischial tuberosities in the seated position.[1] Those patients with upper body strength should be taught to shift weight every 15 minutes to allow for tissue reperfusion. Again, pillows may be used to help position the patient in proper body alignment. Physical therapy and occupational therapy can assist in body alignment strategies with even the most contracted patient. (See Chapter 16 for further discussion on orthotic devices and seating therapeutics.)

Pillow Bridging

Pillow bridging involves the use of pillows to position patients with minimal tissue compression. The use of pillows can help to prevent pressure ulcers from occurring on the medial knees, the medial malleolus, and the heels. Pillows should be placed between the knees, between the ankles, and under the heels.

Clinical Wisdom: *Positioning Pillows*

Five pillows can overcome repositioning pressure point difficulties. Use the pillows in the following positions:

Pillow 1: under legs to elevate the heels
Pillow 2: between the ankles
Pillow 3: between the knees
Pillow 4: behind the back
Pillow 5: under the head

(Use a small pillow for comfort under the arm in sidelying position.)

Pillow use is especially important for reducing risk of development of heel ulcers, regardless of the support surface in use.[42] The best prevention strategy for eliminating pressure ulcers on the heels is to keep the heels off the surface of the bed. Use of pillows under the lower extremities will keep the heel from making contact with the support surface of the bed. Pillows help to redistribute the pressure over a larger area, thus reducing high pressures in one specific area.

Research Wisdom: *Donut Pillow Devices*

One type of pillow device is not recommended for use. Use of a donut type or ring cushion device is contraindicated. Donut ring cushions cause venous congestion and edema, and actually increase pressure to the area of concern.[42]

Use of Pressure-Relief or Pressure-Reduction Support Surfaces

There are specific guidelines for the use of support surfaces to prevent and manage pressure ulcers.[1,79,80] Regardless of the type of support surface in use with the patient, the need for written repositioning and turning schedules remains essential. The support surface serves as adjuncts to strategies for positioning and careful monitoring of patients. The type of support surface chosen is based on a multitude of factors, including clinical condition of the patient, type of care setting, ease of use, maintenance, cost, and characteristics of the support surface. The primary concern should be the therapeutic benefit associated with the surface. Table 15–1 categorizes the types of support surfaces available and their general performance characteristics;[1] Exhibit 15–5 presents

---

Table 15–1 Selected Characteristics for Classes of Support Surfaces

Performance Characteristics	Air Fluidized (High Air Loss)	Low Air Loss	Alternating Air (Dynamic)	Static Flotation (Air or Water)	Foam	Standard Hospital Mattress
Increased support area	Yes	Yes	Yes	Yes	Yes	No
Low moisture retention	Yes	Yes	No	No	No	No
Reduced heat accumulation	Yes	Yes	No	No	No	No
Shear reduction	Yes	?	Yes	Yes	No	No
Pressure reduction	Yes	Yes	Yes	Yes	Yes	No
Dynamic	Yes	Yes	Yes	No	No	No
Cost per day	High	High	Moderate	Low	Low	Low

Source: Reprinted from N. Bergstrom, M.A. Bennett, C.E. Carlson, et al., *Treatment of Pressure Ulcers*, Clinical Practice Guideline No. 15, December, 1994, U.S. Department of Health and Human Services, Public Health Service, Agency for Health Care Policy and Research, AHCPR Publication No. 95-0652.

Exhibit 15–5 Ideal Support Surface Characteristics

- Reduces/relieves pressure under bony prominences
- Controls pressure gradient in tissue
- Provides stability
- No interference with weight shifts
- No interference with transfers
- Controls temperature at interface
- Controls moisture at skin surface
- Lightweight
- Low cost
- Durable

Source: Reprinted with permission from J. McLean, Pressure reduction or pressure relief: making the right choice, *Journal of ET Nursing,* Vol. 20, No. 5, pp. 211–215, © 1993, Mosby Year-Book, Inc.

ideal support surface characteristics. Table 15–1 and Exhibit 15–5 are presented as an overview to the remainder of this section. The information on support surfaces is organized in the following manner: First, information on tissue interface pressure is presented; second, information on pressure-reducing and pressure-relieving support surfaces is presented; finally, this section ends with information and guidelines on how to determine the appropriate surface for specific patients.

Tissue Interface Pressures. Tissue interface pressures are commonly evaluated by using capillary closing pressure (generally considered to be 12–32 mm Hg) as an indirect measure to label effectiveness of support surfaces. The use of capillary closing pressures implies that skin surface interface pressure is equal to capillary closing pressures. Further, as tissue interface (skin surface) pressures approach capillary closing pressures (12–32 mm Hg), the support surface is more effective and less likely to occlude blood vessels (less likely to cause pressure ulcer formation). One of the difficulties with the use of capillary closing pressures is the assumption that capillary closing pressures are absolute values. Capillary closing pressures may be more individualized than absolute values imply. Capillary closing pressures assume that skin interface pressures reflect pressure at the bony tissue interface. Some suggest that pressure on subcutaneous tissues may be three to five times higher than skin interface pressure. Interface pressure is a measurement obtained by placing a sensor between the skin and the resting support surface. It is usually obtained with some type of electropneumatic pressure sensor connected to an inflation system and gauge. Typically, three or more readings are obtained, and the average of the readings is used as the reported value. Instrumentation (size of sensor, shape of sensor, and position of sensor) greatly affects values of pressure readings, so it is difficult, if not impossible, to make comparisons between studies.

Pressure-Reducing Support Surfaces. Pressure-reduction devices lower tissue interface pressures but do not *consistently* maintain interface pressures below capillary closing pressures in all positions, on all body locations.[81] Pressure-reducing support surfaces are indicated for patients who are assessed to be at risk for pressure ulcer development, who can be turned, and who have skin breakdown involving *only one sleep surface.*[40,42] Patients with an existing pressure ulcer who are determined to be still at risk for development of further skin breakdown should be managed on a pressure-reducing support surface. Pressure-reduction devices can be classified as static or dynamic devices.

Static devices do not move; they reduce pressure by spreading the load over a larger area. The easy definition of a static support surface is a device that does not require electricity to function, usually a mattress overlay (lies on top of the standard hospital mattress). Examples of static devices are foam, air, or gel mattress overlays and water-filled mattresses. When considering the foam mattress overlays, the health care provider should consider stiffness of the foam and the density and thickness of the foam. Indentation load deflection (ILD) is a measure of the stiffness of the foam; generally, the ILD should be 25% for 30 pounds. The density and thickness of the foam relate to the foam's ability to deflect the pressure and redistribute the pressure over a wider area. Typically, the density and thickness of a foam product should be 1.3 pounds per cubic foot and 3–4 inches, respectively.[1] Foam devices have difficulties with retaining moisture and heat, and not reducing shear. Air and water static devices also have difficulties associated with retaining moisture and heat.

Dynamic support surfaces move. The easy definition of dynamic support surfaces is that they require a motor or pump and electricity to operate. Examples are alternating pressure air mattresses. Most of these devices use an electric pump alternately to inflate and deflate air cells or air columns, thus the term *alternating* pressure air mattress. The key to determination of effectiveness is the length of time that cycles of inflation and deflation occur. Dynamic support surfaces may also have difficulties with moisture retention and heat accumulation.[1]

Pressure-reduction devices can also be categorized as overlays or replacement mattresses. Mattress overlays are devices that are applied on top of the standard mattress. Most overlays are pressure-reduction devices and require a one-time charge, setup fee, daily rental fee, or a combination of fees. Most are single-use items and may present environmental issues for disposal. When using mattress overlays, the height of the bed is increased, so transfers and linen fit may be complicated. Mattress overlays may be static or dynamic.

Some provide air movement to reduce moisture buildup. Some examples include foam, gel, water, or air-filled mattress, alternating pressure pads, and low-air-loss overlays.

One additional concern when using mattress overlays is the bottoming out phenomenon. Bottoming out occurs when the patient's body sinks down, the support surface is compressed beyond function, and the patient's body lies directly on the hospital mattress. When bottoming out occurs, there is no pressure reduction for the bony prominence of concern. Bottoming out typically happens when the patient is placed on a static air mattress overlay that is not appropriately filled with air or when the patient has been on a foam mattress for extended periods of time. The health care provider can monitor for bottoming out by inserting a flat, outstretched hand between the overlay and the patient's body part at risk. If the caregiver feels less than an inch of support material, the

patient has bottomed out. It is important to check for bottoming out when the patient is in various body positions and to check at various body sites. For example, when the patient is lying supine, check the sacral/coccygeal area and the heels; when the patient is sidelying, check the trochanter and lateral malleolus.[1] Use of a static support surface is warranted if the patient can turn off of the pressure ulcer site without bottoming out.

Replacement mattresses are designed to reduce interface pressures and replace the standard hospital mattress. Most are made of foam and gel combinations. Some are air-filled chambers and foam structures. All are covered with a bacteriostatic cover that can be maintained with standard cleaning. These mattresses involve an initial significant expense, and there are minimal data on long-term effectiveness.

Pressure-Relieving Support Surfaces. Pressure relief devices *consistently* reduce tissue interface pressures to a level below capillary closing pressure, in any position and in most body locations.[81] Pressure-relief devices are indicated for patients who are assessed to be at high risk for pressure ulcer development and who cannot turn independently or those who have skin breakdown involving more than one body surface. Most commonly, pressure-relief devices are grouped into low-air-loss therapy, fluidized air or high-air-loss therapy, and kinetic therapy.

Low-air-loss therapy is a bed frame with a series of connected air-filled pillows with surface fabrics of low-friction material. The amount of pressure in each pillow can be controlled and can be calibrated to provide maximum pressure relief for the individual patient. They provide pressure relief in any position, and most models have built-in scales.

Fluidized air or high-air-loss therapy consists of a bed frame containing silicone-coated glass beads and incorporates both air and fluid support. The beads become fluid when air is pumped through, making them behave as a liquid. High-air-loss therapy has bactericidal properties because of the alkalinity of the beads (pH 10), the temperature, and entrapment of microorganisms by the beads. High-air-loss therapy relieves pressure and reduces friction, shear, and moisture (due to the drying effect of the bed). It is difficult to transfer patients in these devices because of the bed frame. There is increased air flow, which can increase evaporative fluid loss, leading to dehydration. Finally, if the patient is able to sit up, a foam wedge may be required, thus limiting the beneficial effects of the bed on the upper back of the patient.

Kinetic therapy beds are designed to counter the effects of immobility by continuous passive motion. Kinetic therapy is believed to improve respiratory function and oxygenation, prevent urinary stasis, and reduce venous stasis. Multiple body systems are involved in the therapy, and, generally, the patient must have a stable spine. The beds usually are of two types: Either the bed frame itself moves or the air cushions inflate or deflate, rotating the patient from side to side or pulsating. Pressure relief and low-friction surface are provided with repositioning. Most models include built-in scales. Conscious patients may not tolerate the movement of the bed.

The last category of support surfaces includes those designed for obese accommodation. These support surfaces are designed to provide pressure reduction for the severely obese patient and can accommodate extreme loading, as is the case with the obese patient. Obese accommodation devices have features similar to the other support surfaces described. Generally, the bed frame is larger and many include the capability of raising the patient to a standing position while positioned in the bed. There are also chair devices for the obese patient.

Support Surface Selection. Determining which support surface is best for individual patients can be confusing. The primary concern must always be the effectiveness of the surface for the individual patient's needs. The AHCPR guidelines on prevention and prediction of pressure ulcers recommend the following criteria for determining how to manage tissue loading and support surface selection.[42]

- Assess all patients with existing pressure ulcers to determine their risk for developing additional pressure ulcers. If the patient remains at risk, use a pressure-reducing surface.
- Use a static support surface if the patient can assume a variety of positions without bearing weight on an existing pressure ulcer and without bottoming out.
- Use a dynamic support surface if the patient cannot assume a variety of positions without bearing weight on an existing pressure ulcer, if the patient fully compresses the static support surface, or if the pressure ulcer does not show evidence of healing.
- If a patient has large stage III or stage IV pressure ulcers on multiple turning surfaces, a low-air-loss bed or a fluidized air (high-air-loss) bed may be indicated.
- When excess moisture on intact skin is a potential source of maceration and skin breakdown, a support surface that provides airflow can be important in drying the skin and preventing additional pressure ulcers.
- Any individual assessed to be at risk for developing pressure ulcers should be placed on a static or dynamic pressure-reducing support surface.

Use of an algorithm can also be helpful in making clinical decisions. There are multiple decision trees and algorithms available. The algorithm recommended by the AHCPR guidelines (Figure 15–9) is offered as one example of a clinical decision-making tree or treatment algorithm.[1]

There are additional concerns in choosing a support surface. Criteria for choosing support surfaces can be classified as intrinsic and extrinsic. Intrinsic criteria include wound burden (tissue history—previous ulcers, surgical repair, stress, duration of pressure ulcer, number of pressure ulcers present), body build (obese, thin, contractures present), and the magnitude and distribution of interface pressures (location of highest pressures, etc).[84] The following case examples help to illustrate how intrinsic criteria are used for determination of support surface: Patients who undergo specific surgical operative repair of the pressure ulcer may need to be placed on high-air-loss or fluidized air therapy postoperatively. Patients with multiple ulcers involving more than one turning surface also need to be placed on pressure-relieving devices, such as low-air-loss therapy or high-air-loss therapy. Patients with severe contractures may not require a support surface that has good heel pressure readings (with contraction of the legs, the heels do not reach the bottom of the mattress). If the bony prominence of concern is the greater trochanter, the support surface chosen must adequately reduce pressure over the trochanter. Although an algorithm is a helpful tool in choosing a support surface, as these case examples illustrate, the clinician must also evaluate the individual patient's needs.

Extrinsic criteria include all of the following:

- The number of hours spent on the support surface daily (Will product be needed for short- or long-term use?)
- Shear and friction effects
- Environmental factors (temperature, humidity, continence, and moisture)
- Living arrangements (Will patient be in acute care, long-term care, or home care setting?)
- Self-care deficits (Is the risk of pressure ulcer development likely to increase or decrease?)
- Ease of transition and weaning to other products or other health care settings
- Ease of use and manageability
- Cost—reimbursement level
- Service and warranty
- Availability of product
- Scientific validity[80,84]

Evaluation of extrinsic criteria requires the clinician to review the goals for therapy. For example, the patient who uses the support surface only at night and spends most of the day in the chair will require an aggressive approach to seating support surfaces, and a lesser support surface can be chosen for the bed. If the patient spends most of the day in bed, the support surface chosen will be different. For agitated patients (particularly those with continual body motions), the support surface's ability to handle shearing and friction may be critical, and good choices may involve evalu-

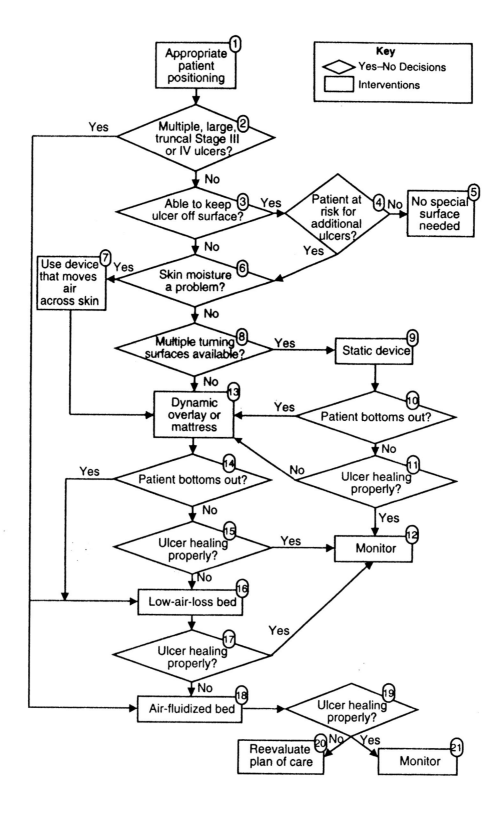

Figure 15–9 Management of tissue loads. *Source:* Reprinted with permission from N. Bergstrom, M.A. Bennett, C.E. Carlson, et al. *Treatment of Pressure Ulcers.* Clinical Practice Guideline No. 15, December, 1994, U.S. Department of Health and Human Services, Public Health Service, Agency for Health Care Policy and Research, AHCPR Publication No. 95-0652.

ation of the support surface covering. The external environment is also essential to include in choosing a support surface. If the patient is at home, with no air conditioning, is incontinent of urine, and lives in a humid environment, the ability of the support surface to breathe and the ability to handle moisture are essential to positive outcomes. Likewise, evaluation of the patient's prognosis is helpful in support surface choice. Is the patient expected to recover and improve? If so, a pressure-reduction or lower-end support surface device may be very appropriate. However, if the patient is expected to decline in function, choosing a support surface that will meet future, as well as present, skin care needs may be prudent. Throughout the decision-making process one thought should prevail: It is important to promote patient independence, not patient dependent behavior. Encouraging patient movement out of bed and, thus, off of the support surface is important for those patients who are able, and this must be considered by the clinician.

Clinical Wisdom: *Reimbursement of Support Surfaces*

Support surfaces are reimbursed in home care under Medicare Part B benefits. Medicare requirements for reimbursement include the following:

- Must be stage III or IV pressure sore
- Must be located on trunk of body
- Must have current Medicare Part B coverage
- Must be in permanent residence (own home, long-term care facility, etc.)

Seating Support Surfaces. Support surfaces for chairs and wheelchairs can be categorized as for the support surfaces for beds. In general, providing adequate pressure relief for chair-bound or wheelchair-bound patients is critical, because the patient at risk for pressure ulcer formation is at increased risk in the seated position because of the high pressures across the ischial tuberosities. Most pressure-reducing devices for chairs are static overlays, such as those made out of foam, gel, air, or some combination. Positioning chair-bound or wheelchair-bound individuals must include consideration of individual anatomy and body contours, postural alignment, distribution of weight, and balance and stability, in addition to pressure relief. Chapter 16 provides additional information on therapeutic positioning.

Evaluating Outcomes of Support Surfaces. To evaluate outcomes from the support surfaces chosen for a particular health care setting, *baseline data must be available on the prevalence and incidence* of the condition in the setting.

Prevalence is the number of all persons with the condition at one particular point in time. Prevalence includes both facility-acquired cases and those admitted with the condition. Prevalence studies can be done on one day (one point in time) and require a team to review all medical records and perform skin inspections of all patients in the organization on that day. *Incidence is the number of new cases developing over a period of time.* Incidence includes only facility-acquired conditions and, as such, reflects the effectiveness of the prevention program in the organization. Incidence studies are done over a period of time (a month, a quarter, a year) and require evaluation of all new patients with the condition (medical record review and skin inspection). The evaluation team reviews all patients (but counts only those with new conditions) at periodic intervals over the time period, eg, once a week for 4 weeks to determine monthly incidence. Many times, prevalence and incidence studies are combined. The team performs a prevalence study on one day, then continues to evaluate the population over a period of time to evaluate the incidence also. Incidence is the most valuable of the two baseline studies because it reflects actual occurrence of pressure ulcer development in the facility. Over time, with an effective prevention program, including availability of the appropriate support surfaces, the incidence of pressure ulcer development in the facility should decline, assuming there are no changes in the patient population.

Clinical Wisdom:
Teaching Wheelchair-Bound Patients

Wheelchair-bound patients with upper body strength can be taught and encouraged to do wheelchair push-ups every 15 minutes to relieve pressure and allow for reperfusion of the tissues in the ischial tuberosity region. Use of a watch with a timer device may be a helpful reminder. The use of a chair support surface can help lessen the burden of wheelchair pushups, but does not eliminate the need for reperfusion of the tissues.

Choosing support surfaces for clients based on algorithms (see Figure 15–9) and predetermined criteria (factors chosen by the clinician, such as the support surface's ability to handle friction, cost, service, etc), use of a multidisciplinary team to finalize selections, and periodic reevaluation of products and patient/institution needs, based on baseline prevalence and incidence data, are the keys to effective support surface use.

Friction and Shear

Measures to reduce friction and shear relate to passive or active movement of the patient. To reduce friction, several interventions are appropriate. Providing topical preparations to eliminate or reduce the surface tension between the skin and the bed linen or support surface will assist in reducing friction-related injury. Use of appropriate techniques when moving patients so that skin is never dragged across linens will lessen friction-induced skin breakdown. Patients who exhibit voluntary or involuntary repetitive body movements (particularly of the heels or elbows) require stronger interventions. Use of a protective film, such as a transparent film dressing or a skin sealant; a protective dressing, such as a thin hydrocolloid; or protective padding will help to eliminate the surface contact of the area and decrease the friction between the skin and the linens.[40] Even though heel, ankle, and elbow protectors do nothing to reduce or relieve pressure, they can be effective aids against friction.

Clinical Wisdom: *Reducing Friction*

Sprinkling cornstarch on the bed linen or use of skin lubricants is helpful in reducing overall friction.

Most shear injury can be eliminated by proper positioning, such as avoidance of the semi-Fowler's position and limiting use of the upright position (positions over 30° inclined). Avoidance of positions greater than 30° inclined may prevent sliding and shear-related injury. Use of footboards and knee Gatches (or pillows under the lower leg) to prevent sliding and to maintain position are also helpful in reducing shear effects on the skin when in bed. Observation of the patient when sitting is also important, because the patient who slides out of the chair is at equally high risk for shear injury. Use of footstools and the foot pedals on wheelchairs and appropriate 90° flexion of the hip (may be achieved with pillows, special seat cushions, or orthotic devices) can help in preventing chair sliding.

Nutrition

Nutrition is an important element in maintaining healthy skin and tissues. There is a strong relationship between nutrition and pressure ulcer development.[60] The severity of pressure ulceration is also correlated with severity of nutritional deficits, especially low protein intake or low serum albumin levels.[60,62,63] The nutritional assessment is key in determining the appropriate interventions for the patient. A short nutritional assessment should be performed on all patients determined to be at risk for pressure ulcer formation at routine intervals. See Chapter 3 for more information on assessment of nutrition.

Malnutrition can be diagnosed if serum albumin levels are below 3.5 mg/dL, total lymphocyte count is less than 1,800 mm,[19] or body weight decreases by more than 15%.[1] Exhibit 15–6 provides an example of a nutritional screening tool. Malnutrition impairs the immune system, and total lymphocyte counts are a reflection of immune competence. If the patient is diagnosed as malnourished, nutritional supplementation should be instituted to help achieve a positive nitrogen balance. Examples of oral supplements are assisted oral feedings, dietary supplements, or tube feedings. Oral assisted feedings and dietary supplements are the first option for intervention, and tube feedings should be tried after other methods have failed. The goal of care is to provide approximately 30–35 kcal/kg of weight per day and 1.25–1.5 g of protein per kg of weight per day.[1] Patients should be encouraged to improve their own dietary habits, and education should focus on healthy nutrition with adequate caloric and protein intake. It may be difficult for a pressure ulcer patient or an at-risk patient to ingest enough protein and calories necessary to maintain skin and tissue health. Oral supplements can be very helpful in boosting calorie and protein intake. Liquid nutritional supplements are designed to be used as an adjunct to regular oral feedings.[85] Monitoring of nutritional indexes is essential to determine effectiveness of the care plan. Serum albumin, protein markers, body weight, dietary intake, and nutritional assessment should be performed at least every 3 months to monitor for changes in nutritional status.

Hypoalbuminemia (serum albumin levels below 3.5 mg/dL) may be associated with pressure ulceration,[60,63] although some have found no relationship and little prognostic value for pressure ulcer healing.[86–88] When protein intake is insufficient, the serum albumin decreases. Serum albumin contributes to the amino acid pool, and amino acids are essential building blocks for new tissue development. Serum albumin also maintains oncotic pressures within the vascular fluid compartment. Colloidal oncotic pressure is the total influence of proteins on the osmotic activity of plasma. When albumin levels decrease, there is a decrease in the oncotic pressure (fewer proteins in the plasma, leading to increased osmotic activity from the vascular bed as the blood vessels attempt to maintain homeostasis by allowing osmosis of water out of the vessels and into surrounding tissues), which leads to edema, further compromising tissue perfusion.[40] Ensuring adequate protein intake is a critical element in nutritional interventions for pressure ulcer patients and those at risk for pressure ulceration.

Dehydration may influence serum albumin levels and tissue health. Nutritional assessment should include assessment of fluid intake, as well as dietary intake. Vitamin and mineral deficiencies may also be present in the patient at risk for pressure ulcer development. Vitamin C and zinc supplements may assist in wound healing when deficiencies exist. Use of a multivitamin for those with deficiencies and supplemental vitamin C, zinc, and iron (if indicated by anemia) can be supportive of skin and tissue health, as well as beneficial

Exhibit 15–6 Example of Nutritional Assessment Guide for Patients with Pressure Ulcers

---

Patient Name: _____ Date: _____ Time: _____

To be filled out for all patients at risk on initial evaluation and every 12 weeks thereafter, as indicated. Trends will document the efficacy of nutritional support therapy.

Protein Compartments

Somatic:

Current Weight (kg)	_____	
Previous Weight (kg)	_____	(_____ date)
Percent Change in Weight	_____	
Height (cm)	_____	
Height/Weight	_____	
Current Body Mass Index (BMI)	_____	(wt(ht)^2]
Previous BMI	_____	(_____ date)
Percent Change in BMI		

Visceral:

Serum Albumin
(Normal ≥ 3.5 mg/dL)
Total Lymphocyte Count (TLC)   _____   (optional)
   (White Blood Cell count × percent Lymphocytes/100)

Guide to TLC:

- Immune competence   ≥ 1,800 mm^3
- Immunity partly impaired   < 1,800 but ≥ 900 mm^3
- Anergy   < 900 mm^3

State of Hydration

24-Hour Intake _____ mL   24-Hour Output _____ mL

Note: Thirst, tongue dryness in non–mouth breathers, and tenting of cervical skin may indicate dehydration. Jugular vein distention may indicate overhydration.

Estimated Nutritional Requirement

Estimated Nonprotein Calories (NPC)	_____/kg	Estimated Protein	_____ (g/kg)
Actual NPC	_____/kg	Actual Protein	_____ (g/kg)

Recommendations/Plan

1.
2.
3.
4.

Source: Reprinted from N. Bergstrom, M.A. Bennett, C.E. Carlson, et al., *Treatment of Pressure Ulcers,* Clinical Practice Guideline No. 15, December, 1994, U.S. Department of Health and Human Services, Public Health Service, Agency for Health Care Policy and Research, AHCPR Publication No. 95-0652.

for wound healing. Clearly, the area of nutritional intervention requires an interdisciplinary approach. Involvement of the dietitian during the early assessment of the patient is important to the overall success of the plan.

Clinical Wisdom: *When To Consult the Dietitian*

General parameters for consultation with the dietitian for a thorough nutritional assessment are:

- Inadequate dietary intake,
- Drop in body weight of 5%, *or*
- Serum albumin level below 3.5 mg/dL

Moisture

The preventive interventions related to moisture include general skin care, accurate diagnosis of incontinence type, and appropriate incontinence management.

General Skin Care

General skin care involves routine skin assessment, incontinence assessment and management, skin hygiene interventions, and measures to maintain skin health. Routine skin assessment involves observation of the patient's skin, with particular attention to bony prominences. Reddened areas should not be massaged. Massage can further impair the perfusion to the tissues.[89] The skin should be evaluated for dryness and cracking. Older adults are at higher risk for dry skin, and dry skin may decrease tissue tolerance to external forces. Lack of moisture in the air may contribute to dry skin and can be counteracted by use of a humidifier in the room.[90] Attention should also be focused on gentle handling to prevent skin tears in older patients. The epidermis and dermis junction is lessened with age, making older patients at higher risk for skin tears. Other factors to include in a skin assessment include temperature, sensory ability, turgor, and texture.[91] Skin should normally be warm to touch. The dorsal aspect of the hand is more sensitive to temperature changes than the palm of the hand; thus, clinicians should use the dorsal aspect of the hand to judge skin temperature. Two-point discrimination is used to evaluate skin sensation. Normally, the patient should be able to distinguish sharp, dull, or pressure sensations against the skin surface. Diminished sensation may be generalized or localized to a specific area, such as the lower extremities. Skin tone should be smooth and elastic. Edema causes the skin to appear taut and shiny, and dehydration is present if the skin is dry, wrinkled, and withered. Observing the skin surface for texture and moisture may reveal signs of excessive moisture or dryness. Most factors in a skin assessment can be reviewed through observation and palpation skills. The information gathered through the simple act of inspection can form a basis for general skin care interventions and for pressure ulcer prevention interventions.

Incontinence Assessment and Management

Specifically related to moisture, the skin should be assessed for signs of perineal dermatitis. Evaluating perineal dermatitis requires understanding of the concepts of tissue tolerance, perineal environment, and toileting ability.[92] (See *Color Plates 14 and 16.*) Objective signs of perineal dermatitis include erythema, swelling, vesiculation, oozing, crusting, and scaling, with subjective symptoms of tingling, itching, burning, and pain.[92] The perineal region is broadly defined as the perineum (area between the vulva or scrotum and anus), buttocks, perianal area, coccyx, and upper/inner thigh regions.[93]

The clinical presentation is variable and may be dependent on the frequency of incontinence episode, rapidity and efficacy of postepisode hygiene, and duration of incontinence. Acute and chronic clinical manifestations of skin reactions in elderly nursing home patients have been described based on clinical experience.[94]

Skin reactions can be divided into acute reactions and chronic changes. Perineal dermatitis may present with acute episode characteristics or with more long-standing chronic skin changes apparent. In acute episodes, the skin characteristics most predominant are erythema, papulovesicular reaction, frank erosions and abrasions, and, in some cases, evidence of monilial infection, due to the moist warm environment. In general, a diffuse blanchable erythema is present involving both buttocks, coccyx area, perineum, perianal area, and upper/inner thighs. The extent of the erythema varies, and the intensity of the reaction may be muted in immunocompromised and some elderly patients. A papulovesicular rash is particularly evident in the groin and perineum areas (upper/inner thigh, vulva/scrotal area). Secondary skin changes include crusting and scaling, and are usually evident at the fringes of the reaction. Erosions and frank denudation of the skin may be more common with incontinence associated with feces. The distribution of the dermatitis differs in men and women, as might be expected. Typically, the more severe damage in male patients occurs on the posterior aspect of the penile shaft and the anterior aspect of the scrotum. More damage is seen in the lower perineal regions, such as the inner thighs and low buttocks, than in the higher perineal regions, such as the sacral/coccygeal area or groin. In women, the skin damage usually involves the vulva and groin areas, and spreads distally from those sites.

Chronic skin changes in elderly patients with long-standing incontinence include a thickened appearance of skin where moisture is allowed to maintain skin contact, and increased evidence of scaling and crusting. The thickened appearance of the skin is similar to the changes seen in peristomal skin of patients with urinary diversions or ileostomies who have pouches with too large an aperture, allowing the urine or fecal effluent to pool around the stoma. This skin is overhydrated and easily abraded, with minimal friction. The reaction is notable at the coccyx, scrotum, and vulva. In a cognitively impaired nursing home sample,[94] there was also evidence of excoriation from patients' scratching at the affected sites. This provides early clinical validation of the symptom of itching in perineal dermatitis.

In many cases, partial-thickness ulcers are present over the sacral/coccygeal area and medial buttocks region, close to the gluteal fold. Although these lesions may present as typical pressure ulcers, the underlying etiology may be the effects of incontinence on the skin. There are some characteristics of these partial-thickness ulcers that assist in differentiating them from true pressure-induced skin trauma. First, the lesions tend to be multiple in nature. The ulcers are almost always partial-thickness or stage II lesions. The lesions may or may not be directly over a bony prominence, and, finally, the lesions are typically surrounded by other characteristics of perineal dermatitis (eg, diffuse blanchable erythema). When caring for patients who are incontinent of urine and feces, health care providers are faced with the challenge of preventing perineal dermatitis and pressure ulceration as a result of the decreased tissue tolerance to trauma. True pressure ulcers result from compression of the soft tissue between the bony prominence and the external surface. When moisture, urine, and feces have caused maceration and overhydration of the epidermis, the skin and tissues are less tolerant of the pressure force. Stage II pressure ulcers and partial-thickness skin lesions, such as abrasions, are most commonly attributed to friction and shearing forces. It is likely that incontinence plays a critical role in the development of stage II pressure ulcers.[54]

Management of incontinence is a huge topic area, and volumes have been written about various management techniques. This discussion is meant to serve as a stepping stone to those resources available to clinicians on management of the incontinent patient. Therefore, the discussion, by necessity, is noninclusive of all management strategies and only briefly addresses several strategies most pertinent to the patient at high risk of developing a pressure ulcer and measures to protect the skin from wetness and irritants. Management of incontinence is dependent on assessment and diagnosis of the problem.

Incontinence Assessment. Assessment parameters to be addressed include history, physical examination, environmental assessment, voiding/defecation diary, laboratory studies, and other diagnostic studies.[95] The history is critical to assessing the problem accurately. History taking should elicit information on patterns of urinary/fecal elimination and past/current management program, patterns of inconti-

nence, characteristics of the urinary stream/fecal mass, sensation of bladder/rectal filling, and a focused review of systems and medical-surgical history.[96] The physical examination is designed to gather specific information related to bladder/rectal functioning and, thus, is limited in scope. A limited neurologic examination should provide data on the mental status and motivation of the patient/caregiver, specific motor skills, and back and lower extremities. The genitalia and perineal skin are assessed for signs of estrogenization, pelvic descent, perineal skin lesions, perineal sensation and bulbocavernosus response in women, and penis/scrotal contents, rectal and prostate, and bulbocavernosus response in men.[95,97]

The environmental assessment should include inspection of the patient's home or nursing home facility to evaluate for the presence of environmental barriers to continence. The voiding/defecation diary is the real tool for management of continence in patients without cognitive impairment. The diary provides baseline data on the problem and so provides a mechanism for determining therapy effectiveness for the future.[95] The diary may provide valuable information for diagnostic purposes. In cognitively impaired patients, the caregiver may complete the diary, and management strategies again can be identified from the baseline data.

Laboratory tests help to rule out infections and other pathology responsible for the incontinence. Some specialized studies are helpful in further evaluation of the condition. Urodynamic studies for urinary incontinence provide valuable data related to the pathology. Even in nursing home populations, simple bedside urodynamics can be a useful clinical tool to elicit more specific data on urinary function.[97] Management strategies for incontinence are grouped into three main areas for this discussion: behavioral management, containment strategies, and skin protection guidelines.

Incontinence Management Strategies. Patients at risk for pressure ulcer development are not candidates for all methods of behavioral management. The most successful behavioral management strategies for the frail, cognitively impaired patient typically at risk of pressure ulcer development include prompted voiding and scheduled toileting programs. Both strategies are caregiver dependent and require a motivated caregiver to be successful. Scheduled intake of fluid is an important underlying factor for both strategies.

Scheduled toileting or habit training is toileting on a planned basis. The goal is to keep the person dry by assisting him or her to void at regular intervals. There can be attempts to match the interval to the individual patient's natural voiding schedule. There is no systematic effort to motivate patients to delay voiding or to resist the urge to void. Scheduled toileting may be based on the clock (toilet the patient every 2 hours) or based on activities (toilet the patient after meals and before transferring to bed). Several studies have demonstrated improvement in continence status in some patients.[96,98]

Prompted voiding has been shown to be effective in dependent and cognitively impaired nursing home incontinent patients.[99,100] Prompted voiding involves use of a toileting schedule (every 2 hours) similar to habit training or scheduled toileting. Prompted voiding supplements the routine with teaching the incontinent patient to discriminate their continence status and to request toileting assistance. The three major elements in prompted voiding include monitoring the incontinent patient routinely, prompting the patient to use the toilet, and praising the patient for maintenance of continence. Prompted voiding results in 40–50% reduction in frequency of daytime incontinence, and between 25% and 33% of urinary incontinent patients in nursing homes respond to the therapy.[99,100] Both of these behavioral management strategies have the added benefit of moving the patient at routine intervals, which should relieve pressure over bony prominences and reduce the risk of pressure ulcer development by allowing reperfusion of the tissues.

Underpads and briefs may be used to protect the skin of patients who are incontinent of urine or stool. These products are designed to absorb moisture, wick the wetness away from the skin, and maintain a quick-drying interface with the skin.[40] Studies with both infants and adults demonstrate that products designed to present a quick-drying surface to the skin and to absorb moisture do keep the skin drier and are associated with a lower incidence of dermatitis.[57] It is important to note that the critical feature is the ability to absorb moisture and present a quick-drying surface, not whether the product is disposable or reusable. Regardless of the product chosen, containment strategies imply the need for a check-and-change schedule for the incontinent patient so that wet linens and pads may be removed in a timely manner. Underpads are not as tight or constricting as briefs. Kemp[54] suggests alternating the use of underpads and briefs if the skin irritation is thought to be related to the occlusive nature of the brief. Her recommendations echo the early work of Willis[101] on warm water immersion syndrome, who found that the effects of water on the skin could be reversed and tempered by simply allowing the skin to dry out between wet periods. Use of briefs when the patient is up in a chair, ambulating, or visiting another department and use of underpads when the patient is in bed is one suggestion for combining the strengths of both products.[54]

External collection devices may be more effective with male patients. External catheters or condom catheters are devices applied to the shaft of the penis to direct the urine away from the body to a collection device. Newer models of external catheters are self-adhesive and easy to apply. For patients with a retracted penis, a special pouching system, similar to an ostomy pouch, is available—the retracted penis pouch.[102]

A key concern with use of external collection devices is routine removal of the product and inspection and hygiene of the skin.

There are special containment devices for fecal incontinence, as well. Fecal incontinence collectors consist of a self-adhesive skin barrier attached to a drainable pouch. Application of the device is somewhat dependent on the skill of the clinician, and the patient should be put on a routine for changing the pouch prior to leakage to facilitate success. The skin barrier provides a physical obstacle to the stool on the skin and helps to prevent dermatitis and associated skin problems. In fact, skin barrier wafers without an attached pouch can be useful in protecting the skin from feces or urine.

The AHRQ panel on guidelines for the prevention and prediction of pressure ulcers in adults[42] recommends use of moisturizers for dry skin and use of lubricants for reduction in friction injuries. The panel also discusses the use of moisture barriers to protect the skin from the effects of moisture. Although the recommendation is made to use products to provide a moisture barrier, the reader is cautioned that the recommendation is derived from usual practice and professional standards, and it is not research based. The success of the particular product is linked to how it is formulated and the hydrophobic properties of the product.[54] Generally, pastes are thicker and more repellent of moisture than are ointments. A quick evaluation is the ease with which the product can be removed with water during routine cleansing. If the product comes off the skin with just routine cleansing, it probably is not an effective barrier to moisture. Use of mineral oil for cleansing some of the heavier barrier products, such as zinc oxide paste, will ease removal from the skin.

The role of incontinence as a risk factor in predicting pressure ulcer formation is somewhat unclear. From a pathophysiologic perspective, creating a skin environment favorable to friction and abrasion makes incontinence a key risk factor for those persons with additional risk for pressure ulcer development. When caring for the incontinent patient, health care providers must address prevention by assessment and treatment of transient causes of the condition. Systematic assessment is the key to defining management strategies. Assessment includes the parameters of patient history, physical examination, environment, voiding/defecation diary, laboratory studies, and other diagnostic studies. Measures to manage incontinence include caregiver-dependent behavioral management therapies of scheduled toileting and prompted voiding, containment devices and products, and skin protection using barriers.

Skin Hygiene Interventions. Skin hygiene interventions involve daily skin hygiene and skin cleansing after fecal or urinary incontinent episodes. The older adult's skin is less tolerant of the drying effects of soap and hot water. Use of warm water and a mild soap (if any soap at all) can limit skin drying. Daily bathing is not necessary for skin health in most older adults. Use of a schedule of twice weekly or every other day bathing or showering is sufficient for most older adults. Daily cleansing of the feet, axilla, and perineal areas is appropriate, but daily showers or baths can be damaging to the skin. Use of solutions designed for incontinence care cleansing can be protective of the skin and can decrease the time and energy involved in postincontinent episode cleansing. These commercially available cleansers include surfactants as ingredients. The surfactants make the removal of urine and stool residue easier, with less abrasiveness. Every attempt should be made to cleanse the perineal skin immediately after an incontinent episode to limit the amount of contact time between the urine or stool and the skin.

Skin Maintenance Interventions. Skin maintenance interventions involve actions to prevent skin breakdown and actions to promote healthy skin. Maintaining skin lubrication is an important skin maintenance intervention. Use of moisturizers on a routine basis can prevent skin drying and cracking. Application of moisturizers immediately after bathing or showering helps to remoisturize and lubricate the skin. There are three main types of moisturizers—lotions, creams, and ointments. Lotions have the highest water content and, therefore, must be reapplied more frequently to be effective. Creams are mixtures of oil and water and, for best results, should be applied four times a day. Ointments (generally lanolin or petrolatum bases) have the lowest water content, are the most occlusive, and have the longest duration of moisturizing action. Special attention to moisturizing the lower legs and feet is often needed to compensate for decreased perfusion and diminished skin health in these areas.

OUTCOME MEASURES

The most appropriate outcome measures to evaluate the effectiveness of prevention programs are incidence and prevalence rates. When a prevention program is successful, the organization's incidence of pressure ulcer development should decrease (if appropriate) or remain at a low level. Incidence and prevalence data should be risk-adjusted by using risk stratification techniques when gathering data. This will allow comparison of data with other health care facilities for benchmarking and adequate evaluation of prevention programs as casemix of the organization varies over time. If a patient already has a pressure ulcer, a successful outcome for pressure ulcer prevention is no further areas of skin breakdown. Again, use of risk stratification techniques should be used so that data can be compared with other facilities and so that severity of pressure ulcers can be truly evaluated.

REFERRAL CRITERIA

Referral criteria for pressure ulcer prevention programs relate to the need for an interdisciplinary approach to prevention of pressure ulcers. Referrals assist with appropriate management of particular risk factors for developing pressure ulcers. Use referral in the following circumstances:

- Nutritional consultation for patients determined at risk for malnutrition or with nutritional concerns
- Enterostomal therapy nurse (or clinical specialist in this area) consultation for patients with urinary or fecal incontinence
- Physical therapy for assistance with correct positioning in seated individuals

SELF-CARE TEACHING GUIDELINES

Patient's and caregiver's instruction in self-care must be individualized to specific pressure ulcer development risk factors, the individual patient's learning style and coping mechanisms, and the ability of the patient/caregiver to perform procedures. These general self-care teaching guidelines must be individualized for each patient and caregiver. In teaching prevention guidelines to caregivers, it is particularly important to use return demonstration by the caregiver as evaluation of learning. Observing the caregiver performing turning maneuvers, repositioning, managing incontinence, and providing general skin care can be enlightening and provides the context in which the clinician provides support and follow-up education. Exhibit 15–7 provides general self-care teaching guidelines.

REVIEW QUESTIONS

1. According to the AHRQ, in general, when should risk assessment for pressure ulcer formation be performed?
   a. according to patient acuity level
   b. on admission to organization, weekly, and when there is a change in patient status
   c. on admission to organization and every two weeks
   d. according to agency protocol and on admission to organization
2. Which of the following extrinsic risk factors decrease the tissue tolerance to pressure?
   a. shear, friction, and moisture
   b. nutrition, age, psychologic issues, and temperature
   c. immobility, inactivity, and loss of sensation

Exhibit 15–7 Self-Care Teaching Guidelines

Self-Care Guidelines Specific to Pressure Ulcer Prevention	Instructions Given (Date/Initials) Return	Demonstration *or* Review of Material (Date/Initials)	Demonstration *or* States Understanding (Date/Initials)
1. Identification of specific risk factors for pressure ulcer development			
2. Immobility, inactivity, and decreased sensory perception strategies a. Passive repositioning			
(1) Demonstrates one-person turning			
(2) Demonstrates two-person turning			
(3) Frequency of turning/repositioning			
(4) Full shifts in position versus small shifts in position			
(5) Avoidance of 90° sidelying position, demonstrates 30° laterally inclined position			
(6) Passive range of motion exercises and frequency			
b. Pillow bridging			
(1) Use of pillows to protect heels			
(2) Pillows between bony prominences			
c. Pressure-reducing/relieving support surface			
(1) Management of support surface in use			
(2) Devices for sitting			
(3) Up in chair for _____ hour(s), _____ time(s) per day			
3. Nutrition strategies a. Provide adequate nutrition			
(1) Small frequent (six meals a day) high-calorie/high-protein meals			
(2) Nutritional supplements provided. Give _____ oz of _____ supplement _____ times per day.			
b. Provide adequate hydration (1) Eight 8-oz glasses of noncaffeine fluids per day unless contraindicated			
c. Provide vitamin/mineral supplements (1) Vitamin C, zinc, iron (Give as ordered.)			
4. Friction and shear strategies			
a. Use of turning and draw sheets			
b. Use of cornstarch, lubricants, pad protectors, thin film dressings, or hydrocolloid dressings over friction risk sites			
c. General skin care (1) Skin cleansing			
(2) Skin moisturizing (Use _____ product on _____ areas of skin, _____ times a day.)			

continues

Exhibit 15–7 continued

Self-Care Guidelines Specific to Pressure Ulcer Prevention	Instructions Given (Date/Initials)	Demonstration *or* Review of Material (Date/Initials)	Return Demonstration *or* States Understanding (Date/Initials)

5. Moisture—incontinence management strategies
  a. Use of absorbent products
    (1) Pad when lying in bed			

(2) Brief or panty pad when up in chair or walking			
b. Use of ointments, creams, and skin barriers prophylactically in perineal and perianal areas (Use _____ product on perineal/perianal areas of skin, _____ times a day.)			
c. Use of behavioral management strategies for incontinence (1) Scheduled toileting: toilet every _____ hours			
(2) Prompted voiding			

d. General skin care
    (1) Skin cleansing
        (a) Cleanser: _____			

(b) Soap: _____			
(c) Frequency: _____			
(2) Skin moisturizing (Use _____ product(s) on _____ areas of skin, _____ times a day.)			
(3) Skin inspection daily			
6. Importance of follow-up with health care provider			

    d. time of pressure, duration of pressure, and compression force

3. Which of the following statements best defines prevalence?
    a. The number of new and old cases at any given point in time requires only one observation with one specific population.
    b. Determination of the rate at which cases develop requires repeated observations on one specific population.
    c. The number of new cases observed over a period of time on one specific population.
    d. The number of old cases at any given point in time requires only one observation with one specific population.

4. A stage II pressure ulcer is best defined as which of the following?
    a. Nonblanchable erythema of intact skin.
    b. Lesions involving only the epidermis and dermis.
    c. Lesions involving the epidermis, dermis, and subcutaneous tissue extending down to, but not through, the fascia.

    d. Lesions involving the epidermis, dermis, subcutaneous tissue, and extending to muscle, bone, joint, and tendon.

5. The clinician is asked to recommend a support surface for P.L., who has three pressure sores, one on the sacral/coccygeal area, one on the left greater trochanter, and one on the right ischial tuberosity. The ulcers range in severity from a clean, healing stage II on the sacral/coccygeal area to necrotic stage III on the left trochanter and clean stage IV on the right ischial tuberosity. Which of the following is the MOST appropriate support surface choice?
    a. a foam gel combination mattress
    b. an alternating air mattress
    c. a mattress replacement
    d. a low-air-loss bed

6. Friction causes what type of skin damage?
    a. superficial abrasion and damage to the epidermis
    b. full-thickness skin loss
    c. skin tears with dermal involvement
    d. stage III pressure ulceration

RESOURCES

National Pressure Ulcer Advisory Panel

11250 Roger Baron Dr., Suite 8
Reston, VA 20190–5202
(703) 464–4849
http://www.npuap.org

Wound Ostomy Continence Society

1550 S. Coast Highway, Suite 201
Laguna Beach, CA 92651
(888) 224–WOCN
http://www.wocn.org

REFERENCES

1. Bergstrom N, Bennett MA, Carlson CE, et al. *Treatment of Pressure Ulcers.* Clinical Practice Guideline No. 15. Agency for Health Care Research and Quality (AHRQ), formerly known as the Agency for Health Care Policy and Research (AHCPR) Publication No. 95–0652. Rockville, MD: AHRQ, U.S. Public Health Service (PHS), U.S. Department of Health and Human Services (DHHS); December 1994.

2. National Pressure Ulcer Advisory Panel (NPUAP). *Pressure Ulcers: Incidence, Economics, Risk Assessment. Consensus Development Conference Statement.* West Dundee, IL: S-N Publications; 1989:3–4.

3. Baker J. Medicaid claims history of Florida long-term care facility residents hospitalized for pressure ulcers. *J Wound, Ostomy, Continence Nurs.* 1996;23(1):23–25.

4. Langemo DK, Olson B, Hunter S, Hanson D, Burd C, Cathcart-Silberberg T. Incidence and prediction of pressure ulcers in five patient care settings. *Decubitus.* 1991;4(3):25,26,28,30.

5. Berlowitz DR, Ash AS, Brandeis GH, Brand HK, Halpern JL, Moskowitz MA. Rating long-term care facilities on pressure ulcer development: Importance of case-mix adjustment [see comments]. *Ann Intern Med.* 1996;124(6):557–563.

6. Bergstrom N, Braden B. A prospective study of pressure sore risk among institutionalized elderly. *J Am Geriatr Soc.* 1992;40(8):747–758.

7. Berlowitz DR, Bezerra HQ, Brandeis GH, Kader B, Anderson JJ. Are we improving the quality of nursing home care: The case of pressure ulcers. *J Am Geriatr Soc.* 2000;48(1):59–62.

8. Hunter SM, Langemo DK, Olson B, et al. The effectiveness of skin care protocols for pressure ulcers. *Rehabil Nurs.* 1995;20(5):250–255.

9. Schue RM, Langemo DK. Pressure ulcer prevalence and incidence and a modification of the Braden Scale for a rehabilitation unit. *J Wound, Ostomy, Continence Nurs.* 1998;25(1):36–43.

10. Hunter SM, Cathcart Silberberg T, Langemo DK, et al. Pressure ulcer prevalence and incidence in a rehabilitation hospital. *Rehabil Nurs.* 1992;17(5):239–242.

11. Baggerly J, DiBlasi M. Pressure sores and pressure sore prevention in a rehabilitation setting: Building information for improving outcomes and allocating resources. *Rehabil Nurs.* 1996;21(6):321–325.

12. Waters RL, Meyer PR Jr, Adkins RH, Felton D. Emergency, acute, and surgical management of spine trauma. *Arch Phys Med Rehabil.* 1999;80(11):1383–1390.

13. Garber SL, Rintala DH, Hart KA, Fuhrer MJ. Pressure ulcer risk in spinal cord injury: Predictors of ulcer status over 3 years. *Arch Phys Med Rehabil.* 2000;81(4):465–471.

14. Eastwood EA, Hagglund KJ, Ragnarsson KT, Gordon WA, Marino RJ. Medical rehabilitation length of stay and outcomes for persons with traumatic spinal cord injury 1990–1997. *Arch Phys Med Rehabil.* 1999;80(11):1457–1463.

15. Whitington K, Patrick M, Roberts JL. A national study of pressure ulcer prevalence and incidence in acute care hospitals. *J Wound, Ostomy, Continence Nurs.* 2000;27(4):209–215.

16. Amlung S, Miller W, Bosley LM, Runfola A, Barnett R. National prevalence pressure ulcer survey: A benchmarking approach. In: 14th Annual Clinical Symposium on Wound Care. *The Quest for Quality Wound Care: Solutions for Clinical Practice;* September 30–October 4, 1999; Denver, CO: Sponsored by the Wound Care Communications Network and University of Pennsylvania Medical Center; 1999:234.

17. Objective 1–16. In: *Healthy People 2010.* Washington, DC: DHHS; 2000.

18. Waite D. Caregiver guilty in fatal neglect of patient's bedsores. *The Honolulu Advertiser.* Saturday, October 28, 2000.

19. Daniel RK, Priest DL, Wheatley DC. Etiologic factors in pressure sores: An experimental model. *Arch Phys Med Rehabil.* 1981;62(10):492–498.

20. Kosiak M. Etiology and pathology of ischemic ulcers. *Arch Phys Med Rehabil.* 1959;40:62–69.

21. Reuler JB, Cooney TG. The pressure sore: Pathophysiology and principles of management. *Ann Intern Med.* 1981;94:661.

22. Seiler WD, Stahelin HB. Recent findings on decubitus ulcer pathology: Implications for care. *Geriatrics.* 1986;41:47–60.

23. Witkowski JA, Parish LC. Histopathology of the decubitus ulcer. *J Am Acad Dermatol.* 1982;6:1014–1021.

24. Lindan O, Greenway RM, Piazza JM. Pressure distributor on the surface of the human body. *Arch Phys Med Rehabil.* 1965;46:378.

25. Scales JT. Pressure on the patient. In: Kenedi RN, Cowden JM, eds. *Bedsore Biomechanics.* Baltimore: University Park Press; 1976.

26. Parish, LC, Witkowski JA, Crissey JT. *The Decubitus Ulcer.* New York: Masson Publishing; 1983.

27. Slater H. *Pressure Ulcers in the Elderly.* Pittsburgh, PA: Synapse Publications; 1985.

28. Walker PM. Ischemial reperfusion injury in skeletal muscle. *Ann Vasc Surg.* 1991;5(4):399–402.

29. Hernandez-Maldonado JJ, Teehan E, Franco CD, Duran WN, Hobson RW. Superoxide anion production by leukocytes exposed to post-ischemic skeletal muscle. *J Cardiovasc Surg.* 1992;33:695–699.

30. Landis EM. Micro-injection studies of capillary blood pressure in human skin. *Heart.* 1930;15:209.

31. Husain T. An experimental study of some pressure effects on tissues, with reference to the bedsore problem. *J Pathol Bacteriol.* 1953;66:347–358.

32. Salcido R, et al. Histopathology of decubitus ulcers as a result of sequential pressure sessions in a computer-controlled fuzzy rat model. *Adv Wound Care.* 1993;7(5):40.

33. Kosiak M, Kubicek WG, Olsen M, Danz JN, Kottke FJ. Evaluation of pressure as a factor in the production of ischial ulcers. *Arch Phys Med Rehabil.* 1958;39:623.

34. Edberg EL, Cerny K, Stauffer ES. Prevention and treatment of pressure sores. *Phys Ther.* 1973;53:246–252.

35. Bennett MA. Report of the task force on the implications for darkly pigmented intact skin in the prediction and prevention of pressure ulcers. *Adv Wound Care.* 1995;8(6):34–35.

36. Graves DJ. Stage I in ebony complexion. *Decubitus.* Letter to the Editor. 1990;3(4):4.

37. Parish LC, Witkowski JA, Crissey JT, eds. *The Decubitis Ulcer in Clinical Practice.* Berlin, Germany: Springer-Verlag; 1997.

38. Meehan M. Multisite pressure ulcer prevalence survey. *Decubitus.* 1990;3(4):14–17.

39. Knight DB, Scott H. Contracture and pressure necrosis. *Ostomy/Wound Manage.* 1990;26(1):60–67.

40. Maklebust J, Sieggreen M. *Pressure Ulcers: Guidelines for Prevention and Nursing Management.* 2nd ed. Springhouse, PA: Springhouse; 1996.

41. Shea JD. Pressures sores: Classification and management. *Clin Orthop.* 1975;112:89–100.

42. Panel for the Prediction and Prevention of Pressure Ulcers. *Pressure Ulcers in Adults: Prediction and Prevention.* Clinical Practice Guideline No. 3. AHRQ Publication No. 92–0047. Rockville, MD: AHRQ, PHS, DHHS; 1992.

43. Maklebust J. Pressure ulcer staging systems: NPUAP Conference Proceedings. *Adv Wound Care.* 1995;8(4):28-11–28-14.

44. Allman RM. Pressure ulcers among the elderly. *N Engl J Med.* 1989;320:850.

45. Braden BJ, Bergstrom N. A conceptual schema for the study of etiology of pressure sores. *Rehabil Nurs.* 1987;12(1):8–12.

46. Bergstrom N, Demuth PJ, Braden BJ. A clinical trial of the Braden Scale for predicting pressure sore risk. *Nurs Clin North Am.* 1987;22:417–428.

47. Exton-Smith AN, Sherwin RW. The prevention of pressure sores: significance of spontaneous bodily movements. *Lancet.* 1961;2:1124–1126.

48. Allman RM, Goode PS, Patrick MM, et al. Pressure ulcer risk factors among hospitalized patients with activity limitations. *JAMA.* 1995;273:865–870.

49. Curry K, Casady L. The relationship between extended periods of immobility and decubitus ulcer formation in the acutely spinal cord injured individual. *J Neurosci Nurs.* 1992;24:185–189.

50. Hammond MC, Bozzacco VA, Stiens SA, et al. Pressure ulcer incidence on a spinal cord injury unit. *Adv Wound Care.* 1994;7(6):57–60.

51. Reichel SM. Shearing force as a factor in decubitus ulcers in paraplegics. *JAMA.* 1958;166:762–763.

52. Bennett L, Kavner D, Lee BY, Trainor FS. Skin stress and blood flow in sitting paraplegic patients. *Arch Phys Med Rehabil.* 1984;65(4):186–190.

53. Dinsdale JM. Decubitus ulcers: Role of pressure and friction in causation. *Arch Phys Med Rehabil.* 1974;55:147–153.

54. Kemp MG. Protecting the skin from moisture and associated irritants. *J Gerontol Nurs.* 1994;20(9):8–14.

55. Bates-Jensen B. Incontinence management. In: Parish LC, Witkowski JA, Crissey JT, eds. *The Decubitus Ulcer in Clinical Practice.* Berlin, Germany: Springer-Verlag; 1997:189–199.

56. Berg RW, Milligan MC, Sarbaugh FC. Association of skin wetness and pH with diaper dermatitis. *Pediatr Dermatol.* 1994;11:18–20.

57. Zimmerer RE, Lawson KD, Calvert CJ. The effects of wearing diapers on skin. *Pediatr Dermatol.* 1986;3:95–101.

58. Buckingham KW, Berg RW. Etiologic factors in diaper dermatitis: The role of feces. *Pediatr Dermatol.* 1986;3:107–112.

59. Maklebust J, Magnan MA. Risk factors associated with having a pressure ulcer: A secondary data analysis. *Adv Wound Care.* 1994;7(6):25–42.

60. Pinchcovsky-Devin G, Kaminsky MV Jr. Correlation of pressure sores and nutritional status. *J Am Geriatr Soc.* 1986;34:435–440.

61. Bobel LM. Nutritional implications in the patient with pressure sores. *Nurs Clin North Am.* 1987;22:379–390.

62. Bergstrom N, Braden B. A prospective study of pressure sore risk among institutionalized elderly. *J Am Geriatr Soc.* 1992;40:747–758.

63. Allman RM, Laprade CA, Noel LB, et al. Pressure sores among hospitalized patients. *Ann Intern Med.* 1986;105:337–342.

64. Jones PL, Millman A. Wound healing and the aged patient. *Nurs Clin North Am.* 1990;25:263–277.

65. Eaglestein WH. Wound healing and aging. *Clin Geriatr Med.* 1989;5:183.

66. Versluysen M. Pressure sores in elderly patients: The epidemiology related to hip operations. *J Bone Joint Surg Br.* 1985;67:10–13.

67. Shannon ML. Pressures sores. In: Norris CM, ed. *Concept Clarification in Nursing.* Gaithersburg, MD: Aspen Publishers; 1982.

68. Anderson TP, Andberg MM. Psychosocial factors associated with pressure sores. *Arch Phys Med Rehabil.* 1979;60:341–346.

69. Vidal J, Sarrias M. An analysis of the diverse factors concerned with the development of pressure sores in spinal cord patients. *Paraplegia.* 1991;29:261–267.

70. Norton D, McLaren R, Exton-Smith NA. *An Investigation of Geriatric Nursing Problems in Hospitals.* Edinburgh, Scotland: Churchill-Livingstone; 1962.

71. Norton D. Calculating the risk: Reflections on the Norton Scale. *Decubitus.* 1989;2(3):24–31.

72. Gosnell DJ. Pressure sore risk assessment: A critique. I: The Gosnell Scale. *Decubitus.* 1989;2(3):32–39.

73. Gosnell DJ. Pressure sore risk assessment: A critique. II. Analysis of risk factors. *Decubitus.* 1989;2(3):40–43.

74. Braden B, Bergstrom N. Clinical utility of the Braden Scale for predicting pressure sore risk. *Decubitus.* 1989;2(3):44–51.

75. Bergstrom N, Braden BJ, Boynton P, Bruch S. Using a research-based assessment scale in clinical practice. *Nurs Clin North Am.* 1995;30:539.

76. Seiler WO, Allen S, Stahelin HB. Influence of the 30 degrees laterally inclined position and the "super soft" 3-piece mattress on skin oxygen tension on areas of maximum pressure: Implications for pressure sores prevention. *Gerontology.* 1986;32:158–166.

77. Lowthian PT. Practical nursing: Turning clock system to prevent pressure sores. *Nurs Mirror.* 1979;148(21):30–31.

78. Smith AM, Malone JA. Preventing pressure ulcers in institutionalized elders: Assessing the effects of small, unscheduled shifts in body position. *Decubitus.* 1990;3(4):20–24.

79. McLean J. Pressure reduction or pressure relief: Making the right choice. *J ET Nurs.* 1993;20:211–215.

80. Krouskop TA, Garber SL, Cullen BB. Factors to consider in selecting a support surface. In: Krasner D, ed. *Chronic Wound Care.* King of Prussia, PA: Health Management Publications; 1990:135–141.

81. International Association for Enterostomal Therapy (IAET). *Dermal Wounds: Pressure Sores. Standards of Care.* Irvine, CA: IAET; 1987.

82. Krouskop TA, Garber SL. Interface pressure confusion. *Decubitus.* 1989;2:8.

83. Bryant RA, Shannon ML, Pieper B, et al. Pressure ulcers. In: Bryant RA, ed. *Acute and Chronic Wounds: Nursing Management.* St. Louis, MO: Mosby-Year Book; 1992.

84. Garber SL, Krouskop TA, Cullen BB. The role of technology in pressure ulcer prevention. In: Krasner D, ed. *Chronic Wound Care.* King of Prussia, PA: Health Management Publications; 1990.

85. Wroblewski JJ. Nutritional aspects of pressure ulcer care. In: Krasner D, ed. *Chronic Wound Care.* King of Prussia, PA: Health Management Publications; 1990:188–193.

86. Berlowitz D, Wilking S. The short term outcome of pressure sores. *J Am Geriatr Soc.* 1990;38:748–752.

87. Hill DP, Cooper DM, Robson MC. Serum albumin is a poor prognostic factor for pressure ulcer healing in controlled clinical trials. *Wounds.* 1994;6(5):174–178.

88. Stotts N. Nutritional parameters at hospital admission as predictors of pressure ulcer development in elective surgery. *J Parenter Enter Nutr.* 1987;11:298–301.

89. Olson B. The effects of massage for prevention of pressure ulcers. *Decubitus.* 1989;2(4):32–37.

90. Franz RA, Gardner S. Clinical concerns: management of dry skin. *Gerontol Nurs.* 1994;20(9):15–18, 45.

91. Gosnell DJ. Assessment and evaluation of pressure sores. *Nurs Clin North Am.* 1987;22:399–416.

92. Brown DS, Sears M. Perineal dermatitis: A conceptual framework. *Ostomy/Wound Manage.* 1993;39(7):20–25.

93. Brown DS. Perineal dermatitis: Can we measure it? *Ostomy/Wound Manage.* 1993;39(7):28–31.

94. Schnelle JF, Adamson GM, Cruise PA, et al. Skin disorders and moisture in incontinent nursing home residents: Intervention implications. *Journal of American Geriatrics Society.* 1997;45(10):1182–1188.

95. Gray M. Assessment of patients with urinary incontinence. In: Doughty D, ed. *Urinary and Fecal Incontinence: Nursing Management.* St. Louis, MO: Mosby-Year Book; 1992:47–94.

96. Urinary Incontinence Guideline Panel. *Urinary Incontinence in Adults: Clinical Practice Guidelines.* AHRQ Publication No. 92-0038. Rockville, MD: AHRQ, PHS, DHHS; March 1992.

97. Kane RL, Ouslander JG, Abrass IB, eds. Incontinence. In: *Essentials of Clinical Geriatrics.* 2nd ed. New York: McGraw-Hill; 1989:139–190.

98. Schnelle JF, Newman DR, Fogarty T. Management of patient continence in long-term care nursing facilities. *Gerontologist.* 1990;30:373–376.

99. Schnelle JF. Treatment of urinary incontinence in nursing home patients by prompted voiding. *J Am Geriatr Soc.* 1990;38:356–360.

100. Ouslander JG, Schnelle JF, Uman G, et al. Predictors of successful prompted voiding among incontinent nursing home residents. *JAMA.* 1995;273:1366–1370.

101. Willis I. The effects of prolonged water exposure on human skin. *J Invest Dermatol.* 1973;60:166–171.

102. Jeter KF. The use of incontinence products. In: Jeter KF, Faller N, Norton C, eds. *Nursing for Continence.* Philadelphia: W.B. Saunders Company; 1990:209–220.

SUGGESTED READING

Bryant RA, ed. *Acute and Chronic Wounds: Nursing Management.* 2nd ed. St. Louis: MO: Mosby; 1999.

Jeter JF, Faller N, Norton C, eds. *Nursing for Continence.* Philadelphia: WB Saunders; 1990:223–240.

Krasner D, Rodeheaver GT, Sibbald RG, eds. *Chronic Wound Care: A Clinical Source Book for Healthcare Professionals*, 3rd ed. Wayne, PA: HMP Communications; 2001.

National Pressure Ulcer Advisory Panel. In: Cuddigan J, Ayello AE, Sussman C, eds. *Pressure Ulcers in Ameica: Prevalence, Incidence, and Implications.* Reston, VA: NPUAP; 2001.

CHAPTER 16

Management of Pressure by Therapeutic Positioning

Laurie M. Rappl

CHAPTER OBJECTIVES

At the completion of this chapter, the reader will be able to:

1. Cite the effects of proper positioning on all systems of the body.
2. Initiate and complete an examination of a patient in sitting and recumbent positions.
3. Prescribe the best positioning options in both sitting and recumbent environments.
4. Evaluate seating and mattress or support surface products for their benefits to patient treatment.

INTRODUCTION

Therapeutic positioning is a dynamic and necessary part of the wound care management program of any person. Without properly positioning a person in bed or in a sitting position, skin management programs can be devastated by inappropriately high carrying loads on improper bony prominences. Persons who become sitting-dependent more than ambulatory, and/or who use the lying down or the sitting position for the majority of the day are at high risk of skin breakdown. Also, for the patient with an existing pressure ulcer, proper positioning in the most active and functional position possible, both in sitting and in recumbent positions, will improve the healing rate of the ulcer and help to minimize the likelihood of recurrence.

Advances in equipment to meet seating needs has, of necessity, elevated therapeutic positioning to a specialty within the therapist and technology supplier ranks. The specialty is as complex as the numbers of people it services, and it is beyond the scope of this chapter to cover all seating/positioning topics thoroughly. Information provided presents (1) an overview of the areas that the clinician should examine to determine the need for intervention, (2) the basics of therapeutic positioning, (3) how therapeutic positioning affects body system impairments, and (4) some specifics in positioning the patient with an existing ulcer, both sitting and lying down. Just as pressure ulcers cross all ages, from pediatrics to young adults to middle aged and older adults, so does the need for therapeutic positioning become appropriate for all age groups.

Although incidence rates of ulcers on specific bony prominences vary, it is conservative to estimate that 50% of all skin breakdown occurs on the sacrum and the ischial tuberosities,[1,2] the major weight-bearing surfaces of the sitting-dependent person. Sacral wounds are most often associated with lying down, whereas ischial ulcers are caused by sitting.[3] It has also been estimated that 75% of the sitting-dependent population will experience the development of pressure ulcers. Of these, 75% will have a recurrence of that same breakdown.[4–6] Recent literature reports failure rates for flap surgeries of 76–91%.[4,5] In addition, it is standard procedure for the plastic surgeon to plan for five more donor sites for flaps on a patient before doing the first one! This confirms what is already known: Treating the symptom does not effect a cure. Therapeutic positioning, using correctly chosen equipment, plays a direct and critical role in reducing these staggering numbers.

The human body requires support for proper balance, both in the sitting position and in recumbent positions. Any person who depends on the sitting position for any part of the day or night should be evaluated to ensure that the optimal position is being attained. The more sitting dependent the person is, the more acute is the need for proper positioning interventions. However, although the full-time wheelchair user is often thought of as the only candidate for therapeutic positioning, the part-time user and the able-bodied who may sit for only relatively short periods of time each day are also candidates. Both full-time and part-time wheelchair users must be evaluated for appropriate support surfaces and positioning in recumbent postures.

THE DIAGNOSTIC PROCESS APPLIED TO THERAPEUTIC POSITIONING

The diagnostic process outlined in Chapter 1 begins with the reason for referral. The clinician should obtain a history of the patient before examination to determine the systems to review. The review of systems will determine the evaluations needed and will dictate the examination strategy. The clinician then collates the information gathered to determine a functional diagnosis that will guide selection of the equipment and positioning interventions required. A prognosis and predicted outcome complete the process.

History

The reason for referral will give the clinician the first clue to the positioning needs. The reason the family, the caregiver, or the person seeks positioning assistance will usually translate into the main goal for positioning, a goal that cannot be subordinate to the clinician's. The goal of the caregiver may be comfort in recumbent positions for an uncommunicative patient, whereas the clinician may want to pursue a more aggressive program to reverse contractures. The clinician's goal may be appropriate, but if the caregiver cannot devote the time or the financial resources to an aggressive program, the clinician may have to consider less aggressive positioning goals.

The medical history is significant for any past surgeries or conditions that would limit the ability of the patient to achieve the "ideal" position or that may need accommodation to help the person maintain that position. Note any conditions that are progressive, such as multiple sclerosis, that would necessitate equipment that can be changed with the changing needs of the patient as the disease progresses and skills decrease. Conversely, conditions may improve with therapeutic positioning intervention, such as a decrease in abnormal muscle tone and a corresponding increase in postural muscle tone; this will also require modification to the seating intervention to match the patient's improvement. Orthopaedic interventions that have been performed and affect normal joint movement or the normal functioning of the skeletal system are of special note. For example, spinal fixation may limit range of motion in the trunk and pelvis and may necessitate equipment that does not force the body to sit in level planes but will accommodate and support a tilted pelvis or curved back posture.

The living situation and the person's level of independence will indicate the level of involvement that the equipment can have. For example, a person in a solid, supportive home environment with a limited number of consistent caregivers may be able to handle more involved equipment than may someone in a group living situation with multiple caregivers. The number of hours spent sitting or lying down will allude to the risk of breakdown; generally, increased time in sitting or lying down equates to higher risk of breakdown and more care in equipment selection and training.

Systems Review

Too often, the wound management program fails to encompass system impairments leading to pressure ulcers, instead focusing on the support surface on the bed and on the direct treatment of the wound through dressings and modalities that affect microcirculation. Impairments to be managed occur in the neuromuscular system, the musculoskeletal system, the cardiopulmonary and vascular systems, the integumentary system, and the psychosocial/cognitive system. Many impairments in all of these systems can be managed by therapeutic positioning in the bed or the chair. Some of these system impairments have been called the *hazards of immobility* and are well known; many, such as respiratory involvement, contractures, slowing of the digestive system, and cognitive changes, will be discussed in the following sections. Therapeutic positioning is a powerful modality to effect changes in treatment programs involving all systems.

Neuromuscular System

Impairment of the central or peripheral nervous system will have profound effects on the development of pressure ulcers. If sensation is diminished, the bony prominences in the insensate areas of the body will have an undue susceptibility to pressure ulceration, especially those that will be weight bearing. Equipment selection and positioning must protect and unweight the skin over bony prominences in the impaired areas as much as possible. In sitting, these are the ischials, sacrum, and coccyx. It is well known that bed rest often leads to breakdown on several bony prominences, including heels, malleoli (ankles), and trochanters (hips). The choice of support surface and instruction in proper recumbent positioning are critical in protecting the insensate patient, especially one with poor self-repositioning abilities.

If there is an insult to the central nervous system, such as a stroke, brain injury, or spinal cord injury, or disease of the central nervous system, there may be a lack of reflex integrity or loss of motor control. A lack of reflex integrity will cause uncontrolled muscular movement patterns, such as posturing or spasticity. A high level of spasticity or a loss of motor control requires equipment that offers more support to the body, because the equipment will give the person the ability to maintain a position. For example, excessive tone in extension will cause the hips to extend out of the ideal 90° position, and the hips will slide forward on the seat. Spasticity, with its uncontrolled, repetitive movements through specific ranges, causes shearing, a major factor in skin breakdown. If not inhibited with appropriate therapeutic positioning in the chair and the bed, spasticity can lead to the development of irreversible muscle and joint contractures. The equipment must support the body in reflex-inhibiting postures (neutral or flexion for extension tone, neutral or extension for flexion tone) to control involuntary movements and the development of contractures. With degenerative diseases of the central nervous system, such as multiple sclerosis, the clinician must select equipment that can be modified as the disease progresses and that can be altered to provide more support.

Musculoskeletal System

The musculoskeletal system is responsible for motor function—strength, ergonomics, and activities of daily living (ADLs). Impairment of the musculoskeletal system, such as fixed or flexible contractures, limitations in range of motion and joint integrity, and skeletal deformities, change strength and ability to perform ADLs. A loss of motor function or muscle strength, revealed in a manual muscle test and ergonomics or mobility assessment, will impair the person's ability to self-position and to maintain correct postures. Incorrect postures are unsafe for skin and will lead to breakdown and deformities, unless accommodated for through positioning. The equipment may again be required to be more supportive than for a person with more intact motor abilities. The degree and location of muscular weakness will also have an impact on the choice of mobility base (wheelchair, scooter, recliner chair, etc.), because powered bases may be required for higher needs, or hemiheight chairs may be required for those who propel with their feet. A firm support surface that enhances mobility may be necessary to assist the person with musculoskeletal impairment in independent repositioning and, thus, enhances the safety of the skin.

The more ADLs that must be done sitting or lying down, the more positioning may be required to ensure proper body function and skin safety. For example, if the person eats in bed or in the mobility base, the positioning system must support safe swallowing. Impairments in range of motion and joint integrity will directly affect the ability of the body to maintain the ideal position and can result in the body's carrying uneven pressures, resulting in skin breakdown. For example, the person who cannot reach 90° of hip flexion will sacral sit and cause excessive pressures on the coccyx and the spinous processes. Equipment must accommodate for the limitations in range by supporting the body at the angle available at the hip with a reclining back and a supportive cushion and/or an angled seat. The person who has had a cerebrovascular accident that resulted in one side of the body having more strength than the other will tend to sit unevenly, thus overweighting one ischium and putting skin in that location at high risk.

When considering skeletal deformities, consider both those induced by trauma (accident) and those induced by surgery (purposeful) and whether they are fixed or flexible. The deformity's effect on achieving the ideal position is the overriding concern. A common example of a purposeful skeletal deformity is a unilateral ischiectomy, resulting in a flexible asymmetric pelvis and scoliosis. The ischiectomy causes the pelvis to sit unevenly on a cushion that works by weighting the ischials and can lead to scoliosis or to skin breakdown on the sitting surface of the lower side, ie, the remaining ischium. A cushion that does not depend on ischial weight bearing, but rather on femoral weight bearing, will accommodate this patient better, because the cushion will not cause the pelvis to sit unevenly, despite the surgical procedure.

A flexible deformity is an impairment that can be corrected by the proper equipment, as described above. A fixed deformity, however, is a disability that must be accommodated by the equipment. Rather than attempting to correct a fixed deformity, the equipment must conform to the deformity and help to hold it in a position as close to proper as possible.

Evaluation or reevaluation for seating needs must be done when significant weight loss is noted. Significant weight loss can make bony prominences that were once fairly protected much more vulnerable to the effects of pressure and shear.

Cardiopulmonary and Vascular Systems

Impairments in the cardiopulmonary and vascular systems directly affect the ability of the blood to carry oxygen and nutrients to the integumentary system. Medical diagnoses such as chronic obstructive pulmonary disease, emphysema, cardiomyopathy, arteriosclerotic vascular disease, and hypertension indicate impairment in these systems and in their ability to deliver oxygen to the tissues, increasing risk of ischemia and pressure ulceration to areas subject to compression of tissues by bony prominences. Therapeutic positioning of those areas of the body affected by the above diagnoses is of paramount importance in helping to avoid skin breakdown in the patient with impairments in these systems.

Inactivity and extended bed rest have several negative effects on these systems. Blood flow will be reduced throughout the body and, therefore, to any wound sites. Decreased total blood volume and decreased hemoglobin concentration, increased resting heart rate, and decreased maximum oxygen consumption (VO_{2max}) have also been documented. Immobility promotes fluid stasis in the kidneys, which can lead to kidney stones and infection.[7] Nutrition intake can be impaired, because the recumbent and inactive positions reduce the appetite. Recumbence inhibits safe swallowing and facilitates aspiration of food, leading to pneumonia. Swallowing occurs 24 hours per day, not just at mealtime. The correct head and neck positions conducive to safe swallowing should be identified and attained in the chair and the bed; consultation with a speech/language pathologist may be necessary for success in this area.

Oxygenation of the blood may be impaired if the person carries any of the cardiopulmonary diagnoses. Proper upright positioning allows greater diaphragmatic expansion, improves breathing patterns and depth (thus improving oxygenation of the blood), and mobilizes pulmonary secretions.[8] Upright positioning in a functional and comfortable position will improve general circulation by placing the patient in a position that encourages activity and movement. Cardiac function is also improved in the upright position. Upright positioning with pressure eliminated on the bony prominences will improve circulation to the ulcer site by gravity, which pulls blood down to the ulcer site.

Clinical Wisdom: *Is Prone Positioning Best?*

It has been suggested that, for the sitting-dependent person with breakdown on the sitting surfaces, the prone position with the wound uppermost actually inhibits circulation to the wound site by assisting blood to flow, as a liquid will, away from the highest point.

Integumentary System

Skin is more susceptible to breakdown if it is dry, flaky, friable, aged, insensate, prone to excessive sweating, or subjected to incontinence, friction, or shear. Positioning can affect the integumentary system by protecting the skin over bony prominences on weight-bearing surfaces, through correct use of the proper equipment to maintain safe postures and to unweight those bony prominences. For some people, an equalization of pressure is sufficient to protect skin from breakdown. For others, complete removal of pressure may be needed for protection, because their combination of risk factors makes them highly susceptible. For example, the skin over the coccyx is prone to breakdown because of the shape of the bone, lack of padding over the coccyx, and frequent use as a weight-bearing surface. Equipment that takes pressure off the coccyx in sitting, used correctly, can help to avoid or treat this breakdown.

Persons who had pelvic irradiation prior to 1980 are at very high risk for skin breakdown over the sacrum, coccyx, and buttocks areas, due to the skin changes that the irradiation used at that time incited.

Psychosocial/Cognitive System

Often overlooked but well known are the hazards of immobility as related to the psychosocial/cognitive system. Extended bed rest or loss of mobility leads to cognitive dysfunction. The recumbent position induces lethargy and inactivity. Often, a patient who refuses to follow prescribed treatments, including extended bed rest, is labeled "noncompliant." In many cases, however, he or she may simply be issuing a cry for help in changing the wound management program because, for the sitting-dependent person, bed rest is a sentence akin to imprisonment.

The patient with impaired cognitive abilities may be unsafe in self-mobility or in the ability to maintain safe postures independently. The equipment for someone with cognitive impairments will probably need to be more supportive than that for one with full abilities to reposition or to ask for assistance in maintaining safe postures. Cognitive and psychologic impairments are definitely affected by inactivity and poor positioning.

Summary

Wound management must be an interdisciplinary team effort. The total wound management program is a combination of the therapist's evaluation of the prominences, the body position, and body movement, along with evaluations by other clinicians with information on medications (eg, steroids), medical status, other health-related conditions (such as diabetes, cancer, and immunosuppressive disorders), nutrition, blood levels of serum albumin and protein, habits that increase risk (such as smoking), choices of clothing that negatively affect skin, excessive sweating, bed mobility, and incontinence.

FUNCTIONAL DIAGNOSTIC PROCESS

The clinician reviews the medical history and systems, then decides on the appropriate examination strategy for the patient. After the examinations are performed and the data collected, the information is reviewed and evaluated. The result of the evaluation is the functional diagnosis. The functional diagnosis will be based on the following:

- The impairments found in the examination that prevent the client from achieving the ideal position, either sitting or lying down
- Identification of the client's preferred position(s)
- Identification of the client's alternative position(s)
- Specific interventions in the form of equipment choices and proper use of that equipment

Tables 16–1 and 16–2 list examples of medical and functional diagnoses relating to need for therapeutic positioning, the prognosis, related interventions, and expected functional outcomes for the sitting-impaired and for the recumbent-impaired client.

Based on the functional diagnosis, the clinician will establish a prognosis and select interventions, with a targeted outcome for each intervention. Interventions include analysis of the most effective forms of equipment required, selection of appropriate equipment to achieve correct therapeutic position, analysis of the patient using the selected equipment, and education of patient and caregivers in correct use. Therapeutic exercise often is another important component of the total therapy plan of care.

RATIONALE FOR INTERVENTION IN THE SITTING POSITION

Sitting can be seen as either the cause of skin breakdown or as part of the solution. In a proactive environment, with an educated clinician with access to the right equipment and armed with techniques in therapeutic positioning, sitting can and should be a part of the healing of skin breakdown and part of a prevention program that can improve the quality of life for the person; it can also decrease medical costs over the course of time.

When the sitting skeleton is viewed from the side, it is apparent that the ischial tuberosities (ITs) extend approximately 1.5 inches past the femurs, making the ITs the major weight-bearing points on the sitting surface. The skin over these points is also the most vulnerable to skin breakdown because of their conical shape and poor natural padding. As a person becomes more sitting dependent, atrophy causes the minimal natural padding to deteriorate, making that person even more vulnerable to skin breakdown. The ITs are the fulcrum, or pivot, points for the pelvis and, when bearing weight, cause the pelvis to rock about a horizontal axis through the frontal plane that leads to anterior or posterior pelvic tilt. Most often, people tend to sit in a posterior tilt, or a slouched position. The act of moving into the slouch causes shearing forces on the ITs, and sacral sitting leads to the formation of pressure ulcers on the sacrum and coccyx, as well.

The goal in seating a client is to help maintain a position that is as close to ideal as possible. Orthopaedic or neurologic limitations may prevent achievement of the ideal position as a realistic goal, but it is the benchmark position.

Ideal is the position that the body should be in to be anatomically aligned for muscle balance, to achieve proper alignment of the bones and joints according to their design, and to take advantage of the most load-tolerant areas of the body in handling pressure to keep the skin safe from breakdown. In the ideal position, viewed from the side, the client should have a 90° angle at the hip, knee, and ankle. The ear should be in line with the acromion process and the hip, and the foot should be positioned under the knee. The thigh should be parallel to the ground so that the hip and knee are in line with each other. The spine should be supported in its natural curves in the cervical, thoracic, and lumbar regions. The face should be vertical (see Figure 16–1). Viewed from the front, the trunk and head should be comfortably upright with shoulders and hips (pelvic crests) level, the thighs in neutral (not internally or externally rotated), feet pointed straight ahead, and arms supported so that the shoulders are not elevated or depressed when the elbows are resting on the armrests. Dignity issues clearly indicate the need for women to be positioned with their legs together, rather than separated.

Sitting Posture Examination and Evaluation

Knowing the ideal position, the clinician then evaluates the patient to determine how closely the patient can come to achieving the ideal position comfortably, what prevents the patient from attaining that position, and what equipment interventions can assist the patient in maintaining a position as close to ideal as is possible or functional.

Neuromuscular System

Reflex Integrity Examination. Nonintegrated primitive reflexes influence seating when central nervous system disorders make them more apparent than in the intact nervous system. One example of the influence of a primitive reflex on function and positioning involves the asymmetric tonic neck reflex (ATNR). This reflex causes the person to extend on the face side when the head is rotated. This can cause the person driving a side-mounted joystick to have difficulty controlling the device. A center-mounted joystick may solve this problem. The symmetric tonic neck reflex (STNR) is influenced by head position; the STNR must be accommodated for by limiting the movement of the head so that voluntary control of the body is maintained. Extensor thrust is evident when the ball of the foot is stimulated and causes extension throughout the body. Limiting contact with the ball of the foot on the foot pedal will help to relax extensor tone and to maintain an upright position. Hypertonicity, spasticity, and athetoid movements all demand stabilization of the body so that extraneous or involuntary movements will be minimized, and the person has some freedom to express voluntary movements.

Sensory Examination. The ability to detect both light and deep pressure must be assessed on all areas of the body that will be weight bearing or that may come in contact with equipment. The inability to detect pain or pressure may lead to skin breakdown. If the person is insensate in the skin over

Table 16–1 Functional Diagnositic—Sitting Position

Medical Diagnosis— Functional Diagnosis	Prognosis	Intervention	Outcome
Kyphosis—Patient cannot maintain 90° hip flexion and keep face vertical due to thoracic kyphosis.	Patient will sit upright with face vertical and as close to 90° hip flexion as possible.	Reclining backrest with stabilizing seat cushion. May need antitippers.	Patient able to sit stabilized as close to 90° back/seat angle as possible with face vertical.
Scoliosis (fixed)—Patient cannot sit with shoulders and hips level due to fixed asymmetric spine or pelvis.	Patient will maintain sitting position with shoulders and hips as level as possible.	Cushion with buildup under higher ischium to accommodate asymmetry; back support to assist in comfortable trunk positioning.	Patient able to maintain upright sitting with shoulders and hips as close to level as possible.
Scoliosis (flexible)—Patient does not but can sit with shoulders and hips level.	Patient will maintain sitting position with level shoulders and hips without strain.	Cushion with pressure elimination at ischials and full femur support or cushion with buildup under lower ischium to raise that side of pelvis.	Patient able to maintain upright sitting with shoulders and hips level and spine straight.
<90° Hip flexion—Patient cannot sit at optimal 90° seat/back angle for maximal functional abilities and mobility.	Patient will maintain correct sitting position with hips on back of seat.	Positioning cushion to stabilize pelvis, with reclining backrest. Reclining angle approximates maximum hip flexion allowed by range of motion limitations.	Patient will maintain upright sitting as close to 90° as is allowed by range limitations.
<90° Knee flexion available—Patient unable to reach standard foot pedals for support.	Provide equipment that supports lower extremity at available range so that patient can maintain proper sitting position.	Elevating leg rest with full calf and foot support, set at full allowed knee flexion.	Patient will maintain upright sitting with hips on back of seat and lower extremities maintained at allowed knee flexion.
Foot propeller—Patient requires use of feet to mobilize chair; unable to reach floor to propel.	Provide equipment that allows efficient heelstrike on the floor.	Hemiheight chair with cushion or drop seat with cushion, so that total seat to floor height is 2 inches less than back of knee to floor measurement.	Patient will be self-mobile via foot propulsion while maintaining proper seating posture.
One-arm driver—Patient can use only one arm for self-mobility.	Provide equipment designed for propulsion with one arm.	One-arm-drive wheelchair.	Patient will be self-mobile using one arm while maintaining proper seating posture.
Above the knee amputee—Patient has limited femur length to support body weight; difficult to maintain posture in sitting; may lead to skin breakdown on ischials due to increased weight on ischials.	Provide firm flat support for femurs, and protection for ischials.	Stabilizing seat cushion; amputee adapters to move rear wheel axle backward from normal position; antitippers.	Patient will maintain upright sitting with full protection of ischials and full femur support.

continues

Table 16–1 continued

Medical Diagnosis—Functional Diagnosis	Prognosis	Intervention	Outcome
Skin breakdown on sitting surfaces (ischials, sacrum, or coccyx)—Patient cannot sit without pressure eliminated at ulcer site.	Pressure elimination on ulcer while maintaining correct postural alignment.	Cushion with selective pressure elimination.	Patient will maintain sitting schedule with pressure elimination provided at the site of breakdown.
Asymmetric tonic neck reflex (ATNR) influence—Patient has difficulty controlling direction with side-mounted joystick when head moves.	Change placement of joystick to decrease influence of ATNR.	Position joystick in center of lap tray.	Patient will drive safely and in control despite movement of head.
Hip fracture—Patient cannot sit with full 90° hip flexion; may lead to skin breakdown due to coccyx weight bearing.	Provide seating arrangement that allows <90° hip flexion with skin protection.	Seat cushion that provides ischial/coccyx pressure reduction or elimination with positioning and can be customized with unilateral sloping to accommodate the lack of hip flexion on the involved side; reclining backrest with sacral protection; solid seat beneath cushion—may require cutout in board.	Patient will maintain upright sitting with maximum allowed hip flexion and no pressure on coccyx.
Trunk/hip extensor tone—Patient cannot maintain hips in proper position on seat due to uncontrolled hip extension; may lead to skin breakdown due to shearing.	Provide seating arrangement that decreases tone and helps maintain as close to 90° hip flexion as possible; antithrust seat assembly with preischial block.	Increase trunk/lower extremity angle past 90°; firm contoured back support; 90° positioning belt.	Patient will maintain proper seated posture with hips on back of seat and trunk upright.

Source: Copyright © Laurie Rappl.

the sitting surfaces, he or she will not know when to shift weight to relieve undue pressure. For the insensate person, great care must be taken to search for and prescribe equipment that not only positions the body but also protects insensate skin (see the section on seat cushion categories).

Musculoskeletal System

Motor Function and Ergonomics Examination. Note how dependent or independent the patient is in self-mobility and what means is easiest for him or her to use. This will determine the mobility base (wheelchair, recliner chair, scooter, etc.) that is prescribed. If the patient does not have the physical, cognitive, or visual perceptive abilities to be safely independently mobile, a total support chair, such as a recliner Geri-chair or recliner wheelchair, may be needed; either one may require additional support devices, such as a commercially available seat and back. If the patient has the cognitive and perceptive skills but not the physical skills, then a powered base, either a power wheelchair or a scooter style, is chosen. If the person can self-propel, the therapist has a choice of a variety of manual chairs, depending on the body parts being used for mobility. The patient who needs one or both feet to propel will require a hemiheight wheelchair, one with a lower-than-standard seat-to-floor height so that the person can contact the ground firmly with the foot without having to scoot the pelvis forward on the chair. The most efficient foot propulsion can be accomplished if the patient can achieve a heel-toe pattern in forward propulsion.

Table 16–2 Functional Diagnostic Process—Recumbent Position

Functional Diagnosis	Prognosis	Intervention	Outcome
Cardiorespiratory or gastrointestinal compromise requiring elevation of the head of the bed.	Patient will assume Fowler's position with proper positioning and skin protection devices to protect heels and sacrum.	Hip aligned at gatch of bed; sacrum protected by lifting under one hip with pillow or foam support; heel protection devices employed; frequent turning/repositioning schedule. Do not substitute elevated head of bed for upright sitting in a supportive chair.	Patient will tolerate head of bed elevated while maintaining safe postures with support devices.
Less than full hip or knee extension allowed due to joint integrity impairment at the knees. Undue susceptibility to pressure ulcers due to potential exposure of heel and sacrum.	Patient will assume supine position with foam support devices in place to accommodate hip/knee flexion requirements, and with protection of occiput, heels, and sacrum.	Foam positioning devices to protect occiput and heels, and to elevate lower extremities to accommodate flexion contractures. One side of pelvis elevated slightly with towel roll or foam to protect sacrum.	Patient will maintain supine position with support devices correctly placed.
Influence of the asymmetric tonic neck reflex (ATNR) causes involuntary movements into trunk extension, and inability to maintain sidelying position.	Patient will be positioned with strong side down and trunk and upper limbs fully supported. Or patient will be positioned with strong side up, body fully supported along full trunk, and the bed situated so that patient is not required to turn the face up to view the room.	Position with stronger side down and trunk fully supported from shoulder to pelvis. Bed is placed so that need for cervical movement is minimized, ie, against far wall, facing door of the room.	30° foam wedge fully supporting trunk, pelvis, shoulders, and uppermost arm and leg supported away from midline in abduction; head supported in midline in both frontal and sagittal planes.
Venous ulcers on lower extremity with edema.	Patient will maintain supine or sidelying positions with lower extremity elevated above midline to reduce swelling, and with ulcer pressure free.	Foam device to support leg above the level of the heart in supine position and in 30° sidelying position.	Patient will maintain safe postures with limb elevated and sacrum protected.

Source: Copyright © Laurie Rappl.

Foot propulsion can cause shearing forces on the skin over the ischials as the person pulls the body forward with the leg. The patient who can propel with only one arm will need a one-arm-drive chair. The patient who will use both arms is a candidate for a standard height wheelchair.

Shear and Friction Examination. While evaluating mobility capabilities, the clinician should pay attention to the quality of those capabilities and assess them for the possibilities of friction and shear. These two causative factors in skin breakdown can become evident during propulsion or when postural changes happen while the patient is seated. Friction and shearing would be evidenced by irregular reddened areas on the weight-bearing surfaces. Proper equipment and positioning can limit trunk and pelvic movement to limit both friction and shearing.

Activities of Daily Living Examination. The more functional activities done in the wheelchair, such as dressing, bathing, eating, and toileting, the more the equipment will

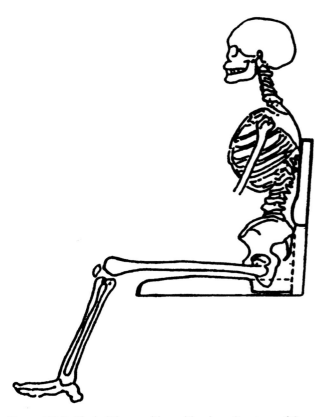

Figure 16–1 Ideal sitting position, side view. Courtesy of Span-America Medical Systems, Greenville, South Carolina.

have to accommodate beyond simple positioning. Waterproof materials will assist in toileting, and noncontoured seating may assist the caregivers in placing the person in many different positions to pull clothing on and off and to bathe the various body parts. Transfers, or the methods used to get the person into and out of the chair, are an important factor in determining seating equipment. Assess for the possibility of shear and friction during the transfer. Try to minimize the number of extra devices, such as abductors and adductors. These tend to get in the way of independent transfers and are cumbersome for the caregivers in dependent transfers.

Clinical Wisdom: *Transfer Technique*

Poor transfer technique is a major contributor to skin breakdown, because the skin is dragged across surfaces or is subjected to sudden overload when the person is set down suddenly.

Range of Motion and Joint Integrity Examination. The spinal curves should be in proper alignment; a fixed, exag-

gerated thoracic kyphosis will limit the person's ability to keep the face vertical. If hip flexion of 90° cannot be attained, the person cannot be accommodated in a chair with a 90° seat/back angle; the back will have to be reclined, and the seat cushion should provide enough pelvic stability to keep the hips from sliding forward. A seat that tilts up in the front may be helpful. If knee flexion is fixed at less than 90° from straight, or more than 90° from straight, the legs will have a tendency to pull the body forward from the back of the seat and out of position. Footrests that support the foot and allow the hip and knee to maintain as close to 90° as possible will be helpful in positioning the lower body.

Stabilizing the pelvis is critical to correct positioning. The pelvis must be evaluated in all planes of movement. The anterior/posterior rotation is assessed from the side. The anterior superior iliac spines (ASIS) should be roughly level with the posterior superior iliac spines (PSIS). A posterior tilt where the PSIS are lower than the ASIS will flatten the lumbar spine, decrease hip flexion from 90°, and cause the body to attain a "slouched" position. An anterior tilt will throw the body forward, making it difficult to attain upright sitting with arms free. A tilt to left or right in the frontal plane is termed a *pelvic obliquity*. This obliquity must be defined as *fixed* or *flexible*. To do this examination, place the person on a firm seat with knees at 90° and feet supported. Note whether one iliac crest is higher than the other, and note the presence of a lateral curvature of the trunk, both with and without upper extremity support. Place a support under the ischium on the lower side of the pelvis to even the iliac crests. If the trunk curvature remains and the person becomes more unstable when the arms are raised, the obliquity is fixed and should be accommodated for by building up the cushion under the opposite ischium. If the trunk curvature decreases and the person is more stable, the obliquity is flexible and can be accommodated for in one of two ways: (1) by putting the person on a firm cushion with both ischials unsupported and both femurs fully supported and at the same height, inducing a level pelvis or (2) by building up the cushion under the lower, supported ischium to even the iliac crests. Pelvic rotation, a twist about a vertical axis, is noted if one iliac crest sits forward of the other.

Limitations in ankle dorsiflexion or plantarflexion or inversion/eversion will affect the support of the lower extremity on the foot pedal. If the ankle cannot be maintained in a neutral (right angle) position with 0° of inversion/eversion, a foot pedal that can change angulation will be needed to accommodate the position of the foot as closely to ideal as possible.

Limitations in the upper extremities are also important to note. A flaccid upper extremity can affect mobility, because that arm will not be useful for propulsion. A flaccid, unsupported arm can also affect positioning, potentially causing the body to sag toward the flaccid side and inducing excessive pressures on that side of the sitting surface. Reflex-inhibiting postures, such as support in elbow flexion and shoulder protraction to break up severe extensor tone, will help the client maintain a forward upright posture.

Skeletal Deformities Examination. Note any limitations in the range of motion that would affect the person's ability to sit upright easily. As previously discussed regarding the pelvis, these problems should be assigned a *fixed*, ie, immovable, or *flexible*, ie, movable or correctable, designation; fixed problems will need to be accommodated for as a disability, whereas flexible problems should be noted as places where the right equipment or positioning can help to correct an impairment.

Integumentary Examination

The clinician must evaluate the status of all skin on the weight-bearing surfaces. The quality of the skin—dry, inelastic, friable, thin—must be noted. Use the bony prominences as anatomic locations under skin to see signs of impairment, eg, change in color (red, blue, purple) from adjacent continuity of skin color. Also record the anatomic locations of each area of breakdown and include the size, date of occurrence, stage, history, and current plan of care of each. Note areas of previous breakdown and any previous surgeries to repair skin, because these areas are at high risk of reopening and must be protected at all costs.

Even if they have not experienced breakdown, any bony prominences on weight-bearing surfaces may be at risk, and palpation will reveal those at highest risk by showing which ones are most prominent, least protected, and bearing the most weight. Muscle atrophy or significant loss of body weight will make the ischium more prominent than usual and may make protection from breakdown a primary need in the selection of seat cushions.

Interface Pressure Examination

With the advent of sophisticated mapping devices that determine interface pressures, many facilities and clinicians are using these measurements as the major factor in determining seat selection. Although pressure is one of the factors that cause breakdown, it is only one of several. The clinician should consider shearing, friction, heat/moisture buildup, and sitting instability as equally important, even though they are more difficult to measure than interface pressure. The clinician must use interface pressure measurements carefully and be sure to look at the total picture of the patient and the equipment.

Pressure measurements can be taken with single-cell, hand-held devices or larger, multiple-cell, computerized mapping devices. The hand-held, single-cell monitors are more portable and less expensive, but the single cell has a tendency to move during the inflation/deflation cycle. It also gives the reading over one small area, when the peak pressure may be somewhere far removed from the placement of the cell. The multiple-cell device gives a better overall picture of the pressures on the entire seating surface simultaneously and prints those pressures out in numeric or pictorial form on a computer screen. These larger, computerized mapping devices are much more expensive and less portable but they are valuable, in that the entire sitting surface is read at the same time, rather than just a single site.

Single-cell meters operate in one of two ways: inflate-placement-deflate-read or deflate-placement-inflate-read. Accurate readings depend heavily on proper placement of the cell under the bony prominence while the person is sitting upright and stable. After taking the first reading, most clinicians will then remove the cell, replace it, and repeat the reading two times to get at least three readings per bony prominence. Some manufacturers recommend taking three readings and averaging the results. Make sure that the cell is not wrinkled during use; that the sitting surface is up to manufacturer's directions for inflation or support, placement on the chair, and support of extra pieces, such as a solid base, a cover, or abductor/adductor/obliquity wedges; and that the sitting surface is smooth and free of wrinkles and excessive layers of padding.

In a recent study conducted by the University of Pittsburgh, higher interface pressures were directly associated with a higher incidence of pressure ulcers on the sitting surfaces of the body.[9] The goal of pressure reading is to find out the location and the value of peak pressures on a particular client on a particular cushion. High pressures on the most vulnerable prominences (ischial, coccyx, sites of previous or current breakdown) may indicate that cushion and client are not an appropriate match. It is preferred that the areas of highest risk (ie, ischials and coccyx) record lower pressures than those at lower risk, such as the femurs; the femurs are load tolerant, can support the majority of the weight, and can, therefore, tolerate higher pressures than can the vulnerable ischials and coccyx.

Intervention Using the Principles of Seating

Therapeutic positioning[10–16] requires skill in evaluation and interpretation of the client's needs and in the matching of equipment to client. This has traditionally been considered the realm of physical therapy and/or occupational therapy; indeed, many physical therapists (PTs) and occupational therapists (OTs) are highly skilled in therapeutic positioning, and there are seating clinics staffed by therapists with a high level of specialization in positioning all ranges of client involvement. Unfortunately, many clinicians and patients do not have ready access to the skilled intervention of knowledgeable PTs and/or OTs. However, proper seating and positioning must be attended to by all clinicians or caregivers involved in health care, and the knowledge and application of the basic principles of seating will benefit the majority of patients. These basic principles of proper positioning can be learned and applied in the home setting, as well as to the nursing home and rehabilitation facility, by all knowledgeable and willing clinical staff.

Clinical Wisdom: *Basic Seating Principles*

The basic seating principles include the following:

- Level cushion and seat upholstery to keep thighs horizontal to the ground; knees and hips even.
- Feet are supported so that the knees are even with the hips.
- Back is supported so that natural spinal curves are maintained; ideally, the ear, shoulder, and hip should be in alignment.
- When the pelvis is properly positioned on the seat, the seat cushion ends 1½ inches from the back of the knee.

The clinician or caregiver should also identify when the basic seating principles will not or cannot help the patient, when equipment will have to accommodate a position that varies from these basic principles as stated in the text, and when referral to a skilled outside source is necessary.

Pelvic Control

Pelvic control is the cornerstone of seating. If the pelvis rolls out of position, the entire sitting posture will be difficult to control. Most seat products control the pelvis by putting some pressure on the most unstable aspect, the ischials, and attempting to control pelvic movement by padding all around the ischials. Others eliminate this unstable point as the control point and use the proximal femurs to control the pelvis. Any chosen cushion requires the assistance of a back support. The top of the back of the pelvis must be supported with the back support so that it cannot rock backward. The back support also fills in the lumbar curve for more supported and comfortable sitting and relieves stresses related to back pain by improving the seating ergonomics.

Thigh Control

Thighs should be parallel to the ground. The seat should be flat, with the hips and knees horizontally aligned. If the knees are lower than the hips, the weight of the legs pulls the body forward and pulls the pelvis into the posterior pelvic tilt that the clinician is trying so hard to avoid, and the patient slouches. This is the position most commonly seen in settings where generic chairs are used, and the footrests

are lengthened as much as possible or have been lost. Conversely, if the knees are higher than the hips, as in the use of a wedge cushion, the lumbar lordosis is lost; the proximal femur, along with the sacrum, coccyx, and ischials, bear an inordinate amount of weight; and the patient is put at high risk of skin breakdown and back pain. These wedge type cushions are typically used in an attempt to keep the person from sliding out of the seat. Wedge cushions cause a number of problems, however, indicating that they should be prescribed with extreme caution, rather than as a general-issue device. These problems can include skin breakdown on the sacrum and spine, due to excessive body weight being forced on those prominences, discomfort in a flexed lumbar spine, difficulties in transferring, and loss of mobility and ADL skills.

Seat Depth

The seat depth, or the length of the seat cushion from backrest to front edge of the seat upholstery, should be about 1½–2 inches shorter than the distance from the seat back to the back of the knee. Seats with less depth than this do not take advantage of the weight bearing or the support that the posterior femur can give; with greater depth than this, the seat will pull the body forward on the chair and out of position. Many people in fleet or institution chairs are sitting on very short seat depths and, therefore, have a tendency to slide about on their chairs and slide out of position. Large recliner-style chairs have seat depths that are too deep, causing pressure on the lower legs and pulling the body forward on the seat.

Footrest

The footrest should support the leg so that the thigh is parallel to the ground. If the footrest is too high, the weight is unevenly distributed across the femur; if it is too low, the weight of the leg pulls the body out of position. To keep the thighs parallel to the ground, simply adjust the foot support or provide a footstool or other support under the feet. Care should be taken to ensure that the individual wears the appropriate supportive footwear to protect the feet from trauma, to evenly distribute pressures across the entire foot, and to assist in decreasing dependent fluid buildup in the feet.

Clinical Wisdom: *Simple Tools*

A simple toolbox is a necessity and a relatively inexpensive investment when working with seating equipment. This should include a variety of screwdrivers, wrenches, and a lubrication agent. For example, a simple wrench is usually all that is needed to change the height of a footrest so that the footrest plate is the proper height for full foot support.

Wheelchair Measurement

Proper wheelchair seating requires that the seat/back angle accommodate the person as close to upright 90° as the person's body will allow. Proper measurements for a wheelchair include seat depth, as described above, back height from seat cushion to the point on the back that gives needed support without hindering function, width from hip to hip and shoulder to shoulder kept as close as is comfortable so that the overall chair is as small as possible, and foot support placed so that the knee is even with the hip. This foot support will be the floor-to-seat height in hemistyle chairs or footrest selection and setting in a manual or power-propelled chair. Measurements must include the cushion when measuring the backrest height, seat to floor, and footrest length (see Figure 16–2).

To choose equipment, match the needs of the client with the features of a product. The client's needs will be assessed in the evaluation; the features of the product are assessed with clinical skills, analytical skills, and common sense. Don't rely strictly on history or manufacturer's claims to determine what products to use; predetermine what features the product should have to fulfill the patient's needs before assessing the benefits of that product for the person.

Wheelchairs or Mobility Bases

The major piece of equipment in seating, the one carrying the highest price tag and acting as the basis for the rest of the seating system, is the chair, sometimes referred to as the *mobility base*. Figure 16–3 is an algorithm to guide the clinician through the decision-making process to determine mobility needs.

The appropriate mobility base must be determined along with the seating system. It is often impossible to make any seating system, even the appropriate one for the patient, work on an inappropriate seating base. For example, many people mobilize their chair by propelling with their feet. If the wheelchair seat is too high to allow the foot to reach the ground, all seat cushions will put the person even higher and further reduce the mobility of the patient. "Quick fixes," such as a drop seat, are often only fair compromises, at best. In the same way, using a seating system on a base for which it is not designed will compromise the effect of the system. Reclining geriatric or Geri-chairs offer little to no support and are not designed to accept most seating systems. However, sometimes these chairs are the only available alternative to bed rest; therefore, it is necessary to attempt to adapt this chair to fit the individual's needs by utilizing the appropri-

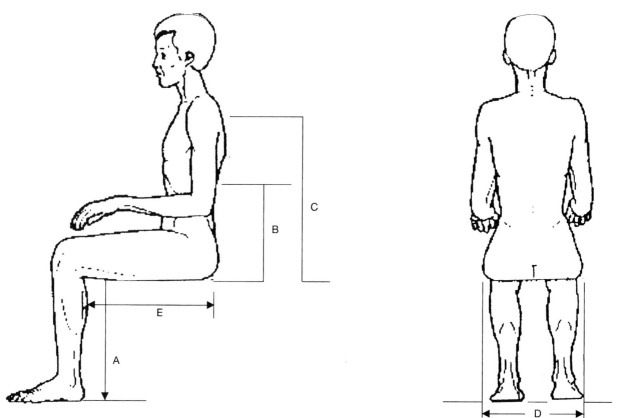

Figure 16–2 Measuring for a wheelchair. A = Seat to foot support height; B = seat to top of sacrum for placement of lumbar support; C = height of backrest needed for back support; D = seat width; E = seat depth, measured from backrest to popliteal fossa less 1.5 inches.

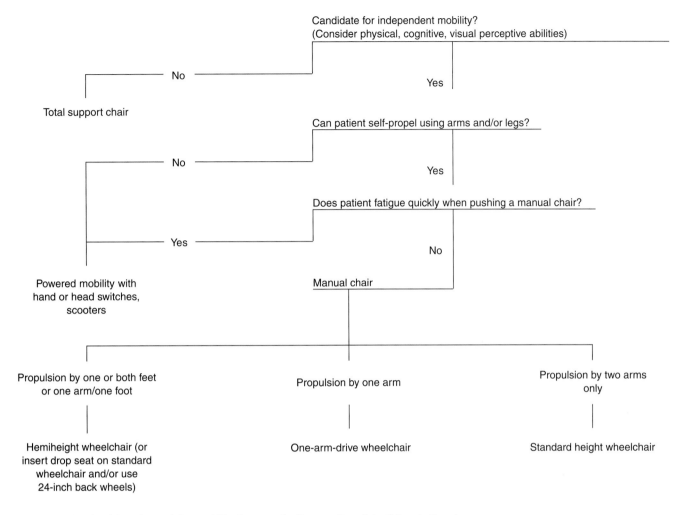

Figure 16–3 Algorithm: determining mobility base needs. *Source:* Copyright © Laurie Rappl.

ate back cushions, head supports, lateral trunk or hip guides, seat cushions, and lower extremity support.

The standard wheelchair—a folding frame style with adjustable or fixed armrests, a seat 18 inches wide by 16 inches deep, and elevating or adjustable footrests—is more for temporary transportation than for all-day every-day mobility and positioning usage. The vast majority of users require more support than these chairs can give. There is a multitude of variations on the standard theme:

- Hemiheight—The axle for the back wheel is fixed higher on the frame than standard, thereby lowering the height of the seat and allowing the user who foot propels to reach the floor with a heel-toe pattern, which is more functional and efficient.
- Sport or lightweight—These chairs are for the very active user who needs the lightest frame possible for transporting and for maximum mobility. They can also

assist the frail elderly to conserve energy and can have a significant impact on overall endurance for activities of daily living.

- Rigid—This is a nonfolding frame style for the very active user; it is less prone to breaking and loosening.
- Pediatric-sized—These chairs are for the child or the child-sized adult.
- Reclining back chairs—These are adjusted by manual releases, hydraulic releases, ratchet-style fixation, or power. The seat-to-back angle can be changed to accommodate the person who cannot attain upright sitting or who needs to recline for some time during the day but not necessarily out of the chair. Similarly, upholstered recliners, such as Geri-chairs or living room reclining chairs, allow the body to relax from upright. However, these chairs cause many positioning problems.
- Power chairs—These are available in wheelchair style or as scooters.

Seat Cushions

Seat cushions are commonly considered to be the primary intervention in positioning the client.[17–19] Products should be evaluated on how they control several physical and physiologic factors that cause skin and seating problems. These factors are pressure, shear, heat and moisture buildup, and postural control and stability.

Pressure. Pressure causes ischemia or loss of circulation to the cells under pressure. Pressure is considered the major causative factor of skin breakdown on the sitting surfaces and has the greatest effect on bony prominences, where high forces are generated on small areas. Large, flat surfaces, such as the posterior femurs, seldom break down because they distribute forces over a larger area. It is generally acknowledged that the ischials can safely tolerate only one-third to one-half of the amount of pressure that the femurs can. Any cushion being considered for a patient must be assessed for its abilities to reduce pressure under the ischials. This can be done with either a pressure-mapping device or a single-

---

Clinical Wisdom: *Seat Cushions Are Not Mattresses in Miniature*

Understand that the seat cushion is not a mattress in miniature! Consider that a mattress has the advantage of the entire weight-bearing surface of the body over which to spread the load. There is more tissue in contact with the bed, so the goal of a mattress can be tissue support, that is, equalizing pressure across the bony prominences and plateaus such that pressures are not high enough to cause breakdown on any one point. Compare this with the seat cushion, which must bear 75% of the body weight on a small area, average size 18 × 16 inches. In seating, that body weight is concentrated on two prominences, the ischials, which are the lowermost skeletal points on the sitting surface. The ischials are small, pointed, and unprotected, and therefore less load tolerant than the large, flat, padded femurs. With this disparity in load tolerance in mind, it is imperative that the seat cushion be examined for the skeletal support it can provide to protect the skin over these at-risk areas, and shift the support to the load-tolerant areas. This is not equalization but load distribution consistent with tolerances. Equalizing the pressure over the sitting surface causes low-tolerance/high-risk prominences (the ischials) to bear the same weight as the high-tolerance/low-risk areas (the femurs). Skin management dictates that the ischials should bear less weight than the femurs, and should not bear any weight in the presence of skin breakdown or for those individuals who are identified as being at high risk for skin breakdown.

---

celled, hand-held pressure meter, as discussed, or by palpation. To palpate, the clinician places the seat cushion on the seat and positions the patient appropriately on the cushion. The clinician inserts a hand, palm up, between the bottom of the seat cushion and the upholstery of the chair, and under the ischium. There should be at least an inch of soft support material (eg, foam, gel, or rubber and air) between the ischium and the seat upholstery to give the skin protection from pressure. Also, beware that muscle tissue is affected by pressure before skin is. This is why pressure ulcers often show deep tissue destruction well before indications on the skin surface appear. "A little bit of breakdown" can be the tip of the iceberg.

Shear. Shear is the distortion force applied to the skin when bone movement pulls the skin one way and the surface pulls the skin the opposite way. The result is a weakening or tearing of the skin and capillaries. Not only does shearing magnify the effects of pressure and cause skin damage, but it also makes it even more difficult to keep dressings on ulcers in place. To address shear, the seat cushion either must eliminate one of the two opposing forces at work on the skin (ie, the force coming from the surface onto the pressure-sensitive prominences) or must provide inherent movement with significant amplitude in individual cells that can shift with the body and decrease drag on the skin.

Heat and Moisture. On cushions that depend on immersion to equalize pressure, sweat and heat are contained around the ischials. This buildup causes maceration of the skin, which puts the skin at even more risk of breaking down. In addition, sweat and heat loosen the adherents that keep dressings in place. Cotton or air-exchange covers help but cannot combat total contact around the ischium. A cushion should provide ventilation of the ischial area.

Postural Control and Stability. No product will help the patient fully if it does not address sitting stability and comfort. The patient must be supported in as close to an upright and aligned posture as possible. This will keep pressures on bony surfaces that can tolerate it (femurs) and off of surfaces that cannot (ischials, coccyx, sacrum, spinous processes). As has been stated throughout this chapter, it also makes the person as functional as possible and helps to prevent further complications, such as contractures and internal organ compression.

It is commonly held that the pelvis is the cornerstone of positioning; stabilizing the pelvis is the foundation for stabilizing the entire body. However, the bases of this cornerstone, the ischials, are also the most vulnerable areas for skin breakdown and the pivot points for pelvic rotation. Most cushions, in equalizing pressure across the sitting surface, maintain pressure on the ischials and address pelvic stability by padding all around the ischials. An alternative way to keep the pelvis in place is to stop the fulcrum action of the ischials by eliminating pressure on them. The pelvis can be stabilized by stabilization of the femurs, because they are intimately connected to the pelvis and provide a larger surface area for the cushion to control. The cushion must match the posterior surface of the femurs with firm, flat support, especially the proximal femur closest to the pelvis. Stabilizing here controls rotation of the entire femur and holds the pelvis on the back of the seat. Movement of the ischials and pelvis is contained within the elimination area (Figure 16–4).

Types of Cushions. Cushions can be divided into groups according to their features and abilities to meet various levels of patient need for both positioning and skin breakdown risk or treatment. Here, cushions have been divided into four groups: simple pressure reduction, generically contoured, selective pressure elimination, and fully customized contouring.

Simple pressure-reduction cushions decrease pressure on the ischials and coccyx (compared with no cushion at all) and attempt to equalize that pressure across the entire sitting surface. They usually do little to address shearing forces and may address heat/moisture via cover materials only. These cushions are for those at low risk for skin breakdown. Users may spend very little time sitting because they are partially ambulatory or may have sensation, the ability to shift weight, adequate nutrition, and skin integrity. There are many cushions in many price levels that satisfy these basic requirements. Most of these cushions are in the lower price levels, under $100. Some are priced very high but still give only basic protection. The clinician must assess the pressure-re-

lieving capabilities of the cushion without regard to price and balance the capabilities of the product with the cost and the acuity of the patient's needs.

Generically contoured cushions are shaped with a depression area under the ischials to assist with pelvic placement and troughing under the femurs to assist in neutral alignment or optimal lower extremity positioning. These cushions are more sophisticated than the simple cushions because they have some means of actively molding to the body to equalize pressure across the ischials and the femurs (air cells, gel or viscous fluids, viscoelastic foam, etc.) while offering contouring for body support. These products are for those who are at moderate risk for skin breakdown and/or for those who require more assistance with positioning than a noncontoured cushion can provide. Understand that the generic contour base is shaped to a muscled bottom, not to the atrophied bottoms of the sitting dependent, and so often do not hold the pelvis as securely as cushions more specifically contoured to fit individual bone structure. Many manufacturers have added the flexibility of providing optional components, such as abductors, adductors, or hip guides that can customize the cushion to control lower extremity positioning further.

A feasibility study recently published by the University of Pittsburgh compared the efficacy of these generically contoured cushions with simple foam slab cushions. Although no statistically significant differences were seen between the groups for pressure ulcer incidence, the generically contoured cushions were more effective in preventing ischial pressure ulcers.[9]

The third category, *selective pressure elimination*, is identified by an area that eliminates pressure on the ischials via a pocket that is sized to the user's ischial span—the mea-

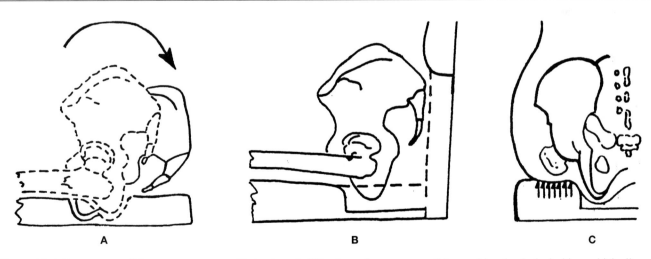

Figure 16–4 Pressure equalizing versus pressure eliminating. **A,** Side view of pressure equalizing cushion; loads the ischium which allows pelvic tilt. **B,** Side view of pressure eliminating cushion. Note pre-ischial bar limiting forward ischial movement. **C,** Rear view of pressure eliminating cushion. Note pressure distribution across full width of femur to support the load of the body. Courtesy of Span-America Medical Systems, Greenville, South Carolina.

surement from the center point of one ischium to the center point of the other. It also offers flat support to the full length and width of the posterior femurs, thereby supporting the body on the femurs, not in the elimination area (see Figure. 16–4B,C). This not only protects the skin over the ischials, but also protects the femurs by pressure distribution. Although appropriate for the moderate-risk patient as well, these products are often used for the highest-needs patients, who may be characterized by some of the following: sitting dependent; minimally ambulatory, if at all; insensate; may have limited abilities to reposition themselves to relieve pressure; have existing or recurrent breakdown on the bony prominences of the sitting surfaces (ischials, sacrum, or coccyx); are in the granulation or remodeling phases of wound healing; or have a history of skin breakdown on those sitting surfaces. Selective pressure elimination at the ischials, shearing elimination, and maximum ventilation puts the skin over the ischials in the healthiest possible environment. These requirements mirror and follow basic medical protocol for pressure ulcer treatment.[6,20–24] The benefits of this cushion design have been well documented.[10,16,19,25–31] This time-tested, fitted cushion design should never be confused with the donut design, which is specifically recommended against by the Agency for Health Care Research and Quality (AHRQ), formerly known as the Agency for Health Care Policy and Research (AHCPR), guidelines. Unlike a true selective pressure elimination cushion, which involves a full seating surface with a small relief area fitted to the user's bone structure, a donut cushion is simply a closed ring of material that cuts off circulation by inducing the tourniquet effect. In addition, the ring forces weight bearing on the area around the ischials, rather than on the femurs, the anatomically load-tolerant areas. For these reasons, the donut cushion should never be used, especially by persons at high risk for or with existing breakdown.

As with any sitting-dependent person, especially those with skin breakdown, maintenance of the properly seated position is essential to enhance function and endurance and to protect the skin under other areas of the sitting surface from breaking down. The pressure elimination cushion positions the pelvis in two ways. First, the ischials are unweighted and cannot act as pivot points for pelvic rotation. Second, the body is controlled by fully supporting the femurs (both length and width) in a nonrotated position and one such that they are even with each other in the horizontal plane. This keeps the pelvis and the trunk level (rather than obliquely inclined), keeps the pelvis toward the back of the seat, and prevents the pelvis from falling into the cutout area. Third, the walls of the elimination area confine movement of the pelvis to a defined area and keep the ischials from sliding forward with an effective preischial block. As with any cushion, the top of the back of the pelvis must also be supported with a back support so that it cannot rock backward. The

back support also fills in the lumbar curve for more supported and comfortable sitting.

The fourth category, *fully customized contouring*, refers to one-of-a-kind cushions fashioned specifically for the individual client. These are usually prescribed for users with severe structural deformities that cannot be accommodated for by off-the-shelf products or for those with excessive trunk and lower extremity tone that pulls them out of other products.

Other features to consider when evaluating cushions include urine-proof surface, stability of the sitting surface, cleanability, weight for portability, leak-proof surface, low maintenance, easy to use correctly, cosmesis, durability, and slip resistance. A representative listing of manufacturing sources for the categories of seat cushion products discussed is found at the end of this chapter.

The algorithm in Figure 16–5 may help the clinician to categorize seat cushion choices. A pictorial comparison of cushions that equalize pressure versus those that eliminate ischial pressure is shown in Figure 16–4.

Back Supports

A seat cushion is a key part, but only a part, of the seating system. To support a body adequately, the proper back support must also be prescribed. Most wheelchairs have a material back that allows the chair to fold. Unfortunately, this material bows in the opposite direction that the back requires. Therefore, almost every patient sitting in a standard folding wheelchair will require some accessory back support as a means of accommodating the lumbar and thoracic curves. The complexity and expense of the back support depends on the needs of the client and the number of roles that the back support must fill. The algorithm shown in Figure 16–6 may help the clinician to categorize equipment when choosing a back support for a patient.

Skin breakdown on the sacrum will be one deciding factor in selecting a back support. Skin breakdown will require that the back support remove pressure from and ventilate the area. Postural support in an upright sitting position may require support on natural spinal curves, accommodation for fixed deformities, or correction of flexible deformities. None of these needs can be overlooked when positioning a patient with sacral skin breakdown in sitting. Look for a commercially available device that is designed to meet all of these goals for the patient.

The patient who can maintain the upright ideal position with little or no assistance may require only minimal back support, perhaps a firm, contoured back that can be slid into the chair with attachment to the upholstery.

If the lumbar spine is flattened and hip range of motion is compromised so that it is less than 90°, a chair fixed at a 90° seat/back angle is inappropriate. This combination of physical factors, often found in the older adult population, can be

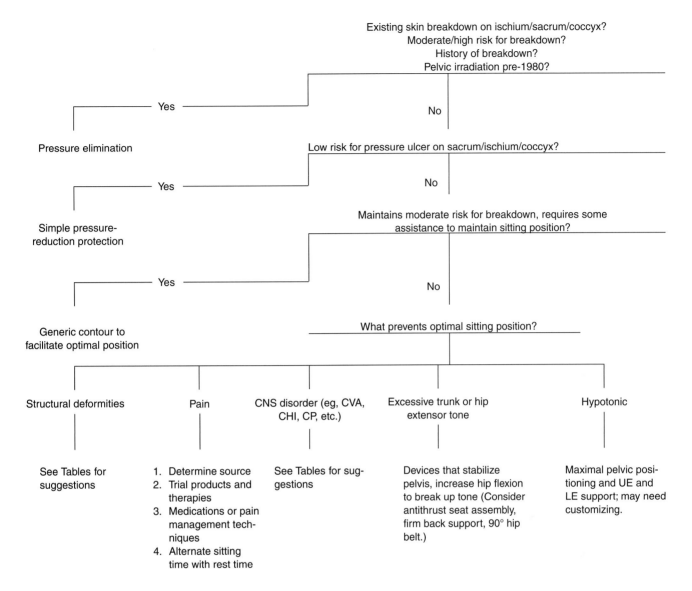

Figure 16–5 Algorithm: determining sitting surface. The surface must work with the mobility base to achieve optimal sitting height. CNS = central nervous system; CHI = closed head injury; CP = cerebral palsy; UE = upper extremity; LE = lower extremity. *Source:* Copyright © Laurie Rappl.

accommodated by a reclining backrest with adjustments to the degree of recline. This allows the patient to be positioned with the hips all of the way back on the seat for full support and the back to be supported at the appropriate degree of recline to facilitate safe swallowing, maximum mobility, and maximum function for the patient.

Those patients who have little inherent trunk support abilities will benefit from back supports that have the flexibility of lateral supports to help maintain the trunk in an upright position. Back supports can also be fully customized to fit the unique contours of an individual. These would be indicated for the patient with fixed trunk deformities or severe trunk weakness. Flexible thoracic or lumbar kyphosis or scoliosis can be handled by correcting the position of the pelvis and possibly using lateral supports on the trunk.

Accessories

The seat, back, and mobility base are the three key elements in a seating system. Many patients require the extra assistance of accessory products that include the following.

Head Supports. Head supports come in a variety of models, depending on the amount of support needed and the ability of the backrest to support the headrest. Models in-

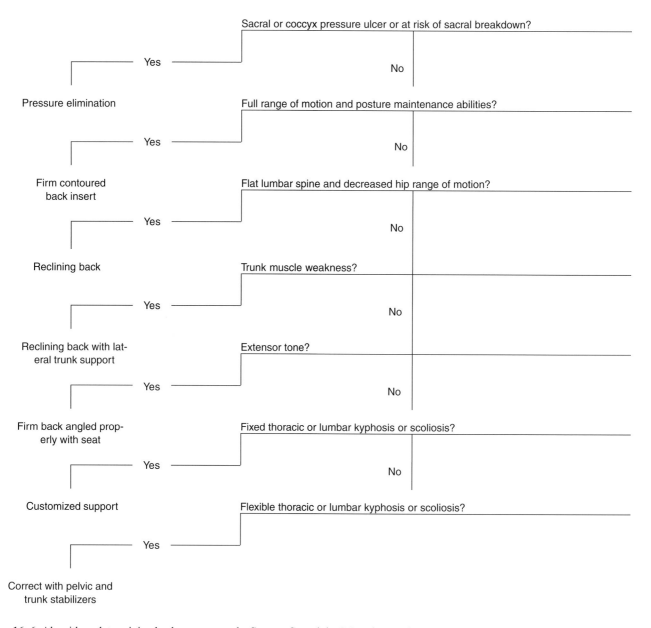

Figure 16–6 Algorithm: determining back support needs. *Source:* Copyright © Laurie Rappl.

clude flat (attached to the seat back uprights of manually reclining chairs), molded around the neck and occipital regions, adjustable in height and angle, and fixed.

Seat Cushion. Seat cushions have already been discussed. When cushions are placed on sagged seat upholstery, many of the positioning effects are negated. The seat support can be stiffened by adding a solid seat or board to the chair or by adding a drop seat that drops the seat pan beneath the level of the seat rails and lowers the patient closer to the floor. Consider adding a cutout seatboard under the seat cushion both to eliminate the sling of the upholstery and to distrib-

ute interface pressure away from the ischial tuberosities. Be aware that, when a solid seat is added, this may increase the interface pressure over the ischial tuberosities if the cushion is inadequate in pressure distribution over time; in other words, if the cushion bottoms out, the ischial tuberosities will be pressing into a solid, unforgiving surface that could then contribute to the formation of a pressure ulcer.

Armrests. Armrests generally come in two styles: tubular with padding or standard with flat metal skirt guards. Either can be attached to the chair in a fixed position or can swing away or be removed for ease of transfers. Standard armrests come in full length, shortened desk length (allows the chair to be pulled up closer to a table or desk), and height adjustable to accommodate the needs of a wide range of patient heights.

Footrests. Footrests are critical pieces in the seating system. As a general rule, the footrests are adjusted so that the knee is even with the hip. Most footrests are adjustable in height, and some allow adjustment in the sagittal plane to change the angle of the ankle. The pedal or platform of the footrest can be ordered in various sizes to support as much of the foot as possible. Elevating-height footrests, although thought useful for edema, often act to pull the body out of position and extend the turning radius of the chair, thus limiting mobility. The elevation has little effect on edema, because the extremity must be positioned above the level of the heart for passive edema control.

Back Wheels. The back wheels of wheelchairs are usually 24 or 26 inches in diameter and come in a variety of widths. The major choice to make is whether to order solid or inflated tires and treaded or nontreaded tires. For everyday, general use, most people use an inflatable tire with moderate tread. There are now solid tires made with treads for those who do not want to deal with the possibility of flat tires. For mainly indoor use, consider a minimal tread. Hint: The height of the seat from the floor—a critical factor in the patient's mobility—can be affected by changing the diameter of the back wheel.

Front Wheels. The front wheels of the wheelchair (casters) come in almost as many varieties as the back wheels—solid or inflatable and in various widths and diameters. The standard caster is 8 inches in diameter, solid rubber, and minimally treaded, if at all. Sport-type chairs are often seen with casters as small as roller blade wheels for increased turning abilities. Outdoor chairs have more substantial casters with larger diameters and widths (and often treads).

Ancillary Devices. Ancillary devices include the following:

- Lap belts or seat belts—usually placed at a 45° angle to the seat/back angle but often more effective when secured to the seat side rail, a few inches in front of the seat/back junction and crossing the proximal femur at a 90° angle, just below the trunk/leg crease.
- Lap trays—full or partial, clear or solid, padded or nonpadded, assist with upper extremity support. These should not be used as a restraint but as an assist to daily living skills, including communication, for support to a flaccid arm or to help provide a point of stability for

hypertonic extremities. Lap trays can also provide trunk support for those who may fatigue over time.

- Antitippers—small wheels that attach to the back of the wheelchair to keep it from tipping over backward, usually used as a safety factor. In everyday life, tipping backward is a necessary ability to lift the front of the wheelchair over small bumps and curbs, and antitippers may limit mobility while providing safety for the patient.
- Amputee adapters—allow the rear wheels to be moved posterior to the seat back upright to keep the user safe from tipping over backward.
- Residual limb support—holds the residual limb of the below-the-knee amputee.
- Chest straps—provide anterior support for the chest and upper trunk.

Working with Suppliers

The supplier is an important resource on the wound care team. A good supplier will help the clinician to match equipment to individual needs. The supplier also should help the clinician to keep abreast of new technology and new items on the market. Do not work with a supplier who limits access to equipment by offering only one or two lines of chairs and seating equipment. Look for suppliers who carry multiple lines and are proactive in assisting with this critical part of patient care—equipment selection. Ultimate accountability for the decision making resides with the clinician working with the patient.

Self-Care Treatment Guidelines

The patient and his or her caregivers must be taught as much as possible about the equipment that has been prescribed, including why each piece was chosen, how to use it properly, from where it was ordered for warranty repair, and how to care for it. The patient may need to follow a weaning-on schedule because new equipment may sit the patient differently or put loads on the skin in patterns different from those of the old equipment. A sample of a weaning-on schedule is as follows:

Day 1: 1 hour in morning and afternoon; assess skin response after each session.

Day 2: 1.5 hours in morning and afternoon; assess skin response after each session.

Day 3: 2.0 hours in morning and afternoon; assess skin response after each session.

Increase the sitting time gradually until a full day of sitting is achieved.

Positioning in the seated position requires constant learning, creativity, and patience. It is up to the responsible clinician to begin and continue the learning process by evaluating new technology as it is developed, determining the client needs, assessing the features of new products, and matching needs with features to benefit clients optimally. Because seating is a dynamic process, a reassessment date should be set so that the therapist can monitor the fit and functioning of the equipment and modify it to match the patient's needs.

RATIONALE FOR INTERVENTION IN THE RECUMBENT POSITION

The average person spends about one-third of life in bed. The client who cannot maintain standing or sitting for normal hours spends increasing amounts of time recumbent. Just as with sitting, choosing the proper support surface and correctly positioning the person on the surface are necessary parts of humane treatment. The human body requires support for proper alignment in the recumbent positions. Technically, any person who depends on the recumbent position for any part of the day or night should be evaluated to ensure that the optimal positions are being attained. The more time spent in bed, the more need there is for positioning intervention. Certainly, the person who has a musculoskeletal or neurologic insult that limits self-mobility, limits sensation to detect the need for position change, and/or makes the bony prominences more prominent and, therefore, at higher risk of breakdown is an uncontested candidate for therapeutic positioning.[32–36]

Bed rest puts many bony prominences of the body at risk of skin breakdown—occiput, shoulders, elbows, trochanters, sacrum, heels, and malleoli—hence the proliferation of "support surfaces" to protect the body in this relatively dangerous but needed environment. Statistics show that the sacrum and the heels are the most likely areas to break down, with references reporting incidence rates of up to 48% and 14%,[1] respectively.

Bed rest causes slowed circulation throughout the body and reduces the functioning of the respiration and elimination systems, as well. Proper utilization of support surfaces, through both proper choice and correct and consistent positioning on the surface, can minimize contractures, minimize the effects of primitive reflexes released during central nervous system insult, affect the integrity of the skin, provide restful sleep, and maximize a person's independence in self-mobility.

Mattresses either equalize pressure by maximum distribution of pressure or alternately remove it from areas at even intervals. The clinician chooses the appropriate surface, determines the therapeutic positions for the patient, chooses the equipment to attain those positions, and instructs caregivers on use of the equipment.

Effects of Lying Down on Pressure Ulcer Formation

No matter how conforming the surface of the bed, when the many contours of the body are placed on a relatively flat bed, bony prominences are likely to endure high pressures and end up with skin breakdown. These prominences—the occiput, shoulder, elbow, lateral trochanter, sacrum/coccyx, fibular head, malleoli, and heels—must be protected when they are on the weight-bearing surface of the client. Supporting body parts so that the major joints are in positions of least stress and highest relaxation will decrease muscle stimulation and, therefore, reduce spasticity and the formation of joint contractures. As with seating, the goal in positioning in the recumbent positions is to help maintain a position that is as close to ideal for tissue load management and muscle relaxation as is possible for the individual client.

In supine position, the head and neck should be centered and the cervical and lumbar curves supported. The trunk should be aligned and straight. Anatomically, the resting position for the hips and knees is not fully extended or straight but bent or flexed 25–30°.[32] Maintaining this slight flexion can put increased pressure on the sacrum and the heels. Therefore, these prominences must be watched carefully and provided with extra protection if the surface itself is not adequate. This protection may take the form of lifting one side of the pelvis so that the sacrum is not directly weight bearing. The heels may be protected by placing a pillow under the calves or by using heel protection devices on the feet to unweight the heels (Figures 16–7A, B). Devices should be chosen that eliminate pressure from or completely unweight the heel, rather than simply putting a layer of padding under the heel.[37] The ankles should be maintained close to 90° (a right angle), and the lower extremities should be maintained in a neutral position, with the knees and toes pointing straight up to the ceiling and about shoulder width apart. Protection in the form of pressure-reducing surfaces or ancillary positioners may be required for the at-risk areas of the occiput, thoracic spinous processes, and elbows.

Many people consider sidelying to be turning the body so that it is at 90° from supine. However, this is documented to put the greater trochanter at tremendous risk of breakdown, and recent documentation advocates the use of a 30° incline, rather than a 90° incline. This position takes direct pressure off the pointed lateral trochanter and distributes weight across flatter areas of the posterolateral femur. In this position, the head and neck should be centrally aligned, with the cervical curve supported. Support will be needed behind the entire trunk and pelvis to maintain the 30° position (Figure 16–8). The uppermost leg tends to adduct and rest on the bed but should be elevated with pillows or with foam positioners, so that it is in a straight line with the trunk and maintained in a neutral rotation, with slight hip and knee flexion for comfort. The lowermost leg must be pro-

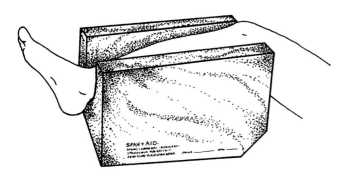

Figure 16–7 A, Limb elevator. Courtesy of Span-America Medical Systems, Greenville, South Carolina.

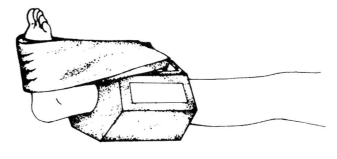

Figure 16–7 B, Footdrop stop. Courtesy of Span-America Medical Systems, Greenville, South Carolina.

tected from pressure from the uppermost leg, so that skin breakdown on the medial knee, malleolus, and foot can be avoided. Protection in the form of pressure-reducing surfaces or ancillary positioners may be required for the at-risk areas of the lowermost ear, shoulder, greater trochanter, lateral knee, lateral malleolus, and fifth metatarsal head, and the uppermost medial knee and medial malleolus. The uppermost arm must be given support as close to the neutral position of the shoulder (55° abduction with 30° horizontal adduction[32]) as can be achieved comfortably, so that it does not fall forward across the body or fall backward, pulling the trunk into a twisted position.

The prone position requires full range of motion of the cervical, thoracic, and lumbar spine and is not well tolerated by most patients. This position requires full extension at the hip and knee, and full external rotation of the shoulders. The trunk should be centrally aligned, with the head turned to the side. The hips should be in neutral rotation and slight abduction, and the ankles plantarflexed. The bony prominences at risk are the ears, patellas, and the dorsum of the feet. Not only does the prone position put the shoulder into its most stressful position of full external rotation with abduction, but it can also encourage footdrop, due to the ankle position.

Examination and Evaluation

As with seating, the clinician must have an understanding of what the optimal or ideal positions are. During the examination, the clinician determines what prevents the patient from attaining ideal, recognizes what may be improved with therapy or other interventions, and accommodates for those factors that cannot be improved upon.

Neuromuscular System

Reflex Integrity Examination. Nonintegrated, primitive reflexes, released after neurologic insult, greatly affect recumbent mobility and positioning. A dominant ATNR will make maintaining a sidelying position very difficult. The strengthening of the face side will cause the client to rotate backward and extend the uppermost leg and arm. The trunk and uppermost side will need to be firmly supported in flexion to overcome the extension tendencies. Approaching the client so that he or she does not have to turn the face over the uppermost shoulder will also help to combat this extension tendency. A dominant tonic labyrinthine reflex (TLR) will cause activation of flexion in prone and extension in

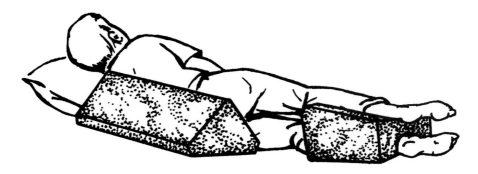

Figure 16–8 30° Wedge for body alignment in sidelying. Courtesy of Span-America Medical Systems, Greenville, South Carolina.

supine. The prone position will cause breathing difficulties, and would be contraindicated without extreme caution to head and neck position. In supine, the TLR and extension tone, in general, may increase the risk of breakdown on the occiput and the heels, and should be broken up with head/cervical support and flexion of the hips and lower extremities. In sidelying, the TLR causes extension on the weight-bearing side and flexion in the uppermost side; therefore, this is the preferred position for the client dominated by the TLR. Break up reflex postures as much as possible with support devices designed for controlling the body position. Usually, pillows are not stable enough to do this; an investment may have to be made in foam positioning aids specifically designed for certain positions and body parts. These may, on first glance, appear more expensive than pillows, but their effectiveness will outweigh cost (see Figures 16–7 and 16–8).

Sensory Examination. Neurologic insults often cause a lack of sensation in some part of the body. Those areas with loss of sensation are obviously at the highest risk of breakdown and will require the greatest care in positioning, support, and protection. Assess for the ability to detect both light and deep pressure and pain throughout the body, especially over the bony prominences. Those patients having a complete sensory, proprioceptive, and visual loss on one side of the body need attention to protect the involved limbs and to position for maximum environmental interaction. For example, position the individual so that he or she can visualize the entrance to the room with ease. This simple act will eliminate much fear and agitation. Caregivers should be instructed to approach from the noninvolved side first, then to move to the involved side as the patient learns to track to and beyond midline visually.

Musculoskeletal System

Motor Function and Ergonomics Examination. Assess for level of skill or assistance required to accomplish rolling right or left from supine, moving from sit to supine, supine to sit, sit to stand (exit from bed), stand to sit (enter into bed), moving body toward head of bed, moving body toward foot of bed, and shifting body side to side. Firmer, stable surfaces that do not move under the patient make bed mobility much easier to accomplish for all patients. Assess for the ability to perform transfers independently, dependently, or assisted in many combinations: bed to chair, chair to bed, commode to bed, bed to commode, sit to stand. The choice of support surface must directly and positively affect functional mobility to be considered a patient benefit and for eligibility for reimbursement of services and supplies. For the patient with skin breakdown, functional mobility occasionally may be compromised in favor of a less stable surface for improved tissue load management. Once the pressure ulcer is closed, a more stable support surface can be evaluated for both the

functional mobility of the patient on the surface and its efficiency in managing tissue loads.

Activities of Daily Living Examination. All ADLs done in bed, such as eating, bathing, and dressing, should be taken into account when determining the support surface and the recommended positions. Eating, especially, requires correct head elevation and cervical support for safe swallowing. The speech therapist should be consulted to determine the best head and neck positions for swallowing. This position may include aligning the ear over the acromioclavicular joint and the face in a vertical plane with the chest. Occupational therapy may be indicated to determine the upper extremity adaptations that can be utilized by the individual. Note that there are serious skin concerns in elevating the head of the bed for extended periods of time without protecting the sacrum or the heels. This position should not be used as a substitute for sitting in a chair properly positioned.

Range of Motion Examination. Note any surgeries that limit mobility or that limit placing the client in the ideal posture in a given position. These would include orthopaedic surgeries that immobilize part of the body and, therefore, limit overall mobility. Note limitations in range of motion in the cervical, thoracic, and lumbar spines, hip extension, hip rotation, knee extension, ankle rotation, and plantar/dorsiflexion. Whether limitations are fixed or flexible, the limitations must be firmly supported as close to anatomically correct as possible to minimize progression of deformities. It is most important to note where limitations affect positioning. For example, a progression in spinal kyphosis will make the supine position dangerous to the skin over thoracic spinous processes and the sacrum/coccyx. One possible solution to this problem is to elevate the head of the bed just enough to accommodate for the kyphosis and to support the head and neck, with or without the use of pillows. Gravity can then assist in at least maintaining the current degree of kyphosis without facilitating increased kyphosis. Consider managing tissue loads over the bony prominences with the effective use of support surfaces.

Another example of accommodation to limitations in range of motion deals with hip extension. Limitations in hip extension will necessitate support under the full lower extremity in supine to maintain the degree of hip extension allowed. This can be most easily accomplished with foam devices designed to position the leg (Figure 16–7A).

Integumentary System Examination

Pay special attention to surgeries and resulting incision or repair sites involving skin breakdown. Any area that has previously broken down or areas that have scar tissue are risk areas that require protection in the recumbent positions. All disciplines should note condition of the skin on weight-bearing surfaces—turgor, elasticity, hydration, edema, and thinness/brittleness. Note any sites with a past history of breakdown. Sites with current breakdown are obvious areas of primary concern in choosing surfaces and using therapeutic positioning. Where moist wound healing is being employed, the potential for low-air-loss or air-fluidized beds to dry out the wound should be considered. The patient should be positioned so that there is no weight bearing on areas of broken skin or on areas of scar tissue that are most vulnerable. If fecal or urinary incontinence is present, it is necessary to cleanse the skin with an appropriate acid-based (4.5–5.5 pH scale) skin cleanser and to protect the skin with a sealant. Be aware that every layer of incontinent liner that is used increases the interface pressure over that part of the body and inhibits the effectiveness of the support surface, both in bed and in the chair.

Interface pressure measurements taken with either a single-cell monitor or a bed-sized computerized model may be helpful in determining areas at risk and effectiveness of the chosen devices or positions. The procedure for performing interface pressure measurements is outlined in the seating section of this chapter. Record measurements at the bony prominences on the weight-bearing surfaces with body positioners in place in all of the positions that the patient will utilize. In sidelying, this includes the ear, shoulder, iliac crest, rib cage, trochanter, fibular head, lateral malleolus, fifth metatarsal, and first metatarsal of the uppermost foot. In supine, these include the occiput, scapulae, spinous processes, posterior iliac crest, rib cage, sacrum, coccyx, ischial tuberosities, and posterior heels. Assess pressures with the head both elevated and flat.

Cardiopulmonary/Gastrointestinal Systems

Involvement of the cardiopulmonary or gastrointestinal systems may require frequent position changes or may require elevation of the head of the bed. Note the reasons why the head of the bed must be elevated, to what degree, and for how long each day. Time in this position should be minimized; people tend to slide toward the foot of the bed when the head of the bed is elevated. This causes shearing forces on the skin, especially over the sacrum and the coccyx. Whenever the patient is in this position, line up the hip with the gatch angle of the bed to minimize sliding of the patient toward the foot of the bed. If this position is necessary for more than half an hour at a time, place a pillow or foam support under one femur, hip, and shoulder to tilt the patient slightly off the sacrum. Alternate the supported side at frequent and even time intervals. Provide support under the plantar surface of the feet, so that slipping down is minimized.

Assess for respiratory movements, level of breathing, and any oral secretions coming from the lungs. Take vital signs in the fully recumbent position and in the head-elevated position. Review the medical history for gastric reflux associated with hiatal hernias that require elevating the head of the bed. A patient taking oxygen probably cannot lie flat; extra care with positioning must be taken with these patients because of breathing difficulties and to ensure transport of oxygen to tissues.

Choosing Equipment

Many factors go into choosing bed support surfaces. Chapter 15 details some of the many positive and negative features of the various surfaces on the skin. Each of these categories also has positive and negative features for maintaining position and maximizing mobility.

Overlays. Whether powered alternating surfaces or contoured foam, all overlays raise the level of the bed surface. Sitting to standing is easier and safer to accomplish when the height of the surface of the bed is equal to the distance from popliteal fossa to the bottom of the foot. Overlays tend to raise this level, making ingress and egress more dangerous. However, overlays are inexpensive, and foam overlays with contoured, cross-cut cells (eg, Geo-Matt) are extremely effective pressure distributors. If the level of the height of the bed can be changed or if ingress or egress is not an issue, an overlay may be a cost-effective and appropriate choice.

Mattress Replacements. Most clinicians prefer a mattress replacement with a stable bolster edge for patient safety when sitting on the edge of the bed. A trapeze setup will help the patient to lift his or her body to move, rather than sliding across the surface. This helps to limit shearing forces.

Static Mattress Replacements. These come in a variety of mediums: all foam, foam/air, foam/water, and foam/gel. These surfaces replace standard mattresses and offer better distribution of pressures than the standard mattress. They eliminate the extra height that an overlay entails and are often purchased as permanent equipment for the patient, rather than as a rental item. However, they are more expensive than an overlay. Static surfaces generally offer a more stable surface to accomplish bed mobility and ingress or egress than do alternating pressure or low-air-loss mattresses.

Powered Dynamic Mattress Replacements. These entail some means of moving air through the mattress to float the body, as in a low-air-loss mattress, or moving air through chambers in the mattress to put pressure on and take pressure off of each area of the body alternately at regular intervals. The air movement is accomplished by electrically powered motors. Although some clinicians feel that these surfaces are safer for the skin than are static mattresses, due to the constant changes in pressure on any one body part, the movement in the surface makes maintaining or changing a position more of a challenge than on a static surface. Surfaces that alternate under the patient may make transfers more dangerous because the bed surface is constantly shifting beneath the patient.

Nonpowered Dynamic Mattress Replacements. A new breed of mattress (eg, PressureGuard CFT) offers the stability of the static mattress replacement for maintaining or changing position, along with the skin protection of a dynamic mattress. Dynamic air movement for self-adjustment to bony prominences is accomplished by elasticized reservoirs that accept air from and release air into the support tubes.

Air-Fluidized. Although felt to be the best surfaces for equalizing pressures across the whole body, air-fluidized surfaces are extremely difficult to maintain therapeutic positions on, and independent ingress or egress is nearly impossible; maximal assist is usually required.

Positioning Supplies

All patients will require the use of positioning devices to help maintain therapeutic and anatomic body alignment, and protection of bony prominences. Pillows are an inexpensive support but only minimally effective. They are puffy rectangles that do not naturally conform to body contours, have a tendency to slide on the surface when body pressure is applied, and are often not readily available for positioning if they have been confiscated for other purposes. Foam positioners are available that are shaped for supporting specific body contours, will not shift on the surface when pressure is applied, and will be less likely to be confiscated for other purposes. These devices are often inexpensive to purchase and more than pay for themselves in the quality of alignment, positioning, and protection they afford the patient. Table 16–3 describes the use and expected outcomes for commonly used and available positioning supplies.

Clinical Wisdom: *Photographs*

The use of photographs of the patient in position with the devices, displayed in a place easily seen by caregivers, is the most helpful way to describe positions and use of devices to all caregivers, so that devices are used consistently and appropriately.

Table 16–3 Positioning Supplies

Device	Function	Action/Outcome
Abduction pillow	Maintains lower extremities in slight abduction, neutral rotation, and knee extension.	Supine—maintains lower extremities (LEs) in neutral positions. Sidelying—maintains separation of LEs to protect medial knee and malleolus of upper leg.
30° Incline wedge (See Figure 16–8)	Supports trunk and pelvis in 30° sidelying position.	Sidelying—protects lower greater trochanter by maintaining 30° incline position.
Cradle Boot or Heel Protector	Keeps heel elevated off surface while maintaining right angle or neutral ankle dorsiflexion.	Supine—Protects heel from breakdown by suspending off surface. Should also protect malleoli, fifth metatarsal heads, and Achilles tendon. Sidelying—suspends lower malleoli and fifth metarsal head.

continues

Table 16–3 continued

Device	Function	Action/Outcome
Limb elevator (See Figure 16–7A)	Uses wedge with leg trough to put LE in slight hip/knee flexion with ankle elevated above knee.	Supine—maintains neutral hip position with slight hip/knee flexion and foot elevation. Sidelying—is used with trough side down to cup the lower leg and maintain leg separation for skin protection.
Flexion/abduction pillow	Maintains slight knee flexion with separation of medial knee surfaces.	Supine—maintains hip/knee flexion while breaking up adduction tone.
Cervical pillow	Is shaped to support cervical curve while cradling occiput.	Maintains cervical curve in supine or sidelying.
Occipital pillow, head-neck cushion, Occi-Dish	Cradles posterior surface of skull to reduce or eliminate pressure on occiput.	Supine—protects occiput by pressure removal, supports cervical curve, inhibits tonic lab reflex. Sidelying—protects lower ear and supports cervical curve.

Source: Copyright © Laurie Rappl.

Case Study: Therapeutic Positioning for Pressure Ulcer Healing

History

The patient is a longtime resident in a nursing facility. Past medical history includes surgical removal of a benign brain tumor 10 years prior to therapy intervention. She has paralysis of the lower extremities and significant cognitive deficits (see Figures 16–9A and 16–9B).

Reasons for Referral

- Right ischial tuberosity pressure ulcer, stage III, increasing in length, width, and depth
- Abnormal extensor tone in trunk and hip musculature with mild flexion contractures in knees
- Sitting in wheelchair for 6 hours, two times per day, for a total of 12 hours daily
- Dependence in position changes in bed and sitting
- Dependence in all transfers, requiring a two-person lift
- Dependence in all ADL (feeding, wheelchair propulsion, personal hygiene, dressing)

Examinations

Neuromuscular

Reflex exam shows severe trunk and hip extensor tone present in recumbent and sitting positions.

Musculoskeletal

Motor Exam. Trunk strength is poor, upper extremity strength is fair. The patient has no volitional movement in lower extremities.

Joint Mobility Exam. All joint ranges of motion are within functional limits with the exception of knee flexion contractures, which measure 20° bilaterally. There is a flexible right pelvic obliquity, 2 inches lower on the right than on the left.

Postural Exam. The patient prefers full fetal positions with flexion of all major joints in sidelying when recumbent; in supine recumbent position, head and neck are hyperextended into the pillow and extensor tone dominates all other major joints. In sitting, she demonstrates trunk, hip, and knee extension with pelvis sliding forward on the seat and into posterior tilt, and the cervical spine is in hyperextension.

ADL. The patient is unable to move or change positions volitionally in the bed or wheelchair. She is dependent in all transfers, requiring total assistance of two persons to transfer, and in feeding, personal hygiene, wheelchair propulsion, and dressing.

continues

Case Study: continued

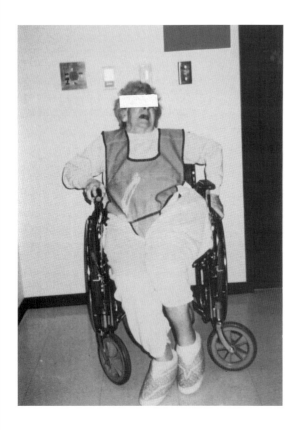

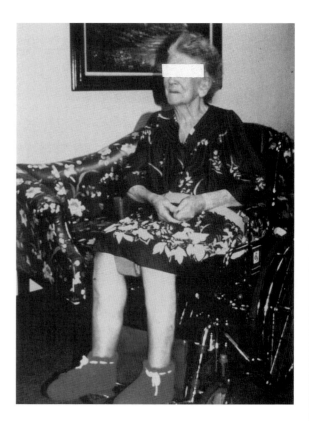

Figure 16–9 A, before. Note cervical and trunk hyperextension, pelvis/chest restraint, right pelvic obliquity, hips forward on seat, lower extremities unsupported. Courtesy of Debby Hagler, Cheyenne Mountain Rehabilitation.

Figure 16–9 B, after. Note that head and neck are in a safe and functional position, and lower extremities are supported. Courtesy of Debby Hagler, Cheyenne Mountain Rehabilitation.

Sensory

The patient is unable to detect deep or surface pressure on sitting surfaces and lower extremities.

Integumentary

The patient has a Braden Scale risk assessment score of 12. She presents with Stage III pressure ulcer on the right ischial tuberosity, measuring 3 cm × 3 cm × 1 cm deep. The pressure ulcer is 50% yellow slough and 50% granulation tissue. The surrounding skin is pale and the perimeter is macerated. Drainage is serosanguineous. No undermining or tunneling is present. Interface pressures over the sacrum, trochanter, heels, and shoulders in the supine and sidelying positions in bed were considered unsafe, as they ranged from 70 to greater than 100 mm Hg. Interface pressures over the right ischial tuberosity and the coccyx in the sitting position in the wheelchair were also considered unsafe, as they were greater than 100 mm Hg.

Evaluation

The patient has impairment of sensory, neuromuscular, and musculoskeletal systems, causing improper positioning and susceptibility to skin breakdown. There are impairments in musculoskeletal and neurologic systems that, in turn, affect the cardiopulmonary and circulatory

continues

Case Study: continued

system function to transport oxygenated blood to the wound site.

Functional Diagnosis

- There is functional impairment of volitional movement.
- There is functional impairment of reflex muscle tone resulting in dysfunctional body positions (postures) in sitting and in recumbent postures.
- The impairments of volitional movement and reflex muscle tone and dysfunctional body positions produce undue susceptibility to unsafe interface pressures on intolerant bony prominences: coccyx, ischial tuberosities, sacrum, heels, trochanter, and shoulders.
- The patient has risk factors of immobility, lack of sensation, joint integrity impairment of the knees, and abnormal extensor tone, which contribute to undue susceptibility to pressure ulceration.

Need for Physical Therapist Services

The patient needs intervention by a physical therapist to achieve the following goals:

1. Heal pressure ulcer
2. Correct impaired postural alignment
3. Position for redistribution of interface pressures from bony prominences to tolerant areas
4. Reduce risk of additional ulcerations

Prognosis

1. The ulcer will heal.
2. The risk of further pressure ulceration will be reduced by intervention with support surface and positioning equipment.
3. The patient will sit in a functional upright position in wheelchair with a 90° hip/back angle with a side-to-side wedged, pressure-eliminating seat cushion and a firm back cushion, with lower extremities supported and protected.
4. The sitting schedule will be 2 hours, three times per day for a total sitting time of 6 hours; the time up in the wheelchair will be coordinated with the meal schedule to facilitate safe swallowing and improved nutritional intake. Sitting time will be increased gradually according to a prescribed sitting schedule.
5. The patient will be positioned in functional positions in supine and 30° sidelying on a prescribed support surface in bed, with safe interface pressure readings on all bony prominences in all positions.

6. Staff will demonstrate correct use of all equipment supplied and in therapeutically positioning this patient at all times, whether in bed or in the wheelchair.

Intervention: Therapeutic Positioning

- Analysis of patient for selection of adaptive seating equipment requirements. The following are recommended:
  1. Side-to-side 5- to 3-inch, side-to-side, wedged seat assembly with full pressure-relief pocket at ischials and coccyx, sized to distribute pressure fully over posterior trochanter and thighs.
  2. Firm back support to maintain 85° seat/back angle to inhibit extensor tone.
  3. A 90° positioning hip belt to facilitate 90° hip angle and keep pelvis in appropriate position.
  4. Padded lap tray to provide upper extremity and trunk support.
  5. Footrests, calf support, and protective footwear to protect and support lower extremities and to facilitate appropriate positioning.
  6. Hip abduction wedge to inhibit adductor and extensor tone and to facilitate positioning and pressure distribution on the seat assembly.
- Analysis of patient using adaptive equipment for appropriateness and safety
- Analysis of patient for recumbent positioning and pressure-relief devices. The following are recommended:
  1. A self-adjusting, dynamic air/foam mattress replacement to encourage mobility and allow skin protection
  2. Positioning in 30° sidelying to distribute interface pressure away from the trochanter and shoulder
  3. Utilization of wedges and a pillow between the knees to maintain the sidelying position
  4. In supine, utilization of a leg-positioning cushion to inhibit hip extensor tone, to accommodate for the knee flexion contractures, and to position heels off the bed
  5. Utilization of a head-positioning cushion to provide occipital and cervical spine support and to inhibit cervical extensor tone in supine
  6. Utilization of an over-the-bed trapeze and side rails to assist patient in self-mobility
- Analysis of patient using recumbent positioning and pressure-relief devices for safety and proper pressure relief
- Staff instruction: Instruction in appropriate usage of all seating and bed-positioning supplies and equipment and in safe and effective position changes, transfers, and positioning in the bed and the wheelchair for two shifts of nursing personnel because of projected

continues

Case Study continued

sitting schedule of 2 hours, three times per day, coordinated with the meal schedule. Increased sitting time according to a prescribed schedule as the patient's strength, endurance for sitting, and tolerance improve over time.

- Follow-up assessment of staff for appropriate and safe use of devices and components of the devices

Functional Outcomes

1. The patient is able to sit in a functional and safe position for a total of 9 hours per 24-hour period (3 hours, three times per day).
2. Interface pressure is eliminated on the ischial tuberosities and coccyx, and the flexible right pelvic obliquity is corrected.
3. Posture is corrected: The extensor tone in the neck, trunk, and hips is inhibited, and the abdominal musculature and cervical flexors are facilitated and strengthened, facilitating wheelchair self-propulsion, and self-feeding.
4. The patient is positioned in a safe and functional position in bed on a nonpowered dynamic air/foam mattress replacement with safe interface pressure on all bony prominences in all positions; in sidelying, using a wedge cushion behind the back, a wedge cushion under the bottom leg, and a pillow between the knees, and in supine, using a leg-positioning cushion and a head-positioning cushion.
5. The patient is able to assist in repositioning self from side to side, using the trapeze and the side rails. No additional ulcers have developed, providing a reduced pressure risk score.
6. The pressure ulcer on the ischial tuberosity is healed.

Note: Case study and pictures provided by Debby Hagler, Cheyenne Mountain Rehabilitation.

REVIEW QUESTIONS

1. It has been noted that bed is the most dangerous place for a patient to be. Discuss the negative effects of prolonged bedrest, and the sites on the body most likely to break down from lying in bed.
2. Describe the best recumbent positions for patients with venous ulcers on the lower extremities.
3. Describe the ideal sitting position.
4. What are the five measurements that must be taken on the body when measuring a patient for a new wheelchair? Why are each of these important to the fit of the wheelchair?

RESOURCES

The following is a representative listing of manufacturing sources for the categories of seat cushion products discussed in the text. Some manufacturers have products in multiple categories.

Simple Pressure Reduction

AliMed
Ken McRight Supplies; Bye-bye Decubiti
Maddak
Skil-Care
Span-America Medical; Geo-Matt

Generic Contour

Cascade Designs; Varilite
Crown Therapeutics; Roho family
Flofit Medical; Flexseat
Invacare; PinDot
Jay Medical; Jay family
Span-America Medical; Geo-Matt Contour
Supracor

Selective Pressure Elimination

Span-America Medical; ISCH-DISH

Customized Contour

Freedom Designs
Invacare

SCI Clinical Practice Guidelines

Paralyzed Veterans of America

Wheelchair Seating Standards

International Standards Organization
Working Group–II

REFERENCES

1. Oot-Giromini B. Pressure ulcer prevalence, incidence and associated risk factors in the community. *Decubitus.* 1993;6(5):24–32.

2. Maklebust J, Sieggreen M. *Pressure Ulcers: Guidelines for Prevention and Nursing Management.* West Dundee, IL: S-N Publications; 1991.

3. Pompeo M, Baxter C. Sacral and ischial pressure ulcers: Evaluation, treatment, and differentiation. *Ostomy/Wound Manage.* 2000;46(1): 18–23.

4. Disa J, Carlton J, Goldberg N. Efficacy of operative care in pressure sore patients. *Plast Reconstr Surg.* 1992;89:272–278.

5. Evans G, Dufresene CR, Manson PN. Surgical correction of pressure ulcers in an urban center: Is it efficacious? *Adv Wound Care.* 1994;7(1):40–46.

6. Curtin I. Wound management care and cost: An overview. *Nurse Manage.* 1984;15(2):22.

7. Ross J, Dean E. Integrating physiological principles into the comprehensive management of cardiopulmonary dysfunction. *Phys Ther.* 1989;69:255–259.

8. Gerhart K, Weitzenkamp D, Charlifue S. The old get older: Changes over three years in aging SCI survivors. Report from Rehabilitation Research and Training Center on Aging with an SCI, Craig Hospital. *New Mobility.* June 1996;18–21.

9. Geyer M, et al. A randomized clinical trial to evaluate pressure reducing seat cushions for at-risk, elderly nursing home residents. *Adv Wound Care.* 2001;May/June.

10. Mooney V, Einbund MJ, Rogers JE, Stauffer ES. Comparison of pressure distribution qualities in seat cushions. *Bull Prosthet Res.* 1971;10(15):129–143.

11. Engstrom B. *Seating for Independence: Manual of Principles.* Waukesha, WI: ETAC USA; 1993.

12. Kreutz D. Seating and positioning for the newly injured. *Rehab Manage.* 1993;6:67–75.

13. Manser S, Boeker C. Seating considerations: Spinal cord injury. *PT Magazine.* December 1993;47–51.

14. Presperin J. Postural considerations for seating the person with spinal cord injury. In: *Proceedings from RESNA Seating Conference*; June 6–11, 1992; Vancouver, BC, Canada.

15. Walpin LA. Posture—The process of body use: Principles and determinants. In: Gelb H, ed. *New Concepts in Craniomandibular and Chronic Pain Management.* St. Louis, MO: Mosby-Year Book; 1994:13–76.

16. Zacharkow D. *Wheelchair Posture and Pressure Sores.* Springfield, IL: Charles C Thomas; 1984.

17. Rappl L. A conservative treatment for pressure ulcers. *Ostomy/Wound Manage.* 1993;39(6):46–48, 50–55.

18. Garber S. Wheelchair cushions for spinal cord injured individuals. *Am J Occup Ther.* 1985;39:722–725.

19. Ferguson-Pell M. Seat cushion selection. *J Rehabil Res Dev.* 1990;(Suppl 2):49–73.

20. Knight A. Medical management of pressure sores. *J Fam Pract.* 1988;27:95–100.

21. National Pressure Ulcer Advisory Panel. Pressure ulcers—Prevalence, cost, and risk assessment: Consensus development conference statement. *Decubitus.* 1989;2(2):24–28.

22. Noble PC. The prevention of pressure sores in persons with spinal cord injuries. In: *International Exchange of Information in Rehabilitation.* New York: World Rehabilitation Fund; 1981.

23. Stotts N. The physiology of wound healing. In: Stotts N, Cuzzell J, eds. *Proceedings from the AACCN National Teaching Institute.* Kansas City, MO: Marion Laboratories; 1988.

24. van Rijswijk L. Full thickness pressure ulcers: Patient wound healing characteristics. *Decubitus.* 1991;6(1):16–21.

25. Ferguson-Pell MW, Wilkie IC, Reswick JB, Barbenel JC. Pressure sore prevention for the wheelchair-bound spinal injury patient. *Paraplegia.* 1980;18:42–51.

26. Key AG, Manley MT. Pressure redistribution in wheelchair cushion for paraplegics: Its application and evaluation. *Paraplegia.* 1978–1979;16: 403–412.

27. Perkash I, O'Neill H, Politi-Meeks D, Beets CL. Development and evaluation of a universal contoured cushion. *Paraplegia.* 1984;22:358–365.

28. Peterson M, Adkins H. Measurement and redistribution of excessive pressures during wheelchair sitting. *Phys Ther.* 1982;62:990–994.

29. Reswick JB, Rogers JE. Experience at Rancho los Amigos Hospital with devices and techniques to prevent pressure sores. In: Kenedi RM, Cowden JM, Scales JT, eds. *Bedsore Biomechanics.* Baltimore: University Park Press; 1976:301–310.

30. Rogers J, Wilson L. Preventing recurrent tissue breakdowns after "pressure sore" closures. *Plast Reconstr Surg.* 1975;56:419–422.

31. Rappl L. Seating for skin and wound management. In: *Proceedings from Thirteenth International Seating Symposium.* Pittsburgh, PA: January 23–25, 1997.

32. Metzler D, Harr J. Positioning your patient properly. *Am J Nurs.* 1996;96:33–37.

33. Plautz R. Positioning can make the difference. *Nurs Homes Long Term Care Manage.* 1992;41:30–34.

34. Cantin JE. Proper positioning eliminates patient injury. *Today's OR Nurse.* 1989;11:18–21.

35. Kozier B. *Fundamentals of Nursing: Concepts, Process and Practice.* 4th ed. Redwood City, CA: Addison-Wesley Publishing; 1991.

36. Magee D. *Orthopedic Physical Assessment.* Philadelphia: WB Saunders; 1992.

37. Pinzur M, et al. Preventing heel ulcers: A comparison of prophylactic body-support systems. *Arch Phys Med Rehabil.* 1991;72:508–510.

CHAPTER 17

Diagnosis and Management of Vascular Ulcers

Carlos E. Donayre

CHAPTER OBJECTIVES

At the completion of this chapter, the reader will be able to:

1. Describe the vascular anatomy of the lower extremity and its relationship to peripheral vascular disease
2. Present signs and symptoms of peripheral vascular disease
3. Analyze ulcer risk factors for patients with arterial occlusive disease
4. Review the pathogenesis of diabetes and foot ulceration
5. Describe the pathophysiology of venous stasis ulcers
6. Provide information leading to differential diagnosis of venous stasis ulcers
7. Describe medical treatment and classification of venous stasis ulcers

INTRODUCTION

When one takes into consideration what feet routinely accomplish, it is not hard to see why they develop so many problems. A man of average weight (160–170 pounds) walks 7.5 miles on an average day. This requires that each foot carry more than 500 tons a day! Women's lighter bodies place fewer demands on the feet than do the usually heavier men's bodies, but fashionable footwear nullifies this weight advantage. High-heeled shoes put 75% more pressure on the balls of the feet than does going barefoot. The constant wear and tear that feet are submitted to daily takes its toll, and the older one gets, the more likely one is to develop foot problems. At one time or another, 85% of all Americans have foot problems serious enough to require professional atten-

tion. In nursing home patients, this figure rises to nearly 100%.[1]

Most people afflicted with foot ailments fail to seek professional help promptly and rely on their self-diagnosis for treatment. The causes of foot problems are rarely obvious, and delays in correcting them give the underlying disorder more time to develop and worsen. Furthermore, when a serious disease is misdiagnosed as a minor foot malady, results are often drastic and costly. Dry skin, brittle nails, numbness, discoloration, and coolness are usually minor signs and symptoms of foot ailments, but they can also be the first indication of vascular insufficiency or diabetes. (See Chapter 19, Management of the Skin and Nails.)

VASCULAR ANATOMY OF THE LOWER EXTREMITIES

To have a clear understanding of the effects of altered circulation to the foot, a basic knowledge of vascular anatomy is needed. Neither the vascular system of the lower extremities nor the task it performs is terribly complicated. The main role of arteries and veins is to provide a pulsatile flow of oxygen-rich blood to the foot and to return the oxygen-depleted blood back to the heart for restoration.

The aorta, the largest blood vessel in the body, divides into two large branches, the right and left common iliac arteries, at the level of the umbilicus (see Figure 17–1). Each of these branches divides again into an external and internal iliac artery. The internal iliac artery, also known as the *hypogastric artery*, supplies the pelvis via a variety of branches. The external iliac artery travels distally and becomes the common femoral artery when it crosses the inguinal ligament. This vessel again divides and gives rise to the superficial femoral and deep femoral arteries. The deep femoral artery, or profunda femoris, supplies the muscles of the thigh and is truly the workhorse of the leg. This vessel becomes a major collateral pathway to the lower extremity in the event that the superficial femoral artery becomes occluded due to atherosclerotic disease. The superficial femoral artery becomes the popliteal artery when it crosses the adductor canal, which is formed by the tendon of the adductor magnus muscle. This is the most common site of atherosclerotic disease in the lower extremity and may be related to local vessel trauma caused by the constant pulsation of the superficial femoral artery against this hard, tendinous structure.

The popliteal artery courses medially and divides below the knee to give rise to its first branch, the anterior tibial artery and the tibioperoneal trunk. This trunk divides into the peroneal and the posterior tibial arteries (see Figure 17–2). The peroneal artery terminates at the ankle, and only the anterior and posterior tibial arteries travel into the foot. The anterior tibial artery continues in the foot as the dorsalis pedis artery, but it is absent or terminates early in 2% of individuals. When this occurs, the perforating branch of the peroneal artery can become the dorsalis pedis artery. In up to 5% of individuals, the posterior tibial artery is either absent or terminates early. In this situation, the communicating branch of the peroneal artery gives rise to the plantar arches.[2] The plantar arch is formed by the lateral plantar artery from the posterior tibial artery and the deep plantar arch from the dorsalis pedis artery. The predominant blood supply to the plantar arch originates from the dorsalis pedis artery. In most individuals, the dorsalis pedis artery and the deep plantar arch give rise to the dorsal and plantar metatarsal arteries, which go on to supply the toes.

The venous system of the lower extremity is, in a sense, more complex to describe because of the numerous vessels involved and the great number of anatomic variants. A short description will suffice to provide an adequate background to the discussion of chronic venous insufficiency that follows later. The veins of the lower extremity are divided into superficial, deep, and perforating veins (see Figure 17–3). The superficial veins are located in the subcutaneous tissues, superficial to the fascial envelope of the thigh and calf muscles. The deep veins accompany the above-mentioned arteries and lie deep to the fasciae and muscles. The perforating veins penetrate the deep fascial envelope to connect the superficial and deep venous systems. Venous flow is normally from the superficial to the deep veins and is directed by a system of one-way bicuspid valves, which are present in all three venous groups. These valves are more numerous in the deep venous system and in the distal veins.[3]

One comment about venous nomenclature needs to be made about the superficial femoral vein, which begins at the adductor hiatus as a continuation of the popliteal vein. It is joined by the deep femoral vein just below the inguinal ligament to form the common femoral vein, which receives the venous drainage from the longest vein of the body, the greater saphenous vein. The superficial femoral vein is not a superficial vein at all, and any evidence of thrombosis or reflux in this vessel must not be ignored.

OCCLUSIVE PERIPHERAL VASCULAR DISEASE—SIGNS AND SYMPTOMS

Intermittent Claudication

Ailments of the lower extremity can usually be diagnosed accurately by obtaining a careful history and performing a detailed physical examination. Intermittent claudication is the most common presenting complaint in patients with chronic arterial occlusion of the lower extremities. The first case of intermittent claudication in man was described by Charcot in 1858. The word *claudication* comes from the Latin word *claudicatio*, which means to limp, but the patient with claudication does not limp; he or she stops to rest. The pain due to intermittent claudication is characterized by a cramping or aching sensation, most often in the calf, that is associated with walking and is relieved by stopping without the need to sit down. Intermittent claudication most commonly occurs as pain in the calf area, but higher vascular obstruction, such as aortic or iliac occlusion, will cause pain in the buttocks and in the upper thigh and is frequently accompanied by impotence in men. This is known as *Leriche syndrome* or *aortoiliac occlusive disease*.

The symptoms of intermittent claudication depend on the degree of ischemia to which the muscles in the legs are submitted. The distance a person can walk will vary from patient to patient, and intermittent claudication can occur after a short distance if a person is walking up a hill, is on a hard surface, or is walking fast. The distance a person walks will be longer if he or she walks more slowly and avoids inclines or hills. People with progressive intermittent claudication note that, over time, they are able to walk only shorter and shorter distances before discomfort develops.

Examination of the patient with intermittent claudication involving the calf muscle may reveal both a femoral and a pedal pulse but no popliteal pulse. In these patients after a brisk walk, the foot will become pale and pulseless because the blood flow bypasses the skin of the foot and tends to flow to the skeletal muscles of the calf instead. Intermittent claudication usually results from a single arterial blockage, which can be predicted accurately by a carefully performed pulse examination. If a femoral pulse is present but a popliteal pulse is diminished or absent, a stenosis or occlusion can be expected in the superficial femoral artery at the adductor canal. Intact pedal pulses in the presence of a popliteal pulse imply disease of the infrapopliteal vessels or trifurcation disease. Physical findings, such as lack of hair growth on the dorsum of the foot, thickening of toenails, and delayed capil-

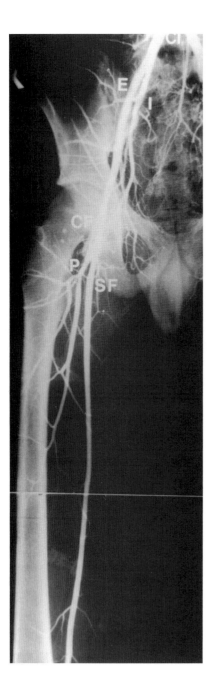

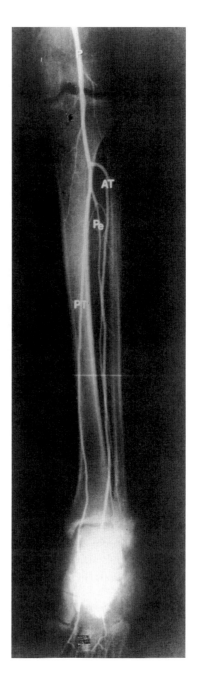

Figure 17–1 Normal arterial anatomy in the pelvic region. An angiogram demonstrates the usual course of the right iliac vessels: common iliac (*CI*), external iliac (*E*), and internal iliac (*I*) arteries. The external iliac artery becomes the common femoral artery (*CF*) when it crosses the inguinal ligament, and gives rise to the profunda femoris artery (*P*) and the superficial femoral artery (*SF*).

Figure 17–2 Normal arterial anatomy in the lower extremity. An angiogram of the left lower extremity demonstrates the usual course of the vessels. The superficial femoral artery traverses the adductor magnus canal to become the popliteal artery (*P*), which bifurcates into the anterior tibial artery (*AT*) and a tibioperoneal trunk. The tibioperoneal trunk also bifurcates to give rise to the posterior tibial (*PT*) and peroneal (*Pe*) arteries. The peroneal artery terminates at the ankle, and only the anterior and posterior tibial arteries travel into the foot. The anterior tibial artery continues in the foot as the dorsalis pedis artery, and the posterior tibial artery bifurcates into the medial and lateral plantar arteries.

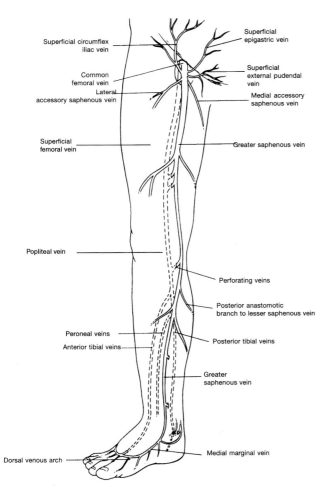

Figure 17–3 Normal venous anatomy. A schematic diagram demonstrates the veins of the lower extremity, which are divided into superficial, deep, and perforating veins.

lary filling, should also be looked for because they point to chronic arterial insufficiency.

Another part of the physical examination that should be routinely performed on patients with suspected vascular insufficiency is the resting ankle-brachial pressure measurement or index. With the patient placed in a supine position, bilateral brachial and ankle (posterior tibial and dorsalis pedis arteries) pressures are measured by obliterating blood flow with a standard adult-size sphygmomanometer (blood pressure) cuff. The exact pressure at which there is cessation of arterial blood flow, as determined by the use of a continuous-wave Doppler instrument placed over the area of maximum audible flow, is recorded. Because systemic blood pressure may vary in patients, the absolute ankle pressure is usually normalized by expressing it as a ratio of the highest obtainable brachial pressure, or ankle-brachial index (ABI).[4] In the normal patient, the ankle pressure is usually greater than or equal to the brachial artery pressure, with an ABI

greater than 1.0. An ABI equal to or less than 0.9 almost always represents some degree of arterial insufficiency. For each major arterial blockage that is present, the ABI will usually be reduced by 0.3. Thus, in the patient afflicted with intermittent claudication, the resting ABI will vary between 0.5 and 0.8 (see Exhibit 17–1).

Rest Pain

Rest pain is caused by nerve ischemia and is persistent in nature, with peaks of increasing intensity. It is worse at night and usually requires the use of narcotics for relief. Rest pain is decreased by dependency of the lower extremities but is aggravated by heat, elevation, and exercise. Because of the relief produced by dependence, these patients often sleep in chairs, and the edema of the legs is secondary to constant dependence.

Nocturnal pain is a form of ischemic neuritis that usually precedes rest pain. It occurs at night, because during sleep, the circulation is essentially of the core variety, with little perfusion to the lower extremity. The pain is classically described as occurring in the toes, across the base of the metatarsals, and in the plantar arches. The ischemic neuritis produced becomes intense at night and disrupts sleep. The patient gains relief by standing up, dangling the feet over the edge of the bed, or, on occasion, walking a few steps. This increases the cardiac output, leads to improved perfusion of the lower extremities, and results in relief of the ischemic neuritis. Thus, in patients with rest pain, a chronically edematous, erythematous foot and ankle may reflect a reliance on dependence for relief of symptoms.

Rest pain usually indicates the presence of at least two hemodynamically significant arterial blocks. The ABI is reduced by 0.6 with two arterial blockages, and these patients usually have an ABI of less than 0.5. If the lesions that produce nocturnal and rest pain are not corrected by vascular surgery, tissue necrosis and gangrene almost always develop, necessitating amputation.

Exhibit 17–1 Noninvasive Evaluation of Arterial Insufficiency: Ankle-Brachial Index

Index	Clinical Description
> 1.1	Calcified, noncompressible vessels must be suspected
0.9–1.1	Normal vessels
0.5–0.8	Intermittent claudication
< 0.5	Rest pain; ulceration and tissue loss

Ulceration and Gangrene

Ulceration and gangrene of the lower extremity represent the most advanced complications of arterial occlusive disease and are generally associated with diffuse, severe, multilevel arterial obstruction (see Figure 17–4). Ischemic ulcers generally occur on the distal portion of the foot, toe, or heel and are particularly painful. These ulcers generally do not bleed and often have a necrotic rim or crater; their associated

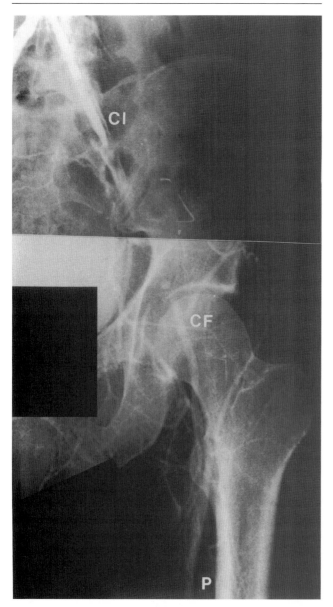

Figure 17–4 An angiogram reveals occlusion of left common iliac artery (*CI*), reconstitution of the common femoral (*CF*) and profunda femoris (*P*) arteries via collateral pathways, and occlusion of the superficial femoral artery. Multilevel atherosclerotic disease is consistent with failure of tissue healing and a decreased ABI. (See *Color Plate 55* for photos of the ulcer on this same patient.)

pain may be relieved by dependence. Just as in patients with rest pain, the ABI is usually less than 0.5 in these patients. Arterial reconstruction, if feasible, must be undertaken in patients with ulceration to prevent limb loss.

Risk Factors

The importance of risk factors in patients with arterial occlusive disease and their order of appearance or development will vary widely from patient to patient. Genetic factors are extremely important risk factors; premature atherosclerosis is frequently seen in family groups, with an age of onset of 40 years or older. However, it is not rare to find significant peripheral vascular disease (PVD) before the age of 40 in the diabetic patient.

Another risk factor of importance is smoking. Clinical experience strongly confirms that patients who smoke and have chronic occlusive arterial disease affecting the extremities do not do well.[5] Among patients under the age of 50 years who quit smoking after they developed intermittent claudication, none progressed to rest pain, as opposed to those who continued to smoke. Smoking causes a decreased blood flow to the extremities and a decrease in the skin temperature of the digits. A single cigarette can cause spasms of the arteries and reduction of blood flow that may last as long as 1 hour or more. The mechanism by which smoking is atherogenic is unknown but may be related to intimal injury caused by increased levels of carboxyhemoglobin, or it may be caused by an effect on platelet function and an increased tendency toward thrombus formation.[6] Another effect of smoking is the influence it exerts on prostacyclin, an important prostaglandin produced by the endothelium of blood vessels that prevents platelet aggregation and promotes vasodilatation. Recent work has shown that cigarette smoking inhibits prostacyclin formation.[7]

Hypertension is another extremely important risk factor in the development of PVD. In the Framingham Study,[8] hypertension imposed a threefold increased risk of developing intermittent claudication during a follow-up period of 26 years. The frequency of hypercholesterolemia and hypertriglyceridemia has also been found to be significant in most clinical diseases of the peripheral vascular system. It has been suggested that a high level of high-density lipoprotein (HDL) cholesterol does not protect the patient if the low-density lipoprotein (LDL) is also inordinately high. It is probably the ratio of HDL to LDL that determines the risk factor, rather than the absolute level of each.

Patients presenting with signs and symptoms of arterial insufficiency should be counseled and educated about risk factor modification if disease progression is to be avoided.

DIABETES AND FOOT ULCERATION

Ulceration and other complications of the foot associated with diabetes are increasing problems of significant epidemiologic proportions. Nearly half of the major amputations performed each year are for patients suffering from diabetes.[9] Only 8% of the overall population in the United States, however, has diabetes at the present time. Each year, 35,000–40,000 diabetic patients undergo major limb amputation at a cost of $1.2 billion.[10] This figure does not include the costs of rehabilitation, prostheses, loss of time from work, loss of jobs, and welfare payments.

The amputation rate in people with diabetes is 15 times that of the nondiabetic population. The initial lesion in most of these cases is painless trauma occurring in a neuropathic, insensate foot. It is the presence of PVD, however, that prevents these lesions from healing. Impaired circulation is a major contributor to infection because the delivery of leukocytes and antibiotic agents is compromised by the lack of sufficient blood flow. The decreased delivery of oxygen to infected tissues further promotes the growth of highly destructive anaerobes. Studies have demonstrated that oxygen is necessary for macrophage mobility in wound debridement and the ingrowth of granulation tissue during wound healing.[11]

The function of some tissue growth factors is oxygen dependent. Furthermore, some antibiotics, principally the aminoglycosides, depend on oxygen for their function. The triopathy of neuropathy, vascular insufficiency, and an altered response to infection makes the diabetic patient uniquely susceptible to pedal complications. Not surprisingly, foot problems remain the most common indication for hospitalization in patients with diabetes mellitus.

Approximately 8% of non–insulin-dependent (type II) diabetic patients have evidence of PVD at the time of diagnosis. The incidence of PVD rapidly increases with age and duration of diabetes. Nearly 45% of patients with diabetes over 20-year duration have evidence of PVD, and this percentage is much higher in those patients who smoke. Vascular disease affecting the lower extremity in diabetic patients has many similarities to that found in the nondiabetic patient. The changes in the vessel wall, in both the media and the intima (consisting of deposits of platelets, smooth muscle cells, lipids, cholesterol, and calcium), are qualitatively the same in both groups, although these changes are quantitatively greater in those with diabetes. There are, however, some important differences. The atherosclerotic process is more commonly seen in diabetic patients than in nondiabetic patients, occurs at an earlier age, advances more rapidly, and is almost as common in women as in men. Differences also exist with regard to the vessels that are involved and the extent of the involvement. The femoral, iliac, and aortic vessels appear to have a similar degree of atherosclerotic changes in diabetic and nondiabetic patients. The profunda femoris artery is affected with greater frequency and extent in diabetics, but the vessels most frequently involved in diabetes are those below the knee—the tibial and peroneal arteries and their smaller branches. In a diabetic patient, multisegment occlusions can be seen with diffused mural changes proximally and distally, whereas, in the nondiabetic subject, the occlusions most often involve a single segment with a normal adjacent arterial tree. Once the process begins in the diabetic patient, both lower extremities are usually involved; in the nondiabetic patient, the lesions are more likely to be unilateral. A summary of 485 patients in five studies showed that, following the initial limb amputation, 42% of diabetics in the first 3 years and 56% in 3–5 years required a contralateral amputation (greater than 10% per year).[12]

Diabetes poses a special risk because diabetic individuals tend to have severely diffused vascular disease; therefore, the diabetic patient must pay particular attention to foot care to ward off ulceration and infection, which mandate an increase in blood flow that their vascular system cannot provide. A major risk factor that has always been considered important in the development of diabetic vascular disease is the control of blood sugar.[13] The Diabetes Control and Complications Trial Research Group in 1993 published a study of 1,444 patients followed for 6.5 years to assess the progression of retinopathy, nephropathy, and neuropathy. Clinical neuropathy was defined as abnormal neurologic examination findings consistent with peripheral neuropathy, plus either an abnormal nerve conduction test result in at least two peripheral nerves or unequivocal autonomic nerve testing. In this multicenter study, patients were randomly assigned to standard insulin control or to an intensive therapy administered by either external insulin pump or by three or more daily injections of insulin, guided by frequent blood sugar monitoring. The developments of neuropathy and nephropathy were each significantly reduced by the strict monitoring of insulin levels. In patients assigned to an intensive management group, the incidence of retinopathy was reduced by 76%, compared with that in patients receiving the usual twice-daily insulin injections. Equally impressive, a 69% reduction in the onset of neuropathy was reported. The findings represent the 3% incidence of neuropathy in those with intensive insulin management versus 10% development in those with the usual insulin management during this 5-year study. The results would support the theory that more stringent insulin management will reduce the onset and progression of neuropathy. The study did note, however, that there was a two- to threefold increase in severe hypoglycemic reactions, which required management in the strict control group. No fatalities and no serious complications were reported, despite this complication. This and other studies support the need for optimum insulin control in diabetic patients. A therapy regimen designed to achieve blood glucose values as close to the normal range as possible would seem to prevent the onset and progression of diabetic complications. Thus, such monitoring should be part of optimum diabetic foot care.

In summary, the risk for developing PVD in the diabetic patient stems from a combination of factors. Heredity, age, and the duration of diabetes are factors that cannot be controlled. Nevertheless, the blood sugar level should be well controlled but balanced against the risk of hypoglycemia. Although each risk factor may have a variable degree of importance by itself, a combination of these factors can become very significant. Therefore, it is extremely important to control hypertension and reduce cholesterol and triglyceride levels. Needless to say, one of the strongest risk factors discussed above is smoking. It is critically important that diabetic patients and certainly all patients who have PVD do not smoke.

A common complaint of patients with peripheral vascular insufficiency is cold feet. It is the discomfort of cold feet that prompts the diabetic patient to resort to the use of hot water bottles, heating pads, or hot water soaks. This practice can result in severe burns to a foot that has become insensitive to heat because of a peripheral neuropathy. At an ambient foot temperature of approximately 70° F, the patient requires 1 mL of blood flow per 100 g of tissue per minute. A patient with even moderate PVD can manage this. Soaking the foot in hot water can quickly raise the skin temperature to 104° F. This requires an increase of 10 times the flow of blood. A patient with PVD cannot achieve this. This results in blistering, ulceration, infection, and gangrene, which not infrequently may lead to an amputation. Another symptom that diabetics complain of is rest pain. In the diabetic patient, rest and nocturnal pain may be absent, despite severe ischemia, because neuropathy has destroyed sensory perception, stressing the need for a careful examination of these patients for vascular sufficiency at every clinic visit.

All of the modern advances in medicine, including sophistication of microbiologic analyses, new and more potent antibiotics with improved antimicrobial activity, advances in radiologic imaging of the foot and leg, and better education and understanding on the part of health care professionals and patients about the etiology and the therapy of the diabetic foot infections, should have reduced the major amputation rate in diabetic patients. Unfortunately, the major amputation rate for diabetic patients has not been significantly reduced. The triopathy of neuropathy, vascular insufficiency, and an altered response to infection makes the diabetic patient uniquely susceptible to foot problems. Diabetics live quite normally with all of these complications until minor trauma results in cutaneous ulceration and the development of an acute infection that may lead to hospitalization and limb loss. Neuropathy probably represents the greatest risk for ulcer development. Diminished or absent proprioception and sensation quite often delay early recognition and treatment of a seemingly benign problem. Autonomic nerve dysfunction, characterized by dry skin, absent sweating, and increased capillary refill secondary to arteriovenous shunting, leads to fissure, cracking, and a false sense of security about the circulation. Motor neuropathy leads to denervation of the intrinsic and skeletal muscles of the foot and leg, resulting in abnormal bone-related problems, due to a compromised foot architecture that is susceptible to traumatic injury.

Ischemia may complicate up to half of the diabetic foot ulcers; 40% of diabetic patients presenting with gangrene or severe limb threat infections will have palpable popliteal pulses. Aggressive vascular evaluation and treatment are essential for healing ischemic ulceration and must be considered for chronic ulcers that fail to respond to treatment. Diabetic patients tolerate infection poorly. Defects in the host defense include altered leukocyte function and wound repair. Most important is the fact that systemic signs and symptoms of a septic process often occur late, making unexplained and uncontrollable hyperglycemia the only reliable sign of a potentially serious limb- and/or life-threatening infection. Less than one-third of patients with pedal osteomyelitis have elevated temperature or white blood cell count. The lack of blood flow reduces oxygen to the afflicted tissue and contributes to the development of foot sepsis. Studies have demonstrated that oxygen is necessary for macrophage mobility in wound debridement and the ingrowth of granulation tissue during wound healing.[11]

Restoration of blood flow with increased oxygen levels to ischemic tissue is of the utmost importance if limb salvage is going to be achieved.[14] The extent and severity of the infected diabetic foot ulcer determines the course of treatment. To determine the severity, one must do a careful initial inspection of the wound, which, because of neuropathy, can usually be done at bedside. Sterile forceps, a probe, scissors, and a good light are all that are needed. The severity of tissue destruction and sepsis may not be totally apparent from simply looking at the ulcer or infected callus, especially in those patients who continue to bear weight on a painless area or who do not have the visual acuity to recognize a problem. One must unroof all encrusted areas and, using a probe, inspect the wound to determine deep-tissue destruction and possible bone or joint involvement. A determination can be made for whether the ulcer is superficial so that treatment can be done at home, or whether there is any limb-threatening potential that requires immediate hospital admission. Patients with superficial ulceration and minimal (less than 2 cm) cellulitis may be treated on the outside initially if there is no evidence of systemic toxicity, if the patient is compliant and reliable, and if the patient has an adequate support system at home. Treatment requires that the patient be non–weight-bearing to provide complete and total rest. Contact casting and other immobilization endeavors do not replace non–weight-bearing and are used only in selected instances. The wound specimen is cultured at initial debridement and broad-spectrum oral antibiotics are begun, with changes made based on sensitivity reports and the response of the wound. Simple dressings appear to work best, with wet-to-dry dressings of either saline or diluted antiseptic solutions applied one or three times per day, depending on the size and the area being treated. Dry, scaly skin is best treated with lubricated creams, and cracks and fissures are best managed with antibiotic ointment. Patients must be examined every 24–48 hours; if there is no improvement, hospitalization is recommended. Once healing is ensured, weight bearing is progressed in modified footwear to protect the high-risk areas. Simply allowing the patient to return to full activity or weight bearing may result in acute Charcot's foot or recurrent breakdown. Shoe modification and periodic follow-up are essential to all patients at risk. Patients with limb-threatening infections are managed with hospitalization. Again, inspection is essential because one cannot rely on systemic signs and symptoms to ascertain severity. Indications for hospitalization are deep ulcers with bone or joint involvement, cellulitis greater than 2 cm, lymphangitis, and systemic toxicity. Initial management includes immediate hospitalization, medical stabilization, control of blood sugar, and complete bed rest.

There is probably no greater controversy right now in the treatment of diabetic infection than the proper diagnosis and treatment of osteomyelitis. One thing is known for certain: Inadequate diagnosis and treatment of osteomyelitis increase the risk for major amputation. Methods to diagnose osteomyelitis include plain radiographs, bone scans, leukocyte scans, computed tomography scans, magnetic resonance imaging, and clinical evaluation. Proponents of each radiologic test quote acceptable sensitivity and specificity but largely without confirmation by microbiologic or histopathologic proof. Whatever test one uses, it should not delay urgent or emergent surgical intervention. Cost is now also an important consideration, with fixed reimbursement the norm. These tests are costly; thus, the use of a sterile probe to examine the wound is very cost-effective. If a sterile probe taps the bone or a joint, there is excellent sensitivity and specificity that the area is involved with osteomyelitis. A plain radiograph should be obtained, with or without magnification views, to look for gas, foreign bodies, associated fractures, or other bony abnormalities. Antibiotics are adjunctive to good surgical debridement and management. At the time of debridement, deep culture specimens are obtained, and bone or biopsy of deep tissue is sent whenever possible to ensure a reliable specimen. The majority of cultures from patients with limb-threatening disease grow Gram-positive bacteria, 50% grow Gram-negative enteric bacteria, and 50–70% of these patients also grow anaerobes. Therefore, antibiotic selection must take this into account, and broad-spectrum intravenous antibiotics or combination therapy to ensure maximum delivery to the infected site are recommended. Antibiotic changes are made only on the basis of the sensitivity reports and the response of the wound.

Except in rare circumstances, antibiotics do not cure osteomyelitis. Studies supporting the use of antibiotics alone for curing osteomyelitis, in general, lack histopathologic or microbiologic proof and accept a major amputation rate of almost 30% after treatment.[15] Opponents also note that bacteremia, open wounds after treatment, gangrene, and ischemia are associated with poor outcome. Courses of antibiotics of 6 weeks or longer are also quite costly, even when delivered on an outpatient basis.

Infected limb-threatening ulcers are a surgical emergency. Surgical debridement and drainage of the infection should be carried out as expeditiously as possible. Diabetics do not tolerate undrained sepsis, and patients with systemic toxicity will not improve until this is done. A good monitor of accuracy of debridement is to follow the blood sugar levels and management, which should improve dramatically as infection is controlled. Incisions are carefully placed, ensuring adequate debridement and conserving as much healthy tissue as possible, such as small skin flaps that may later be used in reconstruction. Any viable area should be left and protected, even if this means multiple trips to the operating room for infection control. Most of the debridement can be done with little or no anesthesia because of the presence of neuropathy.

The location of the ulcer, the extent of the infection and its control, and the adequacy of circulation will determine what the final result will be. It is important to remember that the more ischemic the lower extremity is, the more important it is to close an involved area primarily. A neuropathic foot with excellent circulation is managed differently than the same infection in an ischemic foot. Once sepsis is controlled, evaluation and treatment of the ischemia are the next most important options. The overwhelming success of surgical revascularization, even to the pedal vessels, supports an aggressive approach. Once circulation is reestablished, revisions or more definitive local surgical procedures can be performed. It is important to try to save as much of the weight-bearing part of the foot as possible, especially the first toe and its metatarsal head. Only with an aggressive control of diabetic sepsis and restoration of foot pulses by revascularization can the amputation rate be reduced in this challenging group of patients (see Chapter 18, Management of the Neuropathic Foot.

Clinical Wisdom:

Blood sugar levels should fall as infection is controlled.

VENOUS STASIS ULCERS

Despite decades of clinical and laboratory research, the exact mechanisms by which patients develop venous stasis ulceration remain uncertain. There is little doubt that sustained venous hypertension remains the underlying etiologic factor common to all patients with venous stasis ulcers. Venous hypertension can occur primarily in the deep venous system or may be isolated to the superficial saphenous veins. These entities may also occur in combination. This has been associated with congenital or acquired valvular dysfunction within the deep veins or with valvular incompetence located at the saphenofemoral junction or via incompetent perforators below the knee. Clearly, the underlying pathologic process must be determined in each individual patient prior to embarking on a specific treatment plan.

The Swollen Leg

One of the first complaints of patients with venous insufficiency is swelling of the legs, which, on occasion, is accompanied by discomfort and a heavy feeling in the lower extremities. As opposed to similar complaints in patients with arterial insufficiency, this complaint is readily relieved by leg elevation in the person afflicted by venous disease. A basic understanding of the function and structure of the venous system is needed to comprehend the pathophysiologic derangements that are responsible for the development of lower extremity edema.

The main and foremost task of the venous system is to return blood from the periphery to the heart. In addition, it serves as a storage network intimately involved in blood volume regulation. It also facilitates the exchange of substances between tissue and blood in the capillary region. To carry out these functions and to maintain a vigorous flow of blood in a low-pressure system, the venous vessels have to rely on the elastic components of their walls (see *Color Plate 56*). The walls of veins consist of an intact endothelium that coats a thin basal membrane. An adjoining layer of fibrous connective tissue with strands of collagenous and muscle fibers helps to stabilize the walls of the veins and, in conjunction with a delicate system of valves, is responsible for the return of venous blood to the heart. The slightly helical structure of muscle fibers and collagenous strands enables healthy veins to return to their original position after undergoing distention of length and girth from increased blood volumes. Failure of this collagenous and muscular infrastructure results in veins that become wider, longer, and convoluted, giving rise to the formation of tortuous varices. Progressive venous dilatation can lead to valvular incompetence by interfering with the delicate apposition of venous valve leaflets, which is required for transport of blood up the leg and into the central circulation. Thus, the failure of proper venous valve closure may be the result and not the primary cause of blood vessel widening.

Venous congestion can also alter the delicate balance that exists between arterioles, venules, and the capillaries. About 20 L of fluid are filtered into the interstitial space by this complex system each day, with 18 L (90%) being reabsorbed by the venous branches of the capillary system. The remaining 2 L (10%) return to the circulatory system through lymph drainage. Hydrostatic and colloidal-osmotic forces work together in capillary filtration and reabsorption. Intracapillary pressure drops from 35 mm Hg in the arterial branches to 15 mm Hg in the venous branches. Higher pressure in the arterial side leads to outward filtration, which is counteracted on the venous side by a continuous reabsorption, driven by colloidal and osmotic forces. A delicate balance is maintained as long as the amounts of filtered and reabsorbed fluid remain equal. Altered venous return due to increased venous dilatation and valvular deficiency results in perceptible increases in capillary hydrostatic pressure and permeability of the capillary endothelium. These two factors lead to an enhanced filtration of fluid into the interstitial space and the classic appearance of the signs and symptoms of peripheral edema.

As can be gleaned from the above discussion, the lymphatic system can also be involved in chronic venous insufficiency. Both the lymphatic and venous systems share an early embryologic development and an intimate anatomic relationship. The lymphatic channels course along the pathway of the lesser and greater saphenous veins to drain into the superficial inguinal lymph nodes. The deep lymphatic vessels of the lower extremity likewise accompany the deep vessels of the leg to the popliteal lymph nodes, then continue along the femoral vessels to reach the deep inguinal lymph nodes.

Congenital or acquired insufficiency of the lymphatic transport results in lymph stasis and the accumulation of protein-rich interstitial fluid. Chronic lymphedema, however, develops only if the collateral lymphatic circulation is inadequate or tissue macrophages (which aid in the removal of macromolecules from the interstitial space) are overwhelmed. Impaired lymphatic drainage results in significant structural changes in the lymphatic vessels themselves and the subcutaneous tissues they serve. This leads to fibroblast proliferation, sclerosis of the subcutaneous tissues, and increased vascularity—changes that are usually associated with chronic inflammation.[16] Secondary changes in lymph vessels due to lymph stasis include fibrosis of the wall with loss of permeability and lymph-concentrating ability. Furthermore, just as in the venous system, lymphatic valves may also fibrose or become incompetent as a result of proximal lymphatic obstruction and distal vessel dilatation. The lymph vessel wall loses its intrinsic contractility, and the muscle pump is rendered ineffective. Lymph stasis favors the development of obstructive lymphangitis, with further destruction of the main and collateral lymphatic channels.

Chronic venous insufficiency can lead to recurrent attacks of skin cellulitis, which may result in increased destruction of cutaneous lymphatic channels and subsequent obstructive lymphatic patterns.[17] This is strongly suggested by lymphoscintigraphy, a noninvasive imaging modality used to interpret the morphologic and functional alterations occurring in the lymphatic system. Lymphoscintigraphy has been used to show that the lymphatic system is often impaired in patients with chronic venous insufficiency. This impairment is reflected by the development of anatomic changes in lymphatic vessels, as well as the presence of a delayed lymphatic flow. These changes ultimately may interfere with the absorption of interstitial fluid in the extremities of patients afflicted with chronic venous insufficiency and, thus, contribute to the increased clinical swelling that is seen in them.

Pathophysiology of Venous Ulceration

There are several mechanisms described in the literature that outline the pathophysiologic events leading to skin ulceration. The concept of fibrin cuffs developing at the capillary level was initially described by Browse and Burnand in 1982.[18] These authors suggested that sustained venous hypertension is transmitted to the superficial veins in the subcutaneous tissue and the overlying skin. This, in turn, causes widening of the capillary pores, thus allowing the escape of large macromolecules (including fibrinogen) into the interstitial space. Owing to associated defects in the fibrinolytic process, fibrin accumulates around these capillaries, forming a mechanical barrier to the transfer of oxygen and other nutrients. Ultimately, this leads to cellular dysfunction, which, in turn, leads to cell death and skin ulceration. Unfortunately, there is no published evidence that fibrin provides a barrier to oxygen diffusion.

In more recent years, additional physiologic changes have been noted in the microcirculation of patients with chronic venous hypertension. Specifically, this relates to an altered inflammatory mechanism in these patients. These changes have been linked to the accumulation of white blood cells at the capillary level, which has been termed the *white blood cell-trapping hypothesis*.[19,20] Transient elevations in venous pressures have been shown to decrease capillary blood flow, resulting in trapping of white blood cells at the capillary level. This occurs to a much greater degree in patients with long-standing venous hypertension and liposclerotic skin. These marginated white blood cells, in turn, plug capillary loops, resulting in areas of localized ischemia. These cells may also become activated at this level, which, in turn, causes release of various proteolytic enzymes, as well as superoxide free radicals and chemotactic substances. These substances ultimately lead to direct tissue damage and, thus, to ulceration[21] (see Chapter 2 for a more comprehensive discussion of the mechanisms of ischemia reperfusion injury).

Differential Diagnosis of Venous Stasis Ulcers

All that ulcerates is not venous in origin. The common feature of all ulcerations of the legs is an underlying systemic or local problem that complicates the healing of wounds, which are inevitably traumatic in origin. Once-minor trauma leads to a chronic, recalcitrant wound, which is a challenge to heal. Those ulcerations that are not venous but may mimic or be confused with venous ulcers are to be differentiated on the basis of a different historical evolution, the presence of other systemic or local disease processes, and often subtle but important different physical findings (see Exhibit 17–2).

Medical Treatment of Venous Stasis Ulcers

Definitive treatment of venous stasis ulcers is dependent on the operative repair of the underlying reason for venous incompetence of the affected extremity. This is seldom possible, however, and long-term success is rarely achieved. Excision and grafting of the ulcerated area and surrounding scar tissue, even when accompanied by local and regional subfascial ligation of perforating vessels, does not uniformly result in returning long-standing skin integrity. Therefore, there remain a great many patients whose venous stasis ulcers have to be managed nonoperatively.[22] Before attempting a medical management of a venous stasis ulcer, the diagnosis must be assured. Noninvasive measurements must eliminate a significant ischemic component to that etiology. The ABI must be at least greater than 0.5 and, preferably, greater than 0.75. If transcutaneous oxygen measurements are performed, the foot dorsal pressures should exceed 30 mm Hg. (See Chapter 7, Vascular Evaluation.) Hemoglobin electrophoresis should eliminate sickle cell disease and, if suspected, a biopsy should eliminate vasculitis as the cause of the ulcer.

To allow the ulcer to heal by secondary intention, the wound must be in bacterial balance and contain 10^5 or fewer bacteria per g of tissue; it must not harbor β-hemolytic streptococci. If the biopsy shows the wound to be infected, bacterial balance is best reestablished by a topical antimicrobial. Systemically administered antibiotics do not lower the bacterial count in granulation tissue. However, systemic antibiotics are effective and indicated if the ulcer has an area of surrounding cellulitis. Another method of reestablishing bacterial balance is with the use of temporary biologic dressings, such as allograft skin. Once the ulcer is in bacterial balance, it can heal by secondary intention. The process of epithelialization is more important than the process of contraction for these ulcers.

Clinical Wisdom:

To achieve bacterial balance:
1. Apply topical antibiotics if wound shows signs of infection.
2. Administer systemic antibiotics if periwound shows signs of cellulitis.

Exhibit 17–2 Differential Diagnosis of Lower Extremity Ulcers

	Ischemic	Venous Stasis	Neuropathic
Etiology	Arterial insufficiency	Chronic venous insufficiency	Diabetes
Usual location	Distal to medial malleolus; dorsum of foot or toes	Proximal to medial malleolus; lateral lower leg	Along pressure points; plantar aspect of metatarsal heads (first or fifth)
Pain	Severe; nocturnal, relieved by dependency	Mild; relieved by elevation	None
Bleeding	Little or none	Venous ooze	May be brisk
Lesion characteristics	Irregular edge; poor granulation tissue	Shallow, irregular shape; granulating base with rounded edges	Punched-out; callous edges with deep sinus
Associated findings	Trophic skin changes (dry skin, brittle nails, alopecia); absent pulses	Stasis dermatitis; hyperpigmentation; palpable pulses	Neuropathy; warm skin; pulses may be present or absent

Source: Modified from Rutherford RB. The vascular consultation. In: Rutherford RB, ed. *Vascular Surgery,* 4th ed. Philadelphia: W.B. Saunders Company, 1995, p. 9.

Compression therapy is the cornerstone of effective nonoperative treatment of venous stasis ulcers. Many combination dressings, such as the time-honored Unna boot, have been reported to provide adequate compression if good patient compliance is achieved.[23] The U.S. Food and Drug Administration presently considers compression therapy to be the standard of care for venous stasis ulcers. *Color Plate 57* shows a patient with venous stasis ulceration. *Color Plate 58* shows an ulcer and associated signs of chronic venous insufficiency. Chapter 10 describes the management of edema associated with venous stasis ulcers, and Chapter 12 explains the use of bioengineered skin, a recent addition to the therapeutic agents for venous stasis ulcers of long duration and/or large size.

Recently, a variety of growth factors have been introduced for the treatment of venous stasis ulcers. The trial with transforming growth factor-β (TGF-β) in a collagen sponge delivery system has given the most encouraging data of those trials that have been completed.[24] Interestingly, the topical antimicrobial silver sulfadiazine (Silvadene, SSD) has also shown beneficial results. It is thought that the base of this compound has properties that stimulate wound epithelialization. Contrary to previous experience, many patients who have healed during carefully controlled clinical trials have remained healed, as long as they comply with compression therapy. Because the underlying etiology of the ulcer is not treated with medical therapy, such treatment can be considered only palliative. However, as more is learned about modulating the wound healing process, palliation may be extended for the life of the patient.

To evaluate properly the many therapeutic modalities that are being applied in the treatment of chronic venous disease, the Ad Hoc Committee on Reporting Standards in Venous Disease of the Society of Vascular Surgery and the North American Chapter of the International Society for Cardiovascular Surgery have recommended the use of a classification designed to allow such comparisons.[25] Limbs with chronic venous disease should be classified according to clinical signs (C), etiology (E), anatomic distribution (A), and pathophysiologic condition (P) (see Exhibit 17–3).

Any limb with possible chronic venous disease is first placed into one of seven clinical classes (C_{0-6}) according to objective clinical signs, and is further characterized as being asymptomatic ($C_{0-6,A}$) or symptomatic ($C_{0-6,S}$). Because therapy may alter the clinical category of chronic venous disease, limbs should be reclassified after any form of medical or surgical treatment. The venous dysfunction encountered is then to be classified according to one of three mutually exclusive categories: congenital (E_C), primary (E_P), or secondary (E_S). Next, the anatomic site or sites affected with venous disease are to be described as involving the superficial (A_S), deep (A_D), or perforating (A_P) veins. Finally, the pathophysiologic reason for the development of signs and symptoms of chronic venous disease is to be determined as being the result of reflux (P_R), obstruction (P_O), or both ($P_{R,O}$). Observance of this classification in the clinical arena will lead to an improvement in communications in the field of venous disorders and will help in the evaluation and proper application of therapeutic regimens.

Exhibit 17–3 Chronic Lower Extremity Venous Disease

CLINICAL CLASSIFICATION	
Class	**Clinical Description**
0	No visible signs of venous disease
1	Telangiectasias, reticular veins, malleolar flare
2	Varicose veins
3	Edema without skin changes
4	Skin changes ascribed to venous disease (eg, pigmentation, venous exzema, lipodermato-sclerosis)
5	Skin changes as defined above with healed ulceration
6	Skin changes as defined above with active ulceration

ETIOLOGIC CLASSIFICATION	
Etiology	**Description**
Congenital	Cause of chronic venous disease present since birth
Primary	Chronic venous disease of undetermined cause
Secondary	Chronic venous disease with an associated known cause (postthrombotic, posttraumatic, other)

ANATOMIC CLASSIFICATION	
Veins Involved	**Description**
Superficial	Telangiectasias/reticular veins and greater saphenous veins; lesser saphenous veins and nonsaphenous veins
Deep	Inferior vena cava, iliac, pelvis, gonadal, femoral, popliteal, tibial, and muscular veins
Perforating	Thigh and calf

PATHOPHYSIOLOGIC CLASSIFICATION	
Type	**Description**
R	Reflex
O	Obstruction
R,O	Reflux and obstruction

Source: Adapted with permission from Porter, J.M., Moneta, G.L., and International Consensus Committee on Chronic Venous Disease. Reporting Standards in Venous Disease: An update. *Journal of Vascular Surgery*, Vol. 21, pp. 635–645, © 1995, Mosby, Inc.

REVIEW QUESTIONS

1. Name major arteries and veins of the lower extremity.
2. Describe the three signs and symptoms of occlusive PVD and their significance.
3. List four risk factors for development of arterial ulcers.
4. What clinical signs are reliable indicators of systemic infection in diabetic patients?
5. How do the venous and lymphatic systems relate to the "swollen leg?"
6. What steps must be performed before attempting medical management of venous stasis ulcers?

REFERENCES

1. McGann MM, Robinson LR. *The Doctor's Sore Foot Book.* Avenel, NJ: Wing Books; 1994.

2. Kadir S. Arterial anatomy of the lower extremity. In: Kadir S, ed. *Atlas of Normal and Variant Angiographic Anatomy.* Philadelphia: WB Saunders; 1991:123–160.

3. Lundell C, Kadir S. Lower extremities and pelvis. In: Kadir S, ed. *Atlas of Normal and Variant Angiographic Anatomy.* Philadelphia: W.B. Saunders Company; 1991:203–225.

4. Strandness DE Jr, Summer DS. Application of ultrasound to the study of arteriosclerosis obliterans. *Angiology.* 1975;26:187–189.

5. Jonason T, Rinquist I. Factors of prognostic importance for subsequent rest pain in patients with intermittent claudication. *Acta Med Scand.* 1985;218:27–36.

6. Couch NP. On the arterial consequences of smoking. *J Vasc Surg.* 1986;3:807–812.

7. Hillis LD, Hirsch PD, Campbell WB, et al. Interaction of the arterial wall, plaque, and platelets in myocardial infarction. *Cardiovasc Clin.* 1983;14:31–44.

8. Kannel WB, McGee DL. Update on some epidemiologic features of intermittent claudication: The Framingham Study. *J Am Geriatr Soc.* 1985;33:13–21.

9. Reiber GE. Diabetic foot care. *Diabetes Care.* 1992;15:29–31.

10. Bransome ED Jr. Financing the care of diabetes mellitus in the United States. *Diabetes Care.* 1992;15:1–5.

11. Vogelberg KH, Konig M. Hypoxia of diabetic feet with abnormal arterial blood flow. *Clin Invest.* 1993;71:466–470.

12. Kucan JO, Robson MC. Diabetic foot infections: Fate of the contralateral foot. *Plast Reconstr Surg.* 1986;77:439–441.

13. McDermott JE. *The Diabetic Foot.* Rosemont, IL: American Academy of Orthopaedic Surgeons; 1995.

14. LoGerfo FW, Gibbons GW, Pomposelli FB, et al. Evolving trends in management of the diabetic foot. *Arch Surg.* 1992;127:617–621.

15. Bamberger DM, Daus GP, Gerding DN, et al. Osteomyelitis in the feet of diabetic patients: Long-term results, prognostic factors and the role of antimicrobial therapy and surgical therapy. *Am J Med.* 1987;83(4):653–660.

16. Olszewski W. Pathophysiology and clinical observations of obstructive lymphedema of the limbs. In: Clodius L, ed. *Lymphedema.* Stuggart, Germany: Georg Thieme Verlag; 1977:79–102.

17. Hammond SL, Gomez ER, Coffey JA, et al. Involvement of the lymphatic system in chronic venous insufficiency. In: Bergan JJ, Yao JST, eds. *Venous Disorders.* Philadelphia: WB Saunders; 1991:333–343.

18. Browse NL, Burnand KG. The cause of venous ulceration. *Lancet.* 1982;2:243–245.

19. Thomas PRS, Nash GB, Dormandy JA. White cell accumulation in the dependent legs of patients with venous hypertension: A possible mechanism for trophic changes in the skin. *Br Med J.* 1988;296:1693–1695.

20. Butler CM, Coleridge-Smith PD. Microcirculatory aspects of venous ulceration. *Dermatol Surg Oncol.* 1994;20:474–480.

21. Coleridge-Smith PD, Thomas P, Scurr JH, et al. Causes of venous ulceration: A new hypothesis. *Br Med J.* 1988;296:1726–1772.

22. Robson MC. Medical treatment of venous stasis ulcers. Presented at American College of Surgeons Postgraduate Course 13: *Current Treatment of Venous Stasis Ulcers.* October 22–27, 1995; New Orleans, LA.

23. Villavicencio JL, Rich NM, Salander JM, et al. Leg ulcers of venous origin. In: Cameron JL, ed. *Current Surgical Therapy.* Toronto, Canada: BC Becker; 1989:610–618.

24. Bishop JB, Phillips LG, Mustoe TA, et al. A prospective randomized evaluator-blinded trial of two potential wound healing agents for the treatment of venous stasis ulcers. *J Vasc Surg.* 1992;8:251–257.

25. Porter JM, Moneta GL, International Consensus Committee on Chronic Venous Disease. Reporting standards in venous disease: An update. *J Vasc Surg.* 1995;21:635–645.

SUGGESTED READING

Beitz JM, Burton CS. Kerstein MD, et al. *Venous Leg Ulcer Guidelines.* Philadelphia: University of Pennsylvania; 1997. Print copies and video available from the University of Pennsylvania School of Medicine, Attn: Maryanne McGuckin, MD, 605A Stellar Chance Bldg., 422 Curie Blvd., Philadelphia, PA 19104-6021. Telephone: (215) 573-3066 or (215) 898-4969; fax (215) 573–0826. Summary available at National Guideline Clearinghouse. http://www.guideline.gov/index.asp

Browne AC, Sibbald RG. The Diabetic neuropathic ulcer: An overview. *Ostomy/Wound Manage.* 1999;45(Suppl. 1A):6S–20S.

Falanga V. Care of venous ulcers. *Ostomy/Wound Manage.* 1999;45(Suppl. 1A):33S–43S.

Klucan J. *Lower Extremity Ulceration Guidelines.* American Society of Plastic and Reconstructive Surgeons (ASPRS); 1998. Print copies available: 444 E. Algonquin Rd, Arlington Heights, IL. Outline available at National Guideline Clearinghouse. http://www.guideline.gov/index.asp

CHAPTER 18

Management of the Neuropathic Foot

Nancy Elftman and Joan E. Conlan

CHAPTER OBJECTIVES

At the completion of this chapter, the reader will be able to:

1. Identify patients at risk for foot ulceration due to lack of protective sensation.
2. Understand the relationship between surface temperature and inflammation.
3. Implement off-loading techniques with wound care protocol.

INTRODUCTION

Medical research has provided advancements in medication and technology that now extend the lives of patients with previously fatal diseases: The prognosis has changed from fatality to chronic complications.[1] The chronic disease complication addressed in this chapter is neuropathy. The objective of management of the problem is to control progression and reduce amputations conservatively.

The patient with neuropathy often has dysvascular components that must be addressed by a medical team, rather than one specialty (see Chapter 17, Diagnosis and Management of Vascular Ulcers). With the team approach, the limb can be evaluated, treated, and monitored through follow-up to provide continued ambulation for the patient.[2] The team goal is the prevention or delay of amputation and/or limb salvage of lower extremities. In the formation of clinical teams, there has been a trend to include practitioners of several disciplines, including the wound care, advanced practice, or enterostomal therapy (ET) nurse; diabetologist/endocrinologist; vascular surgeon; physical therapist; orthotist/pedorthist; orthopaedic surgeon/podiatrist; and dermatologist.

The multidisciplinary approach to treating foot problems is an optimum intervention for prevention of amputations. The disciplines playing the most important roles are nurse educators, who encourage high-risk patients to modify their behavior; orthotists, for recommendation of suitable footwear, stockings, and orthoses; and primary care providers, to remove calluses, treat minor trauma, and provide health care. Physical therapists will play a role in all of these aspects of care. Referrals should be available to vascular surgeons and other specialists when specified by a physician.[3]

The multidisciplinary clinic requires special training in treatment of chronic disabilities. Although the individual training programs of professionals include normal foot anatomy and biomechanics, few describe the neuropathic foot and associated complications, leading to inadequate medical advice or treatment.[4] In the clinical setting, no initial problem is too small to address. The clinical team is important and must treat minor trauma immediately to prevent deterioration of the condition. There is a destructive chain of trauma surrounding the neuropathic foot, as follows:

1. Trauma
2. Inflammation
3. Ulceration
4. Infection
5. Absorption
6. Deformity
7. Disability

This chain can be broken with proper objective measurements, treatment, and patient education.[2]

The patient with neuropathy requires a consistent follow-up schedule relating to level of insensitivity, history of complications, and general physical condition. A patient with loss of protective sensation (10 g of force) and no history of ulceration will require less frequent follow-up than will the patient with a chronic breakdown history. Records should reflect as many objective measurements as possible and a method of classification of patient types. Management of the neuropathic and dysvascular limb is a process of continuing evaluation. The process of history, examination, and charting details cannot be overemphasized. All clinical findings should be charted and relayed to the patient's primary care provider.[5]

Although neuropathy exists in many disease processes, there are concerns about the growing number requiring management. When breakdown occurs in one neuropathic limb, the contralateral limb is commonly involved within 18 to 36 months, so prophylactic measures are especially important. Many considerations must be addressed by the team treating the neuropathic and dysvascular limb before a treatment plan is developed. Once the plan is in place, it is imperative to educate and involve the patient in the plan.

PATHOGENESIS

The neuropathic process is poorly understood, and there are many theories regarding its etiology. When evaluating the neuropathic patient, the medical team encounters the following obstacles:

- Lack of clear definition of diabetic neuropathy
- Absence of single repeatable tests of neuropathy that are not dependent on either expensive technology or subjective clinical judgment
- Varied manifestations of neuropathy: distal symmetric, mononeuropathies, autonomic neuropathies
- Separation of diabetes from other potential etiologies of neuropathy

The neuropathic foot is affected by a trineuropathy, which consists of three phases that occur simultaneously; manifestations of two of these phases are shown in Figure 18–1.

1. Sensory neuropathy—loss of sensation, leaving patient incapable of sensing pain and pressure. The patient has no sense of identity with the feet.
2. Motor neuropathy—the loss of intrinsic muscles, resulting in clawed toes (Figure 18–2) and eventual foot-drop. The ankle jerk reflex is absent.[6]
3. Autonomic neuropathy—the loss of autonomic system function, resulting in the absence of sweat and oil production and leaving skin dry and nonelastic.

Until recently, all forms of neuropathy were lumped together. It is now clear that there are different types, which de-

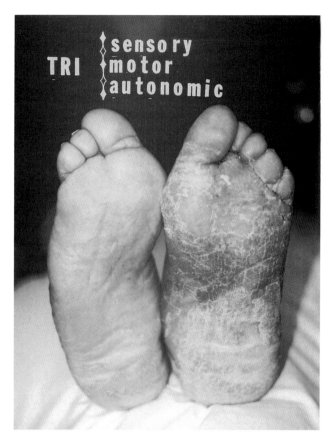

Figure 18–1 Feet of a patient with sensory, motor, and autonomic neuropathies. Manifestations of motor neuropathy (deformity, clawed toes, toe amputation, foot imbalance needing immediate intervention) and autonomic neuropathy (dry, cracked skin) are evident. Note the difference in trophic changes between the feet. *Source:* Reprinted with permission from N. Elftman, Clinical Management of the Neuropathic Limb, *Journal of Prosthetics and Orthotics.* Vol. 4, No. 1. pp. 1–12. Copyright © American Academy of Orthotists and Prosthetists.

velop differently. Peripheral neuropathy can be broken down into two major groups:

1. Gradual onset, those that develop gradually and are usually painless. The exact cause is unknown but may be related to duration of diabetes and level of blood sugar control. Symptoms may include numbness, tingling, burning, and a pins-and-needles sensation.
2. Sudden onset and disappearance, those that develop suddenly (or acutely) and are almost always painful; then the pain disappears, leaving sensory loss.

Many believe that neuropathy is caused by hyperglycemia—high levels of glucose in the blood. Tight control may be the best prevention of severe neuropathy.[7]

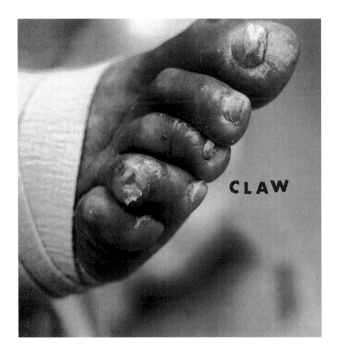

Figure 18–2 Clawed toes. Note the corn on the fourth toe, caused by rubbing top of shoe.

MEDICAL HISTORY

The medical history is a useful way to identify potential neuropathy that may be present in many disease processes. The neuropathy may be isolated (nerve damage or entrapment) but, for most chronic disease processes, the effect is peripheral. The most common disease processes resulting in peripheral neuropathy are the following:

- Diabetes
- Spina bifida
- Hansen's disease
- Systemic erythematosus lupus
- Acquired immune deficiency syndrome (AIDS), human immunodeficiency virus (HIV) infection, AIDS-related complex
- Cancer
- Vitamin B deficiency
- Multiple sclerosis
- Uremia
- Vascular disease
- Charcot-Marie-Tooth muscle disease

Toxins and toxic syndromes can also cause insensitivity in the limbs, including those related to overuse of or exposure to alcohol, arsenic, lead, steroids, gold, and isoniazid.

Many other chronic complications may result in neuropathy, but the above list indicates why all patients must be evaluated for neuropathy, regardless of reported history. Congenital sensory loss, as in spina bifida, is important to the examiner because the patient has never experienced normal sensation and cannot evaluate his or her own sensory status.[8–10]

Diabetic Neuropathy

The most common disease process seen in neuropathy is diabetes, which results in true peripheral neuropathy. Statistics on diabetes are growing, and the medical cost related to diabetes in the United States is currently $14 billion per year. Included in this cost are 54,000 lower extremity amputations per year, of which 50–70% could have been prevented by team management. It is estimated that 50–84% of the lower extremity amputations were preceded by a foot ulcer. More than 14 million Americans have diabetes (half are undiagnosed), with 700,000 cases diagnosed per year. In the general population, 1 in 20 has diabetes. Many diabetics are diagnosed when they present a nonhealing foot ulcer.[11–16] Of major concern is the mortality rate after amputation, which is 50% within 3–5 years. The rate of contralateral amputation is 50% within 4 years.[17]

Although there are several different divisions of diabetes, the two main categories are insulin-dependent diabetes mellitus (IDDM), or type I, and non–insulin-dependent diabetes mellitus (NIDDM), or type II. In IDDM, the insulin deficiency is due to pancreas islet cell loss. It occurs at any age but is common in youth. NIDDM is more frequent in adults but occurs at any age. The majority of patients with NIDDM are overweight.[18]

The dysvascular patient may also be diabetic, which leads to impaired healing of a limb that cannot deliver antibiotics sufficiently to combat extremity infection (see Chapter 17). One limb may be severely insensitive while the other is mildly affected (see Figure 18–1). The loss of vascularity caused by calcified arteries or a disease process is first referred to the vascular surgeon for possible correction or improvement.

The four types of stress that lead to ulceration and destruction of tissue in the neuropathic limb are as follows:

1. Ischemic necrosis is usually seen on the lateral side of the fifth metatarsal head and is due to wearing a shoe that is too narrow. The ischemia is caused by a very low level of pressure (2–3 psi) over a long period of time, causing death of the tissue.
2. Mechanical disruption occurs when a direct injury caused by high pressure (600+ psi) inflicts immediate damage to tissue. This can also be caused by heat or chemicals that damage the skin. Such injuries commonly occur by stepping on a foreign object.
3. Inflammatory destruction occurs with repetitive moderate pressures (40–60 psi). Inflammation develops

and weakens the tissue, leading to callus formation and ulceration from thousands of repetitions per day.

4. Osteomyelitis (and other sepsis) destruction is the result of a moderate force in the presence of infection. Infection is spread as forces are applied by intermittent pressure.[19]

The highest incidence of ulceration occurs at sites of previous ulceration. The history should be reviewed carefully for previous ulcers or infection.[20] A newly healed ulcer is covered by thin skin that is likely to tear. In completely healed ulcer areas, scar tissue may adhere to underlying structures. The healed areas are composed of tissues of different density and, therefore, compress uniquely, causing shear between opposing tissue durometers.[21,22]

The progression of breakdown continues at the metatarsal heads, due to migration of fat pads, leaving bone and skin to absorb shock. The neuropathic limb has lost heat and cold sensation and reflex response. The incidence of ulceration is 71% on the forefoot, with the third metatarsal head most commonly affected, followed by the great toe and first and fifth metatarsal heads. Once breakdown has begun on the foot, 53% of the contralateral limbs follow the progression of breakdown within 4 years.[23] Newly healed wounds need time to mature and become strong, yet there will always be a potential for breakdown in a previous area of ulceration. Scar compresses at a different rate than does other tissue, and the area of adherence will be prone to shear stresses.[23]

Of all amputations, 86% could have been prevented by patient education and appropriate footwear.[3] The aging process alone will produce changes in appearance and alterations in sensitivity, joint motion, and muscle-force production, any of which can lead to dysfunction.[24] Improper nutrition can also delay healing.[25] The majority of amputations are due to gangrene (90%), followed by infection (71%) and nonhealing ulcers (65%).[26] The dry, dark ulcers of gangrene are usually found on toes or bony parts of the foot. Neuropathic ulcers are usually moist and draining.[15] Diabetic neuropathic ulcers occur in a foot with severe sensory impairment, yet they typically have adequate blood supply for healing.[24,27]

There are two types of gangrene: wet and dry. Dry gangrene is due to loss of nourishment to a part, followed by mummification. The area is dry, black, and shriveled, and results in a well-defined line of demarcation with specific localization and self-amputation (autoamputation; Figure 18–3A). Wet gangrene is the necrosis of tissue, followed by destruction caused by excessive moisture. Bacterial gases accumulate in the tissue. The line of demarcation is ill defined, and the limb is painful, purple, and swollen. Wet gangrene is common when infection exists.[28,29] Figure 18–3B shows wet gangrene of the fifth toe. *Do not* debride. The patient needs immediate referral to a surgeon.

SYSTEMS REVIEW AND EXAMINATION

A multisystems review and examination for the patient with neuropathy is required to determine the coimpairments that will affect wound healing and require management. Four systems to review for this patient population are the neuromuscular system, the vascular system, the musculoskeletal system, and the integumentary system.

Neuromuscular System

A foot with neuropathy is dry, with small fissures, has toes that are clawed, and is incapable of sensing trauma. The rigid anesthetic foot is more likely to break down than is a flexible anesthetic foot.[30] The insensitive foot should be evaluated carefully and bilaterally. Any form of peripheral neuropathy can produce the discomfort of paresthesia: prickling, burning, and jabbing sensations.[31,32] The length of this period of discomfort is unknown; it varies among patients. Neuromuscular system examinations to assess for neurologic changes are the focus of the foot screening process and are described in detail later.

Research Wisdom: *Interventions for Paresthesia*

Paresthesia may be helped by use of a transcutaneous electronic nerve stimulator (TENS) unit, which generates small pulses of electricity similar to an electric massage. Another method of controlling the discomfort is with topical creams.[33,34] See Chapter 21, Electrical Stimulation for Wound Healing, for more information.

Vascular System

Peripheral vascular disease (PVD) is a serious complication affecting millions of Americans. Of the 500,000 vascular-related ulcerations, 10% are arterial and 70% are venous ulcerations; some individuals have both venous and arterial diseases.[15] Many patients with neuropathy also have PVD. Therefore, it is critical to review the vascular history before planning any intervention to identify strategies that are being used to manage vascular problems. Some of the related circulatory systems diseases that usually accompany neuropathy and management recommendations are described here. Chapter 17 describes the pathogenesis and management of vascular problems in more detail. Chapter 7 discusses noninvasive vascular testing for patients with diabetes.

Atherosclerosis is also known as hardening of the arteries. The interior wall of arteries is usually smooth but with atherosclerosis platelets, calcium, and connective tissue deposit

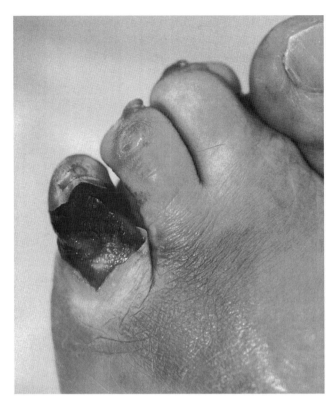

Figure 18–3A Dry gangrene. Such a lesion needs immediate referral to a surgeon. It should not be debrided.

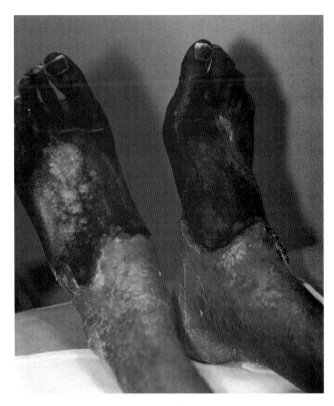

Figure 18–3B Wet gangrene. Such a lesion needs immediate referral to a surgeon. There is probable infection.

on the walls. In early stages, the patient may experience intermittent claudication or cramping in the lower limb, which goes away with rest. As the disease progresses, symptoms appear when the patient is not walking (rest pain).[15] Arterial compromise can be noted by the loss of hair growth, shiny skin, atrophy, and cool skin over the toes.[35] Atherosclerosis leads to impaired circulation in the legs and is one of the most important causes of gangrene, leading to amputation.[36] Arterial ulcers are located on tips or between toes, heel, metatarsal heads, side or sole of foot, and above the lateral malleoli. The ulcer will look punched out, with well-demarcated edges, and be nonbleeding (see *Color Plate 54*). The ulcer base may be deep and pale or black and necrotic. Treatment involves vascular reconstruction, bed rest, and immobilization. Arterial ulcers have a poor prognosis. Misdiagnosis of an arterial ulcer as a venous ulcer can lead to serious complications.

The venous stasis ulceration has a better prognosis for healing than does the arterial ischemic ulceration. Veins are less elastic than are arteries. The valves within veins no longer function to return blood to the heart against gravity, leaving blood to pool in the lower limb. The pooling does not allow new oxygenated blood into the area, and the cell walls of the veins begin to break down. The waste blood products begin to weep through the lower limb. Venous stasis ulcer-

ations are commonly located in the anteromedial malleolus and pretibial areas. The ulcerations are irregular in shape, surrounded by bluish, brown skin. These ulcers are exudative and show evidence of bleeding.

Treatment of venous stasis ulcerations begins with leg elevation.[37] The limb must be treated with compression bandages or an Unna boot. The Unna boot is a semirigid dressing of gelatin and zinc oxide. Its application protects vulnerable skin from the weeping exudate, especially below the ulcer site. The Unna boot is applied wet. When it dries, it forms a nonelastic, nonexpandable, nonshrinkable, porous mold that sticks to the skin. This treatment has been used on venous stasis for 100 years. It is a means of controlling edema when it is applied across a joint. The motion of the joint generates a pumping action.[1]

The chronic venous stasis lower limb without an open ulceration will show signs of edema that must be controlled. The presence of small water blisters or weeping will be a sign that compression should begin (see *Color Plates 59* and *60*). This limb should be treated with pressure-gradiated stockings as daily prevention; an Unna boot with Ace bandage wrap is required for severe edema or periods of breakdown. Pressure-gradiated stockings have a graduated pressure to facilitate pumping action and assist the venous system in removing fluids from the lower limb. Antiembolism stockings are not designed for the ambulatory patient and do not supply the pumping action required. Antiembolism compression is for the recumbent hospitalized patient.

Compression can be ordered to begin at the metatarsal heads and decrease pressure in the calf (neuropathic compression stocking; Figure 18–4) as a further assist to the venous system. Most patients do well with compression in the range of 30–40 mm Hg at the foot and ankle. When using these stockings for the neuropathic/dysvascular patient, remember to avoid seams around bony prominences, and never place a zipper over the malleoli.

When venous stasis ulceration occurs on one limb, begin compression therapy on the contralateral side. The appearance of small water blisters or weeping is a sign that compression should begin. The prosthetic shrinker sock (Figure 18–5) should be used following a major limb amputation to reduce edema and shape the residual limb. The prosthetic shrinker applies both circumferential and vertical (distal to proximal compression).[38] Chapter 10 describes procedures for management of edema.

Musculoskeletal System Examination

The musculoskeletal system examination includes examination of joint integrity, range of motion, skeletal deformity, and muscle strength. Motor neuropathy will distort skeletal alignment, and Charcot joint will leave a foot deformed, as will be shown later in this chapter. An analysis of abnormal gait should also be included. Beginning with the joint range of motion review, it is important that the foot has a dorsiflexion range of at least 10° to allow ambulation without harm to the great toe.[39] The forces on the plantar surface can peak to 275% of body weight when running and 80% when walking.[40] With limited motion in the joints, the trauma can result in ulceration. It is important to test range of motion, as well as to perform manual muscle testing.[2,41] There is an absence of the ankle jerk reflex when neuropathy is advanced to glove-and-stocking distribution.[42]

Leg length discrepancy affects 70–80% of the population and often does not cause pain or deformity. A discrepancy can relate to chronic complications, such as hammertoes, hallux valgus, and referred joint disruption of the ankle, knee, hip, and lower back. A 2-cm discrepancy is sufficient to cause symptoms and requires shoe lifts with physical therapy. Any lift over ¼ inch should be placed on the sole of the shoe and added gradually to allow the body to respond to changes as the pelvis levels.[43]

There is a constant concern with toe deformities that may result in ulceration. In the case of claw toe deformity, the toes are dorsiflexed at the metatarsal-phalangeal joints, with flexion at the interphalangeal joints.[44] The great toe should be examined for deformity. A fibrous proximal joint can cause ulceration that is especially difficult to relieve. Great toe extension can be seen when weight bearing, because the patient will thrust the toe into extension when ambulating, causing calluses and discoloration on the distal tip near the nail from contacting the shoe. Great toe pronation is seen on the medial/plantar surface of the great toe. Hallux rigidus refers to limited range of motion in the proximal great toe metatarsal-phalangeal joint and requires a rigid rocker-bottom shoe to allow ambulation without excessive pressure on

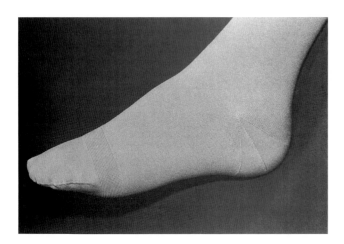

Figure 18–4 The full foot compression stocking begins compression at the metatarsal heads and decreases compression above the ankle to assist in the venous pumping mechanics. Courtesy of Juzo-Julius Zorn, Inc., Cuyahoga Falls, Ohio.

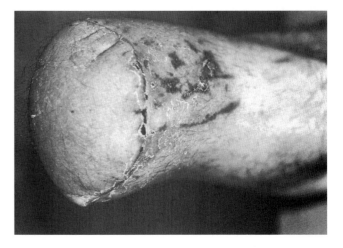

Figure 18–5A The prosthetic shrinker assists in shaping the limb following major amputation surgery. **A,** postop bulbous residual limb of below knee (transtibial) amputee; **B,** application of prosthetic shrinker; **C,** final residual limb shape for prosthetic application.

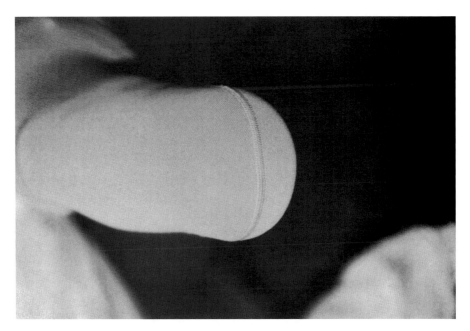

Figure 18–5B
Source: Courtesy of Juzo-Julius Zorn, Inc., Cuyahoga Falls, Ohio.

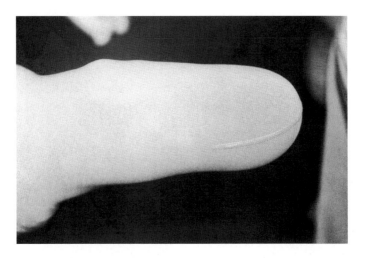

Figure 18–5C
Source: Courtesy of Juzo-Julius Zorn, Inc., Cuyahoga Falls, Ohio.

the great toe. Hallux valgus (bunion) is the increased valgus angle of the great toe in relation to the metatarsal, requiring a shoe that can be modified and molded to conform to the medial bunion formation.

Toe amputations may be for single or multiple toes (see Figure 18–1). The amputation may be a disarticulation or a resection (metatarsal shaft is removed). The distal end of the amputation site must be followed carefully and protected from trauma.

There are common complications to be addressed with the neuropathic limb. Bursa formation over the navicular prominence is due to the constant high forces and must be provided with an area of pressure relief before ulceration occurs. A sinus tract formation will result when previous areas of ulceration heal over a pocket of bacteria instead of healing from internal to external tissues. The small pocket of bacteria will be moved anteriorly through the tissues, causing infection to spread.

A common complication of the neuropathic patient is severe foot deformity following neuropathic fractures or Charcot arthropathy (discussed later in this chapter), including joint subluxation or dislocation. The presence of severe foot deformity has been shown to be predictive of prolonged healing time for patients treated with total-contact casting (TCC). Sinacore et al[45] found that fixed foot deformity prolonged healing of ulcers with TCC when located in the midfoot and rearfoot. Ulcers located in the midfoot healed in 73 ± 29 days, and rearfoot ulcers healed in 90 ± 19 days. Individuals without fixed deformities with chronic diabetes mellitus and those with forefoot ulcers healed in 41 days. Therefore, early detection during the musculoskeletal examination of a fixed foot deformity in a patient with an ulcer located in the midfoot or rearfoot can be used to determine a prognosis that healing time will be significantly longer when a TCC is used as the treatment intervention.

Motor neuropathy produces common abnormal gait characteristics in the neuropathic population. The shoes are worn on the lateral side of the sole because of a varus deformity (see Figure 18–6A). This weakness often causes ankle injuries. After further deterioration, footdrop can occur. The stiffness in the complex joint structures leads to abnormal motion in the foot's function.

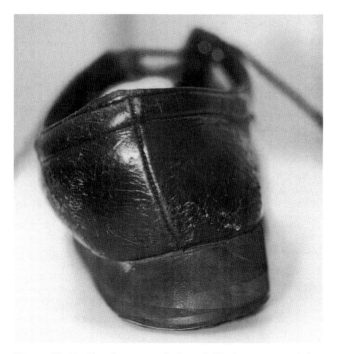

Figure 18–6A Shoe is worn on the lateral side due to a varus deformity. *Source:* Reprinted with permission from R.B. Chambers and N. Elftman, Orthotic Management of the Neuropathic and Dysvascular Patient, in *Atlas of Orthoses and Assistive Devices*, 3rd edition, B. Goldberg and J.D. Hsu, eds., p. 443, © 1997, Mosby-Year Book, Inc.

Clinical Wisdom:
Modification of a Standard-Depth Shoe

To compensate for varus gait abnormalities, shoes need to be modified. The modifications required are (1) a full, lateral-flare sole, as shown in Figure 18–6B, (2) a strong counter to support the heel, and (3) a high top to support the ankle. A standard-depth shoe can be modified by an orthotist, or a shoe repairperson may be able to do the job, if guided. Although not all orthotists will agree to modify an existing shoe, others will. This will save the patient money.

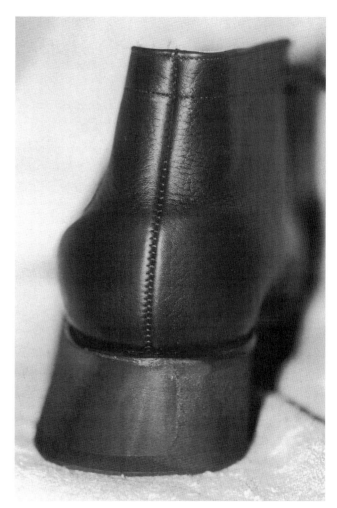

Figure 18–6B Standard-depth shoe with sole modification. The shoe has a full-flare sole, a strong counter, and a high top to stabilize the varus abnormality. *Source:* Reprinted with permission from R.B. Chambers and N. Elftman, Orthotic Management of the Neuropathic and Dysvascular Patient, in *Atlas of Orthoses and Assistive Devices*, 3rd edition, B. Goldberg and J.D. Hsu, eds., p. 433, © 1997, Mosby-Year Book, Inc.

Integumentary System Examination

Integumentary system examination of the foot includes the toenails. Toenail deformities are commonly seen in the neuropathic foot. Hypertrophic nails are caused by onychomycosis (fungus) infection (see Figure 18–7) and are common in the diabetic population. The nails tear shoe lining and create areas of rough surface to abrade the toes. Nail care for fungus, ingrown toenails, and trimming must be performed by trained medical personnel to ensure that injury is not inflicted. Soft corns are hyperkeratotic lesions found between toes (usually between the fourth and fifth toes), due to pressure of an opposing toe in a region that is moist.[29] Injury and maceration of the toes is commonly controlled by the use of lamb's wool between the toes or tube foam to space toes and prevent friction (Figure 18–8A, B, and C, Exhibit 18–1). Buildup of callus is indicative of high pressures and stress of an isolated area that must be relieved. The thickening of the skin in the area of a callus is preceded by abnormal pressure or friction.[29,46] Areas of excess pressure require pressure redistribution in the clinic setting, rather than scheduling additional appointments.

Dryness of the skin is the result of autonomic neuropathy in which the sweat and oil production is decreased and moisture must be replaced. Loss of hair growth may be indicative of vascular impairment. Ulcerations that are necrotic are debrided to allow healing to progress from internal to external tissues for optimum closure of the ulcer site.

> **Clinical Wisdom:** *Tube Foam and Lamb's Wool for Quick Relief of Pressure on Toes*
>
> Claw toes, hammer toes, calluses, corns, and small ulcerations can be relieved of pressure by inserts and shoe modifications and spaced with tube foam or lamb's wool separators to allow air flow. Separators prevent maceration and skin breakdown; they should be removed before and replaced after bathing. In addition, the custom tube foam separator serves as a toe separator, reduces shear from the shoe, cushions metatarsal heads, and can be used as a positioner for overlapping toes. Figure 18–8A shows lamb's wool pieces placed between toes. Figure 18–8B shows a tube foam toe separator in place. Figure 18–8C and Exhibit 18–1 illustrate and describe the diagram of steps to create a tube foam separator. The tube foam is available from podiatric supply companies.

Another common occurrence is burns, due to either heat or chemicals, such as over-the-counter remedies. Soaking the foot in hot water is a specific cause of burns. A common wisdom is that neuropathic patients should *never* soak their

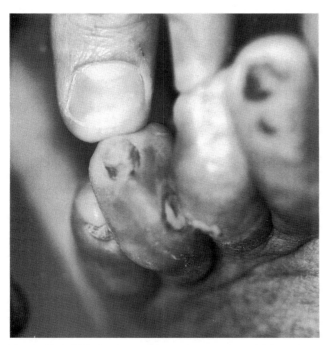

Figure 18–7 This foot has soft corns between toes, thickened toenails, and onychomycosis (fungal) infection.

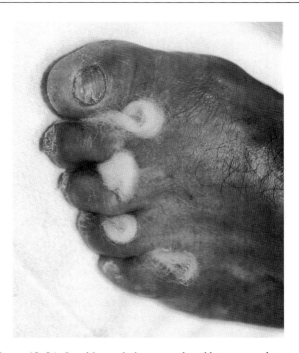

Figure 18–8A Lamb's wool pieces are placed between each toe to prevent maceration. They should be replaced after bathing. *Source:* Reprinted with permission from R.B. Chambers and N. Elftman, Orthotic Management of the Neuropathic and Dysvascular Patient, in *Atlas of Orthoses and Assistive Devices*, 3rd edition, B. Goldberg and J.D. Hsu, eds., p. 441, © 1997, Mosby-Year Book, Inc.

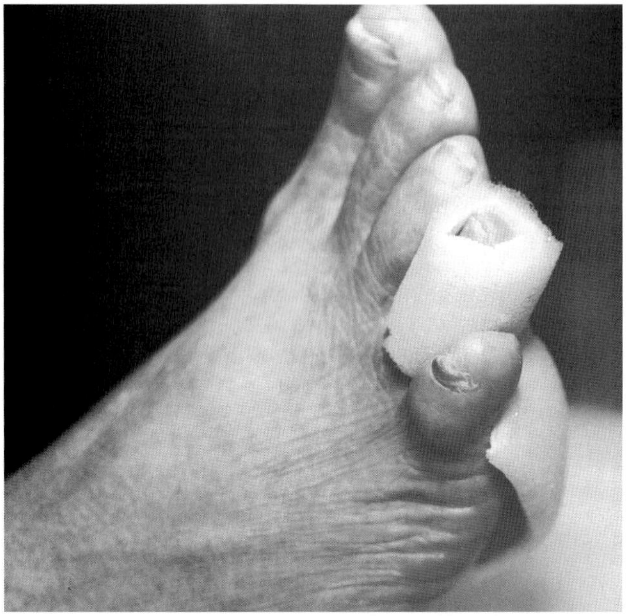

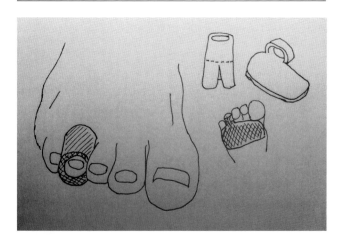

Figure 18–8B A custom tube foam toe separator. *Source:* Reprinted with permission from R.B. Chambers and N. Elftman, Orthotic Management of the Neuropathic and Dysvascular Patient, in *Atlas of Orthoses and Assistive Devices*, 3rd edition, B. Goldberg and J.D. Hsu, eds., p. 431, © 1997, Mosby-Year Book, Inc.

Figure 18–8C Diagram of construction of a tube foam separator.

Exhibit 18–1 Instructions To Make a Foam Toe Separator

Make a custom foam toe separator (Figures 18–8B and 18–8C) by the following steps:

1. Select a size of tube foam with a diameter that will not constrict the toe.
2. Cut a 2 ½–3-inch piece of the foam.
3. To make the toe cuff:
   a. Measure back ½ to ¾ inch from one end of the tube foam and mark.
   b. Cut across the diameter of the tube three fourths of the way through.
   c. Slit up the tube to the marking on the side that is cut to the diameter cut (see diagram)
   d. The foam will flatten out (see diagram).
   e. The tube will slip over the toe and the flat section will be located on the plantar surface of the foot.

feet. The insensitive foot cannot produce the warning signals necessary to prevent severe burns (see Chapter 5).

Dermatologic conditions can affect treatment programs until they are resolved. Necrobiosis lipoidica diabeticorum may be seen on the shin (along tibia) as a dermatologic condition in diabetic patients (Figure 18–9). The condition manifests as irregular patches of degenerated collagen with reduced numbers of fibrocytes. The dry, scaly areas have been infiltrated with chronic inflammatory cells.[47] Necrobiosis can be confused with venous stasis disease but does not require or respond to extensive treatment. The round, firm plaques of reddish brown to yellow are seen three times more often in women than in men.[48,49] These ulcerations are common along the tibia and require only protective dressings.

The callus (or tyloma) is a yellowish-gray lesion that may be flat or raised and spread over a large area. The callus is caused by friction (shear), irritation, and/or pressure. There is hyperemia and thickening of the skin. The skin is compressed, and superficial layers of callus are laid down. The callus may be reduced mechanically with tools and the forces to the area reduced. Many facilities use sanding tools and callus reducers to break the chain of callus buildup. The pumice stone is used as a wet tool on wet skin. The callus reducer debrides dry callus with a dry tool (Figure 18–10).[50]

Keratoderma plantaris, characterized by keratin cracks and ulcerations, is caused by the loss of sweat and oil elasticity in the skin (autonomic neuropathy). As keratin builds up, it creates small fissures that allow entrance of bacteria, and infection begins. The entire sole around the margin of the heel will undergo diffuse thickening and develop painful fissures if the foot is sensate or will go undetected if insensate (see Figure 18–11). Prevention includes reduction of keratin buildup and retention of skin moisture.[29] There are many forms of rashes and dermatologic conditions that must be evaluated and treated in the neuropathic limb. These are usually discovered by inspection, rather than patient discomfort. Typical skin conditions in the diabetic population include shin spots and diabetic bullae (with less frequency than necrobiosis).[48]

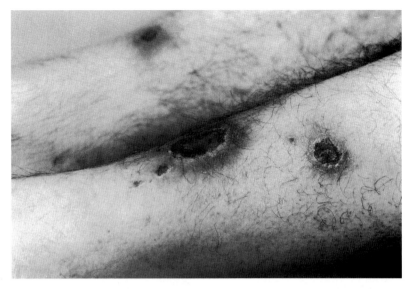

Figure 18–9 Necrobiosis lipoidica diabeticorum: a dermatologic condition often present in the diabetic, neuropathic limb.

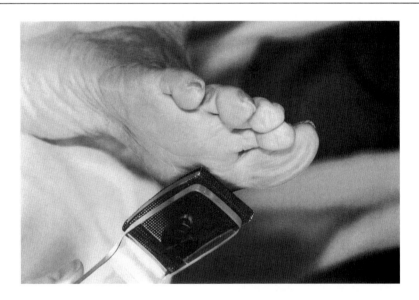

Figure 18–10 Callus reducer: a tool used dry on dry callus to remove buildup and reduce the superficial layers.

Infections are commonly seen in the neuropathic foot, including *Pseudomonas* infection, which is bacterial growth that occurs within a moist environment. Signs and symptoms of infection are usually absent in the neuropathic foot, even though the infection is present and virulent, due to impaired circulation and immunosuppression. Both are other common coimpairments of neuropathy. The problems of infection are identified during the integumentary system review. See Chapter 9, "Management of Exudate and Infection," for

strategies to assess and treat infection and Chapter 23, Ultraviolet Light and Wound Healing.

Dry gangrene is another finding that may be discovered during the integumentary system review. When dry gangrene is present, there is a line of demarcation at which the body will autoamputate the affected area. This process of autoamputation could take weeks to months;[44] it is nature's way of protecting the body from infection and should not be disturbed. Figure 18–3A (Wagner grade 5, discussed below) is

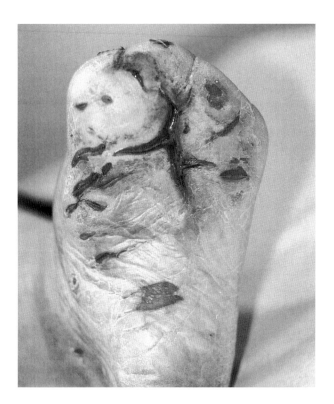

Figure 18–11 Typical neuropathic foot with keratoderma plantaris. Note the dry, cracked skin, dirt imbedded in the skin, open wounds, and the absence of dressing, due to lack of awareness of the condition.

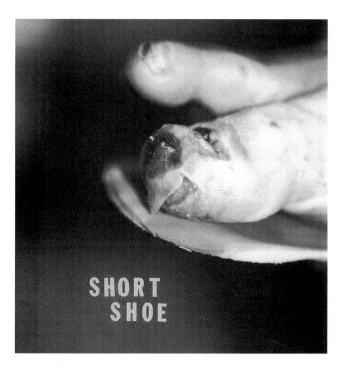

Figure 18–12 Short shoe. The toe extends to the end of the insole. *Source:* Reprinted with permission from N. Elftman, Clinical Management of the Neuropathic Limb, *Journal of Prosthetics and Orthotics*, Vol. 4, No. 1, pp. 1–12, Copyright © American Academy of Orthotists and Prosthetists.

a photograph of a foot with dry gangrene. A patient with dry gangrene needs immediate referral to the surgeon.

FURTHER VISUAL AND PHYSICAL ASSESSMENTS

Examination of the neuropathic limb includes further visual and physical examination to avoid future complications. The patient is never asked for his or her own foot evaluation. The shoes are removed to allow the practitioner to examine the foot. The neuropathic patient will not limp, even with a foot ulceration (see Figures 18–11 and 18–12). Inspection should be both weight bearing and non–weight bearing.

Footwear Assessment

The footwear must be examined for wear of orthosis and sock patterns indicating excessive pressure. The ends of the toes should be examined for injury caused by a short shoe. Figure 18–12 shows a toe wound caused by a short shoe. Notice that the toe extends to the end of the shoe insole. Alignment is required when fitting a shoe for proper weight

distribution and length measurement, and will be discussed later in this chapter. The interventions section of this chapter describes orthotics and adaptive equipment and includes instructions in footwear interventions. Shoes should show a normal wear pattern on the lateral heel of the sole, as contrasted with the pattern in Figure 18–6A. Shoes should be resoled on a regular basis to keep sides from wearing down. Inserts are replaced as required when relief modifications are no longer sufficient and shock absorption is decreased.

Wound Assessment

The Wagner scale[51] for grading neuropathic ulcers classifies ulcer severity in six grades, based on the depth of the ulcer and the presence of infection or necrosis. Ulcer grading is useful for prognosis and for selection of treatment intervention. In addition, the Wagner ulcer grading system is a uniform system that is used by health care practitioners of different disciplines to describe ulcers in neuropathic limbs. Ulcers with low grades are managed by conservative measures, whereas ulcers with higher grades are a direct threat to limb loss and require surgical management. The neuropathic limb often suffers from dysvascularity, as well; therefore, the system is often used for both populations. The Wagner ulcer classification system differs from other grading systems by including a grade of zero, which describes preulcerative skin, healed ulcers, and the presence of a bony deformity where the skin is intact (Figure 18–13A). Preulcerative areas include calluses located under the metatarsal heads or areas of weight bearing.[52] For continuity of documentation and communication, the team must understand the Wagner scale of ulcer grading and use it consistently. Exhibit 18–2 shows the six Wagner ulcer grades. The preferred conservative method of treatment is guided by the Wagner grade. Exhibit 18–3 shows how the different grades dictate different treatment strategies.[53]

Sensation Testing

When evaluated for insensitivity, most patients who had hypoesthesia could sense pinprick and cotton wisp applications. Patients with foot ulcers were observed to have less *pressure sensation* than did those without foot ulcers.[54] In 1898, von Frey attempted to standardize the stimuli for testing the subjective sense of light touch by using a series of horse hairs of varying thicknesses and stiffness. Wienstein used nylon monofilaments mounted on Lucite rods as substitutes for the hairs.[55] The Semmes-Wienstein monofilaments can be obtained commercially in elaborate sets for precise measurement, but research at Carville Hansen's Disease Center in Carville, Louisiana, has consolidated the testing to three sizes of monofilaments for grading the insensitive foot (Exhibit 18–4).[56] The 4.17 monofilament supplies 1 g of force and is indicative of normal sensation. If the patient cannot feel the next monofilament (5.07), he or she does not have the protective sensation level of 10 g and cannot sense trauma to the foot to cease weight bearing. Failure to sense the 10-g monofilament is used as the determining factor for use of protective footwear and accommodative orthotics. No patient with protective sensation can ambulate on an ulcerated foot. A large percentage of patients do not feel the largest monofilament (6.10), which indicates a loss of sensation at 75 g. This largest-diameter monofilament indicates an insensate foot that must be accommodated and followed closely. Use of the monofilament is not to be confused with the testing for sharp/dull sensation. The sharp/dull test stimulates multiple nerves, as opposed to a single-point perception test.

The monofilament is a single-point perception test and requires the examiner to place the monofilament on the skin, press until the monofilament bends (diameter of monofilament controls point of bend), and remove it from the skin surface. The monofilaments are tested and determined to be reliable at the 95% confidence level.[56] The patient is to respond when he or she feels the pressure sensation. To avoid errors in testing, the monofilament is never used in areas of scarring, calluses, or necrotic tissue. The bilateral testing for sensation is especially important for the unilateral and bilateral amputee to determine areas of insensitivity and progression of the neuropathy. Figure 18–14 shows the proper method for the monofilament testing procedure. Note the bend of the monofilament. This must occur to measure correct pressure sensation.

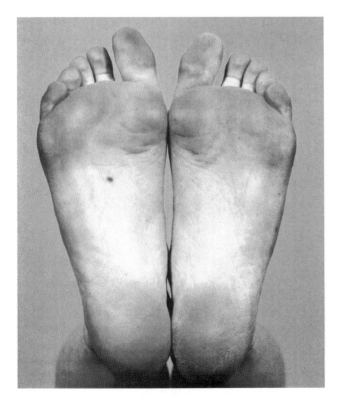

Figure 18–13A Skin intact, Wagner grade 0.

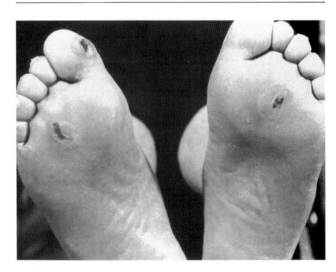

Figure 18–13B Superficial ulcer, Wagner grade 1.

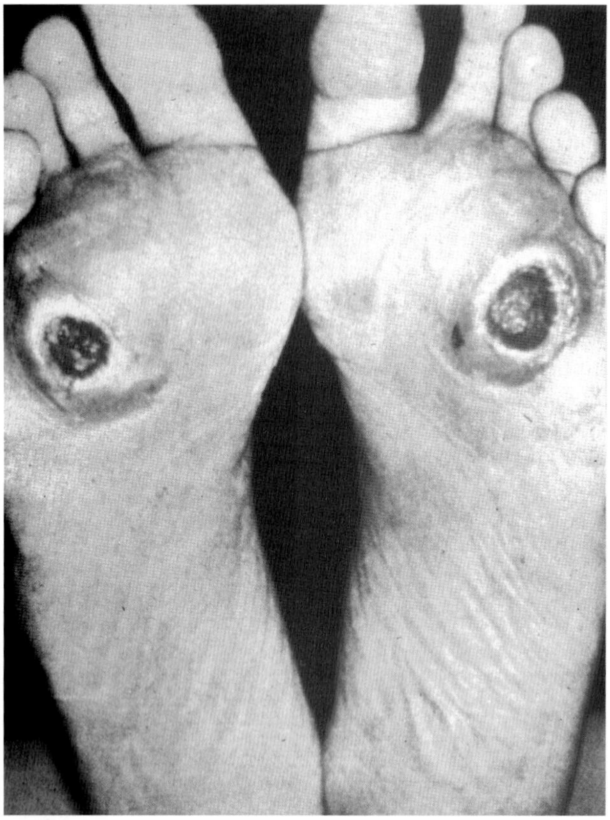

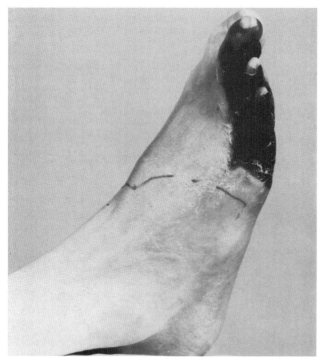

Figure 18–13C Deeper ulcer to tendon or bone, Wagner grade 2.

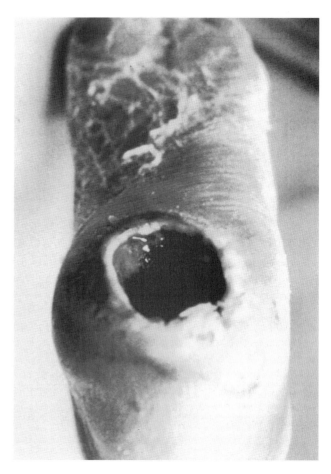

Figure 18–13D Ulcer has abscess or osteomyelitis, Wagner grade 3.

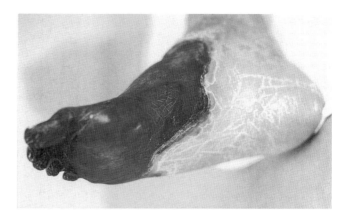

Figure 18–13E Gangrene on forefoot, Wagner grade 4.

Figure 18–13F Gangrene over major portion of foot, Wagner grade 5.

Exhibit 18–2 Wagner Scale

Grade	Description
Grade 0	Skin intact (Figure 18–13A)
Grade 1	Superficial ulcer (Figure 18–13B)
Grade 2	Deeper ulcer to tendon or bone (Figure 18–13C)
Grade 3	Ulcer has abscess or osteomyelitis (Figure 18–13D)
Grade 4	Gangrene on forefoot (Figure 18–13E)
Grade 5	Gangrene over major portion of foot (Figure 18–13F)

Source: Reprinted with permission from F.E.W. Wagner, the Dysvascular Foot: A System for Diagnosis and Treatment, *Foot and Ankle*, 2:64–122, © 1981, American Orthopaedic Foot and Ankle Society.

Exhibit 18–3 Conservative Management by Wagner Ulcer Grade

Wagner Ulcer Grade and Recommended Treatment

Grade 0—may be treated with extra-depth shoe and insert

Grade 1—cast or Plastazote healing shoe, reducing weight to ulceration; antibiotic intervention as required[52]

Grade 2—debridement and cast; antibiotic intervention as required[52]

Grade 3—remove infected tissue and cast; antibiotic intervention as required[53]

Source: Data from M. Glugla and G. Mulder, The Diabetic Foot, in *Medical Management of Foot Ulcers in Chronic Wound Care: A Clinical Source Book for Healthcare Professionals*, D. Krasner, ed., pp. 223–239, © 1990, Mosby/Health Management Publications, Inc., and F.A. Wagner, *A Classification and Treatment Program for Diabetic, Neuropathic and Dysvascular Foot Problems*, pp. 1–47, © 1983.

At Hansen's Disease Center, Birke[57] developed a risk classification system based on the loss of protective sensation. Loss of protective sensation, history of prior ulceration, and reduced circulatory perfusion are important factors in development of foot ulcers. A risk classification system based on these factors is useful in identifying patients who would benefit from different levels of intervention (Exhibit 18–3). Risk is classified by four grades: 0, no loss of protective sensation; 1, loss of protective sensation (no deformity or history of plantar ulceration); 2, loss of protective sensation and deformity or abnormal blood flow without history of plantar ulcer; and 3, history of plantar ulcer. Three interventions have proven effective in reducing risk of ulceration: protective footwear, patient education, and frequent clinic follow-up. For example, when a patient's ulcer is grade 0, preulceration, and the patient can sense the 10-g monofilament (has protective sensation), he or she will sense pain before damage occurs to the feet. Patients in this category usually do well with a standard shoe of correct sizing and a simple shock-absorbing pad.

The patient without protective sensation will not cease ambulating when damage begins to tissues. Patients with feet such as those in Figure 18–11 who walk into the clinic are insensate. They require extra-depth shoes with a total-contact accommodative insert to distribute pressure and reduce forces on areas of potential breakdown. The insert may be molded to the patient or fabricated on a cast. The cast does not have corrective forces added, only accommodation.

The accommodative insert does not apply correction; it fills only the spaces between the flat shoe and the foot contours. Any force added will receive full weight bearing, and breakdown will occur. If the addition of metatarsal head (MTH) pads or scaphoid pads is requested, these pads must

be of a soft durometer. Rigid pad additions will cause excess pressure and ulcerations. The MTH pads are placed proximal to the MTHs to redistribute the weight from the heads to the metatarsal shafts (Figure 18–15).

Testing for vibratory sensation may be accomplished by using the bioesthesiometer. This instrument is essentially an electrical tuning fork that uses repetitive mechanical indentation of skin delivered at a prescribed frequency and amplitude.[58] The simple graduated tuning fork is a rapid means of sensory testing.[59,60] The purpose of all sensory testing equipment is to identify those at risk.[61]

Upper and lower extremity peripheral neuropathy is present when sensation testing reveals that the level of sensation loss is symmetric and equidistant from the spine in both arms and legs. The hands of these patients should be considered in the evaluation process. Physical signs of upper extremity involvement include chaeroarthropathy (motor neuropathy in upper extremity), when the patient cannot touch the palms together in the prayer position. Another physical sign is atrophy of the web space between the thumb and first finger. This is the first sign of motor neuropathy in the hand. Consideration of the hand deficit must be taken into account for donning, doffing, and choice of closures for orthotics and footwear.[41] Little attention has been paid to the diabetic hand syndrome, or limited joint mobility (LJM), in which the joints of the fingers and wrists become limited. This condition occurs in 30–50% of people who have had type I diabetes for more than 15 years. One test for LJM is performed by having the patient place the hands flat on a table. Patients with severe LJM will not be able to flatten the fingers onto the table. The skin will also be thick and can be tented on the back of the metacarpophalangeal (MCP) joint[62] (see Figure 18–16).

Exhibit 18–4 Foot Evaluation Form

PATIENT		DIAGNOSIS
CODE _____ ORTHOTIST		DATE _____

INSENSITIVE FEET WITHOUT ULCERATION

CATEGORY	MONOFILAMENT RESPONSE		ULCER	DEFORMITY	FOLLOW-UP	INSERT
A	+5.07	(10 g)	No	Yes/No	12 Mo	Cushion
B	−5.07	(10 g)	No	No	6 Mo	Molded
C	−5.07	(10 g)	No	Yes	4 Mo	Molded
D	−5.07	(10 g)	Yes	Yes/No	3 Mo	Molded
E	−6.10	(75 g)	Yes/No	Yes/No	2 Mo	Molded

ULCER GRADE

0 Intact Skin
1 Superficial
2 Tendon or Bone
3 Abscess or Osteo
4 Forefoot Gangrene
5 Foot Gangrene

CHARCOT ARTHROPATHY

☐ Active ☐ Hx
L/R
___ Phalanges
___ Forefoot
___ Midfoot
___ Hindfoot
___ Other

FOOT DEFORMITY

__ Pes Cavus
__ Pes Planus
__ Valgus
__ Varus

TOE DEFORMITY

Claw Toe   Hallux
__ Mild   __ Valgus
__ Severe   __ Rigidus
__ Rigid   __ Extension

COMPLICATIONS

Proximal Neuropathy

☐ Calf
☐ Knee
☐ Thigh

Upper Ext. Neuropathy

☐ Fingers
☐ Hands
☐ Forearm

☐ Dialysis
☐ Vascular Impairment
☐ Venous Stasis
☐ Retinopathy
☐ Proprioception
☐ **Dermatologic Breakdown**
☐ **Fungal Nail**

Edema Control
☐ Full Foot
☐ Other

DORSAL

RIGHT   LEFT

Source: Reprinted with permission from R.B. Chambers and N. Elftman, Orthotic Management of the Neuropathic and Dysvascular Patient, in *Atlas of Orthoses and Assistive Devices,* 3rd edition, B. Goldberg and J.D. Hsu, eds., p. 441, © 1997, Mosby-Year Book, Inc.

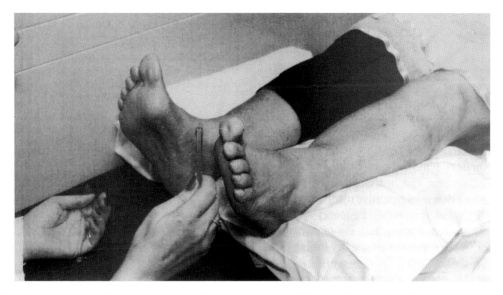

Figure 18–14 Monofilament testing. *Source:* Reprinted with permission from R.B. Chambers and N. Elftman, Orthotic Management of the Neuropathic and Dysvascular Patient, in *Atlas of Orthoses and Assistive Devices*, 3rd edition, B. Goldberg and J.D. Hsu, eds., p. 433, © 1997, Mosby-Year Book.

Body Temperature Testing

Since the time of Hippocrates, physicians have known that body temperature variations offer important clues for diagnosing disease. Diagnostic tools convert infrared radiation and display it on monitors with the use of thermography.[60] There are many methods of acquiring surface temperatures. The objectives and procedure for doing so are listed in the box below.

Thermistors or thermocouples are accurate recording devices that, when touched to the skin for 10 seconds, give a numeric display of temperature.[63] Wound temperature depends on the vascularity of the area and can be measured by thermography. In a study of vascular wounds, vascularity was measured indirectly by measuring skin temperatures. The subject surgical site was measured prior to surgery and postoperatively for 8 days at a specified time. The first- through third-day temperatures increased at the surgi-

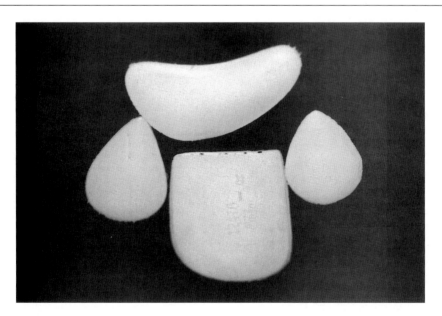

Figure 18–15 Metatarsal pads made of soft durometer to aid in pressure relief of metatarsal heads and increase transverse arch of foot. Courtesy of UCO International, Inc., Wheeling, Illinois.

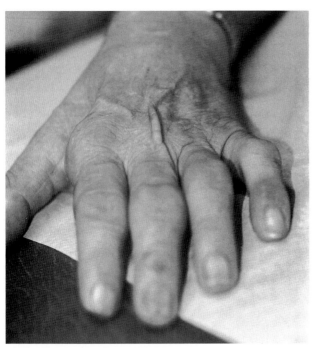

Figure 18–16 Neuropathic hand. Motor neuropathy testing reveals tenting on the back of the MCP joint, clawing of the fingers, and atrophy of the web space between the thumb and the first finger.

cal wound and a wide surrounding area. Days 4 through 8 had lower temperatures, and the zones of warm surrounding area became narrower. The stitches were removed at day 7, and, by day 8, the area assumed preoperative temperatures, except in the very narrow incisional site. Documentation noted that the persistence of a wider zone of increased temperatures after day 4 predicts wound infection and disturbed healing.[64] The infrared scanner thermometer unit (Figure 18–17A and B) allows accurate, immediate spot temperature reading and the feature of scanning the foot quickly.

The use of temperature is valuable as an objective measurement of tissue damage and inflammation produced by repeated mechanical (pressure) trauma.[65] When evaluating the limb, the most distal aspects of extremities are cool. Muscular areas with good blood supply are warmer than bony regions. Arches are several degrees warmer than heels or toes.[63] Excessive heat in an area of the foot is a vascular response to trauma. The trauma may be due to external forces, infection, Charcot joint, or other internal complications. The examiner can feel the increased heat manually and determine where complications may reside, but without instrumentation to record actual numbers, there will not be objective documentation for follow-up and comparison. Using a surface-sensing temperature device (thermocouple or infrared), temperatures are recorded in predetermined areas, usually those related to common areas of breakdown. When there is one definite area whose temperature is 3° F higher than that

of adjacent areas, it can be assumed to be an area of high pressure or stress. If there is no current breakdown, this area must be relieved of pressure and the pressure distributed over the remaining weight-bearing surfaces. Upon follow-up of this same patient, the temperature differentiation should decrease as healing of tissue progresses. In a comparison of contralateral limbs, vascular impairment should be suspected when one limb is significantly colder or distal portions of the foot show an extreme drop in temperature. A chronic hot spot points to the fact that there is a chronic stress or an underlying bone or joint problem. Increased temperature tells that there is a problem and where it is—not what it is![21]

Objectives and Procedure for Taking Temperature

Objectives for taking temperature:

- To evaluate baseline temperature at sites of high incidence of ulceration
- To determine presence of inflammation
- To evaluate sites of baseline elevated temperature for decrease in temperature after intervention to relieve pressure

Procedure for taking and recording temperatures:

1. Expose the bare skin of the foot to the room temperature for 5–10 minutes before recording any temperature.
2. Take temperature at 10 locations on the sole of foot and toes (shown by circles on foot evaluation form Exhibit 18–4).
3. Follow steps for measuring temperature.
4. Record readings in degrees at each location on foot evaluation form and date.
5. Record readings at each location on successive evaluations below the initial reading and date.

Procedure for Use of an Infrared Scanner Thermometer

Follow these steps in measuring temperature with an infrared scanner thermometer:

1. Temperature testing may be done with or without contact of skin.
2. Read the first number seen.
3. Avoid pressure against the skin that causes ischemia.

Courtesy of Measurements, LLC, New Orleans, Louisiana. (See Figures 18–17A and 18–17B.)

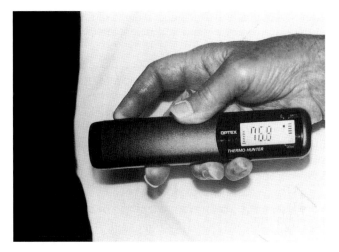

Figure 18–17A Measurements, Inc. infrared thermometer. Courtesy of Measurements, LLC, New Orleans, Louisiana.

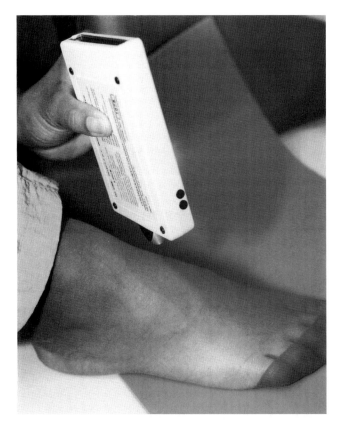

Figure 18–17B Deltatrak infrared thermometer. Courtesy of Measurements, LLC, New Orleans, Louisiana.

Pressure Testing

A rubber mat was developed by R.I. Harris that would print light foot pressures in large, light squares (formed by tall grid ridges) and heavier pressures in darker, smaller squares (deep ridges).[2] The Harris mat will give a grid analysis of pressure distribution at a relatively low cost per patient. The Harris mat can be used for static and dynamic assessment and can provide permanent records. Figure 18–18 shows an imprint on a Harris mat. The darker areas are areas of high pressure.

Force plates have given us valuable information regarding peak pressures during ambulation but represent a single step on the plate. Attempts to place sensors in the shoes have been unreliable because of the sensor structure and attachment within the shoe.[66] The new age of computer-aided documentation provides color replicas of three-dimensional pressure recordings and illustrations that can be used for static or dynamic documentation. Although costs of the computer-aided devices are high, technology is advancing to provide unrestricted data collection.[67] Progress is also being made to produce live scanning of the foot in order to provide a positive mold for orthotics, as well as for custom shoes.[68] Using computed three-dimensional, digital computer graphics, a plastic sock may be molded to the patient and converted to a shoe cast.[69]

Charcot Joint Examination

Charcot joint (Charcot arthropathy) is a relatively painless, progressive, and degenerative arthropathy of single or multiple joints, caused by underlying neuropathy. The neuropathy may be periosteal and not cutaneous. There are several theories behind the causes of Charcot joint, as follows:

- Multiple microtraumas to the joints cause microfractures. These fractures lead to relaxation of the ligaments and joint destruction.[70]

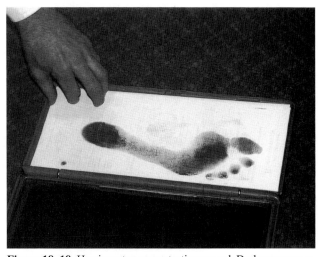

Figure 18–18 Harris mat pressure testing record. Darker areas represent higher pressure.

- There is increased blood flow (osteolysis) and bone re-absorption. Patients with Charcot joints have bounding pulses.
- Changes in the spinal cord lead to trophic changes in bones and joints.
- Osteoporosis is accompanied by an abnormal brittleness of the bones, leading to spontaneous fracture.[71]

In clinical observations, the limb is usually painless, swollen, and red. Unhealed painless fractures are often radiographically present. In advanced Charcot disease, there are multiple fractures, accompanied by extensive bone demineralization and reabsorption. Later stages reveal architectural distortion of the foot, with shortening and widening of the joint.[49] The foot joints most commonly affected are the following:

- tarsometatarsal (30%)
- metatarsophalangeal (30%)
- tarsus (24%)
- interphalangeal (4%)

Charcot joint is frequently misdiagnosed and mistreated, leaving the patient with deformities that require further medical intervention and/or expensive footwear (see Figure 18–19). The acute stage will show a foot that is 5–10° hotter than the contralateral limb in the same area. The red, hot, swollen foot will usually not have a skin opening or ulcer-

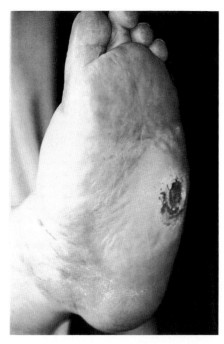

Figure 18–19 Classic Charcot rocker bottom foot deformity. Note ulceration over bony deformity surrounded by callus formation.

ation. Laboratory tests, including radiographs, may not show changes in the acute stage to differentiate Charcot disease from other diagnoses.

The duration of the catastrophic destruction, dissociation, and eventual recalcification found with Charcot joint will vary with the individual, but the average healing time in a cast for the hindfoot is 12 months; for the midfoot, 9 months; and for the forefoot, 6 months. By evaluating with comparative temperature measurements of the contralateral foot, the stages can usually be verified by radiograph. As the involved foot temperature increases, the destruction and dissociation are taking place. The temperature gradually decreases as recalcification is in progress. A radiograph shows that recalcification is complete when temperatures bilaterally are within 3° F.

The treatment plan for acute Charcot joint is the TCC. The cast must be changed in 1 week to accommodate volume changes. Following the period of volume changes, the cast should be changed every 2–3 weeks. When the temperature is equal to that of the other limb, the patient may be weaned gradually from the cast to a splint, then to shoes. Follow-up should continue to ensure that there is no recurrence of an episode of Charcot joint.

Osteomyelitis Examination

The clinical observations for Charcot joint and osteomyelitis are very similar, and the patient should be monitored closely to verify the diagnosis. Laboratory tests will also be similar. The only exception would be the presence of an opening in the skin to allow an entrance for bacteria to infect the bone (see Figure 18–20A). Take the temperature over the best surrounding skin. Refer for immediate medical management. The recalcification would not occur radiographically as in Charcot disease (Figure 18–20B.) Verification may be made for osteomyelitis with a three-phase bone scan or biopsy.[20]

Diabetic patients with foot ulcers that expose bone should be treated for osteomyelitis, even if there is no evidence of inflammation.[72]

INTERVENTIONS

Orthotics and Adaptive Equipment

Treatment of the neuropathic foot requires accommodation, relief of pressure/shear forces, and shock absorption. Regardless of materials used for accommodative inserts, the combination of materials must be compressible by one-half of original thickness to accommodate for pressure relief through the gait cycle.[21] It is important to evaluate the materials you will be utilizing in the manufacture of inserts. Cellular polyethylene foams, such as Aliplast, Plastazote,

---

Case Study: *Charcot Arthropathy*

The patient was a 44-year-old woman with a 15-year history of non–insulin-dependent diabetes mellitus (NIDDM). She had neuropathic extremities to mid-calf bilaterally, loss of sensation and motor function demonstrated by bilateral drop foot. She had a right foot Charcot arthropathy post 4 years. The extremity was treated with a series of total-contact casts for 11 months and gradually weaned to ankle-foot orthotics with shoes. Contralateral side used ankle-foot orthosis to control drop foot.

The patient came to the clinic for an emergency check-up due to weekend traumatic injury to the left foot. She recalls twisting the left ankle and slight discomfort. Within an hour, there was swelling so she went to a local emergency department. The patient was told that she had possibly torn a ligament and was put in a precautionary plaster cast with a rubber walking pad.

When the patient came to the clinic two days later, she was in a great deal of discomfort and the plaster cast seemed to have absorbed exudate. The toes were left exposed in the cast and had swollen beyond the confines of the distal cast edge. When the cast was removed, it was observed that the walking pad had been forced through the plaster on the plantar surface and traumatized the entire plantar midfoot. The patient had Charcot arthropathy of the midfoot that was further destroyed by the nonreinforced walking pad. The edges of the plaster caused open abrasions to the exposed toes, leading to infection.

The patient was treated for abrasions and put into a total-contact cast. After 16 months, the Charcot episode was over but the foot was left with deformities that could not be accommodated in a standard shoe. A custom shoe was ordered for the left foot deformity.

Key Points

1. Immediate total-contact casting could have reduced the deformities and length of treatment.
2. A total-contact cast differs from a standard short leg cast and should be applied by a skilled technician.

---

and Pelite, are composed of a mass of bubbles in a plastic and gas phase. The bubbles are cells with lines of intersection called *ribs* or *strands*, and the walls are called *windows*. In closed-cell materials the gases do not pass freely; open-cell material has no windows, leaving many cells interconnected so that gas may pass between cells. Cell walls are not totally impermeable to the flow of gases. Under a sustained load (especially the heavy patient), gases are squeezed out; when the load is removed, gases are drawn back into the cells.[73] These materials will bottom out from compaction of the materials as cells fracture under repetitive stress. The advantages are low-temperature molding, nontoxicity, water resistance, and washability without absorbency of fluid.[74] Plastazote has a limited effective period of about 2 days; Poron remains effective for 6–9 months. The two materials can be combined for their attributes and perform well as a single unit.[75,76] There are different types of inserts, as follows:

- Soft: cushioning/accommodation, improves shock absorption
- Semirigid: some cushion/accommodation; affords pressure relief
- Rigid: hard, single layer of plastic; it controls abnormal foot and leg motion[77]

The Aliplast/Plastazote insert is an immediate preparation and can be provided within a clinic setting, but it has a relatively short life of compressibility (6–8 months). Plastazote is a closed-cell polyethylene foam that can be heated to 280° F and molded directly onto the patient's foot.[22] Care must be taken never to mold the toes or create ridges that the toes will ride over as the patient ambulates. By combining materials over a cast model of the foot, the composite type of insert can achieve all goals of the accommodative insert and provide a minimum life of 1 year.

An insert with a Plastazote surface in contact with the foot can be used as an excellent diagnostic tool for future follow-up. The self-molding properties of Plastazote reveal deep sock prints in areas of high pressure. These high-pressure areas should be noted and relieved in future insert design for the patient. By using temperature as a tool for evaluation, the areas of high trauma will be noted as increased temperature locations. After the patient has worn accommodative inserts, the temperature differentiation will decrease if the proper accommodation has been achieved. If the temperature has not decreased in the area, the relief may require enhancement, or there may be other underlying complications to be investigated. All relief areas are applied on the underlying surface in contact with the shoe, never in contact with the foot. The surface in contact with the foot is always a solid, uninterrupted surface that will not apply edges for the foot to receive shear forces. Figure 18–21 diagrams the fabrication of several different layers into an accommodative insert.

Shoes for the insensitive foot should be of soft leather that will conform to abnormalities on the dorsal surface and allow for the depth of an accommodative insert. Figure

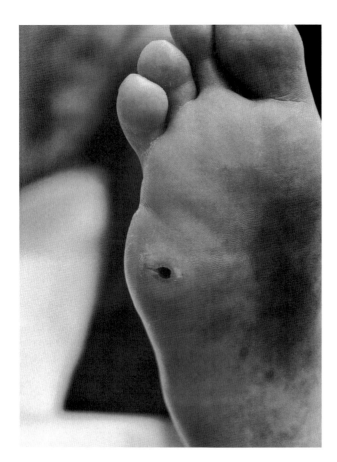

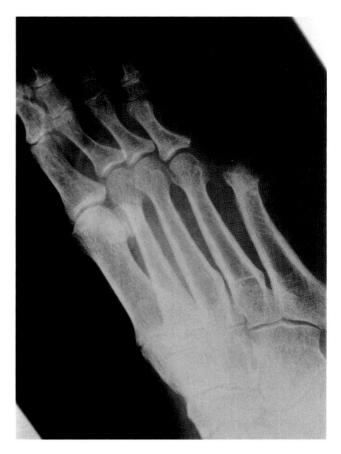

Figure 18–20A Osteomyelitis. Note puncture wound over the fifth metatarsal head, the site of the osteomyelitis. *Source:* Reprinted with permission from R.B. Chambers and N. Elftman, Orthotic Management of the Neuropathic and Dysvascular Patient, in *Atlas of Orthoses and Assistive Devices*, 3rd edition, B. Goldberg and J.D. Hsu, eds., p. 439, © 1997, Mosby-Year Book, Inc.

Figure 18–20B Radiograph of same foot as in Figure 18–20A shows calcification changes at the head of the fifth metatarsal. *Source:* Reprinted with permission from R.B. Chambers and N. Elftman, Orthotic Management of the Neuropathic and Dysvascular Patient, in *Atlas of Orthoses and Assistive Devices*, 3rd edition, B. Goldberg and J.D. Hsu, eds., p. 439, © 1997, Mosby-Year Book,

18–22 shows modifications of the depth shoe appropriate for the insensitive foot.

Clinical Wisdom: *Choose Crepe Sole Shoes for Pressure Relief*

Crepe soles, which are full of air cells, provide pressure relief to the plantar surface, whereas air or water "pillows," which are enclosed in an inflexible compartment, create pressure.

Leather gradually adapts to the slope of the foot and will retain shape between wearings. The leather will breathe and absorb perspiration.[74] The patient should not depend on the "feel" of a shoe for correct size. The shoe must be full width and girth and allow 1/2 to 3/4 inches of space beyond the longest toe to prevent distal shoe contact through the gait

cycle. Standard modifications of extra-depth shoes for the neuropathic patient include stretching of the soft toe box for clawed toes, flared lateral soles to discourage varus instability, and shank/rocker bottom for a partial foot, hallux rigidus, or decreased motion at the metatarsal heads. A rocker bottom should be added to the shoe when metatarsophalangeal extension is to be avoided.[22] When properly fit, the instep leather should not be taut. There are three tests to determine the proper fit of shoes (see Figure 18–23):

1. *Length:* Allow 1/2 to 3/4 inch of space in front of longest toe.
2. *Ball width:* With the patient weight bearing, grasp the vamp of the shoe and pinch the upper material; if leather cannot be pinched, it is too narrow. The ball should be in the widest part of the shoe.[78]
3. *Heel to ball length:* Measure the distance from the patient's heel to the first and fifth metatarsal heads.

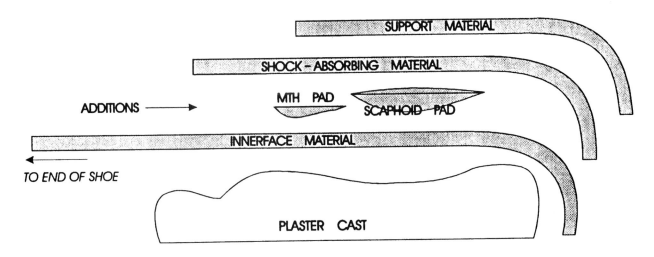

Figure 18–21 Diagram of accommodative insert fabrication. *Source:* Reprinted with permission from R.B. Chambers and N. Elftman, Orthotic Management of the Neuropathic and Dysvascular Patient, in *Atlas of Orthoses and Assistive Devices*, 3rd edition, B. Goldberg and J.D. Hsu, eds., p. 444, © 1997, Mosby-Year Book, Inc.

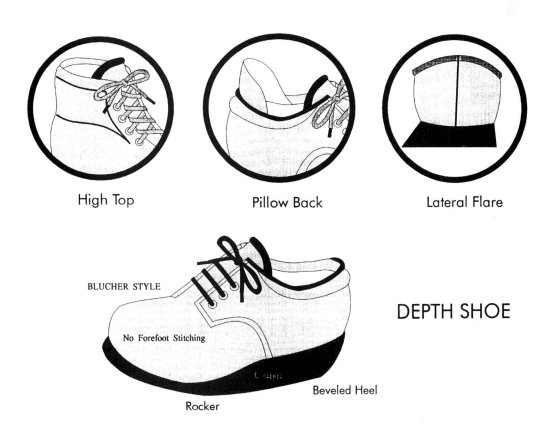

Figure 18–22 Depth shoe modifications. *Source:* Reprinted with permission from R.B. Chambers and N. Elftman, Orthotic Management of the Neuropathic and Dysvascular Patient, in *Atlas of Orthoses and Assistive Devices*, 3rd edition, B. Goldberg and J.D. Hsu, eds., p. 443, © 1997, Mosby-Year Book, Inc.

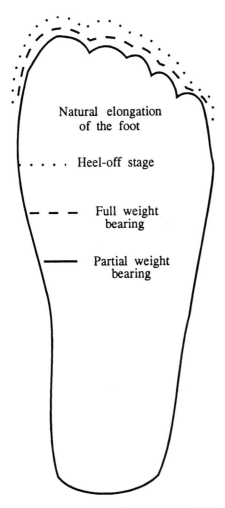

Figure 18–23 How to measure the proper shoe fit. *Source:* Reprinted with permission from R.B. Chambers and N. Elftman, Orthotic Management of the Neuropathic and Dysvascular Patient, in *Atlas of Orthoses and Assistive Devices*, 3rd edition, B. Goldberg and J.D. Hsu, eds., p. 442, © 1997, Mosby-Year Book, Inc.

Bend the shoe to determine toe break, and repeat measurements on the shoe. They should be close to the same measurements.[79]

The simple addition of shoes instead of walking barefoot may correct many deformities.[80] Laced shoes will give the best control, but they must be broken in slowly, beginning with 2 hours per day and slowly adding time.[22] Caution should be taken with cutout sandals for the possibility of irritation along the borders of the sandal and straps.[81] To evaluate pressures within a shoe, there is a pressure-sensitive sock that is coated with dye-filled wax capsules. The capsules fracture when a certain pressure threshold is exceeded, leaving dye stains in areas of high pressure.[74] To protect a heal-

ing area in which dressings will be applied, a healing shoe lined with Plastazote will allow greater circumference and volume adjustability.

Socks for the neuropathic limb should have no mended areas or seams over bony prominences. A cotton/acrylic blend will assist in the wicking of perspiration away from the foot.[82] The sock should be fully cushioned and have a nonrestrictive top. The partial foot requires a sock that will conform to the shape without distal prominent seams or excess material at the distal end. For the active patient, socks can be obtained with silicone over high-stress areas to prevent shear for full or partial feet.

The partial foot may require a block within the shoe for the area of amputation. The purpose of a block is to reduce migration of the partial foot and medial/lateral shear for the toe amputation. No block or "prosthetic toe" is to be used for a central digit amputation. The low pressures applied by a block to central digits cause ischemic ulcerations on opposing surfaces. Medial or lateral amputations (first and fifth toes) may require a block to hold the foot in the correct position within the shoe. The forefoot block holds the shoe leather away from the distal end of the foot and discourages distal migration of the foot. All forms of blocks must have space from the amputation site and be an integral part of the insert, not added to an existing orthotic. Forefoot blocks require a rigid rocker sole to prevent ulceration to distal end.

By utilizing state-of-the-art foams and room temperature vulcanized (RTV) silicone elastomers, shear can be reduced in areas of skin grafts, chronic ulcerations, and calcanectomies within more rigid orthotics. The viscoelastomer gel is a two-part gel that can be adjusted for durometer desired. The mixture can be used for shock absorption and shear reduction. Scar-adherent areas can benefit from a medium durometer mixture. The disadvantage is weight, so it should be used in small areas. Low-density foams can be designed into orthotics, such as toe breaks and forefoot blocks and reliefs. Reliefs for heel pain can be designed into the insert or shoe sole as a Sach heel. Sach heels use soft and medium durometer soling to simulate plantar flexion and provide shock absorption at heel strike.

Total-Contact Casting

The TCC method provides decreased plantar pressures by increasing weight bearing over the entire lower leg. It has been successful as a treatment for plantar ulcerations but requires careful application, close follow-up, and patient compliance with scheduled appointments to minimize complications.[83] Brand introduced the total-contact cast to the United States in the 1950s to redistribute walking pressures, prevent direct trauma to the wound, reduce edema, and provide immobilization to joints and soft tissue. The average healing time for ulcerations treated with the healing cast was 6 weeks.[81] This method has been used for patients with and without evidence of severe peripheral vascular disease.[84] The cast spreads weight evenly over the lower limb so that no part of the foot takes more than 5 psi. There is never a window cut in the cast or there may be localized swelling, shear stresses, and, eventually, a secondary wound (see Figure 18–24).[22]

Application methods of the total-contact healing cast vary with different institutions. The healing cast was originally designed with minimal padding, but padded variations are utilized. Although the steps for application of the Carville-type TCC are given, remember that it is most important to have the cast applied by a skilled technician, because harm can occur from improper application. Following are steps for fabrication of the Carville-type TCC:

1. The ulcer is covered with a thin layer of gauze.
2. Cotton is placed between the toes to prevent maceration.

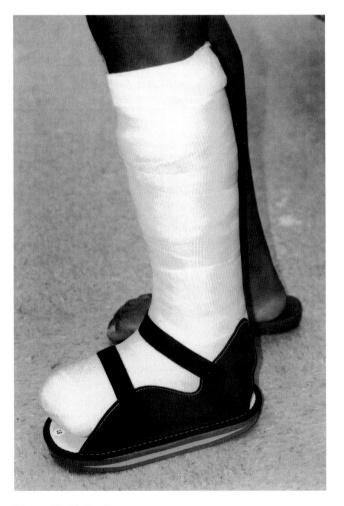

Figure 18–24 Total-contact cast.

3. A stockinette is applied.
4. A 1/4-inch piece of felt is placed over the malleoli and anterior tibia.
5. Foam padding is placed around toes.
6. A total-contact plaster shell is molded.
7. The shell is reinforced with plaster splints.
8. A walking heel is attached.
9. A fiberglass roll is applied around the plaster.

The patient is instructed to ambulate only 33% of usual activity. The cast is removed in 5–7 days and reapplied. New casts are applied every 2–3 weeks.[83] To allow thorough drying, the patient should not stand or walk on the cast for 24 hours.[81]

While not as effective as total contact, a posterior splint covers the posterior lower leg and plantar foot surface, and is held in place with elastic wrap. The splint acts to protect the plantar surface. This casting procedure may be chosen for the patient with a limb compromised by poor circulation or when the patient cannot tolerate the confinement of a cast.[85]

There have also been attempts to heal ulcers by using a healing cast shoe molded of plaster. This healing cast shoe must be changed in 3 days, then reapplied every 10 days. Results have reported healing of plantar ulcers in 39 days.[86] Contraindications for the use of a healing cast shoe include infection (redness, swelling, warmth, fever) and hypotrophic skin (thin, shiny appearance, marked dependent edema).[81]

Orthotic Dynamic System Splint

The orthotic dynamic system (ODS) splint was developed to take advantage of the casting method of a TCC with the inclusion of a custom-molded insert that could be removed and reliefs modified. With all of the advantages of the TCC, the advantages that were added with the ODS splint included the possibilities for daily inspection, regular cleaning/dressings/debridement, and adjustments to areas of excessive pressure and/or friction (see Figure 18–25).

Clinical Wisdom: Bathing While Wearing a TCC Is Simplified by Wearing a Seal Tight Cast and Bandage Protector

This heavyweight plastic vinyl bag slips over the cast and forms a seal that is watertight. The product is convenient to use, durable, and has a sueded sole to minimize slippage in the shower

---

The Plastazote/Aliplast insert is first molded to the patient's foot and trimmed to follow the plantar surface, with 1/4-inch length added beyond toes. A stockinette is placed

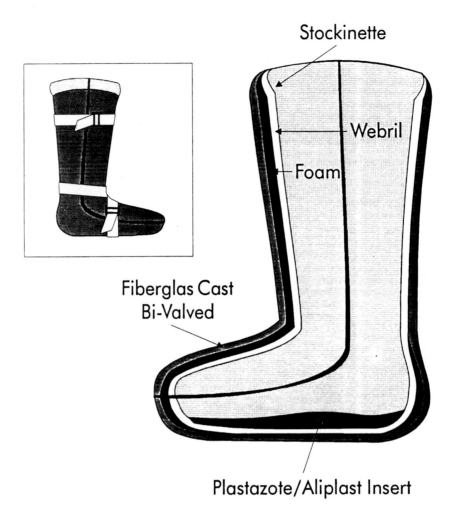

Stockinette

Webril

Foam

Fiberglas Cast
Bi-Valved

Plastazote/Aliplast Insert

Figure 18–25 Diagram of the ODS splint. *Source:* Reprinted with permission from R.B. Chambers and N. Elftman, Orthotic Management of the Neuropathic and Dysvascular Patient, in *Atlas of Orthoses and Assistive Devices*, 3rd edition, B. Goldberg and J.D. Hsu, eds., p. 441, © 1997, Mosby-Year Book, Inc.

on the leg, the insert is positioned, and another stockinette is applied to hold the insert in place. A padded TCC is applied, using Fiberglas only. The cast is bivalved; straps are added; edges are finished; and the insert is removed, relieved, and replaced to unweight the area of ulceration. After insert modification, it is replaced within the splint, and the patient may ambulate with a rocker-bottom cast shoe under the splint. The patient is instructed on volume control with sock thickness.

The disadvantage will lie with compliance of the patient. The splint design allows donning and doffing by the patient, therefore allowing him or her to remove the cast. The total contact of a healing cast cannot be compared in its superiority, but the clinical experience of the author has found the

daily inspection and relief adjustability to be a great asset in the treatment protocol.

Neuropathic Walker

The neuropathic walker is a combination of an ankle-foot orthosis (AFO) and a boot that is custom-designed to be total contact for weight distribution (Figure 18–26). The ankle is locked to reduce force through the Lisfranc joint and/or ankle. The design is indicated for the patient with changes of Charcot joint in the tarsal and ankle joints, chronic recurrence of Charcot disease, and chronic ulcerations. The orthosis is easily donned and doffed, and is fabricated of a copolymer plastic with a closed-cell lining. The remov-

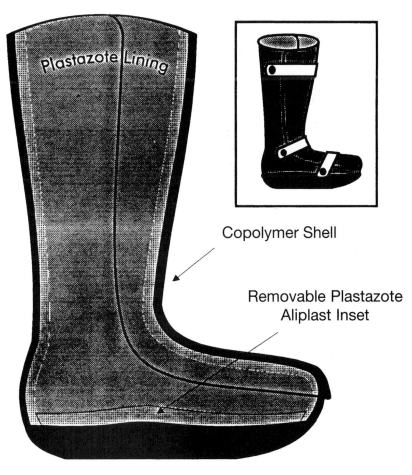

Copolymer Shell

**Removable Plastazote
Aliplast Inset**

Rocker Sole

Figure 18–26 Diagram of the neuropathic walker. *Source:* Reprinted with permission from R.B. Chambers and N. Elftman, Orthotic Management of the Neuropathic and Dysvascular Patient, in *Atlas of Orthoses and Assistive Devices*, 3rd edition, B. Goldberg and J.D. Hsu, eds., p. 448, © 1997, Mosby-Year Book, Inc.

able insert may be adjusted to reassign weight-bearing areas on the plantar surface. The insert may also be formed over chronic breakdown areas, such as the malleoli, posterior heel, and bunions, to reduce pressure. The rocker sole allows for easy ambulation, but the contralateral shoe must be adjusted for height.

When casting for the neuropathic walker, the patient's limb is wrapped and placed on a soft foam block until the plaster is set. The plantar surface will accommodate without excessive pressures on bony prominences. Modifications of the positive model include smoothing the plantar surface but never removing plaster. Any area that has had plaster removed during modification will be an area of excess pressure in the finished orthosis. The distal end is built up at the medial and lateral metatarsal areas and the length is ex-

tended 1/2 inch to allow room for the toes and to decrease the chances of maceration.

Fabrication is completed on the modified positive cast. The insert is first fabricated, finished, and placed in position. The posterior Plastazote lining is pulled over the insert, followed by the copolymer (plastic) vacuum-formed shell. The entire posterior section is finished and trimmed. The anterior Plastazote is positioned, and the copolymer shell is applied over the entire posterior. There should be a 1/2- to 1-inch overlap of copolymer on the finished orthosis. The Velcro straps and rocker bottom are attached (apex of rocker proximal to MTH).

The patient must be instructed to check skin for redness and possible breakdown. The patient should be followed and temperatures of the plantar surface recorded for possible adjustment of insert pressures. Sock management will be very important to continue a snug fit of the orthosis and volume control.

Total-Contact Ankle-Foot Orthosis

Similar to the neuropathic walker, the total-contact AFO is utilized for the patient who has an area of trauma in the mid- or hindfoot. The orthosis includes a custom, removable insert and is lined with Plastazote. This orthosis must be fit within a shoe, which may be difficult in standard shoes. The casting procedure is the same as that for the neuropathic walker. The toes are open, and the anterior shell terminates at midfoot.

Other Devices

Short leg walkers and orthopaedic walkers have been used by some clinics, but they compromise the total-contact fea-

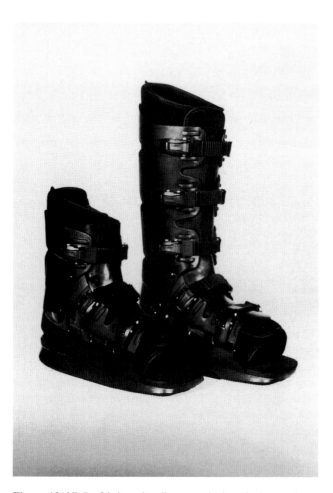

Figure 18–27 Prefabricated walker to assist in reducing motion at the ankle. Courtesy of Darco International, Huntington, West Virginia.

ture. The walkers have become popular as alternatives to cast immobilization but the indications for their use are for foot and ankle fractures, sprains, acute ligament/muscle, and postsurgical immobilization. Although prefabricated walkers (Figure 18–27) are not custom-made to provide total contact, they contain some features that may assist in reducing movement of the limb within the walker.[87] The walkers can be improved in function with the addition of a wide base, rocker sole and custom off-loading insert.[88] The low risk patient does well in the orthosis with a custom insert. The high risk patient with sensory neuropathy may be better served by a custom total contact orthosis.[89]

Patellar tendon-bearing (axial resist) designs are intended to decrease forces on the plantar weight-bearing surface of the foot. With this design as a casting procedure, there have been attempts at its use in place of plaster cast immobilizations.[90] The design transmitted considerable axial forces from the knee region onto the cast, but it did not offer rotary stability. The results offered very little effectiveness in reducing the load off the lower leg.[91] The patellar tendon-bearing design AFO has been used successfully for calcanectomy, plantar skin graft, and heel ulceration. This orthosis is contraindicated in the patient with vascular impairment because of the excess restriction in the popliteal area of arterial flow.

The prosthesis has been the orthotic replacement when the amputation case is complicated and the patient is not a candidate for prosthetic management. The prosthesis becomes a useful device for transfers and limb protection. This is always a creative design, with no two the same, unique to the individual and his or her needs.

The nonambulatory patient must be examined carefully for pressure ulceration due to positioning. Heel ulcers are particularly difficult to off-load in the recumbent position (Figure 18–28A). The prefabricated soft ankle foot orthosis (soft AFO) is constructed of a soft foam over a semirigid posterior/plantar support. The device allows decreased pressure at the posterior, medial/lateral, and plantar areas of the heel (Figure 18–28B). The soft outer construction decreases trauma to the contralateral leg.[87]

Off-Loading of Foot Ulcerations

In the treatment of foot ulcerations, there must be wound care protocol with debridement/cleansing and simultaneous off-loading of the affected area. This combination has shown optimal results in the healing of wounds. There are prefabricated, as well as custom applications that the team must consider for each individual patient. Many patients are given crutches, walker, or wheelchair but they must have the upper body strength, cardiovascular reserves, and/or motivation to use assistive devices.[87] Bed rest eliminates the pressures on the foot but promotes deconditioning of the patient.[88]

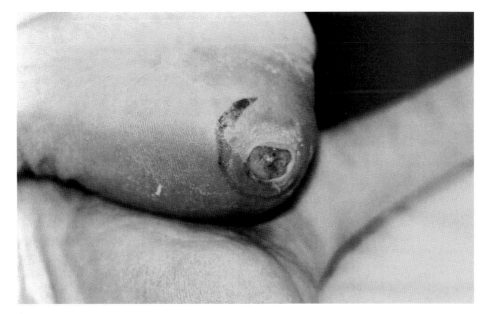

A

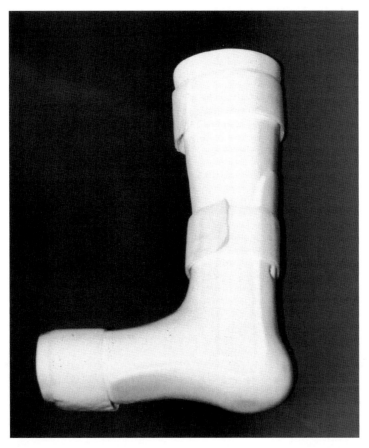

B

Figure 18–28 **A**, Common heel ulceration; **B**, Soft AFO for the recumbent patient to off-load heel ulceration and prevent trauma to contralateral limb. Courtesy of Boston Brace International, Avon, Massachusetts.

Plastazote Healing Sandals

The custom Plastazote sandal contains a molded foot bed and has a rigid rocker sole (Figure 18–29). The device is lightweight but requires considerable time and experience to fabricate.[87] The Carville sandal has been used as a successful off-loading shoe and interim device following the TCC and before definitive shoewear.[92]

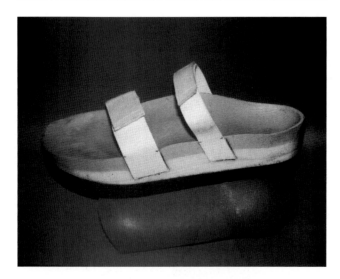

Figure 18–29 Plastazote Healing Sandal developed at Carville to provide a molded foot bed and rigid rocker sole. Courtesy of the Department of Health and Human Services, Division of National Hansen's Disease Program.

Prefabricated Off-Loading Alternatives

There are inexpensive alternatives for off-loading ulcerations with wound care protocol. For optimal healing, the wound must be off-loaded in conjunction with moist healing methods.[93] Over a third of the patients seen by home care practitioners have wounds. There is a low use of specialty dressings in home care, and the methods are usually clean instead of sterile.[94] Introduction of off-loading devices enhances the home care protocol. The following prefabricated products are improved in function by the addition of a customized, accommodative off-loading insert. The area of off-loading can be designed using the patient's floor reaction imprint (Harris mat) as a pattern. Follow-up appointments should include temperature measurements to ensure proper off-loading. If the temperatures have increased, the off-loading area must be increased; if the temperature differential is lower, there is an indication of decreased inflammation, and healing is occurring.[95]

Post Op/Med Surg/Cast Shoe

An inexpensive alternative for wound off-loading would be the postoperative (rigid sole) and cast shoes (roller sole) to contain the ulcerated foot and off-loading insert (Figure 18–30). These shoes adjust for bandage volume but do not offer an intimate fit to control foot motion.[89] These shoes usually require extensions to Velcro straps and minor modifications. Use of the shoes as off-loading devices requires careful monitoring of the patient.

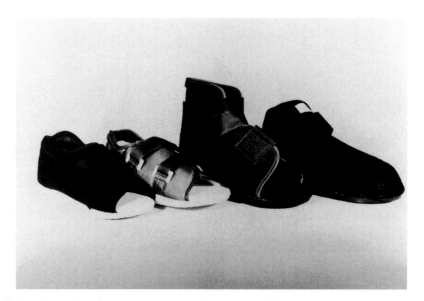

Figure 18–30 Postoperative/med. surg./cast shoes: an inexpensive alternative to off-loading a wound on the plantar foot surface when plantar insert is supplied. Courtesy of Darco International, Huntington, West Virginia.

Wedged Shoe

The wedged shoe (Figure 18–31) has full contact with the plantar surface of the foot but reduces load forces applied from the ground. The sole angle is designed to shift weight bearing away from the ulcerated area. The wedge shoe is contraindicated when the patient does not have the range of motion to accompany the shoe angle. A patient with poor proprioception may not be able to ambulate without assistive devices.

Half Shoes

Many clinics use the half shoe (Figure 18–32) to suspend the ulcerated area, providing complete off-loading of the ulcerated area. The forefoot half shoe provides a pressure-free area for the forefoot, especially for the common ulcerations of the hallux. The heel relief shoe suspends the heel for noncontact. These devices may be contraindicated for the patient with limited ankle motion or balance problems associated with proprioception. Assistive devices may be required to reduce incidence of falls.[87,88]

Wound Healing System

The wound healing system (Figure 18–33) was designed for the practitioner who does not have casting facilities or available support to off-load ulcerations by TCC or ODS splint. The wound care provider can supply off-loading properties in conjunction with the wound care protocol to deliver optimal healing of ulcerations in any environment. The basic wound shoe provides a base that allows relief of pressure for the dorsum, medial, lateral, and posterior ulceration. The plantar contact system (Figure 18–34) enables the practitioner to off-load plantar ulcerations with four layers (multiple durometer) of material (Figure 18–35A). The system is to be worn until the ulceration has healed. On final closure of the wound, a long-term material layer is added, and the wound shoe becomes the casual slipper to be worn at all times when definitive off-loading footwear is not being used (Figure 18–35B). A previous ulceration site is susceptible to

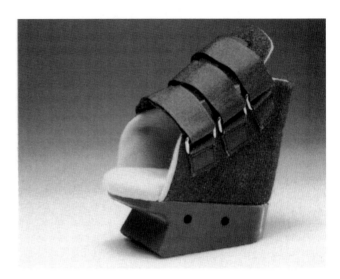

Figure 18–32 Half shoes suspend ulcerated area to eliminate external pressure. Courtesy of IPOS, North America, Niagara Falls, New York.

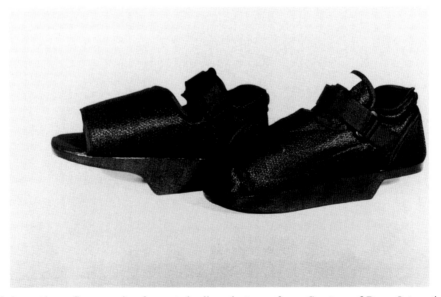

Figure 18–31 Wedged shoe reduces floor reaction forces to healing plantar surfaces. Courtesy of Darco International, Huntington, West Virginia.

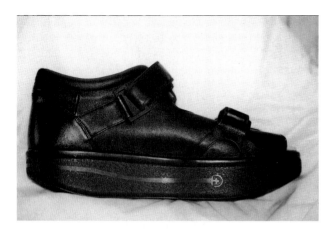

Figure 18–33 The wound healing system provides optimal environment for wound care protocol and simultaneous off-loading to encourage healing. Courtesy of Darco International, Huntington, West Virginia.

breakdown repeatedly, and the wound shoe used as a casual slipper ensures that pressure relief is achieved at all times. The patient must never walk barefooted.

The floor reaction imprint (Harris mat, Figure 18–36) is helpful as a pattern for the off-loading position but is not necessary. The top layer to contact the foot is always a solid interface that will mold to the foot contours. There are two layers of higher durometer that will be relieved using available tools (scissors, scalpel, blade). The lower grades (Wagner 0 and 1) will utilize one off-load layer (Figure 18–35C, whereas the higher grades will have two off-loading layers available (Figure 18–35D). On wound closure, a

shock-absorbing layer is to be added to prolong use of the system as a slipper (Figure 18–35E).

For the ulcerations that are not weight bearing (not plantar surface), the double-layer upper construction can be trimmed to off-load pressure areas without allowing window edema to occur (Figure 18–37A, B). The Velcro system is adjustable for bandage volume. The off-loading system allows for minimal dressings, which will usually add excess pressure areas when the patient is weight bearing. The goal of the wound healing system is to allow partial weight bearing while off-loading the high-risk foot with ulcerations. The combination of state-of-the-art wound care preparations and off-loading delivers optimal outcomes, as well as unlimited adjustments to forces applied.

SURGICAL MANAGEMENT

The most conservative treatment of foot infections will be utilized to rehabilitate, but antibiotic therapy alone is not always sufficient to treat aggressive, virulent foot infections.[96] Surgical intervention may be in the best interest of the patient if conservative therapy is not an option or has proven ineffective. Options should be discussed with the patient and the family, and they should be involved in the final outcome, when possible. Surgical debridement of all osteomyelitis and nonviable tissue must be completed.[97] The surgeon will preserve as much length and width as possible to balance the motor function.[9] The goal of amputation is ambulation and reconstruction. Typical locations of partial foot amputations are shown in Figure 18–38.

Metatarsal osteotomies can eliminate the intrinsic stresses caused by elongated or plantarflexed metatarsal joints in

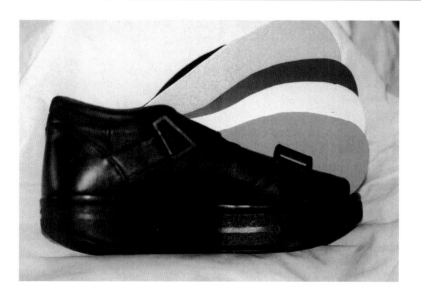

Figure 18–34 The wound shoe system allows off-loading of plantar, as well as dorsal wounds.

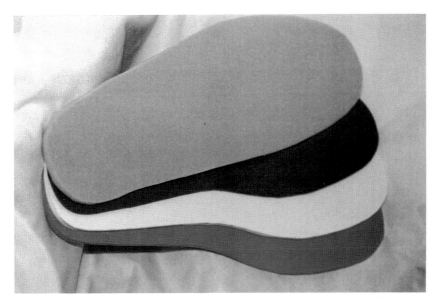

Figure 18–35A Plantar layers provide immediate in-clinic off-loading of wounds using four color-coded materials of varying durometers.

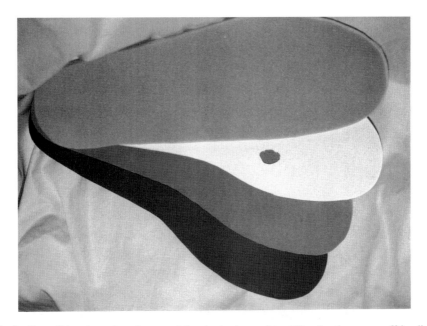

Figure 18–35B Upon the healing of the ulceration, the material order is changed to utilize the shoe as an off-loading house shoe.

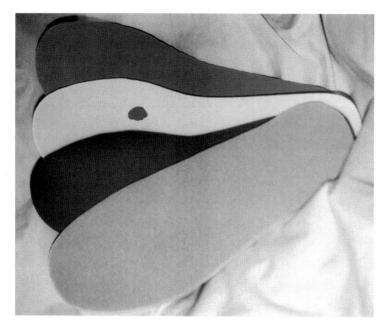

Figure 18–35C Superficial wounds (Wagner grade 0 +1) use one off-loading modified layer.

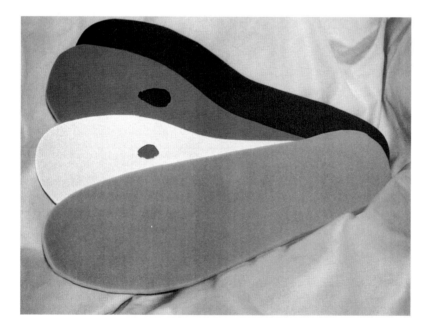

Figure 18–35D Wagner grade 2+ ulcerations will require two off-loading layers.

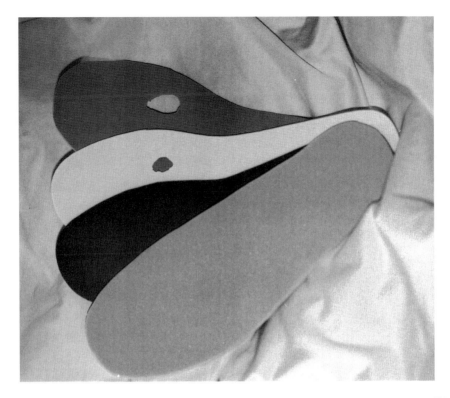

Figure 18–35E Upon healing of the superficial layer, the order of the materials is changed to provide an off-loading shoe for home ambulation.

neuropathic limbs and decrease number of amputations.[98] Toe resections are the most distal amputation choices available. Expected outcomes of each toe resection are as follows:

- First toe—Interphalangeal disarticulation for an infected distal phalanx gives good balance. When possible, a wafer of the proximal phalanx should be left to maintain the position of the sesamoids beneath the first metatarsal head.
- Second toe—Disarticulation results in loss of lateral support of the first toe. A second ray resection is usually better to avoid secondary hallux valgus.
- Third or fourth toes—The remaining toes will tend to shift to close the gap.
- All five toes—A long forefoot lever is left with good weight-bearing properties.[9]

The advantages of the partial foot amputation are the following:

- It preserves end weight-bearing function.
- It preserves proprioception.
- It provides for limited disruption of body image.

- It requires shoe modification/orthosis or limited prosthesis.

Limitations of the partial foot amputation are the loss of normal foot function related to loss of forefoot lever length and associated muscles, and the challenges presented in selecting appropriate adaptive equipment.

The Chopart's amputation is selected when a patient retains sensation in the heel pad. Metatarsals and tarsals are removed, leaving a very short limb. It is difficult to suspend a shoe without the aid of an AFO or prosthesis.

The transmetatarsal/Lisfranc amputation is preferred for the resultant length of foot; amputation is through the metatarsals. The longest partial foot amputation is the distal metatarsal amputation, in which the toes are amputated. This level will require a short shoe or forefoot block to prevent forward motion.

In all partial feet, it is important to watch for an equinus deformity. The toes are no longer present, and visual inspection is more difficult without their reference.

Whether from trauma or chronic infection, the partial removal of the calcaneus is a follow-up challenge for the orthotist. Removing weight bearing from the heel is difficult, and the patient who has had a calcanectomy must be followed carefully.

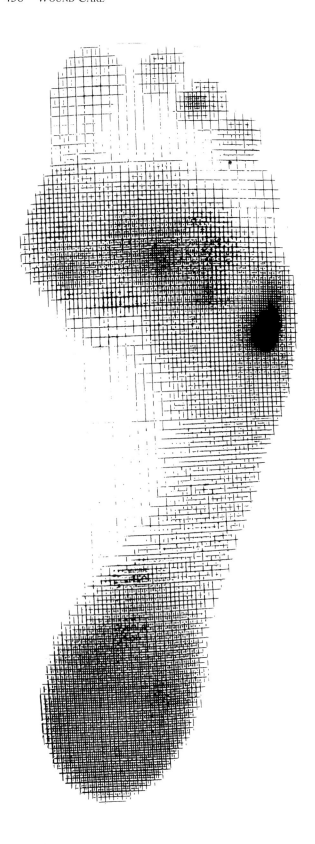

Figure 18–36 Floor reaction imprint (Harris mat) serves as pattern for plantar off-loading. Courtesy of Theradynamics, Milwaukee, Wisconsin.

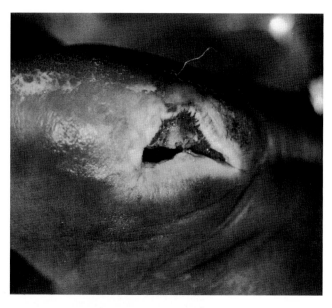

Figure 18–37A **A,** Lateral foot ulceration; not a weight-bearing surface; **B,** Upper construction allows relief of pressure for non-plantar ulcerations without window edema consequence.

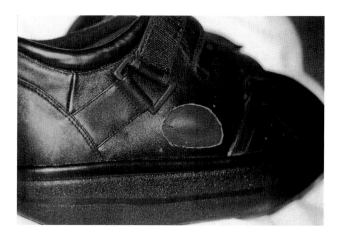

Figure 18–37B

The most successful methods of controlling future breakdown have involved the patellar tendon-bearing (axial resist) orthosis or the neuropathic walker. A soft RTV foam has been used to fill a void between the orthosis and the heel area. The same orthotic treatment is useful for chronic heel ulcers and plantar skin grafts that require reduction in weight-bearing and shear forces.

DOCUMENTATION

Documentation continuity is essential for all patients and requires a standard form to be used for assessment and future

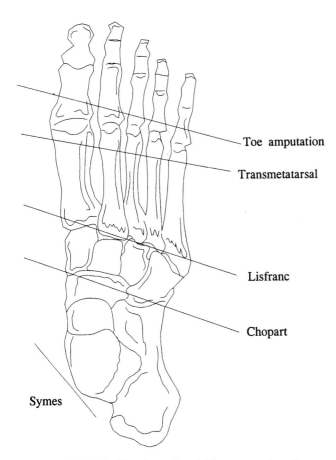

Figure 18–38 Typical locations of partial foot amputations. *Source:* Reprinted with permission from R.B. Chambers and N. Elftman, Orthotic Management of the Neuropathic and Dysvascular Patient, in *Atlas of Orthoses and Assistive Devices*, 3rd edition, B. Goldberg and J.D. Hsu, eds., p. 432, © 1997, Mosby-Year Book, Inc.

follow-up (Exhibit 18–4). Tracing the ulceration on transparent film will allow for accuracy of detailed healing progression. Providing the patient with a duplicate tracing can improve compliance because the patient can follow his or her own progress. Photographs of ulceration sites are important for noting improvement in depth and granulation of ulceration. Methods for making tracings and taking photos are described in Chapter 5.

CARE OF THE SKIN AND NAILS OF THE NEUROPATHIC FOOT

The Skin

Routine noninvasive skin and nail care is an important asset to any clinical team. The basic foot care can also be taught to the patient and family as promotion of foot health, along with daily examination for early detection of complications. This section includes the procedures, implements,

and techniques for optimal results. The professional treatment of skin and nails is vital to the patient with neuropathy. The medical community has recognized the need for this skilled area of clinical expertise. Routine foot conditioning should not include any sharp debridement, which is addressed in other chapters.

Healthy skin is soft, flexible, moist, and acidic. It is the largest organ of the body, covering 3,000 square inches on the average adult. The skin weighs approximately 6 pounds (twice the weight of the brain and liver). The skin receives about one-third of all circulating blood of the body. Its two main parts, the epidermis and the corneum (the dermis), serve as a protective barrier against microorganisms. The skin insulates against heat and cold and helps to eliminate body wastes in the form of perspiration. Its sense receptors enable the body to feel pain, cold, heat, touch, and pressure. The epidermis is thickest on the palms and soles of the feet and becomes thinner over the surface of the trunk. It is important to promote conditions as close as possible to normal skin for the neuropathic patient because he or she already has compromised utility of the skin's attributes. With routine care, the performance of the skin as protection of the body can be improved (see Chapter 4, Assessment of the Skin and Wound).[99]

The Nails

Nails are composed of hard keratin, a modification of the horny epidermal cells of the skin. The white crescent shape of the lunula at the proximal end of each nail is caused by air mixed in the keratin matrix. The nail plate originates from the proximal nail fold and attaches to the nail bed (Figure 18–39A, B). It grows about 1 mm per week unless inhibited by disease. Regeneration of a lost toenail occurs in 6–8 months.[99]

Clinical Wisdom: *Facts about Nails*

- Nails grow approximately 0.1 mm per day, or 3 mm per month.
- Nails grow faster in daytime and summer.
- Fever and serious illness slow growth rates.
- Pregnancy enhances growth.
- Nails grow more rapidly in men and young people than in women and the elderly.
- Toenails grow one-half to one-third the rate of fingernails.[100]

Noninvasive Skin and Nail Care

Before beginning skin and nail care, thoroughly inspect feet and ankles for breaks in the skin. Look for ulcers, heel

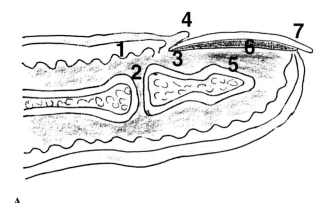

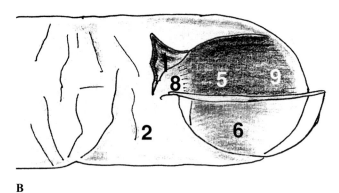

Figure 18–39 Anatomy of the nail. **A,** Cross-section. **B,** Nail diagram. 1, nail matrix; 2, nail root; 3, nail fold; 4, eponychium; 5, nail bed; 6, nail body; 7, free edge; 8, lunula; 9, hyponychium.

fissures, maceration between the toes, or imbedded objects. When nails are neglected and overgrown, they can break the skin of the neighboring toe. Abnormal nails that are not given routine care can accumulate excess keratin and debris under the nails and in the nail folds, creating an ideal environment for bacteria to grow.[101] Poor hygiene necessitates routine foot care. The poorly managed foot will require professional treatment twice a month until the skin and nails are conditioned; routine care can be managed monthly. All tools should be cleaned and sterilized, or disposed of, to reduce cross-contamination. The procedure for basic skin and nail care for neuropathic feet (Figure 18–40A through H) is as follows:

1. Wash hands and prepare sterilized tools. (Figure 18–40A–1 through A–5)
2. Submerge feet into warm water (not to exceed 95° F, use thermometer). You can also use water that is three parts water to one part vinegar in cleaning the feet. Vinegar softens the skin and nails.[102]

3. While wearing gloves, make a paste of baby shampoo (or any mild soap) and baking soda in the palm of your hand and gently massage over the entire foot.
4. Rinse and wrap feet individually in towels.
5. Expose toes and apply Blue Cross cuticle remover.
6. Using the curette, gently remove dead skin and loose cuticle from the toes (Figure 18–40B).
7. Rinse.
8. Using the nail clippers, cut the nail straight across. Don't cut what you can't see. Always have good lighting (Figure 18–40C).
9. Thinner, more fragile nails can be cut using the smaller cuticle nippers (Figure 18–40D).
10. Ingrown toenails are a puncture wound. To prevent them, use the ingrown nail file to smooth sharp corners that can dig into the skin (Figure 18–40E).
11. Smooth rough edges of nails with an emery board. The patient may take the emery board home for self-care (Figure 18–40F).
12. Massage emollient into feet but not between toes. Avoid lotions with fragrance, because they contain alcohol that will dry the skin. Vaseline, lanolin, or even Crisco may be used as a moisture barrier to contain the moisture within the skin. Remind the patient to use caution when using emollient to prevent slipping and falling. Removing excess and covering with socks will help to minimize the hazard.
13. Educate the patient regarding appropriate footwear.

There are nails that are difficult to trim. The safest way to trim the pincer nail is to file it straight across, rather than to risk cutting the skin (Figure 18–40G). Some nails have grown into a "tent" shape. This tenting is usually caused by years of wearing pointed shoes. When trimming this type of nail, be aware of the skin under the nail at the dorsal apex. A condition called *onycholysis*, separation of the nail plate from the nail bed, can be caused by nail traumas and disorders. If onycholysis has been present for an extended period (6 months or more), the structure of the nail bed can change, and the nail plate will no longer attach to the nail bed. At this point, the condition becomes permanent. Keep the patient's nails short to prevent them from catching on surroundings and tearing off.[103] Some patients will have nails that are atrophied, due to their illness. Figure 18–40H reveals an atrophied nail with a hematoma.

Heel Fissures

Patients with autonomic neuropathy can have very dry, nonelastic skin, due to the lack of sweat and oil production. Deep heel fissures develop from the dry skin and may compromise the integrity of the skin. When the fissures occur, there is an opportunity for bacteria and debris to invade the skin, causing ulcerations and infection (Figure 18–41A).

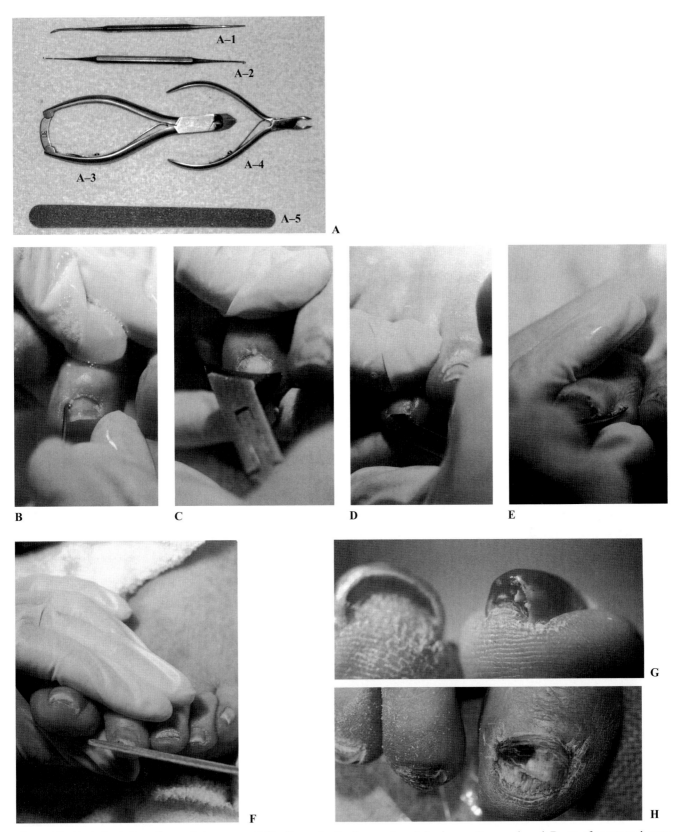

Figure 18–40 A, Tools for nail care: 1, ingrown nail file; 2, curette; 3, clippers; 4, cuticle nippers; 5, emery board; **B**, use of curette to loosen and remove debris; **C**, clippers to cut nails; **D**, cuticle nipper for fragile nails and small spaces; **E**, ingrown nail file to round sharp corner; **F**, emery board to smooth edges; **G**, pincer nail; **H**, nail with hematoma.

Care of heel fissures begins with the basic callus care procedure. Use a dry callus reducer on dry skin with one-directional strokes. When skills for using the Dremel (Moore Medical, New Britain, CT) are developed, the tool can be used in the same fashion for very thick hyperkeratotic skin. Do not attempt to finish a difficult case in one session; several appointments will be required to reduce the buildup.

Heel Fissure Care

1. Wash hands and don gloves.
2. Use the callus reducer (Figure 18–41B) or Dremel (Figure 18–41C) to decrease the hyperkeratotic thickness.
3. Wrap the foot in a warm, moist towel for 5 minutes.
4. Remove towel, apply Vick's VapoRub to heel, followed by Back to Basics Callus Paste (Figure 18–41D, Exhibit 18–5). The paste can be held in place with a plastic heel cup or plastic wrap, followed by a towel wrap, for 10 minutes (Figures 18–41E, F).
5. Unwrap foot and remove paste from the heel with a wet foot file (Figure 18–41G).
6. Rinse the foot and apply a moisture barrier emollient (Figure 18–41H).
7. Wipe excess emollient off and don socks and shoes.

Once the patient's feet are conditioned, routine foot care can be maintained with 4- to 6-week follow-up appointments.

Care of the Hypertrophic Nail (Onychauxis)

The hypertrophic nail may be caused by damage to the matrix, fungal infection, age and/or vascular complications. Hypertrophic nails that have been neglected need to be thinned make shoe fit possible and to prevent secondary infections due to traumatization of the prominent nail.

The most effective and expedient method for thinning the nail is to use the cordless rotary Dremel tool with a disposable abrasive disc. These discs (emery medium 1/8 inch) are easily interchangeable and are discarded after each patient. It is important for the practitioner and the patient to don masks, eye, and hair coverings to protect both from airborne dust. Use of a HEPA air filter device would give added protection.

Procedure for reducing hypertrophic nails:

Exhibit 18–5 Back to Basics Paste

1 cup kosher salt 1/2 cup Epsom salts 8 tbsp baking soda 8 tbsp mineral oil[104]

1. Wash hands, don gloves, have practitioner and patient don hair coverings and masks.
2. Examine the skin around the nail for damage (Figure 18–42A).
3. If there are no signs of broken skin or infection, secure toe with thumb and index fingers and move other toes away from the working area.
4. Turn Dremel on and move sanding disc in a proximal to distal direction, with slow, even strokes until nail is thinned (Figure 18–42B). Caution must be exercised when thinning the nail, due to unanticipated raised nail beds (Figure 18–42C).
5. Wash and dry the thinned nail and apply a conditioning agent, ie, Tineacide. Use of this or comparable product will allow future nail care to be more effective by keeping the nail and surrounding skin conditioned (Figure 18–42D).

Callus (Hyperkeratosis) Care

A callus is located in an area of high pressures and shear forces. It is the body's protective mechanism for an area of chronic irritation. To the neuropathic patient, the callus is indicative of chronic trauma (repetitive stress injury) that may lead to skin breakdown and serious complications.[105] Lack of sensation prevents the neuropathic patient from reacting to high pressures that can produce an ulceration. Reduction of callus is required on an ongoing basis to prevent the callus and eventual ulceration. The majority of plantar ulcerations in neuropathic patients are located in the forefoot, especially at the great toe and first, second, and fifth metatarsal heads.[101]

Clinical Wisdom: *Callus Care*

Avoid corn medications that can produce chemical burns; they contain salicylic acid. Vick's VapoRub will act quickly to soften the hardened skin. Vaseline is the daily treatment to provide a moisture barrier after bathing.

Procedure of callus reduction:

1. Wash hands.
2. Don gloves and hold foot securely with one hand. In the other hand, use the dry callus reducer over the dry callused area in one direction. When the screen fills with debris, tap on a hard surface, clear the screen, and continue the process. After the callus is reduced, give the screen to the patient with instructions on home use.

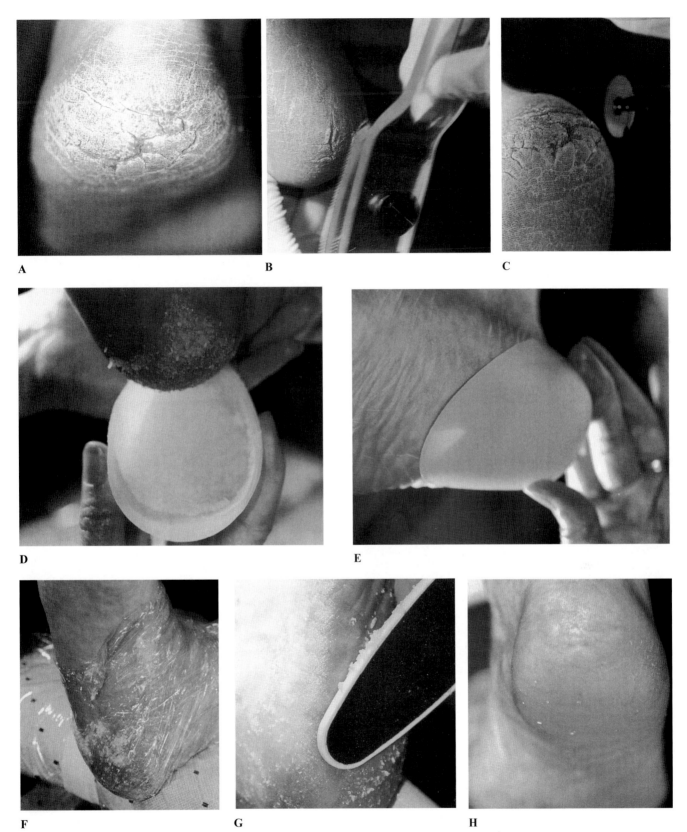

Figure 18–41 Heel fissures: **A**, dry, cracking hyperkeratotic heel; **B**, callus reducer; used dry on dry skin; **C**, Dremel tool to reduce callus; **D**, heel cup to concentrate basic callus paste; **E**, heel cup on foot; **F**, plastic wrap to apply and contain basic callus paste on large areas; **G**, foot file to exfoliate heel callus; **H**, heel fissures after first treatment.

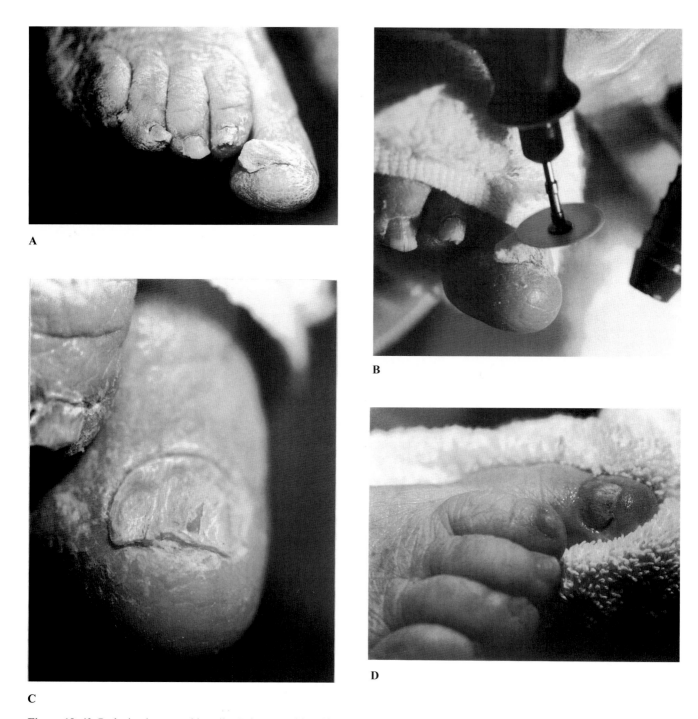

Figure 18–42 Reducing hypertrophic nails: **A**, hypertrophic nails; **B**, Dremel tool to reduce nail thickness; **C**, reduced nail with raised nail bed; **D**, completed nail procedure after conditioning.

3. When the callus is reduced, there may be an ulceration revealed under the callus. Reduce the callus but do not open the skin. An off-loading insole will be necessary to reduce the pressure and shear to the area (Figure 18–43).
4. Once the callus is reduced, wrap the foot in a warm, moist towel for 5 minutes.
5. Remove the towel and apply Vick's VapoRub, followed with Back to Basics Paste (Exhibit 18–5). Cover with plastic wrap and towel for 10 minutes.
6. Gently remove paste with foot file, rinse, and pat dry.
7. The patient may need to be seen weekly to reduce the callus in stages.
8. Assess footwear to determine what is causing callus formation. Therapeutic depth shoes with accommodative inserts should be worn by all patients with neuropathic feet (unable to feel the 5.07 monofilament).[101]

Clinical Wisdom: *Bathroom Surgery*

Remind patients to never perform "bathroom surgery." Self-inflicted wounds due to razor blades and other sharp objects are common with patients who lack protective sensation.

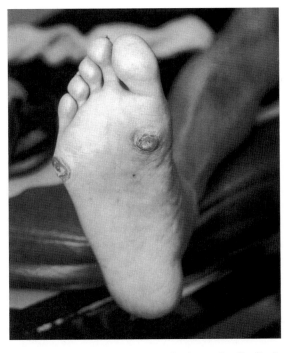

Figure 18–43 Foot requiring callus reduction and redistribution of weight-bearing forces at first and fifth metatarsal head.

Using a cordless Dremel rotary tool to reduce callus:

1. When learning to use the Dremel, begin with the less powerful Mini-mite cordless model until skills are developed. Practicing on hoof trimmings purchased from a pet supply company will give similar experience to working on callus and hypertrophic nails. When proficient, the more powerful Multi-Pro model can be used.
2. When using a Dremel, thin the callus thickness by sanding in one direction (proximal to distal). Do not work in an area for a long period because the prolonged friction can cause overheating at the skin surface.
3. Continue with steps 2 through 7 in the procedure for callus reduction above.

CONCLUSION

As the post-World War II generation ages, the medical community will be faced with the increasing demand for basic, noninvasive foot care with minimal risk of transmitted infections and skin conditions. Attention to foot care has become a recognized requirement for aging and, especially, neuropathic patients. Health care professionals are seeking information and specialized training relating to foot care in the clinical setting. Their efforts are being rewarded with fewer amputations, and patients are being educated in self-care. Self-care has allowed early detection and medical attention to conditions that would otherwise result in catastrophic events. Routine foot care is an integral part of comprehensive care for the neuropathic patient, and its presence will greatly improve the quality of life to those in the greatest need. See Chapter 19 for more information about foot and nail care in the nondiabetic foot.

SELF-CARE TEACHING GUIDELINES

Foot Inspection

The patient is the most important member of a clinical team approach to the treatment of his or her neuropathic limb. There is no complication too small to be addressed, and the patient must bring abnormalities to the team's attention. Self-care begins with daily inspections of the feet, with the help of mirrors, magnifying glasses, and family members, when necessary. Examination includes footwear and orthotics for wear and foreign objects. The diabetic patient must understand that this examination may be complicated by other disease processes, including retinopathy, autonomic neuropathy (loss of smell and sensory signals), and decreased mobility of joints. These patients are handicapped by the lack of pain as a warning signal and require systematic

Exhibit 18–6 Self-Care Guidelines for the Patient with Neuropathic Foot

Self-Care Guidelines for Patient with Neuropathic Foot	Instructions Given (Date/Initials)	Demonstration or Review of Material (Date/Initials)	Return Demonstration or States Understanding (Date/Initials)

1. Foot Inspection Methods
  a. Use mirror to check feet
  b. Use magnifying glass to check feet
  c. If blind, family member performs foot inspection			

2. Foot Inspection Item
  a. Toe nails: check for broken, cracked, or sharp nails
  b. Broken skin: check between toes, along sides of feet, tops and ends of toes, sole of foot
  c. Soft toe corns: check between toes
  d. Callus: check for cracks
  e. Drainage: check for any drainage from a sore
  f. Odor: check for odor from any source on the foot			

3. Patient Understands
  a. Significance of findings of foot inspection: break in nails, skin, or callus
  b. When to notify health care provider if there is break in nails, skin, or callus
  c. To notify health care provider immediately if there is any injury to the feet			

4. Foot Care Routine
  a. Wash feet with nondrying soap and towel dry
  b. Apply coating of petroleum jelly to all skin surfaces of feet
  c. Cover coated feet with clean white socks			

5. Foot Care Precautions
  a. Never walk barefoot
  b. Never use adhesive tape products on the skin
  c. Never put feet in hot water or apply a heating pad or hot pack
  d. Never soak feet
  e. Never apply over-the-counter foot care products to remove corns or callus, or to treat nails			

6. Shoe Wear Orthotic Inspection
  a. Choose shoes that are correct size and width
  b. Make sure there is no stitching over the forefoot of shoe
  c. Check for wear: heels, soles, tops, inside, bottom, edges, counter
  d. Always check shoes, socks, and orthotics for foreign objects; remove objects before donning			

7. Exercise Precautions
  a. Never jog
  b. Walk with short, slow steps			

continues

Exhibit 18–6 continued

Self-Care Guidelines for Patient with Neuropathic Foot	Instructions Given (Date/Initials)	Demonstration or Review of Material (Date/Initials)	Return Demonstration or States Understanding (Date/Initials)

8. Preferred Exercises
  a. Aerobic: low impact
  b. Swimming (wear soft bathing shoes in water to protect feet, dry feet thoroughly following)
  c. Cycling: protect feet and ankles from trauma
  d. Dancing
  e. Chair and mat exercises			

9. Importance of Follow-Up with Health Care Provider			

instruction to educate them in the proper skills required for daily inspection and detection of impending trauma.

Precautions and Risk Reduction Methods

There are several precautions for the patient with a neuropathic limb. The skin is very susceptible to damage and infection, and it must be treated carefully. It is advised that the patient not soak the feet in water because the chance of burns is always present, and the soaking will leave the skin moist and susceptible to fungal infection. Prolonged soaking can remove the natural protective barrier from the skin and lead to other infections. Feet should be washed with a nondrying soap and towel dried. After the foot wash, petroleum jelly can be applied to retain natural moisture and the feet covered with socks. Care should be taken not to use creams with perfumes (alcohol) because they will further dehydrate the skin.

Dehydrated skin is especially susceptible to trauma. Adhesives of any form should never be applied directly to the skin of a neuropathic limb. On removal of the adhesive, there is a risk of loss of the outer layer of skin, leaving an area open to infection. The adhesives could be in the form of tape, a Band-Aid, or over-the-counter self-adhesive pads.

When the patient selects footwear, he or she should choose not only the correct size and width, but also shoes with no stitching over the forefoot. The stitched areas will never mold to the foot; instead, they will cause breakdown of the skin, especially over bony areas.

Socks for the neuropathic foot should be seamless and without holes or repairs (Figure 18–44). Tube socks do not contour to the foot without folds that can cause irritation. The socks should be a blend to wick perspiration and should be nonconstricting at the calf. The use of white or light colors will enable the patient to detect drainage due to trauma easily. With a new shoe, the break-in period should be completed with two thin socks on each foot. The double socks will allow shear to occur between them and will decrease the probability of blistering from new leather.

The partial foot sock is designed of highly elastic fibers. The sock shape will conform to partial foot length and shape. The single size fits a Chopart's amputation, as well as a long transmetatarsal amputation. There are no folds or seams to cause friction.

Toe socks decrease maceration between toes. The moist environment between the toes encourages fungal growth and may lead to ulceration and bacterial infection. The seamless construction helps to reduce overlapping of lesser toes but must be compensated for in shoe size if they are to be worn with shoes.

Keep current on recalled products. For example, one hair removal system published a product alert on its device because of problems occurring with diabetic patients. Small areas were bleeding after hair was removed, leaving an entrance for bacteria and possible infection! Over 50% of the over-the-counter foot care products should never be used by a patient with a neuropathic limb or diabetes. There are occasionally warnings, but they are in very fine print.

Care must be taken with exercise programs. When we walk, each step carries one and one-half times our body weight; jogging increases the force to three times the body weight.[106] The patient with a neuropathic limb would be advised to choose an exercise program that includes aerobics, swimming, cycling, dance, or chair exercises. Even walking should include slow, short steps only—no jogging.[107]

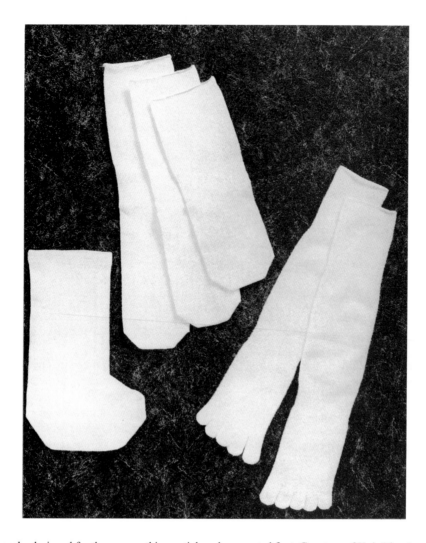

Figure 18–44 Specialty socks designed for the neuropathic, partial, and macerated foot. Courtesy of Knit Rite, Inc., Kansas City, Kansas.

The patient with a neuropathic limb should never walk barefoot. Even in the pool or on the beach, water shoes should be worn. Hot sand can cause burns, and undetected objects in the sand can cause injury. Burns can be caused by the floorboard of an automobile, as well as by any warmth-producing equipment. The interior of the shoe must be examined before every donning. Small objects can easily drop into a shoe.

Compliance Issues

The practitioner must understand compliance problems of patients with neuropathic limbs, especially diabetic patients. They do not willfully neglect self-care activities but simply are not aware of the possible dangers and are not taught adequately or motivated sufficiently.[2] Diabetic patients may have other complications that the practitioner does not consider in the compliance of their activities. Many cannot see (retinopathy), feel (sensory neuropathy), or smell (autonomic neuropathy) that there is an infection or a potential problem. Those with vision impairments will need help from a family member or caregiver to perform self-care guidelines.

Patients with neuropathic and dysvascular limbs require knowledge and skills to administer self-examination and self-care. The medical community must educate the patients, as well as the medical team, to treat conservatively and accommodate the chronic complications that exist in a growing portion of the population. Exhibit 18–6 is a checklist of instructional items with documentation to verify learning and understanding for the patient with neuropathic foot.

REVIEW QUESTIONS

1. Loss of sensation in the upper and lower extremity that is equidistant from the spine is classified as peripheral neuropathy. TRUE
2. A rigid hallux deformity requires a rigid rocker sole on the shoes. TRUE
3. An increase in local surface temperatures indicates that an area has healed and the patient may resume previous activity level. FALSE
4. The acute Charcot foot is cool and blue, and pulses are absent. FALSE

RESOURCES

Acor Orthopedic
18530 South Miles Pkwy
Cleveland, OH 44128
(800) 237-2267 fax (216) 662-4547
Materials/fabrication tools
Prefab orthoses
Custom and diabetic shoes

Alimed, Inc.
297 High Street
Dedham, MA 02026
(800) 225-2610 fax (800) 437-2966
Materials/wound supplies
Wheel chairs/positioning
Specialty diabetic products

Apex Foot Health
170 Wesley St.
South Hackensack, NJ 07606
(800) 526-2739 fax (800) 526-0073
Materials/tools
Prefab orthoses
Modifiable footwear

Boston Brace International
20 Ledin Dr.
Avon, MA 02322
(800) 262-2235 fax (800) 634-5048
Soft ankle foot orthosis (AFO)

Brown Medical Industries
481 South 8th Ave. East
Hartley, IA 51346
(800) 843-4395 fax (712) 336-2874
Cast and bandage protector

Comfort Products, Inc.
705 Linton Ave.
Croydon, PA 19021
(800) 822-7500 fax (215) 785-5737
Diabetic socks

Darco International, Inc.
1327 7th Ave
Huntington, WV 25701
(800) 999-8866 fax (304) 522-0037
Wound healing shoe system
P/O med/surg shoe/cast boot
Neuropathic shoes/walker

Deltatrak, Inc.
5653 Stoneridge Dr.
Pleasanton, CA 94588
(800) 962-6776 fax (925) 467-5949
Infrared thermometer

Hands on Foot, Inc.
2076 Bonita Ave.
La Verne, CA 91750
(909) 596-7674 fax (909) 596-5211
Neuropathic limb courses
Wound off-load courses
Callous reducers

Ipos, North America, Inc.
2045 Niagara Falls Blvd. #8
Niagara Falls, NY 14304
(800) 626-2612 fax (716) 297-0153
Heel and forefoot relief shoes

Juzo-Julius Zorn, Inc.
P.O. Box 1088
Cuyahoga Falls, OH44223
(800) 222-4999 fax (800) 645-2519
Neuropathic/compression stockings
Sleeves/gloves/gauntlets
Prosthetic shrinker/suspension

Knit-Rite, Inc.
120 Osage Ave.
Kansas City, KA 66105
(800) 821-3094 fax (800) 462-4707
Diabetic/partial foot socks
Prosthetic socks/shrinkers
Prosthetic suspension

Measurements, Inc.
2946 Ponce de Leon
New Orleans, LA 70119
(504) 949-1192 fax (504) 943-3489
Infrared thermometer

Moore Medical, Inc.
389 John Downey Dr.
New Britain, CT 06050
(800) 234-1464 fax (800) 944-6667
Wound care supplies/material
Tools/tube foam/crest pad support
Medical supplies

North Coast Medical, Inc.
187 Stouffer Blvd.
San Jose, CA 95125-1042
(800) 821-9319 fax (408) 277-6824
Monofilaments

Theradynamics
7283 W. Appleton Ave.
(800) 803-7813 fax (414) 438-1051
Milwaukee, WI 53216
Floor reaction imprint (Harris)
Material/fabrication equipment
Prefabricated orthoses

UCO International, Inc.
16 E. Piper Ln. # 130
Prospect Heights, IL 60070
(800) 541-4030 fax (847) 541-4144
Material/specialty pads (MTH)
Tools and equipment
Prefabricated orthoses

CARE OF THE SKIN AND NAIL OF THE NEUROPATHIC FOOT RESOURCES

Antoine de Paris
P.O. Box 1310
Solvang, CA 93464
(805) 688-0666 fax (805) 686-00330

(800) 222-3243
Pedicure Tools
Nail Clipper #30
Cuticle Nipper #14
Ingrown Nail File #86

Hands on Foot, Inc.
P.O. Box 7674
2076 Bonita Ave.
La Verne, CA 91750
(909) 596-7674 fax (909) 596-5211
Callus Reducers
Socks
Shoes (Gentle Step)

Moore Medical Products
389 John Downey Dr.
P.O. Box 2740
New Britain, CT 06060–2740
(800) 234-1464 <http://www.mooremedical.com>
Tube foam
Lamb's wool
Curette
Dremel tool

Sally's Beauty Supply (nationwide franchise)
Blue Cross cuticle remover
Foot files
Emery boards

Sussman, C. *Diabetic Foot Care and Ulcer Prevention, Wound Care Patient Education and Resource Manual*, Gaithersburg, MD: Aspen Publishers; 1999.

Tineacide
(800) 307-8818

REFERENCES

1. Brenner M. *Management of the Diabetic Foot.* Baltimore: Williams & Wilkins; 1987.

2. Shipley D. Clinical evaluation and care of the insensitive foot. *Phys Ther.* 1979;59:13–22.

3. Veves A, Boulton A. Commentary. *Diabetes Spectrum.* 1992;5: 336–337.

4. Bowker J. Commentary. *Diabetes Spectrum.* 1992;5:335.

5. Brenner M. Management of the diabetic foot. *Podiatr Products.* May 1988:54–58.

6. Ellenberg M. Diabetic neuropathic ulcer. *J Mt Sinai Hosp.* 1968;35: 585–594.

7. Green D, Waldhausl W. A forum on neuropathy. *Diabetes.* 1988:10.

8. Bowker J. Neurological aspects of prosthetic/orthotic practice. *J Prosthet Orthot.* 1993;5(2):52–54.

9. Bowker J. Partial foot and Syme amputations: An overview. *Clin Prosthet Orthot.* 1987;12:10–13.

10. Letts M. The orthotics of myelomeningocele. In: *Atlas of Orthotics.* St. Louis, MO: CV Mosby; 1985:300–306.

11. Weingarten M. Commentary. *Diabetes Spectrum.* 1992;5:342–343.

12. Pecoraro R, Reiber G, Burgess E. Pathways to diabetic limb amputation: Basis for prevention. *Diabetes Care.* 1990;13:513–521.

13. Fylling C. Conclusions. *Diabetes Spectrum.* 1992;5:358–359.

14. Bamberger D, Stark K. Severe diabetic foot problems: Avoiding amputation. *Emerg Decis.* 1987;3(8):21–34.

15. Olin J. Peripheral arterial disease. *Diabetes Forecast.* October 1992: 78–81.

16. Newman B. A diabetes camp for Native American adults. *Diabetes Spectrum.* 1993;6:166–202.

17. Harkness L, Lavery L. Diabetes foot care: A team approach. *Diabetes Spectrum.* 1992;5:136–137.

18. Robbins D. Office guide to diagnosis and classification of diabetes mellitus and other categories of glucose tolerance. *Diabetes Care.* 1991;14(suppl 2):3–4.

19. Brand P. Neuropathic ulceration. *The Star.* May/June 1983:1–4.

20. Ashbury A. Foot care in patients with diabetes mellitus. *Diabetes Care.* 1991;14(suppl 2):18–19.

21. Brand P. In: *Insensitive Feet—A Practical Handout on Foot Problems in Leprosy.* London: The Leprosy Mission; 1977.

22. Brand P. Management of sensory loss in the extremities: management of peripheral nerve problems. *J Rehab.* 1980;862–872.

23. Myerson M, Papa J, Eaton K. The total contact cast for management of neuropathic plantar ulceration of the foot. *Diabetes Spectrum.* 1992;5:352–353.

24. Edelstein J. Foot care for the aging. *Phys Ther.* 1988;68:1882–1886.

25. Utley R. Nutritional factors associated with wound healing in the elderly: The role of specific nutrients in the healing process. *Diabetes Spectrum.* 1992;5:354–355.

26. Knighton D, Fiegel V, Doucette M. Treating diabetic foot ulcers. *Diabetes Spectrum.* 1990;3:51–56.

27. Ellenberg M. Don't be fooled by peripheral neuropathy. *Diabetes Forecast.* January/February 1983.

28. Yale J. *Yale's Podiatric Medicine.* 3rd ed. Baltimore: Williams & Wilkins; 1980.

29. Cailliet R. *Foot and Ankle Pain.* Philadelphia: F. Davis; 1983: 181–189.

30. Jahss M. Shoes and shoe modifications. In: *Atlas of Orthotics.* St. Louis, MO: CV Mosby; 1985:267–279.

31. Tsairis P. Differential diagnosis of peripheral neuropathies. In: *Management of Peripheral Nerve Problems.* Rancho los Amigos; 1980:712–725.

32. Thomas P. Clinical features and differential diagnosis. In: *Peripheral Neuropathy.* Philadelphia: WB Saunders; 1984;2:1169–1185.

33. Wakelee-Lynch J. Relieving pain with peppers. *Diabetes Forecast.* June 1992:35–37.

34. Dailey G. Effect of treatment with capsaicin on daily activities of patients with painful diabetic neuropathy. *Diabetes Care.* 1992;15:159–165.

35. *Diabetes Mellitus: Management and Complications.* New York: Churchill Livingstone; 1985:234–235, 277–293, 360–361.

36. Apelqvist J, Castenfors J, Larsson J. Prognostic value of systolic ankle and toe blood pressure levels in outcome of diabetic foot ulcer. *Diabetes Care.* 1989;12:373–378.

37. Cherry G, Ryan T, Cameron J. Blueprint for the treatment of leg ulcers and the prevention of recurrence. *Wounds.* 1992;3:1–15.

38. Field M. The use of garments to create compression. *Biomech Desk Ref.* 6:139–140.

39. Perry J. Normal and pathological gait. In: *Atlas of Orthotics.* St. Louis, MO: CV Mosby; 1985:83–96.

40. Mann R. Biomechanics of the foot. In: *Atlas of Orthotics.* St. Louis, MO: CV Mosby; 1985:112–125.

41. Barber E. Strength and range-of-motion examination skills for the clinical orthotist. *J Prosthet Orthot.* 1993;5(2):49–51.

42. Thomas P, Eliasson S. Diabetic neuropathy. In: *Peripheral Neuropathy.* Philadelphia: WB Saunders; 1984;2:1773–1801.

43. Boughton B. Experts debate long and short of limb length discrepancy. *Biomechanics.* 2000;7:139–140.

44. Oakley W, Catterall R, Martin M. Aetiology and management of lesions of the feet in diabetes. *Br Med J.* 1956;56:4999–5003.

45. Sinacore OR, Elsner R, Rubenow C. *Healing Rates of Diabetic Foot Ulcers in Subjects with Fixed Charcot Deformity.* Platform Presentation, Physical Therapy 1997 APTA Scientific Meeting and Exposition; San Diego, CA; May 30–June 4, 1997.

46. Tiberio D. Pathomechanics of structural foot deformities. *Phys Ther.* 1988;68:1840–1849.

47. Yale J. *Yale's Podiatric Medicine.* 3rd ed. Baltimore: Williams & Wilkins; 1980:135–136.

48. Wilson J, Foster D. *Textbook of Endocrinology.* Philadelphia: WB Saunders; 1992:1294–1297.

49. Olefsky J, Sherman R. Diabetes. In: *Insensitive Feet—A Practical Handout on Foot Problems in Leprosy.* London: The Leprosy Mission; 1977.

50. Yale J. *Yale's Podiatric Medicine.* 3rd ed. Baltimore: Williams & Wilkins; 1980:159–160.

51. Wagner FEW. The dysvascular foot: A system for diagnosis and treatment. *Foot Ankle.* 1981;2:64–122.

52. Glugla M, Mulder G. The diabetic foot. In: Krasner D, ed. *Medical Management of Foot Ulcers in Chronic Wound Care: A Clinical Source Book for Healthcare Professionals.* St. Louis, MO: Mosby/Health Management Publications, Inc; 1990:223–239.

53. Wagner F. A classification and treatment program for diabetic, neuropathic and dysvascular foot problems. *Foot Ankle.* 1983:1–47.

54. Sosenko J, Kato M, Soto R. Comparison of quantitative sensory threshold measures for their association with foot ulceration in diabetic patients. *Diabetes Care.* 1990;13:1057–1062.

55. Omer G. Sensibility testing. In: *Management of Peripheral Nerve Problems.* Philadelphia: W. Saunders; 1980:3–14.

56. Birke J, Sims D. Plantar sensory threshold in the ulcerative foot. *Br Lepr Relief Assoc.* 1986;57:261–267.

57. Birke J. Management of the diabetic foot. *Wound Care Manage.* 1995.

58. Ashbury A. Diabetic neuropathy. *Diabetes Care.* 1991;14(suppl 2):63–68.

59. Thivolet C, Farkh J, Petiot A. Measuring vibration sensations with graduated tuning fork. *Diabetes Care.* 1990;13:1077–1080.

60. National Aeronautics and Space Administration. Mission accomplished (thermography aids in the detection of neuromuscular problems). *NASA Tech Brief.* January 1993:92.

61. Apelqvist J, Larsson J, Agardh C. The influence of external precipitating factors and peripheral neuropathy on the development and outcome of diabetic foot ulcers. *J Diabetic Complications.* 1990;4:21–25.

62. Huntley A. Taking care of your hands. *Diabetes Forecast.* August 1991:11–12.

63. Bergtholdt H. Temperature assessment of the insensate. *Phys Ther.* 1979;59:18–22.

64. Horzic M, Bunoza D, Maric K. Contact thermography in a study of primary healing of surgical wounds. *Ostomy Wound/Manage.* 1996;42(1):36–43.

65. Chan A, MacFarlane I, Bowsher D. Contact thermography of painful neuropathic foot. *Diabetes Care.* 1991;14:918–922.

66. Zhu H, Maalej N, Webster J. An umbilical data acquisition system for measuring pressures between foot and shoe. *IEEE Trans Biomed Eng.* 1990;37:908–911.

67. Wertsch J, Webster J, Tompkins W. A portable insole plantar measurement system. *J Rehabil Res Dev.* 1992;29:13–18.

68. Lord M. Clinical trial of a computer-aided system for orthopaedic shoe upper design. *Prosthet Orthot Int.* 1991;15:11–17.

69. McAllister D, Carver D, Devarajan R. An interactive computer graphics system for the design of molded and orthopedic shoe lasts. *J Rehabil Res Dev.* 1991;28:39–46.

70. Sims D, Cavanagh P, Ulbrecht J. Risk factors in the diabetic foot: Recognition and management. *Phys Ther.* 1988;68:1887–1916.

71. DeJong R. *The Neurologic Examination.* New York: Harper & Row; 1969:742–743.

72. Newman L, Palestro C, Schwartz M. Unsuspected osteomyelitis in diabetic foot ulcers: Diagnosis and monitoring by leukocyte scanning with indium in oxyquinoline. *Diabetes Spectrum.* 1992;5:346–347.

73. Kuncir E, Wirta R, Golbranson F. Load-bearing characteristics of polyethylene foam: An examination of structural and compression properties. *J Rehabil Res Dev.* 1990;27:229–238.

74. Levin M, O'Neal L. *The Diabetic Foot.* St. Louis, MO: CV Mosby; 1988.

75. Pratt D. Medium term comparison of shock attenuating insoles using a spectral analysis technique. *J Biomed Eng.* 1988;10:426–428.

76. Pratt D. Long term comparison of shock attenuating insoles. *Prosthet Orthot Int.* 1990;14:59–62.

77. Lockard M. Foot orthosis. *Phys Ther.* 1988;68:1866–1873.

78. Hack M. Fitting shoes. *Diabetes Forecast.* January 1989.

79. McPoil T. Footwear. *Phys Ther.* 1988;68:1857–1865.

80. McPoil T, Adrian M, Pidcoe P. Effects of foot orthoses on center-of-pressure patterns in women. *Phys Ther.* 1989;69:66–71.

81. Coleman W, Brasseau D. Methods of treating plantar ulcers. *Phys Ther.* 1991;71:116–122.

82. Dwyer G, Rust M. Shoe business. *Diabetes Forecast.* June 1988: 60–63.

83. Mueller M, Diamond J, Sinacore D. Total contact casting in treatment of diabetic plantar ulcers. *Diabetes Care.* 1989;12:384–388.

84. Sinacore D, Mueller M, Diamond J. Diabetic plantar ulcers treated by total contact casting. *Phys Ther.* 1987;67:1543–1549.

85. Birke J, Novick A, Graham S, et al. Methods of treating plantar ulcers. *Phys Ther.* 1991;71:41–47.

86. Diamond J, Sinacore D, Mueller M. Molded double-rocker plaster shoe for healing a diabetic plantar ulcer. *Phys Ther.* 1987;67:1550–1552.

87. Armstrong DG, Lavery LA. Healing the diabetic wound with pressure off-loading. *Biomechanics.* 1997;4:67.

88. Fleischli JG, Laughlin TJ. TCC remains the gold standard for off-loading plantar ulcers. *Biomechanics.* 1998;5:51–52.

89. Giacolone VF. Diabetic footwear: Pressure relief modalities. *Podiatr Today.* 1998;10:16–20.

90. Birke J, Nawoczenski D. Orthopedic walkers: Effect on plantar pressures. *Clin Prosthet Orthot.* 1988;12:74–80.

91. Lauridsen K, Sorensen C, Christiansen P. Measurements of pressure on the sole of the foot in plaster of paris casts on the lower leg. *J Int Soc Prosthet Orthot.* 1989;13:42–45.

92. Nawoczenski DA, Birke JA. Management of the neuropathic foot in the elderly. *Top Geriatr Rehab.* 1992;7:36–48.

93. Ovington LG. Wound healing forecast looks wet. *Biomechanics.* 1998;5:39–70.

94. Pieper B, Templin T, et al. Wound prevalence, types and treatments in home care. *Adv Wound Care.* April 1999;117–126.

95. Armstrong DG, Lavery LA, et al. Infrared dermal thermometry for the high-risk diabetic foot. *Phys Ther.* 1997;77:169–171.

96. McIntyre K. Control of infection in the diabetic foot: The role of microbiology, immunopathology, antibiotics, and guillotine amputation. *J Vasc Surg.* 1987;5:787–802.

97. Lai C, Lin S, Yang C. Limb salvage of infected diabetic foot ulcers with microsurgical free-muscle transfer. *Diabeties Spectrum.* 1992;5:356–357.

98. Tillow T, Habrshaw G, Chrzan J. Review of metatarsal osteotomies for the treatment of neuropathic ulcerations. *Diabetes Spectrum.* 1992;5:357–358.

99. Stanley J. *Structure and Function in Man.* 3rd ed. Philadelphia: WB Saunders. 1974; 65–68.

100. Kechiijian P. How do nails grow? *Nails.* May 1993:78–79.

101. O'Neal LW. Surgical pathway of the foot and clinicopathologic conditions. In: Bowker JH, Pfeifer MA, eds. *The Diabetic Foot.* 6th edition. St. Louis, MO: CV Mosby; 2000:501–506.

102. Ruscin C, Cunningham G, Blaylock A. Foot care protocol for the older client. *Geriatr Nurs.* July/Aug 1993;210–212.

103. Sher RK. The nail doctor. *Nails.* December 1977:94–95.

104. Levin SM, Jacoby S. *Your Feet Don't Have To Hurt.* New York: St. Martin's Press; 2000:65–68.

105. Harkless LB, Satterfield VK, Dennis KJ. Role of the podiatrist. In: Bowker JH, Pfeifer MA, eds. *The Diabetic Foot.* 6th ed. St Louis, MO: CV Mosby; 2000:690.

106. Furman A. Give your feet a sporting chance. *Diabetes Forecast.* April 1989:17–22.

107. Graham C. Neuropathy made you stop. *Diabetes Forecast.* December 1992:47–49.

CHAPTER 19

Management of the Skin and Nails

Teresa J. Kelechi

CHAPTER OBJECTIVES

At the completion of this chapter, the reader will be able to:

1. Describe the clinical presentation of three foot problems: tinea pedis, onychomycosis, and plantar fasciitis.
2. List two interventions each for the treatment of tinea pedis, onychomycosis, and plantar fasciitis.
3. Discuss four patient education points related to prevention of foot disorders.
4. List three referral criteria for foot complications.

SIGNIFICANCE OF FOOT PROBLEMS

Foot problems plague approximately 70% of persons 65 years of age and older.[1] Many problems are related to the nails and skin. Nail deformities are among those conditions that require intervention, particularly onychomycosis, or fungal infection of the nail that causes it to discolor and thicken. Loss of nail integrity from a deformed toenail can lead to more serious complications, such as infections, osteomyelitis, wounds, and, in some cases, amputations. Patients with diabetes and impaired circulation may be at greater risk. Skin problems such as xerosis, tinea pedis, and fissures can also place the patient at risk for more serious skin complications. Skin and nail problems can reduce functional ability, thus leading to impairment in quality of life. Therefore, it becomes critical that health care providers address the feet by inspecting the skin and nails and providing interventions to ameliorate or prevent more serious foot problems.

Foot care procedures, such as debriding toenails, paring hyperkeratotic lesions (corns or calluses), and prevention/

management of diabetic foot complications, are not covered in this chapter. The literature is replete with references and texts related to assessment, identification of risk factors, interventions, and patient education specific to the population with diabetes.[2] This chapter discusses common foot problems. See Chapter 18 for care of the skin and nails of the neuropathic (diabetic) patient.

TINEA PEDIS

Tinea pedis is the most common form of dermatophytosis, or fungal infection of the feet. Dermatophytes are aerobic fungi. Tinea pedis, most commonly known as "athlete's foot," is a disorder that can be classified into three categories: interdigital infections, scaling hyperkeratotic moccasin-type infections of the plantar surface, and highly inflammatory vesiculobullous eruptions. Dermatophytes invade, infect, and persist in the stratum corneum and, rarely, penetrate below the surface of the epidermis or its appendages. The skin responds to the superficial infection by increased proliferation, which leads to scaling and epidermal thickening.[3]

The causes of tinea pedis are classified into three anomorphic genera; *Trichophyton*, *Microsporum*, and *Epidermophyton*, depending on their conidial structures. Dermatophytes can be acquired from the soil, animals, and from other humans. The most common source in the United States is infected individuals. A higher incidence in modern times can be attributed to the increased use of broad-spectrum antibiotics, the expanding number of immunocompromised patients, and lifestyle changes. Those with hepatic, renal, and endocrine (diabetes mellitus) diseases are at higher risk. There is also an increased incidence among gardeners and farmers; those who wear boots or sports shoes; and those who frequent sports facilities, pools, and communal leisure facilities. Ten percent of the population is estimated to be infected by a dermatophyte; of these, tinea pedis is the most common, occurring in up to 70% of adults.[1] Contributing factors include warmth and high humidity, with constant occlusion. Exhibit 19–1 presents the clinical findings in tinea pedis. Symptoms include pruritis, painful or uncomfortable breaks in the skin, odor, and disability.[1,4]

Laboratory studies are generally indicated because greater diagnostic accuracy occurs if the clinical diagnosis is verified by laboratory tests. This verification is especially important when the use of systemic therapy is anticipated. Potassium hydroxide preparation (KOH) and fungal cultures may be performed.

KOH specimens should be obtained from the active border or edge of a lesion or scale from the site of infection. If a vesicle or bulla is present, the roof is an appropriate specimen. In pustular lesions, the purulent debris is acceptable. Place the material on a glass slide, add 10–15% KOH, with or without dimethyl sulfoxide (DMSO). If DMSO is added, heating is not necessary. A fungal stain, such as Chlorazol Black E or Parker's blue black ink, may be added to highlight the hyphae. A positive KOH will show multiple septate hyphae.[5]

Fungal cultures are recommended for the persistent and more difficult conditions requiring specific identification. Various methods to obtain the culture have been published, such as using a sterile toothbrush or rubbing moistened sterile swabs or gauze pads over the affected area, then pressing into the surface of the dermatophyte test medium to be cultured. The laboratory should be contacted for the acceptable method for obtaining the culture and which medium is to be used if culture is required.

Exhibit 19–1 Clinical Presentation of Tinea Pedis

1. Whitish, macerated interdigital spaces, most often the fourth and fifth digits.
2. Erythematous skin with vesicles, scales, or fissures.
3. Malodor from bacterial superinfection, which may mask the underlying fungal infection.
4. Thickened, scaly, dry patches on the soles and sides of feet.
5. Lesions may be described as noninflammatory scaly, acute or subacute eczematous-like, chronically lichenified, nodular and granulomatous, bullous and pustular, or resembling pyoderma.
6. Associated findings may include infections involving the hair follicle and nail, persistent hyperpigmentation and/or hypopigmentation, and secondary bacterial infection.

Differential diagnosis is indicated to rule out psoriasis, parapsoriasis, eczema, candidiasis, bacterial infection, and other dermatoses. The diagnosis of tinea pedis is generally classified into three categories: interdigital toe web infections, plantar moccasin-type infection, and vesiculobullous tinea pedis.

Interdigital toe web infections usually start as dermatophyte infections (*Trichophyton rubrum* and *Trichophyton mentagrophytes*) with an interplay between various bacterial species and, although rare, *Candida* species. Scaling is the initial feature, and, when the bacteria proliferate, maceration occurs (see Figure 19–1). The terms *dermatophytosis simplex* and *dermatophytosis complex* have been proposed to address two forms of interdigital infection, where *simplex* refers to features of scaling and, at times, fissures. *Complex* includes a highly macerated, leukokeratotic symptomatic process in which dermatophytes can be recovered in only one-third of patients. This variety of interdigital infection is mainly caused by an overgrowth of a myriad of bacterial species.[6]

Plantar moccasin-type infection results in diffuse hyperkeratotic scaling of the plantar surface and is often associated with toenail involvement. The skin may become red, with severe itching in some cases. The main feature is small scales that often appear as small, round areas of peeling skin (see Figure 19–2).

Lastly, vesiculobullous tinea pedis presents as acute, highly inflammatory eruptions, particularly on the arch and side of the foot. *T. mentagrophytes* is primarily responsible. Persons with recurrent episodes tend to have low-grade scaling between exacerbations of acute inflammation. Differing environmental factors, such as seasonal temperature, sweating from physical activities, and types of shoe wear, influence the growth of the fungus. When sufficient proliferation and penetration of the stratum corneum occur, the epidermis comes into contact with fungal antigens, and a T-cell-mediated immune contact allergic response occurs.[7]

Treatment modalities include general and specific interventions. General interventions involve use of topical antifungal agents. Topical antifungal agents are indicated for the following types of dermatophytoses: simple interdigital, and noninflammatory moccasin-type. Exhibit 19–2 presents common topical products.

Clinical Wisdom

Terbinafine hydrochloride cream (Lamisil Cream 1%, available over the counter) should be applied twice daily until clinical signs and symptoms of tinea pedis significantly improve, usually by day 7. The duration of drug therapy should be for a minimum of 1 week, not to exceed 4 weeks.

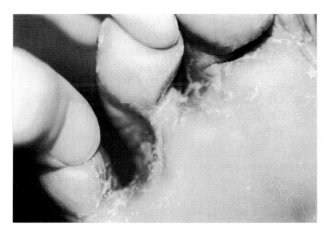

Figure 19–1 Photo of tinea pedis interdigital toe web infection.

Specific interventions for tinea pedis relate to the type of infection. For dermatophytosis complex, the use of a topical fungicidal agent, such as an allylamine (terbinafine) in conjunction (alternated with) a double antibiotic ointment, such as Polysporin, or with broad-spectrum antibacterial agents, such as Castellani's paint, aluminum chloride, and various tinctures of dye (gentian violet) may be used. If the toenails are infected, this reservoir of fungi must also be treated. Topical therapy is often recommended for an indefinite period to eradicate residual fungus and to prevent relapse, but this should be closely monitored.[3,8]

Research Wisdom

Most recently, the literature suggests oral antifungal agents for 1 week[9] are perhaps more effective in treating the skin than are topical agents.

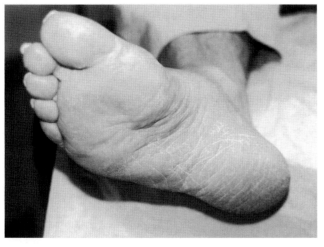

Figure 19–2 Photo of mocassin-type tinea pedis.

Exhibit 19–2 Common Topical Antifungal Products

- Imidazoles (examples include: Clotrimazole, Econazole, Ketoconazole, Miconazole, Oxiconazole, Sulconazole)
- Allylamines (examples include: Naftifine, Terbinafine)
- Ciclopirox olamine
- Miscellaneous (Whitfield's ointment, Tolnaftate, Haloprogin, drying agents, powders, antibiotics [when applicable], salicylic acid, and other keratolytic agents).

A severe moccasin-type or dermatophytosis complex resistant to topical therapy alone requires use of systemic therapy, such as itraconazole (Sporanox) 200 mg daily for 1 week (increase to 12 weeks if toenails are involved—refer to package insert for more detailed prescribing information) or terbinafine hydrochloride 250 mg daily for daily 1 week (protocol will change if the patient has onychomycosis—see prescribing information in package insert).[7,10,11]

Clinical Wisdom

Tinea pedis can mimic dry skin. Dry skin tends to be flaky, whereas the skin, when infected, tends to produce small, round scales that give the appearance of the skin peeling.

Vesiculobullous tinea pedis with acute, highly inflammatory eruptions requires topical or systemic corticosteroids in conjunction with antifungal agents for acute attacks. The choice of topical or systemic therapy depends on the extent and severity of the process. Caution must be exercised in the use of combination topical corticosteriod-antifungal mixtures, which contain potent fluorinated corticosteriods. Steroid therapy is withdrawn once the cell-mediated immune response is curtailed.

Surgical intervention is usually not indicated. However, some clients may elect to have the infected toenail plate permanently removed, due to continuing nail deformity. The complications of both topical and systemic therapy should be discussed with each client. The most common side effects of topical therapy include irritation, burning, itching, and dryness. Systemic therapy side effects may occur with terbinafine (see Exhibit 19–3) and itraconazole (see Exhibit 19–4). Clients who have known hypersensitivities to topical and systemic antifungal therapy should not take these drugs.

Outcome measures for treatment success include skin that is free of scaling, flakiness, and peeling, and symptoms such as itching or discomfort. Treatment failure should be suspected if the skin has not improved after 1 month of treatment. Skin cultures can be obtained if the infection is suspected to be recalcitrant to therapy.

Exhibit 19–3 Side Effects Related to Terbinafine

Terbinafine (Lamisil)
- gastrointestinal symptoms including diarrhea, dyspepsia
- dermatologic symptoms, including rash, pruritus, urticaria
- liver enzyme abnormalities
- taste disturbance
- visual disturbance

Clinical Wisdom

Liver function studies are indicated prior to treatment with oral itraconazole and terbinafine, per package insert.

Prevention of tinea pedis is a lifelong goal. Many individuals experience several acute exacerbations during their lifetimes. The goal of treatment is to minimize damp, moist skin caused by footwear and to avoid environments that promote fungal growth, such as contaminated showers. The following self-care tips may help to prevent recurrences:

1. Dry feet well after bathing and showering, making sure to dry between the toes.
2. Use antifungal powders or sprays twice daily to minimize moisture on the feet and between the toes.
3. Use lambswool or other absorptive product between the toes when maceration, the whitish overhydrated epidermis, first appears.

Exhibit 19–4 Side Effects Related to Itraconazole

Itraconazole (Sporanox)
- gastrointestinal disorders
- edema
- fatigue
- fever
- malaise
- skin, including rash and pruritus
- central and peripheral nervous system, including headache
- psychiatric disorders, including decreased libido
- hypertension
- hypokalemia
- albuminuria
- abnormal hepatic function
- impotence

---

4. Change socks frequently, especially when damp.
5. Wear fabrics that are most conducive to wicking moisture away, which are synthetics such as nylon; cotton tends to absorb moisture and "holds" it next to the skin.
6. Change shoes frequently and apply antifungal powders and sprays to the inside of the shoes, which helps to reduce fungus in the shoes.

Members of households may choose to use separate tubs and showers from those who are affected to prevent the transmission from one to another; the surface should be cleaned after each use with a solution that will kill fungus.

HEEL PAIN PLANTAR FASCIITIS

Plantar fasciitis is the most common form of heel pain and is due to inflammation, microruptures, hemorrhages, and collagen degeneration of the plantar fascia. The sequalae are fibrosis and possible ossification between the origin of the flexor digitorum brevis and the fascia. The cause of plantar fasciitis is variable and multifactorial.[12] The major underlying factor is overuse injury to soft tissue, involving repetitive, excessive loading impact on heel strike over time. Anatomic, biomechanical, and environmental factors contribute to damage. Anatomic risk factors include pes planus, subtalar joint pronation, cavus foot, unequal leg length, tarsal coalition, and low or high foot arch. Biomechanical forces include tight Achilles tendon with inflexibility, weak plantar flexors, weak ankle flexors, weak intrinsic muscles, obesity, sudden weight gain, and sudden trauma. Change in activity level; rapid increase in training activities related to speed, intensity, and duration; running on steep hills, poor/hard surfaces, or barefoot on sand; outworn running shoes; poor shoe supports; inadequate stretching; excessive walking on the job; and excessive standing on hard, unyielding surfaces are examples of environmental risk factors. Athletic activities that have been linked to plantar fasciitis are running, distance running, tennis, gymnastics, and basketball.[13]

The clinical features include subjective symptoms of pain or discomfort. The pain may be described as a slow, dull ache; intense achiness; or burning sensation. The pain may be sharp, pinpoint, knifelike pain. Patients may complain of pain in the heel when standing after periods of rest, especially during the first step in the morning.[14] This pain diminishes with each successive step but may return late in the afternoon after prolonged weight bearing. It is usually described as nonradiating and well localized to the medial aspect of the heel pad. The symptoms are predominantly unilateral, but bilateral involvement occurs in 10% of cases.[15]

Clinical Wisdom

One of the most common complaints of heel pain associated with plantar fasciitis is the report that the pain is often excruciating upon first rising in the morning, when the foot touches the floor. This tends to be a hallmark symptom of fasciitis.

Objectively, pain can be evaluated as localized point tenderness with palpation over the medial calcaneal tuberosity. The pain can be reproduced during passive dorsiflexion of the ankle or toes and when standing on the toes to tighten the plantar fascia. If the condition is chronic, thickening, nodularity, and tautness can be palpated along the fascia. Diagnostic tests such as radiographs, bone scans, and blood studies are generally reserved for ambiguous presentation. A radiograph can be normal or may reveal a horizontal bone spur projecting from the calcaneal tuberosity. The spur is not necessary in making the diagnosis, but its presence indicates chronic inflammation.[16]

Other related problems that can mimic plantar fasciitis include, but are not limited to:

- Heel pad atrophy
- Tarsal tunnel syndrome
- Achilles tendinitis
- Calcaneal fracture
- Stress fracture
- Compartment syndrome
- Complete or partial plantar fascia rupture
- Systemic disorders, such as lupus erythematous, rheumatoid arthritis, ankylosing spondylitis, Reiter's syndrome, gout, or vascular insufficiency

Client assessment and diagnosis include a thorough history (reports of heel pain, as described previously) and physical examination. The procedure for examining the client is as follows:

1. Ask client to stand. Assess for a rigid cavus foot (high arch) or pes planus (flat foot).
2. Ask client to walk. The gait should be observed for any excessive pronation (ankles turning inward) on heel strike. Observe for a limp that might occur with weight bearing when the foot touches down on its lateral (outside) aspect.
3. Ask client to dorsiflex (move foot upward toward leg) and plantar flex (push toes downward toward floor). Assess range of motion of the ankle. The client should also repeat this, using only the toes. The purpose of this is to identify a tight heel cord or limitation in flexing and extending the great toe.
4. Inspect the shoes for any abnormal wear and the quality of arch support within them. Shoes that are ill fitting and in poor condition should be replaced. Athletic-type walking shoes with proper arch supports are indicated.

Interventions address treatment of pain, restoring flexibility to the ankle and arch, strengthening the muscles in and around the foot, and gradual resumption of activities. Conservative measures are described.[17]

General measures include rest, ice application, stretching, and muscle strengthening. A conservative rest program involves a decrease in activity for 6 weeks.[18] Local ice application several times per day (conservative) involves ice massage for 6–7 minutes or application of an ice pack for 20–40 minutes. Ice should be applied long enough to achieve a numbing affect while avoiding any frostbite injury. (It is recommended that a bag of frozen vegetables, such as peas, be placed in a plastic zipper bag and labeled *ice bag*. A paper towel should be placed around this ice bag and applied to the heel several times a day.) Also, the client can be instructed to place a foam cup filled with water in the freezer. When frozen, place in plastic zipper bag and massage the foot with the ice.

Conservative stretching is considered by some to be the most important part of the regimen. Demonstrate gastrocnemius and soleus stretches to the patient and have him or her return the demonstration. Gastrocnemius stretch is performed by having the client lean forward into a wall and placing the affecting foot 12–18 inches from the wall, with the foot flat against the floor and the knee straight. The soleus stretch is performed in the same manner; however, the back knee is slightly bent. The stretch can be obtained in the seated position by placing a towel under the ball of the foot and gently pulling it upward. Proper stretching is gentle pulling pressure in the muscle with the tendon being stretched, not an increase in pain. Ice or medication (nonsteroidal antiinflammatory drugs [NSAIDs] or other antiinflammatory agents) can be used prior to stretching. It is recommended that a 10- to 20-second stretch be done on arising, with 15 repetitions performed at least two to five times per day. Conservative muscle strengthening exercises can also be taught to the patient. Instruct the patient to pick articles off the floor, using only the toes. Patients should observe the clinician demonstrating any exercise and should perform these exercises several minutes each day for at least 6 weeks.

Specific interventions include use of medications, support devices, strapping, shoe wear, and orthotics.[19] NSAIDs may be prescribed for pain management. These are prescribed for acute cases for a 7- to 10-day course up to 1 month, depending on the drug and degree of symptom management required. Currently, some of the drugs of choice are the longer-acting agents, such as oxaprozin (DayPro). Conservative support devices include use of heel cups, pads, lifts, and arch support inserts placed in both shoes.[20] These devices relieve the tension on the plantar fascia by reestablishing the arched shape of the foot. Cups and pads are especially beneficial to the elderly when there is atrophy of the plantar heel pad. If tenderness is localized, a cutout can be made into any of these three types of shoe inserts to relieve pressure over the tender area. Pedorthists, physical therapists, chiropractors, and podiatrists can recommend the proper inserts and orthotics when needed.

Conservative strapping helps to reestablish or maintain the arch of the foot, stabilizes the first metatarsal head and decreases forefoot pronation, controls heel valgus (turning outward), and changes the foot strike position. Strapping is considered to be beneficial in the acute phase of plantar fasciitis. Night splints can be obtained from orthopaedic foot stores and worn at night to keep the foot in proper alignment (dorsiflexed), thus preventing relaxation of the fascia, which, when supported, is less painful. Sports medicine or physical therapy will perform the strapping procedure and can recommend night splints. They can also be obtained from specialty footwear catalogues.[21]

Shoes—good walking shoes and athletic-type footwear—are part of the treatment plan. Shoes with a firm heel, good heel cushioning, and an adequate longitudinal arch support are recommended. Orthotics are devices that relieve symptoms by providing adequate resistance to the mechanical forces applied to the foot. Clients are referred to an orthotist, pedorthist, podiatrist, or other foot care-related specialist.

Clinical Wisdom

Pain on rising from bed in the morning when the affected foot is placed on the floor is a hallmark symptom that can be minimized when the client first stretches and puts on a shoe before walking.

If no improvement is noted within 6 weeks, the client can be referred to physical therapy—there are conflicting data regarding the benefit of physical therapy modalities, such as pulsed ultrasound, phonophoresis, and high-voltage galvanic stimulation. Additionally, contrast soaks may be recommended. Contrast soaks involve using hot and cold soaks for 15 minutes twice a day, beginning with a warm soak for the first half and followed by cold soaks for the remainder.

If improvement is only minimal after another 6–8 weeks, a steroid injection may be necessary. A corticosteroid injection into the calcaneal attachment can help control the inflamma-

tion of plantar fasciitis. The major risks are fascia rupture associated with degeneration of the fascia and fat pad atrophy. These injections tend to be very painful. Measures to reduce the pain associated with injection are use of local anesthetic, along with a corticosteroid cryospray before the injection, and use of medial injection parallel to the fascia. Three injections may be given 2–4 weeks apart. If pain is recalcitrant to treatment after 2 years, surgery may be an option. Candidates for surgery are limited to those with significant pain and disability in activities of daily living. Exhibit 19–5 presents complications related to plantar fasciitis treatment.

Outcomes measures of success include clients who note a reduction in pain after 4–6 weeks of conservative treatment and report a cessation of symptoms after 8 months to a year. Referral criteria include clients whose symptoms last longer than 6 months or who present with chronic symptoms of many months' to years' duration. Consultation to a foot care specialist in sports medicine, orthopaedics, podiatry, pedorthy, physical therapy, etc. is dependent on the client's response to conservative treatment. Follow-up is generally within 6 weeks from onset of treatment.[22]

Self-care strategies for prevention of exacerbations include wearing proper footwear with adequate arch supports and avoiding extreme dorsiflexion of the feet, such as bending down on the forefoot, putting excessive pressure on the toes and metatarsal heads of the feet. This position causes extreme tension on the fascia and can induce microtears. Avoiding excessive trauma from sports-related "pounding" of the feet during running, etc. against hard surfaces, such as concrete, is also recommended. [23]

ONYCHOMYCOSIS

Onychomycosis (tinea unguium) is an infection of the toenails in which fungal organisms invade the nail unit via the nail bed or nail plate, causing insidious, progressive destruc-

---

Exhibit 19–5 Complications of Plantar Fasciitis Treatment

A. orthotics — toe jamming, heel irritation, and slippage from an improper fit
B. nonsteroidal antiinflammatory drugs — gastrointestinal upset most common (see package insert for comprehensive list of adverse reactions)
C. strapping — allergy to tape, prep adhesive; blistering and irritation
D. shoes — ill-fitting footwear, leading to blisters, corns, calluses, and pain
E. steroid injections — fat pad atrophy, pain and degeneration of the fascia, plantar fascia rupture
F. surgery — decrease in strength and function

tion of the nail plate if left untreated (see Figures 19–3 and 19–4). It is precipitated by environmental factors, repeated microtrauma to the nail and its structures, moisture, and skin fungal infection. It is also related to aging, extensive use of chemotherapeutic, systemic antibiotic and immunosuppressive therapies, and the spread of human immunodeficiency virus (HIV). Fungal infections appear more commonly in those 40–80 years of age, in elderly more than in the younger population, and in men more than in women.[22]

There are three main classes of fungi that cause onychomycosis. Dermatophyte fungi account for 90% of fungal infections and include *T. rubrum*, *Epidermaophyton floccosum*, and *T. mentagrophytes*. Yeasts, including *Candida albicans*, account for 8% and nondermatophyte molds, including *Aspergillus* species, *Scopulariopsis brevicaulis*, *Scytalidium dimidiatum*, *Scytalidium hyalinum*, *Fusarium* species, and *Acremonium* species account for 2% of onychomycosis. Mixed infections involving two or more fungi may occur. The initial pathophysiology involves a mild inflammatory response to the fungi, once they have invaded the nail bed, causing hypertrophy of the bed. Hyperkeratosis and hypertrophy of the nail plate results in a deformed, thick, crumbly nail.

There are four patterns of nail infection, each associated with a different entry point of the fungi into the nail unit, as well as a different appearance of the infected nail. Distal subungual onychomycosi is the most common type, and *T. rubrum* is the most common cause. The distal nail plate turns yellow or whitish brown, with hyperkeratotic debris accumulation under the nail. The plate often becomes thickened,

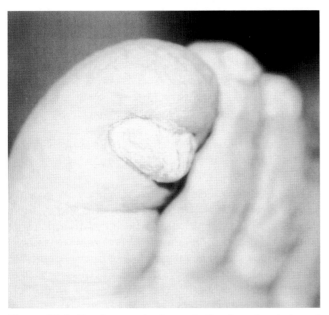

Figure 19–3 Onychomycosis demonstrating hyperkeratosis and hypertrophy of the nail plate with a deformed, thick, crumbly nail. The plate is thickened, deformed, brittle, and crumbly.

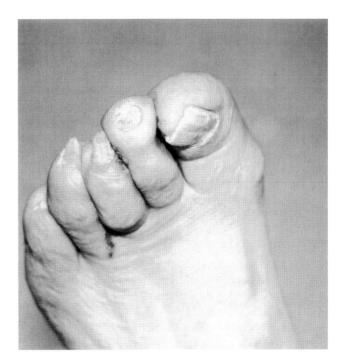

Figure 19–4 Onychomycosis involving multiple nail plates.

deformed, brittle, and crumbly, and can make wearing shoes uncomfortable or painful.[23]

Proximal subungual onychomycosis appears more frequently in immunocompromised patients caused by dermatophytes. Fungi invade the proximal nail fold and cuticle, then infect the deeper portion of the plate. The proximal nail plate develops a white color in patchy areas. The surface remains smooth and intact. Hyperkeratotic debris can accumulate under the plate. The third type, white superficial onychomycosis is most often caused by the dermatophyte *T. mentagrophytes* and a variety of molds. Fungi directly invade the surface of the plate, producing a white, soft, dry, powdery, crumbly appearance. The plate does not thicken and continues to adhere to the nail bed.[24] It may occur in patients with HIV disease. Candida onychomycosis is the fourth pattern of nail infection and is caused mainly by *C. albicans*. It is a rare syndrome, limited to patients with chronic mucocutaneous candidiasis. The nail plate thickens and turns yellow-brown.[25]

The predisposing factors to nail infections include chronic tinea pedis or other foot infections, advanced age with slower growth of the nail and decreased circulation, and athletics where trauma to the nail weakens the seal between the nail plate and nail bed, allowing fungal organisms to penetrate the nail unit. Athletes are at higher risk because of profuse sweating, with runners particularly prone to onychomycosis. Exogenous heat and moisture, which worsen the condition, as well as hyperhydrosis (excessive sweating), as seen in anyone who wears shoes or boots every day for 12 or more hours at a time, also increase risk. Data suggest that people who wear sandals are less vulnerable to fungi because their feet are exposed to the air. Immunosuppressed patients, in whom the body's ability to combat the infection is compromised, are also at risk. Postmenopausal women are affected, because estrogen appears to exert a protective effect in younger women. Onychomycosis seems to manifest itself initially in individuals in their 40s and 50s. It is common in older populations and in those with diabetes and circulatory impairment.[26,27]

Onychomycosis presents with three common signs. The nail plate becomes discolored, with white, brown, or yellow patches or streaks. Resulting subungual hyperkeratosis and debris as the plate loses its structural integrity and onycholysis (loosening or separation of all or part of the nail plate from the bed) are common. Symptoms include pain; trauma to adjacent soft skin folds from the thickened nails; and embarrassment from disfigured, discolored, and deformed nails. Pain can result from the thick nail plate because it causes pressure on the nail bed from ill-fitting footwear.[28]

As a rule, laboratory studies are conducted when onychomycosis cannot be managed by standard mechanical or pharmacologic treatments. Histologic analysis via nail culture should be conducted in resistant clinical situations when fungal infection is suspected. It can take up to 30 days to obtain results. Because processing these specimens may require special techniques, contact local laboratory for requirements. If a diagnosis is still not possible using the microscopic exam or histologic analysis, biopsy of the nail bed is indicated.

Clinical Wisdom

Many other nail conditions can mimic onychomycosis, such as trauma-induced dystrophic nail (abnormal in appearance, shape, and texture), psoriasis, eczema, lichen planus, ischemic conditions, congenital nail disorders, yellow nail syndrome, and pseudomonas.

Treatment measures include general measures of mechanical manual debridement with nippers and/or a rotary grinding tool and more specific measures, such as surgical nail removal (because monotherapy is rare and not recommended), topical nail reduction using urea compound (20–40%) in petrolatum under thin film dressing, and topical antifungal agents. The overall cure rates of topical therapy are relatively low, and relapse rates are relatively high. The duration of topical antifungal monotherapy for onychomycosis is at least 6–12 months, and it may be a lifelong process.[29] Nail lacquers and creams can be used in conjunction with manual debridement and may include (but are not limited to): ciclopirox (Loprox), oxiconazole nitrate (Oxistat), halo progin (Halotex), econazole nitrate (Spectazole), sulconazole nitrate (Exelderm), ketoconazole (Nizoral), naftifine hydrochloride (Naftin), terbinafine hydrochloride (Lamisil), and others (sodium pyrithione, amorolfine, allylamines, bifonazole/urea, propylene glycol-urea-lactic acid, imidazoles, organic acids). Systemic antifungal agents, such as itraconazole (Sporanox) or terbinafine (Lamisil), can also be useful (Exhibit 19–6). Baseline liver function studies are obtained prior to initiation of oral therapy and during its course. Refer to package insert for prescribing information.[30,31,32]

The optimal clinical effect for systemic therapy is seen some months after cessation of treatment and is related to the period required for outgrowth of healthy nail. It may take up to 8–12 months for nail cure.[33] Outcomes measures include a nail free of discoloration, thickness, and crumbly texture.[34] It is important to remind clients that a "perfect" nail may not be an attainable goal. However, a nail plate that is much less thick is cosmetically more appealing and does reduce the risk of injury to the underlying nail bed.[35,36]

Measures to prevent fungal infection or reinfection are critical. Clients should be instructed on the following key points:

A. Wear properly fitting shoes and do not wear the same pair every day. Instruct client to alternate between two pairs. Shoes with a high toe box of extra depth can accommodate thickened nails.
B. Wear thin acrylic or acrylic-blend socks, such as those worn by runners. These wick the moisture away from the skin, rather than absorbing it, keeping the skin less damp. The socks should be changed frequently if they do become moist.
C. Wash the feet daily and pay close attention to drying well between the toes.
D. Trim toenails straight across, smoothing any rough or jagged edges and following the contour or shape of the toe.
E. Instruct the client to alert health care professionals of any changes in the nail or skin.

Referral criteria include treatment failure with systemic agents (after 9–12 months of nail growth, even after systemic therapy has been completed) and client dissatisfaction with mechanical debridement. Those who are unable to take systemic therapy should be referred to foot care specialists for evaluation of more aggressive treatment, such as removal of the nail plate by surgical or chemical methods, particularly when severe toenail deformities exist. Clients who elect conservative measures, such as mechanical debridement, should see foot care professionals every 2–3 months.

Exhibit 19–6 Guidelines for Systemic Antifungal Therapy for Onychomycosis[32]

- Itraconazole, 200 mg twice a day for 7 days per month for 3 months. Advise clients to take with a full meal. Adverse reactions include elevated liver enzymes (> 2 times normal range), gastrointestinal disorders, rash, hypertension, orthostatic hypotension, headache, malaise, myalgia, hypokalemia, albuminuria, vertigo.
- Terbinafine, 250 mg gd for 12 weeks. Adverse reactions include headache, gastrointestinal symptoms such as diarrhea, dyspepsia, abdominal pain, nausea, diarrhea, and flatulence; dermatologic symptoms such as rash, pruritus, and urticaria; liver enzyme abnormalities; taste disturbance; and visual disturbance.

MISCELLANEOUS CONDITIONS

This section presents information on miscellaneous foot conditions. Each condition is defined, brief pathophysiology related to the condition is presented, then key points and general guidelines for management are listed.

Xerosis/anhidrosis—excessively dry, flaky skin that may be particularly severe on the heels and bottoms of the feet. Anhidrosis is often related to autonomic dysfunction due to endocrine or neurologic disorders that cause loss of moisture production in the skin, leading to severe flaking (see Figures 19–5 and 19–6).

1. Teach client to avoid soaking feet in water because it can cause excessive drying by depleting moisture from the skin.
2. Apply topical hydrating products and seal them with petrolatum-based products several times each day and at bedtime—may require a prescription-strength product if symptoms do not resolve after 4 weeks.
3. Wear proper footwear and socks, which are barriers between the skin and shoe.

Hyperhidrosis—excessive moisture production related to endocrine/neurologic or sweat gland disorders.

1. Teach client to change acrylic or acrylic-blend socks several times each day.
2. May use spray antiperspirants on skin and absorptive powders daily or more frequently as needed—prescription-strength antiperspirant (ie, Drysol) may be needed to treat recalcitrant sweating.
4. Footwear should be of leather or canvas/cloth material that is breathable.

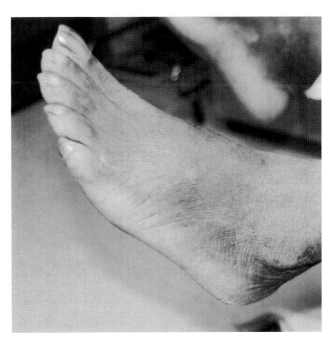

Figure 19–5 Anhidrosis of the foot.

Cellulitis/infection—inflammation and subsequent infection of the connective tissue between adjacent tissues and organs, commonly due to bacterial infection. It gives the overlying skin a reddish appearance. Infection may be in toes, dorsum and plantar surface of the feet, and the lower leg skin. This can be as a result of trauma, wounds, and immunodeficiency syndromes.

1. Order diagnostic testing, such as radiograph, magnetic resonance imaging to r/o osteomyelitis.
2. Initiate proper antibiotic therapy.
3. Initiate wound care, if wound is present.
4. Teach patient to dress wound and prevent mechanical, thermal, or chemical injury to area.
5. Instruct patient to report worsening of symptoms, such as increased size, drainage, redness, pain, or fever.
6. Instruct patient to take pain relievers.

Maceration—macerated toe web spaces result from rigid or fixed toe deformities or functional impairment, such as stiffness, that prevent the client from bending over to dry the feet and areas between the toes. Excessive moisture gets trapped and can lead to fungal and bacterial infections.

1. Implement moisture control practices, eg, drying well between toes after bathing or showering and wiping toe web spaces with dry agents, such as alcohol, for up to 1 week.

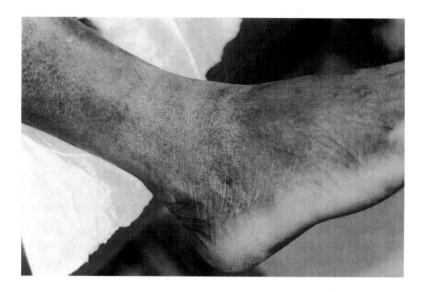

Figure 19–6 Close-up photo of the skin in Figure 19–5. Note the cracking in the skin.

2. Use lambswool, cotton, or other absorptive material between toes to reduce moisture. This should be changed daily.
3. Apply absorptive powder between toes and in shoes to reduce moisture.
4. Instruct client to wear thin acrylic or acrylic-blend socks when wearing shoes.
5. Advise client to change shoes frequently.
6. Once maceration is treated, skin preparation/protectant wipes may be used between the toes as a moisture barrier.

Hyperkeratotic lesions (corns/calluses)—corns (helomas; see Figure 19–7) and calluses (tylomas; see Figure 19–8) are circumscribed masses of a hornlike collection of epidermal cells that are thicker in the center and gradually taper, becoming thinner at the periphery. Hard corns arise on top of or on the sides of the fifth toes; soft corns arise between the toes. Calluses are found on the plantar surface of the feet under prominent weight-bearing areas and on the medial and lateral aspects of the sides of the feet and great toes. Corns and calluses form as a result of abnormal intermittent or chronic weight-bearing pressure and/or shear sliding stresses.

1. Reduce amount of thickened keratoses by either mechanical debridement (buffing) or paring with sharp debridement.
2. Pad with sheet hydrogel and silicon-based products, nonmedicated—may also use foam pads.

3. Recommend pressure relief shoes, such as those with high toe box and padded cushion inserts.
4. Instruct client to gently buff areas 2–3 times per week with pumice stone, file board, etc. before taking shower or bath and to pad with proper over-the-counter pads, as directed (Pedifix Viscogel corn protectors or Dr. Scholl's Cushlin nonmedicated corn and callus pads).

Fissures—cracks in the dermis, causing a partial thickness wound.

1. Reduce keratotic tissue around fissure, if present, by mechanical or sharp debridement
2. Cleanse area and apply dressing such as thin film, thin hydrocolloid, sheet hydrogel, dressing cloth tapes, etc. to close the wound.
3. Change dressing weekly to allow for closure of wound.
4. Instruct client on moisturizing protocol to prevent further fissures.
5. Instruct client to wear shoes at all times and to avoid slippers or sandals that "flop" against the heel, causing excessive friction.

Onychauxis—hypertrophic toenails or excessively thick toenails as a result of trauma, aging, genetic predisposition, etc., not related to onychomycosis.

1. Mechanical debridement is required.

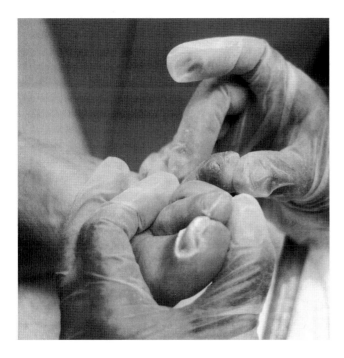

Figure 19–7 Example of corn in the interdigital space.

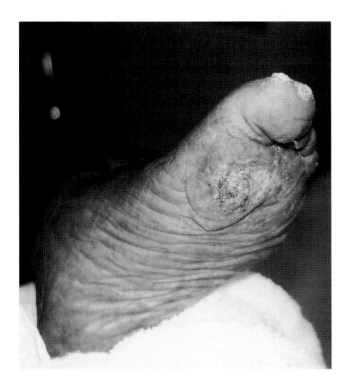

Figure 19–8 Callus formation.

2. Teach client to reduce toenails at home if functionally able, using proper equipment.
3. Instruct client to obtain extra-depth shoes or shoes with a high toe box to accommodate thickened toenails.

SELF-CARE TEACHING GUIDELINES

Specific self-care teaching guidelines are presented under each specific foot problem. General guidelines for self-care are presented here. It is important to instruct clients on purchasing shoes that accommodate structural deformities, offer support and cushion, and are easy to get on. Shoes are important to prevent a variety of complications. Those that are too narrow can cause blisters and corns. Those that are too short can cause toenail injury and hammertoes. Others that offer little support can lead to foot pain. Finally, shoes should be thought of as functional aids, rather than stylish accompaniments to clothing. Unfortunately, culture often dictates dress codes. The health care professional can be very influential in helping clients to understand the need for proper footwear, which can prevent serious foot complications, provide relief from excessive pressure and mechanical stress, and can add to the quality of life by reducing foot pain.

Teaching guidelines for foot care in general should address the following:

1. Proper self-care practices to include general information on bathing, drying well between toes, and avoidance of excessive soaking. No bathroom surgery!
2. Daily self-inspection of feet and the areas between the toes is important. A mirror can be placed on the floor and the client instructed to look at the reflection of the plantar surface of the foot for any cracks, discolorations, etc.
3. Always wear shoes at all times, even when getting up at night to go to the bathroom.
4. Information on purchasing proper shoes to accommodate structural deformities, diabetes, etc.
5. When to report problems to the health care provider, such as abnormal sensations, pain in the legs at night or when ambulating, etc.
6. Reminding the health care provider to inspect the feet routinely during each visit.

REVIEW QUESTIONS

1. How does the clinical presentation of tinea pedis differ from dry skin (xerosis)?
2. What is the hallmark symptom of plantar fasciitis?
3. Why is wearing shoes one of the most important prevention activities for a variety of foot problems?

REFERENCES

1. Aly R. Ecology and epidemiology of dermatophyte infections. *J Am Acad Dermatol*. 1994;31:S21–S25.

2. Mayfield JA, Reiber GE, Sanders LJ, Janisse D, Pogach LM. Preventive footcare in people with diabetes. *Diabetes Care*. 1998;21:2161–2177.

3. Leyden JL. Tinea pedis pathophysiology and treatment. *J Am Acad Dermatol*. 1994;31:S31–S33.

4. Malcom B. Tinea pedis. *Practitioner*. 1998;242:225.

5. Uphold C, Grahm M. *Clinical Guidelines in Adult Health*. Gainesville, FL: Barmarrae Books; 1999.

6. Drake LA, et al. Guidelines of care for superficial mycotic infections of the skin: Onychomycosis. *J Am Acad Dermatol*. 1996;34:116–121.

7. Lesh B. Dermatophytosis. *J Am Acad Nurs Pract*. 1996;8:289–292.

8. Svejgaard E, Avnstorp C, Wanscher B, Nilsson J, Geremans A. Efficacy and safety of short-term itraconoazole in tinea pedis: A double-blind, randomized, placebo-controlled trial. *Dermatology*. 1998;197:368–372.

9. Barnetson RS, et al. Comparison of one week of oral terbinafine (250/mg/day) with four weeks of treatment with clotrimazole 1% cream in interdigital tinea pedis. *Br J Dermatol*. 1998;139:675–678.

10. Patel A, et al. Topical treatment of interdigital tinea pedis: Terbinafine compared with clotrimazole. *Aust J Dermatol*. 1999;40:197–200.

11. Tausch I, et al. Short-term itraconoazole versus terbinafine in the treatment of tinea pedis. *Int J Dermatol*. 1998;37:128–144.

12. Campbell-Giovaniella KJ. Plantar fasciitis. *Am J Nurs*. 1997;97:38–39.

13. Cornwall MW, McPoil TG. Plantar fasciitis: Etiology and treatment. *J Orthop Sports Phys Ther*. 1999;29:756–760.

14. Charles LM. Why does my foot hurt? Plantar fasciitis. *Lippincott's Primary Care Pract*. 1999;3:408–409.

15. Quaschnick MS. The diagnosis and management of plantar fasciitis. *Nurs Pract*. 1996;41:50–65.

16. Barrett SJ, O'Malley R. Plantar fasciitis and other causes of heel pain. *Am Fam Phys*. 1999;59:2200–2206.

17. Lynch DM, et al. Conservative treatment of plantar fasciitis. A prospective study. *J Am Podiatr Med Assoc*. 1998;88:375–380.

18. Tisdel CL, Donley BG, Sferra JJ. Diagnosing and treating plantar fasciitis: A conservative approach to plantar heel pain. *Cleveland Clin J Med*. 1999;66:231–235.

19. Probe RA, Baca M, Adams R, Preece C. Night spline treatment for plantar fasciitis. A prospective randomized study. *Clin Orthop Relat Res*. 1999;368:190–195.

20. Pfeffer G, et al. Comparison of custom and prefabricated orthoses in the initial treatment of proximal plantar fasciitis. *Foot Ankle Int*. 1999;20:214–221.

21. Sykes TF, Dale SJ, David DJ. Effective approaches to common foot complaints. *Patient Care*. March 15, 1997;158–180.

22. Milles CL, Riley PA, Kessenich CR. Onychomycosis: Diagnosis and systemic treatment. *Nurs Pract*. 1998;23:40–51.

23. Schlefman BS. Onychomycosis: A compendium of facts and a clinical experience. *J Foot Ankle Surg*. 1999;38:290–300.

24. Dambro MR, Griffith JA. *Griffith's 5-Minute Clinical Consult*. Philadelphia: JB Lippincott; 1999.

25. DeCuyper C, Hindryckx PH. Long-term outcomes in the treatment of toenail onychomycosis. *Br J Dermatol*. 1999;141:(Suppl 56):15–20.

26. Rich P, Hare A. Onychomycosis in a special patient population: Focus on the diabetic. *Int J Dermatol*. 1999;38:17–19.

27. Albreski DA, Gupta AK, Gross EG. Onychomycosis in diabetes. Management considerations. *Postgrad Med*. 1999;26–30.

28. Elewski BE. Clinical pearl: Diagnosis of onychomycosis. *J Am Acad Dermatol*. 1996;32:500–501.

29. Jain S, Sehgal VN. Onychomycosis: Treatment perspective. *Int J Dermatol*. 2000;39:10–14.

30. Drake LA, et al. Guidelines of care for superficial mycotic infections of the skin: Tinea corporis, tinea cruris, tinea faciei, tinea manum and tinea pedis. *J Am Acad Dermatol*. 1996;34:282–286.

31. Roberts DL. Onychomycosis: Current treatment and future challenges. *Br J Dermatol*. 1999;141(Suppl 56):1–4.

32. Warrick D, Church L. Continuous terbinafine versus intermittent itraconazole for toenail onychomycosis. *J Fam Pract*. 1999;48:492–493.

33. Gupta AK, Shear NH. A risk-benefit assessment of the newer oral antifungal agents used to treat onychomycosis. *Drug Safety*. 2000;22:33–52.

34. Drake LA, et al. The impact of onychomycosis on quality of life: Development of an international onychomycosis-specific questionnaire to measure patient quality of life. *J Am Acad Dermatol*. 1999;41:189–196.

35. Van Laborde S, Scher RK. Developments in the treatment of nail psoriasis, melanonychia striata, and onychomycosis. *Dermatol Clin*. 2000;18:37–46.

36. Lubeck DP, Gause D, Schein, JR, Prebil LE, Potter LP. A health-related quality of life measure for use in patients with onychomycosis: A validation study. *Quality Life Res*. 1999;8:121–129.

CHAPTER 20

Management of Malignant Wounds and Fistulas

Barbara M. Bates-Jensen and Susie Seaman

CHAPTER OBJECTIVES

At the completion of this chapter, the reader will be able to:

1. Explain the significance of symptom assessment in malignant cutaneous wounds.
2. Describe methods of managing bleeding, exudate, and odor in malignant cutaneous wounds.
3. Describe interventions for management of pain related to malignant cutaneous wounds.
4. List and explain factors to be considered when assessing the client with a draining wound or fistula.
5. Examine management methods for the client with a fistula.
6. Design a pouching procedure for a draining wound or fistula.

SIGNIFICANCE OF MALIGNANT CUTANEOUS WOUNDS

Malignant cutaneous wounds, also known in the literature as *fungating tumors/wounds*, *ulcerating malignant wounds*, or *tumor necrosis*, present both a physical and emotional challenge for patients and even experienced clinicians. Fungating or ulcerating wounds are often unsightly, malodorous, and painful (see *Color Plates 61–63*). These wounds are a blow to self-esteem and may cause social isolation at the very time when the patient needs more time with family and friends. In treating patients with malignant cutaneous wounds, the goal of care is to improve quality of life through symptom palliation. Treatment is directed at alleviation of the distressing symptoms associated with these lesions, with attention focused on minimizing pain and infection, manag-

ing exudate and odor, and controlling bleeding. The wound care clinician plays a pivotal role in the development of a treatment plan aimed at decreasing the effect that these lesions have on the patient's quality of life.

Malignant cutaneous lesions may occur in up to 5% of patients with cancer and 10% of patients with metastatic disease. Lookingbill and colleagues[1] retrospectively reviewed data accumulated over a 10-year period from the tumor registry at Hershey Medical Center in Pennsylvania. Of 7,316 patients, 367 (5.0%) had cutaneous malignancies. Of these, 38 patients had lesions as a result of direct local invasion, 337 had metastatic lesions, and 8 had both. A secondary analysis from the same registry found that 420 patients (10.4%) out of 4,020 with metastatic disease had cutaneous involvement.[2] In women, the most common origins of metastasis were breast carcinoma (70.7%) and melanoma (12.0%). In men, melanoma (32.3%), lung carcinoma (11.8%), and colorectal cancer (11.0%) accounted for the most common primary tumors. Although these types of cancer account for the majority of skin involvement, it is important to note that metastatic cutaneous lesions may arise from any type of malignant tumor.[3,4]

PATHOPHYSIOLOGY OF MALIGNANT CUTANEOUS WOUNDS

Malignant cutaneous lesions may be secondary to local invasion of a primary tumor or metastasis from a distant site.[5] Local invasion may initially manifest as inflammation with induration, redness, heat, and/or tenderness. The skin may have a *peau d'orange* appearance, and the area may be fixed to underlying tissue. As the tumor infiltrates the skin, ulcerating and/or fungating wounds develop. In metastatic disease, tumor cells detach from the primary site and travel via blood and/or lymphatic vessels or tissue planes to distant organs, including the skin.[3,4] Infiltration of the skin involves spread of cancerous cells along tissue planes, blood and lymph capillaries, and via perineural spaces because these areas offer little resistance.[6] These lesions may initially present as well-demarcated nodules, ranging in size from a few millimeters to several centimeters. Their consistency may vary from firm to rubbery. There may be pigmentation changes noted over the lesions, from deep red to brown-black. In general, these nodules are painless. Over time, these nodules may ulcerate, drain, and become very painful. Changes in local tissue perfusion at the tumor site lead to both increased tumor growth and tissue death. Altered perfusion in the vascular network results in a constant source of nutrition and oxygen to the tumor, supporting unregulated tissue growth.[7] Additionally, tumor cells secrete growth factors that promote angiogenesis and extracellular matrix deposition and thus, tumor growth. As the tumor grows larger, it is unable to sustain sufficient vascular growth to support the entire mass. This results in fragile capillaries, poor perfusion, altered collagen synthesis, and resultant tissue ischemia and necrosis.[7] Additional tissue destruction occurs secondary to proteolytic enzymes secreted by tumor cells.[8] The resulting lesion may be fungating, in which the tumor mass extends above the skin surface with a fungus or cauliflower-like appearance, or it may be erosive and ulcerative.[8] The wound bed may be pale to pink with very friable tissue, completely necrotic, or a combination of both. The surrounding skin may be erythematous, fragile, and exceedingly tender to touch. The skin may also be macerated in the presence of excessive wound exudate. The ulceration itself results in local infection, offensive odor, and fragile capillaries, with subsequent bleeding. Often, there are large amounts of necrotic material in these wounds, and the necrosis may account for much of the odor.

Heavy bacterial burden in malignant cutaneous wounds leads to significant odor. Typical organisms that infiltrate tumor wounds include *Escherichia coli*, *Pseudomonas aeruginosa*, and strains of *Staphylococcus*, *Proteus*, and *Klebsiella*.[7,8] Necrotic tissue provides an excellent medium for growth of anaerobes, such as *Bacteroides*.[7]

MALIGNANT CUTANEOUS WOUND ASSESSMENT

Assessment of malignant cutaneous wounds includes all parameters of wound assessment, with particular attention to evaluation for potential complications and evaluation of treatment appropriateness. Wound assessment for malignant cutaneous wounds is intended for use not only to document healing but as a precursor to determining treatment needs and evaluation of treatment appropriateness. In particular, attention to size and shape of the lesion; exudate characteristics; wound appearance, including necrotic tissue characteristics and bleeding or ulcerations; odor; presence of infec-

tion; and surrounding skin condition are important wound characteristics to consider in planning for topical dressing application.[9,10] Haisfield-Wolfe and Baxendale-Cox[8] have proposed a staging classification system for assessment of malignant cutaneous wounds. Use of wound classification increases communication effectiveness among health care practitioners and makes treatment evaluation consistent. The proposed classification system was tested in a pilot study with 13 wounds. The wounds were evaluated using wound depth as described with clinical descriptors, predominate color of the wound, hydration status of the wound, drainage, pain, odor, and presence of tunneling or undermining.[8] Use of the Haisfield-Wolfe and Baxendale-Cox classification system provides a basis for a standard set of descriptors that clinicians can use both to understand and to assess malignant cutaneous wounds.

Malignant cutaneous wounds are expected to increase in size over time and to change in appearance. They may occur singly or in groups, and nodules may enlarge and remit, due to treatment.[11] Although chemotherapy may bring about regression of lesions and radiation therapy may achieve healing of some fungating lesions from breast cancer,[12] usual treatment is only palliative to ease suffering. Radiation therapy is used to destroy tumor cells and shrink the lesion. Reduction in the size of the lesion may result in decreased exudate and pain, in addition to decreasing bleeding from lesions.[11]

Assessment is composed of the following categories: location, surface appearance, infection, surrounding skin, symptoms, and potential for serious complications. Location of the wound may impair mobility and functional level of the patient. Occupational therapy can help in facilitating activities of daily living and functional ability. Wound location will impact the dressing selection and dressing fixation because malignant cutaneous wounds may be located in wrinkled skin or highly uneven anatomic sites. The location of the wound also has significant psychologic impact. If the wound is located in an area where it is easily covered from public view, the patient will respond differently than if the wound is located such that hiding the wound is not possible.

Assessment of wound appearance is not so different from assessment of any other wound type. However, there are some special considerations for malignant cutaneous wounds.[9,10] Wound appearance should be evaluated for size, specifically looking for undermining and deep structure exposure. The wound should be assessed as fungating or ulcerative, with objective assessment of the percentage of viable versus necrotic tissue. Assess tissue friability and bleeding. Odor and exudate amount should be monitored and the presence of a fistula documented. Evaluation of the wound appearance also includes assessment of wound colonization versus infection. Identification of heavy bacterial colonization provides information on the deterioration or response of the wound to palliative care and can impact dressing selection. Malignant cutaneous wounds that are heavily colonized require special attention to cleansing, odor-reducing dressing selection, and exudate management. Clinically infected malignant cutaneous wounds with associated cellulitis and fever require systemic antibiotic therapy.

The skin surrounding the wound should be evaluated for color, integrity, and presence of nodules or other signs of progression of malignancy. Typically, the skin surrounding malignant cutaneous wounds is erythematous. The skin may be fragile, macerated, or denuded, as a result of excess exudate. Many times, extension of the wound can be predicted by the presence of nodules or eruptions in the skin surrounding the wound site. Surrounding skin may also exhibit signs of radiation skin damage, with erythema and other evidence of poor tissue perfusion. Tumor extension or metastasis will impact dressing type selection and fixation methods, such as using nonadherent dressings or methods other than tape for affixing the dressing. Significant deterioration in the surrounding skin becomes problematic in determining appropriate dressing selection because of the need for larger and larger dressings and the problems associated with securing the dressing on the site.

Symptom assessment is also important in malignant cutaneous wounds. The symptoms of pain and pruritis are characteristically associated with these wounds. Pain may include deep pain that is characterized by aching or stabbing of a continuous nature and superficial pain, such as burning and stinging, that may be associated only with dressing changes. If pain symptoms are the result of dressing changes, use of a short-acting topical analgesic with a rapid onset will be beneficial for total management of the wound. These fast-acting pain medications make dressing changes more bearable for the patient. If the pruritic symptoms are related to dressings, the remedy may be as simple as trying a different dressing. More typically, pruritis is a side effect of systemic analgesia and, if significant to the patient, may warrant change in pain medication or new systemic medications.

Assessment of the malignant cutaneous wound must include assessment of the potential for serious complications. Evaluation should include potential for hemorrhage, especially for patients in which the lesion is located close to major blood vessels. Lesions in these areas may also lead to blood vessel compression and obstruction. Lesions in the neck and chest area pose the threat of airway obstruction. Assessment includes attention to potential complications of bleeding and hemorrhage, swelling, pain, tissue necrosis, and airway obstruction.

Assessment of potential complications also involves evaluation of the patient's risk for infection and local bleeding from the tumor. Use of extreme care in dressing removal and attention to bleeding preparedness is essential. Infection risk increases with capillary fragility and bleeding. The presence of infection results in increased odor and exudate. Assessment of treatment appropriateness must occur frequently be-

cause, if the prognosis is one of increasing degeneration of the wound site, the treatment may need to be changed more frequently than in other wound types. Pain assessment is critical, because these wounds are often severely painful.

MALIGNANT CUTANEOUS WOUND MANAGEMENT

Control of bacterial colonization, exudate, odor, bleeding, and pain are the cornerstones of management for malignant cutaneous wounds.[5,9,13–18] In determining the appropriate treatment regimen, the abilities of the caregiver must also be considered. The limited information on treatment effectiveness reflects the absence of evidenced-based care in this area and the extreme need for further research and dissemination of findings.[14]

Infection Control: Wound Cleansing and Debridement

Infection control is facilitated by focusing on wound cleansing and wound debridement. Because malignant cutaneous lesions are frequently associated with necrotic tissue and odor, wound cleansing is essential to remove necrotic debris, decreasing bacterial counts and, thus, reducing odor.

Clinical Wisdom

If the lesion is not very friable, the patient may be able to get in the shower. This not only provides for local cleansing, but also gives the added psychologic benefit of helping the patient to feel clean. The patient should be instructed to allow the shower water to hit the skin above the wound, then allow the water to run over the wound.

If there is friable tissue (tissue that bleeds easily with minimal trauma) or the patient is not able to shower, the nurse/caregiver should gently irrigate the wound with normal saline or a commercial wound cleanser. Skin cleansers should generally be avoided because they tend to cause burning. However, for significant odor and to cleanse surrounding skin, skin cleansers may be efficacious because of the antiseptics that they contain and may be considered if they do not cause burning. Wound cleansing should be carried out using low-pressure irrigation with normal saline for those not able to shower and those requiring more aggressive cleansing. Saline has the advantage of not disturbing any tissues that might be healthy, but a disadvantage is the lack of odor-reducing ingredients. Use of the new pulsatile lavage devices has not been described but would appear to be of benefit for malignant cutaneous wound cleansing.

Use of antimicrobial solutions, such as povidone-iodine, sodium hypochlorite solution, chlorhexidine, or hydrogen peroxide is not recommended by some;[5] however, sodium hypochlorite solution and chlorhexidine are recommended by others.[7] The best approach may be short-term use of sodium hypochlorite solution or chlorhexidine for 2 weeks for reduction in odor, followed by reevaluation of treatment effectiveness. The rationale for antimicrobial solution use is the decrease of bacterial burden on the surface of the wound, with resultant decrease in odor. However, the antimicrobial solutions do not inhibit further bacterial proliferation because they are inactivated by body fluids, blood, pus, and slough (all of which are found in abundance in malignant cutaneous wounds).[12,21,22] Wound cleansing is followed by necrotic tissue debridement.

Necrotic tissue in malignant cutaneous wounds is typically dry, encrusted material; slough; or black eschar. Necrotic tissue in malignant cutaneous wounds can be extremely malodorous. Conservative debridement strategies are the basis for odor control. Use of autolytic and enzymatic debridement are the preferred options. Debridement of dry, encrusted material and black eschar may be best accomplished with a protocol described by Collinson,[19] involving warm normal saline cleansing, application of an amorphous hydrogel primary dressing, and covering with a thin film dressing as secondary dressing. The dressing is changed daily at first and less frequently as debridement occurs. It should be noted that use of the thin film dressing will significantly increase wound odor (which may not be tolerable for patients and caregivers), and the adhesive backing may damage the fragile surrounding skin. Collinson[19] describes initiation of liquefaction of necrotic tissue within 24 hours of starting the dressing. The hydrogel dressing allows for rehydration of the necrotic tissue and manages drainage associated with autolytic debridement. Use of hydrogel dressings is a gentle debridement technique with the additional advantage of decreasing pain.[16]

Procedures for sloughy, wet, necrotic tissue differ. Collinson[19] advocates use of calcium alginate dressings as a primary dressing and covering with either a thin film dressing or a foam dressing. The use of the calcium alginate dressing has the additional advantage of controlling bleeding in the wound site. Secondary foam dressings will result in less odor than will use of secondary transparent film dressings; foam dressings will not damage fragile surrounding tissues. Use

of this procedure adequately debrides soft, sloughy, necrotic tissue while protecting surrounding skin from maceration by controlling exudate.

If eschar on the tumor is extensive and thickly adherent to the tissues, surgical sharp debridement may be indicated to allow for infection prevention, odor control, and exudate management. Frank wound infection, as evidenced by wound cultures of 10^5 organisms on wound culture, may be effectively treated with topical antibiotic preparations, in conjunction with systemic antibiotics. The topical preparation may work better in malignant cutaneous wounds, due to the decreased perfusion and vasculature throughout the tumor that impedes systemic antibiotic dissemination, making the combination approach most successful.

Management of Exudate and Odor Control

The goal in management of exudate is to provide a moist wound environment to prevent trauma from drying and fissuring or dressing adherence. Moisture in the wound environment is positive but a wet wound is to be avoided. Dressings should be chosen both to conceal and to collect exudate *and* odor.[10] It is crucial to use dressings that absorb and contain exudate, because a patient who experiences unexpected drainage on clothing or bedding may experience significant feelings of distress and loss of control. Specialty dressings, such as foams, alginates or starch copolymers, are notably more expensive than gauze pads or cotton-based absorbent pads. However, if the use of these dressings reduces costs by reducing the need for frequent dressing changes (improving quality of life for the patient), they are cost-effective, both in terms of dollars spent and quality of care. In wounds with low exudate, the goal is to maintain a moist environment and to prevent dressing adherence and bleeding. Dressing choices for wounds in this category include nonadherent contact layers, such as Adaptic (Johnson & Johnson), Dermanet (DeRoyal), Mepitel (Mölnlycke), petrolatum gauze (numerous manufacturers), and Tegapore (3M Health Care). Amorphous hydrogels, sheet hydrogels, and hydrocolloids may also be helpful for low exudate wounds. Hydrocolloids are contraindicated with fragile surrounding skin and may increase odor. Semipermeable film dressings are also contraindicated with fragile surrounding skin. Nonadherent dressings are best for the primary contact layer because they minimize the trauma to the wound associated with dressing changes.

Wounds with high exudate require attention to absorbing and containing exudate. Dressings such as alginates, foams, starch copolymers, gauze, and soft cotton pads are all possible selections. Seaman[23] suggests nonadherent contact layers, such as Vaseline gauze for the primary dressing on the wound bed, covered with soft, absorbent dressings, such as gauze and abdominal binder dressings, for secondary dressings to contain drainage, changing the dressing one to two times daily. When drainage increases, the use of calcium alginate dressings to decrease the frequency of dressing changes should be considered. Grocott[24] also recommends use of calcium alginate dressings and discusses use of hydrocolloids for less exudative wounds. Hydrocolloids may be difficult to apply to malignant cutaneous wounds because of the uneven wound surface and gel dressings may be easier for caregivers to manage. Protection of the surrounding skin and tissues is another goal with exudate management.

Clinical Wisdom

Use of menstrual pads as wound dressing selection may be helpful for wounds with heavy exudate. These pads have the added benefit of clothing protection because of the outer plastic lining.

Use of skin barriers on the skin surrounding the wound, then taping dressings to the skin barriers (changing the barrier every 5–7 days) is one method of protecting surrounding skin from both excess drainage and tape, and the resultant skin stripping with dressing changes. Another method of protecting the surrounding skin is use of a barrier ointment to the skin surrounding the ulcer. The barrier protects fragile tissue from maceration and the caustic effects of the drainage on the skin. Dressings can then be held in place with Montgomery straps or tape affixed to a skin barrier placed on healthy skin, flexible netting, tube dressings, sports bras, panties, and the like.[10]

Odor control is by far the most challenging management aspect of malignant cutaneous wounds. Literature supports use of metronidazole (Flagyl, Helidac, MetroCream, Metro-Gel, Noritate Cream) topically and systemically in controlling wound odor.[25–32] Application of Metrogel (Galderma Laboratories) (a 0.75% topical antibiotic wound deodorizer gel) to the wound results in a decrease in wound odor in 2–3 days, even in the presence of resistant odor.[12,25–28] Typically, dressings are changed once to twice daily, and the topical gel may be supplemented with irrigant solution and/or systemic metronidazole administration. Topical therapy is available by crushing metronidazole tablets in sterile water and creating either a 0.5% solution (5 mg/cm^3) or a 1% solution (10 mg/cc).[17,29,30] Additionally, as an irrigant solution, 500 mg metronidazole in 100 mL normal saline IV solution can

be used to irrigate the wound and may be used as a wet-to-moist gauze dressing (this may be very effective for packing undermined or tunneled areas of the wound).[31,32] Others have reported odor reduction with use of 0.8% gel metronidazole, with or without systemic therapy (200–400 mg orally three times a day).[12,25] Systemic metronidazole 500 mg two to four times a day may also be administered when clinical infection is suspected or for severe wound odor management, but caution should be used because of the adverse gastrointestinal effects that may occur.[33,34]

Seaman[23] recommends that a gel wound deodorizer be tried prior to instituting use of metronidazole. Puri-Clens gel (Coloplast Corporation) contains benzethonium chloride, a cytotoxic antimicrobial compound that is effective against odor-causing bacteria. Some patients may complain of burning with the Puri-Clens, despite use of topical anesthesia, and this may contraindicate further use.

Another topical antimicrobial agent is Iodosorb gel, an iodine complexed in a starch copolymer (cadexomer iodine). This product contains slow-release iodine and has been shown to decrease bacterial counts in wounds without cytotoxicity.[35,36] Seaman has had clinical experience with this product in reducing odor associated with venous ulcers. Cadexomer iodine is available in a 40-g tube and is applied to the wound in a 1/8-inch layer. An advantage of this product is exudate absorption, in that each gram absorbs 6 mL of fluid. Disadvantages include cost (comparable to metronidazole 0.75% gel) and possible burning on application.

Clinical Wisdom

Use of peppermint oil or other aromatherapy products in the environment around the patient may help in eliminating wound odor. Charcoal also acts to absorb the odor from the wound. A basket of charcoal under the bed or table may also help in ridding the environment of wound odor for the home care patient.[20]

Use of charcoal dressings may also be helpful in odor management. Many charcoal dressings are expensive and less flexible, so their use must be individualized as appropriate. Charcoal dressings typically are applied after the primary and secondary dressing have been applied and may be reused with each dressing change unless strike-through of wound drainage has occurred. Magnesium hydroxide (Maalox) and honey applied to wound beds after cleansing have also been reported to be successful in controlling odor from wounds.[12]

Less conventional methods of odor management are also available. The topical use of yogurt or buttermilk has been reported to be successful in eliminating some malignant cutaneous wounds odors.[33,37,38]

The yogurt or buttermilk is applied topically to the wound after cleansing. The use of yogurt or buttermilk may work by decreasing the wound pH, thus stunting bacterial proliferation and the resultant odor. It is theorized that the low pH of the lactobacilli present in the yogurt and buttermilk are responsible for the alteration in wound pH. There are limited studies supporting the use of yogurt or buttermilk, and none have addressed specific limitations or contraindications for use of the treatment.

Controlling Bleeding

Wound bleeding is common in malignant cutaneous wounds. Prevention is the best therapy for controlling bleeding. Prevention involves use of a gentle hand in dressing removal and thoughtful attention to use of nonadherent dressings or moist wound dressings. Dressings should be soaked off with normal saline for easy, nontraumatic removal.[12] On wounds with low exudate, the use of hydrogel sheets, or amorphous hydrogels under a nonadherent contact layer, may keep the wound moist and prevent dressing adherence. Even highly exudating wounds may require a nonadherent contact layer to allow for nontraumatic dressing removal. When dressings stick to the wound on removal, they should be soaked away with normal saline to lessen the trauma to the wound bed. Even with use of nonadherent or moist wound dressings, bleeding may occur in malignant cutaneous wounds. Applying direct pressure to visible bleeding vessels for 10–15 minutes is the first intervention. The addition of ice packs may be helpful and also contribute to local comfort. If pressure alone is ineffective, several other options exist.

One suggestion is use of calcium alginate or collagen dressings because both have hemostatic properties.[11] Others advise use of gauze soaked in 1:1000 epinephrine over the bleeding point or application of sucralfate (Carafate) paste (crush a 1-g sucralfate tablet in 2–3 mL of water-soluble gel) over widespread oozing.[12,18] As an alternative, use of a topical absorbable hemostatic sponge or foam, such as Gelfoam, may be appropriate. Small bleeding points can be controlled with silver nitrate sticks. If bleeding continues, more aggressive palliation may be necessary. Radiation therapy may be useful in achieving hemostasis.[12] Additionally, super-selective angiography with transcatheter embolization of the arteries supplying the tumor may control bleeding and shrink the lesion.[39] Uncontrolled bleeding, as well as continuous capillary oozing, can result in acute and chronic anemia.

Minimizing Pain

There are several types of pain associated with malignant cutaneous wounds, deep pain, burning sensations, and superficial pain related to procedures. Deep pain should be managed by premedicating patients prior to dressing changes. Opioids for preprocedural medication may be needed, and rapid-onset, short-acting analgesics may be especially useful for those already receiving other opioid medication. Use of nonsteroidal antiinflammatory drugs may be beneficial.[12] For management of superficial pain related to procedures, Seaman[23] recommends use of Hurricaine Topical Anesthetic Aerosol Spray, which is a reasonably priced, over-the-counter aerosol of benzocaine 20%. The onset of action is 15–30 seconds, and the spray is applied after removing the dressing prior to wound cleansing and again after wound cleansing, for residual action. If the spray is applied to chest wall or head/neck wounds, the patient's face should be covered to prevent mouth and throat numbness if inhaled. Use of ice packs over tender areas may be beneficial to some patients for pain relief.[23] Magnesium hydroxide or a similar antacid applied directly to the wound area and allowed to dry may provide temporary relief of burning and superficial pain. Another emerging option for topical analgesia is the use of topical opioids, which bind to peripheral opioid receptors.[40–42] Back and Finlay[41] reported the use of diamorphine 10 mg added to an amorphous hydrogel and applied to the wounds of three patients on a daily basis. Two of the patients had painful pressure ulcers, and the third had a painful malignant ulceration. All three patients were on systemic opioids. The patients noted improved pain control on the first day of treatment. Krajnik and Zbigniew[42] reported the case of a 76-year-old woman with metastatic lesions on her scalp that caused severe tension pain. Ibuprofen 400 mg three times a day was ineffective, and because the pain was in a limited area, the authors applied morphine 0.08% gel (3.2 mg morphine in 4 g of amorphous hydrogel). The patient's pain decreased from 7 on a 10-point visual analogue scale (VAS) to 1 within 2 hours of gel application. Pain increased back to 6 on the VAS at 25.5 hours postapplication. Therefore, the gel was reapplied daily and maintained pain control with no side effects. Nurses should discuss this new option for topical pain relief with the patient and physician. Because wound care is performed frequently in these patients, the addition of topical opioids may be an excellent adjunct to the pain management plan.

Other Management Options

Many patients in the early stages of cutaneous metastasis or local invasion may be candidates for more aggressive care aimed at tumor shrinkage and the resulting decrease in pain, exudate, bleeding, and odor. These treatments may include transcatheter embolization,[39] local radiation therapy,[12] and/or intraarterial chemotherapy.[43] Bufill, Grace, and Neff reported the case of a 59-year-old woman with an extensive fungating chest wall tumor secondary to breast cancer whose tumor completely resolved following local intraarterial chemotherapy.[43] She died 10 months later with only a palpable breast mass but no open wound. Despite the fact that patients may eventually succumb to the underlying cancer and that there may no longer be a curative treatment available, individual patients may benefit from temporary improvement in the lesion through more aggressive palliative treatments. The wound care clinician should speak with the patient's primary provider about the feasibility of these treatments for individual patients.

MALIGNANT CUTANEOUS WOUND OUTCOME MEASURES

The expected outcome for most malignant cutaneous wounds is that the wound will deteriorate and increase in size. Outcome measures are, therefore, related to palliation of symptoms, not wound healing. The major goals of therapy are to reduce odor, manage exudate, minimize pain, and control bleeding. Outcomes of therapy relate to the ability and success of the treatment in meeting these goals. Patient or caregiver reports of wound odor or even of the amount of time family members spend with the patient on a daily basis are good measures of outcomes related to achieving effective odor control. Outcomes related to effective management of exudate include the amount and type of exudate and possibly the number of dressing changes per day to manage exudate. Number of accidental leaks of exudate through to clothing or maceration of surrounding skin due to moisture are other options for outcome measures related to exudate. Pain outcome measures must include patient self-report with an evidence-based tool for assessment of pain. Additional outcomes related to pain and discomfort may be related to the patient's perception of the wound dressing itself. The dressing should be perceived as comfortable, accessible, user-friendly, and as staying in place for the desired time period.[11] Amount of analgesia required by the patient is not a good outcome measure for pain because the implication is that as the analgesia amount decreases as the outcome improves, and this is generally not the case with palliative care. In fact, in many instances, the amount of analgesia will increase over the course of therapy. Outcome measures for controlling bleeding may include monitoring of hemoglobin and hematocrit status and prevention of excessive trauma to the wound by the wound dressing, as well as frequency of bleeding events. Outcome measures typically will reflect the goals of therapy; therefore, with malignant cutaneous wounds, outcomes are focused on alleviation of suffering related to the wound. Achievement of comfort, general psychologic well-being, and a satisfactory level of physical functioning can all be measures of patient outcomes.[11]

PATIENT AND CAREGIVER EDUCATION RELATED TO MALIGNANT CUTANEOUS WOUNDS

The same education provided to the patient and caregiver about basic wound care should be provided to those with malignant cutaneous wounds. Frequency and procedures for dressing changes, including time of premedication for pain management and alternatives for odor control, should be presented and reinforced. Education regarding reportable conditions is important. Patient and caregivers should be taught to report the following conditions to their health care provider:

- excessive or malodorous exudate
- pruritis or cellulitis
- severe emotional distress
- increased or change in pain
- bleeding
- fever
- unusual or major change in the wound appearance
- inability of the caregiver to manage wound care
- inability to obtain needed wound care supplies[11]

Patient and caregiver education must also focus on the psychosocial aspects of malignant cutaneous wounds. Patients are often unable to separate themselves from the wound and may feel as though their body is rotting away. Indeed, patients are often unable to view the wound, may become nauseous or retch when dressing changes are performed, or provide other signs of low self-esteem related to the wound. The clinician can facilitate a trusting relationship with the patient by reviewing the goals of care and by openly discussing issues that the patient may not have talked about with other providers. For example, it is helpful to acknowledge odor openly, then to discuss how the odor will be managed. Attention to cosmetic appearance of the wound with the dressing in place can assist the patient in dealing with body image disturbances. Use of flexible dressings (such as foam dressings and thin film dressings) and use of dressings that can fill a defect (such as pastes or calcium alginates) may be appropriate in restoring symmetry and providing adequate cosmesis for the patient.[11]

Isolation may result from embarrassment, shame, or guilt. Family caregivers may be overcome by the appearance of the wound or the other associated characteristics, such as the odor. Assisting the patient and the caregiver to deal with the distressing symptoms of the malignant cutaneous wounds such that odor is managed, pain is alleviated, and exudate is contained will allow for time to deal with the psychosocial issues related to body image disturbance. Improving cosmetic appearance of the wound, eliminating odor, and containing exudate will help to achieve the goal of satisfactory psychological well-being.

Education must include realistic goals for the wound. Both the patient and the caregiver must understand the realistic goals of care. In malignant cutaneous wounds, the goal of complete wound healing is seldom achievable but, through attention to exudate, odor, and pain, the patient's quality of life can be maintained, even as the malignant cutaneous wound degenerates. Determination of priority goals in palliation may be the first step in patient and caregiver education. For example, if the patient is most disturbed by odor, measures to address wound odor should be foremost in the treatment plan. Continual education and evaluation of the effectiveness of the treatment plan are essential to maintaining quality of life for those suffering with malignant cutaneous wounds.

SIGNIFICANCE OF FISTULAS

A fistula is an abnormal passage or opening between two or more body organs or spaces. The most frequently involved organs are the skin and either the bladder or the digestive tract, although fistulas can occur between many other body organs/spaces. Often, the organs involved and the location of the fistula influence management methods and may complicate care, although the goal of care is fistula closure. For example, fistulas involving the small bowel and the vaginal vault and those involving the esophagus and skin both create extreme challenges in care related to both the location and the organs involved in the fistula. Although spontaneous closure with adequate medical management can occur in 60–70% of all enteric or small bowel fistulas,[44–46] the time required to achieve closure is 4–7 weeks, thus requiring long-term treatment plans for all patients with fistulas. Of those that will close spontaneously, 90% will do so within the 4- to 7-week time frame.[45,47,48] Therefore, if the fistula has not spontaneously closed with adequate medical treatment within 7 weeks, the goal of care may change to palliation, particularly when chances of closure are limited by other factors inhibiting closure. Factors that inhibit fistula closure include complete disruption of bowel continuity, distal obstruction, presence of a foreign body in the fistula tract, an epithelium-lined tract contiguous with the skin, presence of cancer, previous radiation, and Crohn's disease.[49] The goal for fistula care is closure of the fistula (either spontaneous or surgical) through attention to fluid and electrolyte balance, prevention of sepsis and infection control, maintenance of adequate nutrition, and protection of surrounding tissues.[49] Goals of care for palliative fistula management involve containment of effluent, management of odor, increased comfort, and protection of the surrounding skin and tissues.[10] Patients with a fistula demonstrate 6–20% morbidity, despite advancements in care practices, including fluid and electrolyte stabilization, nutritional support, surgical management, and diagnosis and treatment of infection.[44]

Surgical management may be indicated for fistula closure and for palliative care. Optimizing the patient prior to surgical procedures is desired, and the exact timing of the intervention is highly individualized. Management involves surgical resection, bypass, diversion, or, more recently, endoscopic use of fibrin tissue glue. Surgical resection involves removal of the diseased area of the intestine, including the fistula site, with end-to-end anastomosis and temporary di-version to protect the healing site. Surgical bypass involves using end-to-end anastomosis of the intestinal tract, bypassing or going around the fistula site. The intestinal tract just before and just after the fistula opening are attached or anastomosed together, effectively isolating and separating the area of the intestine containing the fistula opening. Surgical diversion involves creation of an ostomy located proximal to the fistula site, thus diverting the fecal stream before it reaches the fistula site. Use of endoscopic procedures and fibrin tissue glue has also been used to seal low-output fistulas, with no adverse effects and early healing reported in small samples.[50] Additional research with use of endoscopy and fibrin tissue glue in fistula management is required for determining the definitive role in fistula management. Fistulas involving the bladder (such as enterovesical fistulas) require surgical intervention for closure.

PATHOPHYSIOLOGY OF FISTULA DEVELOPMENT

In cancer care, those with gastrointestinal cancers and/or those who have received irradiation to pelvic organs are at highest risk of fistula development. Fistula development occurs in 1% of patients with advanced malignancy.[51] In most cases of advanced malignancy, the fistula develops in relation to either obstruction from the malignancy or from irradiation side effects. Radiation therapy damages vasculature and causes damage to underlying structures. In cancer-related fistula development, management is almost always palliative. However, fistula development is not limited to those with cancer.

In addition to cancer patients or those who have received radiation therapy, postsurgical adhesions, inflammatory bowel disease (Crohn's disease), and small bowel obstruction all place an individual at high risk for fistula development. The number one cause of fistula development is postsurgical adhesions. Adhesions are scar tissues that promote fistula development by providing an obstructive process within the normal intestinal passageway. Many have reported the majority of fistula cases as arising from anastomotic breakdown immediately following surgical procedures.[47,52] Inadequate blood supply and aggressiveness of surgical procedure can create vulnerability to fistula formation in surgical patients.

Those with inflammatory bowel disease, Crohn's disease in particular, are prone to fistula development by virtue of effects of the disease process on the bowel itself. Crohn's disease often involves the perianal area, with fissures and fistulas common findings. Because Crohn's disease is a transmural disease, involving all layers of the bowel wall, patients with Crohn's are prone to fistula development. Crohn's disease can occur anywhere along the entire gastrointestinal tract, and there is no known cure. Initially, the disease is managed medically with steroids, immunotherapy, and metronidazole for perianal disease. If medical management fails, the patient may be treated with surgical creation of a colostomy in an attempt to remove the bowel affected with the disease. In later stages of disease, if medical and surgical management has failed, multiple fistulas may present clinically, and the goal for care becomes palliative, with symptom control the primary objective.

Other factors contributing to fistula development include the presence of a foreign body next to a suture line, tension on suture line, improper suturing technique, distal obstruction, hematoma/abscess formation, tumor or additional disease in bowel anastomotic site, and inadequate blood supply.[49] Each of these can contribute to fistula formation by promoting an abnormal passage between two body organs. Typically, the contributing factor provides a path of least resistance for evacuation of stool or urine along the tract, rather than through the normal route. Such is the case with a foreign body next to the suture line and hematoma or abscess formation. In some cases, the normal passageway is blocked, as with tumor growth or obstructive processes. Finally, in many cases, the pathology relates to inadequate tissue perfusion, as with tension on the suture line, improper suturing, and inadequate blood supply.

FISTULA ASSESSMENT

Assessment of the fistula involves assessment of the fistula source, surrounding skin and fistula output, and fluid and electrolyte status. Evaluation of the fistula source may involve use of diagnostic tests, such as radiographs, to determine exact structures involved in the fistula tract. Assessment of the fistula source involves evaluation of fistula output, or effluent, for odor, color, consistency, pH, and amount. These all provide clues to the fistula origin. Fistulas with highly odorous output likely originate in the colon or may be related to cancerous lesions. Fistula output with minimal odor may be from small bowel origins. Color of fistula output also provides clues to the source of the fistula. Clear or white output is typical of esophageal fistulas. Green output is usual of fistulas originating from the gastric area. Light brown or tan output may indicate fistula output from small bowel sources. Small bowel output is typically thin and watery to thick and pasty in consistency, whereas colonic fistulas have output with a pasty to a soft consistency. The volume of output is often an indication of the source of the fistula. For small bowel fistulas, output is typically high with volumes from 500 mL over 24 hours for low-output fistulas to 3,000 mL over 24 hours for high-output fistulas. Esophageal fistula output may be as high as 1,000 mL over 24 hours. Fistulas can be classified according to output, with less than 500 mL over 24 hours classified as a low-output fistula and those with greater than 500 mL over 24 hours classified as high-output fistulas.[53]

Assessment of the anatomic orifice location, the proximity of the orifice to bony prominences, regularity and stability of the surrounding skin, number of fistula openings, and the level the fistula orifice exits onto the skin all influence treatment options. Fistulas may be classified according to the organs involved in the defect and according to the location of the opening of the fistula orifice. Fistulas with openings from one internal body organ to another (such as from small bowel to bladder or from bladder to vagina) are *internal* fistulas, whereas those with cutaneous involvement (such as small bowel to skin) are termed *external* fistulas.[53] Exhibit 20–1 presents common fistula terminology related to internal and external fistula types.

Clinical Wisdom

The location of the fistula often impedes containment of fistula output. Skin integrity should be assessed for erythema, ulceration, maceration, or denudement from fistula output. Typically, the more caustic the fistula output is, the more impaired the surrounding skin integrity will be. Multiple fistula tracts may also hamper containment efforts.

Assessment of fluid and electrolyte balance is essential in fistula assessment, due to the risk of imbalance in both fluids and electrolytes. In particular, the patient with a small bowel fistula is at high risk for fluid volume deficit or dehydration and metabolic acidosis, due to the loss of large volumes of alkaline small bowel contents. Significant losses of sodium and potassium are common with small bowel fistulas. Laboratory values should be monitored frequently. Evaluation for signs of fluid volume deficit is also recommended. Fistulas of gastrointestinal origins are more prone to electrolyte and

Exhibit 20–1 Fistula Terminology

Fistula Name	*Organs Involved/Fistula Type*
Pancreatico-Colonic	Pancreas to colon/Internal
Enterocutaneous	Small bowel to skin/External
Enterovesical	Small bowel to bladder/Internal
Enterovaginal	Small bowel to vagina/Internal
Colocutaneous	Colon to skin/External
Colovesical	Colon to bladder/Internal
Rectovaginal	Rectum to vagina/Internal
Vesicocutaneous	Bladder to skin/External

fluid disruptions. Exhibit 20–2 presents typical composition of output from gastrointestinal organs involved in fistulas.

FISTULA MANAGEMENT

Nutrition management and fluid and electrolyte maintenance are both essential in adequate fistula care. One of the cornerstones of fistula management is attention to nutrition. Most fistula patients are malnourished and become more so as the duration of time with the fistula increases. Fluid and nutritional requirements may be greatly increased with fistulas, and there are difficulties using the gastrointestinal system with gastrointestinal fistulas. Lack of adequate intake of protein and calories, inadequate digestion and absorption of nutrients, extreme losses of nutrient-rich output, and increased metabolic demands from infection also contribute to the nutritional deficits present in patients with fistulas. Consultation with a nutritionist or dietitian is highly encouraged early in the management of the fistula patient. Protein and calorie needs vary, based on the type of fistula, amount of output, status of the patient prior to fistula development, and infection status. The route for nutritional supplementation depends on the anatomic location of the fistula and the patient's ability to take in adequate nutrition orally. As a general guideline, the intestinal system should be used whenever possible for nutritional support. Using the gastrointestinal tract allows the intestines to continue performing usual functions, thus maintaining normal anatomy and physiology of the gastrointestinal tract. When the intestinal tract is not used, there is always the possibility of damage to the intestinal tract from atrophy of the villi, with subsequent loss of absorption capabilities. If nutrition can bypass the fistula site, absorption and tolerance are better with use of the intestinal tract. Enteral nutrition is preferred when the fistula is located in the *most* proximal or distal portions of the gastrointestinal tract. For small bowel fistulas, bypassing the fistula orifice is not always feasible. If the small bowel fistula is located distally, there may be enough of the intestinal tract available to absorb nutrients adequately prior to the fistula orifice. If the fistula is located more proximally, there may not be enough intestinal tract available for nutrient absorption prior to the fistula orifice. Specific solutions or feeding regimens should be ordered in consultation with the dietitian because he or she can recommend the most appropriate supplement. Many of these patients must be managed with intravenous hyperalimentation during the early stages of fistula management. The specific goals of fluid and electrolyte and nutritional support for fistula management must be discussed with the patient and family, particularly with the patient receiving palliative care.

Wherever anatomically possible, the fistula should be managed with an ostomy pouching technique. The surrounding skin should be cleansed with warm water, without soap or antiseptics; skin barrier paste should be used to fill uneven skin surfaces to create a flat surface to apply the pouch, and pouch types should be chosen based on fistula output. Pediatric pouches are often smaller and more flexible, and may be useful for hard-to-pouch areas where flexibility is needed, such as the neck for esophageal fistulas. For example, if the fistula output is watery and thin, choose a pouch with a narrow spigot or tube for closure and, in contrast, a fistula with a thick, pasty output would be better managed with a pouch with an open end and closure clamp for closure. Pouches must be emptied frequently, at least when one-third to one-half full. There are several wound drainage pouching systems that will allow for visualization and direct access to the fistula through a valve or door that allows opening and reclosing of the pouch. These wound management pouches are available in large sizes and often work well for abdominal fistulas.[54,55] Pouching the fistula allows for odor control

---

Exhibit 20–2 Fistula Output Characteristics

Organs Involved	Approximate Amount of Secretions/Output (24 hr)	Characteristics
Esophagus	1,000 mL	Alkaline pH, clear-colored liquid
Stomach	2,000 mL	Acidic pH, green, clear liquid, major losses of Cl and some Na
Duodenum, Jejunum, and Ileum	3,000 mL	Alkaline pH, light brown liquid, major losses of Na, K, & Cl
Pancreas	1,200 mL	Alkaline pH, clear liquid, major losses of Na, Cl, and HCO_3
Gall Bladder	600 mL	Alkaline pH, bile—yellow brown liquid—major losses of Na and Cl
Colon	150 mL	Alkaline pH, brown color, may be soft, pasty consistency

(many fistulas are quite malodorous), containment of output, and protection of the surrounding skin from damage. Gauze dressings with or without charcoal filters may be used when the output from the fistula is less than 250 mL over 24 hours and is not severely offensive in odor.[53] Colostomy caps (small, closed end pouches) may be very useful for low-output fistulas that continue to be odorous.

There are specific pouching techniques that are useful in complex fistula management, including troughing, saddlebagging, and bridging.[49,53] These techniques are particularly helpful when dealing with fistulas that occur in wounds, most commonly the small bowel fistula that develops in the open abdominal wound. Troughing is useful for fistulas that occur in the posterior aspect of large abdominal wounds.[56] Line the skin surrounding the wound and fistula with a skin barrier wafer and seal edge the nearest wound with skin barrier paste. Then apply thin film dressings over the top or anterior aspect of the wound, down to the fistula orifice and the posterior aspect of the wound. Last, use a cut-to-fit ostomy pouch to pouch the opening in the thin film dressing at the fistula orifice. Wound exudate drains from the anterior portion of the wound (under the thin film dressing) to the posterior portion of the wound and out into the ostomy pouch, along with fistula output. The trough technique does not prevent fistula output from contaminating the wound site. Figure 20–1 shows the trough technique.

A similar method of managing fistulas is by a closed suction wound drainage system. Jeter and colleagues[57] describe the use of a Jackson-Pratt drain and continuous, low suction in fistula management. After cleansing the wound with normal saline, the fenestrated drain of the Jackson-Pratt is placed in the wound on top of a moistened gauze opened up to line the wound bed (primary contact layer); a second fluffed wet gauze is placed over the drain, and the surrounding skin is prepared with a skin sealant. Next, the entire site is covered with a thin film dressing, crimping the dressing around the tube of the drain where it exits the wound. The tube exit site is filled with skin barrier paste, and the Jackson-Pratt is connected to low, continuous wall suction. The connection site may have to be adjusted or may require use of a small "Christmas-tree" connector or device and secured with tape. Jeter and colleagues advise changing the system every 3–5 days.[57] Others have used a similar setup for pharyngocutaneous fistulas.[58] Some have reported success with high-output fistulas and suction catheters attached to low, intermittent suction, using the approach described by Jeter and colleagues.[57,59,60] Topical dressings and skin protection around the suction catheter are still required with this approach because the suction catheter will not provide for complete containment of drainage.[59,60] The suction catheter technique is most effective when fistula output is liquid and watery. Fistula output that is pasty, thick, or chunky will clog the suction catheter, making the system ineffective. Insertion of the suction catheter into the fistula opening will prevent fistula closure because the body responds to the catheter as a foreign object. However, laying the catheter in the wound around the fistula opening will not prevent fistula closure. A soft catheter should be used to prevent undue trauma to the wound bed.

The bridging technique will prevent fistula output from contaminating the wound site and allows for a unique wound dressing to be applied to the wound site. Bridging is appropriate for fistulas that occur in the posterior aspect of large abdominal wounds, where it is important to contain fistula output away from the wound site. Using small pieces of skin barrier wafers, a bridge is built by consecutively layering the skin barriers together until the skin barrier has the appearance of a wedge or bridge and it is the same height as the depth of the wound.[49,53] Using skin barrier paste, the skin barrier wedge is adhered to the wound bed (it will not harm the healthy tissues of the wound bed) next to the fistula opening. An ostomy pouch is then cut to fit the fistula opening, using the wedge or bridge as a portion of intact surrounding skin to adhere the pouch.[49,53] The anterior aspect of the wound may then be dressed with the dressing of choice. Figure 20–2 presents the bridging technique.

Saddlebagging is used for multiple fistulas, where it is important to keep the output from each fistula separated and the fistula orifices are close together. Using two (or more for multiple fistulas) cut-to-fit ostomy pouches, the fistula openings are cut on the back of the pouch, off-center or as far to the side as possible; the second pouch is cut to fit the next fistula and is cut off-center as far to the other side as possible. The skin is cleansed with warm water, and skin barrier paste is applied around the fistulas orifices. The ostomy pouches are applied, and, where they contact each other (down the middle), they are affixed/adhered to each other in a "saddlebag" fashion. Figure 20–3 presents the saddlebag procedure, and Figure 20–4 shows the procedure in use. Multiple fistulas can also be managed with one ostomy pouching system accommodating the multiple openings. This method is appropriate when fistula openings are close together and there is no need to separate drainage. Figure 20–5 demonstrates multiple fistulas managed with one large pouching system.

Vaginal fistulas present complex management problems. Whether the fistula involves the bladder or intestine, manifestations are continual leakage of stool or urine (depending on fistula origins) through the vaginal vault, with erosion and denudation of the sensitive vaginal epithelium, as well as perineal skin. Containment of the fistula output is very difficult, due to the anatomic constraints of the perineal area. Female urinary containment pouches can be tried, as can soft, cuplike devices inserted into the vaginal vault to direct output flow into a tube and drainage bag system. Use of skin protector ointments, attention to odor control, and some form of fistula output containment are essential for these

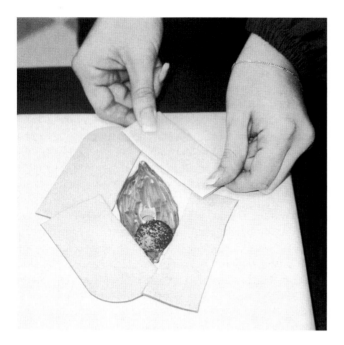

A

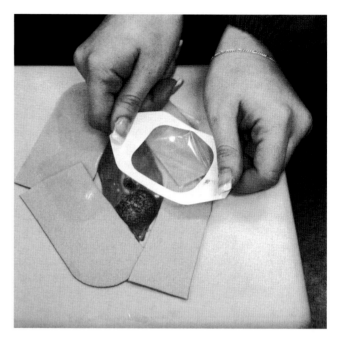

B

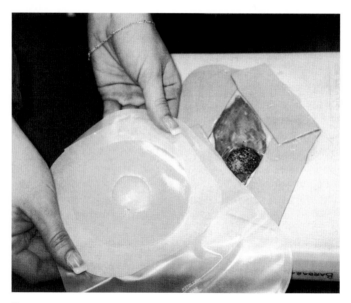

C

Figure 20–1 Photo series depicting the Trough procedure. **A,** Skin barrier wafers on hydrocolloid wound dressings are used to protect the skin surrounding the wound. **B,** Thin film dressings or transparent dressings are applied to the anterior portion of the wound on top of the hydrocolloid dressing or skin barrier wafers. The thin film dressings can be overlapped to obtain continuity and provide adequate coverage. The fistula area is left open and not covered by the thin film dressings. **C,** An ostomy pouch is sized for the fistula opening and prepared appropriately. *Source:* Copyright © Barbara Bates-Jensen.

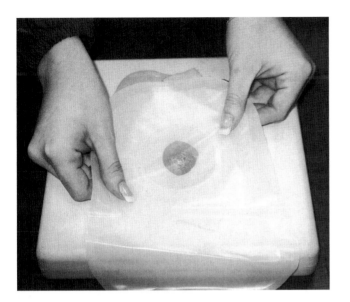

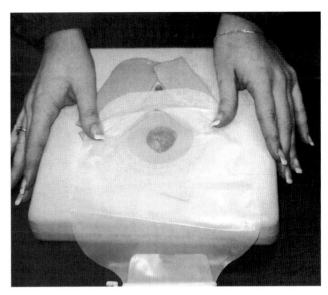

D

E

Figure 20–1 D, The ostomy pouch is applied over the open fistula site. **E,** The ostomy pouch is applied over and on top of the thin film dressing covering the anterior portion of the wound. *Source:* Copyright © Barbara Bates-Jensen.

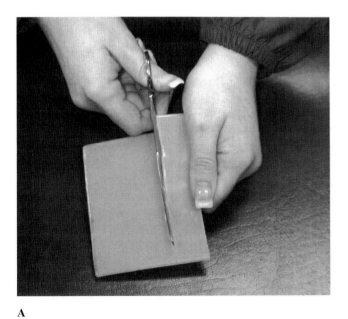

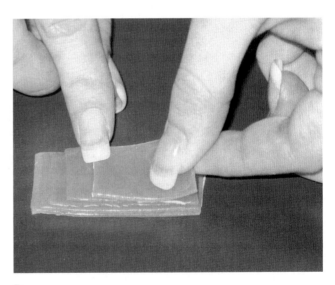

B

A

Figure 20–2 Photo series depicting the Bridging procedure. **A,** A skin barrier wafer is cut into strips. **B,** The strips of skin barrier wafer are applied on top of each other to create a "bridge." *Source:* Copyright © Barbara Bates-Jensen.

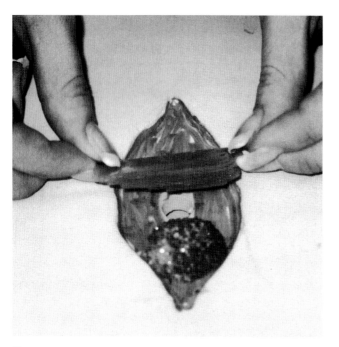

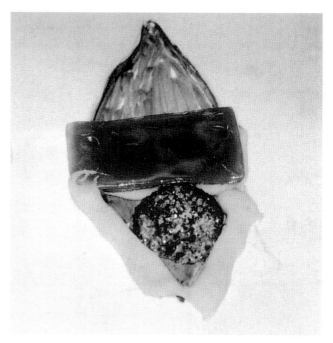

C   **D**

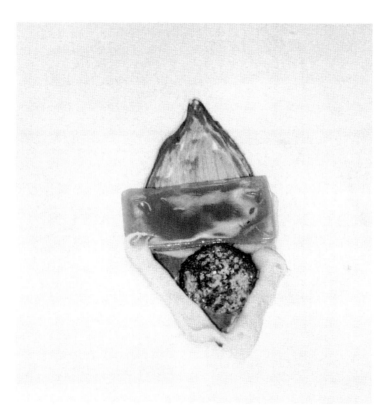

E

Figure 20–2 C, The skin barrier "bridge" is applied to the wound. **D,** The skin barrier "bridge" is secured in the wound bed using skin barrier paste. The paste is also used around the fistula site as necessary to create an even surface. **E,** The skin barrier "bridge" is in place and the anterior portion of the wound can be seen to be clear of the fistula area. *Source:* Copyright © Barbara Bates-Jensen.

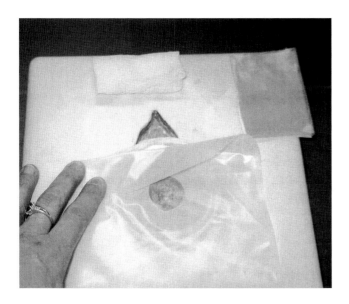

F

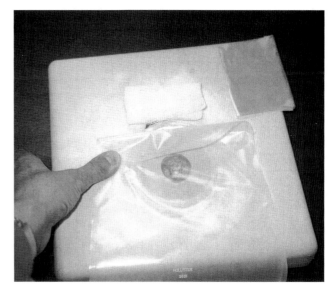

G

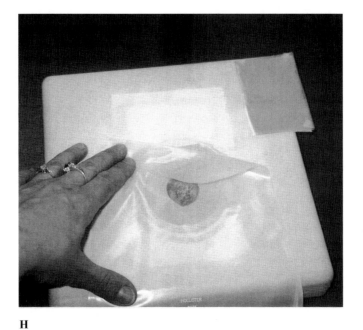

H

Figure 20–2 **F,** An ostomy pouch is sized and cut to fit the fistula area. The ostomy pouch is applied over the fistula, using the skin barrier "bridge" as part of the adhesive surface area for pouch application. **G,** A wound dressing can be applied to the anterior portion of the wound that is now protected from fistula output by the ostomy pouch. **H,** The wound dressing can be changed more frequently than the fistula pouch system if necessary. This system allows the wound to be treated with a different approach than the fistula area. *Source:* Copyright © Barbara Bates-Jensen.

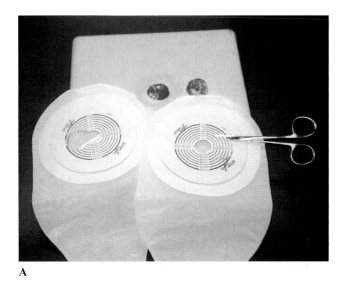

A

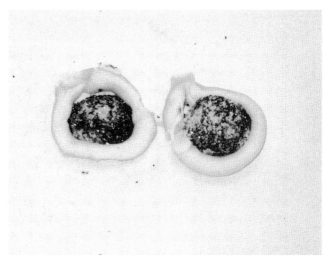

B

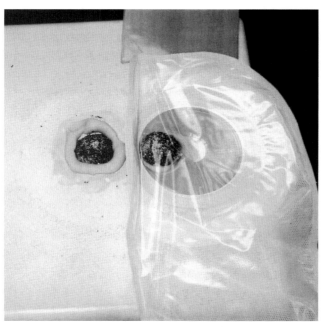

C

Figure 20–3 Photo series depicting the Saddlebagging procedure. **A,** Two ostomy pouches are used to pouch each of the fistulas present separately. This will allow for unique containment of fistula output for each site. Ostomy pouches are sized and cut to fit the fistula openings. The fistula openings are cut off-center, as far to one edge of the pouch skin barrier backing as possible. **B,** Skin barrier paste is used around the fistula openings to provide for a smooth adhesive area and fill in any dips or crevices around the fistula openings. **C,** Each ostomy pouch is applied to the fistula site. The adhesive area of the pouch closest to the second fistula site is not firmly adhered to the skin, rather it is left (or bent up) in a non-adhered manner. *Source:* Copyright © Barbara Bates-Jensen.

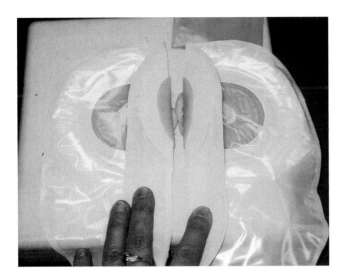 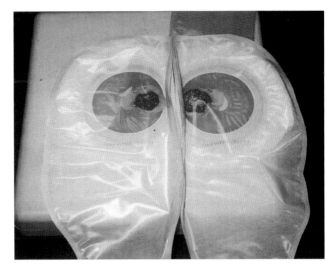

D   **E**

Figure 20–3 D, The second ostomy pouch is applied over the second fistula and, as with the first pouch, the adhesive area closest to the other fistula is left in a non-adhered fashion. **E,** The non-adhered middle sections of the two pouches are adhered to each other to create the "saddle." Both pouches will require simultaneous changing as it is nearly impossible to change one without changing the other due to the adherence of one pouch to the other in the middle section. *Source:* Copyright © Barbara Bates-Jensen.

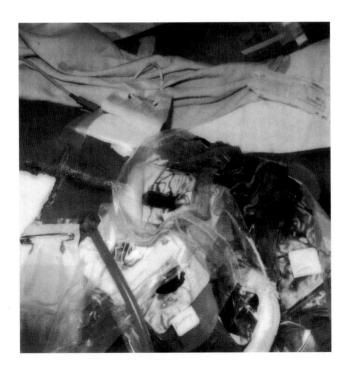

Figure 20–4 Saddlebagging procedure in use. Photo demonstrates abdomen with multiple fistula sites and draining wound sites. Each site was pouched separately with the saddlebagging technique used for most due to the close proximity of many of the sites. The midline abdominal wound shows a posterior fistula that was pouched using the bridging technique. *Source:* Copyright © Barbara Bates-Jensen.

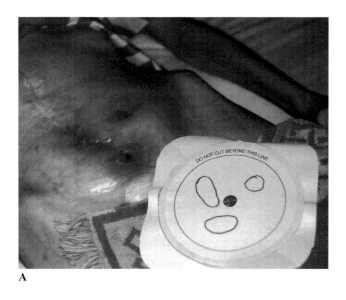

A

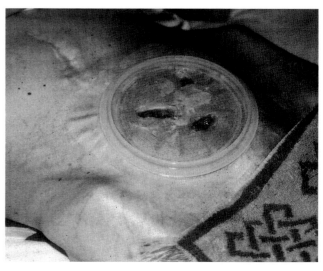

B

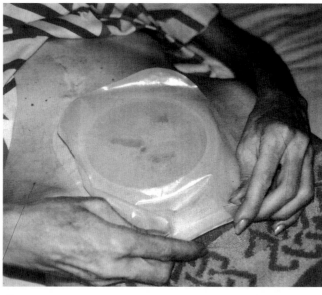

C

Figure 20–5 Photo series depicting the use of one pouch for multiple fistulas. **A,** Three major fistula sites evident on abdomen (from long-standing Crohn's Disease). A two-piece pouch is used and the skin barrier wafer portion is cut to fit the fistula openings. Pouch with large opening has been cut to fit the three fistula sites. Caution must be used to cut the pouch barrier so that the fistula openings are cut with attention to how the skin barrier will be applied on the skin (it is common to accidentally reverse the images if not aware). **B,** Skin barrier portion of two-piece pouch applied. Skin barrier paste has been used around the fistula openings to help apply the pouch. **C,** Pouch has been attached to skin barrier and closure clamp applied. *Source:* Copyright © Barbara Bates-Jensen.

---

patients. Consultation with the enterostomal therapy (ET) nurse or ostomy nurse is extremely advantageous in any of these cases because clinical experience plays a major role in successful management of the complex fistula.

Pouching to contain the fistula output will usually contain odor, as well. If odor continues to be problematic with an intact pouching system, internal body deodorants may be helpful,

such as bismuth subgallete, charcoal compositions, or peppermint oil.[61] Taking care to change the pouch in a well-ventilated room will also help with odor. If odor is due to anaerobic bacteria, some suggest use of 400 mg metronidazole orally three times a day.[51] Management of high-output fistulas may be improved with administration of octreotide acetate (Sandostatin) 300 μg subcutaneously over 24 hours.[51]

OUTCOME MEASURES FOR FISTULAS

Outcome measures for fistula care relate to the potential for fistula closure, maintenance of fluid and electrolyte balance, and management of the fistula output. Of course, for a newly developed fistula, the goals of care are fistula closure, and the major outcome measure is slowing of fistula output, with eventual closure of the fistula site. In some cases, when fistula closure is not likely to occur spontaneously and the patient is not a surgical candidate, outcomes of care become targeted to quality of life with the fistula. The outcome measures may include decrease in fistula output; management of fistula odor, as measured by patient/caregiver self-report; and maintenance of fluid and electrolyte balance, as monitored by frequent laboratory values.

PATIENT AND CAREGIVER EDUCATION FOR FISTULAS

Patient and caregiver teaching first involves adequate assessment of self-care ability of the patient and the caregiver's abilities. The patient and caregiver must be taught the management method for the fistula, including pouching techniques, how to empty the pouch, odor control methods, and strategies for increasing fluid and nutritional intake. Many of the pouching techniques used to manage fistulas are complicated and may require continual surveillance by an expert, such as an ET nurse or ostomy nurse.

CONCLUSION

Fistulas and malignant cutaneous wounds require attention to basic care issues, creativity in management strategies, and thoughtful attention to psychosocial implications of cutaneous manifestations. Both malignant cutaneous wounds and fistulas are often palliative care conditions. Palliative care intervention strategies for both skin disorders reflect a similar approach as nonpalliative care, with the goals of treatment to reduce discomfort, manage odor and drainage, and provide for optimal functional capacity. In each area, involvement of the caregiver and family in the plan of care is important. To meet the needs of the patient and family, access to the multidisciplinary care team is crucial, and consultation by an ET or certified wound, ostomy, continence nurse is highly desirable. Goals of care, although not always to cure the condition, are at all times to alleviate the distressing symptomatology and improve quality of life.

REVIEW QUESTIONS

1. Which of the following areas form the base of palliative care for malignant cutaneous wounds?
   a. pain control, maintaining a moist wound environment, odor control
   b. prevention and control of infection, pain control, maintaining a moist wound environment
   c. prevention and control of infection, pain control, odor control
   d. prevention and control of infection, pain, odor, bleeding, and exudate
2. Describe one method of pain management for the patient with pain from a malignant cutaneous wound.
3. An enterocutaneous fistula is a connection between which structures?
   a. bladder to rectum
   b. rectum to vagina
   c. rectum to skin
   d. small bowel to skin

REFERENCES

1. Lookingbill DP, Spangler N, Sexton FM. Skin involvement as the presenting sign of internal carcinoma. *J Am Acad Dermatol.* 1990;22:19–26.
2. Lookingbill DP, Spangler N, Helm KF. Cutaneous metastases in patients with metastatic carcinoma: A retrospective study of 4020 patients. *J Am Acad Dermatol.* 1993;29:228–236.
3. Rosen T. Cutaneous metastasis. *Med Clin North Am.* 1980;64:885–900.
4. Brodland DG, Zitelli JA. Mechanisms of metastasis. *J Am Acad Dermatol.* 1992;27:1–8.
5. Ivetic O, Lyne PA. Fungating and ulcerating malignant lesions: A review of the literature. *J Adv Nurs.* 1990;15:83–88.
6. Collier M. The assessment of patients with malignant fungating wounds—A holistic approach: Part 1. *Nurs Times.* 1997;93(suppl):1–4.
7. Goodman M, Hilderley LJ, Purl S. Integumentary and mucous membrane alterations. In: Groenwald SL, Hansen-Frogge M, Goodman M, Yarbro CH, eds. *Cancer Nursing, Principles and Practice*, Boston: Jones & Bartlett Publishers; 1997:768–821.
8. Haisfield-Wolfe ME, Baxendale-Cox LM. Staging of malignant cutaneous wounds: A pilot study. *Oncol Nurs Forum.* 1999;26(6):1055–1064.
9. Moody M, Grocott P. Let us extend our knowledge base: Assessment and management of fungating malignant wounds. *Prof Nurs.* 1993;8:586–590.
10. Bates-Jensen BM, Early L, Seaman S. Skin disorders. Skin disorders. In: Ferrell B, Coyle N, eds. *Textbook of Palliative Care in Nursing.* New York: Oxford University Press, Inc.; 2001.
11. Haisfield-Wolfe ME, Rund C. Malignant cutaneous wounds: A management protocol. *Ostomy/Wound Manage.* 1997;43(1):56–66.
12. Waller A, Caroline NL. Smelly tumors. In: Waller A, Caroline NL, eds. *Handbook of Palliative Care in Cancer.* Boston: Butterworth-Heinemann; 1996:69–73.
13. Hallet A. Fungating wounds. *Nurs Times.* 1995;91(39):78–85.
14. Fairburn K. A challenge that requires further research: Management of fungating breast lesions. *Prof Nurse.* 1994;9:272–277.
15. Clark L. Caring for fungating tumours. *Nurs Times.* 1992;88(12):66–70.

16. Young T. The challenge of managing fungating wounds. *Community Nurse.* 1997;3(9):41–44.

17. Whedon MA. Practice corner: What methods do you use to manage tumor-associated wounds? *Oncol Nurs Forum.* 1995;22:987–990.

18. Grocott P. The management of fungating wounds. *J Wound Care.* 1999;8:232–234.

19. Collinson G. Improving quality of life in patients with malignant fungating wounds In: Harding KG, Cherry G, Deale C, Turner TD, eds. *Proceedings of the 2nd European Conference on Advances in Wound Management.* London: MacMillan Magazines; October 20–23, 1992:59–63.

20. Cormier AC, McCann E, McKeithan L. Reducing odor caused by metastatic breast cancer skin lesions. *Oncol Nurs Forum.* 1995;22(6):988–999.

21. Butler GA. Desloughing agents at work. *Nurs Mirror.* 1985;160(13):29.

22. Leaper D. Antiseptics and their effect on healing tissue. *Nurs Mirror.* 1985;82(22):45–47.

23. Seaman S. Home care for pain, odor, and drainage in tumor-associated wounds. *Oncol Nurs Forum.* 1995;22(6):987.

24. Grocott P. Application of the principles of modern wound management for complex wounds in palliative care. In: Harding KG, Leaper DL, Turner TD, eds. *Proceedings of the 1st European Conference on Advances in Wound Management.* London: MacMillan Magazines; 1991:88–91.

25. Newman V, Allwood M, Oakes RA. The use of metronidazole gel to control the smell of malodorous lesions. *Palliative Med.* 1989;3:303–305.

26. Bower M, Stein R, Evans TRJ, Hedley A, Pert P, Coombs RC. A double-blind study of the efficacy of metronidazole gel in the treatment of malodorous fungating tumours. *Eur J Cancer.* 1992;28A:888–889.

27. Poteete V. Case Study: Eliminating odors from wounds. *Decubitus.* 1993;6(4):43–46.

28. Finlay IG, Bowszyc J, Ramlau C, et al. The effect of topical 0.75% metronidazole gel on malodorous cutaneous ulcers. *J Pain Symptom Manage.* 1996;11:158–162.

29. Gomolin IH, Brandt JL. Topical metronidazole therapy for pressure sores of geriatric patients. *J Am Geriatr Soc.* 1983;31:710–712.

30. Rice TT. Metronidazole use in malodorous skin lesions. *Rehabil Nurs.* 1992;17:244, 245, 255.

31. Ashford RFU, Plant GT, Maher J, Teares L. Double-blind trial of metronidazole in malodorous ulcerating tumours. *Lancet.* 1984;1(8388):1232–1233.

32. McMullen D. Topical metronidazole. Part II. *Ostomy/Wound Manage.* 1992;38(3):42–46.

33. Forman WB, Sheehan DC. Symptom management. In: Sheehan DC, Forman WB, eds. *Hospice and Palliative Care.* Sudbury, MA: Jones & Bartlett Publishers; 1996:83–97.

34. Jacob M, Markstein C, Liesse M, Deckers C. What about odor in terminal care? *J Palliative Care.* 1991;7(4):31.

35. Holloway GA, Johansen KH, Barnes RW, et al. Multicenter trial of cadexomer iodine to treat venous stasis ulcer. *West J Med.* 1989;151:35–38.

36. Danielsen L, Cherry GW, Harding K, et al. Cadexomer iodine in ulcers colonised by *Pseudomonas aeruginosa. J Wound Care.* 1997;6:169–172.

37. Welch LB. Simple new remedy for the odour of open lesions. *RN.* 1981;44(2):42–43.

38. Schulte MJ. Yogurt helps to control wound odor. *Oncol Nurs Forum.* 1993;20(8):1262.

39. Rankin EM, Rubens RD, Reidy JF. Transcatheter embolisation to control severe bleeding in fungating breast cancer. *Eur J Surg Oncol.* 1988;14:27–32.

40. Stein C. The control of pain in peripheral tissue by opioids. *N Engl J Med.* 1995;332:1685–1690.

41. Back IN, Finlay I. Analgesic effect of topical opioids on painful skin ulcers. *J Pain Symptom Manage.* 1995;10:493.

42. Krajnik M, Zbigniew Z. Topical morphine for cutaneous cancer pain. *Palliative Med.* 1997;11:325.

43. Bufill JA, Grace WR, Neff R. Intra-arterial chemotherapy for palliation of fungating breast cancer. *Am J Clin Oncol.* 1994;17(2):118–124.

44. Berry SM, Fischer JE. Classification and pathophysiology of enterocutaneous fistulas. *Surg Clin North Am.* 1996;76(5):1009.

45. Rose D, et al. One hundred and fourteen fistulas of the gastrointestinal tract treated with total parenteral nutrition. *Surg Gynecol Obstet.* 1986;163(4):345.

46. Rombeau J, Rolandelli R. Enteral and parenteral nutrition in patients with enteric fistulas and short bowel syndrome. *Surg Clin North Am.* 1987;67(3):551.

47. Fischer JE. Enterocutaneous fistulas. In: Najarian JS, Delaney JP, eds. *Progress in Gastrointestinal Surgery.* St. Louis, MO: CV Mosby; 1989.

48. Kurtz R, Heimann T, Aufses A. The management of intestinal fistulas. *Am J Gastroenterol.* 1981;76:377.

49. Rolstad BS, Bryant RA. Management of drain sites and fistulas. In: Bryant RA, ed. *Acute and Chronic Wounds: Nursing Management.* 2nd ed. St. Louis, MO: CV Mosby; 2000:317–341.

50. Hwang TL, Chen MF. Short note: Randomized trial of fibrin tissue glue for low-output enterocutaneous fistula. *Br J Surg.* 1996;83(1):112.

51. Waller A, Caroline NL. Stomas and fistulas. In: Waller A, Caroline NL, eds. *Handbook of Palliative Care in Cancer.* Boston: Butterworth-Heinemann; 1996:81–86.

52. Chamberlain RS, Kaufman HL, Danforth DN. Enterocutaneous fistula in cancer patients: Etiology, management, outcome and impact on further treatment. *Am Surg.* 1998;64(12):1204.

53. Bryant RA. Management of drain sites and fistula. In: Bryant RA, ed. *Acute and Chronic Wounds: Nursing Management,* St. Louis, MO: Mosby–Year Book; 1992:248–287.

54. Schaffner A, Hocevar BJ, Erwin-Toth P. Small bowel fistulas complicating midline surgical wounds. *J Wound/Ostomy Continence Nurs.* 1994;21(4):161–165.

55. O'Brien B, Landis-Erdman J, Erwin-Toth P. Nursing management of multiple enterocutaneous fistulae located in the center of a large open abdominal wound: A case study. *Ostomy/Wound Manage.* 1998;44(1):20.

56. Wiltshire BL. Challenging enterocutaneous fistula: A case presentation. *J Wound/Ostomy Continence Nurs.* 1996;23(6):297–301.

57. Jeter KF, Tintle TE, Chariker M. Managing draining wounds and fistula: New and established methods. In: Krasner D, ed. *Chronic Wound Care.* King of Prussia, PA: Health Management Publications; 1990:240–246.

58. Harris A, Komray RR. Cost-effective management of pharyngocutaneous fistulas following laryngectomy. *Ostomy/Wound Manage.* 1993;39(8):36–44.

59. Beitz JM, Caldwell D. Abdominal wound with enterocutaneous fistula: A case study. *J Wound/Ostomy Continence Nurs.* 1998;25(2):102.

60. Lange MP, et al. Management of multiple enterocutaneous fistulas. *Heart Lung.* 1989;18:386.

61. McKenzie J, Gallacher M. A sweet smelling success. *Nurs Times.* 1989;85(27):48–49.

Management of Wound Healing with Physical Therapy Technologies

Carrie Sussman

INTRODUCTION

The management of wound healing with physical therapy technologies, including electrotherapeutic modalities and physical agents commonly used by physical therapists, is presented in Part IV. Electrotherapeutic modalities and physical agents are physical therapy technologies with long histories of clinical application and effectiveness, and defined by the American Physical Therapy Association as follows:

"Electrotherapeutic modalities include physical agents that use electricity to modulate or decrease pain, reduce or eliminate soft tissue inflammation caused by musculoskeletal; peripheral vascular or integumentary injury, disease, or surgery; or increase the rate of healing in open wounds."[1(pp746–747)] These modalities include alternating, direct, and pulsed current (eg, high-voltage pulsed current, low-voltage pulsed current, and transcutaneous electrical nerve stimulation (TENS)).

"Physical agents use heat, sound, or light energy to increase the connective tissue extensibility, modulate pain, reduce or eliminate soft tissue inflammation and swelling caused by musculoskeletal injury or circulatory dysfunction, increase the healing rate of open wounds and soft tissue, remodel scar tissue or treat skin conditions."[1(p746)] These modalities include deep thermal modalities (eg, thermal ultrasound, pulsed short wave diathermy), nonthermal modalities, (eg, pulsed ultrasound, pulsed radio frequency energy, ultraviolet light), hydrotherapy (eg, whirlpool, pulsatile irrigation with suction).

Chapters 21 to 26 describe the physical science associated with each technology, the evidence of efficacy and safety and rationale for its use, devices, application of, and case studies for eight modalities: electrical stimulation, pulsed electromagnetic fields (pulsed short wave diathermy, pulsed radio frequency stimulation, and pulsed electromagnetic fields), ultraviolet light, ultrasound, whirlpool and pulsatile lavage with suction.

Interventions include the purposeful and skilled interaction of the skilled physical therapist and the patient and, if appropriate, others who are involved in the patient's care to produce changes in the patient's condition consistent with the diagnostic process as described under the elements of patient/client management in the American Physical Therapy Association Guide to Physical Therapist Practice.[2] The diagnostic process described in Chapter 1 guides the physical therapist to select interventions for the plan of care that will help determine the prognosis. This is a dynamic process that begins with the reason for referral, the history of the patient, and the wound and the physical therapist making clinical judgments based on the data collected. Interventions have three recognized components: 1) direct procedures; 2) patient-related instruction; and 3) coordination, communication, and documentation. The physical therapy education curriculum includes instruction in the selection, protocols, and application of electrotherapeutic modalities and physical agents. Licensing examination includes testing of knowledge in appropriate, safe use; protocols; and interpretation of the results. Liability issues also suggest that physical therapists should be the health care professional responsible for treatment or instruction in the use of these interventions because the physical therapist is the legally licensed and the most qualified practitioner to refer to for these interventions.

Nurses are usually the initial treatment provider and often initiate referral to the physical therapist, as well as serving as case managers and medical reviewers. Therefore, it is very important that nurses understand the candidacy, referral criteria, and clinical outcomes expected from the therapy. The chapters in Part IV contain technical information that may be beyond the interest of most nurses, but there are also clinical decision making sections that will guide the nurse through the rationale for treatment selection used by the physical therapist. Collaborative practice requires mutual understanding of the treatment recommended and the expected results. In addition, nurses, patients, or caregivers may be the individuals who deliver the direct treatment established by the physical therapist. Those modalities suited to self-care or care by a provider other than a physical therapist are explained in each chapter's section on self-care treatment guidelines.

Definition of Standard Wound Care

- Cleansing
- Debridement
- Management of infection
- Occlusion
- Compression for venous ulcers
- Off loading for diabetic neuropathic ulcers
- Pressure relief for pressure ulcers
- Good nutrition

CANDIDACY FOR THE INTERVENTION

Candidacy for application of electrotherapeutic interventions and physical agents is determined by the performance of a thorough diagnostic process described in Chapter 1 to determine those conditions that would benefit from or prevent use of the intervention, and to determine that the body systems lack the ability to perform the necessary process of repair without intervention. The clinical decision-making process used for selecting each of the modalities is related to the system impairments it affects, as well as practical consideration, such as the patient's tolerance of the treatment, and knowledge and comfort level of the clinician. Candidates for physical therapy technologies include patients with observable acute inflammation of the tissues, including pain, chronicity of or absence of any phase of repair, circulatory compromise and edema, as well as impairments of different body organ systems such as the cardiopulmonary, musculoskeletal, neuromuscular, and integumentary systems. The interventions discussed in this part are often classified as adjunctive therapies. Eaglstein suggested to add new, alternative, or adjunctive therapies at four "points" in the course of care: 1) initially when predictors such as ulcer size and duration indicate a likely failure of standard care; 2) when the rate of healing with standard care predicts failure; 3) after failure to heal in the "magic" time (2–4 weeks); and 4) under special circumstances such as unusual diagnosis or patient demand.[3] The mode of intervention best suited to the patient, the treatment setting, and the wound will be determined by the physi-

cal therapist and recommended to the wound management team.

As a guide, the patients should be referred to the physical therapist for intervention with an electrotherapeutic or physical agent modality when the additional following candidacy criteria are met:

- Medical comorbidities exist that predict that a wound needs extra help to heal (eg, insensitivity associated with spinal cord injury, diabetes)
- Healing will be speeded by the therapy
- Wound has large size or long duration
- The wound has been recalcitrant to other methods
- There is an acute wound in a patient with a coimpairment such as chronic obstructive pulmonary disease or impaired circulation, or diabetic neuropathy, indicating a high probability of nonconforming healing
- The acute traumatic wound(s) is associated with neuromuscular or musculoskeletal problems that may require immobilization
- The wounds extend into subcutaneous tissue and deeper underlying structures and interfere with functional activities (eg, the patient is unable to sit up in a wheelchair because of the wounds over the ischial tuberosities or coccyx)
- The patient's functional status is impaired by slow wound healing (eg, gait will be helped if the wound is healed more rapidly, or the patient may be able to return to work)
- Patient or family preference

Reasons for Referral

The patient referred to the physical therapist for wound healing is usually an individual who has not shown signs of normal wound repair. Often other treatment interventions are being used or have been tried with limited or no success. Actually, the very best time for intervening with electrotherapeutic or physical agent modalities is during the first 72 hours immediately after injury. Several recent studies show that intervention by a physical therapist soon after onset of the problem (eg, stroke,[4,5] acute musculoskeletal pain[6,7]) reduces cost. Appropriate early intervention by the physical therapist has a proven track record of significantly reducing the development of costly chronic health problems. A review of the research literature cited in the chapters on electrical stimulation, pulsed electromagnetic fields, pulsed short wave diathermy, and ultrasound all cite research that demonstrates optimal effectiveness when the treatment intervention is applied early. However, since in reality more chronic wounds than acute wounds are referred to the physical therapist, other research cited in the chapters demonstrates efficacy of these technologies for healing of chronic wounds or to alter factors related to chronic wound healing such as circulation, oxygen uptake by cells, and edema. Expected outcomes should be based on the reason for the referral.

Patients, caregivers, and physicians seek care for a wound for many reasons. Although it seems as if the obvious goal of treatment is healing, healing is not the highest priority for everyone with a wound, and that assumption should not be made. It is very important to ask the patient, family, physician, and payer the reason for the referral and base the intervention selected and expected outcomes on meeting those objectives. Most of the time the patient and family are looking for a simple functional outcome. For example, the patient with a foot ulcer secondary to pressure and insensitivity is fearful of amputation and loss of the ability to walk. The patient wants to know if the limb can be saved. The family of a debilitated nursing home patient wants its loved one with a pressure ulcer to be comfortable. The family may realize that closure is not an option. Fear is a concern and creates a reluctance to attend therapy. All of these issues need to be addressed. The physical therapist's first intervention will be to learn as much about the patient and his or her goals and then begin education about the treatment options, effects of the treatment, and the expected outcomes.

Diagnosis

The diagnosis is the synthesis of the information gathered (see Part I chapters). Physical therapists use a functional diagnosis to describe an impairment, disability, or handicap of an associated body function. For example, the patient with a neuropathy as a consequence of alcoholism, diabetes, or spinal cord injury or the immobile or immobilized patient could all have a functional diagnosis of impaired sensation with undue susceptibility to ischemia, tissue anoxia, infection, and pressure ulceration. The impairment is decreased immunity, tissue anoxia, infection, and cell death. The disability is desensitized skin and risk for skin breakdown. The handicap is inability to maintain normal activity and mobility.

Patients with chronic wounds have an absence of progression through the phases of repair, that is, a functional impairment to wound healing at the cellular level or the tissue level. *Absence of inflammation and inability to progress to proliferation* is a functional diagnosis about functional impairment of the process at the cellular level or tissue level. This could be applied equally to a functional impairment of the proliferation phase: absence of proliferation or wound contraction with inability to progress to closure. Chronic wound edges do not produce functional epidermal cells to migrate across the wound to close it. *Absence of epithelialization due to impairment of epidermal cell activity* is a functional diagnosis for absence of wound progression to closure. A poorly healed wound or a minimally healed wound

has a functional diagnosis of *absence of remodeling due to integumentary system impairment.*

Another example of functional diagnosis is *impairment of sensation with undue susceptibility to pressure ulceration.* Reflexive neuronal mechanisms are impaired, and other methods must be used to stimulate circulatory responses; the prognosis for this functional diagnosis would be *adequate circulatory perfusion for delivery of oxygen and nutrients to tissues to progress through phases of repair.* Multiple functional diagnoses may be made that lead to multiple interventions, all of which will affect the outcome with the electrotherapeutic or physical agent modality intervention chosen for the wound. For instance, the patient with an impairment of sensation with undue susceptibility to pressure ulceration must be assessed for pressure risk. An intervention of pressure relief or elimination then must be included in the treatment plan so that the enhanced circulatory perfusion brought about by the selected intervention can reach the tissues. The physical therapist would apply this methodology to predict an outcome. The prognosis for repair of a closed tissue injury would be *accelerated absorption of hematoma, accelerated deposition of collagen, and restoration of normal ranges of motion, tissue extensibility, tissue strength for functional activities* (eg, self-care, work, leisure, or play).

Although traditionally patients with nonhealing wounds are referred for physical therapy, patients with musculoskeletal injuries and soft tissue trauma should also be viewed as patients with a closed wound. Hunt and Hussain found that open- and closed-wound healing physiology are similar.[8] Therefore, it is reasonable to assume that they would respond similarly to the same treatment interventions. Patients with the following types of wounds should be viewed as candidates for intervention with physical agents and electrotherapeutic modalities:

- ligamentous tears
- muscle strains
- sprains
- skin tears
- hematomas
- stage I pressure ulcers
- stage 0 neuropathic ulcers
- superficial and partial thickness burn wounds
- donor sites
- surgical wounds that do not heal in an orderly manner
- abrasions that interfere with one's ability to walk, work, or compete in a sport.

In patients with metabolic diseases (eg, lupus or diabetes) who suffer wounding, acute wounds can, and often do, become chronic. Also, microtrauma resulting from excessive forces and repetition can also lead to closed wounds such as tendinitis and nerve entrapments. In these patients, the impairment is also a closed tissue wound. The disability is pain and usually limitation in range of motion. A handicap would result from prolonged disability and the resulting inability to work or participate in normal activities of daily living or recreation. Early and effective intervention to accelerate repair with the listed interventions should be considered.

In summary, a patient who has a functional diagnosis of impairment of a body system at the cellular, tissue, or organ level (or a combination) related to tissue repair should be considered a candidate for intervention with electrical stimulation, pulsed radio frequency stimulation, pulsed short wave diathermy, or ultrasound. In addition, patients with musculoskeletal injuries in need of accelerated repair should also be considered candidates for the same interventions used for closed wound healing.

Prognosis

Clinical research studies are very useful to guide the clinician in predicted outcomes and can function as a guide for projecting a target due date. Clinical research studies usually identify the wound duration so that acute or chronic status of the patients can be determined. Because clinical research studies are usually carried out in ideal settings under optimal conditions, they should be considered only as *guidelines* that need to be tested in the individual clinical setting to determine the outcomes for the specific program. For example, the literature describes wound healing as closure or improvement. *Improvement* is less clearly defined and usually is described by reduction in depth of tissue loss or size and is listed as incompletely healed. Since most clinical studies of chronic wound healing interventions do not continue until closure, other ways of determining the effectiveness of therapeutic agents have been evaluated. These include construction of a graph of the wound healing to determine if the trajectory of the curve of healing is on a path for healing or nonhealing.[9] This methodology is described in Chapter 5.

Normal wound healing takes 3 to 4 weeks;[10] the definition of a chronic wound is a wound healing that has not occurred in an orderly manner in the expected time without help.[11] Risk factors for slower healing that have been identified include: the depth of tissue involvement (severity); partial-thickness wounds heal faster than full-thickness and deeper wounds;[12] wound size, larger wounds take longer to heal, and wound etiology; venous ulcers heal nearly twice as fast as do diabetic ulcers.[13] The concept of using electrotherapeutic modalities and physical agents is to initiate or accelerate the rate of repair of acute or chronic wounds. For example, Dyson and Young[14] found that application of low-intensity ultrasound during the early inflammatory phase of acute wounds accelerated the inflammatory phase of repair leading to an earlier proliferative phase.

While the functional diagnosis and risk factors are predictive of the need for the intervention, the intervention selected must have a predictable outcome, or prognosis, that will reduce the impairment or alter the consequences of the disease associated with the functional diagnosis in a predictable time period. A wound diagnosis of *absence of the inflammatory phase*, for example, is predictive that the wound needs an inflammatory phase followed by progression through the phases of healing to reach closure. The prognosis is initiation of inflammatory phase followed by progression of the wound through the proliferative phase of healing with reduction of 30% in surface area size in 2–3 weeks.

Multiple clinical randomized controlled studies report a healing rate of 30–47% in 2–3 weeks from start of care is predictive of wound healing, whether the etiology is pressure ulcers, venous ulcers, or diabetic ulcers[15–19] (see Chapter 5, Wound Measurement). Therefore, the wounds that do not meet this target healing rate with standard care should be referred for adjunctive therapy interventions such as those described in Part IV.

The addition of an adjunctive therapy intervention should be expected to speed the healing rate. Electrical stimulation is now being considered as a primary treatment modality rather than adjunctive therapy by some experts.[20]

Choosing between Interventions

A frequently asked question is, How do I know which intervention to choose? There is no single answer to this question. The mechanisms of action on the biologic system are different, but the expected treatment outcomes of progression through the phases of healing are similar for each of the devices presented in Part IV. Chronic wounds usually develop due to underlying problems of inadequate perfusion and ischemia. Therefore, reperfusion of the tissues may be the stimulus needed to reinitiate the inflammatory phase. However, new research shows that when blood flow is reestablished to ischemic tissues, further damage to the tissue from free radicals may occur. This is referred to as "reperfusion injury"[21] (see Chapter 2). Devices described in Part IV are expected to reinitiate a mild inflammatory phase in chronic wounds, usually through increased blood flow to the wound and adjacent tissues. If the intended response fails to occur and signs of tissue die back appear, the cause may be reperfusion injury. Research on how to prevent ischemia and reperfusion injury is receiving attention. Perhaps early intervention after injury with some of these modalities would prevent ischemia and resulting reperfusion injury. This could be a fruitful area for research.

Some modalities have optimal or preferred times for application, however. For instance, ultrasound, as described, is best delivered in the inflammatory phase to early proliferative phase[14] or to restart the inflammatory phase, but it is not effective for speeding wound contraction or improvement of tensile strength if used in the later proliferative or epithelialization phase.[22] Figure IV–1 is an algorithm showing the phases of wound healing with a key to highlight which are the putative effects on the phase or factor of healing of the eight physical therapy technologies described in Part IV. If one or more of the technologies affects the same aspect of the phase, other criteria would be used to choose the modality. For instance, most devices described have the ability to increase tissue perfusion. What differs is mechanism by which it acts. The thermal modalities have the ability to heat and increase circulation to produce a mild inflammatory reaction by vasodilation of the blood vessels of the skin and deeper tissues. Care must be exercised in applying them to ischemic tissues that cannot dissipate the heat. The nonthermal devices are gentler but effective in increasing tissue perfusion.

In evidence base practice, research is highly valued as the basis for selection of an intervention, and consequently the intervention with the most supporting research may be given the nod over less tested devices; however, clinical experience and patient preference must be considered. For example, pulsatile lavage with suction (PLS) has no controlled clinical trials for efficacy of wound healing but has been used in the operating room for many years to cleanse and debride wounds, and studies and clinical experience show that it is effective in removing debris and bacteria. Since wound cleansing and debridement are standards of care, selection of PLS would be use of good clinical judgment to meet this standard. The patient may have a very painful wound, so minimal handling of the wound and surrounding tissues using a treatment like pulsed radio frequency stimulation is indicated for comfort and compliance by the patient and by the facility. Hospitals, nursing homes, and outpatient clinics accredited by the Joint Commission on Accreditation of Healthcare Organizations (Joint Commission) must meet newly established standards requiring that every patient's pain be assessed regularly, managed aggressively and effectively, and be documented.[23] Use of the physical therapy technologies described in Part IV that have pain-modifying capabilities should be considered for incorporation into a nonpharmocologic plan of care for pain managment, along with wound healing as a means of compliance with this standard.

There are also practical considerations in choosing an intervention. These include the treatment setting, the treatment provider, the treatment payer, the treatment availability, medical contraindications, and adjunctive treatments (dressings, multiple technologies). If the treatment provider is to be other than a physical therapist or physical therapist assistant, the treatment must be safely applied by a person not trained in physical therapy. This would involve evaluation of the person and his or her ability to provide the care. For the most predictable outcomes and for patient safety, the physical therapist should be involved throughout the process starting with the assessment, determining candidacy, prescribing the protocols of treatment, and regularly scheduled follow up. This would preclude use of pulsed short wave diathermy or ultrasound, for example.

The treatment payer must be agreeable to paying for the physical therapy intervention selected. For example, Medicare has an exclusion policy for payment of ultraviolet light (UV) to treat wounds. However, now there is evidence that UV is a useful treatment to control infection and to reinitiate an inflammatory response. At this time, the cost of the UV treatment could not be billed separately. Other rationale would be needed to justify its selection such as the short treatment time (eg, 30 seconds) and rapid wound disinfection that would speed healing and reduce long-term costs. Treatment availability is a practical reality. If the preferred intervention is not available and cannot be obtained, then another choice will have to be made. Medical contraindications exist for all of the different technologies, but the medical contraindication that rules out the use of one will not necessarily rule out others. For example, a semicomatose patient should not be seen in the whirlpool, but wound cleansing with pulsatile lavage with suction at bedside would be an appropriate alternative. The following case study illustrates where thoughtful evaluation of the history and systems review narrowed down the choice of treatment intervention to one appropriate technology after considering all the factors.

Treatment Outcomes Management

Clinical managers have an obligation to review treatment outcomes systematically for wound patients referred to physical therapy. Most often the patient population referred are those individuals with complex wounds and comorbidities and many are also very debilitated. Careful screening and monitoring procedures are necessary to utilize treatment effectively. Sussman Physical Therapy, Inc. (SPT), is used to illustrate how a clinical program utilizes a wound database to do program evaluation and quality improvement, and evaluate program outcomes. SPT treated a population of complex and debilitated nursing home patients. SPT developed and conformed to a self-imposed standard of 50% reduction in wound size within a 4-to-6 week period using Sussman's noninvasive, surgery-alternative treatment protocol with debridement, occlusion, pressure relief or compression, and physical therapy technologies. The first requirement was identification, for the patient's medical manager, when the wound was clean and stable. If the wound healing was on target, then the decision would be made to proceed with the protocol until wound was healed. If not on target, then alternative options were considered. The patients in this long-term care facility were not candidates for surgical and other more costly interventions.

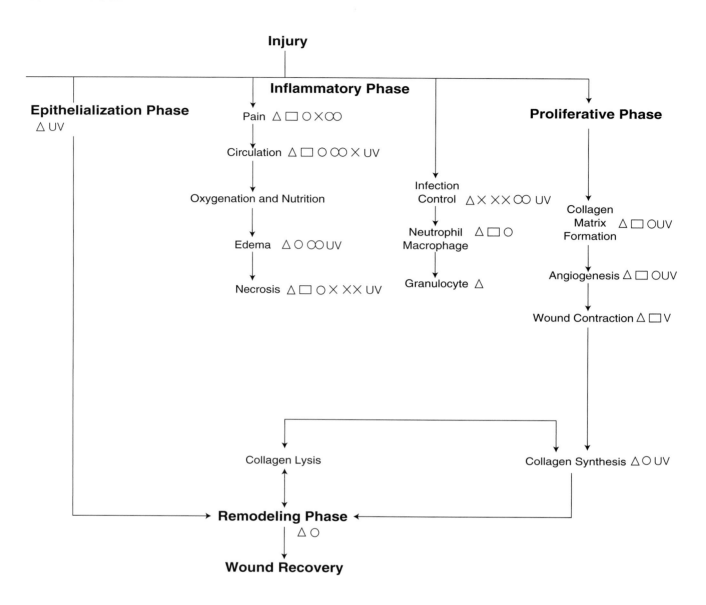

Injury

Inflammatory Phase

Epithelialization Phase
△ UV

Pain △ □ ○ ✕ ∞

Circulation △ □ ○ ∞ ✕ UV

Oxygenation and Nutrition

Edema △ ○ ∞ UV

Necrosis △ □ ○ ✕ ✕✕ UV

Infection Control △ ✕ ✕✕ ∞ UV

Neutrophil Macrophage △ □ ○

Granulocyte △

Proliferative Phase

Collagen Matrix Formation △ □ OUV

Angiogenesis △ □ OUV

Wound Contraction △ □ V

Collagen Lysis

Collagen Synthesis △ ○ UV

Remodeling Phase
△ ○

Wound Recovery

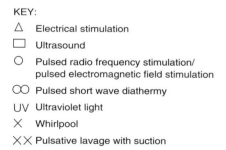

KEY:

△   Electrical stimulation

□   Ultrasound

○   Pulsed radio frequency stimulation/
    pulsed electromagnetic field stimulation

∞   Pulsed short wave diathermy

UV Ultraviolet light

✕   Whirlpool

✕✕ Pulsative lavage with suction

Figure IV–1 Putative treatment effects of physical therapy technologies on phases of wound healing. *Source:* Adapted with permission from C.A. Sussman, The Role of Physical Therapy in Wound Care, *Chronic Wound Care: A Clinical Source Book for Health Professionals*, D. Krasner (ed), pp. 327–367. © 1990, Health Management Publications, Inc.

Case Study: Choosing the Appropriate Treatment Intervention

A case example where multiple factors had to be considered when making a choice of intervention was required for E.F. An elderly lady, E.F. lived in a nursing home because of incompetence related to Alzheimer's disease. She had venous disease and a history of recurrent venous ulcers of the lower leg. A new episode of ulceration occurred, and the patient was referred to the physical therapist. The patient had a pacemaker, would not stay in bed or in a wheelchair for 5 minutes, and would not tolerate dressings or compression devices. The venous disease diagnosis ruled out whirlpool. The pacemaker ruled out any form of diathermy. The low tolerance for compression ruled out compression devices. The inability to tolerate staying in one place more than 5 minutes and intolerance for dressings ruled out electrical stimulation. Pulsatile lavage with suction was not available and would not have been tolerated by the patient. The only choice remaining was ultrasound because she could be kept still and amused for the 5 minutes required for a periwound ultrasound treatment. This was also an appropriate choice because ultrasound is particularly effective during the acute inflammatory phase and effects absorption of hemorrhagic materials. This patient is included as one of the case histories in Chapter 24, Therapeutic and Diagnostic Ultrasound. The results are viewed in *Color Plates 74* to *76*.

SPT staff used paper-and-pencil instruments to record wound data information. The information was then transferred to bubble sheets and scanned into a computer database. Statistical analysis of the SPT wound database was performed by Swanson and Co., Inc.[24] Findings were that SPT had excellent success with chronic leg ulcers with its treatment approach. Patients were referred to SPT when other methods failed. The program evaluation demonstrated that more than two-thirds of the chronic leg ulcers treated by the SPT method healed. This information was of value to the contract facility administrator, to the managed care contract payer, to the total quality assurance committee of the facility, and to the health department survey team. Furthermore, the information derived from the data analysis determined that the average length of treatment for the patients in the healed group was 49 days. This information was then applied to do cost outcomes analysis as described below.[25]

Functional Wound Cost Outcomes Management

In 1992, the cost for treatment of pressure ulcers in all settings in the United States was $1.3 billion.[26] The average cost of treatment of a pressure ulcer in the United States, based on 1990 data, is $2,000 to $30,000. The typical cost for a medical approach to treatment of pressure ulcers by surgical debridement is at least $4,000.[27] How do costs for treatment with physical therapy technologies for wound healing compare? Based on data from Swanson,[28] Maver,[29] and Birke,[30] physical therapy technologies are competitive for certain wounds. Swanson[28] compared the costs of a course of wound care with hydrotherapy (whirlpool) with a high-voltage pulsed-current (HVPC) type of electrical stimulation. She found that the course of 3 months (90 days) of care with hydrotherapy treatment (whirlpool) for necrotic wounds with an unknown outcome was $4,500 compared to $2,100 for a 7.5-week (52 days average) course of care with outcome of wound closure following treatment with HVPC electrical stimulation. Maver[29] compared the cost of conventional treatment for stage III pressure ulcers that did not heal during a course of care with a mean time of 34.62 weeks at a cost of $7,946.33, with 8.5 weeks course of care to healed status with Diapulse, pulsed radio frequency stimulation,[31] combined with conventional care cost of $2,929.62. The reported savings per ulcer in this study was $4,484. Birke[30] reported on numerous studies using total-contact casting (TCC) to heal plantar ulcers in patients with neuropathy. The average time to closure was 42 days. The average cost for a closed wound was $1,250. These cost savings do not include savings derived from reduced mortality, morbidity, and reduction in amputations. Comparative lengths of care and expected outcome for hydrotherapy, HVPC, and TCC are illustrated in Figure IV–2.

Cost comparison allows for a profile of wound cost outcomes and comparative analysis of the results of a course of care. Physical therapy is cost competitive for certain wounds (Figure IV–3). Physical therapist managers and program directors need to understand the information required to predict and manage cost for proper utilization management of services. The necessary information to predict cost and outcome are available from several sources: clinical trials, program evaluation reports, the facility's clinical database, evidence-based clinical practice guidelines, and payer data-based reports.

Does your clinic know your cost outcomes? Cost outcomes are differentiated from the technical outcome for the wound (eg, closure). Cost outcomes are what it costs to provide a course of care compared with the billed charges. That determines the cost to the provider as differentiated from the charges to the payer. The cost outcome is based on all the related costs for providing the service: labor cost, supply cost, and equipment cost. To determine the cost of treating a wound the clinical manager needs to predict the number of expected visits to achieve a predicted outcome. For example, if an outcome of closure is expected in 49 visits, a cost analysis can be done as follows:

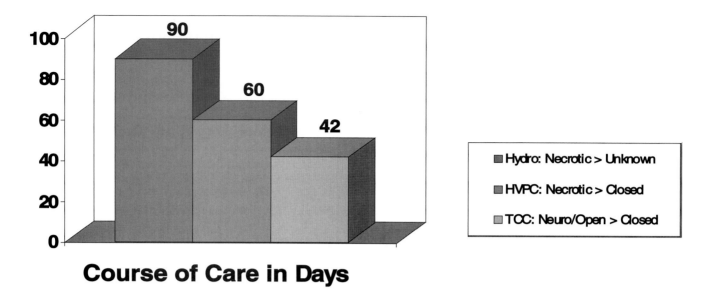

Course of Care in Days

Figure IV–2 Length of stay dependent on wound type and procedure.

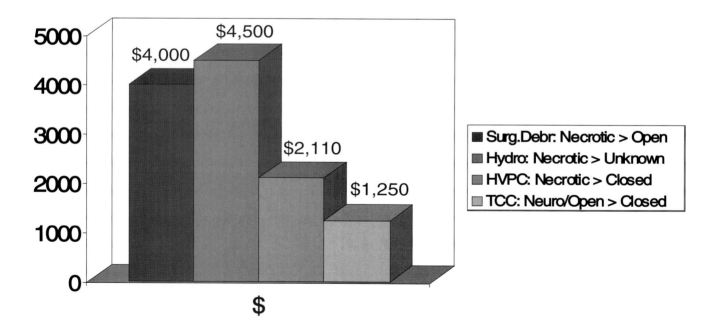

Figure IV–3 Cost comparison for different wound interventions and outcomes. Physical therapy is competitive for certain wounds.

Labor cost at $30/visit × 49 = $1,470
Supply cost at $6.25/visit × 49 = $306.25
Equipment cost at $0.50 × 49 = $24.50
Total cost = $1,800.75
Billed charges at $60/visit × 49 = $2,940
Net profit = $1,139.25

The cost for a different outcome to convert the wound to clean and stable may take half the time to closure. Cost to the payer would be reduced by half to $1,470. The case manager for the payer may be more willing to authorize an interim step for a known cost than an unknown outcome at unmanaged cost.

Reducing variability in healing rates and being able to predict outcomes helps the management of wound care costs. Recent research is there to help with clinic management. For example, Kantor and Margolis[13] found that with good wound care, 56% of venous ulcers healed in 16 weeks, but only 28% of diabetic neuropathic ulcers healed in the same time period. Further results suggest that there was a steady rate of healing for venous ulcers during the first 12 weeks but the linear rate begins to diminish rapidly after that point. For the diabetic neuropathic ulcer group there was little improvement in proportion healed after 16 weeks. Based on these data, an average healing rate for two thirds of the chronic leg ulcers of 49 (7 weeks) days with standard care plus physical therapy technologies was significantly less than the healing rates reported and was cost effective. This is an example of how to compare the results of one clinic outcomes with reports in the literature.

Utilization and Cost Management

Utilization and cost outcomes management mean that continued ongoing evaluation of the patient candidacy be reviewed. Candidacy determined at the initial evaluation may change as the patient experiences a course of care (Figure IV–4). This would initiate a reevaluation to assess appropriateness for further treatment. The Sussman Wound Healing Tool, described in Chapter 5, was developed as a diagnostic tool to evaluate progression through the phases of healing when wounds were treated with physical therapy technologies. For example, reduction in wound depth is a finding that the wound has progressed to the acute proliferative phase. Reduction in size is a measure of wound contraction, also part of the proliferative phase and of the epithelialization phase. If these benchmarks of healing are not occurring in an orderly and timely manner, this may be due to a poor response to treatment or changes in medical status and should trigger a change in the treatment approach. The following are some examples of situations that trigger a change:

- *Failure to progress:* For example, if the wound(s) are not progressing through the biologic sequence of repair and reducing in size significantly after 2–4 weeks of treatment with HVPC, the entire wound management plan needs to be reviewed to determine whether it is the treatment with the HVPC or other factors that are responsible for failure to progress. Since all wounds have multiple associated interventions, including wound cleansing, topical treatments, dressings, and debridement, along with the HVPC, each intervention should be reviewed to determine whether continuation is appropriate or if there needs to be change in these interventions or with the HVPC protocol.

- *Wound regression:* If the wound has gotten larger or deeper or has developed undermining or tunneling from the separation of the fascial planes or is invading named structures or areas or has become infected, this is referred to as wound *regression*. It may be the result of debridement or ischemia or infection. The physical therapist, physical therapist assistant, or nurse should be able to recognize the signs and symptoms of regression and take responsibility to report the change in condition to the physician.

- *Medical instability:* If the patient has become medically unstable (eg, pneumonia, sepsis, renal failure), the body's ability to heal is impaired, and the situation requires a change in medical management before continuing with physical therapy. The physical therapist may determine that the physical therapy intervention may need to be put on hold until the medical condition is stabilized.

- *Other management required:* If the wound has progressed to a clean and stable wound in the proliferative phase, it may indicate that the wound is ready for grafting or artificial skin to cover the wound more quickly and perhaps reduce scarring. It may be the best prognosis for the wound and/or for the patient and may have been the reason for referral, the objective of the patient, the family, the therapist, and the physician.

- *Wound needs less skilled care:* The wound is now at a phase of repair on the trajectory of healing that demonstrates that the healing response is sustained. Now the patient/caregiver or nurse may be able to continue to provide standard wound care procedures until healed and the physical therapist would bow out.

- *Goals met:* Sometimes, the patient and family have reached their goals and do not wish to continue or become noncompliant with treatment. In other cases, the wound has healed.

- *Closure and beyond:* Wound closure may be the intent of the treatment, but closure does not include remodeling. Wounds that are minimally closed are at very high

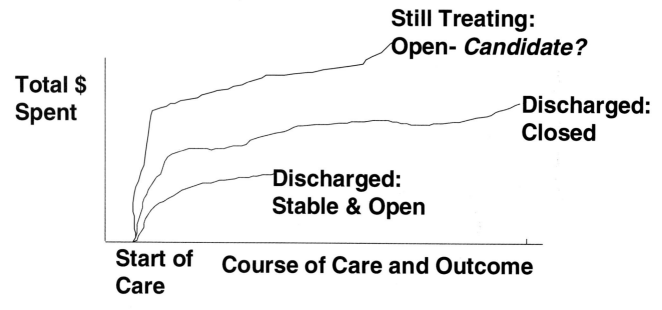

Figure IV–4 Monitor candidacy and outcome throughout course of care.

risk for recurrence, especially when located over areas of friction, shear, and pressure, such as on the seating surface or plantar surface of the foot. Wounds in those areas of high risk would benefit from further stimulation of collagen synthesis by treatment like electrical stimulation or Warm Up therapy until the minimally healed scar is acceptably healed.[11] Acceptable healing is achieved when there is a thickening of the scar formation and the color of the scar blanches from bright red or pink to light pink or white (see Chapter 13 for more about scar).

Plan of Care/Treatment

Part IV focuses primarily on the use of externally applied treatments for wound repair and does not address specific dressings nor does it outline the specifics of an exercise program. It must be reinforced, however, that all of the described technologies are supplemental to standard wound management. It is noted where specific requirements of technology are compatible with the dressing regimen or vise versa. In addition to physical therapy technologies, every patient who is able to participate in exercise must be instructed in an appropriate exercise program. For some, traditional strengthening and conditioning exercises would be appropriate (eg, walking, running, stationary bike). In others it may be active range of motion of the extremities or isometric exercises. Every physical therapist must address the issues

of immobilization and prevention of demineralization, atrophy, and contractures. In some cases, soft tissue mobilization techniques could be used around the wound. In all cases, the patients and caregivers must also be educated about hydration, nutrition, and a balanced lifestyle that addresses stress reduction and positive health. The physical therapist is usually the only team member who can manage the electrotherapeutic modalities and physical agent program, the therapeutic exercises, and appropriate soft tissue mobilization procedures along with the wound care.

CONCLUSION

The rules for selection of treatment interventions include consideration of the medical status of the patient, the status of the wound healing phase, and all treatments used to achieve the expected outcome. Wounds all receive multiple treatment interventions requiring that all treatment interventions must be compatible with the patient, one another, and the wound. Treatment interventions may change during the progression of healing. The most universal treatment intervention is the wound dressing. Modern wound dressings have specific effects and times for reapplication. Because wounds need to be cleansed periodically, the wound cleanser is another common intervention. Topical agents from enzymes to antimicrobials are often added to the wound intervention regimen. Depending on the phase of wound healing,

Exhibit IV–1 Rules of Treatment Selection

---

1. **Medical assessment and tissue assessment determine the selection of treatment.**

   Example: Client has a venous stasis ulcer in inflammatory phase and has a cardiac pacemaker implant. Whirlpool, HVPC, PRFS, and PSWD are contraindicated. Ultrasound would be a good choice for local application.

2. **Treatment changes during the progression of healing so as to affect the recovery process.**

   Example: Client has a necrotic hip ulcer with eschar. Treatment starts with whirlpool, enzymes, and occlusive dressing. Necrotic tissue is removed. Treatment changes.

3. **Each selected treatment is goal-specific based on how it affects the predicted outcome.**

   Example: Client has a clean partial-thickness wound in the acute proliferative phase. Prognosis is wound closure. Treatment selected: clean with normal saline, use hydrogel impregnated gauze dressing, apply HVPC through dressing, and cover with secondary dressing.

   Formula To Select Treatment

   Wound Healing Phase of Tissue + Treatment A + Treatment B + Treatment C = Wound Healing Phase of Tissue in X Period of Time

---

one or more of these interventions will be needed. The addition of an electrotherapeutic modality or a physical agent must be compatible with the other treatment interventions. This will require collaboration of the team members—nurse, physician, pharmacist, and physical therapist—to select interventions that are compatible and efficacious for wound healing. Exhibit IV–1 lists three rules of treatment selection, an example of how each is used, and a formula for selection of treatments to achieve a desire outcome in a prescribed period. The letters "A," "B," and "C," in the formula represent three treatment interventions. The number of treatments usually given is often three, but is not limited to three. Each chapter in Part IV will address the issue of treatment interactions and compatibility with other interventions.

CHAPTER ORGANIZATION

Each chapter in Part IV covers the following information about each modality:

- Related definitions and terminology
- Associated physical science
- The theory and science of the therapy
- Clinical trials when available that relate to efficacy
- Indications, contraindications, and precautions
- Expected outcomes and outcomes measures
- Equipment use and safety
- Procedures, including protocols and patient set-ups
- Clinical and research-related wisdom
- Self-care treatment guidelines, if appropriate
- Case study, using the functional outcome report

REFERENCES

1. American Physical Therapy Association. A guide to physical therapist practice, Vol. 1: a description of patient management. *Phys Ther.* 1995;75:707–764.

2. American Physical Therapy Association. Guide to physical therapist practice, second edition. *Phys Ther.* 2001; 81:9–744.

3. Eaglstein W. What is standard care and where should we leave it? In: *Evidence Based Outcomes in Wound Management.* Dallas, TX: ConvaTec; 2000.

4. General Accounting Office, US Congress, reported in PT Bulletin. American Physical Therapy Association, Vol. 12, No. 10, March 7, 1997.

5. Hayes S, Carroll S. Early intervention care in the acute stroke patient. *Arch Phys Med Rehabil.* 1986;67:319–321.

6. Linton S, Hellsing A, Andersson D. A controlled study of the effects of early intervention on acute musculoskeletal pain problems. *Pain.* 1993;54(3):353–359.

7. American Physical Therapy Association. *Outcome Effectiveness of Physical Therapy: An Annotated Bibliography.* Alexandria, VA: APTA; 1993.

8. Hunt T, Hussain MZ. Can wound healing be a paradigm for tissue repair? *Med Sci Sports Exerc.* 1994;26:755–758.

9. Robson MC, Hill DP, Woodske ME, Steed DL. Wound healing trajectories as predictors of effectiveness of therapeutic agents. *Arch Surg.* 2000;135(7):773–777.

10. Harding K. Wound care: putting theory into clinical practice. In: Krasner D, ed. *Chronic Wound Care: A Clinical Source for Health Care Professionals.* King of Prussia, PA: Health Management Publications Inc; 1990:19–30.

11. Lazarus GS, Cooper DM, Knighton DR, et al. Definitions and guidelines for assessment of wounds and evaluation of healing. *Arch Dermatol.* 1994;130:489–493.

12. Ferrell BA, Osterweil D, Christenson P. A randomized trial of low-air-loss beds for treatment of pressure ulcers. *JAMA.* 1993;269:494–497.

13. Kantor J, Margolis DJ. Expected healing rates for chronic wounds. *Wounds: A Compendium of Clinical Research and Practice.* 2000;12(6):155–158.

14. Dyson M, Young S. Acceleration of tissue repair by low intensity ultrasound applied during the inflammatory phase, APTA/CPTA Joint Congress, Abstract No. R-186, presented in Las Vegas, Nevada, June 1998.

15. Skene AI, Smith JM, Dore CJ, Charlett A, Lewis JD. Venous leg ulcers: a prognostic index to predict time to healing. *British Medical Journal.* 1992;305(6862):1119–1121.

16. Tallman, P, Muscare E, Carson P, Eaglstein WH, Falanga V. Initial rate of healing predicts complete healing of venous ulcers. *Arch Dermatol.* 1997;133(10):1231–1234.

17. Phillips T. Machado F, Trout R, Porter J, Olin J, Falanga V. Prognostic indicators in venous ulcers. *J Am Acad Dermatol.* 2000;43(4):627–630.

18. vanRijswijk L. Full-thickness pressure ulcers: patient and wound healing characteristics. *Decubitus.* 1993;6(1):16–21.

19. Marston W, Carlin RE, Passman MA, Farber MA, Keagy BA. Healing rates and cost efficacy of outpatient compression treatment for leg ulcers associated with venous insufficiency. *J Vasc Surg.* 1999;30(3):491–498.

20. Garber, SL, Biddle AK, Click CN. *Pressure Ulcer Prevention and Treatment Following Spinal Cord Injury: A Clinical Practice Guideline for Health-Care Professionals.* Jackson Heights, NY: Paralyzed Veterans of America; 2000:12–14.

21. Coleridge-Smith, PD. Oxygen, oxygen free radicals and reperfusion injury. In: Krasner D, Kane D, eds. *Chronic Wound Care: A Clinical Source Book for Healthcare Professionals.* Wayne, PA: Health Management Publications, Inc.; 1997:348–353.

22. Hart J. The effect of therapeutic ultrasound on dermal repair with emphasis on fibroblasts activity. PhD thesis, London: University of London, 1993.

23. Joint Commission on Accreditation of Healthcare Organizations (Joint Commission). Pain Management Standards (Standard RI 2.8 and PE 1.4). In: Joint Commission, ed. *Comprehensive Accreditation Manual for Hospitals.* Oakbrook Terrace, IL: Joint Commission; 2001.

24. Swanson G. *Sussman Physical Therapy 1991 Wound Database Report.* Long Beach, CA: Swanson and Co.

25. Sussman C. Functional wound cost outcomes. Presented at the American Physical Therapy Association Combined Sections Meeting, February 1996, Atlanta, GA.

26. Bergstrom N, Bennett MA, Carlson CE, et al. *Treatment of Pressure Ulcers.* Clinical Practice Guideline No. 15. AHCPR Publication No. 95–0652. Rockville, MD: Agency for Health Care Policy and Research, U.S. Public Health Service, U.S. Department of Health and Human Services; December 1994.

27. Wethe J. Sharp debridement of wounds instructional course. Wound Care Management Conference. October 1993.

28. Swanson G. Use of cost data, provider experience, and clinical guidelines in the transition to managed care. *J Ins Med.* 1991;23(1):70–74.

29. Maver RW. An actuarial report on the cost-effectiveness of a new medical technology. *J Ins Med.* 1991;23(2):120–123.

30. Birke J. Management of the diabetic foot instructional course. Wound Care Management Conference. November 1995.

31. Itoh M, et al. Accelerated wound healing of pressure ulcers by pulsed high peak power electromagnetic energy (Diapulse). *Decubitus.* 1991;4(1):24–34.

CHAPTER 21

Electrical Stimulation for Wound Healing

Carrie Sussman and Nancy N. Byl

CHAPTER OBJECTIVES

At the completion of this chapter, the reader will be able to:

1. Discuss the physical properties of electrical stimulation used for wound healing treatment and their significance
2. Describe evidence of the physiologic effects of electrical stimulation on body systems: cellular, circulatory, and neuronal
3. Understand the results of animal and clinical studies using different types of electrical stimulation waveforms
4. Select the appropriate candidates for wound healing with electrical stimulation along with contraindications and precautions
5. Apply electrical stimulation for different wound healing situations including home self-care and evaluate outcomes of care.

INTRODUCTION

Use of exogenous electrical current for wound healing of chronic indolent ulcers of many etiologies has been reported in the literature since the 1960s. There are many descriptive reports, quality assurance documents, case reports, and experimental research, including randomized controlled trials (RCTs) evaluating efficacy and safety. Yet, there remains skepticism about use of this treatment for wound healing. Some reasons for the skepticism include the variation in modes of stimulation delivery, different protocols, and limited data available for each specific electrical stimulation (ES) device. Not all ES procedures are alike, creating confu-

sion about which one to use for wound healing. Two methods of synthesizing the evidence related to use of ES for wound healing are the development of clinical practice guidelines and the meta-analysis of research studies. The findings of both will be discussed.

EVALUATING THE EVIDENCE

In 1993, the Agency for Health Care Policy and Research (AHCPR), now the Agency for Health Care Research and Quality (AHRQ), convened a panel of experts to review the literature related to adjunctive treatments for pressure ulcers. In 1994, this panel published guidelines[1] for pressure ulcer treatment. The literature review by the AHCPR panel (1993) focused on several adjunctive therapies used to facilitate healing of pressure ulcers. Usually, an adjunctive therapy is selected to restart or accelerate wound healing. The adjunctive therapies considered by the panel were: ES, hyperbaric oxygen, infrared, ultraviolet and low-energy laser irradiation, ultrasound, miscellaneous topical agents, and systemic drugs (not antibiotics). At the time of the review, only ES had sufficient supporting evidence to warrant better than a "C" recommendation by the panel. ES was given an evidence rating of "B," based on five clinical trials[2,3,4,5,6] where ES was used to treat pressure ulcers in 147 patients. The recommendation read: "Consider a course of treatment with electrotherapy for Stage II and IV pressure ulcers that have proved unresponsive to conventional therapy. Electrical stimulation may also be useful for recalcitrant Stage II ulcers."[1(p55)] In 1996, the American Medical Directors Association published clinical practice guidelines for pressure ulcers and supported the recommendation of the AHRQ panel to consider a course of electrotherapy.[7]

In an update of the AHCPR *Guidelines for Pressure Ulcers*, Ovington[8] revisited the issue by reviewing the literature through May 1998 to determine the status of adjunctive therapy evidence in the 5 years since the AHCPR review. The goal was to determine whether any new data existed that would change or strengthen the evidence of the AHCPR recommendations. In her review, Ovington[8] changed the designation of "*controlled clinical trials* (CCTs)" for the five studies used by AHCPR to "*randomized controlled trials* (RCTs)" and added one additional RCT study for treatment of pressure ulcers in 74 patients.[9] Based on an additional RCT not included in the 1993 AHCPR evidence review, she recommended that ES be upgraded to an "A" from a "B" for the treatment of pressure ulcers. Further review of the literature (1998 through December 2000) located one additional RCT[10] of individuals with spinal cord injury (SCI) who had a total of 185 pressure ulcers that had a positive treatment effect from a protocol using ES and a CCT with 34 subjects having wounds of mixed etiologies. An RCT of patients with leg ulcers—venous, arterial, and diabetic—has also reported significant treatment effect with ES and is under review for publication.[11] In another RCT study of 37 human subjects with pressure ulcers, the ES group showed significant decrease in volume measurements. This study is also under review for publication.[12] In August 2000, the Consortium for Spinal Cord Medicine published *Pressure Ulcer Prevention and Treatment Following Spinal Cord Injury* clinical practice guidelines.[13] In these guidelines, ES treatment was recommended (grade level A) as primary treatment for use to promote closure of stages III or IV pressure ulcers, along with standard wound care interventions.

Meta-analysis

A meta-analysis is a mathematical synthesis used in statistics to average the findings across multiple studies quantitatively. It is used to estimate better the magnitude of a treatment effect. Gardner and Frantz[14] recognized the problem of analyzing the efficacy of ES for wound healing when the methods are variable. They undertook to examine the entire body of evidence irrespective of device and parameters and performed a meta-analysis to acquire information about the merits of using ES as an adjunctive wound healing therapy. Another goal of the Gardner, Frantz meta-analysis was to provide clinicians and researchers with valuable information about the utility of pursuing further research in this area. Their methods and findings are discussed below.

Efficacy and Reimbursement

Evidence of the efficacy of treatment should be an appropriate standard in reimbursement policies. In 1997, the Health Care Financing Administration (HCFA) reported findings in a review of ES by an independent group, ECRI, a health care technology assessment consulting firm, that ES in all forms is no *more or less* effective than standard care. Based on this report, HCFA announced that it would exclude reimbursement for all forms of ES therapy for wound healing for Medicare recipients. Its findings contradicted the findings of the AHCPR panel. The meta-analysis of ES had not been prepared at that time. Opposition to this decision came from providers, patients, health care professionals, and the American Physical Therapy Association (APTA), which observed the benefits of treatment of chronic wounds with ES. In November 1997, the federal court enjoined HCFA from implementing this policy.[15]

In July 1999, HCFA notified program carriers and intermediaries that the court order remained in effect until further notice and to disregard Section 35–98 of the Medicare Coverage Issues Manual issued in 1997 that excluded ES reimbursement for the treatment of wounds and to pay for claims based on supporting documentation.[16] Still, doubts remain in the health care community about use of ES for chronic wound healing. However, that seems about to change because in October 2000, the tide turned when an HCFA Medical and Surgical Procedures Panel unanimously voted that there was sufficient evidence that ES has obvious public benefits and that they could classify this therapy as *more* effective than standard care alone for the treatment of nonhealing chronic wounds.[2] HCFA is continuing the process, possibly leading to national coverage guidelines in the near future.

The goal of this chapter is to present the evidence based on a review of the current literature (through December 2000) about what is known regarding the efficacy and utility of using ES as adjunctive therapy for wound healing. The chapter begins with definitions and terminology used to discuss and distinguish ES parameters. The second section details the science and theory of the therapy and relates back to the parameters. Clinical decision making applies the science and theory by considering the indications for the therapy, reasons for referral, medical history, and systems reviews that are part of the diagnostic process. This section is followed by description of the equipment and accessories used, the rationale for selection of protocols, the expected outcomes, and the patient set-up. Because ES is a treatment intervention that can be taught to patients or other caregivers, self-care teaching guidelines are included. Case studies applying the functional outcome report (FOR) to document the rationale for selection of ES as the intervention, followed by a discussion revealing the clinical decision-making process and the actual outcomes, conclude the chapter.[17] Chapter 2 describes the FOR.

DEFINITIONS AND TERMINOLOGY

Electrical stimulation for wound healing is defined as the use of a capacitive coupled electrical current to transfer energy to a wound. The type of electricity that is transferred to the target tissue is controlled by the electrical source.[1] Clinicians need to be familiar with the terminology and characteristics associated with ES to better understand the interrelationships between the various stimulation characteristics and the clinical effects desired. This is not meant to be a comprehensive description of all ES characteristics, but to emphasize those that have an evidence-based role in wound healing clinical practice. For more information, see the suggested readings listed at the end of this chapter.

Capacitive Coupling

Capacitively coupled ES involves the transfer of electric current through an applied surface electrode pad that is in wet (electrolytic) contact (capacitively coupled) with the external skin surface and/or wound bed. When capacitively coupled ES is used, at least two electrodes are required to complete the electric circuit. Electrodes are usually placed over wet conductive medium: (1) in the wound bed or on the skin a distance away from the wound—monopolar technique, or (2) straddling the wound—bipolar technique. Bipolar technique along the wound edge has advantages of not having to disrupt the wound bed or dressing, thus chilling the wound, as well as not introducing contaminants into the wound or spreading disease when the electrode is removed. It is the method reported in most of the biphasic studies that will be discussed later in this chapter.

Polarity

Polarity refers to the property of having two poles that are oppositely charged. The positive pole is called the *anode* and the negative pole the *cathode*. The positive pole lacks electrons and attracts electrons from the negative pole, or cathode. If the wound is placed between the poles as in the bipolar technique described above, and the electrodes are relatively close together, no one polarity predominates, and this is referred to as tangential polarity.[18] Polarity can be chosen or emphasized for biologic effects that are described throughout this chapter, by taking into account the placement of the electrodes (see section on active and dispersive electrodes). In a review of the literature,[18] it was concluded that alternating polarity (negative initially) was more effective for potential wound healing results than maintaining either positive or negative polarity throughout the course treatment.

Amplitude and Voltage

Amplitude refers to the measure of the magnitude of the voltage and should not be referred to as the intensity.[19] Voltage is a measure of the force of the flow of electrons, and amperage is the measure of the rate of flow of the current. When voltage is turned up, the current will also go up, and vice versa. Some stimulators provide a readout of voltage and some a readout of current. The relationship between voltage and current is expressed as Ohm's law. The formula for this is current times resistance equals voltage [$V = IR$, where V is voltage, I is current, and R is resistance]. In general, low-voltage devices produce voltages of different ranges from 60 to 100 V. High-voltage devices range from 100 to 500 V. These are peak ranges. Peak amplitude is the highest amplitude of the current or voltage. Amplitude for wound healing is adjusted until the patient with sensation can feel a tingling sensation (paresthesia) at the edge of the wound. Insensate individuals, of course, cannot respond to this sensation. The voltage is usually turned up until there is a mild muscle contraction or fasiculation, and then backed down until that muscle contraction is no longer visible. For wound healing treatment with high-voltage pulsed current (HVPC), the amplitude is usually set between 75 and 150 V to achieve this response.[20]

Amperage

The unit of current is the ampere (A), which is defined as the rate at which electrons move past a certain point. A milliampere (mA) is one-thousandth of an ampere, and a microampere (μA) is one-millionth of an ampere. Microamperage current is usually between 5 and 20 μA of current (less than 1.0 mA).

Waveforms

Different types of current have different characteristic waveforms. Waveforms are the graphic representations of a current on a current/time or voltage/time plot.[21] Waveforms are classified by the direction of current flow. Current flow is either unidirectional or bidirectional. Figures 21–1 to 21–6 show examples of direct current, monophasic square wave pulsed current, twin-peaked pulsed monophasic current, AC, and balanced biphasic and asymmetric biphasic waveforms. Each waveform and related characteristics are described.

Phase Charge and Charge Density

Phase charge and charge density, also known as current density, have not been considered closely in the past. How important are phase charge and current density to tissue healing? Phase and pulse charge refer to the total charge within each phase.[22] Phase charge is a time and amplitude dependent characteristic.[19] It is possible to calculate the pulse charge for any type of electrical waveform if waveform, the frequency (rate) and duration (width) of the pulse, and the amplitude (voltage) are known. The unit of measure for charge is the coulomb. One coulomb is the quantity of electricity transferred by a current of one ampere in one second.

Brighton et al[23] studied the relationship between charge, current density, and the amount of new bone formed in rabbits. They reported that a classical dose–response relationship exists between current amplitude, charge delivered, and biologic effect. At a low, constant DC current regime there is minimal or no effect. A regime of optimal or maximal effect occurs at 20 µA (36.29 C) and a gradual occurrence of cellular necrosis as currents increase significantly higher, 80 µA (145.15 C). The findings indicated that the amount of bone formed by the cathode is related to both the current density and charge. The amount of bone formation by pulsed direct current approached that of constant DC, *only* as the total charge delivered by the pulsed current approached that delivered by the constant current (27.20 coulombs, pulsed vs 36.3 coulombs constant current). To achieve this pulse charge with pulsed current at 20 µA, a frequency of 750 Hz[23] is needed. The relationship between charge delivered and biologic effect has thus been established for bone healing and appears that a significant relationship has been established between charge delivered and biologic effect for soft tissue healing.

Waveforms are either symmetric with equal phase characteristics with respect to the baseline for each phase and thus the phase charges of each are equal. An asymmetric waveform means that the waveform characteristics are unequal with respect to the base line. These waveforms may be either charge balanced or unbalanced with the phase charge being the same or different.[19] For instance, when considering a monophasic square wave pulse (LVPC), the phase charge (q) is represented by the area under the curve and is expressed as the product of the phase duration (t) and the peak current amplitude (I).[22]

In biologic systems, the charges are small and are usually expressed in microcoulombs (µC).[24] One µC is equivalent to 10^{-6} coulombs. To calculate the amount of phase charge per second, the number of µC is multiplied by the frequency of the pulse. See example. A typical high-voltage stimulator with very short duration (5–20 µ sec), twin-peaked (triangular shaped) pulses, for example, has a maximum pulse charge of only 10 to 15 µC, which is very low and within safety limits.[25] One of the deficits of the high-voltage stimulator is that at a tolerable voltage level it has insufficient phase charge to excite skeletal muscle of large muscle groups to produce a vigorous muscle contraction. However, it can cause threshold excitation of sensory, motor, and pain-conducting fibers because at very short phase duration, less charge is needed to cause threshold excitation.[22]

The pulse charge of a sine wave can be compared with the pulse charge of a square wave by doubling the charge delivered by one phase. The result is that the charge delivered by the square wave is significantly greater than that of the sine wave. Thus, more pulse amplitude is required to provide the same charge with a sine wave than a square wave, making it less efficient for excitation.[22] It makes no difference what type of current is used (high or low volt, monophasic, biphasic or AC time, or amplitude modulated), as long as there is sufficient phase charge for a given phase duration, excitation of the nerve and cellular effects will occur.[22]

Kloth presented evidence to the HCFA Medical and Surgical Procedures Panel that the phase charge quantity (dosage) needed to enhance soft tissue healing can be computed for monophasic (triangular) HVPC and square wave (PES or LVPC) pulses using the formula described here to quantify the dose (phase charge) delivered to the tissues across a number of studies, regardless of device used.[20] In his review of the literature, Kloth found that four studies (3, 4, 5, 6) reported the pulse charge. Two of the studies used HVPC (3, 5) and two (4, 6) PES or LVPC. Then he went on to calculate the charge quantity per unit for other studies using the data in those reports. Based on the calculations derived from his review of these studies, Kloth found that the charge quantity varied somewhat, but that the effective "window of charge" dosage is between 200 and 600 µC.[20]

Calculation of Pulse Charge for Monophasic Square Wave Pulse (LVPC)

Amplitude of current (I) X pulse duration (t) X pulse frequency = pulse charge/time
Example: 30 mA X 140 µsec = 4.2 µC X 128 pps = 537.6 µC/ second[26]

Calculation of Pulse Charge for Monophasic Triangular Wave Pulse (HVPC)

Area of one phase = phase charge = (1/2) X phase duration X amplitude = (1/2) X 20 µsec X .325 amp = 3.25 µC. Total charge per second = phase charge X frequency = 3.3.25 microcoulombs X 105 pps = 342 µC/sec[5]

The second measurement of dosage is the current density. Current density is an indicator of the electrochemical effects of stimulation.[27,28] The charge or current density is the electrical charge per cross-sectional area of the electrodes. The larger the size of the electrode, the smaller the charge current density and conversely. Reich et al reviewed 17 studies of pulsed stimulation and computed the absolute spatial current density for each of them.[18] The findings indicated the parameter obtained by multiplying the average spatial current density by the effective duty cycle (duty cycle = 1 for DC) by the total duration of treatment is essential in measuring dosage delivered to the tissues. To perform this calculation it is essential to know the size of the electrode or to have a report of current density (A/cm²) as part of the study methods. A follow-up calculation of importance is to multiply the absolute current density by the time of the treatment. This gives the total amount of charge delivered per unit area (coulombs/centimeter squared).[28] Unfortunately, most researchers fail to provide all of the data needed for these calculations. Most notably the electrode size is omitted.[28,29] These authors went the extra mile and contacted some of the researchers or manufacturers to obtain the information needed to perform the calculations. Based on their review, they found a trend that an absolute charge density transfer (dose) on the order of 0.1–2.0 C/cm² may be effective and that further research is indicated to verify this range.

Example of Calculating Current Density

Current amplitude divided by the area of the electrode
Example: Current amplitude is 10 A and the electrode is 10 cm². Current density equals 1 A / cm².[28]

An adequate but not excessive charge amount must be delivered to stimulate the desired response in the tissues. Different tissues or cells receive different pulse charge per unit area depending on their physical structure. For instance, sensory nerve fibers of the skin may receive up to 100 times more stimulation (pulse charge per unit area) than epidermal cells and fibroblasts due to their physical properties.[30] The sensitivity of the nerve fiber to sensory stimulation may be responsible for the vascular changes associated with ES. On the other hand the weak stimulation of the epidermal and fibroblast cells may be what enhances the metabolism of these cells to speed up wound healing.[30]

Reporting of ES Parameters

In order to use the evidence produced from clinical studies, several parameters have been identified that are needed to help define the effective treatment dose, to make studies reproducible, and to compare studies.[20,28,29] They include

- current amplitude
- pulse frequency and width or duration
- electrode size or average current density/area of the electrode (ie, mA/cm²)
- duty cycle for pulsed currents

- calculation of the phase charge delivered
- treatment time

Direct Current

Unidirectional current is also called *galvanic* or *direct current* (Figure 21–1). Direct current is continuous, uninterrupted, unidirectional current. Direction of the flow is determined by the polarity selected. Direct current waveforms may be subdivided into pulsatile currents (PC).

Monophasic Pulsed Current

Pulsed current is phasic. Monophasic pulsed current is defined as PC that deviates from baseline and returns to baseline after a designated time period. The monophasic pulsed current waveform may be either a square wave or the traditional twin-peaked pulsed wave of the HVPC. Monophasic pulses and phases are identical (Figure 21–2). Monophasic waves are such that, at one electrode, the polarity is positive, and the other is negative. This stays constant throughout the treatment unless changed by the clinician. Polarity appears to have specific effects on biologic responses.

Frequency or Pulse Rate

PC is defined as an electrical current that is conducted as a signal(s) of short duration. Each pulse lasts for a few msec or μsec, followed by an interpulse interval, then repeated.[26]

Pulse rate or frequency is the number of pulses delivered per unit of time. The *rate* of the off and on cycle is defined as pulses per second (pps). Alternating current frequency is usually expressed in Hertz (Hz) and pulsed monophasic current in pps. Thus, Hz and pps represent the same property, ie, the number of pulses delivered each second.[26]

The range of pps is usually from 0.1 to 999 Hz. A pulse of 0.1 Hz is on for 10 seconds, and a pulse of 999 Hz is on for 1 msec. The time between pulses when no electrical activ-

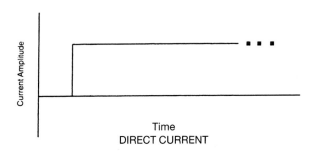

Time
DIRECT CURRENT

Figure 21–1 Graphic representation of the unidirectional flow of charged particles. *Source:* Reprinted with permission from *Electrotherapeutic Terminology in Physical Therapy*, p. 11, © 1990, Section on Clinical Electrophysiology and the American Physical Therapy Association.

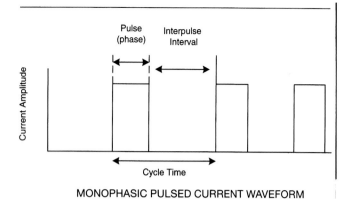

MONOPHASIC PULSED CURRENT WAVEFORM

Note: In a monophasic waveform, phase and pulse are identical.

Figure 21–2 Graphic representation of monophasic pulses. *Source:* Reprinted with permission from *Electrotherapeutic Terminology in Physical Therapy*, p. 13, © 1990, Section on Clinical Electrophysiology and the American Physical Therapy Association.

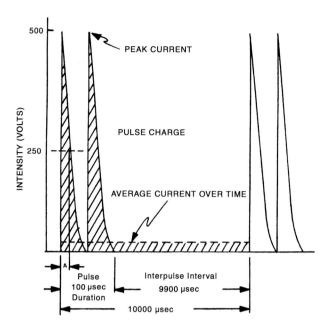

Figure 21–3 Typical pulse characteristics of a high-voltage stimulator. *Source:* Reprinted with permission from Alon G, De Dominico G. *High Voltage Stimulation: An Integrated Approach to Clinical Electrotherapy*, 1st ed., p. 62, © 1987, Hixton, TN: The Chattanooga Group.

ity occurs is the interpulse interval (see Figure 21–3). Pulsed ES (PES) has a train of pulses that are repeated at regular intervals and are termed the *pulse rate* or *pulse frequency*. PC can be either unidirectional or bidirectional.

Pulse Duration

The on time during which current is flowing is the pulse duration. On some stimulators the pulse duration is labeled incorrectly as "pulse width." Pulse duration affects biologic responses. For example, direct current has a continuous duration that can raise tissue temperature and change the pH under the electrode, which can produce blisters under the electrode. However, a short pulse duration (5–100 μsec), typical of HVCP, produces insignificant changes in both tissue pH and tissue temperature.[31–33] Such a current is therefore very safe but raises questions about the effect of polarity when the pulse duration is so short. For purposes of muscle stimulation, the stimulation must be provided at an amplitude and a duration that will stimulate a muscle contraction which is a minimum of 1msec.[33]

If the goal is to keep the stimulation tolerable, the amplitude must be kept as low as possible, forcing the duration of the stimulus to be longer. Because high-voltage pulsed monophasic current has a pulse duration shorter than 1 msec, it cannot be used to stimulate denervated muscle. Even at maximum pulse rates, the phase duration for HVPC represents less than 1% of the on time, and the interpulse interval 99% percent of the total time.[31] Depite this, HVPC stimulators can cause excitation of sensory, motor, and pain-conducting fibers. The laws of excitation state that "at a shorter phase duration, less charge is needed to cause threshold excitation."[22(p106)] For pain management and wound healing, the pulse duration and the amplitude of the current are variable. Some clinicians and researchers suggest that this current must be on for at least 1 second to produce strong polarity effects of the tissue under the electrodes. Yet, even at these very short pulse durations of HVPC, different effects related to polarity are reported. Many of these effects will be presented.

Because high-voltage pulsed monophasic current has a shorter pulse duration, it cannot be used to stimulate denervated muscle. For pain management and wound healing, the pulse duration and the amplitude of the current are variable. Some clinicians and researchers suggest that this current must be on for at least 1 second to produce strong polarity effects of the tissue under the electrodes.

Duty Cycle

The on/off ratio is the ratio of the time the current is on to the time the current is off. A duty cycle is the ratio of *on time* to the *total cycle time*, including both the on and off time (Figure 21–2). A ratio is used to express the relative proportion of the on and off time and can be expressed as a percentage. For instance, if the total cycle is 60 μsec, the on time is 20 μsec, and the off time is 40 μsec, there is a 1:2 on/off ratio and the duty cycle is a 1:3 ratio, or a 33% duty cycle.

The calculation for duty cycle is pulse duration in seconds × frequency (Hz) = fraction of time during which current is actually applied.

High-Voltage Pulsed Current

HVPC typically has a twin-peaked monophasic waveform. HVPC is a misnomer if *galvanic* is used with it. This current was named incorrectly by the manufacturers. The acronym HVPC does not have *galvanic* in the acronym. The pulse rate most frequently used for wound healing is 50–120 pps (0.83–1.25 msec). Each peak or spike has an effective 5- to 20-µsec phase duration. Voltage can be selected with intensity between 100 and 500 V. The amplitude selected for wound healing is usually between 80 and 200 V, and the polarity and pulse rate are varied. There is a long interpulse interval between pulses that makes a low average current. The high-voltage stimulation has a high peak current that means greater penetration into tissue, allowing for stimulation of deep motor points.[31] On the skin surface, alkaline/acidity changes under the electrodes have not been measured.[32,33] Because HVPC is not galvanic, this explains why there are no alkaline/acidity effects. Absence of chemical changes under the electrodes has led to questions about how polarity effects can be the factor that stimulates cellular responses when the duration of the HVPC pulse is so short. However, multiple studies demonstrate different effects on blood flow, edema, and bacteria under the anode and cathode when using HVPC (see Table 21–1). One study showed that fibroblasts were attracted to the cathode of an HVPC stimulator, suggesting that there may be some cellular polarity effects under the electrode.[34] Although multiple studies show cellular effects and responses to HVPC, each study shows something different; therefore, corroborating research would be useful to support the findings of these single studies (see section on Galvanotaxis).

Microcurrent Electrical Stimulation

A pulsed monophasic stimulus is referred to as *monophasic low-voltage microcurrent electrical nerve stimulation* (MENS). This refers to a pulsed current at an intensity less than 1 mA (1–999 µA), and the voltage is less than 100 V. MENS is delivered at amplitudes that have minimal detectable sensation and are incapable of motor nerve stimulation. MENS typically has a single modified monophasic square waveform. The pulse duration of these devices ranges from 0.1 to 999 Hz, equivalent to on time of 10 seconds to 1 µsec. The pulse duration is inversely related to the frequency. Microcurrent stimulation has a prolonged pulse duration at the lower frequencies, which will have a different tissue polarity effect than a shorter-duration pulse, most typically used in high-voltage stimulation. For example, a low-voltage pulsed stimulus at 0.1 Hz is on for 10 seconds, whereas the high-voltage monophasic simulators are used at 80–120 pps and are on for only 0.83–1.25 msec. Thus, pulsed low-voltage current of at least 1 pps can maintain the polarity effect delivered to the tissues under the electrode. The peak amplitude is usually 600 µA/60 V. The average amplitude commonly used is 200–300 µA for soft tissue[35] and 20 µA for bone healing in rabbits.[36] MENS current has been used in bone healing; however, in this clinical application, the amplitude recommended is 20–50 µA.[37–44] When pulsed slowly, there are reported cellular and tissue polarity effects under the electrodes.[45] This type of current may be used to restore the normal bioelectrical resting current or reverse the injury current.[45] There is some concern that the voltage may be too low to push the current through the resistance of the skin and the subcutaneous tissues, but no specific studies could be found to confirm this.

Alternating/Biphasic Current

Bidirectional waveforms are referred to as *faradic* or *alternating*, as well as *biphasic* or *bipolar*. British literature uses the term "*faradic*" for all AC, probably in reference to the scientist Faraday. In the United States, faradic is no longer designed in ES units because it is very uncomfortable. AC is uninterrupted bidirectional current flow. The waveforms may be symmetric, where the shape of the waveform is always balanced (Figure 21–4). Both the shape and size are the same. An asymmetric waveform can be balanced or unbalanced (see Figures 21–5A and 21–5B). One of the most common outputs from an electrical stimulator is balanced asymmetric. A balanced asymmetric waveform is typical of transcutaneous electrical nerve stimulation (TENS) used for pain modulation (Figure 21–5A). Biphasic waves are such that the polarity is constantly changing. They are opposite at any moment in time. However, the waveform can be biased so that one polarity is emphasized. Several studies using this type of current for wound healing have been reported in the literature, which are described in this chapter. The best wound healing effects seem to be achieved when a biphasic waveform is asymmetric and biased, so that the polarity at one pole predominates. Pain modulation and edema reduction in patients with diabetic neuropathy have been reported with a biphasic waveform.[46,47] The effects of stimulation with a biphasic waveform on wound healing are discussed further in following sections.

Transcutaneous Electrical Nerve Stimulation

Except for true DC and subliminal stimulators, most clinical stimulators are TENS. In TENS, the electrodes are applied transcutaneously, with the physiologic objective of exciting peripheral nerves. As long as surface electrodes are

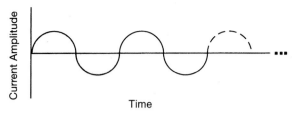

Figure 21–4 Symmetric alternating (biphasic) waveform. *Source:* Reprinted with permission from *Electrotherapeutic Terminology in Physical Therapy*, p. 11, © 1990, Section on Clinical Electrophysiology and the American Physical Therapy Association.

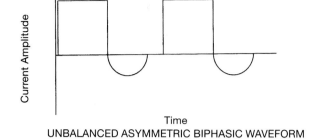

Figure 21–5B Unbalanced asymmetric biphasic waveform. *Source:* Reprinted with permission from *Electrotherapeutic Terminology in Physical Therapy*, p. 15, © 1990, Section on Clinical Electrophysiology and the American Physical Therapy Association.

used and peripheral nerves are excited, the stimulator is a TENS unit, regardless of the names used by commercial companies or the waveforms.[26] However, for clarification, the studies that report use of TENS stimulators are usually using biphasic or modified AC currents. Some stimulators are identified as DC, HVPC, LIDC, PES (also LVPC), or microamperage current.

THEORY AND SCIENCE OF ELECTRICAL STIMULATION

Bioelectrical Systems

The body has its own bioelectrical system. This system influences wound healing by attracting the cells of repair, changing cell membrane permeability, enhancing cellular secretion through cell membranes, and orientating cell structures.

Sodium Current of Injury

The intact skin surface maintains an average constant electronegative charge of approximately –23 mV with respect to the deeper epidermal layers. The negative charge on the surface is created by negatively charged chloride ions (Cl^-), which stay on the surface after positively charged sodium ions (Na^+) are pumped into the inner layers of the epidermis by the sodium ion pump. Thus, the skin has electrical potentials across it, and it acts as a battery. When there is a break in the skin surface, current can flow between the parts of the skin transmitted through the ionic fluids of the tissues between the outer and inner layers of the skin (see Figure 21–6).[48] Regenerating tissues show a distinct pattern of unidirectional current flow and polarity switching. As healing is completed, or *arrested*, these currents disappear. When ulcers become dry, the voltage gradient is eliminated, and the current disappears.[45] This has been suggested as an explanation of why moist wounds heal better than dry wounds.

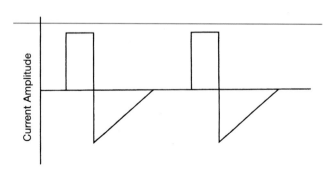

Figure 21–5A Balanced asymmetric alternating (biphasic) waveform. *Source:* Reprinted with permission from *Electrotherapeutic Terminology in Physical Therapy*, p. 12, © 1990, Section on Clinical Electrophysiology and the American Physical Therapy Association.

Clinical Wisdom: *Moist Wounds Promote the "Current of Injury"*

Keeping a wound moist with normal (0.9%) saline (sodium chloride) maintains the optimal bioelectric charge because it simulates the electrolytic concentration of wound fluid. Dressings such as amorphous hydrogels and occlusive dressings help to promote the body's "current of injury" by keeping the wound environment moist.

To test the hypothesis that ulcers kept moist maintain a higher electrical potential than do dry wounds, Cheng[49] measured the electrical potentials of partial-thickness wounds treated with occlusive dressings. He devised a system of

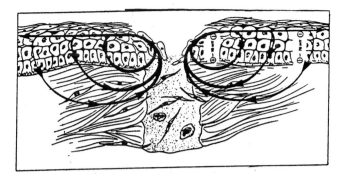

Figure 21–6 Current path in wounded section of the skin. Disruption in epidermis has provided a return path for current driven by transepithelial potential. *Source:* Reprinted with permission from *Clinics in Dermatology*, Vol. 2, L.F. Jaffe and J.W. Vanable, Electric Fields and Wound Healing, 1984, with permission from Elsevier Science.

electrodes connected to a voltmeter that could be used for measuring the electrical potential during the 4 days that it took for the wound to epithelialize. The device was placed with one electrode in the center of the wound and a second electrode placed on the adjacent normal skin surface. He compared the changes in electrical potential between wounds that were occluded to retain moisture and those that were air exposed and allowed to dry out. On day zero, day of wounding, both groups had the identical electrical potential (35–38 mV). The occluded wounds maintained a high electrical potential of 29.6 mV for the 4-day period. The air-exposed wounds' electrical potential dropped to 5.2 mV. After epithelialization was completed in the occlusion group, the electrical potential returned to a similar potential to that of the air-exposed group. This work seems to support the hypothesis that occlusive dressings can help to promote the electrical current of injury.

One rationale for applying ES is that it mimics the natural current of injury and will jump-start or accelerate the wound healing process.[6] Sumano and Mateos[50] applied a protocol of modified biphasic stimulation to recalcitrant wounds and burns. Part of the protocol called for the wounds and burn injuries never to be closely covered with heavy dressings or gauzes, and the patients were instructed to allow air contact to the wounds in the home and minimal coverage outdoors. Of the 44 wounds treated, 41 (93%) had > 90% healing, and 3 (7%) had > 60–90% healing. None of the wounds healed less than 60%. Perhaps the ES that was delivered for 20 minutes on a daily or every-other-day basis imitated the current of injury sufficiently that, even with the dry wound environment, the wounds progressed toward healing. Further investigation is needed to clarify the role of ES in imitating the current of injury and the benefit of maintaining a wound environment that is moist versus dry.

Galvanotaxis and Polarity

Unidirectional electrical current flow in the tissues attracts the cells of repair and is called *galvanotaxis*. There is a significant body of research that demonstrates that polarity influences healing in different ways at different phases. Table 21–1 summarizes the polarity effects on other aspects of biologic systems related to wound healing. Table 21–2 summarizes the cellular effects by phase of wound healing.

Neutrophils, lymphocytes, platelets, and macrophages are early responders to injury and start the inflammatory response. The neutrophils are attracted to the negative pole if the wound is infected, to the positive pole if not infected.[59] Lymphocytes and platelets are attracted to the negative pole.[34] Macrophages are attracted to the positive pole.[60] These cells fight infection and produce chemotactic and growth-stimulating cytokines needed to repair or regenerate the tissue. Autolysis and phagocytosis are mediated by the macrophages and neutrophils. Thus, a suggested clinical application of electrical current that integrates these principles would be as follows: for a wound that is necrotic but not infected, use a positive electrode over the wound to promote autolysis, and put the negative electrode over the wound if it is infected.[61] However, for the treatment of diabetic ulcers, Alon et al[62] used positive polarity with HVPC throughout the course of care.

Fibroblasts are key cells in contraction and connective tissue formation. Fibroblasts are attracted by the negative pole to proliferate and synthesize collagen and to contract the wound rapidly.[34] Protein and DNA synthesis are enhanced by negative stimulation. Under similar parameters, calcium ion (Ca^{2+}) or uptake by fibroblast cells is increased, which immediately produces an increased exposure of insulin receptors on the fibroblast cell surface. If insulin is available to bind, the additional receptors on the fibroblasts will significantly increase protein and DNA synthesis. If insulin is added after exposure to HVPC stimulation, further increase in Ca^{2+} uptake and a twofold increase in protein and DNA synthesis occur. Therefore, timing of insulin delivery and HVPC treatment to diabetic patients with wounds may have a different outcome. Conversely, these same receptors are inhibited by Ca^{2+} channel blocker medications.[34] Slower healing can be expected in wounds if the patient is taking Ca^{2+} channel blocker medication. Studies with guinea pigs showed that pulsed low voltage microamperage direct cur-

Table 21–1 Polarity Effects of Electrical Stimulation

Effect	Pole	Researcher	Type of Current
↑ Blood flow	Negative	Mohr et al[72]	HVPC
		Politis et al[74]	PES
		Pollack[75]	PES
		Gentzkow et al[6]	PES
↓ Edema	Negative	Mendel and Fish[101]	HVPC
		Reed[100]	HVPC
		Ross and Segal[99]	HVPC
Debridement	Negative	Sawyer and Deutch[109–111]	DC
Thrombolysis	Negative	Sawyer and Deutch[109–111]	DC
Thrombosis	Positive	Williams and Carey[56]	DC
Oxygen	Anode	Byl et al[117]	MENS, 100 µA low volt
Oxygen	Negative Bias	Baker et al[57]	Asymmetric biphasic
Wound contraction	Alternating (±) every 3 days	Stromberg[64]	PES
Tendon repair	Positive	Owoeye et al[58]	HVPC
Bacteriostatic effects	Both	Barranco et al[112]	DC
		Rowley et al[113]	DC
		Kincaid and Lavoie[115]	HVPC
		Szuminsky et al[116]	HVPC

Table 21–2 Galvanotactic Effects on Cells by Phases of Healing

Effect	Cells	Pole	Type of Current	Researcher
Inflammatory: autolysis and phagocytosis	Macrophages (+)	Anode	DC	Orida and Feldman[60]
	Neutrophils (±)	Anode/cathode	DC	Fukushima et al[59]; Kloth[61]
	Mast cells (decreased) (−)	Anode	PES, 35 mA, 128 pps	Weiss et al[67]; Gentzkow and Miller[48]
Proliferative: fibroplasia (collagen formation)	Fibroblasts (+)	Cathode	HVPC, 50 V, 100 pps	Bourguignon and Bourguignon[51]
			DC, 10–100 µV/cm	Canaday and Lee[52]; Erickson and Nuccitelli[53]
			DC, 1,500 mV/cm	Yang et al[54]
Wound contraction	Myofibroblasts (+)	Alternating	HVPC	Stromberg[64]
Epithelialization	Epidermal cells (−)	Anode	DC, 50 mV/mm	Cooper and Schliwa[55]

rent (LIDC) caused a rapid calcium flux in the epidermis. The researchers concluded that the growth of fibroblasts and keratinocytes may be enhanced by pulsed LIDC, due to changes in calcium homeostasis.[9] LIDC clinical study results are presented in Table 21–3.

When the clinician is taking a medical history, the pharmaceutical history should be reviewed with these factors in mind. Drug effects could change the prognosis for healing.

The use of ES to enhance the benefits of antibiotics is being researched.[63] Research to investigate timing of drug delivery and physical therapy modality treatment to enhance effects of both could open a new approach to interventions.

Research on rapid wound contraction can also provide clinical guidance for treatment selection. Stromberg[64] found that pulsed monophasic current, alternating polarity every 3 days at 128 pps and amplitude at 35 mA accelerated wound contraction during the first 4 weeks after injury. Conversely, he found that constant polarity, either negative or positive, was less effective. Thoughtful application should be considered in areas where rapid wound contraction would not be desirable, such as in the hand or neck.

Epidermal cells have been reported as migrating toward the positive pole. Animal studies demonstrate that, in the early acute inflammatory phase of healing, the rate of epidermal cell migration in dermal wounds is enhanced by 3 days of stimulation with a negative pole, followed by stimulation with the positive pole for 4 days. Closure was achieved in 100% of the treatment group and only 87% of control group. Comparison of tensile strength and mitotic activity between treated and control groups was comparable.[65,66] This corresponds to a 0- to 3-day inflammatory phase and a 4- to 7-day repair phase of healing.

The goal of wound healing is a scar whose characteristics are most like the original skin. Mast cells regulate this process throughout the healing cycle. A large number of mast cells in the healing wound are associated with diseases of abnormal fibrotic healing, such as keloid and hypertrophic scar formation (see Chapter 13). After exposure to positive polarity current (PES 150 μsec, 128 pps, peak current 35 mA), a decrease in mast cells, decreased scar thickness, softer scar, and better cosmetic results were observed in donor sites used for partial-thickness skin grafts. Control scars on the same patients showed evidence of hypertrophy. Differences were clinically apparent at 1 month postoperatively, and subtle differences persisted after 6 months. A side benefit of the ES treatment was the reduction in pruritus in the treated wounds, compared with intense pruritus in the control scar on the same patient.[67]

Refining the choice of polarity for specific effects has been the subject of many research studies (Tables 21–1 and 21–2). There will always be a need for additional research to explain and validate the efficacy of procedures and protocols. Meanwhile, reading and interpreting the current literature builds understanding and professional judgment. The physical therapist (PT) is the best-trained practitioner to understand and interpret the research pertaining to electrotherapeutic modalities. As such, the PT has an obligation to understand the physiologic implications of each treatment intervention selected and to be responsible for accurately predicting outcomes.

In practice, the issues of polarity and wound healing are appropriate when referring to continuous or monophasic pulsed current. Even though the electrodes are marked as positive and negative for units that deliver AC and biphasic current, the imbalance of the charge of the electrodes is very small and not enough to affect the movement of the ions under the electrodes. When using continuous current, a change in polarity is a change in the direction of the current and a change in the flow of the ions under the electrode. The studies demonstrating these polarity effects have been done with continuous and pulsed currents, usually with the current on for more than 1 second. One of the concerns in wound healing research is whether the polarity effects of monophasic pulsed current predictably occur under the electrodes when the duration of the current is on for such a very short period of time. For example, with high-voltage stimulation, the monophasic waveform is on for less than 1 second (80–120 pps), and no measurable changes occur relative to alkalinity (H^+) or acidity (OH^-).[32] The question is whether some cell migration is still facilitated by the polarity of the electrodes at the wound site or whether some other factors explain the physiologic effectiveness of externally applied HVPC for healing wounds. More research is needed to show that high-voltage stimulation creates measurable polarity effects or that other physiologic processes of healing are facilitated.

Although the effects of polarity and wound healing have focused primarily on the movement of ions under the electrodes, there are other issues about current flow that could facilitate healing. For example, Wolf's law[68,69] states that, under conditions of repetitive stress, collagen is remodeled. One type of stress on a tissue is a mechanical force, such as weight bearing. This weight bearing facilitates the deposition of collagen in soft tissue and bone along the lines of the force on the tissue. Mechanical forces on the tissue can also be created when other types of energy are delivered to the tissue, such as ultrasound or electricity. When a sound wave pulsates or an electrical current pulsates, a force is created on the cell, and it expands and contracts, creating a piezoelectric effect. It has been suggested that this piezoelectric effect accounts for the increased collagen deposition.[70,71] Thus, in pulsed current, it is possible that wound healing repair (collagen deposition) measurement is facilitated by this mechanism, independent of the polarity effects of the electrode. If this is true, biphasic current should have a piezoelectric effect. However, at this time, biphasic current is rarely used

Table 21–3 LIDC Clinical Study Protocols and Results

Investigator	Type of Study	Polarity	Amplitude/ Rate	Frequency and Duration	Disease State	Mean Healing Times
Wolcott et al[86]	Uncontrolled clinical trial	3 days cathode followed by anode; reversed daily or every 3 days if wound plateaus	200–800 µA	2 hr twice or three times daily	Ischemic dermal ulcers	9.6 weeks 10.4%/week
Gault and Gatens[130]	Uncontrolled clinical trial	3 days cathode followed by anode; reversed daily or every 3 days if wound plateaus	200–800 µA	2 hr twice or three times daily	Ischemic skin ulcers	5.0 weeks 20%/week
Carley and Wainapel[2]	Randomized controlled clinical trial	3 days cathode followed by anode; reversed daily or every 3 days if wound plateaus	200–800 µA pulsed	2 hr twice daily	Pressure ulcers	8 weeks for 58% of group treatment 12.5%/week
Katelaris et al[131]	Comparative clinical study	Negative throughout	20 µA	Not stated	Venous leg ulcers	No significant difference between groups except much longer mean healing rate for ES/ providone-iodine group (12.2 weeks) 8.2%/week
Wood et al[9]	Randomized clinical trial	Starting negative	300–600 µA; .8 Hz	3 times/week, duration not stated	Pressure ulcers	6.5–7 weeks 14.3%/week

Note: Calculations of mean healing times based on study data.

Source: Data from reference #'s 2, 9, 86, 130, and 131.

for wound healing. In the future, this may change, given that recent results of several studies document significant healing effects with biphasic current.

Blood Flow, Oxygen, and Edema

Blood Flow Studies

Numerous studies in the literature that have looked at the effects of ES on blood flow in animals and humans, both healthy and with disease, are described in this section. The results reported are inconsistent. Reasons for the inconsistencies are related to the dissimilarity of study populations, electrical current characteristics (polarity, frequency, waveform), and methods of recording measurements. Standardization from one study to another is lacking. This section will look at and evaluate the evidence presented in several studies. Human studies are summarized in Table 21–4.

Animal Studies. Treatment with HVPC with negative polarity induced greater blood flow in rats than did positive polarity. The blood flow volume was increased nearly instantaneously at the pulse rates tested: 2, 20, 80, and 120 pps. In addition, blood flow was enhanced by increasing the amplitude of the current (up to stimulating muscle contraction). In a small number of cases, however, blood flow volume increased without visible muscle contraction. Blood flow velocity remained elevated from 4 to 20 minutes after treatment.[72]

Merhi et al[73] showed that there is an age-related decline in skin vascular reactivity by the sensory nerves that correlates with a decline in wound repair efficacy. They used low-frequency TENS (20 V, 5 Hz for 1 minute) and compared the effect on blood flow, using laser Doppler flowmetry (LDF), with high frequency (20 V, 15 Hz for 1 minute). At the high frequency, the vascular response in old rats was significantly reduced (46%) compared with young controls. At low frequency, however, older rats produced similar vascular responses to the young. Results suggest that sensory nerves respond preferentially to low-frequency ES.

Necrosis of skin flaps and free full-thickness skin grafts are a major problem following plastic surgery. Two skin flap studies in rats and pigs showed greater blood flow increases and improved survival of anode-treated flaps than did controls or those treated with the cathode.[74–76] Another study[77] with pigs used PES (128 pps, 35 mA, 30 minutes twice daily) and a protocol of alternating polarity every 3 days. Treated flaps that were given PES twice on the first day postoperatively had a 92% survival rate, compared with those treated only once on that day (19% survival). None of the control flaps survived.

Human Studies. LDF, laser Doppler imaging (LDI), intravital video microscopy, and computerized image analysis technologies have made it possible to evaluate and quantify circulatory changes induced by ES at the microcirculatory levels. Earlier researchers used a variety of methods to report results of blood flow following ES, including photoplethysmography, cutaneous thermistors, transcutaneous oxygen partial pressure ($tcPO_2$) measurement, and laboratory tests for vasodilator substances.

Hecker et al[78] chose to look at the effects of pulsed galvanic stimulation on peripheral blood flow in 10 healthy adult volunteers. They systematically varied both current polarity and frequency to maximize the likelihood of observing blood flow and/or temperature effects. The electrodes were placed over the left brachial artery in the axilla, negative polarity, and over the left radial artery at the wrist, positive polarity. Stimulation was given for 1 hour at each of five frequencies: 2, 8, 32, 64, and 128 Hz. A 30-minute period between changes in frequency was allowed to return to baseline. Current amplitude was adjusted to the highest level attainable, not exceeding the subjects' perceived discomfort. Testing was repeated on two separate occasions. On the second test, polarity was reversed. Measurements were made with thermistors attached to fingers and photoplethysmography. Results showed that current frequency, polarity, and varying combinations of the two had no significant effect on blood flow. A trend toward greater blood flow corresponded to the highest frequencies (32, 64, 128 Hz) with negative polarity. No significant temperature variations, compared with baseline, were found. The authors postulated that healthy individuals may have transient blood flow increases but that they rapidly return to baseline.

Cramp et al[79] compared the sensitivity to change in blood perfusion during treatment with TENS, using LDF and a skin thermistor. Low- and high-frequency (4 and 110 Hz) TENS was applied to the forearm skin of 30 healthy human volunteers. Double blind conditions were implemented. Blood flow and skin temperature readings were recorded before, during, and for 15 minutes after TENS application. Analysis of the results showed significant increases in blood perfusion during the treatment period in the low-frequency group, when compared with the other two groups, and no significant changes in skin temperature.

Wikstrom et al[80] quantified blood flow changes at two different frequencies (2 Hz, 100 Hz, and sham) when TENS was applied to nine healthy adults. Changes in blood flow were measured, using LDI every 5 minutes. Results showed mean blood flow increases of 40% during low-frequency TENS, compared with 12% increase at high frequency and no change during sham stimulation. In the second part of this study, Wikstrom and associates looked at circulatory changes in blister wounds of the leg induced in the same nine healthy adults before and during 45-minute application of TENS (2 and 100 Hz). The blister wound is a new standard wound used for clinical studies. Microcirculatory blood flow

Table 21-4 Effects of Electrical Stimulation on Blood Flow in Human Subjects

Researcher	Hecker et al[78]	Cramp et al[79]	Dodgen et al[89]	Forst et al[90]	Gilchreast et al[92]	Peters et al[91]	Kaada[82]	Cosmo et al[83]	Mawson et al[85]
Type Stimulator	PES	TENS	TENS HVPC	TENS	HVPC	DC	TENS	TENS	HVPC
Frequency Low / High	2 Hz, 8 Hz / 32 Hz, 64 Hz, 128 Hz	4 Hz / 110 Hz	Not stated	Not stated / Not stated	100 pps	N/A	2 Hz	2 Hz / Not tested	10 pps
Polarity	Negative/positive	Biphasic	Biphasic positive/negative	Biphasic	Negative		Biphasic	Biphasic	Biphasic
Amplitude	Mean 22.56 mA	Not stated	Not stated	Not stated	100 V	Not stated	15–30 mA	10–45 mA	75 V
Duration of stimulation	60 min at each FQ	15 min	30 min	Not stated	30 and 60 min	4, 60-min periods	30 min 3 times daily	60 min	30 min
Effect during Rx	High ↑ BF trend at 32, 64, 128 Hz, negative polarity; no temperature variations from baseline	Low ↑ BF High, no change; no change skin temp	Both stimulators produced ↑ tcPO₂ levels Response not polarity dependent	↑ BF axon reflex vasodilation in neuropathic group; induced hyperemia associated with suppressed sweat response in all groups	Bimodal response ↓ BF (73%) (N = 35) Oxygen response higher at baseline than later responders; olders with neuropathy ABI <>	No significant increase unless PVD present; transient rise in PVD group	Widespread vasodilation; release of vasoactive polypeptide	35% ↑ BF in ulcer 15% ↑ BF periwound skin	35% ↑ sacral TcPO₂ supine
Effect post Rx (15–30 min)	Not stated	Not stated	Rose further for 30 min	Not stated	Not tested	No increase in BF	30–45 min poststimulation increase in skin temperature (5.2°C)	29% ↑ BF in ulcer 9% ↑ BF periwound skin	Fell slightly after 15 min
Method of measurement	Photoplethysmography and cutaneous thermistors	Laser Doppler flowmetry and thermistor	TcPO₂	Laser Doppler flowmetry	TcPO₂	TcPO₂	Skin temperature	Laser Doppler imaging	TcPO₂
Population tested and N	Healthy adults (N = 10)	Healthy adults (N = 30)	Diabetes (N not stated)	Controls: (N = 21) Diabetics: (1) without complications (N = 14), (2) with neuropathy and without retinopathy (N = 14), (3) with retinopathy and without neuropathy (N = 8), (4) with neuropathy and retinopathy	Diabetics (N = 132)	Diabetics (N = 19)	Diabetes; Raynaud's disease; mixed etiologies Note: Stimulation given at HoKu point between first and second metacarpals	Chronic leg ulcers (N = 15)	Spinal cord injured (N = 29)

Source: Data from reference #'s 78, 79, 82, 83, 85, 89, 90, 91, and 92.

was measured, using intravital video microscopy and computerized image analysis, as red blood cell velocity (RBC-V) in 5–14 individual capillaries in each wound. Mean RBC-V increased by 23% during low-frequency TENS (n = 6) and by 17% during high-frequency TENS (n = 8).

Kaada[81,82] reported a causal relationship between TENS and mechanisms involved in widespread microvascular cutaneous vasodilatation. Results showed that a 15- to 30-minute period of TENS-induced vasodilatation produced a prolonged vascular response with a duration of several hours or longer, potentially indicating the release of a long-lasting neurohumoral substance or metabolite. Kaada attributed the effects to three possible modes of action: inhibition of the sympathetic fibers supplied to skin vessels; release of an active vasodilator substance, vasoactive intestinal polypeptide; or a segmental axon reflex responsible for affecting local circulation. The Kaada studies included reports of clinical results, wherein patients served as their own controls of stimulation-promoted healing in cases of chronic ulceration of various etiologies.[82]

LDI was used to study the effects of TENS in and around chronic lower leg ulcers. Cosmo et al[83] enrolled 15 older adult patients with chronic leg ulcers of various causes in the study. Duration of the ulcers ranged from 3 months to 16 years. Low-frequency TENS (2 Hz , 10–45 mA) was applied for a 60-minute period. The changes in blood flow were measured every 5 minutes by LDI. After the treatment period, mean blood flow had increased in the ulcer by 35% and in the intact skin surrounding the ulcer by 15%. Mean blood flow increases of 29% in the ulcer and 9% in the skin were measured 15 minutes after the cessation of TENS treatment.

Oxygen Studies

Oxygen is critical for wound healing. Constant delivery of oxygen is required to meet high metabolic demands of the tissues, oxidative killing of infectious organisms, protein and collagen synthesis, and hydroxylation of proline to make useful collagen. Blood flow is the mechanism of oxygen transport to the tissues. Treatment interventions that increase blood flow consequently will enhance oxygen delivery to the tissues, improve healing, and possibly prevent tissue damage from tissue loads.

Mawson et al[84] wanted to determine whether tissue oxygenation at the sacrum is reduced in individuals with SCI, due to the interactive effects of prolonged immobilization and injury related to autonomic nervous system dysfunction. This group of investigators compared the $tcPO_2$ levels in 21 subjects with SCI and 11 able-bodied subjects lying prone and supine on egg-crate mattresses. $TcPO_2$ levels of SCI individuals were lower than those of controls in prone position (65.3 ± 16 mm Hg versus 76.4 ± 13 mm Hg; p # .053) and markedly lower in supine position (49.1 ± 26 mm Hg

versus 74.2 ± 13 mm Hg; p # .004). $TcPO_2$ levels were monitored following supination, and the results showed that the levels of oxygen in controls fell slightly after supination but returned to previous levels within 15 minutes. In contrast, the oxygen levels of the SCI group fell rapidly by 18 mm Hg and stabilized after 15 minutes at a level 27 mm Hg below that of controls. Next, SCI subjects above and below the median supine $tcPO_2$ value were compared in terms of presence or absence of pressure ulcers. Five of the 10 (50%) of SCI subjects with $tcPO_2$ levels below the median supine $tcPO_2$ level had a pressure ulcer, compared with one among the 11 (9%) SCI subjects with $tcPO_2$ levels above the median (p = .055 by Fisher's exact test) These findings suggest the need for further studies on the role of reduced oxygen in the etiology of pressure ulcers.

Mawson et al[85] next looked at the possibility of developing a new way of preventing pressure ulcers in SCI individuals. They chose to study whether HVPC could increase sacral $tcPO_2$ levels in SCI persons lying prone and supine. They conducted four experiments, with the following results:

1. When HVPC was applied to the back at the spinal level T6, dose-related increases in sacral $tcPO_2$ were measured in three subjects lying prone.
2. In the second experiment, carried out on 29 subjects lying supine on egg-crate mattresses, HVPC (75 V, 10 Hz) produced a 35% increase in sacral $tcPO_2$ from baseline level (mean ± SD) or 49 ± 21 mm Hg to 66 ± 18 mm Hg after 30 minutes of stimulation (p = 0001).
3. Simulated HVPC was found to have no effect on sacral $tcPO_2$ in five subjects lying supine.
4. HVPC was repeated on 10 subjects, and its effects were found to be highly reproducible. The mode of action attributed by the researchers to these effects is that the HVPC restores the sympathetic tone and vascular resistance below the level of the spinal cord lesion, thereby increasing the perfusion pressure gradient in the capillary beds.

Lack of adequate oxygen could be a partial explanation for difficulty in healing diabetic ulcers.[86] Baker et al[87,88] measured oxygen enrichment to the cells of wound repair in a study of age-matched older normal adults and diabetic subjects. Oximetry readings of $tcPO_2$ were taken 30 minutes prior to stimulation, during 30 minutes of stimulation, and 30 minutes after stimulation. The ES waveforms used were monophasic-paired spikes with negative polarity and a compensated monophasic waveform. Both waveforms were introduced with the cathode over the wound. The older normal adults showed higher $tcPO_2$ levels at the end of 30 minutes of stimulation, regardless of waveform used. However, there were differences in response time for the diabetics. The normal adults showed increased oxygen levels earlier in the treatment period than did the diabetics. Diabetic subjects showed measurable but not significant increases in tcPO$_2$ at the end of the 30 minutes of stimulation but did show significant increases 30 minutes after cessation of the stimulation with the monophasic and submotor compensated monophasic waveforms. The authors' analysis of the study was that diabetic subjects demonstrate a compromised ability to increase transcutaneous oxygen during submotor stimulation, *regardless* of the waveform used. When trace level muscle contraction was elicited with the compensated monophasic waveform, there was no change in the tcPO$_2$ levels in the diabetics. For some reason, the trace muscle contraction blunted the tcPO$_2$ response in the diabetics. The same effects were found for both waveforms and with stimulation by either the positive or the negative pole.

In another study of diabetics, Dodgen et al[89] compared the effects of a monophasic paired spike waveform, using both negative and positive polarity, with a symmetric biphasic waveform. Measurements of tcPO$_2$ from baseline 30 minutes prior to stimulation, during 30 minutes of stimulation, and 30 minutes after treatment were compared. The findings showed that the tcPO$_2$ levels were significantly increased, regardless of waveform or polarity. Increases were present at the end of the stimulation period and continued to rise during the next 30 minutes after stimulation. Therefore, researchers concluded that the mechanism of action of ES on increasing transcutaneous oxygen was unrelated to polarity and did not require any net ion flow. Both the Baker and Dodgen studies cited here were reported as abstracts. Details about the variables of frequency and amplitude are missing from these reports.

Comparison of the microvascular response to TENS and postocclusive ischemia in the diabetic foot was reported by Forst et al.[90] LDF was used to measure the "flare" response (hyperemia) following TENS and to compare this axon reflex vasodilatation with postischemic hyperemia in the skin of the foot of diabetic and nondiabetic subjects. Twenty-one control subjects and 57 diabetic subjects were enrolled. The diabetics were stratified into 4 groups:

1. 24 without complications
2. 14 with neuropathy and without retinopathy
3. 8 with retinopathy and without neuropathy
4. 21 with both neuropathy and retinopathy

Following TENS, there was increased skin blood flow across all groups. However, compared with the control group, axon reflex vasodilatation was significantly reduced in groups 2 and 4. All groups had equivalent increased blood flow after arterial occlusion. There was a good association observed between postocclusive and TENS-induced hyper-

emia at the dorsum of the foot but poor association at the base of the big toe. An observation reported was that the TENS-induced hyperemia was associated with a diminished sweat response but not with pathologic cardiovascular function tests. The conclusion reached was that electrical axon reflex vasodilatation is diminished in diabetic patients suffering from peripheral autonomic C-fiber injury, especially in skin rich in thermoregulatory blood flow. The diminished neurovascular response is independent of vascular alteration due to diabetes mellitus.

Peters et al[91] evaluated the effects of galvanic ES on vascular perfusion in 19 diabetic subjects. Eleven of these were diagnosed with impaired peripheral perfusion, based on their initial tcPO$_2$ values (< 40 mm Hg). Stimulation was given at the lateral side of one leg, and measurements were taken at the dorsum of the foot and at the base of the great toe of *both* feet. On the first day, one foot was treated with ES for four 60-minute periods and vascular perfusion assessed before and after the stimulation session. Measurements were taken for 1 hour on day 1 of the experiment. Methods of measurement were transcutaneous oximetry and LDF. Findings were that, during the first 5 minutes of stimulation, there was a significant rise in tissue oxygenation, as compared with the control measurements in the group of diabetics with impaired vascular perfusion. However, for those without vascular disease (tcPO$_2$ levels > 40 mm Hg), there was no significant increase, compared with baseline. Also, after the stimulation periods, the stimulated feet did not show any significant increase in blood flow over the control feet. The data suggest to the researchers that external subsensory ES induces a transient rise in skin perfusion in persons with diabetes and impaired peripheral perfusion.

Gilcreast et al[92] tested the effect of HVPC (100 pps, 100 V, negative polarity) on foot skin perfusion in diabetics at risk for foot ulceration. A sample of 132 subjects was tested. Baseline tcPO$_2$ levels were obtained, stimulation applied, and the repeat tcPO$_2$ measurements recorded at 30- and 60-minute intervals. Initial tcPO$_2$ levels were significantly higher than subsequent readings. However, the oxygen response was distributed bimodally: 35 (27%) subjects showed increased tcPO$_2$, and 97 (73%) experienced a *decreased* tcPO$_2$ reading. This treatment appears to increase blood flow in a subset of diabetics.

Byl et al[93] found that, when supplemental oxygen was given by mask prior to and during microamperage stimulation (100 μA for 45 minutes), there were significant increases in subcutaneous oxygen measured. Maximal oxygen saturation may be necessary prior to and during ES in order to facilitate the dissociation of oxygen from the hemoglobin.[93]

In transferring technology from the lab bench to the bed, the PT could take the information from these research studies and formulate and test a protocol for wound healing for diabetics. For example, nasal supplementation of oxygen could be provided during ES treatment for patients with diabetes to accelerate the oxygen uptake. A trial to evaluate the difference in wound healing outcomes for diabetics treated with ES while breathing room air or supplemental oxygen could yield useful clinical data. The result would be development of a new clinical protocol for treating diabetic wounds.

Venous System Response. Alon and De Domenico[31] reviewed the literature on the effects of ES on venous circulation. As yet, ES is not used extensively for management of venous circulation problems but merits inclusion in this section for thoughtful application. There is no support for intervention in the acute phase of varicose hemorrhage or deep vein thrombosis, but ES can effectively treat chronic conditions, including deep vein thrombosis and venous stasis. When muscle groups in the calf and posterior thigh are stimulated to produce intermittent tetanic muscle contraction, there is very effective enhancement of venous return in cases of venous insufficiency or deep vein thrombosis. The required stimulation parameters are those needed to provide motor excitation leading to evoked intermittent tetanic muscle contraction. Augmentation of the venous return initiates a response of vasodilatation of the arterioles to bring blood flow to the muscles.

In SCI-injured individuals, there is a loss of normal vasomotor tone in the abdomen and lower extremities. Peripheral edema and high incidence of deep vein thrombosis have been associated with the circulatory stasis that occurs. One case study of a patient with edema, cyanosis of the feet, and toe ulcers demonstrated the benefits of using computer-controlled neuromuscular ES to stimulate numerous muscle groups, resulting in reduced edema, improved skin color, and healed ulcers by the fifth week of the treatment regimen.[94] The use of the ES-induced leg muscle contractions in individuals with paraplegia to augment cardiovascular responses, probably via reactivation of the skeletal muscle pump and resulting increased venous return, has been reported in several studies.[95–97] Benefits include ameliorating blood pooling in the lower extremities and prevention of edema in the extremities by promoting lymph flow. Use of ES as a preventive treatment is being investigated, and results indicate that it may be useful in situations where the motor pump function is lost, due to paralysis or other lifestyle situations.[98]

Enhanced blood flow to tissues will support tissue demands for increased oxygen and nutrients required for healing. In the case of the patient with venous insufficiency, stimulation of enhanced blood flow will need to be evaluated and may require aftercare of compression to avoid pooling of blood at the ankles, due to the incompetent valves (see Chapter 10). If the arterioles are severely occluded, the vasodilatation response may not occur, and electrically evoked muscle contraction may not be desired. In fact, the muscle contraction may cause severe pain by curtailing limited blood flow to the area, leading to ischemia. There are very limited clinical data to support specific protocols for this effect. Therefore, it is up to the PT to evaluate the vascular impairments, based on the diagnostic process, and to select a protocol to support the desired effect. The section on protocols and procedures provides an example for guidance.

Summary. To summarize, transcutaneous application of ES has been shown in several studies to increase blood flow, microcirculation of the skin, and tissue oxygen levels (Table 21–4) in animals, healthy individuals, diabetics, patients with SCI, and around chronic ulcers of the lower extremity. Blood flow increases in most studies were greatest when low-frequency stimulation was applied. There are conflicting reports about the effects of ES on circulation in healthy adults, SCI, those with vascular disease, and diabetics that merits further investigation. The bimodal effects reported by Gilcreast et al[92] may be explained by use of high-frequency stimulation (100 pps) and/or the impairment of the electrical axon reflex vasodilatation in diabetics with neuropathy and not in others without neurologic complications, as described by Forst et al.[90]

Increasing oxygenation of tissues for healing and prevention of tissue damage are important reasons to consider treatment intervention with ES. In light of the accumulating body of evidence that low-frequency ES is a potent enhancer of blood flow, randomized CCTs are needed to verify the benefits of using ES for preventing pressure ulcers, as has been suggested by Mawson et al,[85] and to determine the best treatment protocols to take advantage of the information now available about enhancement of microcirculation with low-frequency stimulation.

Edema and Pain Studies

Edema is a consequence of disruption in circulation and blood flow to the tissues. Following traumatic injury, there is hemostasis and margination to halt bleeding. The biologic events that follow (see Chapter 2) result in edema formation as a component of the acute inflammatory phase of repair. In systemic breakdown, such as loss of valvular competency in venous disease or loss of autonomic nervous system function in SCI, edema results. Use of ES as a modality to reduce edema has many anecdotal reports. However, evidence of the efficacy of ES to reduce or prevent edema is limited to a few animal studies, some human subject case studies, and limited clinical trials.

Edema reduction under the negative pole is attributed to a phenomenon called *cataphoresis*.[99] Cataphoresis is the movement of nondissociated colloid molecules, such as droplets of fat, albumin, particles of starch, blood cells, bacteria, and other single cells, all of which have an electrical charge, due to the absorption of ions, under the influence of a direct current toward the cathode.

Animal Studies

Several attempts have been made to learn whether edema reduction occurs with application of HVPC.[100] Reed[100] reported reduction of posttraumatic edema in hamsters following HVPC and attributed the effect to reduced microvessel leakage. Posttraumatic edema was curbed in frogs treated with HVPC when the cathode was used. There was no effect if the anode was applied. Treatment effect was significant from the end of the first treatment session until the end of data recording 17 hours later.[101] A similar study using HVPC on rat hind paws found significant treatment effects after the second 20-minute treatment with the cathode.[72] The above studies showed efficacy in curbing posttraumatic edema in one species of rat and one species of frog. Thornton and colleagues[102] found that edema formation was curbed in Zucker-Lean and Brown Norway rats but not in Sprague-Dawley rats when cathodal HVPC (120 pps) at 10% less than needed to induce visible muscle contraction was applied. The fact that not all species of rat react the same suggests a caveat in extrapolating data to human subjects.

Matylevich et al[103] observed the effect of 40 mA DC on plasma albumin extravasation after partial-thickness burn injury in Sprague-Dawley rats. Silver nylon wound dressings were used as the anodes. Burn rats with no treatment or treated with silver-nylon dressing without current were used as controls. Quantitative analysis of fluorescein isothiocyhanate (FITC)-albumin leakage and accumulation in the wound tissue was performed using confocal fluorescence microscopy. When DC was applied, leakage was reduced by 30–45% and approached normal rates by 8 hours postburn. FITC-albumin concentration peaked at 4 hours postburn, was 18–48% less than in burned control, and approached the level observed in unburned control by 18 hours postburn. The conclusion of the study was that DC has a beneficial effect in reducing plasma protein extravasation after burn injury. Chu et al,[104] who worked with the Matylevich group on the study reported above, then considered the effect of DC on wound edema after full-thickness burn injury in the same rat species. Using the same study design as described, the main results were that continuous DC reduced burn edema by 17–48% at different times up to 48 hours postburn. Neither reversal of electrode polarity nor change in current density had any significant effect on the results of treatment. Starting treatment during the first 8 hours postburn produced the least edema accumulation, but the reduction was significant even when DC was applied 36 hours after burn. If started immediately after injury, treatment had to be continued for a minimum of 8 hours to be most effective.

Human Studies

There is a paucity of human studies on the effects of ES on edema and pain. The few studies located are described in this section. Albumin is a colloidal protein found in blood, is negatively charged, and is repelled by negative polarity, causing a fluid shift and, thereby, a reduction of edema. Ross and Segal[99] claimed benefit in treating postoperative edema, healing, and pain with HVPC in 25 postoperative patients. Effects of direct current on edema were attributed to cataphoresis, based on the effects of direct current. They formulated a protocol based on the use of the cathode to reduce edema. The treatment parameters were negative polarity, four paired pulses per second for 15 minutes. After 15 minutes, the polarity was switched to positive and pulse rate increased to 80 paired pulses per second for another 15 minutes. Treatment was over the surgical site.

Griffin et al[105] compared the efficacy of intermittent pneumatic compression (IPC) and HVPC in reducing chronic posttraumatic hand edema in an RCT. Thirty patients were assigned to one of three groups (10 to each) to receive a single treatment for 30 minutes of IPC, HVPC, or sham HVPC. Chronic edema was defined as edema following traumatic injury persisting for 14–21 days. The HVPC stimulator was set at 8 pps, with a reciprocal mode of stimulation alternating between the ulnar and median nerves at the elbow. Intensity was adjusted to produce minimal muscle contraction of thumb flexion and finger abduction, and polarity was set at negative for the active sites. The results reported were that there was no significant difference between HVPC and IPC ($p = .446$), and the difference between the HVPC and placebo HVPC groups did not quite reach statistical significance. The single 30-minute IPC session produced significant reduction in edema. There was also wide variability reported between the HVPC and IPC groups.

Kumar et al,[46] in a randomized controlled, single-blinded trial with biphasic TENS and amitriptyline (Elavil, Etrafon, Limbitrol) (N = 23), found that there was a beneficial effect from TENS for relief of painful diabetic peripheral neuropathy beyond the effect of the amitriptyline. The treatment unit used was a proprietary device called *H-wave* (Electronic Waveform Laboratory, Huntington Beach, CA), with characteristics of biphasic exponentially decaying waveform with pulse widths of 4 msec, < 35 mA, <35 V, and 2–70 Hz. Treatment was applied at the knee region but treatment effect was in the foot. Results of a survey of patients using H-Wave TENS showed the following: 41 patients reported a 44% ±4% subjective reduction in pain; 13 patients had no improvement.[47] Those who had no improvement also reported significantly higher incidence of foot ulcers than did the responder group. Nineteen patients reported swelling over the ankles. Twelve reported some decrease in the swelling with the TENS treatment, six claimed no change, and one had an increase. Only one of the 12 responders was using compression stockings. However, four of six of those who reported no change were wearing compression stockings. Data from this survey suggest that the beneficial effects of electrotherapy for neuropathic pain continues with prolonged usage. Why the nonresponders had more foot ulcers than the responders deserves further investigation. Pruritis is also classified as pain treatment with PES, effectively reducing pruritis associated with healing of donor sites.[67]

Dobbins et al[106] reported no statistically significant decreases in acute knee edema pain or function after use of HVPC on postoperative days 1–4 following total knee arthroplasty in an RCT with 32 patients. All participated in an exercise protocol daily. The methodology for determining the difference in volume was the truncated cone equation but, because the knee is not really a cone, the results may have been flawed. Using this methodology, the study reported a clinical significance—65 cm^3 less volume in the treatment group than in controls. The treatment may be effective in decreasing post-surgical knee edema and pain, and in increasing function. Treatment parameters, supplied by personal communication with the researcher, were 120 pps and amplitude to patient tolerance but below muscle contraction. In some cases, the amplitude was almost 200 V. The negative pole was used for 20 minutes daily.[107] Based on the studies of effect of ES frequency on blood flow already discussed, perhaps a lower frequency would have improved the outcomes. Further work is needed to determine the most effective parameters.

Fakhri and Amin[108] reported that, if edema was present around a burn wound, there was an immediate discharge of pus and tissue fluids during application of the low-voltage DC that ceased when the current was terminated. Sumano and Mateos[50] included a case study as part of their clinical trial report. Using modified biphasic stimulation on a patient with a second-degree burn wound, there was significant reduction of the signs of inflammation, including edema and pain, after three treatments. Investigation on a larger scale on the efficacy of ES in reducing edema in humans is needed to verify this phenomenon and to determine the effective treatment parameters.

Debridement and Thrombosis

Review of the research is a guide for the clinician and provides evidence to support a protocol for wound healing initiated with the negative pole at the wound site. Debridement is facilitated if the tissue is solubilized or liquefied, such as occurs with enzymatic debriding agents or autolysis. For example, necrotic tissues are made up of coalesced blood elements. ES using negative current can solubilize this clotted blood.[109–111]

Reperfusion of tissues is rapidly followed by autolytic debridement. Increased blood flow, stimulated by ES at the

negative pole, has been attributed to having this effect. When the clinical studies are compared, it becomes clear that the negative pole has been used to initiate treatment in all reported controlled clinical studies. Many of the wounds in the treatment groups included necrotic wounds.

The positive electrode has been found to induce clumping of leukocytes and forming of thromboses in the small vessels. These clumping and thrombotic effects can be reversed with the negative electrode.[6] This may explain a clinical observation, where hematoma and hemorrhaging at the wound margin or on granulation tissue are dissolved and reabsorbed following application of HVPC with the negative pole. Hemorrhagic material goes on to necrosis if not dissolved and reabsorbed quickly. Perhaps continuous use of positive polarity produces the clumping of leukocytes, as well as explaining why a protocol of intermittently changing polarity restarts the healing process. These are critical issues that need to be researched.

Antibacterial Effects

Because infection is a contributing factor in chronic wound healing, methods to control infection are of clinical importance. Bactericidal effects have been attributed to ES. Research suggests that there is evidence to support this theory. In vitro and in vivo studies applying DC have both been shown to inhibit bacterial growth rates for organisms commonly found in chronic wounds at the cathode.[112,113] Passage of positive current (anode) through silver wire electrodes was found to be bactericidal to Gram-negative bacteria in wounds and inhibitory to Gram-positive wound bacteria.[114] At low levels of amplitude, 0.4–4 µA, there were negligible bactericidal effects.[112] Kincaid and Lavoie[115] tested in vitro stimulation, using HVPC at the cathode and anode, and Szuminsky et al[116] tested HVPC in vitro at the cathode. Both studies found inhibition of *Staphylococcus aureus*, *Escherichia coli*, and *Pseudomonas aeruginosa*. However, the amplitude of the stimulation reported by Kincaid and Lavoie was at an amplitude of 250 V, and Szuminsky et al reported 500 V. Patients would likely find this voltage amplitude intolerable. Because there is inconsistency in these findings and because there are no chemical changes (acidity or alkalinity) measured under the electrodes of HVPC, it is not clear whether the antibacterial effects are due to polarity or another mechanism. For example, increased subcutaneous oxygen was found under the anode when a microamperage current (at 0.3 Hz) was passed through the electrode.[117] It is possible that the oxygen, rather than the polarity, is the variable that is responsible for the bactericidal effects on pathogens.

Chu et al[118] used microamperage current (0.4–40 µA) conducted through a silver nylon dressing placed in the wound of male Sprague-Dawley rats. Chu induced burn wounds in rats, then inoculated them with a lethal dose of *P. aeruginosa* bacteria. Treatment with the silver nylon dressing as the anode was effective as a barrier to infection. Even the silver nylon dressing alone, without the current applied, had a significant protective barrier effect. However, when the silver nylon dressing was used with the cathode or just the nylon cloth without a metal coating, an effective protective barrier did *not* occur.

Thurman and Christian,[119] Gault and Gatens,[120] Webster et al,[121] Fitzgerald and Newsome,[122] and Sumano and Mateos[50] published case studies of patients with infected wounds who had positive outcomes following treatment with ES. Organisms mentioned in the studies included *S. aureus and P. aeruginosa*. Infectious conditions reported included septic abscess, chronic osteomyelitis, infected burn, and thoracic spinal infection. Stimulation types used were low-intensity pulsed direct current, constant current, HVPC, and modified biphasic. Wound asepsis was normally accomplished within 3–7 days, using negative polarity.[120] Concurrent use of antibiotics and alternating the polarity during the treatment session with HVPC (negative 20 minutes, followed by 40 minutes of positive polarity) was mentioned by Fitzgerald and Newsome.[122] Webster used electrically activated silver dressings with the dressing as the anode to treat chronic osteomyelitis wounds. Sixteen (64%) of the cases resulted in closed, stable, pain-free wounds, and 9 of 12 cases, complicated by nonunion, achieved union. The authors suggest that the silver *anode* dressing is an effective treatment for chronic bone infection, when combined with surgical debridement, and reduces the need for prolonged systemic antibiotics.

Sumano and Mateos[50] reported that use of antiseptics and antibiotics was precluded in all cases enrolled in their study and attributed the reduction in observable signs of infection to the ES treatment. One case included was a patient who had recurrent osteomyelitis. The patient response to the ES protocol was fair (> 60–90% healing) but complete recovery was not achieved. These authors suggest that, under these circumstances, ES may be regarded as beneficial and harmless, and may even have a preparatory role for further medical care. Presence of osteomyelitis has long been considered a contraindication for ES therapy. After review of the cases reported, further investigation of the use of ES for bactericidal effects in human subjects should be undertaken. Table 21–5 summarizes the beneficial results of ES on infected wounds.

Pain

A large body of literature supports the use of TENS for both acute and chronic pain management. Techniques for pain modulation can be used, along with the wound healing protocols. For example, one electrode may be placed on the painful area, which includes the wound and adjacent tissues,

and the indifferent electrode over the related spinal nerve. The electrodes can also be bracketed proximal and distal to the areas of pain around the wound, such as with a bipolar technique described later in this chapter.[123] Pain management would be a good reason to use electrodes of equal size so that there would be sufficient current density at the dispersive electrode.

Sensory Nerve Activation

Khalil and Merhi,[124] as a second part of their study, induced thermal wounding of aged rats. One group received TENS stimulation twice daily for 5 days, and the second group received sham TENS stimulation. Using healing, full wound contraction as the outcome measure, they found a statistically significant improved rate of healing for the TENS group (14.7 ± 0.2 days versus 21.8 ± 0.3 days). Their contention is that TENS can accelerate peripheral activation of sensory nerves at low-frequency ES parameters. Khalil and Merhi[124] and Mawson et al[85] may be talking about the same or similar mode of activation of the sensory nerves.

Scar Formation

In animal and human studies, flaps and grafts treated with monophasic pulsed current ES heal without ischemia and result in flatter, thinner, and more resilient scars than in controls.[2,64,65] Pulsed ES was used to stimulate healing of burned rat skin.[125] The repaired skin of the electrostimulated group had an appearance similar to that of the control skin, and the overall appearance of the repaired skin was compatible with a well-organized healing process.

Adamian et al[126] report that 12 patients with slow healing postburn wounds received local ES treatment. Morphologic and biochemical studies confirmed marked stimulating effects of local ES-associated acceptance of dermal autografts and healing. Fakhri and Amin[108] reported a descriptive study where they treated 20 indolent burn wounds with DC stimulation twice a week for 10 minutes per session until healed or ready for regrafting. All patients had failed one or two surgical skin grafts and served as their own controls. The wounds were deep dermal wounds or full-thickness or mixed. Epithelialization began by day three after start of the ES treatment. The largest wounds took the longest to heal (up to 3 months). Autologous skin grafts were successful after 2–4 weeks of ES treatment. The paper particularly cites the appearance of islands of epithelial cells in full-thickness skin burns that would have been expected to be destroyed. Benefits to scar formation from the treatment were better elasticity, more durability to stress, better cosmesis, and better regeneration of the skin pigments.

From case studies and clinical trials evidence is being compiled to look at the outcomes of the treatments with ES

Table 21–5 Case Study Reports of Beneficial Results of ES on Infected Wounds

Source	Infection Type	Stimulation Type Used	Results
Thurman and Christian[119]	Abscess in diabetic	HVPC	Healed
Fitzgerald and Newsome[122]	Spinal wound with *Staphylococcus aureus*	HVPC	Healed
Webster et al[121]	Chronic osteomyelitis	DC	Healed
Sumano and Mateos[50]	Osteomyelitis	Modified biphasic	Improved
	Infected burn		Healed

Source: Data from reference #'s 50, 119, 121, and 122.

on all phases of wound healing. Currently, there is a positive trend to treatment with ES, with an expected outcome of a functional, improved quality scar. More studies with human subjects are needed to compare different current waveforms and treatment parameters and their effects on collagen formation and scar.

Comparison of Monophasic and Biphasic Stimulation Effects

Animal Studies

A comparison of biphasic with monophasic stimulation of acute incisional wounds in rats by Bach et al[127] showed that both types of current caused significant increase of collagen content around the incision line, compared with controls, but did not affect the tensile strength or the energy absorption of the collagen formation in the early postoperative period. Reger et al[128] also compared biphasic and monophasic stimulation of wounds induced in new monoplegic pigs with wounds in normal pigs and denervated controls. When compared with controls, both biphasic- and monophasic-stimulated wounds showed reduced healing time and increased perfusion in the early phases of healing. Monophasic stimulation reduced the wound area more rapidly than did biphasic, but biphasic stimulation reduced the wound volume more rapidly than did monophasic. Their impression was that the applied current appears to orient new collagen formation, even in the absence of neural influences. Collagen organization is considered an important factor in improved tensile strength of the scar. This study found that the ES did not reduce the strength of the healing wounds below those of the nonstimulated controls.

Human Studies

Stefanovska et al[129] compared the efficiency of monophasic (600 µA, 2 hours daily) and biphasic (40 Hz, 15–25 mA to produce minimal muscle contraction, 2 hours daily) in healing pressure ulcers in 150 patients with SCI. Treatment was applied across the wounds using a bipolar technique. As in the Reger study,[128] monophasic was less effective for reducing the depth of deep wounds than was biphasic, and bi-

phasic was less effective for reducing wound area of large wounds. Frantz[12] reported that full-thickness pressure ulcers had a statistically significant reduction in depth but not in surface area, when treated with biphasic.[48] Table 21–6 summarizes the treatment effects attributed to biphasic and monophasic.

CLINICAL STUDIES

Since the 1960s, a series of clinical trials has been undertaken to evaluate the effect of ES on wound healing. The early studies are classics in this field.

Low Voltage Microamperage Direct Current Studies

LIDC was used in six clinical studies. Wolcott et al,[86] Gault and Gatens,[130] Carley and Wainapel,[2] Katelaris et al,[131] and Wood et al[9] studied treatment of ischemic and indolent ulcers. In the first three studies, a positive (anode) polarity was used after a period of three or more days at the cathode. The polarity was reversed every day or every 3 days if wound healing did not progress. Rationale for initial cathode application was the solubilization of necrotic tissue[61] and bactericidal effects.[112,113] All studies except the Katelaris study used an amplitude of 200–800 µA. Duration of treatment was very long: 2 hours, two or three times per day, or 42 hours per week for the first two studies, and 20 hours per week for the third study. Treatment in the Wood study was administered three times per week, but length of treatment was not stated. Katelaris et al incorporated ES treatment with dressings, do not state how long current was applied, and used negative polarity throughout. A combined total of 225 patients were treated, and 75 served as controls. In most cases, the patient served as his or her own control. Mean healing times reported were 9.6 weeks, 4.7 weeks, 5.0 weeks, 8 weeks, and 6.5–7 weeks, respectively, for the five studies (Table 21–3). The difference in healing time between these studies is not clear. Perhaps in the Wolcott et al study the wounds were more extensive. Carley and Wainapel[2] noted that the pulsed LIDC treatment group healed 1.5–2.0 times faster than did

Table 21–6 Summary of Treatment Effects Attributed to Direct Current and Alternating Current

Investigator	Subjects and Disease States	Direct Current	Alternating Current (Biphasic)
Stromberg[64]	Healthy pigs	Faster wound contraction if polarity alternated	
Reger et al[128]	Spinal cord injury, pigs	Faster wound contraction	Faster volume reduction
Stefanovska et al[129]	Spinal cord injury, humans	Less effective for deep wounds	Less effective for large wounds
Frantz[12]	Pressure ulcers, humans		Fast volume reduction; slow wound contraction

Source: Data from reference #'s 12, 64, 128, and 129.

the controls, who were treated with wet to dry dressings and whirlpool. Katelaris et al[131] found no statistical difference in healing times between normal saline, normal saline with electrode, and povidone-iodine-treated wounds. However, results when povidone-iodine was used with the negative electrode showed that the mean healing rate was statistically longer, 85.3 days (12.2 weeks). The researcher theorized that the retardation effect may be due to the negative pole ionization of the iodine and forcing iodine ions down an electrochemical gradient into the cell, where they act as intracellular toxins.

> **Research Wisdom**
>
> Make certain that any form of iodine, if used to treat a wound, is thoroughly removed before application of electrotherapy.[131]

Microcurrent stimulation has been studied in animal models in which current was applied only one or two times per day for 30 minutes for 1–2 weeks; no significant clinical effects were demonstrated on wound healing.[117,132] In another study, there were significant increases in subcutaneous oxygen measurements when supplemental oxygen was given by mask during the MENS stimulation.[93] There was no acceleration in healing.

Modified Biphasic Stimulation Studies

Barron et al[133] reported a study of six patients with pressure ulcers who were treated three times a week for 3 weeks, for a total of nine treatments with microcurrent stimulation. The waveform was a modified biphasic square wave. The treatment characteristics were 600 µA, 50 V, and 0.5 Hz. The electrode probes were placed 2 cm away from the edge of the ulcer, then moved circumferentially around the ulcer. Each successive placement of the probes was 2 cm from the prior

placement. In this small study, two ulcers healed 100%, three healed 99%, and one decreased in size 55%.

Sumano and Mateos[50] reported the use of acupuncture-like ES for the treatment of unresponsive wounds of mixed etiologies and burns. In this clinical trial, where patients served as their own controls, the device used had the parameters of 300 mV, 67 Hz, 0.04 mA, and a calculated absolute charge density of 0.4–0.8 C/cm^2. The method of delivery for most wounds was via electrodes clipped to stainless steel acupuncture filiform needles that were inserted subcutaneously along the edges of the lesion and placed to form an almost complete, closed peripheral circuit. In very large burn wounds, the current was applied by means of covering the wound with saline-soaked gauze, then randomly attaching alligator clips from the stimulator to the gauze, maximally separating the positive and negative electrodes. Delivery of current through the gauze in this manner without a conductor is problematic. Treatments were administered either daily or every other day, based on the severity of the lesion and compliance of the patient. Throughout the course of the treatment protocol, no local antiseptics or antibacterials (either systemic or local) were administered. Dry wound healing methods, as described in an earlier section, were used. Only normal saline was used to cleanse wounds. Forty-four wounds (34 wounds/10 burns) were treated. Patients and wounds were assessed using a stratified classification method of lesion and medical condition severity. When wounds were classified according to their severity, as well as the overall condition of the patient, a closer statistical correlation between the lesion grade and number of treatments to total cure was observed (r = 0.98). Number of treatments were less (8.4 ± 2.3) for grade I severity lesions (N = 10) than for those of grade III severity (N = 17)(41.38 ± 6.58). The authors reported a positive correlation between the severity grade and the time of the first visit for alternative treatment. Mean time from lesion identification to first presentation was 11.8 ± 4.49 days for grade I, 15.44 ± 8.58 for grade II, and 24.5 ± 5.21 days for grade III. This study was conducted in Mexico, where patients are familiar with acupuncture. All patients in the study requested this alternative type of medical treatment when their wounds/burns did not heal quickly (2–4 weeks) with conventional wound healing procedures and drugs. Although this procedure uses acupuncture needles, it is not an orthodox acupuncture procedure. Authors reported that the patients were compliant with the treatment and attributed the compliance to high patient satisfaction, with the evident improvement seen from the first treatment session. Early intervention with the ES procedures seems to have accelerated the healing process, reduced risk for increased wound severity, and required less treatment interventions to achieve an excellent outcome. In all patients, healing proceeded in a thoroughly organized manner, almost regardless of the severity of the type of wound or burn treated.[50]

High-Voltage Pulsed Current Studies

Five random controlled and controlled clinical studies have been reported by Kloth and Feedar,[5] Griffin et al,[3] Unger et al,[134] Gogia et al,[135] and Houghton et al,[11] using HVPC. In the study by Kloth and Feedar,[5] wounds of mixed etiologies had a mean healing time of 7.3 weeks, and 100% of the treatment group healed. Positive polarity was used initially, then switched to negative if the wound plateaued. Unger et al[134] reported on a controlled study of nine subjects in the treatment group and eight controls. The average wound size in the treatment group was 460 mm[2], compared with the control group, whose average wound size was 118.5 mm[2]. Mean healing time was 7.3 weeks for the treatment group, with 88.9% completely healed. The protocol started with negative polarity for 3 days or until the wound was clean, then switched to positive. Griffin et al[3] demsonstrated an 80% reduction in size of pressure ulcers in SCI-injured patients in 4 weeks, when treated with negative polarity, but ulcers were not treated until healed. The Houghton et al[11] RCT focused on treatment of leg ulcers. The leg ulcers were stratified into three groups: diabetic, arterial, or venous. Then the ulcers were randomly assigned to one of two treatment groups. One group received HVPC treatment and the other placebo treatment. All HVPC treatment was given at negative polarity. In all the studies except the Gogia and Houghton studies, the treatment frequency was five to seven times per week for 45–60 minutes. Gogia et al[135] treated for 20 minutes following a 20-minute whirlpool session 5 times a week, beginning with 4 days of negative polarity, then switched to positive polarity. The rate of healing in the experimental group was particularly high during the first 2 weeks of treatment (31.45%), then slowed considerably and was not statistically different from the control group after 5 weeks. The Houghton et al[11] study groups received treatment for 45 minutes three times weekly. Wound size in the experimental group decreased 44.3 mm[2] (± 8.8%) or 11% per week. Unger[136] reported an uncontrolled study

using HVPC treatment and the same protocol as above for 223 pressure ulcers. The mean healing time for the 223 wounds in the uncontrolled study was 10.85 weeks (Table 21–7).

Two additional published uncontrolled studies included 30 patients. Alon et al[62] used positive polarity and stimulated wounds three times a week for 1 hour; 12 of the 15 (80%) of the ulcers treated healed. One patient died, one did not respond, and the ulcer in one decreased significantly in size but did not heal in 21.6 weeks. Akers and Gabrielson[137] published a study that compared (1) HVPC direct application to the wound; (2) application of HVPC using the whirlpool as a large electrode; and (3) whirlpool alone. The direct application of the active electrode to the wound site had the best outcome, followed by HVPC using the whirlpool as an electrode. Whirlpool alone was the least effective.

Low-Voltage Pulsed Electrical Current Studies (LVPC)

Two CCTs with low-voltage pulsed current, labeled PES, were located in the literature. Gentzkow et al[6] reported a study of 40 ulcers in 37 patients. Nineteen pressure ulcers were stimulated, and 21 were sham stimulated. The trial lasted for 4 weeks. The treated ulcers healed more than twice as much as the sham-stimulated ulcers (49.8% versus 23.4%), healing at a rate of 12.5% per week, compared with 5.8% for the sham-stimulated group. Crossover results for 15 of the 19 sham-treated ulcers showed a fourfold greater healing during the 4 weeks of stimulation, compared with 4 weeks of sham treatment. This difference was statistically significant.[6] Feedar et al[4] published a study on pressure ulcers. The 61 patients served as their own controls. The treatment phase of the study was preceded by a 4-week control phase of optimal nonelectrically stimulated wound care. Only the stage III or IV ulcers with need of surgical debridement, necrotic/purulent drainage, or exudate seropurulent drainage that did not improve during the control phase went on to the treatment phase. After 4 weeks of treatment, 58.8% of the wounds had improved. After an average of 8.4 weeks, 23% completely healed and 82% improved significantly.

Clinical Wisdom:
Best Method for Effective HVPC Treatment

Apply HVPC directly to the wound for best expected outcome. Conducting current to the tissues during whirlpool is not recommended because it is less effective, and some clinicians report that stimulator leads have become entangled in the agitator. There have even been stories of stimulators falling into the water.

Table 21–7 HVPC Clinical Studies

Researchers	No. of Patients	% Healed	Mean Time To Heal
Alon et al[62]	15 Treated, 0 controls (diabetic)	80%	10.4 Weeks (9.6%/week)
Kloth and Feedar[5]	9 Treated, 7 controls, 3 crossovers (mixed wound etiology)	100%	7.3 Weeks (13.7%/week)
Griffin et al[3]	8 Treated, 9 controls (pressure ulcers)	80% Reduction in size	4-Week treatment period (20%/week)
Unger[136]	223 Treated, 0 controls	89.7%	10.85 Weeks (9.27%/week)
Unger et al[134]	9 Treated, 8 controls (pressure ulcers)	88.9%	7.3 Weeks (13.7%/week)
Gogia et al[135]	6 Controls treated with sterile whirlpool 6 Treated with sterile whirlpool and HVPC	35% (ES with whirlpool) vs 28% (whirlpool) area reduction 30% (ES with whirlpool) vs 58% (whirlpool) depth reduction	20 Days (20%/week)
Houghton et al[11]	43	44.3% Reduction in size	4-Week study (11%/week)

Source: Data from reference #'s 3, 5, 11, 62, 134, 135, and 136.

Biphasic Stimulation Studies

Controlled Animal Study

Khalil and Merhi[124] decided to test the effect of frequency on wound healing in aged rats. Aged rats were wounded, then divided into an active treatment group and a sham treatment group. Low-frequency TENS (20 V, 5 Hz for 1 minute) was applied twice daily to the treatment group and sham treatment to the controls. The active group required 14.7 ± 0.2 days for complete healing, which was a significant improvement over the sham group (21.8 ± 0.3 days). The conclusion reached was that wound healing in aged rats can be accelerated by peripheral activation of sensory nerves, using low-frequency parameters.

Human Studies

There are reports in the literature by Kaada,[82] Lundeberg et al,[138] Stefanovska et al,[129] and Baker et al[10,139] of clinical trials of wound healing with biphasic waveforms. Frantz's[12] RCT has been submitted for publication. Kaada,[82] Lundeberg et al,[138] and Frantz[12] each used biphasic symmetric waveforms with significant improvement in both ulcer area and healed ulcers. Kaada[82] reported results of TENS on 10 subjects, who served as their own controls, with recalcitrant ulcers of different etiologies. Stimulation was provided indirectly over the web of the thumb daily (HoKu point) during three 30-minute sessions with rests of 45 minutes between, for a total of 1½ hours of stimulation. Stimulation was below visible muscle contraction. Lundeberg et al[138] conducted an RCT on 64 patients with chronic diabetic ulcers due to venous stasis. All patients received standard treatment with paste bandage, in addition to the sham or TENS treatment. Asymmetric biphasic stimulation was determined to produce significant wound healing effects, whereas the other waveforms did not increase the healing rate. The RCT study by Stefanovska et al[129] compared direct current and asymmetric biphasic current. In two RCTs, Baker et al[10,139] compared asymmetric biphasic, symmetric biphasic, and microcurrent (DC). The asymmetric biphasic waveform has a potential for some polar effect that should not be discounted. The polar effect may explain why it was more effective than the symmetric biphasic waveform. However, another likely explanation of the effects is stimulation of neural mechanisms that effect healing.[10] In all of the studies except Kaada, stimulation was delivered to the skin at the wound perimeter, rather than into the wound bed. An advantage of the perimeter stimulation was less disruption of the wound bed, less cross-contamination of the wound, and less interference with the dressing. Benefits were found in patients with spinal cord injury who had pressure ulcers[10,129] and in patients with diabetic ulcers, including those with peripheral neuropathy[139] and venous stasis.[138] Franz[12] combined the indirect stimulation over the web of the thumb daily (HoKu point) protocol of Kaada with a protocol of bipolar biphasic stimulation on either side of the wound at the wound perimeter. The patients were elderly nursing home patients with pressure ulcers. The number of days to achieve a 50% or greater reduction in wound size was chosen as the outcome measure using two measurements of the size of wound surface area and wound volume. The 50% closure was selected as the study outcome, rather than 100% healing, due to the relatively short study period of 8 weeks and the chronicity of the wounds entered in the study. Based on surface area measurements, the median time to 50% healing was 42 days for the TENS group and 54 days for the control group. The rate failed to reach significance based on surface area. However, according to volume measurements with stereographic photography, there were significant differences in the time to 50% closure, with a median time of 28 days for the TENS group and 53 days for the control group. Volume data were applicable only to full-thickness ulcers (N = 31). Complete healing was reported for 8 of 20 (40%) of the TENS group and 5 of 17 (29.4%) in the control group. Six of the 17 full-thickness ulcers in the TENS groups healed, compared with 2 of 14 in the control group. Another research finding has been made in this study that more rapid reduction in wound depth occurs when AC is used. One animal RCT[128] and two human RCTs[12,129] have noted this observation. Table 21–8 summarizes the protocols used and results for all of the biphasic studies.

Meta-analysis of Effect of ES on Chronic Wound Healing

Gardner and Frantz[14] used meta-analysis to average quantitatively the findings across multiple ES studies. The meta-analysis for ES for wound healing was undertaken by the authors for three purposes: (1) to quantify the effect of ES as an adjunctive therapy for chronic wound healing, (2) to explore the influence that the type of ES may have on efficacy of the ES treatment, and (3) to explore the influence that the wound etiology may have on ES effectiveness for healing. To achieve these goals, the meta-analysis estimated the rate of healing of chronic wounds treated with ES. To be included in the meta-analysis, the following criteria had to be met: (1) the study was on the use of ES for ulcer or periulcer stimulation, (2) the subjects were humans, and (3) reports would include all types of chronic wounds (arterial, diabetic, pressure, and venous). The outcome measure chosen for evaluation was the percentage of healing per week because it was the most common measurement either reported or that could be calculated from study data. Fifteen studies, which included 24 ES and 15 samples, were analyzed and the average rate of healing per week calculated for each sample.

The 15 studies included have been described in the preceding text. Ninety-five percent confidence intervals were also calculated. The 95% confidence intervals of the ES (18–26%) and control samples (3.8–14%) did not overlap. Then the samples were grouped by type of ES device and chronic wound, and reanalyzed. The rate of healing per week was 22% for ES samples and 9% for control samples. The net effect of ES was 13% per week. Net increase in rate of healing was 10.9%. DC healing rate was 12.6%/week vs pulsed current healing rate net increase of 15.5%. ES treatment was most effective for treatment of pressure ulcers (net effect =13% per week). Findings regarding the relative effectiveness of different ES devices were inconclusive. The authors felt that the problem was extensive overlap in the confidence intervals. The conclusion reached by these authors was that ES produces a substantial improvement in the healing of chronic wounds, and further research is needed to identify which ES devices are most effective and which wound types respond best to this treatment. Evaluation of the meta-analysis showed that the studies chosen for the meta-analysis were both published and unpublished, randomized and nonrandomized clinical trials, and descriptive studies. Only three were reports of TENS, alternating was classified separately, and the rest were either DC or pulsed DC. Many of the studies chosen for this analysis had very small subject samples (3–7). Controls received a variety of treatments, including moist dressings (13), antiseptics (4), and whirlpool (4). However, the evidence of effectiveness of this adjunctive therapy compares favorably or surpasses treatment with other interventions used for wound healing.

Summary

Electrical stimulation studies have varied from continuous waveform application with direct current to pulsed short-duration monophasic pulses to biphasic pulses. What is known and acknowledged is that ES seems to have positive effects on wound healing or on the components necessary for wound healing (eg, blood flow and oxygen uptake, DNA and protein synthesis), but there is still ambiguity about the type of ES characteristics that are most important or critical. For instance, polarity has played an important role in protocols used, even though the likelihood of polarity effects of currents with pulses of very short duration is questionable. One possible reason for the wound healing effects of ES with any type of current may result from the effect of low-level sensory stimulation on the peripheral nerves, which is not wholly dependent on the polar nature of electrical current. Kaada[81] describes effects that include inhibition of sympathetic input to superficial vessels, release of an active vasodilator, and axon-reflex stimulation. Study results are beginning to show evidence that stimulation with DC, AC, and pulsed current have somewhat different physiologic effects.

Table 21-8 Biphasic Treatment Protocols and Results

Parameters	Kaada[82]	Lundeberg et al[138]	Stefanovska et al[129]	Baker et al[10,139]	Frantz[12]	Barron et al[133]	Sumano and Mateos[50]
Phase Duration	Not reported	1 msec	0.25 msec	100 μsec	150 μsec	Not stated	Not stated
Pulse Rate	100 Hz	80 Hz	40 Hz	50 Hz	85 Hz	0.5 Hz	65 Hz
Waveform	Symmetric	Symmetric	Asymmetric, charge balanced	Asymmetric	Symmetric square	Modified square	Symmetric square
Amplitude	15–30 mA muscle contraction	15–25 mA evoking parasthesias	15–25 mA below contraction	24–25 mA below contraction	10 mA	600 μA/50 V	0.04 mA current charge density: 0.4–0.8 C
Frequency and Duration	Daily; three 30-min sessions (off 45 min between sessions)	Twice daily for 20 min	Daily for 2 hours	Daily; three 30-min sessions (short break between sessions)	Three times daily 30 min	Three times per week	Daily or every other day 20 min
Location	Negative electrode Web between 1st and 2nd metacarpal bones	Wound edge	Wound edge	Less than 1 cm from edge; proximal and distal to ulcer	(1) web space both hands (2) + approximal to wound edge (3) – distal to wound edge	.2 cm from ulcer edge, moved around wound edge	Along wound edges
Patient population	Multiple diagnoses (N = 10) CCT	Diabetics with venous stasis ulcers (N = 64) RCT 7%/week decrease in size	Spinal cord injury with pressure ulcers (N = 150) RCT	Spinal cord injury (SCI) with pressure ulcers (N = 185) RCT Diabetic ulcers (N = 80) RCT	Pressure ulcers (N = 37) RCT	Pressure ulcers (N = 6)	Mixed wounds and burns (N = 44) CCT
Results of treatment	Healing of chronic ulcers	42% Healed in treatment group vs 15% healed in control 4.25%/week decrease in size	Monophasic less effective for reducing depth than biphasic Monophasic more effective for reducing area than biphasic Experimental 25.2%/week decrease in size Control 15.4%/week decrease in size	Asymmetric biphasic significantly improved healing rates by 60% over controls SCI experimental controls Diabetic experimental controls	Median time to closure using volume measurements for TENS group: 28 days; controls 53 days. No statistical difference in surface area change	Healing and decreased size	Healing in organized manner

Source: Data from reference #'s 10, 12, 50, 82, 129, 133, 138, and 139.

As identification of the specific effects of different currents is more thoroughly tested, the clinician will be able to choose the type of stimulation and a protocol to derive a specific outcome for prevention or healing.

CHOOSING AN INTERVENTION: CLINICAL REASONING

Applying Theory and Science to Clinical Decision Making

The previous section evaluated the efficacy of ES on many components of healing, as well as clinical trials of wound healing. The studies basically looked at six components:

1. Galvanotaxis and effect at the cellular level
2. Circulatory effects
3. Effects on edema
4. Antibacterial effects
5. Effects on pain
6. Effects on repair, regeneration, and completeness of healing

The clinician should consider these variables when selecting ES intervention and choosing a protocol.

The specific medical diagnosis may not be a significant factor in selecting ES for wound healing. The medical diagnoses of patients in the studies included burns, pressure ulcers, diabetic ulcers (vascular and neuropathic), vascular ulcers, and vasculitic ulcers. The surgical wounds included in the studies were acute incisions, skin flaps, donor sites, and dehiscence. Acute and chronic wounds were included. Electrical stimulation had demonstrated efficacy for wound healing across diagnoses and pathogeneses. Reported effects were related to the stimulation of the mechanisms of healing at the cellular, tissue, and/or systems level. Healing follows a predictable pattern, regardless of etiology; what affects the outcome are the intrinsic, extrinsic, and iatrogenic factors that alter healing, described in Chapter 2. The PT intervenes in wound management specifically to facilitate the functional mechanisms of healing. Electrical stimulation is just one of the interventions that can be used.

Wound attributes that have positively responded to electrical stimulation were necrotic tissue, inflammation, wound contraction, infection, and wound resurfacing. Wounds of all depths, from partial-thickness to full-thickness and deeper, have been successfully treated with electrical stimulation (eg, stage II to stage IV pressure ulcers). Wounds have traditionally been classified by medical diagnosis, by depth of tissue disruption, and/or by phase of wound healing. Depth of tissue disruption is a description of the tissue loss and function that is broader and more generic than that in the medical diagnosis system. The depth of tissue disruption

system can be used for wounds, regardless of the wound etiology, and is referred to as wound severity diagnosis. Classification by phase of wound healing is also independent of the medical diagnosis. This is the wound healing phase diagnosis. Change in wound phase is an outcome of the process of wound healing (see Chapter 4 and Table 21–9).

The typical subjects selected for clinical trials with ES had nonconforming wound healing with long chronicity. The chronic wounds were the reason for referral for ES. There is significant scientific evidence to support that early intervention with externally applied electrical currents will also accelerate healing for the acute healthy wound. Early intervention with ES could be a useful method to prevent chronicity and return the individual earlier to a functional status. This is consistent with other areas of physical therapy practice, such as stroke and low back rehabilitation, where early intervention can reduce the development of costly chronic health problems.

In summary, selection of ES for wound healing is not dependent on the medical diagnosis. Select ES intervention and treatment characteristics when there are impairments to the systems that interfere with healing at one or more levels: cellular, tissue, or organ. Functional loss at any of these levels suggests that the wound will not or has not healed with the current level of intervention. The reason for referral to the PT is for the development of another strategy to facilitate healing. The use of externally applied currents is one such strategy.

Precautions

Signs of adverse effects using ES for wound healing were evaluated in the various clinical trials. The only two adverse signs were some skin irritation or tingling under the electrodes in a few cases and pain in some other cases. Patients with severe peripheral vascular occlusive disease, particularly in the lower extremity, may experience some increased pain with ES, usually described as throbbing. An alternative acupuncture protocol has been suggested in these cases— placing the active electrode on the web space of the hand between the thumb and first finger instead of over the ulcer located on the leg.[81,82] Young children under the age of 3 years should not be considered candidates for intervention with ES. Healing mechanisms for this group are not well understood and, although there are no known adverse effects, the benefits are not defined. However, older children may benefit from use of an ES intervention to stimulate sensory nerves and accelerate the rate of healing.[140]

Contraindications

Contraindications for the use of ES as described are from various sources and fall into the following categories:

Table 21–9 Appropriate Wound Classifications for Electrical Stimulation

Level of tissue disruption (wound severity)	Superficial, partial thickness, full thickness, subcutaneous and deep tissues
Etiologies/diagnostic groups	Burns, neuropathic ulcers, pressure ulcers, surgical wounds, vascular ulcers
Wound healing phase diagnosis	Inflammatory phase: acute, chronic, absent Proliferative phase: acute, chronic, absent Epithelialization phase: acute, chronic, absent Remodeling phase: collagen organization
Age	Older than 3 years

(1) when stimulation of cell proliferation is contraindicated (eg, malignancy); (2) where there is evidence of osteomyelitis; (3) where there are metal ions; (4) where the placement of electrodes for treatment with ES could adversely affect a reflex center; or (5) where electrical current could affect the function of an electronic implant.[61,123] Carefully evaluate the medical history and review body systems when considering candidates for use of this intervention.

Presence of Malignancy

When there is a malignancy in the area to be treated, ES should not be used (eg, malignant melanoma, basal cell carcinoma). Electrical stimulation stimulates cell proliferation and could lead to uncontrolled cell growth. If the malignancy is distant from the wound (eg, breast cancer in a patient with a pressure ulcer on an ankle), however, local use of ES would be a precaution but not a contraindication, although this is not consistent with required manufacturer labeling.

Active Osteomyelitis

There has been a concern that stimulation of tissue growth with ES may cause superficial covering of an area of osteomyelitis. This could blind the site from observation. If the medical record documents a history of a bone infection, that should trigger an investigation of the current status of the infection. If the osteomyelitis is being treated actively with antibiotic therapy, some clinicians are recommending that treatment with ES may be started. It is not unusual for the osteomyelitis to be resolved but not to be noted in the medical record. The contraindications listed here have been included in physical agent texts and manufacturer literature for many years. Based on the publication of the case studies reported earlier, where patients with osteomyelitis were treated successfully with ES, it is time to reevaluate the contraindication to use of ES in an area of osteomyelitis. Controlled clinical trials are indicated to test the benefits of ES for treating wounds where there is evidence of osteomyelitis.

Clinical Wisdom: *Identification of Osteomyelitis*

If a wound penetrates to the bone, as determined by inserting a probe, it must be assumed that osteomyelitis is present, and the patient should not be treated with ES. An immediate referral to a surgeon for evaluation[141] must be initiated.

Topical Substances Containing Metal Ions

Topical substances containing metal ions (eg, povidone-iodine, zinc, Mercurochrome, and silver sulfadiazine (Silvadene, SSD) that may be used as part of the wound treatment regimen) should be removed before the application of ES. Direct-current ES has the ability to transfer ions into the tissues by iontophoresis. Heavy metal ions may have toxic properties when introduced into the body. If removal of the topical substance is not appropriate, however, ES could be used on other areas of the skin where the topical agent has not been applied.

Electronic Implants

Demand-type cardiac pacemakers and other electrical implants raise concerns regarding the use of electrical current. Electrical stimulation is contraindicated *over* electrical implants because the current and electromagnetic fields could disrupt the function of the implant. Use of ES with a demand-type cardiac pacemaker is one of its contraindications. Studies to evaluate safe utilization of TENS in the presence of a cardiac pacemaker report mixed results. Application of TENS in 51 patients with 20 different cardiac pacemakers at four sites (lumbar area, cervical spine, left leg, and lower arm area ipsilateral to the pacemaker) without episodes of interference, inhibition, or reprogramming of the pacemakers was reported by Rasmussen et al[142] Shade[143] reported successful use of a TENS unit in conjunction with a temporary cardiac pacemaker. No interference was seen on the EKG readout. Sliwa and Marinko[144] reported an EKG artifact with routine EKG produced by surface TENS electrodes applied to the thoracic and lumbar regions. Chen et al[145] reported two cases where cardiac pacemaker dysfunction occurred and was undetected by electrocardiograms. It showed up with extended cardiac monitoring with the Holter monitor.

The pacemaker sensitivity was then reprogrammed, and the abnormalities did not recur. The recommendation was extended cardiac monitoring for patients with cardiac pacemakers during prolonged use of TENS to ensure safety and to determine any need for reprogramming of the pacemakers. Patients with cardiac pacemakers should not be excluded from the use of TENS but require careful evaluation and extended cardiac monitoring. Risk-benefit of using ES for wound healing needs to be carefully weighed.

Natural Reflexes

There are areas of the body that are particularly sensitive to any stimulation (eg, carotid sinus, heart, parasympathetic nerves, ganglion, laryngeal muscles, phrenic nerve). Sensory levels of ES might create a vasospasm or some type of vasoconstriction that could lead to a vasovagal response and other neural responses that could interfere with the function of vital centers and be harmful to the patient. Thus, ES is contraindicated to run current through the upper chest and anterior neck.

Equipment

Regulatory Approval

Under what is called *premarket approval* (PMA), manufacturing companies are allowed to make claims of effectiveness and safety about medical devices. PMA requires extensive clinical trials, typically 2,000–3,000 cases for approval. "Off label" means treatment not approved by the U.S. Food and Drug Administration (FDA). No electrical stimulators have received PMA by the FDA for wound healing. Externally applied currents for wound healing are considered as "off-label" use at this time. Off-label use for medical devices is an accepted and common practice in medicine as innovative therapy, as long as the participants are not closely associated with the manufacturer.[146] For example, the "on-label" uses for neuromuscular stimulators, such as HVPC, include application for increased circulation, relaxation of muscle spasms, and muscle reeducation. The on-label use for TENS is pain management.

Expect to find an FDA-mandated instruction manual accompanying each electrical stimulator. Listed in the manual are labeled indications, contraindications, warnings, and precautions (see box). The FDA indications and contra-indications do not exactly match what is described in the previous text. The PT must be aware of these limitations when selecting a protocol with ES and use thoughtful clinical judgment.

Devices

Electrical stimulators have three basic components: a source of power, an oscillator circuit, and an output amplifier. There are two size ranges: clinical models and portable models. The latter may be as small as a beeper. Two basic power sources are used: batteries and house line current. Batteries are used in portable stimulators. House line current is usually used in the clinic setting. Batteries need to be fully charged to deliver the output expected. A spare battery should be kept on hand. Rechargeable batteries may be more cost-effective than single-use types. House line current is usually available.

Many electrical stimulators now use microprocessors with a choice of several waveforms and pulse rates, and even include preset protocols for wound treatment. The clinician should not assume that this is the "correct" protocol for the wound. It is the clinician's responsibility to know the rationale for protocol characteristics and what the settings are on the chosen stimulator. Most programs allow clinicians to override the preset programs.

Select a stimulator based on the available waveform, pulse characteristic, and ability to adjust intensity and polarity. A desirable stimulator should allow for flexibility to set up and deliver a variety of protocols, based on changes dictated by clinical trials and current concepts of physiologic rationale. Manufacturers are an important source of helpful information about the characteristics of their devices.

Testing Equipment

Meters are very useful to the clinician to check on the current flow between two electrodes. Use the device meter if available; if no meter is available on the stimulator, go to other options. Patient sensation is always a good indicator, if the patient can give a report. The use of ES for wound healing is usually done at a sensory level, but many of the patients are insensate or unable to communicate, or the wounds are deep and below the level of sensation and the patient will not be able to indicate if the current is not felt. Another test method is to position the dispersive/indifferent electrode over a muscle motor point to see whether there is a muscle twitch or tingling under the electrode. The electrode pads can be checked by the PT by placing a wet contact on both positive and negative electrodes, then resting the forearms on each electrode pad. Ask a colleague to turn up the device until a sensation of prickling is felt.

Electrical stimulation equipment should have regular calibration checks. In between checks, a multimeter can be used for periodic spot checking to see that the equipment is functioning properly. Multimeters, which are a combination of volt-ohm-milliammeter, have the ability to determine current flow. They are inexpensive, easy to use, and readily available. A broken lead wire, weak battery, or resistant electrode may not be apparent because the stimulation in the wound bed is below the level of sensation or the patient is insensate or cognitively impaired and cannot report changes in sensation. Checking for good electrical conduction is the responsibility of the clinician.

Electrodes

Electrode Materials

The electrode is the contact point between the electrical circuit and the body. The electrode must be a good conductor, provide very little resistance to the current, and conform well to the surface. All metals are good conductors of electricity. Aluminum foil is an excellent conductor to use for electrodes (Figures 21–7A and 21–7B). It is nontoxic, inexpensive, disposable, conformable, and can be sized as needed. Carbon-impregnated electrodes are sold to go with most electrotherapeutic devices. They are designed for multiple uses and are relatively inexpensive, but they need to be disinfected between uses, even if restricted to a single patient. They are less conformable than aluminum foil and will become resistive over time as they lose carbon and accumulate body oils and cleaning products.

Electrode Arrangements

Size and Shape of Electrodes.
Size, shape, and arrangement of electrodes affect the current density and depth. Current density as described is the amount of current flow per unit area. Current density is a measure of the quantity of charged ions moving through a specific cross-sectional area of body tissue. The unit of measurement is mA or mA/cm^2. This measure will affect the reaction of the tissues being stimulated. In general, the greater the current density, the greater will be the effect on the tissue biology. Two determinants of current density are *size* of the electrode and the *amplitude* of the current applied,[147] and for pulsed currents, it is also important to know the duty cycle. Small electrodes concentrate the current for local effects more than do larger electrodes, which tend to disperse the charge. Also, the farther apart the electrodes, the deeper the current penetrates.

Active and Dispersive Electrodes.
For monophasic stimulation, the small electrode is commonly referred to as the *active or treatment electrode*, and the large electrode is called the *dispersive electrode*. If the two are of nearly equal size or have equal current, the current will be divided between the two, with the current density at the two treatment sites the same. If the two are not of equal size, the larger electrode will have less current density than the smaller electrode. A rule of thumb is that the combined area of the active electrodes should not exceed the overall area of the dispersive electrode. Usually, a larger size dispersive electrode is used because it's more comfortable due to the less charge density and perception under it. The effects of the tangential electric field extends and affects events from 2 to 3 cm up to 11+ cm beyond the edge of the stimulating electrodes.[148] Maximum tangential electric field occurs on the body surface in the edge regions where the two electrodes of oppo-

FDA Indications and Contraindications for Electrical Stimulation

- Relaxation of muscle spasms
- Prevention or retardation of disuse atrophy
- Increasing local blood circulation
- Muscle reeducation
- Immediate postsurgical stimulation of calf muscles to prevent venous thrombosis
- Maintaining or increasing range of motion
- Pain
- Edema

FDA Contraindications for Electrical Stimulation

- Should not be used on patients with demand type cardiac pacemakers
- Should not be used on persons known to have cancerous lesions
- Should not be used for symptomatic pain relief unless etiology is established or unless a pain syndrome has been diagnosed
- Should not be used over pregnant uterus
- Electrode placements must be avoided that apply current to the carotid sinus region (anterior neck) or transcerebrally (through the head)

site polarity faced each other and maximum tangential fields are stronger than the perpendicular fields directly under the stimulating electrodes.[148] Therefore, to achieve polarity effects, avoid placement of the active and dispersive electrodes so that they touch each other or are too close to avoid the possibility that the wound is receiving stimulation from both poles. Wounds treated with tangential fields and those treated with perpendicular fields had nearly the same rate of healing.[149] Studies that report patients having two wounds, one of which is used as the control and the second treated with ES, may report results that are better than studies when external controls are used.[130]

At times in clinical practice, it is necessary to treat multiple wound sites with a single electrical circuit, using one or two bifurcated lead wires (Figure 21–8). The advantage of bifurcation is that more sites can be treated simultaneously. A disadvantage is that, although the same amount of current and charge per phase passes through all the bifurcated leads, the physiologic responses may vary significantly because of the different skin impedances. Physiologic reactions may be very different when subliminal stimulation is perceived under one electrode and the sensory stimulation under the other. Also, significant levels of stimulation may affect the healing results of wounds that are distant from each other but on the same body.[18] Another disadvantage is that, if there is a difference in the total surface area of the electrode(s)

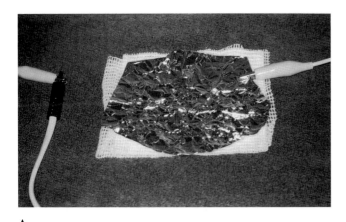

A

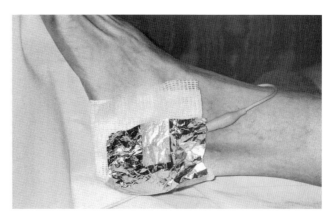

B

Figure 21–7 A and B　Aluminum foil electrode with alligator clip

connected to one lead compared with the other, the stimulation will be stronger under the electrode with the smaller total surface area because there will be greater current density under that electrode. Often, the wound sites are different sizes. It is very important to recognize that the depth and undermining may make the effective electrode size of a small wound significantly larger than the surface area appears. The PT must consider these physical properties of electric current when planning treatment and must correct them in order to provide the "window of charge" (200–600 μC) dose identified by Kloth[21] and the current density recommended by Reich.[18] It may be prudent to use a stimulator with two chan-

nels or to have two treatment sessions if there are multiple wounds with a large discrepancy in wound sizes or if there are different phases of healing. In these situations, it would be important to optimize the phase charge and current density.

Dispersive Pad Placement.　Attempts have been made to apply scientific findings to electrode placement. Most studies use the active electrode for direct application (Figure 21–9A) to the site,[5,11,134,136] but some use the bipolar technique (Figure 21–9B) at the wound edges.[10,129,138,139] The dispersive electrode placement has more variation. For example, in two similar studies, the dispersive electrode was placed differently. In one study,[5] it was placed cephalad on the neural axis, whereas, in the second study, it was placed 30.5 cm from the wound.[4] One study on SCI patients with pressure ulcers in the pelvic region used a protocol where the dispersive was always placed on the thigh. Another method is to place the dispersive proximal to the wound.[134,136] Current thinking suggests that the dispersive should be moved around the wound to induce the current to enter the wound from different sides. At this time, there is not an established, proven method that has been shown to change the effect of the treatment. All reported treatment methods had statistically significant treatment results. The amount of separation of the poles may have been contributory to these effects.

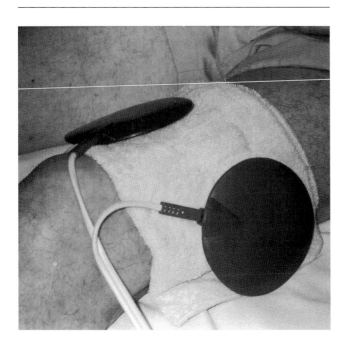

Figure 21–8　Bifurcated leads.

Monopolar Technique.　Monopolar technique is used with monophasic continuous or pulsed waveforms. With the monopolar technique, an electrode is placed to control the polarity at the wound site. Usually, one active electrode is placed on a wet, conductive medium in the wound bed, and the dispersive electrode, in a wet conductive medium at a distance from the wound site, is placed on the intact skin (Figure 21–9A). Polarity for the two electrodes will be opposite. Current will flow through the intervening tissues between

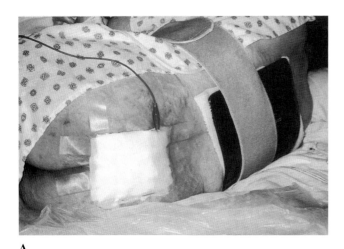

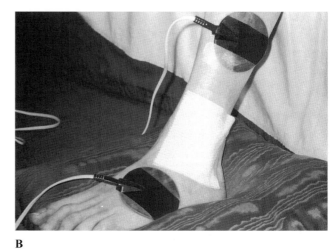

A   B

Figure 21-9 A, Monopolar technique. **B,** Bipolar technique.

the two electrode poles. The current under the active electrode will reflect the polarity selected on the stimulator provided that there is adequate separation of the poles. There is a uniform electrical potential with strong electrical field at the edges of the electrodes and perpendicular to them. However, the amplitude of the electrical field has been found to decrease as the distance between the electrodes increases. The electrical field has maximum value at the edges of the electrodes where the positive and negative stimulating electrodes face each other.[148] As stated before, the farther apart the two electrode poles are, the deeper the current will flow into the intervening tissues. Current will flow through the tissues by following the path with the lowest resistance, which is usually through the muscles and nerves and deeper tissues. More research needs to be done that examines current amplitude in the tangential fields at different depths. Increasing the distance between the electrodes is a good position choice if wounds are deep and extend into underlying tissues, such as stage III and stage IV pressure ulcers, and/or having tunneling and undermined spaces.

Research Wisdom

For polar effects, separate the active and dispersive electrode poles by at least 20-30 cm.

The electrodes can be arranged to target the stimulation to specific tissue sites. Remember to visualize the path of the current flow when placing the dispersive pad. The poles are usually set up in parallel fashion, enabling current to flow between the positive and negative electrodes, no matter how many electrodes are used at either pole. When the surface area of the electrodes is unequal, the current density will

not be the same under the two sites. Current density will also vary, according to the impedance of the intervening tissues and the size of the electrodes. Impedance is the opposition to current flow within the circuit. Different body tissues have different impedances to current flow. Skin, bone, and fat have high impedance and are poor electrical conductors. When there is a break in the skin, however, there is a significant lowering of the skin impedance to current. Techniques to reduce skin impedance include abrasion of the skin surface to remove the hard layers of keratin on the surface, tissue warming, and hydration. High-voltage currents of approximately 100 V have the demonstrated ability to cause sudden, spontaneous breakdown in skin impedance.[147] Because of the fluid in muscles and blood vessels, these tissues are good electrical conductors, and it can be expected that current will flow directly through them, with little impedance.

It is important to understand these principles of tissue impedance and current flow, and then to apply them correctly to derive the optimal benefits from treatment with ES. For example, if the dispersive electrode is to be placed on the back, place it *below* the scapula to avoid the impedance to current flow by the bone. Patients with thick layers of callus on the feet will have high impedance to current. Paring the callus should precede ES treatment, or another placement must be found where the electrode does not lie on callus. A good placement for the dispersive electrode when treating wounds of the lower leg or foot is the muscular tissue of the thigh. One suggestion is to switch the dispersive electrode for each treatment so that the current flows into the wound from each side of the wound through different surrounding tissues and through a different wound edge.[148,150] It is not only the active electrodes that can be bifurcated; the dispersive electrode can also be bifurcated. This allows use of a pair of smaller electrode pads that can be made to conform to smaller body parts, such as an arm or a lower leg (see Figure 21–8).

Clinical Wisdom: *Enlarging the Dispersive Electrode*

If the dispersive electrode area size needs to be increased, this can be accomplished by using a wet washcloth wrapped around a limb or extending a wet washcloth out from the edges of the dispersive electrode to cover a larger skin area. If the wound area size is nearly as large as or larger than the skin area under the dispersive electrode, it will be more comfortable for the patient, but the amplitude of the current or the treatment time may need to be increased to deliver the same total amount of current.

Bipolar Technique. The definition of bipolar technique is the placement of the two leads with their respective electrodes on either side of the target area. This brackets the stimulation to the area associated with the clinical problem.[26] For instance, the two electrodes with opposite polarity may both be placed on the intact skin adjacent to the wound site so that the current passes between the electrodes through the wound tissue. The closer they are together, the more superficial will be the effect; the greater will be the effects of the electric fields of positive and polarity negative at electrode facing edges, and the more the two fields will overlap. This is a reasonable choice for superficial or partial-thickness wound disruptions. The bipolar technique is used with either monophasic or biphasic waveforms. An application of the bipolar technique is to place the electrodes on either side of the wound or to place the treatment electrode in the wound and use four bifurcated dispersive leads connected to electrodes placed around the wound so that current will flow through the wound from all sides at once. Finally, one active electrode could be placed in the middle of the wound and a dispersive electrode fashioned like a donut, made from aluminum foil, slipped over the treatment electrode with an intervening space between so that stimulation would flow into the wound bed from all sides of the wound edges simultaneously. The foil electrode would connect to the dispersive lead with an alligator clip, just like the active leads (see Figure 21–9B).

Clinical Wisdom

Aluminum foil may be used as the dispersive as well as active electrode material. It can be cut to size and conforms easily to all body contours.

WOUND HEALING PROTOCOL SELECTION FOR ELECTRICAL STIMULATION

Aspects

There are many different ES protocols for wound healing. This section first describes some of the aspects of the protocols described, including electrode polarity, rationale, frequency, and amplitude, as described by the researchers.

Polarity

Polarity must be considered when using galvanic and monophasic pulsed current. Electrode polarity varies, depending on the protocol selected. Most researchers studying ES for wound healing start their protocols with the negative pole as the active electrode, then change the polarity after a period of treatment.[2,64,65,99] Griffin et al[3] maintained negative polarity to the wound site throughout the assessment period of 4 weeks. The other researchers recommend using negative polarity for 3–7 days, then change polarity. Another recommendation is to use negative polarity until the wound is cleansed of necrotic tissue and drainage is serosanguineous, and then to continue with the negative polarity for three additional days or change to the positive pole.[134,136] If the wound is not infected, positive polarity can be used to start the treatment.[5] Some researchers suggest that the polarity should be changed back to negative for 3 days when the wound plateaus. Another method is to change the polarity every 3 days until the wound is healed to a partial-thickness depth. Once that outcome is achieved, change the polarity by alternating daily until the wound is closed. Several animal studies demonstrate better healing when polarity is initiated at the negative pole, then switched to positive.[65,66,151] See earlier sections on theory and science for additional rationale for selecting polarity.

Rationale

Usually, the negative electrode is used as the active electrode when infection is suspected. The polarity is often switched back and forth during the course of healing. Electrode polarity switching accommodates the variability in the skin battery potentials that occurs during the course of healing. Thus, electrode polarity may need to be alternated during treatment to achieve an optimal rate of healing. Additional research is needed to ascertain whether wound healing with ES is dependent on matching treatment electrode polarity with fluctuations in wound injury potential polarity.[5] So far, studies have not reported on this important issue. Still, the idea of polarity switching has some demonstrated merit.

Biphasic Protocols

Protocols demonstrating significant benefit for wound healing with biphasic current are now appearing regularly in the literature.[10,49,129,130,133,138,139] The eight studies reported in this chapter have similar protocols, except that the two studies by the Baker et al[10,139] research group found that the best outcome was achieved when the biphasic waveform was asymmetric and biased toward the negative pole. Sumano and Mateos[50] used filiform needles to conduct the current and not carbon electrodes. Biphasic treatment protocols and the results are shown in Table 21–8.

Frequency Pulse Rate

Frequency, or pulse rate, is another variable that varies from study to study without much explanation. Several studies used a pulse rate of 100–128 pps for treatment with HVPC.[5,3] One investigator starts treatment at 50 pps.[134,136] The author uses 30 pps based on the effect of lower frequency on blood flow. In several ES research studies, lower-frequency pulse rates produced higher mean blood flow velocity than did higher pulse rates and had a longer mean recovery time following cessation of ES, compared with control levels.[72] Frequency rate switching during the healing process is also not well understood but becomes more relevant as more information about pulse charge is discovered. For example, in one study, the rationale given for reducing the pulse rate for final phase of healing from 128 to 64 pps was "because we believed the higher pulse frequency might be harmful to the newly healed tissue."[4(p648)] This concern is probably due to the higher pulse charge delivered to the tissue at the higher pulse rate.

Amplitude

Wound healing protocols for amplitude are usually constant, repeated in either milliamperes or voltage. The HVPC protocols all report amplitudes of 100–200 V, the low-voltage DC protocols call for a 35-mA amplitude, and the low-voltage microamperage stimulation units have an amplitude less than 1 mA. The ability of the patient to tolerate high-intensity current will depend on the sensory perception of the individual. For example, in superficial or partial-thickness tissue disruption, if there is intact sensation, an amplitude above 100 V may be very uncomfortable. In deeper wounds or in cases of impaired sensation, these higher amplitudes are well tolerated. Adjust the amplitude to patient comfort. It has been suggested to test the amplitude by stimulating until there is a visible muscle contraction under the electrode. This is not practical if the active electrode is located in a wound within a muscle because the sensory nerves will not be stimulated. If the dispersive electrode is secure over a large body area, the intensity of the stimulation required to cause a muscle contraction will be very high and probably uncomfortable, and may not be visible to the PT.

Conclusion

Clearly, more investigation is needed to achieve an optimal treatment protocol with ES. In the meantime, the protocols and dosage presented in this chapter are for use with

low- and high-voltage monophasic and biphasic waveforms, which represent these authors' interpretation of the literature and the application to clinical treatment. The authors have used these protocols for several years, with good clinical results. Protocols are listed for wound healing for the three phases of repair and for the treatment of an edematous limb where the edema extends beyond the wound area. Protocols change for each phase of repair and have expected outcomes for each. Expected outcomes are based on the literature and clinical experience.

Selecting the Device and Treatment Protocol

The PT is now ready to select the electrical stimulator for treatment. Depending on the stimulator selected, the protocol for treatment will vary. In some cases, the characteristics of ES for different current type may not always be based on the wound healing phases. For example, asymmetric biphasic stimulation parameters are not varied during the progression through the phases of healing.[10,139]

The most common stimulator used for wound healing today is probably the HVPC neuromuscular stimulator. However, now there are more RCTs and CCTs showing efficacy using biphasic and LVPC (TENS) than using HVPC. Protocols and results for using biphasic (TENS) are found in Table 21–8. Depending on the wound status (full versus partial thickness), different stimulator current effects should be considered. The protocols presented below are based on use of the HVPC stimulator. Because the protocol and dosage are similar to the studies reported with low-voltage pulsed electrical current,[4,6] the protocol would also be appropriate to use with those stimulators. The protocols are based initially on the wound healing phase diagnosis, and there are changes in polarity and pulse rate as the wounds progress through the phases of healing.

Sussman Wound Healing Protocol

Sussman uses a wound healing protocol for HVPC, based on the completed diagnostic process (see Chapter 1). Table 21–10 lists the Sussman Wound Healing Protocols for HVPC for all four phases of wound healing and edema control. In using this method, the clinician initiates an HVPC treatment protocol based on the assessed wound healing phase diagnosis and predicts an expected outcome for that protocol. Because the polarity of the healing wound changes during the phases of healing, different treatment characteristics are used as wound healing progresses. In the protocol given below, the stimulation selected for treatment is a monophasic current and monopolar technique used with HVPC. For wounds in the acute inflammatory phase, with an absence of inflammation phase, or in a chronic inflammatory phase, the therapist would start treatment with parameters to stimulate circulation and cellular responses for healing that induce an in-

Table 21–10 Protocols for HVPC Treatment

Parameters	Edema	Inflammation	Proliferation	Epithelialization	Remodeling	Venous Return[4]
Polarity	Negative	Negative	Alternate negative/ positive every 3 days	Alternate daily	Alternate daily	Not critical; adjust for patient comfort
Pulse rate (frequency)	30–50 pps	30 pps	100–128 pps	60–64 pps	60–64 pps	40–60 pps
Intensity	150 V or less depending on patient tolerance	100–150 V	100–150 V	100–150 V	100–150 V	Surge mode, on time, 3–15 sec; off time, 9–40 sec (1:3 on/off ratio) to motor excitation
Duration	60 min	60 min	60 min	60 min	60 min	5–10 min, progress to 20–30 min
Treatment frequency	5–7 times/ week for first week, then 3 times/week for 1 week	5–7 times/ week, once daily	5–7 times/ week, once daily	3–5 times/week, once daily	3 times/week, once daily	Daily; modify to biweekly

flammatory phase. The protocol calls for change of parameters as the wound healing phases progress. Likewise, for a wound healing phase, diagnosis of the repair (proliferative) phase, and a wound in the remodeling phase, the therapist would start treatment using a different set of parameters, as outlined.

Predictable Outcomes with Sussman Wound Healing Protocol

Predictable outcomes are expected for each protocol, which are equivalent to a change in the wound phase characteristics. For example, if the wound healing phase diagnosis is *acute inflammatory phase*, the *expected outcomes* are hemorrhage free, necrosis free, erythema free, edema free, exudate free, red granulation, and progression to the next phase—the proliferative phase. If there is absence of inflammation or chronic inflammation, an acute inflammatory phase needs to be initiated, to restart the healing process. Expected outcomes would indicate change to an acute inflam-

matory phase, described as increased erythema (change in skin color), edema, and warmth. The phase change outcome predicted is *initiation of acute inflammatory phase*. Each wound healing phase has its own diagnosis and expected outcomes that are independent of wound etiology.

When the wound healing phase diagnosis is *acute proliferative phase*, the *expected outcomes* are reduction in size (eg, open area, depth, undermining/tunneling), red granulation tissue-filled wound bed, minimal serous or serosanguineous wound exudate, odor free, adherence of wound edges, and, at the end of the phase, a change in wound healing phase to the epithelialization phase. When the wound healing phase diagnosis is absence of or chronic proliferative phase, the predicted outcome must be acute proliferative phase: reduction in depth, reduction in open area size, and closing of tunnels or undermining. Chronic proliferation may be due to infection of the granulation tissue. There would be clinical signs of infection, including purulent exudate, malodor, and change in appearance of the granulation tissue from beefy red to dull pink. The additional expected outcome for a chronic proliferative phase would then enable the wound to become infection free and to restart the proliferative phase.

A wound healing phase diagnosis of *acute epithelialization phase* has the *expected outcome* of resurfacing and a change in wound healing phase to *remodeling*. A wound in the remodeling phase has an immature scar formation that lacks optimal healing and could benefit from continued stimulation with ES to enhance the migration of the epidermal cells and the maturation of the vascular system of the scar tissue. Absence of an epithelialization phase may result from a drying out of the wound tissues, due to either a poor dressing choice or an absence of dressing. Epidermal cells require a moist environment to migrate across the wound surface. Correction of the inadequate wound treatment would be a necessary part of the plan of care. Chronic epithelialization is associated with rolled wound edges that have become fibrotic and stuck without resurfacing the wound. Other adjunctive measures may be required to reinitiate an inflammatory response in the wound edges that, in turn, will reinitiate the epithelialization process.

Once closure is achieved, the patient is usually discharged from a treatment protocol, including ES. However, the remodeling phase is often overlooked as a point at which treatment with ES can be beneficial in reducing the risk of immature scar breakdown. The remodeling phase is the longest of all the phases of healing, lasting from 6 months to 2 years. A scar that is thicker, better vascularized, softer, and flatter is more resistant to stress from shearing, friction, and pressure, all of which account for a high incidence of recurrence of ulceration on the seating surface or plantar surface of the foot. Electrical stimulation enhances the remodeling of the scar.[67] Of course, other methods also need to be considered to protect the new scar tissue, including pressure-relief devices and dressings. The PT also would include a program of stretching, exercise, and soft tissue mobilization techniques to enhance the elasticity of the mature scar. *Color Plates 1–6* illustrate a case taken through the four phases of healing with ES.

Procedures for High-Voltage Pulsed Current

The procedure section of this chapter is outlined in a stepwise fashion to help the PT and PT assistant deliver the treatment intervention with ES in a systematic and time-efficient way for both the patient and the clinician. Unfortunately, treatment with ES requires a number of supply items and steps. First of all, consider having a PT aide set up the treatment station where the equipment and supplies are available (see list of equipment and supplies needed). The same set of instructions would be useful to give to a patient or caregiver for home treatment. The PT aide can also be responsible to see that the supplies are ordered and available in the department. Always have enough supplies on hand so that treatment is not delayed while someone is running around chasing down the needed equipment.

Clinical Wisdom: *Ultraviolet Light Stimulation To Restart Epithelialization Phase*

One method suggested to restart the epithelialization phase is to use ultraviolet C light stimulation to create an erythema of the wound edges.[153] By using a dosage that produces a second-degree burn, there is a burning back of the leading edge of the cells that have stopped migration. The erythema response to ultraviolet light may lead to shedding of the outer layer of the skin, followed by a mild inflammatory response that includes vasodilatation and capillary permeability and reinitiates the epithelialization process. Ultraviolet light also has the benefit of being bactericidal (see Chapter 23). Another approach is use of topical or oral vitamin A to stimulate an erythema in the tissues. Treatment with electrical stimulation should cease if a method to restart the epithelialization process is not also attempted.

Protocol for Wound Healing

Equipment Needed:

- Normal saline (0.9%)
- Clean gloves
- Irrigation syringe, 35-mL with 19-gauge needle or angiocatheter
- Clean gauze pads
- Aluminum foil electrode or carbon electrode
- Alligator clips or electrode lead
- Bandage tape
- Nylon stretch strap
- Wet washcloth
- Dispersive pad
- HVPC machine leads
- Infectious waste bag

Instructions for Patient and Caregiver:

1. Explain the procedure, the reason for treatment, and how long it will last. Explain that a mild tingling will be felt and where it will be felt.
2. Advise the patient not to handle, replace, or remove electrodes during the treatment. Patients who cannot understand these directions or will not cooperate need to be monitored closely.
3. Give patient a call light to use.

Procedure for Setting Up the Patient for HVPC Wound Treatment:

1. Have supplies ready before undressing the wound.
2. Position the patient for ease of access by staff and for the comfort of both.
3. Remove the dressing and place in infectious waste bag (usually a red bag).
4. Cleanse wound thoroughly to remove slough, exudate, and any petrolatum products.
5. Sharply debride necrotic tissue, if required, before HVPC treatment.
6. Open gauze pads and fluff, then soak to moisten in normal saline solution; squeeze out excess liquid before applying.
7. Fill the wound cavity with gauze, including any undermined/tunneled spaces. Gauze pad can be opened to full size, then pulled diagonally to form a thin "spaghetti" strip. Insert into undermined/tunneled spaces like roller gauze. Pack gently.
8. Place electrode over the gauze packing; cover with a dry gauze pad and hold in place with bandage tape.
9. Connect an alligator clip to the foil.
10. Connect to the stimulator lead to output device.
11. Place the dispersive electrode.
    a. The dispersive electrode is usually placed proximal to the wound (see section on electrode placement for alternative locations).
    b. Place over soft tissues; avoid bony prominences.
    c. Place a moist washcloth over the dispersive electrode.
    d. Place a washcloth against the skin and hold it in good contact at all edges with a nylon elasticized strap. (Covering the wet dispersive set-up with a plastic sheet to separate it from the bed and the patient's clothing to keep them dry will be appreciated by the patient and the nursing staff.)
    e. If placed on the back, the weight of the body plus the strap can be used to achieve good contact at the edges.
    f. Dispersive pad should be larger than the sum of the areas of the active electrodes and wound packing.
    g. The greater the separation is between the active and dispersive electrode, the deeper will be the current path. Use greater separation for deep and undermined wounds.
    h. Dispersive and active electrodes should be at least 20–30 cm apart for monopolar effects. Current flow will be more shallow when they are closer together.

Additional Treatment Methods:

- Up to four wounds can be set up with a single-channel stimulator, using double bifurcated leads from the stimulator to the electrodes. However, this will not provide maximum current density at the treatment sites. For a patient with multiple wounds, it is not practical to run several series of treatments. An alternative is to use two HVPC stimulators, if available. Electrode placement will require careful planning so that the current flows through target tissues. For example, if there is a wound on the right hip, coccyx, left foot, and right heel, the dispersive electrode should be placed on either the right or left thigh. The thigh has a good blood supply and good conductivity. This setup will send the current flowing through the deep tissues to the feet, the hip, and the coccyx.
- Alternating placement of the dispersive electrode for each treatment, if possible, to direct current flow to opposite sides of the wound has been suggested.[131] This will be more difficult when wounds are located in the feet.
- If a limb is involved, the circumference may be too small to wrap with the large dispersive electrode and maintain good contact. An alternative is to use bifurcated leads, which are available to use with the dispersive cable for some stimulators. When using this setup, attach two round, carbon-impregnated electrodes to make the surface area of the dispersive electrode larger than the active electrode. Place the electrodes on either side of the limb. It is easier to conform the two pads to a small limb segment than the large rectangular dispersive electrode, standard with most stimulators. Use wet gauze under the electrodes; if a greater conductive surface is required, extend the wet gauze out from the edges of the electrode over the surrounding skin. Hold the dispersive electrode in place with nylon elasticized straps. If the patient complains of excessive tingling under the dispersive setup, check for good contact and see whether the size can be increased further (see Figure 21–8, which shows bifurcated leads spread out on a washcloth for dispersive electrode).

Alternative Methods of Conducting Current to the Wound. Alternative methods of conducting current to the wound using dressing products have been of interest for a number of years. A recent study of conductivity of different wound dressings reported that: (1) transparent films are poor conductors, (2) fully hydrated hydrocolloids and alignates[152] will conduct current very well, (3) hydrogel amorphous gels and sheet forms are good conductors because of their high water content,[156] and (4) silver dressings have demonstrated benefits when used in animal and human studies for bactericidal effects and reduction of edema that has been enhanced with the addition of anodal DC electical current.[103,104] Silver dressings should be discontinued when infection is controlled; they are not appropriate dressing choice for wounds with eschar. The eschar must be debrided first (see Chapter 12 for indications and contraindications and evidence about the application of silver dressings). While silver dressings are in clinical use for wound treatment, use with ES has not been clinically adapted. There is a definite need to advance this technology for the treatment of infected and edematous wounds. An animal study using pigs with burn wounds demonstrated that use of a hydrogel dressing with PES delivered through the dressing increased the levels of collagenase during the critical period of epithelialization initiation. Collagenase enhancement may be one mechanism by which the ES accelerated the wound healing of these burns.[157] See Chapter 11 and Table 11–1 for a description of amorphous and sheet hydrogel characteristics.

Hydrogels. Use an amorphous hydrogel-impregnated gauze to conduct current. This type of dressing is used for partial-thickness, full-thickness, and subcutaneous lesions extending into deep tissue wounds. Hydrogels can be left in the wound for up to 3 days. This product class can benefit the wound management by:

- Conducting electrical current when covered with an electrode.
- Promoting the "sodium current of injury."
- Absorbing light to moderate wound exudate.
- Maintaining a moist wound environment.
- Gradually absorbing wound moisture (is also a moisture donor to the wound).
- Retaining the cell growth factors in the wound bed.
- Reducing trauma and cooling of the wound, through less handling.
- Reducing product and labor costs by serving a dual purpose.

Hydrogel sheets also have high water content and can also be used to conduct current when placed under the electrode.[156] They have benefits similar to the amorphous hydrogels, except that they should not be left on an infected wound. They are used for lightly exuding wounds and are best used for superficial partial-thickness wounds, such as donor sites after skin grafting.

Amorphous hydrogel-impregnated gauze or a hydrogel sheet can be used as the wet contact coupler under an electrode. Although manufacturers say that all that is required is to clip the alligator clips to the dressing to conduct current, Alon[63] explained that this will focus the current at one small area of the dressing and not disperse it throughout the wound area unless the entire dressing surface is covered with a conductive electrode. Follow the setup steps described above, but substitute the saline-soaked gauze with the amorphous hydrogel-impregnated gauze or hydrogel sheet. Dressings may be left in place for up to 3 days. The amorphous hydrogel should be warmed before application, but be careful not to overheat the product and cause burns. Check temperature with a digital thermometer. Temperature should not be greater than 97° F. If wound conditions permit, cover with a moisture/vapor-permeable transparent film or another dressing to retain moisture without maceration and to maintain body warmth. For amorphous hydrogel-impregnated gauze, on the second day, lift the secondary dressing and slip an aluminum foil electrode underneath; connect an alligator clip lead to the dressing and the stimulator. Replace secondary dressing. Repeat on the third day. The same approach would apply to the hydrogel sheet.

Clinical Wisdom:
Remove Petrolatum before Stimulation

All petrolatum products, including enzymatic debriding agents, such as collagenase (Santyl) and Papain urea (Accuzyme), which are petrolatum-based products, must be removed before treatment or current will not be conducted into the wound tissues.

Protocol for Treatment of Edema

Soft tissue trauma and a closed or minimally open wound would benefit from ES to control, eliminate, or reduce edema formation. Edema stimulates pain receptors because of the tension in the tissues, blocks off circulation inflow to the tissues, and impairs mobility. Edema eliminated, controlled, or reduced would be the expected outcome from this intervention. Table 21–10 shows a protocol for treatment for edema reduction using HVPC stimulation. There are limited reports and no clinical trials to support this treatment.[99–101,109,110]

Procedure for Setting Up the Patient for Treatment of Edema:

1. Use the method for setting up the wound described under protocol for wound healing.
2. Elevate the limb and support it on a pillow or foam wedge, above the heart if possible.
3. Use three or four electrodes.
4. Place one electrode over the wound and arrange the other electrodes over the vascular areas of the limb.
   a. If the wound is in the lower leg, place the second electrode over the medial aspect of the foot and the third over the popliteal area.
   b. If the edema is in the foot distal to the wound, a "foot sandwich" can be made by surrounding the foot with a foil electrode that wraps around the top and bottom of the foot.

Note: Apply the same clinical reasoning for the upper extremity.

Protocol for Circulatory Stimulation in Spinal Cord Injured Patients

Procedure for sacral and lower extremity circulatory stimulation of spinal nerves in spinal cord injured persons:

Preliminary testing found that use of HVPC for increasing circulation and oxygenation of tissues of the sacrum may have a preventive effect on pressure ulcer formation in spinal cord injured patients.[85] Motor stimulation of an SCI patient with acryocyanosis (cyanosis of the extremity) also reversed some circulatory problems of the lower extremity.[94] Rationale for this application is that ES restores the sympathetic tone and vascular resistance below the level of SCI. Vasodilator polypeptides have also been identified in the blood following ES.[81,82] The following procedure is based on the Mawson et al[85] methods. Further testing and reporting are recommended.

1. Clean the skin surface where electrodes will be placed to remove oils and sweat. Alcohol can be used.
2. Use bipolar technique.
3. Use a sponge or gauze pad moistened with water under the electrodes to conduct the current.
4. Place one electrode or bifurcated electrodes over the pad on the soft tissue adjacent to the T 10 spinal level. Bifurcated electrodes could be used on either side of the spinal column.
5. Place second single or bifurcated electrodes on the soft tissue of the buttocks, adjacent to the sacrum.
6. Frequency: 10 pps
7. Amplitude: 75 V (below muscle contraction)
8. Duration: 30–60 minutes daily or 5x/week

Protocol for Infection Control and Disinfection

A clean technique is recommended for treatment of chronic wounds. The use of aluminum foil electrodes is a good method of controlling infection and eliminates the need for disinfection of the electrode pads. If carbon electrodes or electrodes with sponges are used over the wound, they need to be disinfected between each use, even if used for a single patient. A cold disinfection solution, such as Cydex+, will disinfect for all organisms within 10 minutes, according to the material data sheet. Cydex+ comes with an activating solution that is added to the main solution when the bottle is opened. The activated solution can be reusable for up to

28 days. The product is available in quart and gallon sizes. Unless large quantities of electrodes are going to be disinfected at one time, the quart solution has been found to be most cost-effective.[158]

Another cold disinfectant, Milkro-Quat, at the dilution of 18.6 g (2/3 oz) in 3.8 L (1 gal) of water, has been tested for disinfection of electrodes and electrode sponges after treatment of colonized wounds. The electrodes and sponges were soaked in the disinfecting solution for 20 minutes, then tested for bacterial counts. Both the efficacy of the disinfectant and the protocol for disinfection were evaluated. Samples taken from 92% of the post-treatment electrode sponges after they were disinfected contained no bacterial growth. The remaining 8% contained two or fewer colonies. The results were the same for samples cultured anaerobically.[158] The dispersive pad, which is placed on intact skin, should be cleaned between uses with soap and water or wiped with an alcohol-soaked pad. Alligator clips that come in contact with wound contaminants should be disinfected between uses. One company furnishes alligator clips with packs of hydrogel-impregnated gauze that can be kept for single patient use. Over time, the carbon electrodes will absorb oil and detergent products and will become resistant to current flow. A periodic check (eg, every 30 days) of the conductivity of the electrodes is highly recommended.

Clinical Wisdom:
Benefits of Aluminum Foil Electrodes

Aluminum foil electrodes are very cost-effective and time-efficient for treatment of open wounds. They are easily made, are good conductors, can be molded to fit the body part, can be sized for maximum current density to the wound, and are disposable. Saline-soaked gauze packed in the wound and covered with an electrode is also cost-efficient and is particularly good on deep lesions.

Aftercare. After the ES treatment is complete, slip the electrode out from between the wet and dry gauze. The wound can be left undisturbed. If saline-soaked gauze is the conductive medium, it should be changed before it dries or be covered with an occlusive dressing. If additional topical treatments are required, such as enzymatic debriding agents or antibiotics, the packing will need to be removed. Frequent dressing change is being discouraged because it disturbs the wound healing environment by removing important substances in wound exudate and cooling the wound. It takes 3 hours for a chilled wound to rewarm and slows leukocytic and mitotic activity.[159–161]

Protocol for Treatment of Chronic Venous Insufficiency or Chronic Deep Vein Thrombosis

This protocol from Alon and De Domenico[31] is based on using HVPC to elicit the pumping action of skeletal muscles (see Table 21–10, showing HVPC protocols). The best muscle-pumping action is achieved from active exercise, but for some patients, this is not an option or is inadequate to facilitate the venous pump mechanisms. Therefore, ES can be used as an intermittent method for stimulation of muscle pump action. Patients with chronic lymphedema may also benefit.

Setting Up the Patient:

1. A bipolar technique is usually used.
2. Place both electrodes over the plantarflexors, one proximal and one over the muscle bellies.
3. Use a surge or interrupted mode, with an on time of 3–15 seconds and an off time of 9–40 seconds. This 1:3 on/off ratio is essential to avoid muscle fatigue.
4. Begin with shorter on/off time, then increase the stimulation time as patient accommodates.
5. Polarity is not critical and can be adjusted for patient comfort.

Case Study 1

RR, a 50-year-old male, 15 years post-SCI quadriplegic, has had two flap procedures for ischial tuberosity pressure-related ulcers. Wound healed slowly. Cyanosis over the ischial tuberosity occurred when sitting on his pressure relief cushion in his wheelchair for 1 hour and took about 2 hours to resolve. He had been confined to very short trips out of the house to the doctor. Reason for the referral: (1) concern that he would have a reoccurrence of skin breakdown, and (2) bed-bound status was interfering with his social interaction with family and friends and ability to go out into the community. A program of preventive ES was initiated to resolve the cyanosis and increase tissue perfusion and oxygen. After 5 days of 60-minute per day ES with HVPC using the procedure described here, up time in his wheelchair increased to 3 hours and cyanosis was 50–75% less intense and resolved in about 30 minutes. By day 10, he was able to be up in the wheelchair for 6 hours with pressure relief of 5 minutes per hour, and resolution of the cyanosis occurred consistently within 30 minutes. Further testing is indicated to determine efficacy of ES as a preventive procedure for pressure ulcers.

6. Pulse rate is between 40 and 60 pps and can be adjusted for patient comfort.

7. Intensity that will produce intermittent, moderate *tetanic* muscle contraction is required. Increase intensity gradually for patient comfort and compliance.

8. Expect that a few treatment sessions will be required to reach the desired level of muscle contraction.

9. Treatment time is pathology dependent.
   a. Chronic thrombophlebitis: 30–60 minutes biweekly
   b. Venous stasis: commence 5–10 minutes daily; progress to 20–30 minutes biweekly

10. Precaution: Plantarflexors have a tendency to cramp; proceed slowly to avoid cramping. Such cramping must be avoided. To avoid cramping, place the feet against a footboard that limits full range of plantar flexion.

11. Expected outcome: enhanced venous return, measured by reduced edema. May facilitate healing of venous ulceration.

SELF-CARE TEACHING GUIDELINES

Selecting the Candidate for Self-Care

HVPC stimulation and TENS are very safe and easy-to-apply treatments that a patient or caregiver can be taught for self-treatment at home. HVPC stimulators, as described, are available as portable, battery-pack units. Some units come with compliance meters. TENS are also portable. This is a simple treatment, but it requires several steps and clear instructions. Review the procedures with the person who will deliver the care to ensure that adequate care will be given to achieve the predicted outcomes. If the PT does not believe that the person is able to be taught safe, appropriate procedures, this should be documented and may be a rationale for skilled services or another intervention.

To achieve success in a self-care program, psychosocial concerns need to be addressed before establishing the program. Select the patient and/or caregiver who is alert, motivated, and able to learn the directions for application. It will require clinician support and encouragement to convince the patient/caregiver to accept the responsibility for self-care. Patients and caregivers are accustomed to receiving medical care at the clinic or by a home care practitioner, rather than doing self-care. The concept of sharing the problem between patient and clinician is new to many people. It takes a step-by-step process to gain patient cooperation. Begin in the clinic or at the home visit by encouraging and teaching the patient and/or the caregiver to participate in the setup process. Many people are repulsed by the sight of a dirty, smelly, ugly wound. That is often the first hurdle. Take it slowly, with patience and understanding of these feelings. Explain in simple language why the wound is dirty, smelly, and ugly, and how the treatment will improve the problem. Wound measurements and pictures can be used as motivation to encourage continued participation. Before-and-after pictures of other cases treated in this way are particularly effective ways of showing the patient/caregiver how other wounds improved. Move the patient or caregiver increasingly into the role of treatment provider as soon as possible. Observe, instruct, and offer words of support and praise.

Instructions

Independence in the treatment routine must be established before dispensing electrical stimulator for self-care at home. Although it may seem overwhelming to give five steps of instructions for a single treatment protocol, understanding the five steps of instructions listed here will ensure that the patient or caregiver is able to achieve the goal of independence in the treatment routine. Keep instructions as simple as possible so that the responsible party will not be overwhelmed. Because of the number of steps required, prepared instruction sheets listing the five steps would be helpful. Stick-figure drawings can be helpful in teaching the proper placement of the electrodes. Don't assume that the patient will know where to place the electrodes or how to put on the dressing when he or she arrives home. Two or three visits with the PT may be necessary to complete the instruction. Schedule regular follow-up assessments, usually weekly to evaluate outcomes and change protocols.

The Five Steps of Instruction Are as Follows:

1. The list of needed supplies: Make sure that the patient can acquire all the necessary items or help make arrangements to acquire those that are needed (eg, a portable HVPC stimulator with dispersive pad and nylon stretch strap).

2. Setup of the patient and the wound for treatment, including all the steps listed: Review what is on paper, then do a demonstration and return demonstration to confirm understanding.

3. The treatment protocol: Review the treatment protocol by dialing in the characteristics for the selected protocols on the stimulator to be used. The dials can be left at the correct setting to help the patient, but they may be moved and should be rechecked at each treatment session. Give *only* the treatment protocol for the current wound healing phase. Tell the patient or caregiver what outcomes to expect and what findings should be reported promptly. Change instructions as the wound heals.

4. The aftercare procedures: Aftercare procedure instructions should include how to apply the prescribed

Case Study 2: Pressure Ulcer Treated with ES

Patient ID: A.S.   Age: 85   Onset: May

Initial Assessment: Brief Medical History and Systems Review

Reason for Referral

The patient has developed pressure ulceration along the lateral border of her left foot. She is not a candidate for surgical intervention because of multiple comorbidities.

Medical History

The patient is an 85-year-old woman who is unresponsive, with fetal posture and fixed contractures of all four extremities. She has a history of multiple cerebrovascular accidents. She does not reposition herself in bed and cannot sit up in a wheelchair. She is on nasogastric tube feeding for nutrition; a Foley catheter is in place to control incontinence of urine. The wound onset was 2 weeks prior to referral to physical therapy. The wound has deteriorated and become necrotized. The nursing staff has been using enzymatic and autolytic debridement methods.

Systems Review

Circulatory System. The patient has systemically impaired circulation due to arteriosclerotic vascular disease. The circulation to the lower extremity is further impaired as a result of contractures of the hips and knees.

Respiratory System. The patient has shallow, impaired respiration due to inactivity and her bed-bound status.

Musculoskeletal System. The patient has impaired joint mobility due to contractures, resulting in severe disability of the musculoskeletal system.

Neuromuscular System. The patient lacks the ability to respond to the need for self-repositioning and is cognitively unaware.

Examinations Indicated and Derived Data

Vascular Examination

Palpation of pulses indicates a weak dorsal pedal pulse. Determination of the ankle-brachial index is not possible

due to contractures at the elbow. Pulse oximetry of the great toe shows an oxygen saturation of 96%.

Musculoskeletal Examination

There is limited passive range of motion (less than 90° at either the hips, knees, or elbows). There is no active motor movement.

Integumentary Examination

The surrounding skin is erythematous, seen as red glow under darkly pigmented skin. The tissue is edematous. The temperature of the wound is elevated compared with surrounding tissues. There are hemorrhagic areas along the wound margin, and necrotic tissue covers the wound surface.

Evaluation of the Examination Findings and Relationship to Function

The specific dysfunction that generated a referral for the services of the physical therapist is loss of wound healing capacity. The patient's loss of function is due to generalized impairments (circulatory, cardiopulmonary, musculoskeletal, and neuromuscular). Limited bed mobility and limited cognitive ability further complicate the ability to heal without physical therapy intervention for integumentary management.

Diagnosis

Musculoskeletal Disability

Impaired flexibility and strength lead to increased susceptibility to pressure ulceration of the feet.

Neuromuscular Disability

The patient has neuromuscular disability associated with insensitivity and inability to reposition and make needs known.

Wound Healing Impairment

The signs and symptoms identified by the wound assessment, including edema, erythema, heat, and the

continues

Case Study 2 continued

presence of necrotic tissue, indicate that the wound healing phase diagnosis is a chronic inflammatory phase of healing and impaired wound healing associated with a chronically inflamed wound.

Functional Diagnosis

- Undue susceptibility to pressure ulceration on the feet
- Impaired wound healing
- Chronic inflammatory phase
- Insensitivity to need for position change

Need for Skilled Services: The Therapy Problem

The patient has failed to respond to interventions with dressing changes for the last 2 weeks. She now requires the following four interventions:

1. Debridement of the necrotic tissue from the wound bed to determine level of tissue impairment and to initiate the healing process
2. HVPC to enhance circulation to the foot, facilitate debridement, and restart the process of repair
3. Therapeutic positioning to remove pressure trauma on the foot
4. Range-of-motion exercises to all four extremities to maintain tissue extensibility and increase circulation

Prognosis

Healing is not expected without intervention; however, the prognosis is good for a clean, stable wound. Initiation of the acute inflammatory phase with electrical stimulation is expected in 2 weeks with progression to a proliferative phase in 4 weeks, and a clean, stable wound in 6 weeks.

Treatment Plan

- Instruction will be given to nurses' aides in range-of-motion needs of the patient; it will include initial instruction and follow-up for two different shifts (four visits).
- Instruction will be given to the nursing staff in therapeutic positioning; it will include initial instruction and follow-up for two different shifts (three visits).
- HVPC parameters:
  1. The active electrode will be placed on the wound site.
  2. The dispersive electrode will be placed on the thigh.
  3. Polarity initially will be negative, then alternated between positive and negative, as described under the Sussman Wound Healing Protocol, as the wound changes phases.
  4. The pulse rate will be changed from 30 pps to 120 pps to 64 pps as phases change.
  5. The current intensity will be set at 150 V throughout.
  6. HVPC will be of a 60-minute duration, seven times a week.
- Debridement will be achieved by HVPC, enzymes, and sharp instruments daily as needed to remove necrotic tissue.

Interventions

Passive Range-of-Motion Exercises

Passive range-of-motion exercises will be performed to all four extremities, ranged twice daily by the restorative nurses' aide as instructed by the physical therapist.

Targeted Outcome. The nurses' aide will be able to provide the optimal amount of range of motion for all four extremities; increase tissue extensibility at elbows, hips, and knees; and increase perfusion to the lower extremities; due date: 2 weeks.

Healing Pressure Relief

Therapeutic positioning with adaptive equipment will be used to keep feet off the bed, and a pressure-relief mattress replacement will be provided.

Targeted Outcome. The nursing staff will be able to use therapeutic positions to reduce the risk of pressure ulcer formation on the feet, including elimination of pressure on the lateral border of the foot with pressure ulcer; due date: 1 week.

Electrical Stimulation with HVPC 7 Days per Week

Targeted Outcome. The intervention will stimulate perfusion and cellular responses of the inflammatory phase, and wound debridement will progress to the acute inflammatory phase followed by progression to the proliferative phase; due date: 6 weeks.

continues

Case Study 2 continued

Debridement

Sharp debridement will be used for nonviable tissue; enzymatic debridement will be used to solubilize the necrotic tissue between sharp debridement sessions.

Targeted Outcome. The wound will be necrosis free; due date: 4 weeks.

Discharge Outcome

Within 4 weeks the wound was clean, granulating wound edges were contracting, and epithelialization was starting. Because it was now evident that there was potential for wound closure, the prognosis was changed to healed wound from clean and stable; HVPC treatment was continued, and at 12 weeks the wound was fully epithelialized and closed.

Case Study 3: Vascular Ulcer Treated with ES

Patient: C.Z.   Age: 80
(Color photos of the case are *Color Plates 55* and *56*.)

Initial Assessment

Reason for Referral

The patient came to the physical therapist because a vascular ulcer on the posterior right calf would not heal. The patient and his wife reported that they had been caring for the ulcer for more than 6 months, and they wanted it to heal so they could resume their usual activities in the community.

Medical History

The patient has a history of severe arterial vascular occlusive disease of the lower extremities. Old World War II burn scarring covered the surrounding area of the calf, with hyperkeratotic scarring that kept breaking down. The recurrent skin breakdown on his leg resulted in protracted periods of healing (eg, more than 1 year). One ulcer had healed in 6 months after a course of care using electrical stimulation (HVPC). The previous ulcer took more than a year and did not heal. The patient was ambulatory and alert, with mild confusion. His wife reported that any moisture left on the surrounding skin caused maceration and skin breakdown. A femoral angioplasty had been done the week before the patient was seen in the outpatient clinic.

Functional Diagnosis and Targeted Outcomes

Integumentary Examination

Adjacent Skin. Hyperketotic; scar tissue; flaky, friable, dry skin; and pallor are present.

Functional Diagnosis. The patient has loss of functional mobility due to integumentary impairment.

Targeted Outcome. The patient will have improved skin texture and integrity; due date: 6 weeks.

Wound Tissue Examination

The wound edges are poorly defined. There is necrotic tissue along the margins. There is a small island of skin in the middle of the wound bed. The wound has partial-thickness skin loss with moderate exudate. The wound is about 200 cm^2.

Functional Diagnosis. There is absence of an inflammatory phase.

Targeted Outcome: Acute inflammation will be achieved; due date: 2 weeks.

Associated Impairment. Necrotic tissue is present.

Targeted Outcome: A clean wound bed will be achieved; due date: 4 weeks.

Functional Diagnosis. There is absence of a proliferative phase.

Targeted Outcome: The wound will exhibit granulation tissue and be ready for grafting; due date: 6 weeks.

Vascular Examination

Medical Diagnosis. The patient has severe arterial vascular occlusive disease, status postangioplasty.

Functional Diagnosis. The patient has vascular impairment contributing to impaired healing.

Targeted Outcome: Perfusion will be enhanced; due date: 2 weeks.

continues

Case Study 3 continued

The patient's loss of function in these systems is responsible for the undue susceptibility to skin breakdown on the legs and inability to heal without integumentary intervention. The patient has improvement potential. The wound will heal partially, and the wound bed will be prepared for grafting following intervention.

Need for Skilled Services

The patient has failed to respond to treatment with wound dressings and conservative management of the leg ulcer. It requires debridement of necrotic tissue to initiate the healing process and HVPC to initiate the healing phases and to enhance perfusion so that the wound bed is prepared for grafting.

Treatment Plan

- The patient and wife will be instructed to perform HVPC as a daily home treatment program with a portable HVPC rental unit.
- Wound debridement will be performed to remove necrotic tissues; methods will include autolysis, sharp debridement, and enhanced perfusion with the use of HVPC.
- The wife will be instructed in wound dressing changes with alginate to absorb moderate exudate, including how to cut the dressing to fit the wound to avoid maceration.

Discharge Outcomes

- The patient started care in mid-December.
- The wound was necrosis free.
- The wound phase changed to both proliferative and epithelialization. The wound size was reduced to less than half the original area.
- The wound was grafted at the end of February.
- The wound graft was successful. A smaller graft was needed than originally expected because of the epithelialization. Surrounding integumentary integrity was improved: the skin was softer and smoother, and no new hyperkeratosis developed in the scar tissue area.

General Comments

The patient and his wife were very compliant with the home treatment regimen. The femoral angioplasty apparently opened the vessels enough to permit the enhanced perfusion from the HVPC to reach the tissues. Grafting was the best option for this couple because it provided faster closure and allowed them to live more functional lives without having wound care duties. It also provided a better covering with healthier skin from the opposite thigh to cover the open area. New scar tissue was better-quality tissue than that surrounding older scars, possibly due to the improved collagen organization and vascularization associated with the HVPC.

---

dressing product and disposal of the disposable waste products from the treatment in the home setting (see Chapter 11). It is important to make sure that the patient or caregiver understands the proper use of the prescribed aftercare dressing products. Damage to the wound and failure to achieve predicted outcomes can be avoided by instruction in use of products. Again, practice and a return demonstration are proven methods of teaching new techniques.

5. A list of expected signs and symptoms: The patient and the caregiver need to be aware of the importance of any expected changes in signs and symptoms related to the treatment and must know when to report any undesirable results.

DOCUMENTATION

Documentation validates the treatment intervention. Documentation is required to show treatment characteristics and to track responses to treatment, such as described in Chapter 5, Wound Measurements, and Chapter 6, Tools To Measure Wound Healing. Case Studies 2 and 3 use the documenta-

tion methodology described in the FOR. The FOR explains the PT's rationale for selecting the intervention, based on the patient evaluation and wound diagnosis, and the target outcomes expected from the intervention, as shown in Chapter 1, The Diagnostic Process. Data obtained during documentation about treatment outcomes should be done in a systematic manner; they can then be entered into a database to evaluate the program in the clinic, report success of the therapy, and predict outcomes and management costs.

REVIEW QUESTIONS

1. What is a current of injury and galvanotaxis?
2. In what ways do exogenous electrical currents influence healing?
3. What would the expected response of the circulatory system be to different electrical current parameters?
4. Based on the evidence presented, what different effects are attributed to biphasic and monophasic currents?
5. What three suggested areas of research are still needed to support use of electrical currents for wound healing?

REFERENCES

1. Bergstrom N, Bennett MA, Carlson CE, et al. *Treatment of Pressure Ulcers.* Clinical Practice Guideline No. 15. AHCPR Publication No. 95–0652. Rockville, MD: Agency for Health Care Policy and Research, U.S. Department of Health and Human Services; December 1994.

2. Carley PJ, Wainapel SF. Electrotherapy for acceleration of wound healing: low intensity direct current. *Arch Phys Med Rehabil.* 1995;66(7):443–446.

3. Griffin JW, Tooms RE, Mendius SK, Clifft R, Vander Zwaag R, El-Zeky F. Efficacy of high voltage pulsed current for healing of pressure ulcers in patients with spinal cord injury. *Phys Ther.* 1991;71:433–444.

4. Feedar JA, Kloth LC, Gentzkow GD. Chronic dermal ulcer healing enhanced with monophasic pulsed electrical stimulation. *Phys Ther.* 1991;71(9):639–649.

5. Kloth LC, Feedar J. Acceleration of wound healing with high voltage, monophasic, pulsed current. *Phys Ther.* 1988;68:503–508.

6. Gentzkow GD, Pollack SV, Kloth LC, Stubbs HA. Improved healing of pressure ulcers using dermapulse, a new electrical stimulation device. *Wounds.* 1991;3(5):158–170.

7. Taler G, Bauman T, Breeding C, et al. *Pressure Ulcers.* Clinical Practice Guideline. Columbia, MD: American Medical Directors Association; 1996:10.

8. Ovington L. Dressings and adjunctive therapies : AHCPR Guidelines Revisited. *Ostomy/Wound Manage.* 1999;(45A)99S:100S.

9. Wood JM, Evans PE III, Schallreuter KU, Jacobson WE, Sufit R, Newman J. A multicenter study on the use of pulsed low intensity direct current for healing chronic Stage II and Stage III ulcers. *Arch Dermatol.* 1993;130(5):660–661.

10. Baker LL, Rubayi S, Villar F, Demuth SR. Effect of electrical stimulation waveform on healing of ulcers in human beings with spinal cord injury. *Wound Rep Reg.* 1996;4:21–28.

11. Houghton PE, Kincaid CB, Lowell M, et al. Effect of electrical stimulation on chronic leg ulcers. *Phys Ther.* 2000;80(5):S71. Abstract.

12. Frantz RA. Nursing intervention: healing pressure ulcers with TENS, submitted.

13. Garber SL, Biddle AK, Chick CN, et al. *Pressure Ulcer Prevention and Treatment Following Spinal Cord Injury.* A clinical practice guideline for health-care professionals. Washington, DC: Paralyzed Veterans of America; 2000:43.

14. Gardner SE, Frantz RA. Effect of electrical stimulation on chronic wound healing: a meta-analysis. *Wound Rep Reg.* 1999;7:495–503.

15. Anonymous. *Aitkin, Noecker, Heyen, Langill, Sharp, Turner and American Physical Therapy Association vs Shalala.* United States District Court, District of Massachusetts, Civil Action No. 97–11726-GAO, November 18, 1997.

16. Administration HCFA. Suspension of national coverage policy on electrostimulation for wound healing. Baltimore, MD: Department of Health and Human Services; 1999.

17. Swanson G. Functional outcomes report: the next generation in physical therapy reporting. In: Stewart DL, Abeln SH, eds. *Documenting Functional Outcomes in Physical Therapy.* St Louis, MO: Mosby-Year Book; 1993:101–134.

18. Reich J, Cazzaniga A, Tarjan P, Mertz P. The reporting and characterization of exogenous electric fields. In: Brighton C, Pollack SR, eds. *Electromagnetics in Biology and Medicine.* San Francisco, CA: San Francisco Press, Inc.; 1991:355–60.

19. Alon G, Robinson A, Spielholz N, Kloth L, Selkowitz D, Gersch M. *Electrotherapeutic Terminology in Physical Therapy.* 2nd ed. Alexandria, VA: American Physical Therapy Association; 2000.

20. Medical and Surgical Procedures Panel. Medicare Coverage Policy—MCAC: Electrical Stimulation for the Treatment of Wounds. Baltimore, MD: Health Care Financing Administration; 2000:1–73.

21. Kloth L, Alon G, Baker L, et al. *Electrotherapeutic Terminology in Physical Therapy.* Alexandria, VA: Section on Clinical Electrophysiology, American Physical Therapy Association; 1990.

22. Alon G. Principles of electrical stimulation. In: Nelson R, Hayes KW, Currier DP, eds. *Clinical Electrotherapy.* 3rd ed. Stamford, CT: Appleton & Lange; 1999:55–124.

23. Brighton CT, Friedenberg ZB, Black J, Esterhai. JL Jr, Mitchell JEI, Montique F Jr. Electrically induced osteogenesis: relationship between charge, current density and the amount of bone formed: introduction of a new cathode concept. *Clin Orthop Relat Res.* 1981;161(124):131.

24. Kumar D, Alvaro MS, Julka IS, Marshall HJ. Diabetic peripheral neuropathy effectiveness of electrotherapy and amitriptyline for sympotomatic relief. *Diabetes Care.* 1998;21(8):1322–1325.

25. Julka IS, Alvaro MS, Kumar D. Beneficial effects of electrical stimulation on neuropathic symptoms in diabetes patients. *The Journal of Foot and Ankle Surgery.* 1998;37(3):191–193.

26. Alon G. Principles of electrical stimulation. In: Nelson R, Currier D, eds. *Clinical Electrotherapy.* Norwalk, CT: Appleton & Lange; 1991:35–114.

27. Newton RA, Karselis TC. Skin pH following high voltage pulsed galvanic stimulation. *Physical Therapy.* 1983;63(10):1593–1596.

28. Reich J, Tarjan P. Electrical stimulation of skin. *International Journal of Dermatology.* 1990;29(6):395–400.

29. Mertz PM. Electrical stimulation and wound healing: commentary. *Wounds: A Compendium of Clinical Research and Practice.* 2000;12(6):172–173.

30. Cheng K, Mertz PM, Tarjan P. Theoretical study of rectangular pulse electrical stimulation (RPES) on skin cells (in vivo) under conforming electrodes. Paper presented at: Biomedical Sciences Instrumentation; April 2–3, 1993.

31. Alon G, De Domenico G. *High Voltage Stimulation: An Integrated Approach to Clinical Electrotherapy.* Hixton, TN: The Chattanooga Group; 1987.

32. Newton RA, Karsellis TC. Skin pH following high voltage pulsed galvanic stimulation. *Phys Ther.* 1983;63:1593–1596.

33. Newton RA. High-voltage pulsed current: theoretical bases and clinical applications. In: Nelson R, Currier D, eds. *Clinical Electrotherapy.* Norwalk, CT: Appleton & Lange; 1991:201–220.

34. Bourguignon CJ, Bourguignon LYW. Electric stimulation of human fibroblasts causes an increase in Ca^{2+} and the exposure of additional insulin receptors. *J Cell Physiol.* 1989;140:379–385.

35. Gersh M. Microcurrent electrical stimulation: putting it in perspective. *Clin Manage.* 1989;9(4):51–54.

36. Friedenberg ZB, Andrews ET, Smolenski BI, et al. Bone reaction to varying amounts of direct current. *Surg Gynecol Obstet.* 1970;131:894–899.

37. Bassett CAL, Becker RO. Generation of electric potentials by bone in response to mechanical stress. *Science.* 1962; 137:1063.

38. Friedenberg B, Roberts PG, Didizian NH, Brighton CT. Stimulation of fracture healing by direct current in the rabbit fibula. *J Bone Joint Surg.* 1971;53A:1400–1408.

39. Bassett CAL. Electromechanical factors regulating bone architecture. In: Fleish R, Backwood HJJ, Owen M, eds. Third European Symposium on Calcified Tissues. New York: Berlin, Springer-Verlag; 1966:78.

40. Bassett CAL, Pawluk RJ, Becker RO. Effects of electric currents on bone in vivo. *Nature.* 1964; 204:652–654.

41. Friedenberg ZB, Kohanim M. The effect of direct current on bone. *Surg Gynecol Obstet.* 1968;127:97–102.

42. Friedenberg ZB, Harlow MC, Brighton CT. Healing of nonunion of the medial malleolus by means of direct current: a case report. *J Trauma.* 1971;11:883–885.

43. Brighton CT. Current concepts review: the treatment of nonunions with electricity. *J Bone Joint Surg.* 1981;63-A:847–851.

44. Goh JCH, Bose K, Kang YK, Nugroho B. Effects of electrical stimulation on the biomechanical properties of fracture healing in rabbits. *Clin Orthop.* 1988;233:268–273.

45. Jaffe LS, Vanable JW. Electric fields and wound healing. *Clin Dermatol.* 1984;3:34.

46. Kumar D, Alvaro MS, Julka IS, Marshall HJ. Diabetic peripheral neuropathy: effectiveness of electrotherapy and amitriptyline for symptomatic relief. *Diabetes Care.* 1998;21(8):1322–1325.

47. Julka IS, Alvaro M, Kumar D. Beneficial effects of electrical stimulation on neuropathic symptoms in diabetes patients. *J Foot Ankle Surg.* 1998;37(3):191–194.

48. Gentzkow G, Miller K. Electrical stimulation for dermal wound healing. *Clin Podiatr Med Surg.* 1991;8:827–841.

49. Mertz P, Davis SC, Oliveira-Gandia M, Eaglstein WH. The wound environment: implications from research studies for healing and infection. In: Krasner D, Kane D, eds. *Chronic Wound Care.* 2nd ed. Wayne, PA: Health Management Publications; 1997:58.

50. Sumano H, Mateos G. The use of acupuncture-like electrical stimulation for wound healing of lesions unresponsive to conventional treatment. *Am J Acupuncture.* 1999;27(1/2)5:14.

51. Bourguignon CJ, Bourguignon LYW. Electrical stimulation of protein and DNA synthesis in human fibroblasts. *FASEB J.* 1987;1:398–402.

52. Canaday DJ, Lee RC. Scientific basis for clinical application of electric fields in soft tissue repair. In: Brighton CT, Pollack SR, eds. *Electromagnetics in Biology and Medicine.* San Francisco: San Francisco Press; 1991.

53. Erickson CA, Nuccitelli R. Embryonic fibroblast motility and orientation can be influenced by physiological electrical fields. *J Cell Biol.* 1984;98:296–307.

54. Yang W, et al. Response of C3H/10T1/2 fibroblasts to an external steady electric field stimulation. *Exp Cell Res.* 1984;155:92–104.

55. Cooper MS, Schliwa M. Electrical and ionic controls of tissue cell locomotion in DC electrical fields. *J Cell Physiol.* 1985;103:363–370.

56. Williams RD, Carey LC. Studies in the production of "standard" venous thrombosis. *Ann Surg.* 1959;149:381–387.

57. Baker L, Dogen P, Johnson B, Chambers R. The effects of electrical stimulation on cutaneous oxygen supply in diabetic older adults. *Phys Ther.* 1987;67:793.

58. Owoeye I, Spielholtz NI, Fetto J, et al. Low intensity pulsed galvanic current and the healing of tenotomized rat Achilles tendons: preliminary report using lead to break measurements. *Arch Phys Med Rehabil.* 1987;68:415–418.

59. Fukushima K, Senda N, Inui H, Miura H, Tamai Y, Murakami Y. Studies of galvanotaxis of leukocytes. *Med J Osaka Univ.* 1953;4:195–208.

60. Orida N, Feldman J. Directional protrusive pseudopodial activity and motility in macrophages induced by extracellular electric fields. *Cell Motil.* 1982;2:243–255.

61. Kloth LC. Electrical stimulation in tissue repair. In: McCulloch J, Kloth L, Feedar J, eds. *Wound Healing Alternatives in Management.* 2nd ed. Philadelphia: FA Davis; 1995:275–310.

62. Alon G, Azaria M, Stein H. Diabetic ulcer healing using high voltage TENS. *Phys Ther.* 1986;66:77. Abstract.

63. Alon G. Antibiotics enhancement by transcutaneous electrical stimulation. Presented at Symposia, "Future Directions in Wound Healing"; American Physical Therapy Association Scientific Meeting; June 1997; San Diego, CA.

64. Stromberg BV. Effects of electrical currents on wound contraction. *Ann Plast Surg.* 1988;21(2):121–123.

65. Brown M, McDonnell M, Menton DN. Polarity effects on wound healing using electrical stimulation in rabbits. *Arch Phys Med Rehabil.* 1989;70:624–627.

66. Alvarez O. The healing of superficial skin wounds is stimulated by external electrical current. *J Invest Dermatol.* 1983;81(2):144–148.

67. Weiss D, Eaglestein W, Falanga V. Exogenous electric current can reduce the formation of hypertrophic scars. *J Dermatol Surg Oncol.* 1989;15:1272–1275.

68. Wolf J. *Das Gesetz der Transformatin der Knochen.* Berlin, Germany: Hirschwald; 1897.

69. Forrester JC, et al. Wolf's law in relation to the healing of skin wound. *J Trauma.* 1970;10:770–778.

70. Byl NN, McKenzie A, Wong T, West J, Hunt TK. Incisional wound healing: a controlled study of low- and high-dose ultrasound. *JOSPT.* 1993;18(5):619–627.

71. Byl NN, McKenzie A, West JM, Whitney JD, Hunt TK, Scheuenstuhl HA. Low-dose ultrasound effects on ultrasound healing: a controlled study with Yucatan pigs. *Arch Phys Med Rehabil.* 1992;73:656–664.

72. Mohr T, Akers T, Wessman HC. Effect of high voltage stimulation on blood flow in the rat hind limb. *Phys Ther.* 1987;67:526–533.

73. Merhi M, Helme RD, Khalil Z. Age related changes in sympathetic modulation of sensory nerve activity in rat skin. *Inflamm Res.* 1998;47(6):239–244.

74. Politis MJ, Zankis MF, Miller JE. Enhanced survival of full-thickness skin grafts following the application of DC electrical fields. *Plast Reconstr Surg.* 1989;84(2):67–72.

75. Pollack S. The effects of pulsed electrical stimulation on failing skin flaps in Yorkshire pigs. Paper presented at the Meeting of the Bioelectrical Repair and Growth Society; 1989; Cleveland, OH.

76. Lundeberg T, Kjartansson J, Samuelsson U. Effect of electrical nerve stimulation on healing of ischemic skin flaps. *Lancet.* 1988;2:712–714.

77. Im MJ, Lee WPA, Hoopes JE. Effect of electrical stimulation on survival of skin flaps in pigs. *Phys Ther.* 1990;70:37–40.

78. Hecker B, Carron H, Schwartz DP. Pulsed galvanic stimulation: effects of current frequency and polarity on blood flow in healthy subjects. *Arch Phys Med Rehabil.* 1985;66:35–37.

79. Cramp AF, Gilsenan C, Lowe AS, Walsh DM. The effect of high and low-frequency transcutaneous electrical nerve stimulation upon cutaneous blood flow and skin temperature in healthy subjects. *Clin Physiol.* 2000;20(2):150–157.

80. Wikstrom SO, Svedman P, Svensson H, Tanweer HS. Effect of transcutaneous nerve stimulation on microcirculation in intact skin and blister wounds in healthy volunteers. *Scand J Plast Reconstr Surg Hand Surg.* 1999;33(2):195–201.

81. Kaada B. Vasodilation induced by transcutaneous nerve stimulation in peripheral ischemia (Reynaud's phenomena and diabetic polyneuropathy). *Eur Heart J.* 1982;3(4):303–314.

82. Kaada B. Promoted healing of chronic ulceration by transcutaneous nerve stimulation (TNS). *Vasa.* 1983;12:262–269.

83. Cosmo P, Svensson H, Bornmyr S, Wikstrom SO. Effects of transcutaneous nerve stimulation on the microcirculation in chronic leg ulcers. *Scand J Plast Reconstr Surg Hand Surg.* 2000;34(1):61–64.

84. Mawson AR, Siddiqui FH, Connolly B, Sharp CJ, Sammer WR, Bjundo JJ. Sacral transcutaneous oxygen tension levels in the spinal cord injured: risk factors for pressure ulcers. *Arch Phys Med Rehabil.* 1993;74(7):745–751.

85. Mawson AR, Siddiqui FH, Connlly BJ, et al. Effect of high voltage pulsed galvanic stimulation on sacral transcutaneous oxygen tension levels in the spinal cord injured. *Paraplegia.* 1993;31(5):311–319.

86. Wolcott L, Wheeler P, Hardwicke H, et al. Accelerated healing of skin ulcers by electrotherapy: preliminary clinical results. *South Med J.* 1969;62:795–801.

87. Baker LL. The effect of electrical stimulation on cutaneous oxygen supply. *Rehabil Res Dev Prog Rep.* 1988;176.

88. Baker LL, Chamber R, Merchant L, Park D, Sokolski D, Yoneyama C. The effects of electrical stimulation on cutaneous oxygen supply in normal older adults and diabetic patients. *Phys Ther.* 1986;66:749.

89. Dodgen PW, Johnson BW, Baker LL, Chambers RB. The effects of electrical stimulation on cutaneous oxygen supply in diabetic older adults. *Phys Ther.* 1987;67(5):S4.

90. Forst T, Pfutzner A, Bauersachs R, et al. Comparison of the microvascular response to transcutaneous electrical nerve stimulation and postocclusive ischemia in the diabetic foot. *J Diabetes Complications.* 1997;11(5):291–297.

91. Peters EJ, Armstrong DG, Wunderlich RP, Bosma J, Stacpoole-Shea S, Lavery LA. The benefit of electrical stimulation to enhance perfusion in persons with diabetes mellitus. *J Foot Ankle Surg.* 1998;37(5):396–400.

92. Gilcreast DM, Stotts N, Froelicher ES, Baker LL, Moss KM. Effect of electrical stimulation on foot skin perfusion in persons with or at risk for diabetic foot ulcers. *Wound Rep Reg.* 1998;6(5):434–441.

93. Byl N, McKenzie A, West J, Whitney J, Hunt T, Scheuenstuhn H. Microamperage stimulation: effects on subcutaneous oxygen (II). Presented at the Annual Conference of the California Chapter of the American Physical Therapy Association; 1990; San Diego, CA.

94. Twist DJ. Acrocyanosis in a spinal cord injured patient: effects of computer-controlled neuromuscular electrical stimulation: A case report. *Phys Ther.* 1990;70:45–49.

95. Thomas AJ, Davis GM, Sutton JR. Cardiovascular and metabolic responses to electrical stimulation-induced leg exercise in spinal cord injury. *Methods Inf Med.* 1997;36(4–5):372–375.

96. Raymond J, Davis GM, Bryant G, Clarke JE. Cardiovascular responses to an orthostatic challenge and electrical-stimulation-induced leg muscle contractions in individuals with paraplegia. *Eur J Appl Physiol Occup Physiol.* 1999;80(3):201–212.

97. Phillips W, Burkett LN, Munroi R, Davis M, Pomeroy K. Relative changes in blood flow with functional electrical stimulation during exercise of the paralyzed lower limbs. *Paraplegia.* 1995;33:90–93.

98. Faghri PD, Votto JJ, Hovorka CF. Venous hemodynamics of the lower extremities in response to electrical stimulation. *Arch Phys Med Rehabil.* 1998;79:842–848.

99. Ross C, Segal D. HVPC as an aid to post-operative healing. *Curr Podiatry.* May 1981;19–25.

100. Reed BV. Effect of high voltage pulsed electrical stimulation on microvascular permeability to plasma proteins: a possible mechanism in minimizing edema. *Phys Ther.* 1988;68:491–495.

101. Mendel F, Fish D. New perspectives in edema control via electrical stimulation. *J Athlet Train.* 1993;28:63–74.

102. Thornton RM, Mendel FC, Fish DR. Effects of electrical stimulation on edema formation in different strains of rats. *Phys Ther.* 1998;78:386–394.

103. Matylevich NP, Chu CS, McManus AT, Mason AD Jr., Pruitt BA Jr. Direct current reduces plasma protein extravasation after partial thickness burn injury in rats. *J Trauma.* 1996;41(3):424–429.

104. Chu CS, Matylevich NP, McManus AT, Mason AD Jr., Pruitt BA Jr. t al. Direct current reduces wound edema after full-thickness burn injury in rats. *J Trauma.* 1996;40(5):738–742.

105. Griffin JW, Newsome LS, et al. Reduction of chronic posttraumatic hand edema: A comparison of high voltage pulsed current, intermittent pneumatic compression and placebo treatments. *Phys Ther.* 1990;70:279–286.

106. Dobbins GM, Henderson RJ, Schuit D. Effects of high voltage pulsed current on acute edema following total knee arthroplasty. Abstract. *Section on Clinical Electrophysiology Newsletter.* January 1999.

107. Dobbins GM. Personal communication. August 30, 2000.

108. Fakhri O, Amin MA. The effect of low-voltage electric therapy on the healing of resistant skin burns. *J Burn Care Rehabil.* 1987;8(1):15–18.

109. Sawyer PN. Bioelectric phenomena and intravascular thrombosis: the first 12 years. *Surgery.* 1964;56:1020–1026.

110. Sawyer PN, Deutch B. The experimental use of oriented electrical fields to delay and prevent intravascular thrombosis. *Surg Forum.* 1955;5:163–168.

111. Sawyer PN, Deutch B. Use of electrical currents to delay intravascular thrombosis in experimental animals. *Am J Physiol.* 1956;187:473–478.

112. Barranco J, Spadaro J, Berger TJ. In vitro effect of weak direct current on *Staphylococcus aureus. Clin Orthop.* 1974;100:250–255.

113. Rowley B, McKenna J, Chase GR. The influence of electrical current on an infecting microorganism in wounds. *Ann NY Acad Sci.* 1974;238:543–551.

114. Kloth LC. Bactericidal effect of passing an electrical current through a silver wire [poster presentation]. Presented at the Symposium on Advanced Wound Care; April 1996; Atlanta, GA.

115. Kincaid C, Lavoie K. Inhibition of bacterial growth in vitro following stimulation with high voltage, monophasic, pulsed current. *Phys Ther.* 1989;69:29–33.

116. Szuminsky NJ, Albers AC, Unger P, Eddy JG. Effect of narrow, pulsed high voltages on bacterial viability. *Phys Ther.* 1994;74:660–667.

117. Byl N, McKenzie A, West JM, et al. Pulsed microamperage stimulation: a controlled study of healing of surgically induced wounds in Yucatan pigs. *Phys Ther.* 1994;74:201–218.

118. Chu CS, McManus AT, Pruitt BA Jr, Mason AD Jr. Therapeutic effects of silver nylon dressings with weak direct current on Pseudomonas aeruginosa-infected burn wounds. *J Trauma.* 1988;28(10)81488–1492.

119. Thurman BF, Christian EL. Response of a serious circulatory lesion to electrical stimulation. *Phys Ther.* 1971;(51)10:137–140.

120. Gault WR, Gatens PF. Use of low intensity direct current in management of ischemic skin ulcers. *Phys Ther.* 1976;56(3):141–145.

121. Webster DA, Spadaro JA, Becker RO, Kramer S. Silver anode treatment of chronic osteomyelitis. *Clin Orthop Relat Res.* 1981;161:106–114.

122. Fitzgerald GK, Newsome D. Treatment of a large infected thoracic spine wound using high voltage pulsed monophasic current. *Phys Ther.* 1993;73(6):355–360.

123. Barr JO. Transcutaneous electric nerve stimulation for pain management. In: Nelson R, Currier D, eds. *Clinical Electrotherapy.* Norwalk, CT: Appleton & Lange; 1991:280.

124. Khalil Z, Merhi M. Effects of aging on neurogenic vasodilator responses evoked by transcutaneous electrical nerve stimulation: relevance to wound healing. *J Gerontol Biol Sci Med Sci.* 2000;55(6):B257–263.

125. Castillo E, Sumano H, Fortoul TI, Zepeda A. The influence of pulsed electrical stimulation on the wound healing of burned rat skin. *Arch Med Res.* 1995;26(2):185–189.

126. Adamian AA, Shloznikov BM, Muzykant LI, Zaidenberg MA. Clinico-morphological changes in a burn wound after electric stimulation with pulsatile current. *Khururgiia(Mosk).* 1990;(9):77–81.

127. Bach S, Bilgrave K, Gottrup F, Jorgensen TE. The effect of electrical current on healing skin incision. An experimental study. *Eur J Surg.* 1991;157(3):171–174.

128. Reger SI, Hyodo A, Negami S, Kambic HE, Sahgal V. Experimental wound healing with electrical stimulation. *Artif Organs.* 1999;23(5):460–462.

129. Stefanovska A, Vodovnik L, Benko H, Turk R. Treatment of chronic wounds by means of electrical and electromagnetic fields, 2: value of FES parameters for pressure sore treatment. *Med Biol Eng Comput.* 1993;31:213–220.

130. Gault W, Gatens P Jr. Use of low intensity direct current in management of ischemic skin ulcers. *Phys Ther.* 1976;56:265–269.

131. Katelaris PM, Fletcher JP, Little JM, McEntryre RJ, Jeffcoate KW. Electrical stimulation in the treatment of chronic venous ulceration. *Aust NZ J Surg.* 1987;57(9):605–607.

132. Leffmann DJ, Arnall DA, Holmgren PR. Effect of microamperage stimulation on the rate of wound healing in rats: a histological study. *Phys Ther.* 1994;74:195–200.

133. Barron JJ, Jacobson WE, Tidd T. Treatment of decubitus ulcers. *Minn Med.* 1985;68(2):103–106.

134. Unger P, Eddy J, Raimastry S. A controlled study of the effect of high voltage pulsed current (HVPC) on wound healing. *Phys Ther.* 1991;71(suppl):S119.

135. Gogia PP, Marquez RR, Minerbo GM. Effects of high voltage galvanic stimulation on wound healing. *Ostomy/Wound Manage.* 1992;38(1):29–35.

136. Unger PC. A randomized clinical trial of the effect of HVPC on wound healing. *Phys Ther.* 1991;71(suppl):S118.

137. Akers T, Gabrielson A. The effect of high voltage galvanic stimulation on the rate of healing of decubitus ulcers. *Biomed Sci Instrum J.* 1984;20:99–100.

138. Lundeberg TCM, Eriksson SV, Mats M. Electrical nerve stimulation improves healing of diabetic ulcers. *Ann Plast Surg.* 1992;29(4):328–330.

139. Baker LL, Chambers R, Demuth S, Villar F. Effects of electrical stimulation on wound healing in patients with diabetic ulcers. *Diabetes Care.* 1997;20(3):1–8.

140. Alon G, Smith GV. Kid Care: Helping heal with E-Stim. *Adv Directors Rehabil.* 1999;March:47–50.

141. Donayre C. Diagnosis and management of vascular ulcers: arterial, venous and diabetic. Presented at Wound Care Management 96; Torrance, CA; October 1996.

142. Rasmussen MJ, Hayes DL, Vlieststra RE, Thorsteinson G. Can transcutaneous electrical nerve stimulation be safely used in patients with permanent cardiac pacemakers? *Mayo Clin Proc.* 1988;63:443–445.

143. Shade SK. Use of transcutaneous electrical nerve stimulation for a patient with a cardiac pacemaker. A case report. *Phys Ther.* 1985;65(2):206–208.

144. Sliwa JA, Marinko MS. Transcutaneous electrical nerve stimulator-induced electrocardiogram artifact. A brief report. *Am J Phys Med Rehabil.* 1996;75(4):307–309.

145. Chen D, Philip M, Phillip PA, Monga TN. Cardiac pacemaker inhibition by transcutaneous electrical nerve stimulation. *Arch Phys Med Rehabil.* 1990;71(1):27–30.

146. Eaglestein W. Off-label uses in wound care. Paper presented at the Symposium on Advanced Wound Care; Atlanta, GA; April 1996.

147. Cook T, Barr JO. Instrumentation. In: Nelson R, Currier D, eds. *Clinical Electrotherapy.* Norwalk, CT: Appleton & Lange; 1991:11–33.

148. Brown M. Electrical stimulation for wound management. In: Gogia PP, ed. *Clinical Wound Management.* Thorofare, NJ: Slack, Inc; 1995;176–183.

149. Cheng K, Tarjan P, Thio Y, Mertz P. In vivo 3-D distributions of electric fields in pig skin with rectangular pulse electrical stimulation (RPECS). *Bioelectromagnetics.* 1996;17:253–262.

150. Kloth LC. Electrical stimulation for wound healing. Exhibitor presentation at American Physical Therapy Association Conference; Minneapolis, MN; June 1996.

151. Davis S. The effect of pulsed electrical stimulation on epidermal wound healing. *J Invest Dermatol.* 1988;90:555.

152. Selkowitz DM. Electrical currents. In: Cameron MH, ed. *Physical Agents in Rehabilitation.* Philadelphia: WB Saunders; 1999:402.

153. Cummings J, Kloth LC. Role of light, heat and electromagnetic energy in wound healing. In: McCulloch J, Kloth L, Feedar J, eds. *Wound Healing Alternatives in Management.* 2nd ed. Philadelphia: F.A Davis; 1995:275–314.

154. Myer A. Observable effects on granulation tissue using warmed wound care products. Presented at Symposia, "Future Directions in Wound Healing"; American Physical Therapy Association Scientific Meeting; June 1997; San Diego, CA.

155. Beltran, KA, Thacker JG, et al. Impact pressures generated by commercial wound irrigation devices. Unpublished research report. Charlottesville, VA: University of Virginia Health Science Center; 1994.

156. Bourguignon GL, et al. Occlusive wound dressings suitable for use with electrical stimulation. *Wounds.* 1991;3(3):127.

157. Agren MS, Mertz MA. Collagenase during burn wound healing: influence of a hydrogel dressing and pulsed electrical stimulation. *Plast Reconstr Surg.* 1993;94:518–524.

158. Kalinowski DP, Brogan MS, Sleeper MD. A practical technique for disinfecting electrical stimulation apparatuses used in wound treatment. *Phys Ther.* 1996;12:1340–1347.

159. Lock PM. The effect of temperature on mitosis at the edge of experimental wounds. In: Lundgren A, Sover AB, eds. *Symposia on Wound Healing: Plastic, Surgical and Dermatologic Aspects.* Sweden: Molndal; 1980.

160. Myers JA. Wound healing and the use of modern surgical dressing. *Pharm J.* 1982;229:103–104.

161. Thomas ST. *Wound Management and Dressings.* London: The Pharmaceutical Press; 1990.

CHAPTER 22

Pulsed Electromagnetic Fields

Carrie Sussman

CHAPTER OBJECTIVES

At the completion of this chapter, the reader will be able to:

1. Discuss the physical properties of pulsed electromagnetic fields: thermal and nonthermal
2. Identify and differentiate between the physiologic effects of three different pulsed electromagnetic fields used for wound healing
3. Evaluate two radio frequency devices with respect to their different potential to produce the desired physiologic responses
4. Review animal and clinical studies relating to efficacy of the three different pulsed electromagnetic field therapies for factors associated with wounding and wound healing
5. Evaluate the patient's candidacy for pulsed short wave diathermy and pulsed radio frequency stimulation, based on indications, precautions, and contraindications
6. Prepare a patient for treatment and evaluate outcomes of care

INTRODUCTION

Short wave diathermy was introduced in Germany in 1907 and spread throughout Europe and the United States. The word *diathermy* was introduced by Nagelschmidt to describe the relatively uniform heating produced in the tissue by the conversion of high-frequency currents into heat.[1] In the next decades, diathermy was used to treat all types of illnesses and injuries. The stimulator used electromagnetic short waves from the short wave radio portion of the spectrum and was called *continuous short wave diathermy* (CSWD). CSWD was an application of electromagnetic energy to medicine. It became popular because it was then possible to target deep tissue structures and produce subcutaneous tissue heating, rather than superficial heating with hot packs and infrared, where heat is rapidly dissipated by the superficial vasculature.

In the 1960s and 1970s, there were many clinical studies on animals and on biologic systems to determine possible biologic mechanisms of action of electromagnetism on tissues, many of which were not blinded, controlled, or randomized. In the 1980s and 1990s, there have been case studies, clinical trials, and some randomized clinical trials with both animal and human subjects to determine effects of nonthermal pulsed radio frequency stimulation (PRFS) and pulsed electromagnetic fields (PEMF). Study designs have improved over the decades, with better controls concerned with determining the cause and effect relationships of the device and the disease state. A number of these reports will be reviewed in this chapter.

The goal of this chapter is to present the evidence based on a review of the literature about what is known regarding the benefits and disadvantages of using pulsed short wave diathermy (PSWD), PRFS, and PEMF as adjunctive therapy for patients with chronic wounds. The chapter begins with definitions and terminology related to the properties of the devices. The next section details the science and theory of the therapy and the studies that support its use. Clinical reasoning relating to selection of the candidate for treatment and the device, including the reasons for referral, medical history, and systems reviews that are components of the diagnostic process follows. Procedures and protocols for application, precautions, and contraindications are included, along with expected outcomes.

DEFINITIONS AND TERMINOLOGY

Electromagnetic Fields

CSWD, PSWD, PRFS, and PEMF medical equipment operates in one small portion of the electromagnetic spectrum (sometimes referred to as the *radio, radiation,* or *frequency spectrum*). The entire spectrum goes from below power transmission waves (very-low frequency) to above cosmic rays (very-high frequency) and includes radio waves, microwaves, visible light, infrared, ultraviolet light, and X-rays. All frequencies within the spectrum have certain characteristics in common. For example, they all travel at the speed of light, which is 300,000 km (186,000 miles) per second. They all travel unimpeded through a vacuum. They all consist of two parts, a magnetic field, and an electrostatic field, traveling at right angles to each other. One of many important differences between waves from different portions of the spectrum is what happens when they encounter an object. Are they absorbed (like heat waves)? Do they have some other effect on the object? Are they reflected (like light waves striking a mirror)? Or do they ignore the object (like cosmic rays passing through Earth)?

It should be noted that electromagnetic waves discussed here are not sound or ultrasonic waves, which require a physical medium through which to travel. They are "pure energy" and do not have any mass. Also, the equipment and techniques for using the equipment discussed in this chapter are not the same as the high- or low-voltage electrical stimulation equipment, which operates on pulsed direct current, not the 27.12 MHz of the typical CSWD or PRFS equipment discussed in this chapter. At the 27.12 MHz used by short wave diathermy and pulsed radio frequency medical equipment, some of the energy will pass through a patient's body, some will be reflected from a patient's skin, some will be absorbed by the tissue and converted to heat, and some will cause the tissue cells within the patient's body to react in a certain way. The effect that will be produced on the tissues depends on the extent of absorption and energy release in the tissues, and this depends on the wavelength. It is also important to note that, when an electrical field reacts with body tissues, a magnetic field is created, and, similarly, a magnetic field produces an electrical field. Exhibit 22–1 is a reference list of the devices discussed and their acronyms. Table 22–1 shows a comparison between the four types of stimulators and their effects. Exhibit 22–2 lists identified factors that affect the effectiveness of electrotherapeutic devices that are explained in the following sections.

Units of Measurement

There are several units of measurement associated with electromagnetic fields (EMFs) of which the reader should be

Exhibit 22–1 List of Devices and Their Acronyms

Acronym	Device
CSWD	Continous Short Wave Diathermy
PSWD	Pulsed Short Wave Diathermy
PRFS	Pulsed Radio Frequency Stimulation

aware. The frequency of a wave may be expressed in two manners: first, as a frequency, or how many cycles occur within a 1-second period (eg, 27.12 million cycles for a 27.12-MHz wave), and second, the same frequency may be expressed as a wave length, which is how far the wave has traveled (while moving at the speed of light) during one cycle. For our 27.12-MHz example, this would be 11 m. Signal (or wave) strength is measured in volts per meter (V/m). This unit represents how much voltage would be induced by the magnetic flux portion of the wave while traveling through free space and going through a 1-m-long wire.

Carrier Frequency and Waveforms

In studying diathermy equipment, there are two frequencies of which one must be aware: the carrier frequency and the waveform, or modulation frequency. The carrier frequency is the basic operating frequency of the equipment. For example, the carrier of a radio station is the frequency at which the station broadcasts. For PSWD equipment, the carrier (or broadcast) frequency is 27.12 MHz. The waveform or modulation frequency is the frequency at which the carrier frequency is modulated (ie, the music from the radio station). For PSWD and PRFS equipment, modulation frequency is the rate at which the carrier frequency is turned on and off (ie, 600 pulses per second [pps]). For the pulsed high-voltage equipment of Chapter 21, the waveform is monophasic pulsed current. The waveform frequency may be the same as that used for PRFS equipment.

When radio frequency is transmitted as a continuous wave (or signal), enough energy can be absorbed by the body to cause noticeable heating (eg, the microwave oven effect). To control these heating effects and still maintain the tissue-stimulation benefits of the EMF stimulation, several manufacturers developed a pulsed short wave radio frequency generator that delivers bursts or trains of radio frequency pulses. These bursts are another example of modulating frequency.

Diathermy equipment, including CSWD, PSWD, and PRFS, operate at a frequency specified by the Federal Communications Commission, which allows use of radio frequencies of 13.56, 27.12, and 40.68 MHz for these medical devices. Typically, PSWD and PRFS use 27.12 MHz. Signals at these frequencies can travel through the body rela-

Table 22–1 Comparison of Characteristics of Electromagnetic Field Devices

Device	Signal	Typical Pulse Duration	Induced Voltage	Effects
Continuous Shortwave Diathermy (CSWD)	13.57, 27.12, 40.68 MHz sinusoidal	Continuous	V/cm	Tissue heating, no off time for heat dissipation. Unable to depolarize nerve
Pulsed Shortwave Diathermy (PSWD)	27.12 MHz sinusoidal; Duty cycle 3.9%	95 μsec	V/cm	Tissue heating allows for heat dissipation. Unable to depolarize nerve
Pulsed Radio Frequency (PRF)	27.12 MHz 80–600 pps sinusoidal	65 μsec	V/cm	Nonthermal, cellular and circulatory effects. Unable to depolarize nerve
Pulsed Electromagnetic Field (PEMF)	1–100 pps sinusoidal low energy	1–100 msec	mV/cm	Nonthermal, cellular effects

tively uninterrupted, without contact between the applicator and the body. This is an important attribute for treatment. Radio frequency waves transport electromagnetic energy through air or a vacuum without the need for a conductive medium, such as water or air. The energy delivered to the tissues is reduced, however, as the air gap between the tissues and the applicator head increases because a portion of the energy is dispersed away from the target. For example, a clinical application is to increase the air gap between the applicator head and the tissues to reduce the heating effects of PSWD for patients with heat sensitivity or where mild heating is required. When using PRFS, the distance should be *small*, 0.5 cm, so as *not* to reduce energy delivered significantly. Radio waves can interact and influence matter with which they contact, because matter contains electrical charges affected by electromagnetic waves.

Clinical Wisdom: *Using the Air Gap To Modify Heating Effects*

Increase the air gap when using PSWD for patients with heat sensitivity or where mild heating effects are desired.

Greater Pulse Frequency and Width ⇒
More Energy ⇒ More Heat

Pulse Rate and Pulse Duration (Width)

PSWD and PRFS use radio waves that are interrupted (eg, pulsed) at regular intervals. The pulse rates for PSWD vary from 1 to 7,000 pps. The pulse duration (or width) varies from 65 to 400 μsec (1 μsec = 10^{-6} seconds). While the pulse is on, the signal is generated. For example, during a 65-μsec pulse period, some 1,763 waves of 27.12-MHz energy are generated. During the intervals between pulses, no energy is generated.

Longer pulse duration, coupled with greater pulse frequency, delivers more energy to the tissues and has more thermal effect. With high pulse rates (which results in short interpulse intervals), heat builds up in the tissues because the short interpulse interval does not allow heat to dissipate. Conversely, a low-frequency pulse rate, along with a short pulse duration (which means a long interpulse interval), pro-

---

Exhibit 22–2 Factors That Affect the Effectiveness of Electrotherapeutic Devices

- Waveform Shape
- Amplitude
- Pulse shape and duration
- Pulse frequency and repetition rate
- Exposure time in each 24-hour period
- All of the above must be adequate and matched to the biologic needs of the tissues.

Source: Adapted with permission from M.S. Markov and A. Pilla, Electromagnetic Field Stimulation of Soft Tissues: Pulsed Radio Frequency Treatment of Postoperative Pain and Edema, *Wounds*, Vol. 7, No. 4, pp. 143-151, © 1995, Health Management Publications.

duces insignificant tissue heating because the interpulse interval is long enough to allow heat dissipation.

Nonthermal PRFS medical devices generally have a fixed pulse duration of 65 μsec (of the basic 27.12-MHz wave), with pulse rates that can vary from 80 to 600 pps. They are classified as low frequency. This type of signal does not have adequate intensity to heat tissues.

It is very important for the physical therapist (PT) to be familiar with the device to be used. Some devices offer a large range of variability of pulse rates and pulse durations from which to choose. Treatment effects will be different, depending on the parameters selected. Read and understand the instruction manual that comes with the device and choose parameters that provide the physiologic response required.

Clinical Wisdom: *Testing Thermal and Nonthermal Effects at Different Settings*

Try the different combinations of on/off time and different pulse rates on normal subjects over superficial tissues. Evaluate by measuring the surface temperature changes of the skin with a liquid crystal skin thermometer or deeper tissue with infrared scanner before and after the treatment at different time intervals to determine heating effects.

Duty Cycle

The duty cycle is the ratio of on time to total cycle time, which includes both the on and off times. As an example, at a pulse duration having an on time of 65 msec and a pulse rate of 600 pps, each complete period lasts 1/600, or 1,667 msec. The interpulse interval, or off time, is then 1,667 − 65 = 1,602 msec. At 600 pps, the duty cycle is 65 msec/1,667 μsec = 3.9%.[2] This means that, in a 30-minute treatment (30 × 60 seconds × 3.9%), a total of only 70 seconds of energy is delivered.[3]

Amplitude

Historically, power was the way in which the amplitude of the generated field was measured, but this has nothing to do with what is delivered to the tissues. For example, 1,000 watts (W) of generated power is transferred to the drum applicator, where it undergoes significant transformation to the EMF that is then delivered to the patient. Until the transformation into an EMF, it is appropriate to speak of power, but at the last step, it is more correct to speak of the amplitude of the EMF delivered to the tissues. Power driving the applicator coil can be measured either as peak pulse power (which, for Diapulse and MRT SofPulse, range from 185 to 075 W) or as mean power, which (for both devices) ranges from 7.5

to 38 W. These values are determined by settings of peak power and pulse frequency. Thirty-eight W or more mean power is the benchmark for measurement of heating effects. Less than 38 W is, therefore, used as an indicator of minimal heating or nonthermal therapy.[2]

The heating effect of the PSWD is related to the magnitude of the mean power output and can be adjusted to achieve appropriate treatment effects by either direct or indirect application. Treatment outcome can be measured by measuring the skin temperature where heating is desired or by measuring skin blood flow with a laser Doppler.

Commonly, the amplitude of the EMF is described in terms of flux density with the units in gauss (G) or tesla (T), where 10,000 G = 1 T. For example, the magnetic resonance imaging device operates on the order of 1–2 T.[4] Manufacturers include tables in their instruction manuals, listing the approximate values of average output power in watts at different pulse rates and widths. This information should be used only as a guide, not as a definite amount of power delivered to the tissues. The electric or magnetic field itself can be measured, but it is not yet possible to measure the intensity *received* by the tissues.

Comparison of Electromagnetic Field Devices

The devices have been labeled in the literature as PEMF, pulsed electromagnetic induction, pulsed electromagnetic energy, and pulsed radio frequency (PRF). However, these terms are not synonymous, nor should they be considered interchangeable because they have significantly different characteristics. Electromagnetic field modalities used for medical purposes can be categorized into four groups:

1. Static magnetic fields
2. Low-frequency sine waves
3. PEMF
4. PRF

Low-frequency sine waves have a very low signal (smaller than 1 G) and induce 1–10 mV/cm electric field at frequencies below 100 Hz. PEMF waveform is considered relatively low frequency, pulse duration 1–100 msec and a repetition rate of 1–100 pps, and the PRF signal may be a rectangular envelope of sinusoidal waves with a duration of 65 μsec. PRF repetition rate varies between 80 and 600 pps, and the duty cycle is less than 4%. The signals of PEMF are in the mV/cm range and those of PRF in the V/cm range.[3] PEMF signal has been used primarily for osteogenesis, although soft tissue repair studies with this signal have been published recently.[5–10] PRF is used mainly for the treatment of pain, edema, and soft tissue injury and cellular stimulation. Several differences in the signal characteristics exist, the main difference being the signal shape. PEMF waveform is typically an asymmetric train of pulses, whereas the PRF signal represents a burst of pulses within a rectangular envelope (Figure 22–1). Asymmetry of the stimulus pulse was thought to be necessary for therapeutic effect. Asymmetric pulses require significant electrical energy that constrains clinical delivery systems to suboptimal designs. The results of a study on rabbit fibula osteotomy suggest that asymmetry is not necessary for clinical therapeutic effect.[11] The repetition rate of the PRF pulsed signal is 80–600 pps, which is classified as high frequency.[3] The PEMF signal is longer than that of the PRFS.[3]

Thus, it is important to recognize that the acronym *PEMF* is not generic for all EMF devices and that there are important differences between the therapeutic modalities. These distinctions are relevant to the PT when reviewing studies reporting on use of these different EMFs and when selecting therapeutic devices.

The Health Care Financing Administration in 1997 included PEMF in an exclusion policy for reimbursement of wound treatment with electrical stimulation for wound healing of Medicare beneficiaries.[12] Because that policy was stalled by a court injunction,[13] reimbursement for Medicare beneficiaries has been made on a case-by-case basis. Published treatment guidelines for pressure ulcers have not distinguished PRFS-induced current from capacitive electrotherapy as an adjunctive treatment.[14–16] Electrical stimulation is included as recommended modality for best practice in recommendation No. 9 of the *Canadian Association*

of Wound Care Guidelines: Pressure Ulcer Prevention and Treatment following Spinal Cord Injury.[16]

PEMF studies have primarily been conducted or reported in the literature outside of the United States, and only since communication has improved across borders, as a result of the Internet and clinical databases, has this information become available to other clinicians. PEMF devices have been used in the United States primarily for osteogenesis, but several studies on soft tissue repair for venous ulcers have been reported (they are reviewed in the clinical section). Equipment to provide this type of treatment is not readily available in U.S. therapy clinics at this time. Magnatherp electromagnetic (PEMF) unit, 3–50 Hz an amplitude up to 200 Gauss (Meditea Electromedica, Buenos Aires), was the type of equipment used by researchers in some of the animal studies discussed in this chapter (see Figure 22–2). The information is included so as to acquaint the reader about this alternative delivery method for electrotherapy.

Comparison of PSWD and PRFS Equipment

Both PSWD and PRFS apply radio waves from the short wave range of the spectrum at 27.12 MHz. Both modulate the 27.12-MHz carrier frequency with square or pulse bidirectional waveforms (see earlier discussion regarding carrier frequency and waveforms). Like all radio wave signals, the 27.12-MHz signal travels through air and is not impeded by nonmetallic structures (eg, otherwise, your radio would not play indoors). Heating effects are adjusted by changing pulse rate and intensity. Higher pulse rates are thermal. Low pulse rates in the 90- to 200-pps range produce mild heating and are nonthermal at lower rates. Both transmit radiation from a coil contained in the drum head to the target tissues. This method of energy transfer to the tissues is called *induction*. An electrical current is induced in the tissues, as described above. Both types of stimulation penetrate deeply into the tissues and most affect those tissues with good conductivity. Because they are so similar, it is easy to equate them; however, they are not synonymous—the effects are based on two different physiologic phenomena. PSWD has the ability to heat the tissues, whereas PRFS affects the tissues at the cellular level. Further investigation may find that PSWD has cellular effects also. Because PSWD energy penetrates deeply, it heats from the inside out, just as, when cooking food in the microwave, the center is heated first. Heating effects may continue, even after the stimulation is removed. Delayed response to stimulation is an important concept to remember; the patient may not report heating right away because the skin is not heated first, such as when a hot pack is applied. Follow the guidelines listed in the protocols for treatment parameters to use.

Because both PSWD and PRFS deliver a signal at 27.12 MHz to the tissues, this signal has equal ability to penetrate

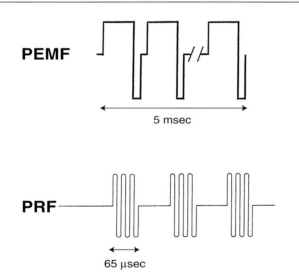

Figure 22–1 Pulse electromagnetic field (PEMF) signal was designed for bone growth stimulation, whereas pulse radio frequency (PRF) waveform is mainly used in treatment of soft tissues. Note: PEMF signal is asymmetric, whereas PRF represents rectangular envelope of pulse burst of 65 µsec. *Source:* Reprinted with permission from *Wounds: A Compendium of Clinical Research and Practice*, Vol. 7, No. 4, © 1995, Health Management Publications.

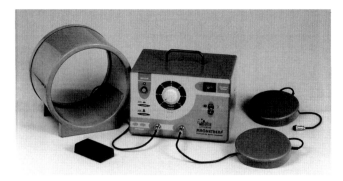

Figure 22–2 Magnatherm electromagnetic (PEMF) unit (3–50 Hz) and amplified up to 200 Gauss. Courtesy of Meditea Electromedica, Buenos Aires, Argentina.

tissues. The depth of penetration of the magnetic field decreases by approximately the square of the distance as it moves away from the surface of the applicator. Guy et al[1] measured thermal changes in the tissues at a depth of 5–6 cm up to 15 cm from the applicator. Markov and Pilla[3] found that the magnetic field of 27.12 MHz radio waves is 30% of the initial value at 5 cm distance from the applicator, 10% at 10 cm, and 3–5% at 15 cm. As already described, treatment effect would be expected to be altered by the distance of the applicator from the target tissues.

Distance from Applicator	Magnetic /Field Value
Surface	100%
5 cm	30%
10 cm	10%
15 cm	3% to 5%

Comparison of PRFS and High-Voltage Pulsed Current Fields

PRFS induces electrical currents in the body through the action of an electromagnetic or a radio field. As such, it has no positive or negative poles, and the current goes in concentric circles (see Figure 22–3 [current in the leg]).[4] This induced alternating current is not related to intervening tissue but is related to the distance from the coil, with the current intensity being greatest just beneath the coil edges.

For treatment purposes, high-voltage pulsed current (HVPC) has, in general, the same amplitude as does PSWD/PRFS. HVPC, however, has a unidirectional flow, with a specific polarity (Figure 22–4),[17] whereas the electromagnetically generated current is a circular flow of current without polarity, as shown in Figure 22–3. The mechanism of action for PSWD/PRFS is a direct effect of magnetic field and induced electric current on the cells. HVPC, on the other hand, has a negligible magnetic field, and the method of cel-

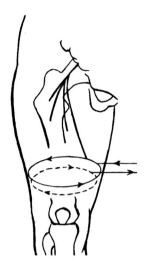

Figure 22–3 A PSWD or PRFS coil placed over the anterior thigh, showing the exciting current (solid line) and the resultant induced current (broken line). *Source:* Reprinted with permission from R. Kellogg, Magnetotherapy: Potential Clinical and Therapeutic Applications, in *Clinical Electrotherapy*, D.P. Currier and R.M. Nelson, eds., pp. 390–391, © 1991, Appleton & Lange.

lular stimulation is by electric current. The direct effect of magnetic and electrical fields in the tissues cannot be distinguished because they come together with high-frequency fields. Methods of delivery are different. PSWD/PRFS is delivered without skin contact; the signal is "broadcast" through the air (Exhibit 22–3). HVPC is delivered by capacitative coupling from an electrode, through a wet contact medium to the skin. HVPC has a negligible magnetic field (Figure 22–4). This stimulation is mainly by electric current.

Exhibit 22–3 PSWD/PRFS Characteristics

- 27.12-MHz radio waves
- Modulation waveform square or pulse bidirectional
- Signal travels through air
- Not impeded by nonmetallic structures
- Pulse rates: 1–7,000 pps maximum; PR = maximum average intensity
- 200 pps → moderate to vigorous heating
- 90–200 pps → mild heat
- <90 pps → nonthermal
- Applicator: wire coil covered by housing
- Uniform magnetic field
- Induce electric current in tissues
- Deep penetration 5–6 cm up to 15 cm (MF value decreased by approximately the square of the distance)

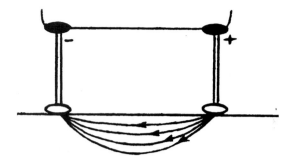

Figure 22–4 A pair of direct-contact electrodes used for HVPC and placed over the skin, showing the resultant current flow through the skin. *Source:* Reprinted with permission from R. Kellogg, Magnetotherapy: Potential Clinical and Therapeutic Applications, in *Clinical Electrotherapy*, D.P. Currier and R.M. Nelson, eds., pp. 390–391, © 1991, Appleton & Lange.

PRFS delivers a more uniform and predictable signal to the tissues than do capacitive coupled electrodes.[3]

Attributes of PSWD and PRFS stimulation that make them useful for treatment of wounds are as follows, and their effects are detailed in Exhibit 22–4.

1. The penetration of the magnetic field into the tissues is not restricted by impedance from intervening structures, such as skin, bone, or plaster. However, metal (eg, rings) will alter penetration and/or localized heating (see safety issues, later).
2. The stimulation at the skin level is not sufficient to depolarize the pain nerve endings in the skin and is painless.
3. Another important aspect of PRFS is that it is non-disruptive. Treatment may be made over a bandaged wound; thus, the dressing need not be changed just because of the PRFS treatment. This decreases the possibility of infection and tissue cooling.
4. There is relative uniformity of the induced magnetic field in the entire volume of the wound.[3]
5. Relatively good dosimetry can be achieved because the magnetic field lines are essentially parallel and remain in this alignment throughout the healing process.[3]

THEORY AND SCIENCE OF THE THERAPY

Both PSWD and PRFS send EMF signals to the tissues, but they are not considered synonymous therapies. Both are classified as diathermy by the Food and Drug Administration (FDA) but in two separate classes: thermal and nonthermal. The cellular effects of PSWD have not been reported in the literature, but ongoing research is being conducted using

Exhibit 22–4 Wound Healing-Related Effects with PSWD/PRFS

- Perfusion of tissues is increased, either directly or indirectly.
- Deep tissue heating with PSWD allows heating within deep wounds and tunnels, including areas with abscess or infection.
- PSWD raises tissue temperatures.
- Painful wounds and associated soft tissue can be treated without direct contact.
- PSWD and PRFS provide analgesia of pain endings.
- PSWD and PRFS produce edema reduction.
- PRFS stimulates cellular activity and cell wall permeability.
- PRFS stimulation can take place over clothing, wound dressings, elastic wraps, and casting materials.
- No disruption of the wound healing environment is needed with PRFS.
- Stimulation of deep structures with PSWD, including nerves and blood vessels, can effect physiologic changes.
- PSWD and PRFS provide relative uniformity of the induced magnetic field in the entire volume of the wound.
- PSWD and PRFS provide relatively good dosimetry.

radio frequency in the thermal range for treatment of tumors; however, there are numerous reports about PRFS and PEMF cellular effects. This is not to say that PSWD does not have similar effects on cells that are as yet uninvestigated. CSWD and PSWD are consider thermotherapy but PRFS and PEMF are classified as nonthermal induced electrotherapy.

Thermotherapy

Warming wounds to promote healing has been practiced since ancient times, and warm soaks and warm compresses are still used for healing. Only recently are scientists beginning to understand and explain why wounds respond to warmth. Under normal conditions, the skin is always colder than the core. The average periwound and wound temperature has been measured to be 4.5–5.6° F lower, respectively, than core temperature, so core temperature may not actually reflect the temperature of the wound bed.[18] Core hypothermia has been recognized as a factor in inhibition of platelet activation, decreased resistance to wound infection, and slowed wound healing. Inhibitory effects of hypothermia on platelet activation is completely reversed by warming the blood to 37° C.[19] Heat has also been attributed to countering the inhibitory effects of chronic wound fluid on fibroblasts. Modalities that can counteract this inhibitory effect could potentially be of therapeutic value. Raising the temperature of the wound by a degree or more could reduce the wound fluid inhibitory activity and assist in the healing of chronic wounds.[20]

Continuous Short Wave Diathermy

The primary benefits of CSWD are attributed to the deep heating effects on muscle and joint tissues, which has subsequent effect on tissue physiology. Early experimental and clinical research was focused on the effects associated with tissue heating that can occur when tissue temperatures are raised to 41–45° C in the deep tissue structures. CSWD and PSWD can be used to raise deep tissue temperature 5° C for therapeutic effects.[21] This was determined to be a safe tissue temperature range when the body could respond to pain stimuli and when there was sufficient reservoir of blood with adequate cooling capacity to dissipate the heating through blood flow. Where circulatory occlusion is present, however, heating is contraindicated because, in limited circulatory systems, there is poor heat dissipation and subsequent high risk for burns.[22]

Researchers in the 1930s, 1940s, and 1960s were interested in testing indirect diathermy application (abdomen and sacrum) to effect peripheral blood flow dynamics in the feet and hands, resulting in several published studies. One study of blood flow changes in normal adult women was published by Wessman and Kottke.[23] Parameters of the treatment were not stipulated. They found statistically significant heating at the hands and toes but less marked in the calf from 13 to 37 minutes after CSWD, with effects lasting up to approximately 80 minutes after application of the diathermy. Heating was noted in the calf later than in the foot and in a two-step pattern. Researchers attributed the results to the ways that circulatory control of the two areas functions. In the foot, there are many arterioanastomoses, allowing greatly increased blood flow to occur in the foot. This shunting with indirect heating occurs to a lesser extent in the calf. It was apparent that changes of blood flow in the hand and foot do not represent changes of cutaneous flow throughout the body, nor do changes of blood flow to the calf or forearm indicate changes of muscular flow only.[23] Clinical application of these findings suggests the use of indirect heating when direct application of heat to patients with peripheral vascular disease (PVD) may be dangerous. However, conversely, heating of the torso may be dangerous for patients with cardiac disease. The fact that indirect heating effects lasted an average of 80 minutes after application of diathermy demonstrates that there is a long-lasting effect on the metabolism of the limbs.[23]

Early CSWD did not have a pulsed option and was, therefore, contraindicated for impaired circulatory conditions. In response, there was an effort to reduce the effects of continuous heating by developing pulsed short wave equipment. The equipment developed allowed adjustment of the pulse rate, the interpulse interval, and the energy output, so that the heat created in the tissues during the on time would dissipate during the off time. Because the signal was pulsed, it was called *pulsed short wave diathermy* and was described in early literature as "athermal." *Diathermy*, which means "heat through," is an inappropriate descriptor for a phenomenon without heat. Despite use of the term *athermal* that appears in the literature, this is not scientifically accurate. The biophysicists suggest that a better descriptor is the term *nonthermal* because the movement of atoms and molecules in all bodies produces some heat.

Tumors are more sensitive to heat than is normal tissue because they are hypoxic, acidic, and poorly nourished. Hypoxic cells, as well as cells in the late S phase of mitotic cycle (DNA synthesis), are normally more resistant to ionizing radiation but are vulnerable to hyperthermia. There are reports of complete regression or partial regression of cancerous tumors when direct thermotherapy with radiofrequency, 8 or 13.6 MHz for 30–60 minutes, is used to raise local tissue temperatures to 41–44° C following radiation therapy. Tissues can be targeted and treatment methods adjusted, depending on the depth and size of the tumor. Currently, hyperthermia is being used only as an experimental treatment in late stages of cancer.[24] Irradiated tissues often develop fibrosis and are subject to skin breakdown, even many years after radiation therapy. Irradiated tissues treated with low frequency (8 MHz) high intensity (1.5 kW) CSWD for 30–60 minutes show an increase in blood flow and cell membrane permeability, resulting in increased ability to revascularize, repair, and prevent ischemia and fibrosis.[25]

Pulsed Short Wave Diathermy

As described, PSWD is a thermal agent that can heat both deep and superficial tissues. Silverman and Pendleton,[25] and Santoro et al[26] wanted to know whether indirect tissue heating in the abdomen and lumbosacral areas would raise the distal tissue temperature in the foot and the calf. PSWD, CSWD, and placebo were used to treat young adults by placing the treatment head over the lower abdomen. Silverman and Pendleton's treatment protocol lasted 20 minutes at a high average power setting of 65 W and low average power of 15 W for both treatment machines. To achieve the high power, the pulse rate was 2,400 pps, and the low power pulse rate was 600 pps. Peripheral circulation was then measured in the calf and in the foot. The result was that the change in circulation was most prominent in the foot and occurred only with high average power. The mean increase was 165% with pulsed high power and 195% with continuous high power. No circulatory effects were found in the foot with low power of either type. Temperatures were recorded under the treatment head. The mean increase in skin temperature was 5.3° C with continuous treatment and 5.8° C with pulsed treatment.

The foot temperature increased 1.9° C and 2.2° C, respectively. Local heating occurred on the abdomen of the subjects who received low power, with mean changes of 3.1° C and 3.4° C for CSWD and CSWD. Subjects reported a comfortable sensation under the treatment heads. These are statistically significant changes in temperature and blood flow but not between the pulsed and continuous generators, confirming the ability of a PSWD generator to heat tissue.

In Santoro's study,[26] 10 patients with moderate to severe arterial PVD were treated with PSWD 5 days a week for 20 days, spread over the period of 1 month. The treatment consisted of a 30-minute, two-part protocol. During the first 20 minutes, the treatment was at maximum amplitude for the unit, which is a high-dose heating level. The parameters were 95 µsec at a rate of 7,000 pps. During the last 10 minutes, the intensity was reduced to a low heating level. The parameters were 95 µsec at a rate of 700 pps. This was called the *cooling phase*. Two applicator heads were used, with one placed over the plantar surface of the foot and the second over the area of the anterior thigh. In cases where both limbs were affected, both applicators were placed over the plantar surfaces of the feet. Variables measured included surface temperature, transcutaneous partial pressure of oxygen ($tcPO_2$), segmental Doppler blood pressure, superficial blood flow (measured with a laser Doppler flowmeter), and patient perceptions. Findings were that temperature peaked at the end of the 20 minutes of high heat, and then gradually reduced. The $tcPO_2$ readings increased in the treated and the untreated limbs. They were insignificant in the treated limbs but significant in the untreated limbs, possibly because of reflex vasodilatation from the warm circulating blood and sympathetic nervous system activity. Sixty percent of the patients reported subjectively that they felt that the treatment had improved their quality of life. No adverse effects were reported.[20]

Exhibit 22–5 lists the effects of PSWD, and Table 22–2 summarizes clinical study reports on the effects of PSWD and PRFS on circulation.

Further study is needed to determine the efficacy of thermotherapy (CSWD and/or PSWD) in prevention of tissue fibrosis and enhancement of healing of irradiated tissues. Like tumors, the chronic wound environment is often hypoxic, acidotic, and poorly nourished. Application of thermotherapy should be investigated clinically for the effects on chronic wound healing. At this time, the reports of successful outcomes for wound healing remain anecdotal. For more information on thermotherapy for wound healing, see Chapters 12, Management of the Wound Environment with Advanced Therapies, and 25, Whirlpool.

Nonthermal Pulsed Radio Frequency Stimulation and Pulsed Electromagnetic Field Stimulation

Pulsing the radio waves did not solve all the problems of creating a truly nonthermal device. The next modifica-

Exhibit 22–5 Summary of Effects of PSWD

↑ Perfusion
↑ Local tissue $tcPO_2$
↑ Tissue metabolism
↑ Antibiotic delivery to tissue
↑ O_2 antimicrobial effect

tion was to change the signal so that the signal was pulsed at lower rates and longer intervals. PRFS, nonthermal, was introduced in the late 1950s, just as use of diathermy was waning. The first device that was approved by the FDA for medical use and appeared on the market was the Diapulse. The FDA allows the Diapulse Corporation to market the device as a short wave diathermy class III device. Diathermy class III devices that are currently being marketed are described in the equipment section later in the chapter. What needs to be clear is that, although there are similarities between PSWD (thermal) and PRFS (nonthermal), they are not synonymous (Table 22–3).

Several studies of effects of nonthermal PRFS using two available commercial PRFS devices, Diapulse and MRT SofPulse, are reviewed in this section. The way in which these two manufacturers handle the technical specifications for their devices is the way in which the outputs are reported. Diapulse is constructed with vacuum tubes. MRT SofPulse is a solid-state analogue of Diapulse. These devices use fixed pulse duration, 65 µsec, with pulse rate adjustable from 80 to 600 pps at the maximum generated power. When pulsed at the maximum rate, power is applied only 3.9% of the time. This equipment was designed to allow for dissipation of heat and to reduce its accumulation. The FDA has designated these two devices as equivalent.

Basic Science of PRFS (Nonthermal) and PEMF

The EMF has been identified as the signal to the tissues that is the therapeutic factor with the ability to modulate biologic phenomena.[3] EMF modulation of biologic processes depends first on the physiologic state of the injured tissues, which establishes whether or not a physiologically relevant response can be achieved and, second, by using effective dosage of the magnetic and electrical fields to that target site.[3] Effective dosimetry is achieved by configuring the waveform to satisfy the target response time and minimum amplitude required for nonthermal effects.[3] Cellular activity can be modified by induced changes in the electrical status of the cell, the cell membrane, and the cell-to-cell communications. Cell-to-cell communications via electrically conducting gap junctions increase the EMF sensitivity by several orders of magnitude versus a single cell exposed to the

Table 22–2 Clinical Studies of the Effects of PSWD and PRFS on Circulation

Researcher	Silverman and Pendleton[25]	Santoro et al[26]	Erdman[40]	Mayrovitz and Larsen[41]	Mayrovitz and Larsen[42]
Type of study	Case series	Uncontrolled	Case series	Controlled	Controlled
Type of stimulator	PSWD	PSWD	PRFS (Diapulse)	PRFS (MRT Sofpulse)	PRFS (MRT Sofpulse)
Frequency	80–2600 pps	7000 pps 90 µsec; 700 pps 95 µsec	400 pps; 500 pps; 600 pps 65 µsec	600 pps, 65 µsec	600 pps 65 µsec
Amplitude	Average high power 65 W; Average low power 15 W	Maximum power	Moderate power level (4) to peak (6) Av power 16 W at (4) Max of 40 W at (6)	Peak power 35 W	1 Gauss at skin surface Peak power
Duration of stimulation	20 min indirect heating at abdomen	20 min max amp indirect heating; 10 min mod amp direct heating	Indirect stimulation at epigastrum	45 min 1x direct stimulation at the arm	45 min 1x direct stimulation of lower limb
Effect of Rx	Average increases tissue temp with pulsed high power at abdomen 5.8° C At foot 2.2° C Increase of 165% at foot Average increases tissue temp at low power at abdomen 3.1–3.4° C at foot no significant change	Insignificant temp increase in tx limb; Significant temp increase contralateral limb Increased tcPO$_2$ both limbs (Note: Temp peaked at 20 min)	↑ Av temp at foot 2.0° C ↑ Volume increase of 1.75 at max power	Blood flow: Mean group increase: 29% in treated limb Untreated: no change Skin Temp: Mean group 1.8° C ↑ skin temp treated limb Untreated limb: 0.5° C ↑ skin temp	↑ Blood flow volume at tx site; No increase at contralateral control site (Note: at baseline the ulcerated limb had higher BFV than contralateral) No increase in skin temp
Effect post Rx (15–30 min)	Not reported	Not reported	↑ Volumetric change Returned to baseline within 30 min post	Not reported	Not reported
Method of Measurement	Temperature	Temperature tcPO$_2$	Volumetric plethysmography Skin temperature readings	Skin temperature (thermistor) Laser Doppler Flowmeter	Skin temperature (thermistor) Laser Doppler Flowmetry
Disease State Tested and N	Healthy young adults N not stated	Arterial PVD N = 10	Healthy young adults N = 20	Healthy adults N = 9	Diabetics N = 15 with foot ulceration, 9 with PVD

Source: Data from reference #'s 25, 26, 40, 41, and 42.

Table 22–3 Comparison of CSWD, PSWD, and PRFS Characteristics

Device	Signal	Pulse Rate	Effect
Continuous short wave diathermy	27.12 MHz	Continuous	No heat dissipation
Pulsed short wave diathermy	27.12 MHz	High repetition rate, moderate repetition rate	Limited heat dissipation, moderate heat dissipation
Pulsed radio frequency stimulation	27.12 MHz	Low repetition rate	Heat dissipation, cellular effects

same EMF source.[3] Understanding the mechanisms of action induced by applying PRFS to tissues has generated interest in the effects on different cellular systems. This section presents a synopsis of the effect of PRFS and PEMF on some cellular systems studied.

Basic science research findings show that, by applying nonthermal PRFS to cells, the energy modulates Ca^{2+} binding kinetics, stimulates all types of cell proliferation, affects the cell membrane diffusion and/or permeability, and moves negatively charged plasma proteins toward lymph capillaries. Cellular changes following treatment with PRFS have been observed to alter processes that are essential to tissue repair, including proliferation of parenchymal and connective tissue cells, synthesis of extracellular matrix proteins, collagenization, and acquisition of wound strength.[3] Because an electrical field is induced, it has been proposed that PRFS energy and PEMF probably affect the body's bioelectric system. One theory is that the sodium ions in the cell build up during the inflammatory phase, and the action of the sodium pump is reduced. This results in a decrease in the cell's negative charge that, in effect, reduces the action of the sodium pump. Under the influence of the EMF from the PRFS energy source, the sodium pump is reactivated, and the cell's ionic balance can be restored.[27]

Like PRFS, PEMF affects calcium (Ca^{2+}) binding kinetics.[28] This process has been identified as one mechanism involved in osteogenesis stimulation with PEMF. Exogenous application of PEMF is designed to mimic the asymmetric waveform that has been detected when bone is dynamically formed.[28] Different energy patterns result in different effects. For example, a burst elevates calcium content, and a single pulse lowers it. Selected pulse modifications appear to activate gene-specific transcription and translation. PEMF thresholds appear to encompass more factors than does dose response alone. Frequency, amplitude, and timing, singly or in combination, appear to be involved in many of the experimental studies.[28] PEMF safety appears to be well established. No toxicologic or teratologic effects have been demonstrated by in vitro or in vivo safety testing.[28]

Hematoma Absorption

Rupture of small or large vessels accompanies both surgical and traumatic wounding and produces hematoma in the tissues. Hematomas produced by pressure are often referred to as "purple ulcers."[29] Hematoma is normally absorbed slowly and often goes on to tissue necrosis. Fenn[30] found that hematoma absorption in rabbit ears was accelerated, compared with the control group, and the acceleration became statistically significant on the sixth day after initiation of treatment with Diapulse PRFS.

One nonthermal phenomenon observed after application of PRFS with Diapulse was called a *pearl chain phenomenon*. When fat globules in milk were exposed to PRFS, the fat globules aligned into an order array of pearl chains and remained in that formation until the energy was removed. A second test using thermal energy caused agglomeration of the fat particles that was irreversible. This pearl chain phenomenon is also reproducible with blood and lymph cells.[31] Cameron[32] looked at wound healing in 20 dogs, comparing a control group of untreated animals with a Diapulse PRFS-treated group. He took specimens from 24 hours to 10 days after wounding and studied the tissues under the microscope. At 48 hours, the hematoma had been absorbed and replaced by fat that was arranged in strands migrating toward the ends of the wounds. By comparison, the control animals had minimal fat activity by day 4 postwounding.

Sambasivan[33] treated four cases of extradural hematomas with Diapulse PRFS. Treatment was applied twice daily for 10 days at a maximum pulse rate of 600 pps and a 65-μsec duration for 30 minutes per session, alternating right and left sides of the head. The treated cases showed clearance of hematoma. If the results are reproducible, this could have tremendous potential for shortening healing times. Clinicians can begin gathering data about wounds that are treated in the clinic that have hemorrhagic areas and are treated with PRFS. Rapid reabsorption of clotted blood is one way to prevent tissue death. The FDA allows PSWD to list hematoma as an indication for application of SWD, although no further evidence to support the efficacy was found in the literature review.

Effects on Attributes of the Inflammatory Phase

The following clinical studies investigated the role of an intervention with PRFS and PSWD on attributes of the inflammatory phase: edema, pain, circulation, and tissue oxygen.

Edema and Pain

Ionescu et al[34] observed that, when burn wounds were treated with PRFS, there was prevention of edema formation, pain, and reduction in local symptoms. These observations led to further investigation to understand the mechanisms involved and to demonstrate objective proof. Local skin enzymatic activity was chosen as an indicator of the viability of the tissue. Samples of proteins and some principal enzymes in normal and burned tissue were compared before and after PRFS therapy. The enzymatic activities of the skin decrease when traumatized or burned. The data showed that, compared with normal skin, the enzymatic activity was significantly modified after the treatment. The earlier the application of treatment, the sooner the normal enzymatic activities will be restored.

Reduction of soft tissue edema resulting from trauma has been reported following treatment with PRFS for 20–30 minutes and has persisted for several hours after treatment. The mechanism by which it is postulated that this occurs is that the PRFS affects sympathetic nervous system outflows to induce vasoconstriction and restriction of blood flow from blood vessels to the interstitial areas around the wound site.[3]

Some PSWD devices can be set at a protocol that is mildly thermal. The Magnatherm and the Curapulse are such devices. A study on 25 podiatric surgical patients was conducted by Santiesteban and Grant[35] at a dosage of 700 pps and a power setting of 12, or approximately 120 W. This intensity, however, is now called *mildly thermal* but was reported in the study as *athermal*. A control group of 25 did not receive this treatment. Two electrodes were used, one over the plantar aspect of the postoperative foot and the other on the inguinal region. If both feet were operated on, the electrodes were placed over the plantar aspects of both feet. Two treatment sessions were given. One was given as soon after surgery as possible and the other 4 hours later. Nurses noted the number and types of pain medications used and the length of the hospital stay, measured in hours. There were significant differences between the treatment group and the control group. The former had an 8-hour shorter length of stay and used weaker analgesic medication.[35]

Early intervention with PRFS (Diapulse) in the treatment of hand injuries was studied by Barclay et al[36] to compare the effects on edema, pain, and improvement of function. Sixty matched pairs of patients who had hand injuries within 36 hours of admission for treatment were evaluated. In the treated group, with the exception of two cases, there was a complete resolution of edema by the third day, compared with the controls, in whom swelling greatly increased. The 17 patients in the treated group were symptom free by the third day, and by day 7, only one in the treated group had slight loss of function; the 29 other patients had been discharged. By contrast, in the control group of 30 patients, 3 had been discharged, and the remaining 27 were still symptomatic with edema, pain, and loss of function.[36]

Acute ankle sprains have a rapid onset of edema and pain and are common injuries in athletes and in the military. Pennington et al[37] studied the effect of PRFS (Diapulse) on 50 patients with grade I and II ankle sprains at 1–24 hours, 25–48 hours, and 49–72 hours after injury and found a statistically significant decrease in the edema (0.95% versus 4.7%) and pain in the treatment group. Reduced pain was reported for 64% of the treated patients, compared with 33% for the control group. Because of the small sample size in the three different time-elapsed groups, no analysis was performed on this component but, overall, those patients who were treated within the 72-hour time frame had a statistically significant effect, including a significant decrease in the time lost from military training.[37]

Two hundred acute head trauma patients with a Glasgow Coma Scale 8 or less were alternately assigned to treatment with PRFS or to serve as controls.[33] The patients in this category had diffuse brain damage, multiple contusions, and brain edema, and were in poor states of consciousness. Except for the addition of the PRFS stimulation, the same management protocol was followed in the intensive care unit (ICU). PRFS stimulation at 600 pps for 30 minutes was given every 12 hours, with the drum alternating on the right and left sides of the head. Treatment began at the time of admission into the ICU. Serial computed tomography scans were done to evaluate the outcomes and for comparison with controls. In all cases, on the first day of admission to ICU, there was clear evidence of edema, and the ventricles appeared slitlike. By the tenth day, for those in the PRFS treatment group, the edema had disappeared, and the ventricles were seen well. However, in the control cases, it took 12–15 days to see the ventricles. Another measure reported for 20 cases was intracranial pressure (ICP). In the 10 cases receiving PRFS, the ICP diminished by the fifth postinjury day and by day 7 came to near normal levels. Controls' ICP began to diminish by day 7. Mortality at the end of one month for the PRFS group was 24% in the PRFS group and 29% among controls.[33]

Early intervention during the inflammatory phase of healing was attributed to the successful outcomes of reduced swelling and pain and early return to functional activities in the studies by Barclay et al,[36] Pennington et al,[37] and Ionescu et al.[34] Research information such as this can be used as a clinical guide for referral to the PT for evaluation of the appropriateness of this treatment following acute trauma. Then it is up to the PT to evaluate the treatment outcomes and to compare them with the research studies.

Research Wisdom: *Early Intervention with PRFS Hastens Recovery*

Intervention during the acute inflammatory phase—the first 72 hours postinjury (eg, trauma including burns, pressure, contusion, etc)—with PRFS has demonstrated reduction of edema, pain, and enhanced perfusion of the tissues, with resulting acceleration through the phases of repair and early return to work.[34,36,37]

Circulatory Effects

Increased blood flow benefits wound healing by autolytic debridement of necrotic tissue, delivering critically needed oxygen and nutrients and removing metabolites. Local application of heat causes vasodilation of the vasculature and allows for increased blood flow. Infection rates are inversely proportional to blood flow and oxygen levels because, in this situation, oxygen functions equivalent to an antibiotic by oxygenation of the leukocytes, which are critical to fighting infection.[38] All of the processes of wound healing are oxygen dependent, including collagen deposition. Heat is a simple and effective method to enhance blood flow.[17,39] For example, if blood flow can increase to the lower extremities without elevating body heat and if it can be maintained, it can then be applied as a helpful treatment of vasospastic PVD and could be beneficial in controlling infection. Treatment interventions that can increase perfusion to the tissues are important tools. The following studies report on the effects of CSWD, PSWD, and nonthermal PRFS on blood flow to the extremities. Table 22–2 summarizes studies on circulatory effects.

Erdman[40] studied the effect of the Diapulse PRFS device, with the inductive head placed over the epigastrium, in a study measuring changes in blood flow to the feet of 20 normal young adults. The findings were mean increase in foot temperature of 2.0° C and an average volume increase of 1.75-fold at the maximum generated power. Rectal temperatures did not change, nor did pulse rates. Furthermore, in all 20 cases, increased blood flow was directly proportional to the energy applied at the three highest settings. A short period of effect followed cessation of the treatment.

Mayrovitz and Larsen[41] reported that treatment with PRFS increased skin blood perfusion in the treated region. PRFS stimulation with the MRT SofPulse at 65 μsec at a pulse rate of 600 pps and peak power, applied for 40 minutes on the forearm skin of nine healthy men and women, produced enhanced microvascular perfusion, averaging 30%, compared with pretest levels. Skin temperature was increased by an average of 1.8° C, but the rise occurred ahead of the measured increased perfusion. This is similar to the study by Erdman.[40] The mechanisms of action are not readily understood.

Mayrovitz and Larsen[42] conducted another study using the MRT SofPulse, also to study effects on perfusion. Laser Doppler red blood cell (RBC) perfusion, volume, velocity, and skin temperatures were evaluated for the effects of PRFS on 15 subjects, each of whom had had diabetes for at least 5 years and each of whom had an ulcer on the foot or toe of one limb. Ulcer duration was a minimum of 8 weeks. The contralateral limb was intact and served as the control. Nine subjects had PVD, as confirmed by noninvasive vascular testing. Baseline data were collected for the multiple variables. The ulcerated limb had pretreatment perfusion and volume much greater than the control limb. A single treatment was administered at the periulcer site. The result was an increase in perfusion, measured by a laser Doppler, and increased skin temperature related to PRFS treatment. These preliminary findings suggest that, if the resting perfusion is marginally inadequate for healing, giving this small boost in perfusion may be sufficient to aid the healing of the ulcer. Parameters of the stimulation were 65 μsec, 600 pps, at peak power, with the head 1.5 cm above the surface of the ulcer.[42] Table 22–4 summarizes changes in tissue temperature after application of PSWD/PRFS.

Wound Healing Clinical Studies

The only studies on the efficacy of PSWD have been described under changes in tissue temperature and blood flow. There are no controlled clinical trials specifically investigating the efficacy of PSWD for wound healing. Several randomized, double-blind, controlled, and case study reports on PRFS efficacy for wound healing in animals and humans will be reviewed. A significant problem with the studies that was identified while reviewing the literature on electromagnetic radiation therapy for wound healing and related systemic factors was the inability to compare or combine results of these studies because, in most cases, the study results reported are subjective, observational, qualitative data, rather than quantitative, statistically analyzed data. For example, most of the studies reviewed did not have data about percentage of change in wound size per unit of time reported or data from which that information can be calculated. Systematic reviews of the literature are usually quantitative. No such reviews of the literature on use of PSWD, PRFS, or PEMF have been made. The data from clinical studies are presented by disease state and intervention used. Using the

Table 22–4 PSWD/PRFS Change in Tissue Temperature

Device	Area Stimulated	Pulse Rate	Intensity	Tissue Temperature
PSWD	Abdomen	2,400 pps	High dose	↑ 1.5°C at abdomen[34]
				↑ 2.2°C at foot[36]
PRFS	Abdomen	600 pps	Peak power	↑ 2.0°C at foot[20]
PRFS	Arm (normal subjects)	600 pps	Peak power	↑ 1.8°C[21]
PRFS	Foot (diabetics)	600 pps	Peak power	↑ 0.5°C[22]

levels of evidence and grades of recommendations quality ratings, PRFS would have levels II, III, IV, and V evidence and a recommendation grade of "B."

Researchers have branched out from investigating effect of PEMF on osteogenesis to look at its effects on soft tissue healing in animals and human subjects. However, stimulation periods using very low-frequency devices that demonstrate efficacy have been much longer than other treatment, up to 3 or 4 hours per day. Treatment at higher frequency and shorter duration had similar effects. Need for longer treatment period or higher frequency and shorter duration is probably due to the need to accumulate sufficient pulse charge in the tissues to have a biologic effect on the target tissues. There is a positive trend to the results for healing of venous ulcers. Although PEMF is not yet a typical application for wound healing, the results of the studies will be presented.

Additional quantitative studies are needed to support the limited evidence presented here. Several of the studies located were performed in countries outside of the United States, some were reported in peer-reviewed U.S. journals, and others were published in the journals of other countries. They are presented here for thoughtful consideration.

Animal Studies

Studies on nerve regeneration in rats treated with Diapulse (30 minutes daily for 3 weeks) showed that the surgical incisions healed in 4 days in the treated rats and in 7 days in the controls. Early recovery of mobility (weight bearing) occurred in the treated group (10 days), compared controls (21 days). Nerve conduction as evidence of tissue regeneration of peripheral nerves in the active treatment group was accelerated, and there were less scar tissue and fibrosis.[43]

Randomized controlled studies of the effects of PEMF on healing of cutaneous surgical wounds in animals (rats,[44–46] dogs,[47] rabbits[48]) demonstrate that PEMF significantly enhances wound epithelialization and provides significant short-term changes in other variables indicative of healing. In one study, PEMF was able to significantly reverse the impaired healing effect of corticosteroids.[44] In another study comparing PEMF and pulsed magnetic field (PMF) therapy

(17 Hz), there was better collagen alignment in repaired tendons in the PMF (17 Hz) group than in a group treated with PEMF, and the PMF group suppressed extravascular edema better during early inflammation.[49] PEMF at different intensity was tested on ligament wound healing. Tissue stimulated by PEMF showed earlier increase in capillaries and fibroblasts, with better organization of collagen than controls. Amongs three intensities tested, the group treated with 50 G had the best results consistently during the study period.[49]

Human Clinical Studies

Human clinical studies reported in this section have been sorted by etiology of the wounding and include: pressure ulcers, postsurgical wounds, and venous ulcers. Studies within each subsection are described in chronologic order, from oldest to most recent. Venous leg ulcer studies all have in common the use of PEMF. However, the parameters for treatment vary. Tables 22–5 (pressure ulcer clinical studies), 22–6 (postsurgical clinical studies), and 22–7 (venous ulcer clinical studies with PEMF) summarize the studies for each section.

Pressure Ulcers. Pressure as the wound etiology was the criteria for participation in the following clinical studies. Itoh et al[50] studied effect of PRFS on stage II partial-thickness and stage III full-thickness ulcers. Comorbidities included cerebrovascular accidents, multiple sclerosis, organic brain syndrome, spinal cord tumor, diabetes, spinal cord injury, and spinal stenosis. Conventional treatments of dressings and topical agents were continued. In all, 22 patients were included during the 9-month study. All ulcers healed. Stage II ulcers healed in 1–6 weeks (mean 2.33 weeks), and all stage III ulcers healed in 1–22 weeks (mean 8.85 weeks). Treatment was provided using the Diapulse PRFS device at a setting of 600-pps pulse frequency and a setting of 6 (peak power) for 30 minutes twice daily. Treatment sessions were scheduled at approximately 8-hour intervals.[50]

Wilson[51] reported on results of recalcitrant pressure ulcers treated with PRFS (Diapulse). Twenty-five stage II, 11 stage III, and 14 stage IV pressure ulcers affecting 32 patients were enrolled in the uncontrolled study. Duration of ulcers was reported to be up to 2 years. Individuals ages ranged from 77

Table 22-5 Pressure Ulcer Clinical Studies

Researcher	Itoh et al[50]	Wilson[51]	Salzberg et al[52]	Seaborne et al[53]
Type of study	Uncontrolled Unblinded Observational	Uncontrolled Observational	DB-RCT	B-RCT
Type of stimulator	PRFS (Diapulse)	PRFS (Diapulse)	PRFS (Diapulse)	ES Vs PEMF
Frequency	600 pps 65 μsec	Not stated	600 pps 65 μsec	20 pps ES 110 pps ES 20 pps PEMF 110 pps PEMF
Amplitude	Peak power	Not stated	Peak power	
Duration of stimulation	30 minutes BID	Not stated	30 minutes BID × 12 weeks	
Effect during Rx	All patients healed Stage II healed mean 2.33 weeks Mean size: 5.56 cm² ± 4.18 — Stage III healed mean 8.85 weeks Mean size: 8.78 cm² ± 11.96 — *Mean healing/week: Stage II 57% Stage III 8.87%	Initial increase in wound exudate (1–2 days) All wounds healed except 1	Stage II Active group: 84% healed at 1 week Median no. days to complete healing: 13.0 Placebo: 40% healed at 1 week Median no. days to complete healing: 31.5 — Stage III Ulcer area Active group: decreased average of 70.6% (*5.9%/week) Placebo: 20.7% (*1.7%/week)	All groups showed highly significant reduction in surface area size. No statistical difference between groups
Method of Measurement	Size measurement Photographs	Observational	Prospective Size measurement	Reduction in surface area size Pressure ulcers
Disease state tested and N	Pressure ulcers N = 9 stage II 13 stage III	Pressure ulcers N = 25 stage II 11 stage III 14 stage IV	Pressure ulcers/SCI N = 10 stage II 10 stage III	N = 20 (4 groups of 5)

* Percentage size change per week calculated from the study data.

Table 22–6 Postsurgical Clinical Studies

Researcher	Goldin et al[55]	Cameron[54]	Santiesteban and Grant[35]	Kaplan and Weinstock[56]	Aronofsky[57]	Comorosan et al[59]
Type of study	DB-RCT	Study I DB Controlled Study 2 Uncontrolled	RCT	DB-RCT	CT (nonrandomized, unblinded)	CT
Type of stimulator	PRFS (Diapulse)	PRFS (Diapulse)	PSWD	PRFS (Diapulse)	PRFS (Diapulse)	PRFS (Diapulse)
Frequency	400 pps/600 pps 65 μsec	400 pps 65 μsec	700 pps 95 μsec	400 pps/600 pps 65 μsec	600 pps 65 μsec	400 pps/600 pps 65 μsec
Amplitude	25.3 W/38 W	Med power (4)	120 W (max power setting)	Peak power (6) Med power (4)	Peak power	Peak power (6) Med power (4)
Duration of stimulation	10 min (hepatic) 20 min (wound) every 6 hours × 7 days	Study 1 20 min (hepatic) 20 min over wound BID × 4 days Study 2 Same as in study 1	30 min after surgery and 4 hrs later	Before surgery 10 min BID post 15 min to wound and 15 min epigastrium (hepatic)	Gr 1: 15 min 24 hr preop and 10 min just preop Postop: 24 hr, 48 hr, 72 hr / Gr 2: 10 min postop Postop: 24 hr, 48 hr, 72 hr / Gr 3: no PRFS	10 min (hepatic) 15 min (wound)
Rx Effect	90% or greater healing for 59% of tx group 29% healing for sham group Degree of pain Evaluated but not reported statistically significant results for healing	Study 1 Tx group little improvement for abdominal incision with regard to suture removal; all other had sutures removed on day 5 postop Study 2 Shorter hospital stay for tx group	Active group had 8 hr shorter length of hospital stay than controls and significantly less pain medication	Postop day 3: Severe/moderate edema Placebo 80% PRFS 58%	Inflammation and pain 72 hr post: Gr 1: None 75% Mod 20% High 3.% Gr 3: None 2% Mod 57% High 37% Pain: Gr 1: None 63% Mod 30% High 6.7% Gr 3: None 7% Mod 57% High 37%	Plasma; fibronectin concentrations ↑ on postop day 7 in tx group; lower than baseline in control group

continues

Table 22–6 continued

Researcher	Goldin et al[55]	Cameron[54]	Santiesteban and Grant[35]	Kaplan and Weinstock[56]	Aronofsky[57]	Comorosan et al[59]
Method of measurement		Retrospective review of medical records Subjective measurements	Retrospective review of medication and length of stay records	Likert-like scale grading for edema, erythema, and pain	Healing in group 1: 3–5 days postop Group 2: 5–7 days postop Group 3: 10–12 postop	Observation of inflammatory and infectious process and scar formation Lab measurements
Disease state tested and N	Split-thickness skin graft donor sites N = 29 active 38 sham	Heterogenous surgical patients Study 1 N = 100 Study 2 N = 81	Post podiatric foot surgery N = 25 active 25 control	Postsurgical podiatric patients	Oral surgery N = 90 (30/group)	Heterogenous surgical wounds N = 15 active 10 control

Source: Data from reference #'s 35, 54, 55, 56, 57, and 59.

Table 22–7 Venous Ulcer Clinical Studies with PEMF

Researcher	Ieran and Zaffuto[60]	Todd et al[62]	Duran et al[61]	Stiller et al[63]	Kenkre et al[64]
Type of study	DB CT	DB-RCT	Observational	DB-RCT	DB-RCT
Type of stimulator	PEMF	PEMF	PEMF	PEMF	PEMF
Frequency	75 Hz	5 Hz	Not available	25% duty cycle	600 Hz / 800 Hz
Amplitude	28 mT	Field strength 60	Not available	0.06 mV/cm / 22 Gauss	25 µT
Duration of stimulation	4 hr daily × 90 consecutive days	15 min twice weekly	15 min × 10 treatments	3 hr daily × 8 weeks	30 min 5×/week × 30 days
Effect during Rx	Healing of exp group Av 71 days 30% decrease in size of ulcers in controls	• Mean reduction of ulcer size: 7% was the same for treatment and control groups • Girth of affected leg: Active: decrease 2.77% Control: increase 1.16%	33% reduction in mean surface area	• Wound surface area: 47.1% decrease for active 48.7% increase for placebo • Wound depth decrease: 46% for active; 3.8% for placebo • Granulation tissue: quantity and quality 14.1% decrease in unhealthy granulation in active 0% decrease for placebo • Clinical Assessment based on 8-pt scale: 50% of active group healed or markedly improved 54% of placebo group rated worse 0% of active group rated worse	Wound surface area: Gr A Placebo ↓ 14.2% (20 days) ↓ 21.8% (30 days) Gr B1 600 Hz ↑ 28.15% (20 days) ↑ 76% (30 days) Gr B2 800 Hz ↓ 24.7% (20 days) ↓ 38% (30 days)
Effect post Rx	Healing continued post-tx period for the tx group 25% reoccurrence in tx group vs 50% in controls				4 week observation period. Day 50 B2 800 Hz group had significantly greater healing (63% vs 34% Gr A) + improved mobility
Method of Measurement	Healing	Reduction in surface area size	Reduction in surface area of ulcer	Wound characteristics	Reduction in surface area size Pain reduction; QOL
Disease state tested and N	Venous leg ulcers N = 44	Venous ulcers N = 19	Venous ulcers N = 18	Venous ulcers N = 31	Venous leg ulcers N = 19

Source: Data from reference #'s 60, 62, 61, 63, and 64.

to 88 years. All received conventional treatment for several weeks up to 2 years prior to inclusion in the PRFS study. Significant wound healing was observed on the most difficult ulcers in 3–7 days. Initially, wound exudate increased for 1–2 days, then ceased by the third day. All but one patient completely healed, and that individual's wound showed marked improvement before the patient expired from other causes.[45]

Salzberg et al[52] studied 20 patients with spinal cord injuries, 10 of whom had stage II pressure ulcers and 10 who had stage III pressure ulcers. The group was randomized to 10 treated and 10 sham-treated groups. Again, the device tested was the Diapulse. Although the study did not list the treatment parameters, an inquiry to the principal author and the Diapulse Corporation provided the information that the settings were 600-pps pulse frequency and 6, peak power. The treatment lasted for 30 minutes twice daily for 12 weeks or until the ulcers healed. Results were that the active treatment group with stage II ulcers had a shorter mean time to complete healing than did the control group (13.0 days versus 31.5 days). The stage III ulcers also healed faster than the controls, but the size of the group was very limited. The study authors' conclusion was that the treatment significantly improved healing.[52]

Seaborne et al[53] randomized 20 nonambulatory individuals with pressure ulcers of the trochanter and sacrum into four groups of five subjects each for a study with PSWD. Allocations were concealed and assessors blinded. Each group was treated with one of four different protocols. Protocols were electrostatic field (electrical stimulation) at 20 and 110 pps, and PEMF nonthermal at 20 and 110 pps. An ABAB repeated measures experimental design was used, with each treatment regimen lasting one calendar week. Multifactorial analysis showed highly significant reduction in the pressure ulcer surface area in all treatment groups, without significant difference between the groups.[53]

Postsurgical Wounds. Cameron[54] undertook three studies on the effect of PRFS (Diapulse) on postsurgical wound healing. Study 1 was a 100-patient, double-blind study of postsurgical patients, study 2 was an observational uncontrolled study of 81 postsurgical and orthopaedic patients, and study 3 was a 465-patient observational uncontrolled study of nonsurgical orthopedic patients. In studies 1 and 2, each patient was treated twice daily for 20 minutes over the liver and 20 minutes over the wound (400 pps, 4-inch penetration) for 4 days postoperatively. Patients in the third study were outpatients and were given the regimen twice daily 3 days a week for 2 weeks, then twice a day on Monday and Friday, then once weekly (twice a day). The PRFS was used as an adjunctive treatment to other standard methods of care. Outcomes were evaluated by the surgeon, who was asked to complete a questionnaire rating whether the patient's condition was the same, better, or worse, as compared with other patients in their experience. The groups analyzed by same, better, or worse showed no statistically significant difference in the treatment and control groups. There was a moderate reduction in length of hospital stay in the treatment group except in those with back surgery. The 81-patient study results demonstrated short hospital stays, despite the fact that some of the patients had osteomyelitis. The outpatient study of 465 patient results showed that acute trauma and inflammatory processes responded the best, but less than 20% were well within 3–4 weeks, which is what would have been expected normally. There also appeared to be no significant benefit from the PRFS treatment of chronic cases. There were some methodologic problems with the Cameron studies. Too much emphasis was placed on subjective clinical findings. Use of other treatment modalities along with the PRFS did not allow for an accurate evaluation of the PRFS stimulation, and absence of inferential statistics further compounds the methodologic problems associated with this study.[35]

A double-blind, controlled clinical trial by Goldin et al[55] used Diapulse PRFS to study the effects on healing and pain in medium-thickness split-skin grafts. The patients were randomized into two groups, 29 in the active treatment group and 38 in the sham treatment group. The parameter for the treatment group was peak output frequency, 400 pps. The average pulse was fixed at 65 μsec. Mean energy output was nonthermal, 25.3 W. Treatment was given preoperatively and postoperatively every 6 hours for 7 days. Two variables were evaluated: the stage of healing and the degree of pain during the healing phase. Healing rates on day 7 were 90% or greater healing for 59% of the treatment group and 29% of the sham-treated group. Mechanisms of healing are not clear. The theories to explain the results include increased blood flow and reduced incidence of edema. The stimulation of cells of repair and repolarization of the depolarized cell membranes of damaged cells that reversed the "injury potential" and the electrical field were thought to be the mechanisms of action.[55]

A double-blind randomized clinical evaluation of PRFS (Diapulse) following foot surgery in 100 patients was reported by Kaplan and Weinstock.[56] Average number of surgical procedures performed was nearly five. As in other studies with Diapulse, the protocol called for 400 pps over the epigastrium and 600 pps over the surgical site. Power level was at 4 for 15 minutes and 6 for 15 minutes to the respective areas. Treatment began before surgery with a 10-minute treatment. A Likert-type scale was used to grade the tissue for symptoms of edema, erythema, and pain. Results reported were statistically significant reduction in severe to moderate edema in the treatment group at the third postoperative day (80%) versus controls (58%); however, the data were reported descriptively.

Dental surgery procedures are often the cause of pain, edema, ecchymosis pressure, and disfigurement. In a nonrandomized controlled clinical trial, 90 dental surgery patients were divided into three groups of 30 each.[57] They were treated with Diapulse at 600 pps peak power preoperatively and postoperatively 72 hours, or just postoperatively 72 hours, or with placebo. Results reported were statistically significant absence of inflammation and pain at 72 hours postoperatively for the pre/post operative treatment group.

Children undergoing orchidoplexy were treated in a double-blind clinical trial. A total of 50 paired boys were involved in the trial. Circumferential measurements of the scrotum were made pre- and postsurgery and treatment of the scrotum, and photographs were taken. Repeat measurements and photographs were taken, with the objective of reducing subjective observation reports of edema and bruising. Treatment was with Diapulse at 500 pps and level 5 intensity for 20 minutes over the scrotum and at 500 pps level 4 intensity over the epigastrium for 10 minutes. The treatment regimen was repeated three times daily for the first 4 postoperative days. Matched pairs of boys were used, with one as the control. Investigators chose this operation as a model because of its classic edema and bruise formation. Results suggest that there was a trend toward improvement in edema formation, and resolution of posttraumatic bruising was found to be significantly accelerated.[58]

Another study of postsurgical wounds treated with Diapulse over the wound site and over the hepatic area was reported by Comorosan et al.[59] Fifteen patients were selected for treatment, and 10 served as the control group. The local application was at 600 pps at maximum power output for 20 minutes and the hepatic application at 400 pps at a power setting of 4 for 10 minutes. Treatment started on the second postoperative day and continued for 5 days. Comorosan et al[59] reported that the results of this protocol were evaluated by looking at the clinical criteria for wound healing, including the disappearance of edema, hematoma, and parietal seroma; the lack of inflammatory and infectious processes; the suppleness and presence or absence of keloids in the scar; and the degree of postoperative sensitivity. All clinical wound attributes evaluated showed clear-cut improvement. An additional analysis of the effects of the hepatic stimulation showed increased fibronectin levels in the treated patients and lower fibronectin levels in the controls. This is another measure of healing.

Venous Leg Ulcers. No clinical studies reporting results of PRFS or PSWD on treatment of venous ulcers were located, but the results of PEMF stimulation of venous ulcers have been reported in several studies. The nature of PEMF stimulation is that it is undetectable by the patient or the clinician. Ieran and Zaffuto[60] carried out a double-blind study of 44 patients with skin ulcers of venous origin using a coil electrode to generate a PEMF with 75 Hz and 2.8 mT intensity for 4 hours daily for 90 consecutive days. Healing was within 71 days, on average. Success was significantly higher in the experimental group, both on day 90 and in the follow-up period. Twenty-five percent of the patients in the experimental group and 50% in the control group experienced recurrence of the ulcer.[60]

A review of 18 cases by Duran et al with venous ulcers who were treated 10 times with PEMF, each session lasting 15 minutes, found that there was a significant reduction in the mean surface area of 33% by reepithelialization following treatment with PEMF.[61] A double-blind randomized controlled clinical trial of 19 patients with venous ulcers used a protocol applying PEMF two times weekly over a 5-week period.[62] Treatment parameters were field strength of 60, 5 Hz intensity duration of 15 minutes. Treatment was carried out by placing coils on either side of the ulcer over the wound dressings. Parameters measured were ulcer size, lower leg girth, degree of pain, and presence of infections. The findings were that there was no statistically relevant difference noted between the active and inactive treatment groups. However, there was a trend in favor of a decrease in ulcer size and lower leg girth in the active treatment group and no proliferation of bacterial populations. No effect was noted on report of pain. One patient in the study in the active treatment group had an initial ulcer size that was so large that it skewed the mean ulcer pre- and posttreatment areas. Removing this patient's ulcer from the study group reflected truer results that showed a trend toward improved healing but was not statistically significant (17.5% in active treatment versus 7.1% in sham treatment). Another study defect was the mean initial duration of the venous ulcer, which ranged from a mean 3.5 years for the active treatment group to a mean of 18.3 years for the sham group.[62] The results of this pilot study are inconclusive, due to the small sample size and lack of rigor in selecting the patients. Also, the duration and frequency of the treatment were perhaps too minimal to have a more statistically significant treatment effect.

Thirty-one patients were enrolled in a prospective, randomized, double-blind, placebo-controlled multicenter study by Stiller et al of venous ulcer healing to determine the efficacy of PEMF treatment.[63] Recalcitrant venous ulcers showed after 8 weeks that the active treatment group of 18 had a 47.7% decrease in wound surface area versus 42.3% for the placebo group of 13 ($p < .0002$). A global evaluation of the wounds indicated that 50% of the ulcers in the active group healed or markedly improved versus 0% in the placebo group. None of the active group of ulcers worsened versus worsening in 54% of the placebo group ($p < .001$). Likewise, there were statistically significant decreases in wound depth and pain intensity in the active group. Results were achieved using a portable home device that the patient or caregiver applied for 3 hours daily for 8 weeks or until the ulcer healed, if prior to 8 weeks. Treatment parameters were 3.5-msec pulse width, bidirectional delta B of approximately 22 G. The protocol was derived from the study of PEMF used effectively to treat nonunion fractures. Conclusion was that PEMF is a safe and effective nonsurgical therapy for recalcitrant venous leg ulcers. Perhaps the reason that the subjects in this trial did so much better than the earlier group was that the duration of the stimulation, given on a daily basis, allowed for enough pulse charge accumulation to reach the target tissues and produce a biologic effect.

Kenkre reported results of a study with 19 patients with venous leg ulcers enrolled in a prospective, randomized, double-blind controlled clinical trial.[64] Outcome measures were rate and scale of ulcer healing, changes in pain levels, quality of life, degree of mobility, side effect profile, and acceptability to patients and staff. Device used was the Elmedistraal electromagnetic device (available in the United Kingdom) that delivered perpendicular electric and magnet fields through a pulse generator, creating a frequency of 100, 600, and 800 Hz. The magnetic field produced was 25 µT. These parameters appear to be similar to PRFS, although the study is called *electromagnetic therapy*. Sixty-eight percent of the active treatment group achieved improvement in ulcer size, and 21% of those healed 100%. Reduction of pain levels was also statistically significant, despite the chronicity of the ulcers. Those treated at 800 Hz were found to have statistically greater healing and pain relief than those in the 600-Hz group or the control group at day 50. However, the treatment phase ended at day 30, and, at that time, the trend for healing was better in the control group and the 800-Hz group, compared with the 600-Hz group but reduction of pain scores was greatest in the 600-Hz group. In all three groups, some ulcers with long history of chronicity healed. It appears that, as in the Ieran study,[60] effects of the treatment continued after cessation of the treatment. Adverse effects reported were sensations of heat, tingling, pins and needles in the lower half of the limb, and headaches (unusual for two patients), but patients who experienced these sensations continued with the study. Psychosocial benefits of improved mobility and community activity were reported. These studies represent a small sample of patients with venous ulcers. More work is needed to establish treatment parameters and utility of this treatment for venous ulcers.

CHOOSING AN INTERVENTION: CLINICAL REASONING

Applying Theory and Science to Clinical Decision Making

The prior section reviewed and evaluated the scientific studies of the mechanisms and efficacy of PSWD, PRFS, and PEMF on components related to tissue repair and clini-

cal trials of wound healing. PSWD studies described the thermotherapy effects on the body. PSWD effects are attributed to changes to the circulatory system and the autonomic nervous system, whereas the effects of PRFS and PEMF are attributed to changes in the cellular activity of the tissues and mechanisms that control blood flow and edema that are not heat related. PRFS and PEMF studies reported effects on the cells' and the body's bioelectric systems. Both PSWD and PRFS devices showed that they can increase blood flow, which increases oxygen transport essential to support the metabolic demands of the tissues and to control infection. All three modes of electromagnetic stimulation affect pain and edema during the inflammatory phase. Because the treatment outcomes desired are edema free and pain free and these are benefited by enhanced circulation, it is logical to choose a treatment approach with demonstrated outcomes for these aspects of the inflammatory phase. If the circulatory effects desired require deep heating such as to raise core body temperature, then PSWD would be the first choice. A protocol for PSWD is given that is based on the circulatory effect on acute, subacute, and chronic inflammation. How PSWD or PRFS could effect ischemia reperfusion injury (see Chapter 2) would be a useful study. The effects on the inflammatory phase of healing are well established, but information about the effect on phases of healing following inflammation until closure is very limited. Enhanced circulation and oxygen are requirements of all the phases of healing, so continuation during all phases is appropriate. PRFS is the preferred choice if the objective is to stimulate the body's bioelectric system at the cellular level, over a dressing, cast, or bandage; to increase peripheral microcirculation; to prevent or minimize edema; to avoid and relieve pain; or if the patient has a medical history that rules out heat (see "Selection of Candidates" section, later). Treatment effects should be seen within hours for acute wounds and in 3–7 days from the start of the protocol for chronic wounds.[51–53] Reported effects include increased wound exudate for the first 1–3 days. Progress through the phases of healing should continue throughout the episode of care.

PSWD and PRFS are similar but not identical. They both are radio wave signals from the short wave spectrum. PSWD has the ability to heat tissue; PRFS does not. Both have reported increased perfusion and blood flow in normal adults. Only two studies by Santoro et al[26] and Mayrovitz and Larsen[42] looked at the effect of PSWD and PRFS on blood flow changes in individuals with PVD. Cellular changes are reported for stimulation with PRFS but not for PSWD, although that does not rule them out. They should be investigated. Exhibits 22–3 and 22–6 list the characteristics and rationale for selecting PSWD and PRFS. PEMF stimulators have distinctly different parameters than the radio frequency stimulators and are not found in PT clinics or wound clinics

Exhibit 22–6 Wound Classification and Characteristics

Wound Classification	PSWD/PRFS
Level of tissue disruption	Superficial, partial thickness, full thickness, subcutaneous and deep tissues
Etiologies/diagnostic groups	Burns, neuropathic ulcers, pressure ulcers, surgical wounds, vascular ulcers
Wound phases	*Inflammatory phase:* necrosis, exudate, edema, pain *Proliferative phase:* Granulation, contraction, collagen synthesis, angiogenesis *Epithelialization phase:* epidermal migration *Remodeling:* collagen organization

because they are typically used by orthopedic surgeons for nonunion fracture healing. Initially used for osteogenesis of nonunion fractures, PEMF has now been tested for soft tissue wound healing in venous ulcers with good outcomes in pilot studies. More research with PEMF is needed to standardize the methodology of treatment, to produce objective data about healing, and to verify results.

A limited number of studies have been reviewed, and the most recent are animal and PEMF studies. Although the results presented look promising, more new studies are needed to answer questions about the effects of PSWD, PRFS, and PEMF on wound healing. There remain many unknowns about mechanisms of action, and there is a need for improved study designs and reporting of the data with objective quantitative results. For example, the rate of healing has been identified as a predictor of healing outcome[65–69] and the trigger for referral for adjunctive therapy. The study data for most of the research projects testing these interventions did not provide quantitative information about the rate of healing of the control or the treatment groups, making it impossible to compare rate of healing between study intervention and controls and between other adjunctive therapy interventions. Except for two studies where the percentage of change could be derived from the data reported, the best available data are the percentage of patients that healed in a study and those that did not. One factor is evident from compiling the matrices of studies for different applications of PRFS: The Diapulse protocol, 400 pps, power level 4 over the epigastrium, and 600 pps peak power over the target tissue, has been followed consistently, with treatment efficacy reported for each application. Although many of the studies are reported as double-blind randomized controlled trials, it is also evident that many of the data reported are observational descriptive data, rather than quantitative.

To review, the studies looked at seven components that the PT should consider when selecting this intervention.

1. PRFS and PEMF stimulate cellular activity and cell permeability.

2. PRFS and PEMF affects the body's bioelectric system.
3. PSWD and PRFS affect edema formation but possibly through different processes.
4. PSWD, PRFS, and PEMF prevent or modulate pain.
5. PSWD and PRFS affect circulation, as measured by increased blood flow and $tcPO_2$, but through different processes.
6. PRFS promotes absorption of hematoma.
7. PSWD heats tissue; PRFS does not.

Patients who were treated in the clinical studies were postsurgery, including split-thickness skin grafts or posttrauma, and had pressure ulcers or venous ulcers. The wounds were either partial- or full-thickness tissue disruption, extending into deeper tissues (eg, stages II through IV pressure ulcers). None of the effects of treatment described are dependent on the medical diagnosis, the wound etiology, or the depth of the wound. However, wounds that are deeper, larger, or of long duration have been identified as slower to heal. Those wounds will probably heal faster with one of these adjunctive therapy interventions.

Selection of Candidates

A comprehensive patient history, systems review, and examination are very important in making a clinical decision to choose either PSWD or PRFS. Review the history and systems for information about sensation, circulation, edema, metal and electronic implants, acute osteomyelitis, cancer, and pregnancy. According to the manufacturer's labeling requirements, PSWD is contraindicated for all conditions for which heat is contraindicated. PSWD should not be used over areas of insensitivity that prevent the patient from reporting sensation of heating. One way to mitigate the heating effect of PSWD is to leave a greater air gap or more toweling between the applicator and the tissues. Check pulses and perform other visual examinations to detect circulatory deficits. If findings show diminished circulation, noninvasive vascular testing may be required. Do not use PSWD over ischemic tissue (eg, an ankle-brachial index of less than 0.8) because the body requires adequate perfusion to regulate tissue temperature. If circulatory perfusion is obstructed, it may not allow for the heat to dissipate and result in burning. However, consider indirect heating with PSWD or PRFS over the lumbar area or the abdomen that will produce reflex vasodilatation in areas remote from the site of heating, eg, the foot.[40,42] This is also suggested for patients with vasospasm.

Do not use PSWD over metal, including surgical metal hardware; foreign bodies, such as shrapnel, bullets, or metallic sutures; or intrauterine devices. The metal may become heated and reflect high levels of energy that will cause burns. Do not use PSWD if the patient has electronic implants or is connected to electrical or electronic equipment because the EMF of the PSWD may cause interference with these electronic devices. PSWD is contraindicated over any area where there is primary or metastatic malignant tissue growth or over organs or tissues containing high fluid volumes (eg, the heart, edematous extremity, and over the abdomen and lumbar areas during pregnancy). Treatment over an area with acute osteomyelitis without adequate drainage or before drainage has been established is contraindicated. A diagnosis of active tuberculosis would be a contraindication for PSWD. Review the patient's vital signs. Patients who are febrile should not be treated with additional heat; however, nonthermal PRFS could be used. Check the pharmacy history for blood-thinning medications and tendency for hemorrhage. Patients during the first 24–48 hours after traumatic injury should not be selected for treatment with PSWD because the treatment may increase bleeding and edema. Hemorrhaging tendency, including heavy menstruation, is a precaution for use of PSWD. Changing the parameters of the treatment would be indicated to modify the amount of heating. If wound examination findings are acute inflammation, direct heating should be avoided, but indirect heating could be useful (eg, inflammation in the foot can be treated with PSWD or PRFS applied over the abdomen or sacrum).

Examination for wound drainage is important. If PSWD is used, wounds that have a heavy amount of wound exudate would require special handling to absorb all of the moisture before treatment, to avoid burns.[2,70] Because treatment with PRFS is reported to increase wound exudate significantly for the first 1–3 days, management of the wound exudate should be planned by either changing the dressing more frequently or using more absorbent dressing materials. The surrounding skin may also require protection from maceration by application of a skin barrier.

Age should be considered when selecting candidates for PRFS or PSWD. Application of PRFS or PSWD over growth plates is probably not harmful because of the short duration of the wound healing treatment application, compared with the lengthy period of stimulation required to alter bone for-

mation in bone healing studies using pulsed EMFs. Children have growth plates until about 16 years of age, depending on race, sex, and the bone involved (use over immature bone is a listed contraindication). Children usually do not have the underlying comorbidities that lead to chronic wounding, but forced immobility due to pain would be detrimental to a child. Some of the most common wounds in children are burns. A child with burn wounds would benefit from PRFS early intervention to normalize skin enzymes and to eliminate edema and pain, resulting in less scarring and quicker return to play and school activities. Sometimes, the risk is insignificant, compared with the benefit. For example, children were treated for subdural hematoma with PRFS without complications and had more rapid resolution of edema and hematoma than did controls, who were not treated.[33] If the benefit of accelerated wound healing outweighs the small risk of interference with a bone plate, prudent judgment should be used. Heat applications must always be applied carefully to the elderly because of impairments of circulatory system functions and changes in sensory perceptions. Exhibit 22–7 shows a list of contraindications, warnings, and cautions to be taken when using PSWD and PRFS equipment.

PRFS has fewer precautions and contraindications because it does not heat tissues. Key information to check in the medical history is the presence of electronic or metal implants (including intrauterine devices), osteomyelitis, cancer, or pregnancy. Avoid using this intervention in the presence of any of these conditions.[2,71] Metals reflect radio frequency energy common to both PSWD and PRFS, so application over metal implants will reflect the energy back into the tissues, creating more intense energy levels in the tissues over the implant than usual, or the energy may be blocked from reaching the target tissues. Location of the metal should guide the PT to consider an alternative method of application, such as moving the applicator head above or below the area of metal (whichever is closest to the wound) to treat the surrounding wound tissues. Contrary to the recommendation to wait until the acute hemorrhaging or acute inflammation have passed to treat with PSWD, PRFS should be applied early after wounding. As described, studies have shown that application of PRFS during the first 72 hours reduces pain, posttraumatic edema, and, in burn patients, the enzymes associated with trauma.

Safety Issues

PSWD

Contact with any metal (eg, jewelry, zippers, brassiere fasteners, and brassiere underwires) should be avoided when using PSWD because of the risk of burns and distortion of the EMF is possible from metal objects placed near the

Exhibit 22–7 FDA Contraindications, Warnings, and Cautions for PSWD and PRFS

PSWD	*PRFS*
• Do not treat over ischemic tissue with inadequate blood flow • Do not treat over or near metallic implants • Do not use with patients with cardiac pacemakers • Do not treat in any region where presence of primary or metastatic malignant growth is known or suspected • Do not treat over immature bone • Do not treat over acute osteomyelitis without adequate drainage or before adequate drainage has been established • Do not treat patients who have a tendency to hemorrhage (including menses) • Do not treat over pelvic or abdominal region or lower back during pregnancy • Do not treat transcerebrally • Do not use over anesthetized areas • Avoid situations that could concentrate the field, including moist dressings, perspiration, adhesives • Use caution when treating patients with heat sensitivity • Use caution when treating patients with inflammatory processes	• Do not use as a substitute for treatment of internal organs • Do not use over metal implants • Do not use with patients with cardiac pacemakers • Do not use with patients who are pregnant • Do not treat over immature bone

Source: Data from International Medical Electronics, *Magnatherm® Model 1000 Instruction Manual* and Electropharmacology, *MRT® sofPulse™ User's Manual.*

cables. Also avoid contact with metal furniture or parts (eg, mattress springs). PSWD should not be used over synthetic materials that may melt and cause burns.[1] Electronic devices (eg, hearing aids, watches) should not be worn during treatment with these devices because the EMF may cause disruption of the device. Hearing aids may produce annoying noise feedback.

PRFS

Electronic devices (eg, hearing aids, watches) should not be worn during treatment with PRFS devices for the same reasons cited above. Do not administer PRFS directly over metal (eg, jewelry, zippers) because the energy will be reflected and not reach the target tissues.

Personnel Safety

Many sources of EMFs are present in the environment, and most do not affect the human body. By the nature of the PSWD and PRFS devices described in this chapter, the EMFs do not pass 100% of the energy into the tissues being treated. Some energy is dissipated into the area close to the equipment. Operators and persons close to the equipment will absorb a small amount of EMFs. EMFs from PSWD at distances of 0.5 m from the cables and 0.2 m from inductive applicators are low at low and medium pulse settings.

A study of PT work habits found that most remain at least 1 m from the applicator and 0.5 m from the cables during the operation of PSWD equipment. At those distances, there is little danger of excess absorption.[72] However, some older-model PSWDs may not have shielded cables. The device should be checked for leakage of EMF energy. For personnel working with this equipment who have electronic implants, however, it would be prudent not to be exposed to the EMF because the stray radiation can affect the operation of those devices. The same holds true for other patients or family members occupying the same treatment areas. A timer is usually part of the equipment, and it will turn the equipment off automatically, but if the patient needs to be assisted during the treatment, the staff member can approach the console without standing close to the cables. Several studies have attempted to measure the effects of EMFs on personnel working in areas where frequent exposure to SWD occurs. An epidemiologic study looked at the risk of birth defects, perinatal deaths, and late spontaneous abortions affecting fetuses of female therapists working with SWD. The result of this retrospective study showed that the risk of a miscarriage was not associated with reported use of SWD.[73] Patients, except as mentioned, have no measurable risk from the EMF associated with this equipment, and the benefits probably outweigh any negative effects.

EQUIPMENT

Regulatory Approval

The PSWD generators are classified as Class II short wave diathermy devices, used for therapeutic deep heating for purposes of treatment of pain, muscle spasms, and joint contractures. PRFS generators are classified as Class III short wave diathermy for all other uses (except treatment of malignancy), intended to treat medical conditions by means other than deep heating as nonthermal units, and are sold to control pain and edema.[74] State licensing agencies regulate what is physical therapy. Medicare guidelines state that the use of diathermy should always be by or under the supervision of a licensed PT. Exhibit 22–7 lists FDA contraindications, and Exhibit 22–8 lists FDA indications.

Devices

Pulsed Short Wave Diathermy

A PSWD generator uses a coil mounted within a case (called a *head*) as the radiating element. This coil is driven by a crystal-controlled amplifier contained within the main chassis of the unit. The output of this head is an EMF with a radio frequency of 27.12 MHz. The head is mounted on a movable, adjustable arm. Depending on the unit design, the head may be rectangular or round. Some devices allow the frequency to be delivered continuously or pulsed. The range of heating and nonthermal effects will depend on the pulse rate and duration. A PSWD device that can be operated at a broad range of pulse rates and pulse durations will have the most potential clinical applications. Heating effects are the principal action of the device at high pulse rates of long duration, and nonthermal effects are achieved at the low pulse rates and short duration. At the nonthermal settings, the PSWD may have effects equivalent to those of the PRFS devices, which are limited to this range. PSWD devices are on the market, including the Magnatherm (International Medical Electronics, Kansas City, MO), the Curapulse (Enraf Nonius, Delft, The Netherlands and Henley International, Sugarland, TX), and Megapulse (Electo-Medical Supplies, Ltd, UK and PTI Corporation, Topeka, KS). They are considered equivalent; however, there are differences in available pulse rates, pulse duration, and average outputs. The Curapulse method of creating the electric and magnetic fields uses a different technology than do the other devices described. Each field is delivered in isolation by means of the condenser electrodes and a monode head, and transformation to an EMF occurs within the body tissue. Curapulse is available with either one or two electrodes that can be operated with different protocols. For example, the pulse rate and the duration of treatment must remain constant for both

Exhibit 22–8 FDA Indications

PSWD	PRFS
Improved blood flow	Relief of pain and edema
Improved oxygenation	
Increased metabolic rate	
Inflammatory conditions	
Relief of pain and edema	

heads, but the other parameters can be set separately for each. Two models are available: (1) Model 670 allows for variation of pulse duration from 65 to 400 μsec, adjustable in seven steps, and an adjustment of frequency from 26 to 400 Hz, adjustable in 10 steps, that can be used for both thermal and nonthermal effects; (2) Model 970 has a fixed pulse duration of 400 μsec and a frequency of 15–200 pps, and is considered a thermal device. Maximum outputs are also different. Table 22–8 shows the available parameters for these different models.

The Megapulse pulse width settings range from 25 to 400 μsec. Three pulse modes are offered with the device on: off cycles consisting of one-third on time and two-thirds off time; two-thirds on time and one-third off time; and continuous. The pulse duration and frequency can be changed during those three modes. When longer on time and shorter off time are selected, there will be more thermal effects. Shorter on and longer off time will be less thermal, and the effects will be stimulation of the cells, rather than heating. It can be used like a PSWD or PRFS device. The wide range of settings may be confusing to new users, but they enhance the choice and variety of applications and conditions that can be treated.

The Magnatherm SSP unit is designed so that each of the two round inductive treatment heads can be set at the same or different settings to deliver controlled dosages for individualized treatment effects. Each is controlled and monitored from its own panel. There is a full range of pulse rates to choose from (see Figure 22–5). The unit is designed to be used on a cart for mobility or to be lifted off the cart and packed in its own carrying case for portability. However, the 25-pound weight would be a real workout for a therapist carrying it from car to house several times a day. A wheeled attachment would facilitate this application.

Research Wisdom: *Pattern of Treatment Effect*

The pattern of treatment effect for PSWD and PRFS stimulators is in the form of the shape and size of the applicator head.

Table 22–8 Typical Equipment Parameters

Device	Operating Frequency (MHz)	Pulse Rates (pps)	Pulse Widths (μsec)	Generated Power (W)
Magnatherm	27.12	700–7,000	95 Fixed	0.2–100% (1,000 peak)
Megapulse	27.12	50–800	20–400	150 Peak, 5–40 average
Nonthermal mode		< 200	< 200	
Thermal mode		> 200	> 100	
Curapulse				
Model 970	27.12	15–200	400 Fixed	1,000 Peak, 80 average
Model 670	27.12	26–400	65–400	200 Peak, 32 average
Diapulse	27.12	80–600	65 Fixed	293–975 Peak, 1.5–38 average
MRT SofPulse, model 912	27.12	80–600	65 Fixed	174–373

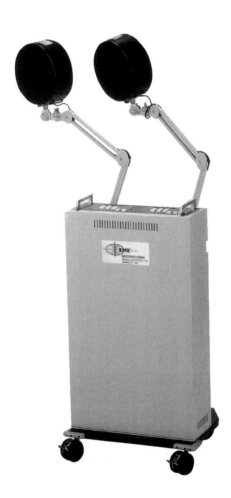

Figure 22–5 Shortwarp diathermy unit (Magnatherm SSP). Courtesy of Meditea Electromedica, Buenos Aires, Argentina.

Pulsed Radio Frequency Stimulators

PRFS generators, like PSWD generators, consist of a radiating treatment head or applicator and an electronic console. The output of this head is also an EMF with a radio frequency of 27.12 MHz. The Diapulse has a pulse length of 65 μsec and an interpulse interval that can be varied from 12.4 to 1.6 msec by altering the pulse frequency. This allows ample time for heat to be dissipated.[75] Electromagnetic effects at the cellular level are the actions to expect from these devices, not heating.[2] The Diapulse has a stronger magnetic field and a weaker electrical field, and both are emitted simultaneously.[76] The frequency can be set in six steps (80, 120, 200, 300, 400, 500 pps) in conjunction with six intensity settings. Peak power output is 38 W delivered to the tissues. The devices on the market, which are deemed by the FDA as equivalents, include the Diapulse (Diapulse Corporation of America, Great Neck, NY) and the MRT SofPulse (AA Northvale Association, Northvale, NJ).

PROCEDURES

Protocols

Protocols are established to achieve a predictable outcome. PSWD is a thermal agent and, as such, has predictable effects on tissue temperature and blood flow. Normal resting body temperature is between 36.3° C and 37.5° C. PSWD at thermal levels has the ability to raise deep tissue temperature to 45° C. Vigorous heating is defined as raising tissue temperature to between 40° C and 45° C.[21] This is estimated to be the maximum safe upper limit to raise tissue temperature and corresponds to the pain threshold of the skin. Maintaining the tissue temperature of 45° C for a sufficiently long period will result in irreversible tissue damage. Three factors influence the maximum tissue temperature reached: the square of the intensity, the tissue impedance, and the length of time the tissue is heated. Also, tissue perfusion determines how quickly the blood flow will dissipate the heat.[2] The observable effect of heating is hyperemia due to increased blood flow. This is a mild inflammatory response, initiating the biologic cascade associated with the process of inflammation (see Chapter 2). Vasodilatation occurs, along with increased capillary hydrostatic pressure and vessel permeability. This promotes movement of fluid from the vessels into the interstitial spaces. Symptoms associated with this process are *edema*, *pain*, and *warmth*. Raising the tissue temperature within a 5- to 15-minute period will raise the tissue temperature to the maximum range. The resulting vasodilatation will produce a marked increase in blood flow that will then dissipate the heat and decrease the temperature by several degrees. A total exposure period of 20–30 minutes is described in the literature as the required time for the optimal therapeutic benefits of heating to occur. Studies show that this can be achieved with inductive coupling using PSWD while avoiding excessive heating of the superficial tissues and subcutaneous fat.[1] Tissue heating below 40° C temperature is considered mild.[17]

PRFS protocols used in the reported studies have a single set of parameters, regardless of whether perfusion, reduction of edema or pain, or tissue healing was the outcome. It is not currently known, however, what may be the optimal parameters of dosage that affect different levels of tissues at different stages of repair. This determination requires further research. In the current situation, the experimental protocols have validity and reliability, and can be used safely. These are listed below, in the "Setup for Treatment" sections.

Expected Outcomes

A change in temperature is not a functional outcome, just as a change in range of motion is not a functional outcome because in neither case are the effects of the measured change related to a change in an impairment. The change in temperature measures the change in tissue perfusion after the treatment. How the tissue responds functionally to the enhanced perfusion is the functional outcome (eg, progression to the proliferative phase—red, neovascularized granulation tissue). The sequence of predictable biologic events occurs during the process of healing. This sequence progresses from an initial phase of healing (inflammatory) to a later phase of healing (epithelialization or contraction). The steps of the progression are outcome measures for measuring and predicting wound healing. See Chapter 1 for possible

wound outcomes and prognoses. The expected outcome for a chronic wound treated with a physical agent such as PSWD or PRFS should progress from one phase to the next phase in a 2- to 4-week period. Research evidence can be used as a guide for the mean time for healing. For example, in two pressure ulcer studies using PRFS (Diapulse),[50,52] closure was reported at a rate of 8.7% and 5.9% per week for stage III pressure ulcers. The healing time will be at the end of the range for patients with the factors that affect healing, such as older age, immobility, comorbidities, long duration of wound, large wound size, and the depth of tissue involvement. If the reassessment does not confirm the expected outcomes, treatment must change. Change can be a change in protocol (eg, mild heating changed to vigorous heating), an increased length of treatment time, a change in frequency from three times per week to daily, or a change in dressing or topical agent. Any or all of the above are ways to consider changing the treatment to affect the wound status and reach a predictable outcome. Below are expected outcomes for the protocols for both PSWD and PRFS.

Wound Healing Phase Diagnosis: Acute or Chronic Inflammation

Expected Outcome Protocol for Acute or Chronic Inflammation

- Hyperemia: change in skin color to red, blue, or purplish, depending on color of surrounding skin
- Temperature: increased temperature, due to increased tissue perfusion
- Edema: resolution or prevention and restoration of tissue turgor
- Wound progression to the proliferative phase

Wound Healing Phase Diagnosis: Subacute Inflammation

Expected Outcome Protocol for Subacute Inflammation

- Skin color: change to that of surrounding skin
- Temperature: change to that of adjacent tissues or same area on corresponding opposite side of the body
- Edema: free
- Necrosis: free
- Wound progression to the proliferative phase

Magnatherm PSWD Protocol

The protocol used by Sussman and reported in Case Study 1 at the end of this chapter was for treatment of a patient with a pressure ulcer, and parameters were proposed by the manufacturer (International Medical Electronics) of the Magnatherm. This protocol called for a short initial phase (5 minutes) of heating at a high pulse rate and peak power output, followed by a reduction in the pulse rate to the lowest level, which also reduced the heating effect (see Table 22–11). The lower pulse rate was maintained for 25 minutes. The total treatment time was 30 minutes. The rationale was that the effects of the high-dose heating treatment would rapidly raise the tissue temperature and cause vasodilatation. The lower pulse rate produced mild heating, and the longer interpulse interval would allow for heat dissipation. Additional rationale for this setting was that this would sustain the vasodilatation effects of the high heating phase throughout the duration of the treatment.

Change Moist Dressing during PSWD Treatment

According to the PSWD instruction manual, it is necessary to remove wound dressings before PSWD.[70] To avoid burns of wound tissue during treatment with PSWD, replace any moist wound dressing with a dry sterile gauze pad. Check the gauze pad during the treatment when there is much wound exudate observed during the setup. If dressing is moist, remove and replace it with another dry gauze.

There are anecdotal clinical reports that the use of PSWD over wound dressings does not have harmful effects. Also, clinical practice for wound management has changed since the PSWD instruction cautions were first issued in 1981. Further evaluation of the effects of PSWD on wound fluids and dressing adhesives is needed to update this position.

Table 22–9 PSWD Power, Effects, and Application

Dose	Level	Effect	Phase of Healing
I (¼ power)	Lowest	Below sensation of heat	Acute inflammation
II (½ power)	Low	Mild heat sensation	Subacute, resolving inflammation
III (¾ power)	Medium	Moderate, comfortable heat sensation	Subacute, resolving inflammation
IV (full power)	Heavy	Vigorous heating, well tolerated; reduce to just below maximum tolerance	Chronic conditions

Source: Reprinted with permission from L. Kloth and M. Ziskin, Diathermy and Pulsed Radio Frequency Radiation, in *Thermal Agents in Rehabilitation*, 3rd ed, S. Michlovitz, ed., © 1996, F.A. Davis Company Publishers.

Table 22–10 PSWD Dosage, Duration, and Outcomes

Dose	Duration*	Outcome
I	15 min one or two times daily for 1–2 weeks	Temperature ↑ 37.5–38.5°C
II	15 min daily for 1–2 weeks	Temperature ↑ 38.5–40.0°C
III	15–30 min daily for 1–2 weeks	Temperature ↑ 40.0–42.0°C
IV	15–30 min daily or two times per week for 1 week to 1 month	Temperature ↑ 42.0–44.0°C

*Continue for 2 weeks. If outcomes are achieved through the phases of healing, continue.

Source: Reprinted with permission from L. Kloth and M. Ziskin, Diathermy and Pulsed Radio Frequency Radiation, in *Thermal Agents in Rehabilitation*, 3rd ed, S. Michlovitz, ed., © 1996, F.A. Davis Company Publishers.

Table 22–11 Magnatherm Protocol Used by Sussman for Case Study 1

Magnatherm Settings	Duration	Effect
PR 5,000 pps power level 12 (thermal)	5 min	Vigorous heating—warm up
PR 700 pps power level 12 (nonthermal)	25 min	No perceived sensation of heat

Setup for Treatment with Pulsed Short Wave Diathermy

1. Explain the procedure to the patient and caregiver.
2. Inspect and remove all metal items, including jewelry, wristwatches, brassieres with metal fasteners, and clothing with zippers.
3. Remove hearing aids and external electronic devices.
4. Place the patient on a nonmetal surface.
5. Avoid contact with synthetic materials, including pillows.
6. Remove clothing from body area.
7. Position the patient for comfort in a position that can be maintained for 30 minutes.
8. Remove the wound dressing and absorb excess exudate; cover with dry gauze.
9. Cleanse the wound of debris and metallic and petrolatum-based products; blot dry.
10. Cover the wound and surrounding skin with a ½-inch thickness of toweling.
11. Cover the drum with a disposable surgical head cap or terry cloth towel for hygiene.
12. Place the drum 0.5–1 cm above the terry cloth.
13. Set the protocol and treatment duration. Start.

Patient Monitoring

- Never leave a patient who is confused or disoriented alone and unsupervised while receiving treatment.
- When using PSWD, remember that pain is a warning that excessive heating is occurring. Give the patient a call light and pay immediate attention to a call. Reduce power level. Increase air space, either by positioning the drum farther from the target tissue or by layering towels between the drum and the body area.
- Check skin before application for unguents that may have been applied (eg, oil of wintergreen, Ben-Gay); clean thoroughly, and dry.

Aftercare for Pulsed Short Wave Diathermy

Because the dressing is always removed before this treatment, it is important that the wound be dressed with the appropriate dressing as soon as possible after conclusion of the treatment. A dressing should be selected that will match the frequency of the PSWD treatment and other components of the wound healing. Rapid redressing of the wound safeguards against wound contamination and desiccation of the wound tissues, sustains the warmth of the wound that has occurred from the increased profusion, and promotes optimal cell mitosis.

Clinical Wisdom: *Tissue Perfusion*

When tissue perfusion is the treatment effect, the wound will be warmed, and the cells will divide and proliferate faster in the warm environment. Therefore, dress the wound *immediately after* PSWD and *before* PRFS.

Clinical Wisdom: *PSWD (Magnatherm) for Venous Disease*

Patients with venous disease do not tolerate high heating and subsequent effects of vasodilatation. Two phases are used. For the first phase of treatment, energy is adjusted to deliver a pulse rate of 1,600 pps for 15 minutes. This is followed by a second phase at 700 pps for a 15-minute period. Power levels are kept at power level 12.[77]

Pulsed Radio Frequency Stimulation Protocol

The protocol suggested for PRFS is based on the parameters used in the several controlled clinical trials with the Diapulse, described earlier. These are nonthermal parameters but have a demonstrated ability to enhance microvascular tissue perfusion. Mechanisms of action may be different. Consider this therapy intervention if microvascular perfusion is desired and/or heating is contraindicated, if wound dressing is to be left intact during the treatment, or if the wound is inside a cast and is painful.

Setup Treatment with Pulsed Radio Frequency Stimulation

1. Explain the procedure to the patient and caregiver.
2. Position the patient for comfort, with the treatment site accessible, so that it can be maintained for 30 minutes.
3. Cover the drum with a disposable surgical head cap or terry cloth towel for hygiene.
4. Place the drum 0.5–1 cm above the terry cloth over the wound site.
5. Leave the dressings in place unless there is strike-through or it is time to change dressing.
6. Set the protocol and treatment duration. Start.

Protocol for PRFS

Pulse rate: 600 pps
Intensity: peak power
Duration: 30–60 minutes
Frequency: twice daily or every day three to seven times per week

Adjunctive Treatments

PSWD and PRFS can be used in conjunction with the other adjunctive treatments, such as whirlpool or pulsatile lavage with suction (PLS). Either whirlpool or PLS would be useful to cleanse the wound, soften necrotic tissue, and flush out wound debris and exudate. The combination of therapies could enhance results. It may be preferable to treat with PSWD or PRFS immediately after the other interventions to keep the wound temperature from declining. Another choice could be to treat the wound with ultraviolet light for bactericidal effects or to initiate a mild inflammatory process, then follow with either PSWD or PRFS to enhance the circulation. Benefits of multiple treatments with different physical agents and electrotherapeutic modalities have not been proven. The PT should assess whether the addition of another of these interventions is needed and support it with a rationale. This is an area that merits further research for best utilization management of services and best efficacy for the patient.

Another adjunctive treatment with well-established effect on circulation is exercise. Exercise following PSWD or PRFS would use the muscle pump for exchange of nutrients and oxygen brought to the tissue by the PSWD or PRFS treatment and removal of waste products, as well as to help dissipate the effects of heating and avoid burning. Exercise encourages movement of fluids from the venous system into the lymphatics and is a way to avoid stasis in the area of heating. For those patients who are unable to exercise actively, assisted or passive range of motion would encourage change in fluid dynamics in the affected area. Therapeutic position-ing should also be considered as an adjunctive treatment because improper positioning may have blood flowing away from the target tissues or applying pressure to the area that is to be perfused.

SELF-CARE TEACHING GUIDELINES

Both PSWD and PRFS labels state "federal law restricts the sale and use of this equipment to a licensed health practitioner."[32,71] However, the manufacturers and distributors of the PRFS nonthermal devices report that patients are using them as home therapy units under physician prescription. MRT SofPulse comes in a portable home care model. PSWD should not be used unsupervised because of the hazard potential.

DOCUMENTATION

The functional outcome report (FOR) described in Chapter 1 is an accepted method to meet Medicare and third-party payer guidelines for documentation of the need for physical therapy intervention for wound healing. The two cases presented as examples of the use of PSWD and PRFS are documented by using the FOR method. A sample form and case are found in Chapter 1. Also, try to apply the method to wound cases in the clinic.[78] Data collected about treatment outcomes in a systematic manner can be of great value to report the success of the therapy and to predict outcomes.

Discussion

The use of PSWD was selected to bring enhanced perfusion to the left leg. Care had to be taken to position the applicator head at a distance away from the metal internal fixation devices at the hip. The patient was not a candidate for whirlpool to soften the eschar because the hip deformity made it difficult to position her in the whirlpool. Electrical stimulation was ruled out because more vigorous perfusion to the foot was desired. Debridement by several methods was selected for the fastest relief of the wound bioburden (see Chapter 8). Immobility limits blood flow to the area and increases risk of ischemia from pressure. Therapeutic positioning for pressure elimination was essential to avoid repetitive trauma from pressure to the wounded areas and to allow the wound to heal (see Chapter 16).

REVIEW QUESTIONS

1. Discuss how PRFS differs from electrical stimulation. Should PRFS and electrical stimulation be considered equivalent modalities? Provide rationale.
2. Describe the benefits of using PRFS.

Case Study: *Pressure Ulcer Treated with Pulsed Short Wave Diathermy*

Patient ID: S.D. Age: 86

Functional Outcome Report: Initial Assessment

Reason for Referral

The patient is minimally mobile and has developed a pressure ulcer on the left heel and fifth metatarsal head. She is alert but lacks the ability to reposition. Autolytic debridement with occlusive dressing has not been successful.

Medical History and Systems Review

The patient experienced a left fractured hip with open reduction and internal fixation 3 years ago. She never regained the ability to ambulate after the hip fracture. She also has a history of multiple cerebrovascular accidents that shows that her circulatory system is impaired. She is placed in a wheelchair for a few hours a day. She takes food orally and eats most of the diet offered. There has been no recent loss of weight. She is incontinent of bowel and bladder and has a Foley catheter in place.

Evaluation

The patient has an impaired healing response that is due to impairment of the circulatory and musculoskeletal system. This functional loss causes the inability to progress through the phases of repair without intervention. The patient has improvement potential for the wounds but will remain at risk for future pressure ulceration. The following examinations are indicated:

- Joint integrity
- Mobility
- Circulatory function
- Integumentary system: surrounding skin and wound

Examination Data

Joint Integrity. The patient has a fixed varus deformity of the leg, and no active mobility of the left hip joint exists. There is minimal mobility of the left knee, and a knee flexion contracture at 75° limits function of the left leg. The hip and knee deformities have created a positioning problem, with the left ankle crossing over the right leg and the lateral aspect of the foot, from toes to heel, in a position that is subject to pressure. Ankle joint mobility is also severely impaired.

Mobility. The patient is immobile. She does not attempt to self-reposition in either bed or wheelchair.

Circulation. There is edema of the left foot, extending to the ankle. The foot is warm (98.6° F), with 1+ palpable pulses. No dependent rubor is noted when the patient is seated in a wheelchair.

Integumentary System. There is an ulcer on the left lateral heel; it has eschar necrosis, inflammation signs of changes in skin color (red), warmth (98.6° F), and local edema. The whole foot to the ankle is edematous. There is an ulcer on the left fifth metatarsal head with eschar necrosis, signs of mild inflammation, no pain, changes in skin color (red), and warmth (98.6° F) and edema. It is 6.9 cm². (See *Color Plates 66* and *67* for pictures of the wounds.)

Functional Diagnosis

- Undue susceptibility to pressure ulceration on the feet
- Both wounds chronic inflammatory phase
- Initial associated impairment status eschar

Need for Skilled Services: The Therapy Problem

The patient has failed to respond to interventions with dressing changes for the last 2 weeks. She now requires debridement of the eschar from both wounds to determine the extent of tissue impairment and to initiate the healing process; PSWD to enhance circulation to the foot, facilitate debridement, and restart the process of repair; and therapeutic positioning to avoid trauma from pressure to the foot.

Targeted Outcomes

- The wound bed will be clean.
- There will be an enhanced inflammatory response: erythema, edema, and warmth.
- The patient will progress through the phases of healing from inflammation to epithelialization.
- The patient will be properly positioned to remove pressure from the left foot.

Treatment Plan

Debridement Strategy

Score eschar and use an enzymatic debriding agent and occlusion for autolysis. Sharply debride when eschar is softened. Apply PSWD for perfusion.

continues

Case Study continued

Prognosis. Clean wound bed; *due date:* 21 days.

PSWD

Apply PSWD for increased circulation to the foot, using the protocol of one applicator over the abdomen and the second applicator over the plantar surface of the foot. Use the device at the vigorous heating setting for 5 minutes, followed by mild heating (nonthermal) for 25 minutes.

Prognosis

- Acute inflammation; *due date:* 14 days.
- Progression through phases to closure; *due date:* 8 weeks.

Frequency. Apply PSWD daily seven times per week, twice daily for 30 minutes.

Therapeutic Positioning

Use therapeutic positioning with pillows to keep pressure from the left foot; instruct nurses' aides in proper positioning.

Discharge Outcome

The wound on the fifth metatarsal head was healed by day 15. The wound on left heel had full-thickness skin loss after removal of eschar and necrotic tissue. The wound had a clean bed by week 4. Closure was achieved by week 7. (See *Color Plate 68.*)

3. Explain how PRFS and PSWD differ and when you would choose each.
4. Describe the putative effects of PRFS. Is this supported by evidence?

5. What treatment outcomes would you expect from PSWD? From PRFS?

REFERENCES

1. Guy A, Lehmann J, Stonebridge J. Therapeutic applications of electromagnetic power. *Proc IEEE.* January 1974:55–75.
2. Kloth L, Ziskin M. Diathermy and pulsed radio frequency radiation. In: Michlovitz SL, ed. *Thermal Agents in Rehabilitation.* Philadelphia: FA Davis; 1996:213–254.
3. Markov MS, Pilla A. Electromagnetic field stimulation of soft tissues: pulsed radio frequency treatment of postoperative pain and edema. *Wounds.* 1995;7(4):143–151.
4. Kellogg R. Magnetotherapy: potential clinical and therapeutic applications. In: Nelson R, Currier D, eds. *Clinical Electrotherapy.* Norwalk, CT: Appleton & Lange; 1991:390–391.
5. Skerry TM, Pead MJ, Lanyon LE. Modulation of bone loss during disuse by pulsed electromagnetic fields. *J Ortho Res.* 1991;7:600–608.
6. Blumlein H, McDaniel J. Effect of the magnetic field component of the Kraus-Lechner method on the healing of experimental nonunion in dogs. In: Burny F, Herbst E, Hinsenkamp M, eds. *Electric Stimulation of Bone Growth and Repair.* New York: Springer-Verlag; 1978:35–46.
7. Herber H. Cordey J, Perren SM. Influence of magnetic fields on growth and regeneration in organ culture. In: Burny F, Herbst E, Hinsenkamp M, eds. *Electric Stimulation of Bone Growth and Repair.* New York: Springer-Verlag; 1978:35–40.
8. Mooney V. A randomized double-blind prospective study of efficacy of pulsed electromagnetic fields for interbody lumbar fusion. *Spine.* 1990;15:708–712.
9. Sharrard WJ. Double blind trials of pulsed electromagnetic fields of delayed union of tibial fractures. *J Bone Joint Surg.* 1990;72-B:347–355.
10. Skerry TM, Pead MJ, Lanyon LE. Modulation of bone loss during disuse by pulsed electromagnetic fields. *J Ortho Res.* 1991;9:600–608.

11. Pienkowski D, Pollack SR, Brighton CT, Griffith NJ. Comparison of asymmetrical and symmetrical pulse waveforms in electromagnetic stimulation. *J Orthop Res.* 1992;10(2):247–255.
12. Medicare Coverage Issues Manual (MCIM)—Medical Procedures, Section 35–98, 5 Medicare and Medicaid Guide (CCH). In: *Health Care Financing Administration (HCFA).* Baltimore: Department of Health and Human Services; 1997:35–98.
13. *Anonymous, Aitken, Noecker, Heyden, Langill, Sharp, Turner and American Physical Therapy Association vs Shalala.* Civil Action No. 979-1127. United States District Court, District of Massachusetts: 1997.
14. Bergstrom N, Allman RM, Alvarez OM. *Treatment of Pressure Ulcers.* Clinical Practice Guideline. Rockville, MD: Agency for Health Care Research and Quality (AHRQ), formerly known as the Agency for Health Care Policy and Research (AHCPR), U.S. Department of Health and Human Services, Public Health Service; 1994.
15. Ovington LG. Dressings and adjunctive therapies: AHCPR guidelines revisited. *Ostomy/Wound Manage.* 1999;45(Suppl 1A):94s–106s.
16. Dolynchuk K, Keast D, Campbell K. Best practices for the prevention and treatment of pressure ulcers. *Ostomy/Wound Manage.* 2000;46(11):38–52.
17. Rabkin J, Hunt TK. Local heat increases blood flow and oxygen tension in wounds. *Arch Surg.* 1987;122:221–225.
18. Bello YM, Lopez AP, Philips TJ. *Wound Temperature is Lower than Core Temperature.* Abstract. In: Symposium for Advanced Wound Care and 8th Annual Medical Research Forum on Wound Repair. Miami, FL: Health Management Publications; 1998.

19. Michaelson AD, MacGregor H, Barnard MR. Reversible inhibition of human platelet activation by hypothermia in vivo and in vitro. *Thromb Haemost*. 1994;71(5):633–640.

20. Park H-Y, Shon K, Phillips T. The effect of heat on inhibitory effects of chronic wound fluid on fibroblasts in vitro. *Wounds*. 1998;10(6):189–192.

21. Lehman JF, deLateur BJ. Therapeutic heat. In: Lehmann JF, ed. *Therapeutic Heat and Cold*. 4th ed. Baltimore: Williams & Wilkins; 1990.

22. Brown G. Diathermy: a renewed interest in a proven therapy. *Phys Ther Today*. Spring 1993:78–80.

23. Wessman HC, Kottke FJ. The effect of indirect heating on peripheral blood flow, pulse rate, blood pressure and temperature. *Arch Phys Med Rehabil*. 1967;48:567–576.

24. Tortorici L, Purdy S. Laser and electromagnetic fields in the treatment of cancer. *Rehabil Oncol*. 2000;18(3):18–22.

25. Silverman D, Pendleton L. A comparison of the effects of continuous and pulsed short-wave diathermy on peripheral circulation. *Arch Phys Med Rehabil*. 1968;49:429–436.

26. Santoro D, Ostranderl, Lee B, Cagir B. *Inductive 27.12 MHz: Diathermy in Arterial Peripheral Vascular Disease*. 16th International IEEE/EMBS Conference; October 1994; Montreal, Canada.

27. Sanservino EG. Membrane phenomena and cellular processes under action of pulsating magnetic fields. Presented at the Second International Congress for Magneto Medicine; November 1980; Rome, Italy.

28. Bassett C. Low energy pulsing electromagnetic fields modify biomedical processes. *BioEssays*. 1987;6(1):36–40.

29. Witkowski JA. Purple Ulcers. *J ET Nurs*. 1993:132.

30. Fenn JE. Effect of pulsed electromagnetic energy (Diapulse) on experimental hematomas. *Can Med Assoc J*. 1969;100:251.

31. Ginsberg AJ. *Pearl Chain Phenomenon*. Abstract. Presented at the 35th Annual Meeting of the American Congress of Physical Medicine and Rehabilitation; 1958;36:112–115.

32. Cameron BM. Experimental acceleration of wound healing. *Am J Orthop*. November 1961:336–343.

33. Sambasivan M. Pulsed electromagnetic field in management of head injuries. *Neurol India*. 1993;41(Suppl):56–59.

34. Ionescu A, Ionescu D, et al. *Study of Efficiency of Diapulse Therapy on the Dynamics of Enzymes in Burned Wound*. Presented at the Sixth International Congress on Burns; August 31, 1982; San Francisco.

35. Santiesteban J, Grant C. Post-surgical effect of pulsed shortwave therapy. *J Am Podiatr Med Assoc*. 1979;75:306–309.

36. Barclay V, Collier R, Jones A. Treatment of various hand injuries by pulsed electromagnetic energy (Diapulse). *Physiotherapy*. 1983;69(6):186–188.

37. Pennington G, Daily D, Sumko M. Pulsed, non-thermal, high-frequency electromagnetic energy (Diapulse) in the treatment of grade I and grade II ankle sprains. *Mil Med*. 1993;158:101–104.

38. Knighton D, Halliday B, Hunt TK. Oxygen as antibiotic: A comparison of inspired oxygen concentration and antibiotic administration on in vivo bacterial clearance. *Arch Surg*. 1986;121:191–195.

39. Jonsson K, Jensen J, Goodson WH III. Tissue oxygenation, anemia, and perfusion in relation to wound healing in surgical patients. *Ann Surg*. 1991;214(5):605–613.

40. Erdman W. Peripheral blood flow measurements during application of pulsed high frequency currents. *Orthopedics*. 1960;2:196–197.

41. Mayrovitz H, Larsen P. Effects of pulsed electromagnetic fields on skin microvascular blood perfusion. *Wounds*. 1992;4(5):197–202.

42. Mayrovitz H, Larsen P. A preliminary study to evaluate the effect of pulsed radio frequency field treatment on lower extremity peri-ulcer skin microcirculation of diabetic patients. *Wounds*. 1995;7(3):90–93.

43. Wilson D, Jagadesh P, Newman P, Harriman D. The effects of pulsed electromagnetic energy on peripheral nerve regeneration. *Ann NY Acad Sci*. 1974;230:575–585.

44. Dindar H, Renda N, Barlas M. The effects of electromagnetic field stimulation on corticosteroids-inhibited intestinal wound healing. *Tokai J Exp Clin Med*. 1993;18(1–2):49–55.

45. Patino O, Grana D, Bolgiani A. Effect of magnetic fields on skin wound healing. Experimental study. *Medicina (B Aires)*. 1996;56(1):41–44.

46. Patino O, Grana D, Bolgiani A. Pulsed electromagnetic fields in experimental cutaneous wound healing in rats. *J Burn Care Rehabil*. 1996;17(6 Pt 1):528–531.

47. Scardino M, Swaim SF, Sartin, EA. Evaluation of treatment with a pulsed electromagnetic field on wound healing, clinicopathologic variables, and central nervous system activity of dogs. *Am J Vet Res*. 1998;59(9):1177–1181.

48. Lin Y, Nishimura R, Nozaki K. Effects of pulsing electromagnetic fields on the ligament healing in rabbits. *J Vet Med Sci*. 1992;54(5):1017–1022.

49. Lee E, Maffuli N, Li CK, Chan KM. Pulsed magnetic and electromagnetic fields in experimental Achilles tendonitis in the rat: a prospective randomized study. *Arch Phys Med Rehabil*. 1997;78(4):399–404.

50. Itoh M, Montemayor J, Matsumoto E, Eason A, Lee M, Folk F. Accelerated wound healing of pressure ulcers by pulsed high peak power electromagnetic energy (Diapulse). *Decubitus*. 1991;4(1):24–34.

51. Wilson CM. *Clinical Effects of Diapulse Technology in Treatment of Recalcitrant Pressure Ulcers*. In: Clinical Symposium on Pressure Ulcer and Wound Management. Orlando, FL: Silver Cross Hospital and Decubitus; 1992.

52. Salzberg A, Cooper-Vastola S, Perez F, Viehbeck M, Byme D. The effects of non-thermal pulsed electromagnetic energy (Diapulse) on wound healing of pressure ulcers in spinal cord-injured patients: a randomized, double-blind study. *Wounds*. 1995;7(1):11–16.

53. Seaborne D, Quirion-DeGirardi C, Rovsseau M, Rivest M, Lambert J. The treatment of pressure sores using pulsed electromagnetic energy (PEME). *Physiother Can*. 1996;48(2):131–137.

54. Cameron BM. A three phase evaluation of pulsed high frequency radio short waves (Diapulse), 646 patients. *Am J Orthop*. 1964:72–78.

55. Goldin JH, Broadbent JD, et al. The effects of Diapulse on the healing of wounds: A double-blind randomised controlled trial in man. *Br J Plastic Surg*. 1981;34:267–270.

56. Kaplan EG, Weinstock R. Clinical evaluation of Diapulse as adjunctive therapy following foot surgery. *J Am Podiatr Assoc*. 1968;58(5):218.

57. Aronofsky DH. Reduction of dental postsurgical symptoms using non-thermal pulsed high peak power electromagnetic energy. *Oral Surg Oral Med Oral Pathol*. 1971;32(5):688–696.

58. Bentall R, Eckstein H. A trial involving the use of pulsed electro-magnetic therapy on children undergoing orchidoplexy. *Hippokrates Verlag Stuttgart*. 1975;17(4):380–388.

59. Comorosan S, Paslaru L, Popovici Z. The stimulation of wound healing processes by pulsed electromagnetic energy. *Wounds*. 1992;4(1):31–32.

60. Ieran M, Zaffuto S. Effect of low frequency pulsing electromagnetic fields on skin ulcers of venous origin in humans: a double blind study. *J Orthop Rev*. 1990;8:276–282.

61. Duran V, Zamurovic A, Stojanovk S, Poljaicki M, Jovanovk M. Therapy of venous ulcers using pulsating electromagnetic fields—personal results. *Med Pregl*. 1991;44(11–12):485–488.

62. Todd D, Heylings D, Allen G, McMillin W. Treatment of chronic varicose ulcers with pulsed electromagnetic fields: a controlled pilot study. *Ir Med J*. 1991;84(2):54–55.

63. Stiller M, Pak G, Shupack J, Thalgr S, Kenn YC, Jondreau L. A portable pulsed electromagnetic field (PEMF) device to enhance healing of recalcitrant venous ulcers: a double-blind, placebo-controlled clinical trial. *Br J Dermatol.* 1992;127(2):147–154.

64. Kenkre J, Hobbs F, Carter Y, Holder R, Holmes E. A randomized controlled trial of electromagnetic therapy in the primary care management of venous leg ulceration. *Fam Pract.* 1996;13(3):236–240.

65. Bates-Jensen B. *A Quantitative Analysis of Wound Characteristics as Early Predictors of Healing in Pressure Sores.* Dissertation Abstracts International, Vol. 59, No. 11. Los Angeles: University of California; 1999.

66. Margolis DJ, Gross EA, Wood CR, Lazarus GS. Planimetric rate of healing in venous ulcers of the leg treated with pressure bandage and hydrocolloid dressing. *J Am Acad Dermatol.* 1993;28(3):418–421.

67. Robson MC, Hill DP, Woodske ME, Steed DL. Wound healing trajectories as predictors of effectiveness of therapeutic agents. *Arch Surg.* 2000;135(7):773–777.

68. Van Rijswijk L. Full-thickness leg ulcers: Patient demographics and predictors of time to healing. Multi-center leg ulcer study group. *J Fam Pract.* 1993;36(6):625–632.

69. International Medical Electronics. *Megatherm (Model 1000) Short Wave Therapy Unit Instruction Manual.* Kansas City, MO: International Medical Electronics LTD; 1981.

70. Van Rijswijk L, Polansky M. Predictors of time to healing deep pressure ulcers. *Ostomy/Wound Manage.* 1994;40(8):40–42, 44, 46–48.

71. Electropharmacology. *MRT SofPulse User's Manual.* Pompano Beach, FL: Electropharmacology, Inc.; 1994.

72. Martin CJ, McCallum HM, Strelley S, Heaton B. Electromagnetic fields from therapeutic diathermy equipment: A review of hazards and precautions. *Physiotherapy.* 1991;77:3–7.

73. Ourllet-Hellstrom R, Stewart. Miscarriages among female physical therapists who report using radio- and microwave-frequency electromagnetic radiation. *Am J Epidemiol.* 1993;138:775–786.

74. 21 CFR Ch. 1 (4-1-93 Edition). Device described in paragraph (BX1); see section 890.3, 48 FR 53047, Nov. 23, 1983, as amended in 52 FR 17742, May 11, 1987, Document No. A779269 (PSWD Instruction Manual).

75. Low JL. The nature and effects of pulsed electromagnetic radiations. *NZ J Physiother.* 1978(November):18–22.

76. Hayne CR. Pulsed high frequency energy—its place in physiotherapy. *Physiotherapy.* 1984;70:459.

77. Frankenberger L, *personal communication.* 1997.

78. Swanson G. Functional outcomes report: The next generation in physical therapy reporting. In: Stewart DL, Abeln SH, eds. *Documenting Functional Outcomes in Physical Therapy.* St. Louis, MO: Mosby-Year Book; 1993.

CHAPTER 23

Ultraviolet Light and Wound Healing

Teresa Conner-Kerr

CHAPTER OBJECTIVES

At the completion of this chapter, the reader will be able to:

1. List and describe the three bands of ultraviolet (UV) radiation
2. Identify immediate and late cutaneous effects of UV radiation
3. Identify the peak wavelengths of UV radiation for erythema and germicidal activity
4. List indications and contraindications to UV treatment of a wound
5. Describe the procedure for applying an UV treatment to a wound

INTRODUCTION

Ultraviolet (UV) radiation, a component of sunlight, has been used for healing since the dawn of primitive man. However, the antimicrobial effects of UV were just recognized during the past two centuries.[1,2] Because of its antimicrobial properties and its ability to increase blood flow by inducing an erythematous reaction in the skin, controlled UV exposure has been used by a variety of disciplines, including dermatology, physical medicine, and physical therapy, to treat a plethora of skin and wound pathologies. The goals of this chapter are to 1) describe the biological effects of UV, 2) provide an overview of UV preclinical and clinical studies, and 3) present a new treatment paradigm for UV radiation in the C band.

DEFINITIONS

UV light is a form of radiant energy that falls between X-rays and visible light on the electromagnetic spectrum (see Figure 23–1). However, UV light is a misnomer because this portion of the electromagnetic spectrum is largely invisible to the human eye. UV light is more appropriately described as UV energy or radiation. UV energy encompasses the wavelengths between 180 nm and 400 nm and has been commonly separated into three distinct bands, UVA, UVB, and UVC.[3–6] According to the International Commission on Illumination (CIE), UV wavelengths can be subdivided as follows: 400–315 nm (UVA), 315–280 nm (UVB), and 280–100 nm (UVC).[3] The World Health Organization (WHO) definition of the three UV bands differs somewhat, compared with that of the CIE. The WHO defines UVA as wavelengths 400–320 nm, UVB as wavelengths 320–280 nm, and UVC as wavelengths 280–200 nm. Recently, UVA has been subdivided into UVA1 and UVA2 because UVA2 rays are thought to have actions more similar to those of UVB. UVA1 encompasses wavelengths from 340–400 nm, whereas UVA2 encompasses wavelengths from 320 to 340 nm.[4]

HISTORICAL PERSPECTIVE

Interest in the effects of sunlight on humans has followed a long and circuitous route. The first documented uses of UV energy, in the form of sunlight, can be traced back to the time of primitive man. The sun and the light that it provided were recognized, if not worshiped, for their ability to give and maintain life. Because of the sun's integral role in ancient societies, many of the ancient gods were named for the sun. One such god was Helios, Greek god of physical light and sun.[1,2] Evidence of the role that the Greeks believed that the sun god played in healing can be seen in ancient stone inscriptions.

One of the first pieces of early evidence that demonstrated a biologic effect of exposure to sunlight included an observa-

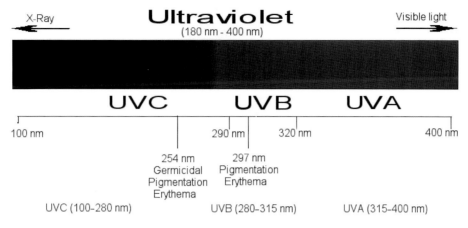

Figure 23–1 UV spectrum

tion by Herodotus, known as the "father of history."[1,2] He was credited with having observed the difference in degree of calcification between the skull bones of vanquished Egyptian and Persian soldiers. He ascribed this difference to the increased exposure of the Egyptians' scalps to the sun because of the cultural practice of shaving the scalp from an early age. As a result of these observations, Herodotus and others became advocates of sun therapy, and sunlight was prescribed for numerous ailments, including epilepsy, paralysis, asthma, malnutrition, and obesity, among others.

However, with the advent of Christianity, little was written about heliotherapy or sun therapy until the eighteenth century.[1,2] It was not until 1796 that significant attention was refocused on the question of whether sunlight was beneficial to humans. At this time, a prize was offered by the University of Gottingen for the best essay on the effects of light on the human body. The winning essay by Ebernaier was the first to propose a relationship between the lack of sun exposure and the development of rickets. Some years later, Niels Finsen prepared a paper on the influence of light on skin. Using his own forearm, he demonstrated the ability of sunlight to induce a delayed erythema on unprotected skin exposed to sunlight.

It was also around this time that the germicidal properties of sunlight were discovered. The bactericidal properties of light were first demonstrated in 1877.[1,2] Using an unboiled Pasteur's solution, Downes and Blunt showed that sunlight could prevent the growth of bacteria. In later experiments, Downes and Blunt were able to demonstrate that light near the violet end of the electromagnetic spectrum had the greatest bactericidal potency. However, it was not until Duclaux in 1885 and Ward in 1892 demonstrated the bactericidal effects of sunlight in the absence of heat generation that the bactericidal properties of sunlight became generally accepted.

Some years later, Bernhard and Morgan were the first to show that UV radiation below 329 nm was bactericidal.[1,2]

Between 1890 and 1909, UV energy was shown to be bactericidal to many bacteria, including *Mycobacterium tuberculosis*, *Staphylococcus*, *Streptococcus*, *Bacillus*, and *Shigella dysenteriae*. It was during this time that UV radiation became a common treatment for tuberculosis of the skin. In fact, the Nobel Prize for Medicine and Science was awarded to Finsen in 1903 for his work on the treatment of tuberculosis-induced skin lesions.

In the following decades, much of the UV research focused on the use of UV radiation to control or prevent surgical wound infection.[1,2,7] This interest continues today, with several groups investigating the utility of using UV radiation to prevent or control infection of orthopaedic surgical wounds.[8–12] Additionally, with the emergence of antibiotic-resistant wound pathogens, the role of UVC radiation in treating infected acute and chronic wounds is being reexamined, along with its putative ability to stimulate wound healing processes.[13–17]

PHYSICAL SCIENCE OF UV RADIATION

Longwave UV radiation, or UVA, is referred to as *black light* or *near UV radiation*. These wavelengths are the closest to visible light. The middle band of UV radiation, or UVB, is known as *sunburn radiation* and is thought to mediate most of the harmful effects of sunlight on human skin, including photoaging and carcinogenesis.[4,18,19] UVA and UVB account for approximately 6.3% and 0.5% of sunlight during the summer, respectively.[5] On the other hand, UVC, or shortwave UV radiation, is known for its germicidal effects, and almost all of these rays are prevented from reaching the earth by the ozone layer.[4,5]

The three bands of UV radiation differ in their ability to penetrate human skin (see Figure 23–2) and to produce certain biologic effects.[20] The UVA band constitutes the longest wavelengths of the UV energy spectrum, and these rays

UVC   **UVB**   **UVA**

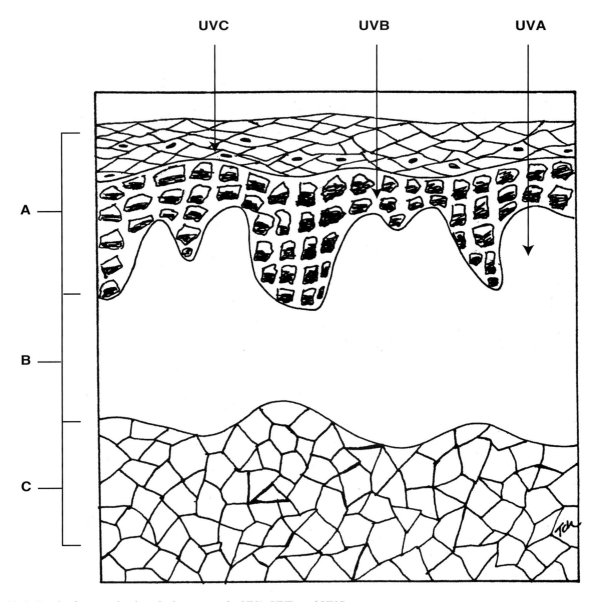

Figure 23–2 Depth of penetration into the integument by UVA, UVB, and UVC rays.

are known to penetrate human skin to the level of the upper dermis. In contrast, UVB rays penetrate only to stratum basale, the lowermost level of the epidermis, whereas UVC rays, which have the least ability to penetrate human skin, reach only the upper layers of the epidermis.

Specific UV wavelengths have been associated with particular biologic responses (see Figure 23–1). For example, the germicidal effects of UV radiation are associated with UV wavelengths from 250 to 270 nm,[5] whereas UV wavelengths of 254 nm and 297 nm have the greatest ability to induce an erythematous, or reddening, reaction in the skin.

The tanning response, on the other hand, is predominantly associated with wavelengths of 254 nm and 299 nm.

Biologic Effects of Ultraviolet Radiation

UV energy has been used to treat a variety of skin conditions, including open wounds, because of its biologic effects.[21] UV radiation is known to promote exfoliation of the outer skin layers, enhance healing through the induction of an erythematous response in the skin, and inactivate a variety of microorganisms. The biologic effects of UV have been classified as immediate or long term (see Exhibit 23–1).[18,19,22] Stenback[22] lists the induction of erythema and its accompanying inflammatory changes, along with increased pigmentation, as examples of acute skin reactions to UV exposure (see Exhibit 23–1). In comparison, late cutaneous effects are identified as elastosis, or the loss of skin elasticity, and carcinogenesis.

Early Cutaneous Effects

Skin reddening, or erythema, is a well-known effect of UV at certain exposure levels. UV radiation produces this reddening of the skin via stimulation of an inflammatory response that leads to increased vascularity of the dermis.[5,18,19,22] Erythema is most effectively produced by the 297-nm and 254-nm UV wavelengths. These wavelengths encompass both the B and C bands of UV. Erythema that results from the longer wavelengths has a greater latency and lasts for a longer period of time than that produced by shorter wavelengths. However, the shorter wavelengths have a greater potency.

UV-induced erythema is associated with a latent period of 2–3 hours.[18] The exact mechanism that underlies this latent appearance of erythema is unknown but several theories have been offered. The latent development of the erythemal response has been ascribed to the production of some diffusible biologic mediator from damaged epidermal cells.[23,24] It is thought that this mediator then diffuses to the dermis, where it enhances blood vessel permeability. The identity of this diffusible mediator is unknown. Several substances, including histamine, bradykinin, and prostaglandins, have been implicated in this role. In the past, prostaglandins were thought to be the most likely candidate for this role as diffusible mediator. However, work by Hensby et al[25] utilizing

prostaglandin antagonists has been inconclusive, and the role that prostaglandins play in mediating erythema is unclear.

Recent studies by Brauchle et al[26] have demonstrated a significant increase in vascular endothelial growth factor (VEGF) expression in cultured keratinocytes after irradiation with both sublethal and physiologic levels of UVB. Irradiation of quiescent keratinocytes leads to both an increase in mRNA levels, as well as increased levels of VEGF. Because VEGF is known to enhance vascular permeability, it is thought that VEGF may be a potential target for the above-described diffusible mediator. However, the identity of this diffusible mediator(s) remains unknown. Congruent with the findings of Brauchle et al,[26] Holtz[27] has shown that UV-induced erythema is accompanied by an intercellular edema in the prickle or spiny cell layer of the skin and an accumulation of white cells in local blood vessels. The development of this intercellular edema is also consistent with the separation of upper and lower epidermal layers that occurs upon exposure to high-intensity UV radiation. These effects on the skin most likely underlie the ability of UV radiation to stimulate debridement. Debridement would result from this sloughing of the upper layers of the epidermis, as well as from recruitment of phagocytic white blood cells. Increased lysosomal activity and leakage of lysosomal enzymes that has been detected with UV exposure may also contribute to this debridement effect.

Research Wisdom: *Use of UVA/UVB Radiation for Wound Debridement*

UVA/UVB radiation has been shown to induce intercellular edema in the upper and lower epidermal layers, as well as to enhance both white blood cell accumulation and lysosomal activity. These biologic effects may be advantageous in stimulating autolysis in wounds that require debridement due to the presence of necrotic tissue.

Exhibit 23–1 Immediate and Long-Term Effects of High-Level Exposure to UVB Radiation

---

Immediate
    Early (0–60 hours)
        Immediate hyperpigmentation
        Epidermal hyperplasia
        Inflammatory reactions
    Late (60–336 hours)
        Secondary hyperpigmentation
        Hyperplasia
        Fibrosis
    Long-term (chronic exposure)
        Elastosis
        Carcinoma

Source: Data from reference #'s 18, 19, and 22.

Another immediate effect of UV exposure includes skin thickening, or hyperplasia.[21,22] UV rays induce a hyperplasia or cellular proliferation in the stratum corneum, or the outermost layer of the skin. This process is thought to be protective against subsequent sunlight-induced skin damage. Research indicates that DNA changes are seen within 4–7 hours after irradiation of the epidermis. Epidermal cells in stratum basale have been shown to accumulate glycogen at 12 hours, and increased RNA levels are seen at 24 hours in both the basal and lower prickle cell layer. These increased levels of RNA are thought to reflect an increased rate of transcription, indicating ongoing repair. They are consistent with the finding that UV radiation stimulates the production of interleuken 1α (IL-1α) by keratinocytes.[28] IL-1α is known to play a role in enhancing wound epithelialization.[29] Work by Kaiser et al[28] demonstrated that UVB stimulated epithelialization, thus providing further evidence of a role for UVB in stimulating epidermal migration by enhancing IL-1α production. This work supports the current treatment approach of utilizing UV to enhance epithelialization, especially with indolent wounds that exhibit fibrotic edges. In these wounds, UV may stimulate or restart the epithelialization process.

When low-level UV radiation exposure occurs, it is thought that the above-described effects are confined to the upper third or half of the epidermis.[23] As a result, no long-lasting effects are thought to occur because the cells in these layers are differentiating in transit to becoming part of the outer dead layer of the skin. Therefore, these data, among others, lend support to the supposition that UV radiation stimulates repair processes and that these effects may be harnessed at a low enough level to prevent long-term damage. The wound clinician may find the induction of epidermal hyperplasia by UV radiation to be beneficial in promoting rapid epithelialization in acute and chronic wounds.

High levels of UVB exposure have also been shown to affect Langerhans cells.[23,30,31] These cells inhabit the middle region of the epidermis and appear to have an immune function. They are part of the macrophage lineage and are derived from the bone marrow. High-level UVB exposure is known to produce Langerhans cell necrosis within 24 hours. This pattern of cellular necrosis is seen in both experimental rodent models and humans. The destruction of these cells is thought to account for the immunosuppressive ability of high levels of UVB. Interestingly, this immunosuppressive effect of high-level UVB exposure has been harnessed by researchers to enhance graft take in individuals with burn wounds.[32] However, because the Langerhans cells are derived from the bone marrow, no long-term effects are expected as a result of this local immunosuppression of the treated skin. Furthermore, the effects of short treatment times at low intensities with UVB or UVC are unknown. It is possible that the effects may be different from those seen with high-level UV radiation.

Late Cutaneous Effects

Late cutaneous effects include elastosis,[23] or loss of skin elasticity, and carcinogenesis.[4,19,23] Elastosis has been observed traditionally in the skin of individuals who labor in the sun for most of their lives. It is characterized by the degeneration of collagen and elastin fibers in the dermis. Histologic analysis of skin that exhibits elastosis includes basophilic degeneration and enlarged, blunted elastic fibers. These changes are not found in adjacent skin areas that have been protected from prolonged exposure to the sun.

Prolonged or lifetime exposure to UV radiation, particularly rays in the B band, is well accepted as a causative factor in certain types of skin cancers. According to Moseley,[18] supporting evidence for UVB-related carcinogenesis includes:

1. Increased number of skin cancers on sites exposed chronically to the sun.
2. Decreased numbers of certain types of skin cancers with increased natural pigmentation.
3. Increased incidence of skin cancer in light-skinned people, especially those who spend significant time outdoors.
4. Increased incidence of skin cancer in light-colored people who live near the equator.

UVB readily produces skin cancer in experimental animal models with prolonged continuous exposure (hours). Individuals with deficient DNA repair mechanisms in the skin are more prone to skin cancers. However, these effects are associated with prolonged exposure to sunlight, particularly high-intensity UVB over a period of years. Therefore, the relevance of these concerns when deciding whether to employ short-duration, low-intensity UV radiation for stimulation of wound healing or treatment of wound infection, especially with UVC rays, should be questioned. Additionally, these carcinogenic effects are linked to cellular changes in the epidermis, and the greatest number of wounds that are candidates for UV treatment are of at least partial thickness. If warranted with this low level of UV energy exposure, the periwound could be protected with draping or an UV-blocking ointment, such as petrolatum.

Bactericidal Effects

Research has shown that UV radiation from all three bands—A, B, and C—has the ability to kill a plethora of microorganisms. As a result of its effectiveness in killing microorganisms, UV light has been used in a variety of ways, including water purification, serum sterilization, and pharmaceutical clean room and surgical theater decontamination.[21] It has also been used to treat a variety of skin infections and heavily contaminated wounds.

Due to continuing issues with surgical infections, there has been renewed interest in the potential role of UV light in preventing surgical wound infections. Taylor et al,[11,12] in the United Kingdom, examined the effectiveness of UVC radiation on reducing bacterial numbers in individuals undergoing total joint arthroplasty. UVC energy was delivered by tubing placed overhead in a conventional plenum ventilated surgical theatre. The UVC tubes were activated 10 minutes after the surgical procedure was initiated. Results of the study showed that the UVC application was effective in significantly reducing bacterial levels in the theater air as well as in the surgical wounds. Bacterial levels in the surgical wounds fell 87% with UVC delivered at 100 μW/cm^2 (N = 18) and 92% with UVC delivered at 300 μW/cm^2 (N = 13).

In a similar study, Moggio et al[10] also found that UV irradiation significantly lowered the average number of airborne bacteria detected over the surgical site. The rate of infection for 1,322 individuals who underwent hip arthroplasties was found to be only 0.15% with application of UVC. Once again, similar findings were obtained by Berg et al[8] when UVC application in operating rooms was compared to a sham blue light application. These authors concluded that the air quality was similar to that produced by ultraclean air ventilation systems. It is also interesting to note that both Berg et al and Taylor et al recorded no adverse effects of UVC exposure on operating room personnel.[8,11]

A growing interest in the use of UV energy for treatment of established wound infections has also been seen in the past two decades. This renewed interest in UV comes at a time when antimicrobial resistance is rampant among common wound pathogens and when the health care community is increasingly under pressure to find the most cost-effective and time-efficient method of treatment for various health care problems.

The effectiveness of UV radiation in killing microbes has been demonstrated by many researchers using in vitro testing. High and High[33] demonstrated that broad spectrum UV radiation delivered by the Kromayer lamp (model 10), which produces wavelengths from all three UV bands, was effective in eliminating a wide range of wound pathogens in vitro. Exposure times tested in this study are consistent with treatment times that have been recommended in the past for skin and wound infections. The times were based on the previously described classification of erythemal responses with E2, E3, and E4 doses (see section on UV treatment times for a description) being effective in killing common wound pathogens. Complete eradication of all wound pathogens tested was obtained only at an E4 dose. In contrast, Nordback et al[34] did not find a difference in colonization levels in rats with acute surgical wounds that were exposed to broad spectrum UV radiation. Because the UV radiation source emitted a broad spectrum of UVA, B, and C wavelengths and the proportion of each type of wavelength is not described, it is difficult to determine whether the wavelengths that are known to have the greatest germicidal activity (UVC at 250–270 nm) were present at adequate doses.

Using a halogen lamp that emits predominantly UVC, it has been shown that a broad range of wound pathogens, including those expressing antibiotic resistance, can be effectively eliminated with short treatment times (see Exhibit 23–2).[13,14,35,36] Using the V-254 lamp, which selectively emits UVC energy, it has been possible to obtain a 99.99% kill rate for all tested common wound pathogens. Using an *in vitro* model with optimal growth characteristics for the microorganisms tested, UVC irradiation has been shown to be effective in eradicating both procaryotic organisms, such as bacteria, and eukaryotic organisms, such as yeast or multicellular fungi, at short exposure times. In fact, UVC was found to be effective in killing multicellular eukaryotic wound pathogens at treatment times shorter than those currently advocated for prokaryotic (bacterial) organisms. However, these data do indicate that multicellular eukaryotic organisms require 10 times the exposure time (30 seconds) for 99.9% kill, as compared with the most susceptible eukaryotic organism (3 seconds).

Research has also demonstrated that short UVC exposure times can produce a 99.99% kill rate for common antibiotic-resistant bacterial pathogens in vitro and in vivo.[13,14] Using an optimal growth model in vitro, 99.99% of methicillin-resistant *Staphylococcus aureus* (MRSA) and vancomycin-resistant enterococcus (VRE) are eliminated with only 5 seconds of exposure to UVC. Additionally, data indicate that once-daily exposure to UVC for 5 days is adequate to produce 100% eradication of MRSA from acute rat surgical wound tissue.

Studies by Taylor et al,[37] using an *in vitro* model, also found UVC to be effective in killing bacteria. In this study, the effects of UVC on bacteria alone and in combination with pulsed jet lavage was compared with commonly used antiseptics. All of the tested topical agents, including 3% hydrogen peroxide, 1% and 10% povidone-iodine, and 0.05%

Exhibit 23–2 Exposure Times for 99.99% Inactivation of Common Prokaryotic and Eukaryotic Wound Pathogens by UVC Radiation

	UVC Treatment Times (seconds)				
	in vitro				*in vivo*
	3	5	15	30	30
Prokaryotes *(bacteria)*					
MRSA		*			*
VRE		*			
Group A Streptococcus		*			
Pseudomonas aeruginosa	*				
Mycobacterium abscesses		*			
Unicellular Eukaryote *(yeast)*					
Candida albicans			*		
Multicellular Prokaryote *(fungi)*					
Aspergillus fumigatus				*	
Mixed Cultures			*		
P. aeruginosa					
C. albicans					
A. fumigatus					

Source: Data from reference #'s 13, 14, 35, and 36.

chlorhexidine were found to reduce bacterial numbers on agar. However, the bactericidal effects of only hydrogen peroxide and povidone-iodine were effectively eliminated when tested on muscle tissue treated with whole blood or plasma. The effects of UVC application and pulsed jet lavage were found to be additive, suggesting a clinical role for coapplication of these modalities in treating wound infection.

UV Preclinical Studies

The effects of UVA and UVB radiation on wound healing has been examined using a number of different animal models, including the rat, hairless guinea pig, and rabbit (see Exhibit 23–3). Positive effects of UVB on wound healing were observed in both the rat[34] and rabbit[38] animal models but not in the hairless guinea pig[39,40] model. Irradiation of the acute surgical wound bed of rats with a UVA and UVB energy source resulted in a significantly increased rate of wound closure between the fourth and fifteenth days of treatment, compared with untreated controls on the contralateral side of the animal. Additionally, no decrement in wound tensile strength was found at either day 7 or 15, compared with the untreated controls. The results from this study also suggest that the effects of UVA and UVB are localized and not systemic because healing of the contralateral wounds was not enhanced.

Similarly, El-Batouty et al[38] found a modestly higher rate of tissue regeneration in acute full-thickness wounds to the pinna of rabbit ears, using a hot quartz lamp (UVA and UVB). UV-treated wounds healed more rapidly than did their untreated controls. Additionally, histopathologic analysis demonstrated significant increases in epithelialization rates and collagen deposition, as compared with untreated controls.

In contrast, acute surgical wounds induced in hairless guinea pigs that had been pretreated with UVA or UVB radiation every other day for 16 weeks did not exhibit enhanced wound closure rates.[39,40] Additionally, wound tensile strength was found to be significantly less in both the UVA- and UVB-treated animals. Histopathologic analysis also demonstrated marked endothelial swelling and eosinophilic infiltration in the irradiated group. Similar findings for decreased wound tensile strength were found using hairless guinea pigs pretreated with pure UVA radiation prior to wounding. Due to the extraordinarily long duration of treatment (16 weeks in the first study and 21 weeks in the second study) and the use of a pretreatment UV paradigm, rather than UV treatment postwounding, the relevance of these findings is not clear. Furthermore, additional work by the same investigators found that there were no significant differences in tensile strength of wounds made to UV-treated versus untreated skin by recovery day 90.[41]

At this point, examination of the effects of UVC on wound healing rates in both the pig and rodent models (see Exhibit 23–3) has shown no grossly detectable facilitation of wound closure. In the porcine model, no significant effect of UVC radiation on wound tensile strength was detected.[42] However, recent studies in our laboratory demonstrated that a 30-second UVC treatment once daily for 5 days in a rodent model resulted in a cleaner and smoother transition area between the periwound and the wound bed, with no tissue curling.[43] This treatment paradigm also produced a change in wound morphology, due to altered wound contraction. The induction of a change in wound contraction by UVC is consistent with the findings of Morykwas et al.[17] Using cultured fibroblasts, researchers demonstrated increased secretion of fibronectin into the culture medium after UVC irradiation. Fibronectin is an extracellular matrix protein that appears to play a role in wound contraction.

UV Clinical Studies

Although there are significant experimental data to suggest a positive role for UV radiation in enhancing wound healing, relatively few clinical studies have been conducted. However, the majority of studies that have been conducted have found positive effects of UV radiation on wound healing (see Exhibit 23–3). Documented positive effects of UVA and UVB on wound healing can be found in the literature as far back as 1945. Stein and Shorey[44] published an article detailing the increased rate of wound healing and reduction of wound infection in two soldiers, one with a traumatic wound and the other with a pressure wound. Both wounds had been resistant to healing prior to the institution of UV radiation. The traumatic wound healed within 10 days of the initiation of UV therapy, and the pressure wound healed in less than 2 months.

A randomized controlled trial examining the effects of both UVA and UVB energy on superficial pressure sores in the elderly has also demonstrated enhanced healing rates.[45] In this study, UV-treated ulcers closed in an average time of 6.25 weeks, compared with an average of 10 weeks for control wounds. Additionally, a clinical study by Crous and Malherbe[46] also examined the effects of UVA and UVB on wound healing in individuals with venous insufficiency. Treatment parameters were based on the commonly accepted method of determining UV dosage by determining the degree of erythemal response by the skin on exposure to successively longer treatment times (see Table 23–1). An E_1 dose was used for periwound skin and granulation tissue and an E_4 dose for necrotic tissue. At these doses, UV radiation appeared to facilitate wound healing but wound closure was not achieved with any of the wounds.

The effects of UVC on chronic wound healing have also been examined. A study by Nussbaum et al[47] examined the effects of UVC combined with ultrasound on pressure ulcer healing. Their treatment parameters were similar to those used with the Crous and Malherbe[46] study. The treatment

Exhibit 23–3 Preclinical and Clinical Studies of the Effects of UVA/UVB or UVC on Wound Healing

Preclinical Studies

UVA/UVB

	In vivo	Healing
	Rat	+
	Rabbit	+
	Hairless Guinea Pig	–

UVC

	In vivo	Healing
	Rat	+
	Pig	–

Clinical Studies

UVA/UVB

Study Type	Number of Studies	Infection Healing	Control
Case Study	1	+	
Clinical Study	1		+
Randomized Placebo-Controlled Trial	1	+	

UVC/Ultrasound

Study Type	Number of Studies	Infection Healing	Control
Clinical Study	1		+
Randomized Controlled Trial	1	+	+

+ = facilitory effects
– = no facility effects detected
clinical study = nonrandomized study with comparison to pretreatment base line.

parameters included E_1 for clean/granulating wounds, E_3 for purulent/slow-healing wounds, E_4 for heavily infected wounds, and $2E_4$ for necrotic wounds. Combination of the UVC and ultrasound treatment was found to enhance healing over that of cold laser or moist wound healing. However, it is difficult to ascribe the enhanced healing effects observed in this study to a UVC-mediated effect because the UVC treatment employed was delivered in combination with ultrasound. Therefore, it is not clear as to what effect either of the modalities had separately.

Taylor[48] also examined the effectiveness of UVC in treating 56 individuals with infections of the skin, including the following lesions, tinea pedis, tinea capitis, sporotrichosis, and tinea corporis. The treatment times were between 2 and 5 minutes, with individuals receiving an average of 3.2 treatments over a period of 5–7 days. Fifty patients showed a good response to therapy, with most showing significant clearing of the infection within 1 week.

CURRENT RECOMMENDED TREATMENT APPROACHES

UVC Treatment Algorithm

Based on recent work[13,14,35,36] performed in the Collaborative Laboratory for Wound Healing, the use of the algorithm found in Figure 23–3 was proposed to determine treatment times for infected wounds when using UVC radiation. This algorithm is based on a review of the available research. This approach would be in place of the older system that utilized degree of skin erythema to determine treatment times. The algorithm is based on the theoretical principle of choosing UVC treatment times according to minimal lethal dose for the infecting organism. The author advocates this approach because it specifically addresses the susceptibility pattern of the infecting organism to UVC and not the response of the host to UVC. As a result, an adequate dose

Table 23–1 Erythemal Dosages Used with UV Radiation Exposure

Dose	Skin Reaction	Time to Development	Time to Resolution
SED	none noted		
E_1	subtle reddening	4–6 hr	24 hr
E_2	similar to mild sunburn skin exfoliation and pigmentation	4–6 hr	3–4 days
E_3	similar to severe sunburn intense erythema marked increased in exfoliation and pigmentation	2 hr	several days
E_4	same as E_3 with significant tissue swelling and exudate	2 hr	several days

SED = suberythemal dose
E_1 = first-degree erythemal dose
E_2 = second-degree erythemal dose
E_3 = third-degree erythemal dose
E_4 = fourth-degree erythemal dose

for killing or inactivation of a particular pathogen can be selected while preventing or minimizing any damage to host cells. As outlined in the previous sections, longer treatment times, especially those used with UVB, are known to produce deleterious effects.

Procedure for Administration

Equipment Selection

The primary decision to be made concerning equipment selection is whether a UVA/UVB or UVC energy source is to be utilized for treatments. Presently, research appears to indicate that either source is germicidal, although the peak germicidal wavelengths are in the UVC band from 250 to 270 nm. *In vitro* testing has shown that 99.99% killing or inactivation of common prokaryotic wound pathogens occurs at 5 seconds with a UVC energy source,[13,35,36] compared with greater than 180 seconds (an E_4 dose) with a UVA/UVB source.[33] Additionally, once-daily treatments for 30 seconds by UVC has been shown to produce greater than 99.99% eradication of MRSA in living tissue.[14] Furthermore, the role of UVC in preventing surgical wound infections during operative procedures has been demonstrated.[11] Therefore, it is recommended that a UVC source be utilized for wound infections because it appears to be more effective than the broad spectrum UVA and UVB lamps in eliminating common wound pathogens.

The greatest number of wound healing studies (many of which are cited in this text) have been conducted using UVA and UVB radiation. Results from both preclinical and clinical studies indicate that UVB, in particular, stimulates wound healing through the promotion of increased epithelialization rates and increased dermal vascularity. Recent molecular studies suggest a role for UVB radiation in facilitating wound healing. As outlined previously, a putative mechanism for the effects of UVB on wound healing may be through the stimulation of cytokines, such as IL-1α or VEGF.[15,16]

Data from several studies also support a role for the use of UVC radiation in stimulating healing. Nussbaum et al[47] demonstrated increased rates of pressure ulcer healing in individuals treated with UVC and ultrasound combined. Healing rates obtained by Nussbaum et al in this study were greater than those seen in a randomized controlled clinical trial using UVB radiation.[45] However, it is difficult to compare these two studies because of the age difference between the two subject groups.

Positive effects of UVC treatment on wound healing has also been seen in the laboratory, using an acute surgical wound model.[43] Once-daily treatments of UVC radiation for 30 seconds were found to produce a more organized transitional area between the periwound and wound tissue, with no apparent rolling over of the wound margins. Changes in the pattern of wound contraction were also noted with UVC treatment of these acute wounds. This finding is consistent

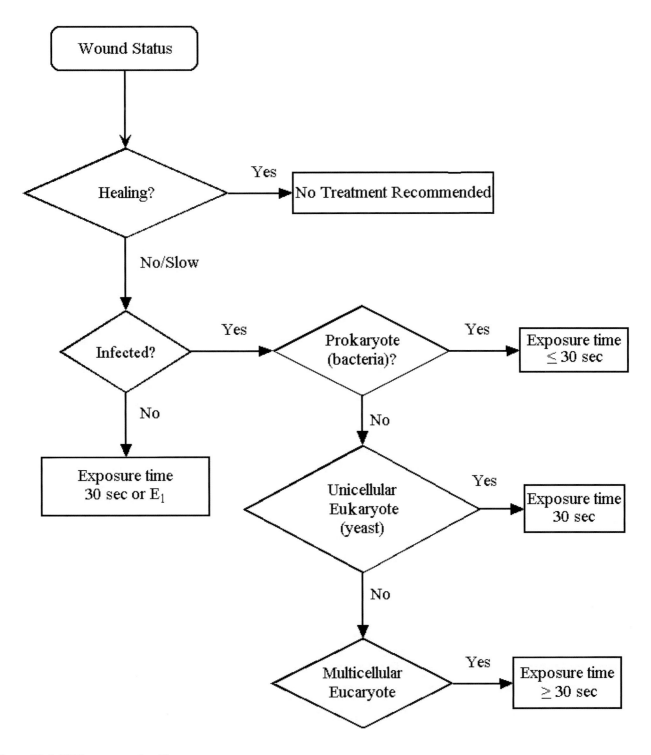

Figure 23–3 UVC treatment algorithm.

with results from an *in vitro* study that showed increased fibronectin secretion by cultured fibroblasts and enhanced lattice contraction after UVC irradiation.[17]

Therefore, the decision to use one particular UV energy source for wound healing is less clear than that for germicidal effects. Because most of the literature has linked chronic exposure to high-dose UVB to carcinoma formation,[19,23] the author recommends that low-dose or MED (E₁) UVB be utilized for treatment and that treatment sessions be limited in number. Individual response to therapy should dictate length and number of treatments, with the minimum number of treatment sessions conducted to stimulate angiogenesis or reepithelialization. Observation of increased rates of granulation tissue formation and/or reepithelialization supports cessation of therapy.

Research Wisdom: *Select a UVC Lamp for Clinical Infections*

The peak germicidal effects of UV radiation are seen with wavelengths 250–270 nm. These wavelengths are found in the UVC band. Therefore, when treating fungal or bacterial skin or wound infections, use low-dose UVC radiation.

Several different lamp types are available that selectively emit UVC radiation; an example can be seen in Figure 23–4. One of the early UVC generators commonly used by physical therapists and physical medicine physicians was the Birtcher cold quartz lamp. The cold quartz lamps emit better than 90% UVC at approximately 254 nm.[5] This emission falls within the peak germicidal range for UV radiation. The V-254 lamp also has a similar emission range. Either of these lamps will provide a good germicidal effect. However, the halogen lamp is lighter and has a larger faceplate that allows for more rapid treatment of larger wounds.

Preparation of Wound and Periwound Area for UV Treatment

A variety of approaches have been used in the past to prepare the wound bed for treatment with UV radiation. Most authorities recommend protecting the periwound and any nontreatment area with draping materials (see Figure 23–5). UV-resistant ointments, such as petrolatum jelly, may also be used to protect the periwound area that is immediately adjacent to the wound bed. On the other hand, it has been argued that protecting the adjacent periwound eliminates a potential source of epithelial cells and wound healing factors that would also be stimulated with the treatment. The author recommends protecting the periwound area if high-level (greater than E₂) UV radiation is to be used. It is not clear as to whether periwound protection is warranted with very low UV exposure times in the clinical situation because most of the information available on carcinogenic potential of UV radiation addresses chronic or high-level exposure times. Furthermore, most of the research has examined the carcinogenic potential of UVB and not UVC. Presently, low-dose UVC appears to be a relatively safe treatment alterna-

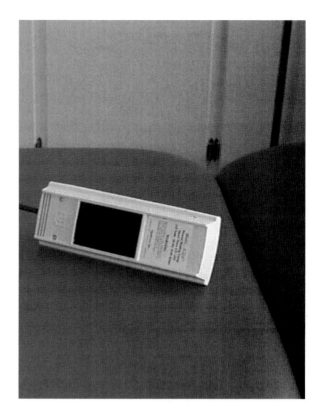

Figure 23–4 Germicidal UVC lamp: the Med Faxx halogen lamp. Courtesy of Med Faxx, Inc., Wake Forest, North Carolina.

---

tive, especially in the treatment of antibiotic-resistant pathogens.

Other considerations for preparation of the wound bed are removal of all dressing materials and cleansing of particulate matter in the wound bed. This can be accomplished by a variety of mechanisms, including pulsatile lavage or normal saline flush. At this point in time, there is one study that found added benefit to decreasing microorganism numbers in an *in vitro* wound model when coadministering jet lavage and UV radiation.[37] Cleansing of the wound bed is also important because the depth of penetration for all UV wavelengths is only, at best, less than 100–200 μm.[18] Therefore, cleansing of particulate increases wound bed exposure.

Clinical Wisdom: *Cleanse Wounds*

Cleanse wound and remove necrotic tissue prior to UV treatment. To maximize exposure of the wound bed to the UV rays, the wound should be cleansed with a gentle cleanser, such as normal saline, and debridement performed to remove as much necrotic tissue as possible.

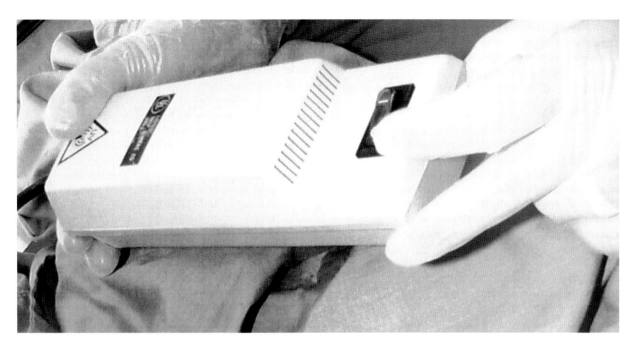

Figure 23–5 UVC treatment of infected sacral pressure ulcer.

It is also recommended that all dressings be removed for treatment. Mackinnon and Cleek[49] had previously suggested that UV radiation could be used with transparent dressings. However, we were unable to detect any bacterial inactivation or killing when bacterial cultures covered with either Tegaderm or Bioclusive were irradiated with UVC for treatment times as long as 120 seconds.[36]

> **Clinical Wisdom:** *Remove Wound Dressings*
>
> Remove all wound dressings prior to treatment with UV. All moist wound dressings should be removed prior to treatment of the wound bed with UV radiation in order for the UV rays to reach the wound tissue.

Treatment Times

In the past, UV dose has been calculated according to the MED response (see Table 23–1) of each individual client.[5,6,18] However, the author questions the appropriateness of this system for determining UVC treatment times because the recommended treatment times for necrotic and/or infected wounds are at levels high enough to produce significant cellular necrosis. Laboratory findings using both in vitro and in vivo modeling indicate that many wound patho-

gens, especially MRSA, can be eradicated at very low treatment times (see Exhibit 23–2).[13,14,35,36]

Therefore, the author advocates the use of the shortest exposure time that has been shown to be effective in eradicating the offending wound pathogen (see Exhibit 23–2). Clinicians are also encouraged to use the shortest treatment times (MED; ~ 30 seconds) or lowest UV dosages that have been found to stimulate the synthesis or secretion of biologic factors[15–17] involved in wound healing or that have been found to induce positive wound healing effects[43] (see Table 23–1).

At this time, it is also recommended that treatment times be considered in relation to the existence of UV recovery mechanisms. Recovery and repair after UV radiation exposure has been documented in many different types of organisms, including viruses, bacteria, fungi, protozoa, and vertebrates, among others.[50] Recovery or photoreactivation of an organism that has been damaged by exposure to UV radiation is defined as the ability of an organism to regain its propagative potential. One of the primary mechanisms by which photoreactivation appears to work is the induction of a repair enzyme upon exposure to near UV- or short wavelength-visible light. This enzyme effectively reconnects two components of DNA that had been cleaved during exposure to UV radiation. The effectiveness of photoenzymatic repair is expressed by a single numerical index called the *fluence-reduction* or *fluence-modification factor*. The fluence reduction factor indicates the degree to which UV radiation-induced damage is reversed as a result of photoenzymatic repair.

It is important for the clinician who is considering using UVC for wound infections or to stimulate healing to recognize the presence of this UV recovery mechanism. Treatment times should be designed to exceed the ability for pathogens to reactivate but not for mammalian cells to recover from any detrimental effects of UV exposure. Because research has shown that increasingly complex organisms[35] are less susceptible to the detrimental effects of UVC radiation at a given dose, theoretically, it should be possible to design a treatment paradigm for wound infections that would prevent or minimize host cell damage. A recent study found that multicellular eukaryotic organisms required 6–10 times the UVC exposure time for 99.99% eradication, as compared with common bacterial wound pathogens, when tested in vitro. Another study[14] showed that UVC decreased the bacterial load in living tissue by 99.99% with once-daily treatment for 30 seconds over a 5-day period.

It is also thought that many of the positive biologic responses elicited by UV radiation can be effected by lower doses than are currently recommended. Therefore, it is recommended that an initial low dosage (MED, 30 seconds of UVC or UVA/UVB) be used in the treatment of wounds.

Treatment Distance

Recommended treatment distances for the UVC lamps are 1 inch or 2.54 cm from the UVC source to the wound bed.[5,6] UVC lamps are available with built-in spacers or the clinician can simply attach spacers made of 1-inch portions of sterile swabs or tongue depressors. The UVC energy should be delivered perpendicular to the wound bed to maximize delivery according to the cosine law.

Similar placement of the UVA and UVB lamp should be utilized to take advantage of the cosine law. However, treatment distances vary, with a general distance from UVA or UVB source to the skin surface being 30 inches.

Step-by-Step Guide to UVC Application

1. Cleanse faceplate of UV lamp with antimicrobial agent per manufacturer's guidelines.
2. As client comfort permits, position client for maximal exposure of the wound.
3. Remove all dressings.
4. Cleanse wound with normal saline.
5. Remove excess wound fluid and loosen particulate matter.
6. Drape periwound area or coat with nontoxic UV-blocking ointment (avoid getting it into the wound bed).
7. Protect clinician and client eyes from UV radiation with UV-protective goggles for clinician and goggles or draping for the client.
8. Place UVC lamp source 1 inch or 2.5 cm from wound.
9. Irradiate wound according to UVC algorithm (see Figure 23–3).
10. Remove UV blocking ointment and redress wound.

Step-by-Step Guide to UVA/UVB Application

1. Allow UVA/UVB lamp adequate time to warm up, according to manufacturer's guidelines.
2. Determine MED or E_1 dose with erythrometer over a nonpigmented area, such as the inner arm, starting with 30 seconds of exposure.
3. Then follow steps 2–7 above.
4. Place UVA/UVB source 30 inches from wound bed.
5. Irradiate wound according to UVC algorithm (see Figure 23–3), using an E_1 dose initially to stimulate epithelialization and increased vascularity.
6. Remove UV blocking ointment and redress wound.

Clinical Wisdom: *Orientation*

Orient UV lamp parallel to wound bed. Observing cosine law, orient UV lamp parallel to wound bed, with UV rays delivered perpendicular to wound in order to maximize energy delivery.

Indications

As outlined in the preclinical[14,37,38] and clinical[44,45,46,47,48] studies sections, UV radiation appears to be indicated for the following:

1. slow or nonhealing wounds
2. necrotic wounds
3. purulent, infected acute or chronic wounds

Contraindications

Commonly cited contraindications[21] to treatment include the following:

1. diabetes
2. pulmonary tuberculosis
3. hyperthyroidism
4. systemic lupus erythematous
5. cardiac, renal, and hepatic disease

6. acute eczema or psoriasis
7. herpes simplex

However, these contraindications may need to be reexamined in light of the recommendations to decrease treatment times significantly.

Adverse Reactions

With any adverse reaction, such as severe pain due to itching or burning, UV therapy should be discontinued. Hydrogel moist wound dressings or other products that have been shown to decrease the pain associated with radiation or burn wounds may increase client comfort and speed healing.

SELF-CARE TEACHING GUIDELINES

Administration of UV energy should be performed by a skilled individual licensed in the application of physical agent modalities. To prevent the occurrence of overexposure to the wound bed and inappropriate exposure to other skin areas, UVC treatment should not be administered by the individual receiving treatment or the responsible caregiver.

Additionally, as with all physical agent modalities or procedures, the clinician should evaluate the necessity of using this modality on a frequent and regular basis to ensure optimum treatment outcomes.

DOCUMENTATION

Treatment times, durations, and angle of incidence should be documented, along with distance that the UV energy source is placed from the wound bed. Client position during treatment, specific lamp model, and serial number of the lamp used should also be documented, as well as treatment outcomes.

REVIEW QUESTIONS

1. What are the early cutaneous changes induced by UV radiation?
2. Describe the mechanism whereby UV radiation facilitates epithelialization.
3. What wavelength range has peak germicidal activity? In what band of UV radiation is this range found?
4. List two ways to protect the periwound from UV exposure.

Case Study: *Decontamination of a Wound Infected with MRSA Using UVC Radiation*

Individual: M.G.

Age: 79
Start of Care Date: 4/98

Medical History

M.G. was a 79-year-old nonambulatory female resident of a long-term care facility with a sacral wound. Her medical diagnoses included CHF with end-stage renal disease. She required mod-max assist of two therapists for all bed mobility. She had no prior history of pressure ulceration.

Reason for Referral

Client was referred to physical therapy due to impaired bed mobility and the presence of a nonhealing stage 3 sacral pressure ulcer.

Functional Diagnosis and Targeted Outcomes

Wound Examination

The wound was a stage 3 pressure ulcer located over the sacrum. Wound margins were indurated, and the peri-

wound expressed moderate erythema. The periwound was also noted to be warmer than adjacent tissues. The wound bed was fully granulated and friable on manual examination, and a distinctive odor of ammonia was detected on initial examination. Semiquantitative swab cultures of this wound indicated that it contained high numbers of MRSA.

Functional Diagnosis

Impaired integumentary integrity secondary to full-thickness skin involvement and scar formation (from Guide to PT Practice, pattern 7D), chronic inflammation phase; *Targeted outcome*: Wound decontamination for progression through stages of wound healing and resolution of chronic inflammation.

Need for Skilled Services: The Therapy Problem

The client had a nonhealing stage 3 pressure ulcer and exhibited clinical signs of wound infection. Wound required decontamination and appropriate moist wound therapy to stimulate the healing process.

Treatment Plan and Outcome

A single application of UVC was applied to the wound bed to determine whether one application of UVC for 30

continues

Case Study continued

seconds was effective in immediately reducing the bacterial load. The wound was initially cleansed with normal saline, then a semiquantitative swab culture was obtained, using the 10-point culturing method. UVC was then applied to the wound bed with a V-254 halogen lamp, with a calibrated output of 15 mW for 30 seconds. The periwound was completely covered with draping materials, and the UVC lamp was placed parallel to the wound bed at a distance of 2.5 cm. Immediately after the UVC treatment, a second semiquantitative swab culture was performed. Both cultures were immediately sent for processing in the clinical laboratory. The laboratory report derived from the swab culture taken immediately prior to the UVC treatment showed high numbers of MRSA present. Results from the swab culture taken immediately posttreatment of the wound bed for 30 seconds with UVC demonstrated very low growth. This case study demonstrates the utility and immediacy of UVC in decontaminating the surface of the wound bed.

REFERENCES

1. Licht S. History of ultraviolet light therapy. In: Licht S, ed. *Therapeutic Electricity and Ultraviolet Radiation.* 2nd ed. New Haven, CT: Elizabeth Licht; 1967:191–212.

2. Licht S. History of ultraviolet therapy. In: Stillwell GK, ed. *Therapeutic Electricity and Ultraviolet Radiation.* 3rd ed. Baltimore, MD: Williams & Wilkins; 1983:228–261.

3. Moseley H. Sources of ultraviolet radiation. In: Moseley H. *Non-ionising Radiation: Microwaves, Ultraviolet and Laser Radiation.* Philadelphia: IOP Publishing Ltd; 1988:110.

4. Schwarz T, Urbanski A, Luger TA. Ultraviolet light and epidermal cell-derived cytokines. In: Luger TA, Schwarz T, eds. *Epidermal Growth Factors and Cytokines.* New York: Marcel Dekker; 1994:303.

5. Weisberg J. Ultraviolet irradiation. In: Hecox B, Mehreteab TA, Weisberg J, eds. *Physical Agents: A Comprehensive Text for Physical Therapists.* Norwalk, CT: Appleton & Lange; 1994:377–378.

6. Hayes KW. Ultraviolet radiation. In: Hayes KW, ed. *Manual for Physical Agents.* 5th ed. Norwalk, CT: Appleton & Lange; 1999.

7. Hart D. Sterilization of the air in the operating room by special antibacterial radiant energy. *J Thorac Surg.* 1936;6:45.

8. Berg M, Bergman BR, Hoborn J. Shortwave ultraviolet radiation in operating rooms. *J Bone Joint Surg.* 1989;71(3):483–485.

9. Lowell JD, Kundsin RB. The operating room and the ultraviolet environment. *Med Instrum.* 1978;12(3):161–164.

10. Moggio M, Goldner JL, McCollum DE, Beissinger SF. Wound infections in patients undergoing total hip arthroplasty. Ultraviolet light for the control of airborne bacteria. *Arch Surg.* 1979;114(7):815–823.

11. Taylor GJS, Bannister GC, Leeming JP. Wound disinfection with ultraviolet radiation. *J Hosp Infect.* 1995;30:85–93.

12. Taylor GJ, Chandler L. Ultraviolet light in the orthopaedic operating theatre. *Br J Theatre Nurs.* 1997;6(10):10–14.

13. Conner-Kerr TA, Sullivan PK, Gaillard J, Franklin ME, Jones RM. The effects of ultraviolet radiation on antibiotic-resistant bacteria in vitro. *Ostomy/Wound Manage.* 1998;44(10):50–56.

14. Conner-Kerr TA, Sullivan PK, Keegan A, Reynolds W, Sagemuehl T, Webb A. UVC reduces antibiotic resistant bacterial numbers in living tissue. *Ostomy/Wound Manage.* 1999;45(4):84.

15. Mertz PM, Davis SC, Oliveira-Gandia M, Eaglstein WH. The wound environment: implications from research studies for healing and infection. In: Krasner D, Kane D, eds. *Chronic Wound Care: A Clinical Source Book for Healthcare Professionals.* 2nd ed. Wayne, PA: Health Management Publications; 1997:57–58.

16. Mertz PM, Davis SC, Oliveira-Gandia M, Eaglstein WH. The wound environment: implications from research studies for healing and infection. *Wounds.* 1996;8(1):1–8.

17. Morykwas MJ, Mark MW. Effects of ultraviolet light on fibroblast fibronectin production and lattice contraction. *Wounds.* 1998;10(4):111–117.

18. Moseley H. Photomedicine. In: Moseley H. *Non-ionising Radiation: Microwaves, Ultraviolet and Laser Radiation.* Philadelphia: IOP Publishing Ltd; 1988:155–182.

19. Harm W. UV carcinogenesis. In: Harm W. *Biological Effects of Ultraviolet Radiation.* New York: Cambridge University Press; 1980:191.

20. Weisberg J. Electromagnetic spectrum. In: Hecox B, Mehreteab TA, Weisberg J, eds. *Physical Agents: A Comprehensive Text for Physical Therapists.* Norwalk, CT: Appleton & Lange; 1994:50.

21. Scott BO. Clinical uses of ultraviolet radiation. In: Stillwell GK, ed. *Therapeutic Electricity and Ultraviolet Radiation.* 3rd ed. Baltimore, MD: Williams & Wilkins; 1983:228–261.

22. Stenback F. Health hazards from ultraviolet radiation. *Public Health Rev.* 1982;10:229.

23. Daniels F. Ultraviolet light and dermatology. In: Stillwell GK, ed. *Therapeutic Electricity and Ultraviolet Radiation.* 3rd ed. Baltimore, MD: Williams & Wilkins; 1983:263–303.

24. Van der Leun JC. On the action spectrum of ultraviolet erythema. *Res Prog Organ Biol Med Chem.* 1972;3:711–736.

25. Hensby CN, Plummer NA, Black AK, Fincham N, Greaves MW. Time-course of arachidonic acid, prostaglandins E_2 and F_2 alpha production in human abdominal skin following irradiation with ultraviolet wavelengths (290–320 nm). *Adv Prostaglandin Thromboxane Res.* 1980;7:857–860.

26. Brauchle M, Funk JO, Kind P, Werner S. Ultraviolet B and H_2O_2 are potent inducers of vascular endothelial growth factor expression in cultured keratinocytes. *J Biol Chem.* 1996;271(36):21793–21797.

27. Holtz F. Pharmacology of ultraviolet radiation. *Br J Phys Med.* 1952;15:201.

28. Kaiser MR, Davis SC, Mertz PM. The effect of ultraviolet irradiation-induced inflammation on epidermal wound healing. *Wound Repair Regen.* 1995;3:311–315.

29. Sauder DN, Kilian PL, McLane JA, et al. Interleukin-1 enhances epidermal wound healing. *Lymphokine Re.* 1990;9(4):465–473.

30. Fan J, Schoenfeld RJ, Hunter RA. A study of the epidermal clear cells with special reference to their relationship to the cells of Langerhans. *J Invest Dermatol.* 1959;32:445–450.

31. Bergstresser PR, Toews GB, Streilein JW. Natural and perturbed distribution of Langerhans cells: Responses to ultraviolet light, heterotopic skin grafting and dinitrofluorobenzene sensitization. *J Invest Dermatol.* 1980;75:73–77.

32. Wu J, Barisoni D, Armato U. Prolongation of survival of alloskin grafts with no concurrent general suppression of the burned patient's immune system: A preliminary clinical investigation. *Burns.* 1996;22(5):353–358.

33. High AS, High JP. Treatment of infected skin wounds using ultra-violet radiation: An in vitro study. *Physiotherapy.* 1983;69(10):359–360.

34. Nordback I, Kulmala R, Jarvinen M. Effect of ultraviolet therapy on rat skin wound healing. *J Surg Res.* 1990;48:68–71.

35. Sullivan PK, Conner-Kerr T. A comparative study of the effects of UVC irradiation on select procaryotic and eucaryotic wound pathogens. *Ostomy/Wound Manage.* 2000;46(10):44–50.

36. Sullivan PK, Conner-Kerr TA, Smith ST. The effects of UVC irradiation on group A streptococcus in vitro. *Ostomy/Wound Manage.* 1999;45(10):50–58.

37. Taylor GJ, Leeming JP, Bannister GC. Effects of antiseptics, ultraviolet light and lavage on airborne bacteria in a model wound. *J Bone Joint Surg Br.* 1993;75(5):724–730.

38. El-Batouty MF, El-Gindy M, El-Shawaf I, Bassioni N, El-Ghaweet A, El-Emam A. Comparative evaluation of the effects of ultrasonic and ultraviolet irradiation on tissue regeneration. *Scand J Rheumatol.* 1986;15:381–386.

39. Das SK, Brantley SK, Davidson SF. Wound tensile strength in the hairless guinea pig following irradiation with pure ultraviolet-A light. *Br J Plast Surg.* 1991;44(7):509–513.

40. Davidson SF, Brantley SK, Das SK. The effects of ultraviolet radiation on wound healing. *Br J Plast Surg.* 1991;44(3):210–214.

41. Davidson SF, Brantley SK, Das SK. The reversibility of UV-altered wound tensile strength in the hairless guinea pig following a 90-day recovery period. *Br J Plast Surg.* 1992;45(2):109–112.

42. Basford JR, Hallman HO, Sheffield CG, Mackey GL. Comparison of cold-quartz ultraviolet, low-energy laser, and occlusion in wound healing in a swine model. *Arch Phys Med Rehabil.* 1986;67:151.

43. Sullivan PK, Conner-Kerr TA, Dixon S, et al. The effect of UVC irradiation on wound closure. Presented at the 2000 Symposium on Advanced Wound Care & Medical Research Forum on Wound Repair, April 2000; Dallas, TX.

44. Stein I, Shorey MM. Ultraviolet radiation in the treatment of indolent, soft-tissue ulcerations. *Physiotherapy Rev.* 1945;25(6):272–274.

45. Willis EE, Anderson TW, Beattie BL, Scott A. A randomized placebo controlled trial of ultraviolet light in the treatment of superficial pressure sores. *J Am Geriatr Soc.* 1983;31:131.

46. Crous L, Malherbe C. Laser and ultraviolet light irradiation in the treatment of chronic ulcers. *Physiotherapy.* 1988;44:73.

47. Nussbaum EL, Biemann, Mustard B. Comparison of ultrasound/ultraviolet-C and laser for treatment of pressure ulcers in patients with spinal cord injury. *Phys Ther.* 1994;74(9):812–825.

48. Taylor R. Clinical study of ultraviolet in various skin conditions. *Phys Ther.* 1972;52(3):279–282.

49. MacKinnon JL, Cleek PL. Therapeutic penetration of ultraviolet light through transparent dressing. *Phys Ther.* 1984;64:204.

50. Harm W. Recovery and repair. In: Harm W, ed. *Biological Effects of Ultraviolet Radiation.* New York: Cambridge University Press; 1980:76–123.

CHAPTER 24

Therapeutic and Diagnostic Ultrasound

Carrie Sussman and Mary Dyson

CHAPTER OBJECTIVES

At the completion of this chapter, the reader will be able to:

1. Recognize the terminology used to describe the properties of therapeutic and diagnostic ultrasound and the significance of each
2. Understand and analyze the present evidence of physical and physiologic effects of therapeutic ultrasound related to wound healing
3. Choose the most appropriate ultrasound therapeutic device for the intended intervention and the most appropriate transmission medium to achieve the desired outcome
4. Evaluate the appropriateness of choosing ultrasound treatment based on the patient, the wound, and the evidence
5. Explain recent advances in high resolution ultrasound to monitor the extent of soft tissue injury and repair

INTRODUCTION

The goal of this chapter is to present evidence of physical and physiologic effects through the comparison and contrast of megahertz (MHz) and kilohertz (kHz) ultrasound (US), demonstrating the rationale for using their physical properties and physiologic effects to accelerate the healing of skin and other forms of tissue repair. Clinical studies where US has been used for healing of animals and humans and a meta-analysis report on effect of US on chronic leg ulcers will be presented. For therapeutic US, the therapist is provided with sufficient information to select the most appropriate method of treatment for tissue repair of injuries of different etiolo-

gies and in different locations. For high-resolution diagnostic US, this chapter describes recent advances in the use of this modality, coupled with fractal analysis, to monitor the extent of soft tissue injury and its repair in a quantitative, objective manner.

EVALUATING THE EVIDENCE

Ultrasound as a treatment for many disorders came into vogue about 1950. After an extensive review of the literature, Gam and Johannsen[1] identified over 300 published papers on US treatment that appeared in the literature from 1949 to 1993, including clinical trials, experimental trials, and review articles. After reviewing the literature, they identified two categories of treatment objectives that met the criteria for inclusion in a meta-analysis: treatment effect on pain associated with musculoskeletal disorders and treatment effect for tissue repair of chronic leg ulcers. Subsequently, they have performed and published a meta-analysis of the studies in each of these categories.[1,2] Their conclusion, based on the results of the pain meta-analysis, was that US used in the treatment of musculoskeletal disorders is based on empirical experience but lacks firm evidence and well-controlled studies.[1] A possible reason for the poor results shown with the meta-analysis for pain is the wide variety of musculoskeletal disorders evaluated in the studies, some of which were acute and others chronic. The meta-analysis included 22 trials, where 12 different musculoskeletal diseases were treated with US.[1] Similar findings were reported by Falconer, Hayes, and Chang[3] in a quantitative synthesis of the literature, addressing the effectiveness of US on pain in acute and chronic inflammatory conditions. Thirty-five studies were identified, and 28 of the studies (16 papers) were published before 1970; five were published during the 1980s. All of the studies included human subjects with musculoskeletal disease. Also, like the findings of the Gam and Johannsen review, uncontrolled or unblinded studies more frequently reported positive outcomes.[1]

The findings regarding the use of US for tissue repair of chronic leg ulcers were more positive but mixed. Six studies met the criteria for this meta-analysis, and the meta-analysis showed significant treatment effect versus placebo or other treatment after 4 and 8 weeks (16.9% mean difference after 4 weeks and 14.5% mean difference after 8 weeks). These investigators found that there was great variability in reporting and treatment methods in both categories. Most studies in both categories were found lacking in reporting the descriptions of dropouts, randomization methods, US apparatus used, mode of treatment delivery, description of sham apparatus, size of the treatment head, dosage, number of treatments, sonation time, methods of blinding, etc.[2] Therefore, it is difficult to make definitive judgments about efficacy without well-designed controlled clinical trials.

If assignment of a grade level, according to the Sackett scheme,[4] is based on the strength of evidence of efficacy, then a grade level of "B" would probably be appropriate for treatment of chronic leg ulcers with US because evidence of efficacy has been demonstrated in several small randomized trials. Pressure ulcer treatment shows mixed and limited supporting evidence. More about the evidence of these clinical trials is presented later.

A 1993 review of the literature by the Agency for Health Care Research and Quality, formerly known as the Agency for Health Care Policy and Research, in preparation for the publication of guidelines for treatment of pressure ulcers in 1994 and Ovington's[5] 1999 literature review and update of these pressure ulcer guidelines considered US as an adjunctive therapy to accelerate or restart healing. Findings of both were that there was not sufficient evidence to permit recommending its use for the treatment of pressure ulcers, and US was assigned a grade "C" recommendation.[5,6]

The literature about US therapeutic efficacy for human tissue repair is inconclusive. Further investigation with well-designed clinical trials is needed to resolve the questions. For now, attention of the research community has shifted to researching the use of mHz US for diagnostic purposes to determine efficacy of wound healing interventions, to diagnose depth of tissue impairment, and kHz US for wound debridement and treatment. The new applications of kHzUS show great promise.

DEFINITIONS AND TERMINOLOGY

Ultrasound

Ultrasound is a mechanical vibration transmitted at a frequency above the upper limit of human hearing (ie, above 20 kHz, where 1 Hertz [Hz] = 1 cycle per second and 1 kHz = 1,000 cycles per second). It causes the molecules of media that can transmit it (eg, biologic tissues) to oscillate or vibrate and can be used therapeutically to accelerate wound healing and diagnostically to assess the extent of soft tissue injuries and to monitor their repair in a quantitative manner.

Megahertz US, typically between 0.5 and 3 MHz (ie, between 0.5 and 3 million cycles per second) has been used for more than 40 years to stimulate healing. During the last 5 years, 30- and 50-kHz US, also known as *long-wave US*, has been demonstrated to have therapeutic effects; this new form of therapeutic US is growing rapidly in use, particularly in Europe, but has not been adapted in the United States for wound healing. Hydrosound (Arjo, Roselle, IL), a product that incorporates 30-kHz US, is sold for hygiene use in the United States but is not approved by the U.S. Food and Drug Administration for wound healing effects.

Frequency

Many of the clinically relevant properties of US are related to its frequency (*f*). This is the number of times per second that a molecule displaced by the US completes a cycle of movement and returns to its original position. Frequencies are expressed in Hz, where 1 Hz = one cycle per second. The time taken to complete a cycle is termed a *period* (*T*).

Attenuation

Attenuation refers to the lessening of the force of the US wave as the sound energy is absorbed into, scattered by, or reflected by the tissues. At higher frequencies, more of the energy is absorbed by superficial structures than penetrates into deeper structures. For example, US units offering 3 MHz are now becoming widely available and are used for wound healing when superficial tissues are to be treated. For decades, 1-MHz US has been useful for deep penetration into tissues. This additional option provides opportunities to select devices with higher and lower frequencies for different treatment protocols and applications. With kHz units, there is even less attenuation and, therefore, greater penetration.

Half-Value Thickness

When US is transmitted through tissue, its intensity gradually decreases as a result of absorption, scattering, and reflection. The thickness of tissue necessary for the intensity applied to it to be reduced to one-half of the level applied to it is termed the *half-value thickness*. The intensity available at any depth within the tissue is inversely proportional to the depth of penetration (ie, the greater the depth, the less will be the remaining available intensity). For example, if 1 W/cm² of 1-MHz US is applied to the skin at a depth of 5 cm, only

0.25 W/cm² would be available. Absorption, which is a major cause of attenuation (eg, loss of intensity), is frequency dependent. The greater the frequency, the shorter the wavelength; the shorter the wavelength, the greater the absorption. For a US beam of 3 MHz, the wavelength is shorter than that at 1 MHz, and, therefore, absorption occurs more readily than at 1 MHz, reducing the half-value thickness by 3. Thus, in the example above, the half-value thickness would be 5/3 = 1.7 cm. A frequency of 3 MHz is an efficient one to use to treat superficial regions, such as injured skin, but lower frequencies are indicated for deeper targets, such as injured muscle or bone.

The amount of absorption varies with the composition of the tissues, as well as with the wavelength, which, as described above, is inversely related to frequency. Bone is more absorptive than highly proteinaceous tissues (eg, dermis and muscle); protein is more absorptive than fat (eg, adipose tissue); and fat is more absorptive than water-rich materials (eg, plasma, edematous tissues). Because of this, the half-value thickness of bone is less than that of muscle, which is less than that of fat, which is less than that of edematous soft connective tissue. US can, therefore, penetrate skin, fat, and edematous tissues to reach a deeply located injury in, for example, a joint capsule or a muscle. With kHz US, even bone and metal can be penetrated, with sufficient energy remaining to have an effect on injured tissue deep to the bone or metal.

Clinical Wisdom: *Use the US Unit Available*

If a 3-MHz US unit is not available, good results can be had with a 1-MHz unit. Part of the US wave will still be absorbed by the superficial tissues, just a lesser amount. As 3-MHz units become more widely available in the clinic, the options for treatment will be enhanced. In the meantime, do not hesitate to use what is available, but for best results, start as soon as possible after injury.

Wavelength

The *wavelength* (λ) is the shortest distance, measured parallel to the direction of wave propagation, between molecules that are at equivalent points of vibration in the repeated cycle of movement, which constitutes a wave. It is related to the frequency and *velocity* (c) of the wave by the equation: $\lambda = c/f$. The velocity of US in water, blood, interstitial fluid, and soft tissues is approximately 1,500 m/s. The higher the frequency, the shorter the wavelength. This is important diagnostically, because the shorter the wavelength, the greater the degree of resolution. The frequency of 20 MHz that is used by a prototype soft tissue scanner, developed at Guy's Hospital in London and tested at West Jersey and West

Hudson Wound Healing Centers, produces a wavelength that is sufficiently short to allow collagen fiber bundles and other acoustically different components of intact and damaged soft connective tissues to be distinguished. The prototype provided the model for the Longport Digital Scanner, which is now being marketed in the United States.

High frequencies are more readily absorbed by tissues than are low frequencies and produce a greater thermal effect in the tissues. Lower frequencies produce cavitation and the microstreaming associated with it more readily than do higher frequencies; there is evidence that many of the biologic effects produced by therapeutic US are caused by cavitation and microstreaming.[1]

Equipment for Generation of Ultrasound

The equipment used to produce therapeutic levels of MHz US typically consists of a microcomputer-controlled high-frequency generator linked by a coaxial cable to an applicator or treatment head. The treatment head contains a disc of a piezoelectric material, such as lead zirconate titanate, which acts as a transducer to change one form of energy into another, in this case, into US. When an alternating voltage is applied across such a disc, it expands and contracts at the same frequency as the oscillation, transducing electrical energy into US. A similar system is made use of for kHz US, but the frequency of vibration is much lower, and the transducers have a different composition and mode of operation.

The Ultrasonic Field

The ultrasonic pressure field generated by the transducer depends on the size and shape of the transducer and on how it is mounted in the applicator. The pressure varies across the surface of the applicator, as well as with the distance from it. The pressure changes experienced by the tissues being treated, therefore, depend in part on their position relative to the applicator. Ultrasound is emitted from a disc-shaped transducer of the type used with MHz therapeutic US as a beam, which is at first cylindric; this region is termed the *near field*, or *Fresnel zone* (generally within 10–30 cm of the sound head surface), and the energy distribution in it is extremely variable, meaning that the energy may vary from little or no intensity to very high peak intensities. Beyond this, the beam starts to diverge and the energy distribution with it becomes more regular; this region is termed the *far field*, or *Fraunhofer zone*. The distance (d) from the transducer to the beginning of the far field is related to the radius (a) of the transducer and the wavelength (λ) of the US: $d = a^2/\lambda$. Unless the part to be treated is immersed in a water bath in which the transducer and target tissue can be separated by a distance sufficient for the target tissues to be in the far field,

US therapy usually involves treatment of tissue in the non-uniform near field. The *beam nonuniformity ratio* (BNR) is a measure of this nonuniformity and is the ratio of the spatial peak intensity (I[SP]) to the spatial average intensity (I[SA]). These terms are defined below. Applicators with low BNRs have more homogeneous beam patterns that give more *predictable* results and are *safer* than those with higher BNRs, because the higher spatial peak intensities of the latter are potentially damaging.[7]

Selection of Equipment

The selection of US equipment should be based on the following considerations:

1. Select a transducer with low BNR.
2. Select a transducer that is water immersible.
3. Select one transducer that is < 2 cm² and another 5 cm². Avoid large transducers with small effective radiating area (ERA).
4. Chose an ergonomically designed transducer that is comfortable to hold.
5. Select a unit with multiple frequencies for optimal treatment options, depending on desired depth of penetration.
6. Select a unit with a built-in test feature that tests output performance every time the unit is powered up.
7. Recalibrate the unit at least twice a year. If there is significant drift, more frequent recalibration is required. If that does not take care of the problem, consider repair or replacement of the device.

Intensity

Intensity (I) is the amount of energy (in watts) per unit area per unit time. Applicators typically have an ERA of a few square centimeters. The ERA is always less than the size of the transducer surface, so the size of the transducer is not a true indicator of the actual radiating surface. Individual transducers should be scanned to ensure proper calibration of intensity in w/cm². The intensity can be averaged in space over the face of the applicator (termed *spatial average* [SA]) or in time (termed *temporal average* [TA]). When pulsed US is used, pulse average (PA) intensity (this is the TA during the period of the pulse) should be noted, as should the TA during the full pulse repetition cycle. The type of intensity should be specified as either I(SATA), if continuous, or both I(SATA) and I(SAPA), if pulsed. Information provided about the SATA is useful in comparing US dosage reported in studies. Exhibit 24–1 summarizes US intensity terminology and gives examples.[8]

Exhibit 24–1 Summary of Ultrasound Intensity Terminology

Intensity = total power output at a given setting of amplitude divided by the ERA in cm², measured in W/cm²

Spatial average (SA) intensity: intensity averaged over the surface area of the transducer

Temporal average (TA) intensity: intensity average over the time of treatment

Pulse average (PA) intensity: temporal average during the period of the pulse

Spatial peak intensity (SP): peak intensity over the surface area of the transducer

Beam Nonuniformity Ratio (BNR): ratio of the spatial peak intensity to the spatial average intensity.

Most units sold have BNR of 5:1 or 6:1 but may be as low as 2:1. Example: Transducer with BNR of 5:1 SA set at 1 W/cm² SP may be as high as 5 W/cm.²

Spatial Average Temporal Peak Intensity (SATA): spatial average intensity of the US during the on time of the pulse. Clinical US units display the SATP intensity and the duty cycle.

Spatial Average Temporal Average Intensity (SATA): spatial average intensity averaged over the on and off time of the pulse (SATA = SATP × duty cycle). Example: 1 W/cm² SATP at 20% duty cycle = 1 × 0.2 = 0.2 W/cm² SATA. SATA is amount of energy delivered to the tissues. For continuous US, the SATA is equal to the SATP.

Source: Adapted with permission from Michelle Cameron, Ultrasound, *Physical Agents in Rehabilitation*, pp. 275–76, © 1999, W.B. Saunders Company.

Thermal and Nonthermal Effects

A medium-intensity range required to elevate tissue temperature to a range of 40–45° C is 1.0–2.0 W/cm² continuously for 5–10 minutes.[7] This is acceptable only in inadequately vascularized tissues. Temperatures above this cause thermal *necrosis* and *must be avoided*. Thermal effects occur with both 1-MHz and 3-MHz US when continuous wave US is applied, but at different tissue depth. In contrast, therapeutic kHz US can be used in continuous mode without physiologically significant heating. At a frequency of 3 MHz, energy absorption occurs mainly in superficial tissues (1–2 cm beneath the surface). At a frequency of 1 MHz, less energy is absorbed by the superficial tissues, provided that there is an adequate output from the transducer. This frequency also penetrates into deeper tissues, with effective energy levels being available up to 5 cm below the surface. Nonthermal effects are reduced by pulsing the wave, because this reduces the temporal average intensity. Whenever US is absorbed, heat is produced, but if the temperature increases less than 1° C, this is not considered to be physiologically relevant; in such circumstances, therapeutic effects are due primarily to nonthermal mechanisms.

Because many wounds occur in ischemic tissues, care must be used when applying thermal US in the presence of arterial occlusive disease. In these areas, there is reduced ability to dissipate heat, and burns can result. Ultrasound is contraindicated in the presence of arterial occlusion. Nonthermal application is safer over areas of impaired circulation.

Stable Cavitation and Microstreaming

Nonthermal effects of US occur at a low spatial average intensity, which can be achieved by pulsing at, for example, a 20% duty cycle and are attributed to two different mechanisms: *cavitation* and *acoustic streaming*. Cavitation involves the production and vibration of micron-sized bubbles within the coupling medium and fluids within the tissues. The US beam affects small gaseous bubbles that move within the tissue fluids. As the bubbles collect and condense, they are compressed before moving on to the next area. The movement and compression of the bubbles can cause changes in the cellular activities of the tissues subjected to US. Stable cavitation occurs when the bubbles in the field do not change much in size. The effect of stable cavitation can result in diffusional changes along cell membranes, thereby altering cell function. Stable cavitation is potentially beneficial because of its ability to initiate cellular changes within the tissues. Unstable or transient cavitation refers to collapse of the bubbles mentioned above. Transient bubbles implode, causing local mechanical damage and free radical formation. This is potentially very hazardous. It occurs at high intensities, particularly when the sound head is not moved during treatment and standing waves develop.

A second nonthermal effect of US is acoustic streaming. This is defined as the movement of fluids along the acoustic boundaries (eg, bubbles or cell membranes) as a result of the mechanical pressure wave associated with the US beam.[7] Outcomes attributable to this effect include increased cell membrane and vascular wall permeability and increased protein synthesis.

It is suggested that stable cavitation and microstreaming are responsible for the stimulatory effects of low-intensity US, acting as a stimulus that reversibly modifies plasma membrane permeability and, thus, modulates cellular activity. Transient cavitation and standing wave formation are potentially damaging but are readily avoided by using low intensities and keeping the applicator moving during treatment.

HIGH-RESOLUTION DIAGNOSTIC ULTRASOUND

Ultrasound, a mechanical vibration transmitted at a frequency above the limit of human hearing, ie, in excess of 20 mHz, is widely used as both a diagnostic and therapeutic agent. As previously described, the US is generated by the electrical stimulation (ES) of a piezoelectric material termed a *transducer*. Ultrasound has an excellent safety record and is considered sufficiently safe to use to image sensitive structures, such as the developing fetus.

Imaging

Ultrasound imaging depends on the principle that different tissue components reflect and absorb the waves of US to varying degrees, depending on their acoustic properties, which, in turn, depend on their structure. For example, tissues rich in fat absorb less US than do tissues rich in protein. Reflection occurs at the interface between materials that differ in their acoustic properties, specifically in their acoustic impedance. Piezoelectric materials not only transduce electrical signals into mechanical vibrations, but also transduce mechanical vibrations into electrical signals. In US imaging, the reflected US is detected by the same transducer that produced it during the short intervals between the pulses of US emitted by the transducer. The transducer converts the reflected mechanical vibrations into electrical signals, which are used to visualize structures deep to the surface by converting the digitized data from consecutive A-scans (scans of echo amplitude) into a two-dimensional image, termed a *B-scan* or *brightness scan*. Movement of the transducer allows a series of scans produced consecutively to be used to form an image analogous to that of a multielement transducer. The reflections or echoes received at each beam position are displayed as spots on the display screen of the scanner, the brightness of each spot being related to the echo amplitude as a gray-scale display. The position of the spots is determined by the orientation of the beam and the time of arrival of the echoes. The gray scale can be replaced by different colors to assist in visual interpretation of the image, the colors representing differing levels of echogenicity from different tissue components. These components—and, hence, the pattern and brightness of the reflections from them—vary with the tissue and are modified by injury and during repair. When high-resolution diagnostic US is used, the resultant image, which superficially resembles a histologic section, can be thought of as a noninvasive biopsy produced in a nontraumatic, painless manner with no damage to the tissues that interact with the low-intensity US.

Visual Details

The detail that can be visualized ultrasonically is dependent on the resolution of the imaging equipment used, and this depends mainly on the wavelength of the US, which is determined by the frequency; the higher the frequency, the shorter the wavelength and, therefore, the greater the resolution. There is an inverse relationship between frequency and depth of penetration, higher frequencies being less penetrative than lower frequencies. In 1991, US at a frequency of 5 MHz (ie, 5 million cycles of vibration per second) was described as providing "high resolution"[9] and was considered to be adequate to view, for example, the plantaris tendon, provided that this was at least 2 mm thick, when the aim was merely to demonstrate whether it was present and whether it was thick enough to be used as a graft. Plantaris is a vestigial muscle; its elongated tendon is an excellent source of tendon graft, being long enough to be used for a wide range of tendon and ligament reconstructions. However, cadaveric studies, cited by Simpson et al,[9] have shown that it is absent from 7% to 20% of human legs, and, if absent from one leg, there is only a one in three chance that it will be present on the contralateral side. In some other limbs, it may be too small to be surgically useful. Ultrasound imaging is, therefore, of clinical value in determining in a noninvasive manner whether the plantaris is present and whether it is of a suitable thickness for use as a graft.

More recently, improved instrumentation, coupled with the use of higher frequencies and image analysis, has resulted in the effective use of US to visualize noninvasive changes in tissue associated with the presence of injury or its development and with its repair. In 1993, O'Reilly and Massouh[10] published a pictorial essay in which they compared the ultrasonic appearance of normal and damaged Achilles tendons, using a real-time scanner equipped with a 7.5-MHz linear transducer and a 5.0-MHz sector transducer. They were able to detect and distinguish between tenosynovitis, acute and chronic tendinitis, peritendinitis, nodular tendinitis, and partial or complete tendon rupture on the basis of differences in echogenecity and measurements of tendon thickness, the changes detected ultrasonographically being confirmed invasively by fine-needle aspiration and histologic examination.

Higher frequencies, permitting greater resolution, can be used for more superficial structures, such as the components of skin, where less depth of penetration is required. In 1994, 20-MHz US was used by Karim et al[11] to image skin from various parts of the body, and it was demonstrated that mathematical algorithms could be used to characterize and classify the dermal monograms as to their site of origin. Two analytic techniques were investigated—fractal analysis and fast Fourier transform—the aim being to develop image analysis techniques sensitive enough to detect minute changes in the pattern of the ultrasonically produced images and to avoid interobserver differences in interpretation of these images.

Fractals

Fractals are a language of geometry, fractal structures being those that have a characteristic form that remains constant over a range of magnifications. A dichotomously branching tree is an example of a fractal structure, maintaining a self-similarity independent of the scale at which it is viewed. The fractal texture analysis program operates by first representing the region of interest selected as a three-dimensional landscape, with lateral and axial dimensions on the horizontal plane and the intensity of the reflections that comprise the image on the vertical axis. The program then calculates the area of the landscape.[12] The area of the image is measured at different resolutions, from 1 to 20 pixels. At a given resolution, the rate of change of this area with respect to resolution is related to the estimated fractal dimension at that resolution. This set of fractal dimensions defines the fractal signature. It describes the manner in which any pattern varies from a fully fractal pattern, the fractal signature of which would be a horizontal line, because true fractals have a constant fractal dimension at all resolutions; the fractal signatures of partially fractal structures are complex curves, any horizontal region indicating the range of resolutions at which the structure is fractal. B-scans of skin from different regions of the body have different fractal signatures, as do scans of damaged and repairing dermis. Williams et al[13] and Karim et al[11] found that Fournier analysis, which models the ultrasonic image by mathematically decomposing it into a series of periodic functions (sine waves) of different frequencies and phases from which the original can be reconstructed, was somewhat less consistent than fractal analysis in distinguishing between scans of dermis from different regions of the body. Fourier analysis has not yet been used to analyze damaged and repairing dermis, although its ability to do this should be investigated.

Longport Diagnostic US Scanner

Most recently, a new generation of high-resolution diagnostic US equipment has been developed at the United Medical and Dental Schools of Guy's and St. Thomas's Hospitals in London. This is now a commercial product, marketed as the Longport Digital Scanner that is currently being used in the United States, Europe, and Australia to monitor changes in soft connective tissues associated with damage and its repair. A patent was applied for to cover this equipment in 1995, the final version of the patent being provided by Dyson et al in 1996. The prototype is portable and is fitted with a polyvinylidene difluoride piezoelectric polymer transducer incorporated into a handset filled with distilled water. It can emit a single cycle pulse at a frequency of between 10 and 50 MHz, although it is generally used at a frequency on the order of 20 MHz. This allows the production of images of the interfaces between acoustically different materials, with a resolution such that structures separated by approximately 65 μm in the direction of US transmission can be distinguished. The transducer is moved within the probe by a stepper motor, producing pulses of US with a repetition frequency of 1 msec. The system has been designed to emit an ultrafast rise and fall time pulse of duration of less than 50 nsec. These sharp pulses allow excellent detection of reflected signals, which, after transduction, pass through a preamplifying unit in the probe before passing to the main unit. As with other US imaging devices, including those operating at lower frequencies, time-gain compensation is used to control for the attenuation that occurs as the US is reflected back to the transducer. Digitization of the reflected signals produces data that can be stored and used for statistical analysis.[14,15] A digital scan converter stores information in the US scan format and displays it in the video format.

Practical Implications

Practically, the system allows the epidermis to be distinguished from the dermis. Differences in the pattern of the reflections distinguish the papillary from the reticular layers of the dermis, and blood vessels, tendon sheaths, tendons, ligaments, and adipose tissue can be identified, as can the interfaces between soft tissue and calcified tissue. Cross-sectional images of the skin produced by this high-resolution, B-mode, 20-MHz US scanner have a very characteristic appearance. The epidermal/dermal interface is clearly identifiable as a hypoechoic zone, deep to which is a highly reflective band, followed by the highly echogenic dermis,[16] the pattern of echoes varying from a speckled appearance in the papillary zone of the dermis to a linear appearance in its deeper reticular zone, where the collagen fiber bundles are thicker. Fluid-containing spaces within the dermis appear to be less echogenic, as does subcutaneous fat, although this produces some thin linear echoes that may represent strands of collagenous fibrous connective tissue *(Color Plate 71)*. The scanner allows changes in soft tissue associated with the development of injury and its repair to be monitored *(Color Plates 72 and 73)* and subjected to fractal analysis, producing fractal signatures that can be compared, as did earlier, less informative and versatile instrumentation.[17,18] Most recently, it has been used to detect dermal changes associated with exposure to pressure[19] and as a means of quantifying the irritant response.[20] Its ability to detect and possibly quantify muscle inflammation remains to be investigated; in 1990, Van Holsbeek and Introcaso[21] demonstrated echogenic differences between normal and inflamed muscle with the less sensitive instrumentation then available.

Other uses are as a means of monitoring changes in the thickness of the epidermis and of underlying soft connective tissues, and in detecting lesions such as melanomas, potentially when as small as approximately 70 μm in thickness. As long ago as 1984, Shafir et al[22] indicated that what were then considered to be high-resolution US scanners could measure precisely the thickness of melanomas. Accurate measurement of thickness can provide useful prognostic information, because this dimension is directly related to metastatic potential.[23] Also of importance is the potential of fractal analysis of these high-quality images to provide quantitative data for comparison and assessment of the effectiveness of various therapies in the treatment of injured tissues. Fractal analysis of the images may also be an aid to the diagnosis of a variety of skin pathologies, but this possibility remains to be examined critically.

One area of concern is about the inability of clinicians to detect stage I pressure ulcers accurately in people with darkly pigmented skin.[24-27] This is due to the reliance on the assessment parameter of color change—specifically, redness (unblanchable erythema)—for all patients, rather than considering the different color change hues of blue-purple in people with darkly pigmented skin. Because the assessment of color is affected by the quantity and quality of the light source used, its value as the only indicator of stage I pressure ulcers in persons of color is questionable. Therefore, inclusion of other characteristics, such as skin temperature, stiffness, and sensation, has been proposed,[27] together with the use of high-resolution US B-scans.[28,29]

Although the specific characteristics of early pressure-related injury are yet to be defined, awareness of the need to educate clinicians in culturally sensitive assessment techniques is growing.[15] Use of the US scanner described above greatly increases both the sensitivity and specificity of correctly identifying stage I pressure ulcers, particularly in darkly pigmented skin. Dependence on less accurate measure to identify stage I pressure ulcers in skin, regardless of its level of pigmentation, could be eradicated by the use of this equipment. The implementation of appropriate preventative measures and treatment, such as the use of physical modalities described in this section, could significantly decrease the incidence of pressure ulcers in those at risk, leading to improvement in the quality of life and savings in the cost of health care. The effectiveness of these measures can now be assessed readily, objectively, and without damage or discomfort to the patient.[28]

The clinical future for high-frequency, high-resolution, diagnostic US is of considerable importance and will grow as more uses are demonstrated for it. What is now required is more research of a high quality; this is being organized internationally.

THEORY AND SCIENCE OF EFFECT OF ULTRASOUND ON WOUND HEALING

Cells close to stable bubbles are subject to bubble-associated microstreaming that has been shown to increase their plasma membrane permeability to calcium ions, temporarily acting as a stimulus to cell activity (eg, cell migration, proliferation, synthesis of intracellular and extracellular materials) and synthesis and release of growth factors. All of these activities would be expected to accelerate wound healing. In cells treated in suspension, the suppression of cavitation also suppresses this stimulation of cellular activity. It should be noted that the ultrasonic stimulus is perceived by the cells and transduced by them; an amplified response then occurs of a type that varies according to the cell type involved.

Clinical Wisdom

The portability of the Longport Scanner and its ease of use makes it ideal for use in every care setting: home, clinic, hospital, hospice, and as an important component of telemedicine. The B-scans of pressure ulcers or of the skin and subcutaneous soft tissue at each pressure point take only a few seconds to produce; they are stored electronically and can be either interpreted on the spot or transmitted elsewhere via the internet for detailed analysis and comparison.[28]

Source: Reprinted from Mary Dyson and Courtney Lyder, Wound Management: Physical Modalities, *The Prevention and Treatment of Pressure Ulcers*, Moya Morrison, ed., pp. 189–191, © 2001, by permission of the publisher Mosby.

Effect on the Phases of Healing

Wound recovery occurs as a series of overlapping biochemical responses to injury. Recovery normally concludes in approximately 21 days. Inflammation occurs in the first 72 hours. In these early hours, epithelial cells begin migration and reproduction to restore the skin integrity and to protect the body from infection or admission of foreign substances.

Inflammatory Phase

In normal wounding, the acute inflammatory state occurs following an initial clotting response that initiates a vascular response involving the arterial and venous systems. This, in turn, leads to vasodilatation and invasion of the area by a large number of white blood cells that release growth factors necessary to initiate repair. (See Chapter 2 regarding physiology of wound healing.) These white blood cells include macrophages, polymorphonuclear leukocytes, and mast cells. The mast cells degranulate, releasing histamine hyaluronic acid and other proteoglycans that bind with the watery wound fluid to create a gel. Coagulated wound gel will later be replaced by a dense, binding scar. The massive vascular incursion into the periwound tissues produces the symptoms associated with the inflammatory phase: calor, dolor, rubor, and turgor. This is a critical period of repair. Ultrasound delivered at this time stimulates the release of growth factors from platelets, mast cells, and macrophages, which, in turn, are chemotactic to the fibroblasts and endothelial cells that later form collagen-containing vascular granulation tissue. Early intervention with US accelerates the inflammatory phase, leading to more rapid entry into the proliferative

phase of repair. It is not antiinflammatory. Therefore, US treatment should begin as soon as possible, ie, during the acute inflammatory phase.

Research and Clinical Wisdom:
Use US To Restart the Inflammatory Phase

- Use US as soon as possible after injury to accelerate the inflammatory phase, leading to more rapid entry into the proliferative phase of repair.
- A single thermal treatment with US has been shown to induce the inflammatory phase in chronic wounds.
- In the clinic, chronic diabetic foot ulcer and pressure wounds that have a diagnosis of "absence of inflammatory phase" (see Chapter 4 for information about diagnosis of absence of inflammatory phase) responded with restarting of the inflammatory phase, including periwound erythema and a gellike serous exudate within 2–3 days after this application of US. In the next 2–3 weeks, there were measurable decreases in wound size, depth, and undermining, indicating an increase in fibroplasia and wound contraction. No adverse reactions occurred. This is a topic for further research. The protocol used involved 1 MHz, 0.5 W/cm² (SATP), 20% duty cycle, daily for 5 minutes to periwound area.[29]

Proliferative Phase

Following the acute inflammatory phase, the proliferative phase begins about 72 hours after injury and overlaps the late inflammatory phase. Proliferative phase is divided into two stages: fibroplasia and contraction. New tissue has a pink granular appearance and is called *granulation tissue*. Granulation tissue builds on the collagen matrix laid down by the fibroblasts. Granulation tissue will remodel into tissue with mechanical properties similar to those of the uninjured tissue. Ultrasound stimulates fibroblast migration and proliferation. Dyson[30] reports that fibroblasts exposed to therapeutic levels of US in vivo were stimulated to synthesize more of the type of collagen that gives soft connective tissue most of its tensile strength. Endothelial cells, responsible for vascularization of the granulation tissue, are also affected by US at this stage to produce more prolific growth. Under histologic examination, more angiogenesis is seen in granulation tissue that has been sonated at 0.75 MHz and 0.1 W/cm² than in untreated tissue.[30–32]

The late phase of proliferation is wound contraction. During this process, the wound is pulled together by the centripetal movement of the surrounding tissue. This results in less scar tissue formation. Fibroblasts transform into specialized contractile cells called *myofibroblasts* for this process. Myofibroblasts at this phase resemble smooth muscle cells.

In some experiments, smooth muscle cells are reported to contract when treated with therapeutic levels of US. It is postulated that myofibroblasts are similarly affected. US, applied during the inflammatory and early proliferative phases, may accelerate wound contraction by causing those cells to develop earlier and increasing their efficiency. At this time, however, the mechanisms by which this occurs are not fully understood. Dyson states that no reports have been found of excessive pathologic contraction (ie, contracture) following treatment with therapeutic US.[30,31] Therefore, intervention with low-intensity, nonthermal US within 72 hours following injury can be used to promote wound contraction, which results in a reduction in size of the resulting scar.[33]

Clinical Wisdom: *Ultrasound and High-Voltage Pulsed Current for Dual Purpose*

Ultrasound has been useful in the clinic to treat over periwound tissue above undermined and tunneled areas because 1 MHz can penetrate up to 5 cm. This treatment has been given in conjunction with high-voltage pulsed current (HVPC) to the wound bed. Response has been decreased size of depth and undermining measurements within the first 2 weeks from start of this treatment. No adverse reactions occurred. This is a topic for further research. Protocol used involved 1 MHz, 0.5 W/cm² (SATP), 20% duty cycle, daily for 5 minutes to periwound area for 2–3 weeks.[29] High-resolution diagnostic US can be used to visualize the extent of tunneling and its resolution.

Epithelialization Phase

Epithelialization begins concurrently with inflammatory and proliferative phases. The epithelial cells begin moving and reproducing within a few hours of injury. These cells require an environment that is warm, moist, free of infection, and provides a supply of nutrients and oxygen in order to move and to multiply.[34–36]

Ultrasound stimulates the release of growth factors necessary for regeneration of the epithelial cells. Ultrasound has the capability of increasing the vascularity of the tissue and may in this way improve nutrient and oxygen delivery. Ultrasound, therefore, appears to stimulate epithelialization and hasten it, associated with granulation, by application to the periwound areas.

Remodeling/Maturation Phase

This phase is affected by low-intensity US *only if* treatment is commenced in the inflammatory phase. If so, the effects are more rapid entry into the remodeling phase, increased wound tensile strength, increased capacity to absorb energy without mechanical damage, increased elasticity, and deposition of collagen fibers in a pattern closer to that of intact tissue. Several researchers have reported the application of thermal US during the remodeling phase to affect collagen extensibility and enzyme activity mechanically. Frieder et al[37] reported improved collagen organization, and Jackson et al[38] reported improved tensile strength in tendon repairs of US-treated animals. Hart[33] demonstrated that treatment with low-intensity nonthermal US in the early inflammatory phase influences the outcome of the scar collagen density and organization. Later treatment is less effective.

Pain and Edema

Pain is a symptom associated with the inflammatory phase due to the influx of blood; the release of chemicals such as histamine, prostaglandins, and bradykinin; and the associated pressure from posttraumatic edema on surrounding nerve endings. Reduction of pain is an essential part of wound healing, resulting in reduced muscle guarding and increased activity that, in turn, enhances circulation to the area of wounding. Pain also stimulates the sympathetic nervous system, producing a reactive hyperemia. The result is an increased area of inflammation. This enhances the metabolic requirements of the surrounding tissue for more nutrients and oxygen. Pain relief can reduce the area of involvement and decrease the bioburden. Theoretically, pain threshold has been raised with thermal application of therapeutic US, due to a rise in the nerve conduction velocity of the C fibers.[39] However, after careful examination of the published reports, there is no conclusive theoretic explanation of how pain is relieved by US.[31]

Clinical Wisdom: *US for Skin Tears*

Skin tears are a common problem for the elderly. They are often painful and surrounded with edema and ecchymosis. Application of nonthermal US with an US conductive gel/lotion over a hydrogel transmission sheet or a transparent film dressing produces reduction in pain and edema after one or two treatments and dispersal of the ecchymosis within 6–10 sessions, depending on the size of the area involved. This method allows the dressing to remain in place between treatments and will not disrupt the wound or cause skin damage. As healing progresses, expect the patient's mobility to increase. Protocol used involved 1 MHz, 0.5 W/cm² (SATP), 20% duty cycle, daily for 5 minutes to periwound area; a setting of 3 MHz is preferable.[29]

Enhanced blood flow creates greater capillary pressure and fluid shift into the interstitial tissues, and this creates edema. Acoustic streaming, described earlier, may affect the vascular permeability and help to control periwound edema. Edema-free and pain-free outcomes are highly desirable because they accelerate and decrease the duration of the inflammatory process.[7]

Circulation

Transcutaneous partial pressure of oxygen (tcPO$_2$) can be measured before and after treatment as a method of monitoring changes in blood flow (see Chapter 7). Byl and Hopf[40] found that, following pulsed low-intensity, 0.5 W/cm^2, 1-MHz US, little increase in tissue temperature or oxygen transport occurred unless the individual was both well hydrated (three to four glasses of water) and receiving supplemental oxygen by nasal cannula. Those subjects then had an increase in subcutaneous oxygen four times higher than that measured when the same subjects were breathing room air. Thermal application with high-dose 1.0 W/cm^2, low-frequency, 1-MHz US produced vasodilatation and raised tissue oxygen levels and temperature significantly. Care must be taken to avoid excessive thermal effects whereby circulation is diminished and heat cannot be dissipated rapidly.[40] Increased circulation brings nutrients and oxygen to the tissues and removes waste products that can impede healing. Because increased circulation and oxygen are such critical components of wound healing and are dose dependent, this needs to be considered in the use of protocols for healing.

Clinical Wisdom:
Increasing Circulation with High-Dose US

Ischemic tissues surrounding a chronic wound, which have not responded to other types of wound treatments, may benefit from periwound US. If the wound bed is clean, expect increased serosanguineous exudate from the wound base to appear in 3–5 days. If the wound has necrotic tissue, expect to see lysis of the necrotic tissue, increased periwound erythema, and temperature due to the increased circulation associated with change in wound phase to acute inflammatory phase. If this does not occur, repeat the single higher-intensity treatment and follow with lower-intensity treatments. Parameters of treatment are 1.0 to 1.4 W/cm^2 (SA, TP), 1 MHz or 3 MHz, continuous 5- to 10-minute duration, depending on the size of the area. Reduce intensity to 0.5 W/cm^2 (SA, TP), pulsed 20%, three to five times per week after one treatment.[18]

Research Wisdom:
Supplement Patient's Hydration and Oxygen

See that patients are well hydrated before US treatment. Add supplemental oxygen by nasal cannula at 5 L/min, which has been shown to prevent infection in surgical wounds[41] and to raise tissue oxygen levels when used in conjunction with US. Both will improve outcome of healing.

Bruising/Hematoma

Ultrasound has been described as increasing dispersal of hemorrhagic material associated with bruising.[42] Ultrasound treatment may increase the efficiency of the phagocytic cells, which remove this material.

Hemorrhagic materials in the tissues can lead to tissue death from hypoxia and ischemia in the surrounding tissues, resulting in ulceration following a tissue trauma (eg, a stage I pressure ulcer). US can accelerate the absorption. *Color Plates 74* through *80* show case examples of absorption of hemorrhagic material following the use of US. In both cases, *no* other treatment intervention was given.

Clinical Wisdom: *US and Absorption of Hematoma*

Stage I pressure ulcers are associated with the rupture of small capillaries and venules, producing a hematoma in the tissue.[43] Treatment with US has been observed by the author to promote absorption of hematoma after two to four treatments. Depending on depth of tissue involvement and size of the area, the hematoma resolves in about 2 weeks without ulceration. Protocol: 1 MHz, 0.5 W/cm^2 (SA, TP), pulsed 20% for 5–10 minutes, depending on size of area sonated. Apply with conductive gel/lotion five to seven times per week for 1–2 weeks or until color returns to that of surrounding skin.[29]

Clinical Studies

Animal Studies

Moderate frequency, 5-MHz US was selected to determine whether there was a beneficial effect from US when applied daily for short periods to postsurgical incisional wounds.[44] Subjects were Fischer F344 male rats. The US frequency was chosen because less than 20% of the power would penetrate deeper than 1 cm below the surface of the skin, so that most of the US energy would be absorbed in the vicinity of the wound. Intensity for a 5-minute exposure was 0.05 or 0.075 W/cm^2. Several experiments were performed at different thermal intensities (ranging from 0.05 to 0.15 W/cm^2). Sonation was continuous. The extent of heat production by insonation and the effect on healing were the study variables. Results of temperature measurements at all intensities following 5 minutes of continuous sonation showed an increase in subcutaneous tissue temperatures that were progressively larger with higher intensities of insonation.[44] At lower intensities (0.025 and 0.05 W/cm^2), 10 minutes of insonation produced only a small additional elevation in subcutaneous tissue temperature, indicating that a plateau in temperature had been approached by 5 minutes.[44] Treatment of the surgically induced incisional wounds began on the fourth postoperative day, when clips could be removed. The clips would have interfered with the US beam, and, at that time, the wounds were entering the proliferative phase of healing. Expectation was that this was the optimal time to stimulate the fibroblasts to augment healing. Findings were that the breaking strength of the sonated wounds was equivalent but not greater than that of those treated by direct heating of the tissues. At the higher intensities (0.1 and 0.15 W/cm^2), healing was impaired, and dermal burns occurred.[44] In other studies, described below, treatment began within 24 hours of surgery; signs of healing were reported by the fourth postoperative day.

In another study of burn-induced wounds in rats, two groups of animals were treated with pulsed (SATP 0.25 W/cm^2) and continuous US (0.3 W/cm^2).[45] No stimulating effects of US were demonstrated in either US treatment group or against controls, when evaluated by change in size and histologic examination. The investigators questioned the relevant clinical benefit of treatment of burn wounds with US. There is no indication in the study report as to how soon after burn-induced wounding the US treatment commenced.

Dosimetry for treatment with US is an area that lacks consensus. To learn more about dosage and wound healing, Byl et al[46] made incisional wounds in miniature Yucatan pigs, and treatment was applied at different doses for different lengths of time. The tensile strength of wounds treated with different intensities, called *high-* and *low-dose US*, was tested. Two variables were evaluated: the breaking strength of the incision and the deposition of hydroxyproline, which is a measure of collagen deposition. High-dose US was classified as 1.5 W/cm^2, continuous mode. Low-dose US was 0.5 W/cm^2, pulsed mode, 20% duty cycle. Both treatment groups received a frequency of 1 MHz for 5 minutes. The wounds were sonated for approximately 1.25 minute/cm of incisional length, beginning 24 hours after surgery. The wounds were covered with a moisture- and vapor-permeable adhesive dressing (Tegaderm, 3M Medical-Surgical Division, St. Paul, Minnesota) that was left in place for up to 1 week. The dressing was found to permit transmission of

US energy and could be left in place, avoiding disruption of the wound between treatment sessions. Forty-eight wounds were made, and the wounds were divided into three groups: 12 for control and 18 each for high-dose US and low-dose US. The groups were subdivided into two groups of 12 that received low dose or high dose for 5 days and two groups of six that received high dose or low dose for 10 days. Results were that the tensile strength for all treatment groups was significantly higher than that of the controls, but there was no difference in hydroxyproline deposition. A significant interaction was found between the number of days of treatment and the US dose. Hydroxyproline deposition was significantly higher and the breaking strength was higher for the low-dose group, compared with the high-dose group, after 10 days of treatment. During the first week, the study findings suggest that either low or high dose will enhance wound breaking strength but, to facilitate collagen deposition and wound strength, low-dose US should be used if treatment is to continue for 2 weeks or more.[46]

A comparative study of the effect of US (0.1 W/cm^2 pulsed) and ES (300 µA direct current, 30 minutes/day) on incisional wound healing in rats found that both US and ES had positive effects on the proliferative phases of healing but that ES was superior at the maturation phase.[47] Treatment started within 2 hours of the surgical procedure. ES treatment allowed the wound to lead to the proliferative phase earlier than in the US group, as indicated by the presence of more fibroblasts on the fourth day. Although density and arrangement of collagen was greater in the US group on the seventh day, the collagen was more regular in the ES group on the same day. Breaking strength was higher in the US group than in the sham US group but not as great as the ES group. Ultrasound affects the early phases of wound healing but ES causes a beneficial effect on all phases. US is more useful for the acute, uninfected, well-perfused wound, but ES is more useful for treatment of chronic or infected wounds, or wounds likely to be infected.[47]

Human Studies

Pressure Ulcers. In 1960, Paul et al[48] published a report of clinical observations of 23 patients with pressure ulcers, suggesting that ultrasonic therapy is effective in reducing the tissue congestion, cleansing necrotic tissue, and promoting healing and return of skin function to a near normal state and that a "scientifically controlled study would be richly rewarding."[48(p440)]

Twenty-five years later, based on the scientific evidence that nonthermal therapeutic US affects the biologic processes of repair through stable cavitation and/or acoustic streaming described above, a double blind randomized study was undertaken by McDiarmid et al[49] to determine whether these nonthermal therapeutic effects could be used to treat soft tissue wounds. Patients with partial-thickness skin loss caused by pressure ulcers but not extending beyond the dermis were selected. Forty patients were entered into the study and randomized into a US treatment and a sham US treatment group. Treatment parameters for the US treatment were 3 MHz, 0.8 W/cm² (SATP), pulse duration 2 msec, duty cycle 20%, SATA intensity, 0.16 W/cm², effective radiating surface area 5.2 cm². Treatment duration was a minimum of 5 minutes for all pressure ulcers up to 3 cm². One additional minute was added for each 0.5-cm² area, for a maximum of 10 minutes. Frequency was three times per week. The insonated ulcers tended to heal more quickly, but the difference was not statistically significant. However, when comparing clean ulcers with infected ulcers, the mean healing time for the clean ulcers was 30 days versus 40 days for the infected ulcers. Although US had little effect on the healing of clean pressure ulcers, there appeared to be a statistically significant effect of US on the healing of infected pressure ulcers, implying that the major factor influencing healing is whether the ulcer is clean or infected. McDiarmid et al[49] speculated that, if the clean wound was already healing at an optimal biologic rate, addition of a therapy such as US would not make a significant difference, but slower healing of infected ulcers may benefit from the effect of US stimulation of the large number of macrophages—the pivotal cell of the inflammatory phase and repair—present in infected wounds, with resulting release of "wound factors" from those cells and other cells of repair.[49]

Nussbaum et al[50] conducted a comparison study of nursing care alone, nursing care with laser, and nursing care with an alternating protocol of US and ultraviolet C (UVC) on 20 spinal cord-injured patients with 22 pressure ulcers. Of the initial group, four subjects dropped out, leaving 16 subjects with 18 wounds considered for the analysis. Nursing care consisted of moist dressings and continuous pressure relief. The laser regimen was provided three times per week. The US/UVC regimen consisted of US treatment five times weekly, alternating the US and UVC daily, 5 days per week. If the ulcer had purulent drainage, the UVC was used three times per week; if not, US was used three times per week. US protocol was frequency 3 MHz and intensity (SATA) of 0.2 W/cm² (1:4 pulse ratio) for 5 minutes per 5 cm² of wound area delivered to the periwound area. Results showed that the US/UVC treatment had a greater effect on wound healing than did the other treatment regimens.[50] The mean treatment time to wound closure was 4.1 weeks. The trend was for ulcers to heal faster in sites where wound contraction was the primary mode of closure (eg, over the coccyx). The conclusion was that this regimen of US/UVC may decrease the healing time for spinal cord-injured patients with pressure ulcers.[50] This was a small study that combined two interventions, making it impossible to demonstrate efficacy of each. Questions remain about whether the combination was essential and the effects of each.

Pressure ulcers were the subject of another study using US by ter Riet et al.[51] Eighty-eight subjects were randomized into two groups—45 for the treatment group and 43 for the control group. The trials lasted 12 weeks. Sixteen ulcers were stage IV, extending into muscle tissue; 72 had less depth of tissue involvement. Treatment was given directly to the wound surface (although how this was accomplished for the stage IV ulcers is not described) and to an extended radius 0.75 cm beyond the wound edge. Treatment parameters were frequency 3.28 MHz, pulse duration 2 msec, SATA 0.1 W/cm², BNR < 4. Minimum treatment duration was 3 minutes, 45 seconds. Wounds with treatment areas larger than 5 cm² were treated longer. A wound with an area of 10 cm² was treated for 7½ minutes. Local wound care included once- or occasionally twice-daily cleansing or rinsing with sterile saline or chlorhexidine (0.1 %) on gauze or in a syringe. Chlorhexidine is a cytotoxic agent to cells of repair, and using it for wound cleansing may have affected treatment results. Four wound characteristics (color of surrounding skin, necrotic tissue, granulation tissue, and deepest tissue involved) were each marked on a four-point scale, with grading from 1 = bad to 10 = excellent. Two outcome variables were end points: surface area reduction (in cm²) and wound closure (yes or no). After 12 weeks, 40% of the ulcers (18/45) in the US group and 44% of the ulcers (19/43) in the sham US group were closed. The results showed a tendency for the US to be more effective in small wounds than in larger wounds, which could not be explained.[51] This multicenter clinical trial of the efficacy of US therapy carried out on patients with pressure ulcers by ter Reit et al and published in 1996[51] did not support the hypothesis that US speeded up healing. However, examination of the methodology reveals that, although the US parameters were suitably controlled and described, there was a large variation in ulcer size and depth, patient health, and wound cleansing methods. The surface area of the pressure ulcers varied at the outset, from less than 1 cm² to more than 10 cm². Ulcer severity ranged from grade II to grade IV. The study sample had 16 patients with grade IV ulcers. Partial-thickness grade II ulcers heal faster than do full-thickness ulcers. To combine the two would bias the results. Furthermore, the patients were elderly (75–87 years); some were terminally ill and many incapacitated, those in the US-treated group being confined to bed for from 14.4 to 24 hours per day and those in the sham-irradiated control group from 14 to 20.5 hours per day. Therefore, it is perhaps unreasonable to expect a significant improvement in healing to occur following US therapy (or possibly any other type of physical therapy). Ideally, variability of both treatment parameters and patient characteristics should be minimized, and the physical condition of the patients should be such that healing is likely to occur. Only then can the efficacy of procedures aimed to speed up healing rather than initiate it be adequately assessed.

Chronic Leg Ulcers. Ultrasound was used as a periwound treatment for a controlled trial for patients with chronic varicose ulcers by Dyson et al.[52] Two groups received either sonation or sham sonation three times per week for 4 weeks. Treatment parameters for the US treatment were 3 MHz, 1.0 W/cm² (SA, TP), pulse duration 2 msec, delivered to the tissues every 10 msec for up to 10 minutes. The treatment technique involved moving the head of the device over the skin immediately adjacent to the ulcer. At the end of 4 weeks, the experimental, sonated group had statistically significant reduction in wound size, compared with the control group (experimental group 66.4 ± 8.8%; control group 91.6 ± 8.9%). No adverse effects of treatment were found.[52]

Application of continuous 30 kHz US at an intensity (SATA) of 0.1 W/cm² via a water bath for 10 minutes three times weekly showed significant healing of chronic venous leg ulcers when Peschen et al[53] treated 24 patients with chronic venous ulceration.[53] All study and control patients were randomized and received conventional therapy of hydrocolloid dressings and compression or conventional therapy plus US treatment for a 12-week period. At the end of the 12-week period, the experimental group showed an average decrease in ulcer area of 55.4%, compared with only 16.5% in the control group—a highly significant decrease ($p = .007$). The water bath method of delivery of therapeutic US has had acceptance in Europe, but not in the United States.[53]

A meta-analysis of studies on the use of US therapy in the treatment of chronic leg ulcers was published recently.[2] Of the 14 studies found during a literature review, 6 were selected for inclusion. The meta-analysis demonstrated a significant effect of US therapy in decreasing ulcer surface area, when compared with sham-irradiated controls. It was suggested, on the basis of the meta-analysis, that US had its best effect when delivered in "low doses" around the edge of the ulcer, but it was noted that further studies would be required to confirm this possible effect and to evaluate a possible dose–response relationship. The authors did not specify what they meant by a low dose. Of the six studies selected for inclusion, five used MHz US,[52,54–56] whereas the sixth used kHz US.[53] It should be noted that kHz US is more penetrative than MHz US, having the ability to pass through bone and metal, but it is less readily absorbed. The frequency of US used was not listed as a treatment variable in the meta-analysis. A statistically significant increase in the healing response, as demonstrated by reduction in the surface area of the ulcers, was reported in four of the six studies. The chapter authors reviewed the two studies that found no significant effect with the following findings. The study of Lundeberg et al,[55] who used an unusual pulsing regimen (1:9), found no significant difference. The use of longer gaps between the pulses than were used in the other studies would reduce the temporal average intensity to 0.05 W/cm²; it is possible that such a low temporal intensity is below the level required to stimulate wound healing in chronic venous ulcers. Also, the study of Eriksson et al[57] failed to show statistically significant healing between controls and the US treatment group. Pulsed US was used but pulsing ratio was not stated. The six studies are summarized in Tables 24–1 and 24–2.

It is suggested that future studies take the form of multicenter trials in which not only are the treatment parameters controlled but also patient variability is minimized. The results of such trials will be of greater clinical relevance than meta-analyses, where the variables are such that valid predictions of the outcome of future treatment cannot be made confidently.

Scar. Ward et al[58] evaluated the therapeutic effect of US on scar contracture after burn injury, as well as the effect of response to standard burn physical therapy of stretching. Greater elongation of collagen tissue following a combination of stretching and heat has been reported to be greater than stretching alone. Therefore, the study investigators wanted to determine whether topical US would benefit patients with burns to progress to healed scar tissue. Joint range of motion and pain were the study variables chosen. The joints to be treated were randomized, and the patients and therapists were blinded to the treatment group. All treatments were performed every other day over a 2-week period with continuous US, 1 MHz, at 1 W/cm². Analysis of the data revealed no statistically significant differences in the two groups in either pain perception or joint range of motion. The lack of significance may be due to the fact that US has been demonstrated to be most effective during the inflammatory phase of healing, before scar formation is established, and to affect scar formation at that time by accelerating the healing response and the deposition and organization of the collagen. It is unlikely that US will be useful for healed scars.

CHOOSING AN INTERVENTION: CLINICAL REASONING

The prior section of this chapter evaluates the efficacy of US on the phases of wound recovery and in clinical trials. To summarize, the studies looked at seven important physiologic effects of US therapy that the physical therapist (PT) should consider when selecting US intervention. Ultrasound has the following effects:

- It affects all phases of wound recovery at the cellular level if applied during the inflammatory phase.
- It accelerates the rate of progression through the phases of repair.
- It affects different tissue types differently, according to the tissues' ability to absorb energy. More tissue absorption requires lower-intensity application.

Table 24–1 Protocols and Results of Studies Used in Meta-analysis[2] of US Effects on Chronic Leg Ulcers

Study Variable	Treatment	Roche and West[54]	Lundeberg et al[55]	Callam et al[56]	Dyson et al[52]	Ericksson et al[57]	Peschen et al[53]
Ulcer etiology		Venous	Venous	Venous predominately (94/108)	Venous	Venous	Venous
Method of randomization		Random allocate	Permuted blocks	Permuted blocks	Alternately	Alternately	Alternately
Number of subjects	Control	13	15	41 (15 dropouts)	12	13	12
	US	13	17	41 (11 dropouts)	13	12	12
Area treated		Periwound	Wound surface	Periwound	Periwound	Wound surface	Wound surface and periwound
Frequency of treatment		3 x/week	3 x/week	1 x/week	3 x/week	2 x/week	3 x/week
Frequency of device		3 MHz	1 MHz	1 MHz	3 MHz	1 MHz	30 kHz
Intensity		1.0 W/cm²	0.5 W/cm²	0.5 W/cm²	1.0 W/cm²	1.0 W/cm²	100 mW/cm²
Pulsed or continuous		1:4	1:9	Pulsed	1:5	Not stated	Continuous
Time		5–10 min	10 min	1 min/probe head area	5–10 min	Max 10 min	10 min
% Healing Results							
4 weeks	Control	↓28% SD 27.3	↓19 SD 9 1 healed	↓30% SD 61.6 5 healed	↓7.4% SD 8.9	↓27 SD 12 1 healed	↓8 SD 20
	US	↓35% SD 21.9	↓24 SD 12 2 healed	↓48 SD 49.8 6 healed	↓34% SD 8.8	↓35 SD 14 2 healed	↓27 SD 24
8 weeks	Control	↓7% SD 36.7	↓47 SD 10 3 healed	↓60 SD 41.9 6 healed	Not reported after 4 weeks	↓52 SD 13 4 healed	↓20 SD 24
	US	↓35.3 SD 30.1 # healed ulcers not reported	↓53 SD 8 5 healed	↓80 SD 24.6 14 healed	# healed ulcers not reported	↓68 SD 9 5 healed	↓40 SD 23 # healed ulcers not reported

Source: Data from reference #'s 52, 53, 54, 55, 56, and 57.

Table 24–2 Intensity Levels for Therapeutic Ultrasound[1]

Intensity Levels	Range	Area
Low	< 0.3	W/cm^2
Medium	0.3–1.2	W/cm^2
High	> 1.2–3.0	W/cm^2

- It promotes absorption of hemorrhagic materials.
- It increases circulation and $tcPO_2$ if the patient is well hydrated and oxygenated.
- It enables noninvasive, nontraumatic treatment of deep or superficial tissue, depending on frequency.

Information about the effects of US on wound healing is less clear because of the limited number of clinical trials, the different parameters used for each study, the small sample sizes, and perhaps because the intervention was not appropriately applied. For example, it was applied to chronic wounds at intensities that would not restart the inflammatory phase of healing, leading to progression through the phases of repair. One study included two interventions, US and UVC, with good outcomes. Two studies included subjects who had pressure ulcers; six studies included patients with chronic leg ulcers. The biologic effects described are independent of the wound etiology. The pressure ulcers ranged from partial-thickness to full-thickness, extending to muscle levels of tissue involvement. Partial-thickness ulcers heal by reepithelialization, deep ulcers by contraction. The results for infected ulcers were better than were those for clean ulcers. Infected ulcers are usually in an inflammatory phase of healing, which is when US is known to be most effective. Would a different protocol be better for a different phase of healing, and would that affect the outcome? More evaluation of the dosimetry parameters on the efficacy of US is still required. In the meantime, US may be the treatment of choice for some patients. Two examples are described in the case studies at the end of this chapter.

Candidacy for the Intervention

With any interactive treatment, the benefit to the patient must outweigh any possible risk. The PT must, therefore, be able to assess both benefit and risk. The potential benefits have been described above. Knowledge of the mechanisms by which US interacts with tissue aids the PT in risk assessment. There is a long list of contraindications in the literature,[31] and the excellent safety record of US owes much to the constraints on treatment that these have engendered (Exhibit 24–2). However, not all contraindications listed have been verified experimentally, and it is possible that some patients who could have benefited from US treatment have

Exhibit 24–2 Contraindications for US[31]

DO NOT USE US	
Over the uterus during pregnancy	
Over the gonads	
Over malignancies and precancerous lesions	
Over tissues previously treated with deep X-ray or irradiation	
On patients with vascular abnormalities	
	Deep vein thrombosis
	Emboli
	Severe atherosclerosis
Over the cardiac area in advanced heart disease	
Over the eye	
Over the stellate ganglion	
For hemophiliacs not covered by factor replacement	
Over the spinal cord after laminectomy	

been denied it. To ensure continued safe use, basic precautions must be considered (Exhibit 24–3).

Basic precautions start by selection of the right candidates for the treatment. The medical history of the patient, the onset date, location of the injury, depth of the injury, and size of the area to be treated will all guide the PT in the selection of US. For example, review the medical history for information about the circulatory system. Look for information about arteriosclerotic vessels, ischemia, and occlusion from reports of vascular studies, or plan to do a noninvasive vascular examination. Ultrasound is not recommended over deep vein thrombosis or thombophlebitis because of the risk of dislodging thrombi. Likewise, hemophiliacs should not be treated with US because of the risk of disturbing clot formation. Check for information about diabetes mellitus, type I or type II; patients with type I diabetes are likely to have vascular and sensory impairments. Diabetes is an impairment to the repair process; expect slower healing. Ultrasound should

Exhibit 24–3 Precautions for Use of US[31]

EXERCISE CAUTION IN USE OF US
In acute infections
Over subcutaneous bony prominences
Over epiphyseal plates
Over subcutaneous major nerves
Over the cranium
Over anesthetic areas

be used in the pulsed mode over areas of poor circulation. Loss of sensation due to many pathologic causes (eg, spinal cord injury and alcoholic neuropathy; see Chapter 18 for a more complete list) means that the patient is not a candidate for thermal US. Treatment over anesthetic areas is a risk because malfunction of the equipment could lead to exposure to intensities that would normally induce pain and be indicative of tissue damage. The insensate patient will not be able to indicate pain during the treatment; therefore, pulsed low-dose US should be used for those cases. If the patient has a history of spinal laminectomy, do not treat with US over that area because of effects on the spinal cord that have not yet been determined but may be harmful. A history of malignant or precancerous lesions or tumors in the area to be treated would be a contraindication because therapeutic levels of US could stimulate cellular proliferation.[59] Sometimes, injuries occur around the eye, but this is a location that should *not* be treated with US because the sensitive retina may be affected by it. Metal implants, including foreign objects, are often described in the medical history or by the patient. Use only kHz US over metal implants. Do not treat over the uterus during pregnancy to ensure that no embryo or fetus is exposed to the intensities used in therapeutic US, which are higher than those used diagnostically. Do not treat over the gonads. After a thorough review, consider whether US therapy is indicated. If in doubt, do not irradiate.

PROCEDURES

Protocol Considerations

Review the history for onset of the wound and prior treatment interventions. This will determine both the candidacy and the appropriate treatment parameters. If the wound is acute, make use of the nonthermal effects of US. If chronic, use a protocol of one upper-medium-intensity treatment and subsequently treat at lower intensity. If the wound is located over a bony prominence, the PT must consider a method of sonation that will avoid increasing periosteal temperature. There are several ways to accomplish this objective: (1) select a high frequency (3 MHz), which is absorbed in the more superficial tissues; (2) move the treatment head continuously to avoid standing waves; (3) treat through water for a more uniform far field; or (4) for deeper wounds, select a lower frequency (1 MHz). If the local circulation is poor, use pulsed US to avoid excessive heating because it will take longer for heat to be dissipated from the area. Assess the size of the area to be treated. Use this assessment to determine the duration of the treatment and the size of the applicator to select. Note that an applicator with a larger ERA will allow treatment of a large wound more rapidly than if an applicator with a smaller ERA is used. Small applicators, however, are very useful for being more selective in treating specific tis-

sues. Select the coupling medium, depending on whether the skin is intact or broken (coupling media are described later). Intensity selection for acute conditions is the upper end of the low range; for chronic conditions, the middle range (see later). The anatomic location of the wound is a very important consideration when using US. For example, be aware of the location of major subcutaneous nerves, which absorb US energy very well and can become overheated, and epiphyseal plates, if treating young people prior to the termination of growth of the plate concerned. This varies with the bone and with the sex. There are also racial differences.

To ensure the continued safe use of US, the following basic precautions are recommended:

- Use US only if adequately trained to do so.
- Use US only to treat patients with conditions known to respond favorably to US therapy, unless it is being used experimentally with the understanding and approval of the patient, his or her medical advisors, and the local medical ethics committee or internal review board.
- Use the lowest intensity that produces the required effect, because higher intensities may be damaging. Burns, for example, occur when the intensity is too high or the frequency is low, and when the treatment head is not moved continuously or is moved too slowly.
- Move the applicator constantly throughout treatment to avoid the damaging effects of standing waves and of high-intensity regions when treating in the nonuniform near field.
- Make sure that there is adequate couplant and that it is free of air bubbles.
- Make sure that the equipment is calibrated regularly. A broken crystal, for instance, may occur if the applicator head is dropped. Staff must report any dropping of the applicator head so that it can be tested before reuse. A faulty piece of equipment can result in inadequate treatment for the patient or can produce shear waves and standing waves that can cause burns or other harmful effects.[31]

Expected Outcomes

Ultrasound is most effective when treating in the acute inflammatory phase of healing. During this phase, expect an acceleration of the inflammatory phase and early progression to the proliferative and epithelialization phases of healing (Exhibit 24–4). In chronic wounds, the first outcomes to treatment will be increased perfusion, observed as warmth, edema, and darkening of tissue color, compared with adjacent skin color tones (Exhibit 24–5). In necrotic wounds, expect to see autolysis of the necrotic tissue; the outcome will be a clean wound bed. Wounds in two clinical trials progressed to closure in a mean time of 4–6 weeks.[49,50] These

Exhibit 24–4 Outcomes: Acute Wound

Wound healing phase diagnosis: acute inflammatory phase

Expected outcome:
    Skin color: change to that of surrounding skin
    Temperature: change to that of adjacent tissues or same
       area on corresponding opposite side of the body
    Edema free
    Necrosis free
    Wound progressed to proliferative phase

---

times could be longer for patients with intrinsic and extrinsic factors that limit healing. Published research is a valuable guide to the clinician in prediction of outcomes, but it must be supported by the experience of the program where the treatment is used.

Reassessment should confirm the predicted outcomes. If the wound does not change phase and/or reduce the size of surface area or overall size estimate within 2–4 weeks, the treatment regimen must change. There are several changes to US treatment to consider: Enhance the inflammatory phase or restart it with the protocol for chronic wounds; change the frequency of the transducer; use a different size transducer for better ERA, or increase the treatment time; or recalculate the area if the wound has been debrided and the wound is larger than initial size.

Typical Protocol

Acute Wounds

Onset. Begin as soon as possible—ideally, within a few hours of injury but always during the inflammatory phase of healing, when treatment with MHz US has been shown to result in the liberation of stimulatory growth factors from platelets, mast cells, and macrophages, with the result that inflammatory phase is accelerated, the proliferative and remodeling phases occur earlier, and the scar tissue is stronger than that of controls (Exhibit 24–6). If treatment is delayed beyond the inflammatory phase, the strength of the scar tissue is not affected.[33]

Duration. Duration is usually based empirically on the surface area to be treated. The area is divided into zones, each 1.5 times the area of the ERA of the applicator, with 1–2 minutes being allowed for treating each zone. Some PTs recommend 1 min/cm². For the sake of the therapist, the maximum treatment time should be no longer than 15 minutes. If the wound is large, two sessions per day, one to each section of the wound, would be preferable. Three treatments per week have been found to be effective.

Intensity. In the interests of safety, the lowest I(SATA) should be used. This is usually near the upper end of the low range (see Table 24–3). Note that, to obtain a significant increase in temperature, an I(SATA) of at least 0.5 W/cm² is required, but that primarily nonthermal effects can be achieved with lower SATA intensities, obtained by pulsing I(SATP) 0.5 W/cm² at, for example, 2 msec on, 8 msec off. Treatments should be pulsed if the local circulation is compromised and might be unable to dissipate heat efficiently.

Chronic Wounds

Onset. Begin as soon as possible.
Duration. Duration is the same as for acute wounds.
Intensity. I(SATA) at approximately the middle of the medium range is generally recommended (eg, 0.5–1.0 W/cm² SA, TP). Pulsing should be used. Repair can be initiated by using *one* treatment at the upper end of the medium range (eg, 1.2 W/cm²), after which, lower intensities in the medium range are used, as described above. It is suggested that the higher intensity may produce local trauma, followed by acute inflammation, which is necessary to initiate healing in any postnatal wound. Note that this is a hypothesis that requires testing.

Frequency Selection

The PT should consider the following when selecting a frequency for treatment:

Exhibit 24–5 Outcomes: Chronic Wound

Wound healing phase diagnosis: chronic inflammatory phase

Expected outcome:
    Hyperemia: change in skin color to reddish blue or
       purplish, depending on color of surrounding skin
    Temperature: increased temperature of tissue, due to
       enhanced perfusion
    Edema: hardness, tightness, and shiny skin
    Wound progressed to proliferative phase

Exhibit 24–6 Nonthermal US Protocol: Acute Inflammatory Phase

Frequency	1 or 3 MHz
Pulsed duty cycle	20–50%
Intensity	0.1–0.2 W/cm² (SATA)
Treatment frequency	3 times per week
Time	1 min/cm², max 15 min total

Table 24–3 Wound Dressing US Transmission Rates

Dressing Product	US Transmission Rate
Hydrogels	
Nu-Gel	77.2% (±4.6%)
ClearSite	72% (±2.2%)
Aquasorb Border	45.3% (±2.1%)
CarraDress	42.8% (±5.9%)
Film Dressings	
CarraSmart Film	60.5% (±4.4%)
J & J Bioclusive	53.2% (±2.4%)
Tegaderm	47.1% (±2.3%)
Opsite Flexigrid	31.5% (±4%)

Source: Reprinted from Klucinec, B., et al., Effectiveness of Wound Care Products in the Transmission of Acoustic Energy, *Physical Therapy*, Vol. 80, No. 5, pp. 469–76, © 2000, with permission of the American Physical Therapy Association.

- If the lesion is superficial, a higher frequency is appropriate because high-frequency US is absorbed superficially.
- Although it is not readily available in many clinics, kHz US is another frequency that may be considered more in the near future. Differences between kHz and MHz US are that kHz US is less attenuated, being less readily absorbed than MHz, and is readily transmitted through metal implants and bone; however, sufficient absorption occurs to produce a stimulatory effect.
- High frequencies (more than 1 MHz) are more appropriate than lower frequencies if thermal changes are required in the tissues.
- Lower frequencies (1 MHz or less) are more appropriate than higher frequencies if primarily nonthermal effects, such as stable cavitation and/or microstreaming, are required in the tissues. Equipment now on the market allows more flexibility to choose US frequencies and provides additional choices for the PT. The PT must know what each frequency is best suited to treat.

Coupling Media

Megahertz US requires a coupling medium that displaces air. This is essential because MHz US is reflected from air/water or air/tissue interfaces. The greater the difference in *acoustic impedance* (z) between the two materials forming the interface, the greater the amount of energy is reflected. The acoustic impedance of a medium is the product of its density (p) and the velocity of US through it (c). With MHz US, only 0.2% reflection occurs at the interface between soft tissue and water, more than 50% between soft tissue and bone, and virtually complete reflection (99.9%) between soft tissue and air. Reflection reduces the amount of energy reaching the target tissues; if this falls below the stimulatory threshold (approximately 0.1 W/cm² I[SATA]), the US will be ineffective. The ideal coupling medium would:

- have the same acoustic impedance as skin
- also act as a wound dressing
- be sterile, thixotropic, nonstaining, nonirritant, and chemically inert
- be slow to be absorbed and to evaporate
- be free from gas bubbles and other inclusions
- not break down when the US energy is transmitted through it
- be inexpensive

Hydrogel sheet and transparent film dressings are commonly used by PT clinicians for treatment of full- and partial-thickness wounds, and many US treatments are performed over these dressings. The transmissivity of wound care dressings would affect the efficacy, the efficiency of delivery, and the cost of US treatment. A study of wound care products identified four sheet hydrogels and four transparent film dressings with different transmission rates.[60] Intensities from 0.2 to 2.0 W/cm² were tested. Frequency was 3.3 MHz. US transmission gel was used on the skin and on top of the dressing to remove air. Plastic sheets were removed from the tops and bottoms of the hydrogel sheets that could have interfered with the sound energy transmission. Findings that will help to guide the clinician in selecting the dressing that will optomize treatment effects are listed in Table 24–3. For quick reference, sources for the dressing products are found in Appendix B at the end of this book.

Suitable coupling media that displace air and that can be used along the wound perimeter are commercially available US transmitting gel and over the wound, sterile, transparent, US-transmitting wound dressings with a high water content, eg, Geliperm (Geistlich Sons Ltd., Newton Bank, Long Lane, UK) and Hydroscan (Echo Ultrasound, Reedsville, PA). Hydroscan (Figure 24–1A, B) is not labeled for use as a dressing but is used for diagnostic US transmission and is an excellent transmitter of US energy, as long as there are no bubbles of air (N. Byl, *personal communication*, 1994). Geliperm is available in Europe but not in the United States at this time. Tegaderm, which was used in another study, was tested for transmission of US energy and found to transmit 40% of the acoustic energy.[46] Tests of the results of US stimulation on tcPO₂ measurements when energy was transmitted through Tegaderm showed no significant differences in the measurements, with or without the Tegaderm.[40] Tegaderm and similar transparent film dressings are useful for treating full-thickness wounds because the film will stretch down into the wound bed under the pressure of the US head. Make sure that the size of the film dressing is larger than the wound, so that the stress of the stretching doesn't pull the adhesive away from the skin. Using US transmission gel on the surface of the film makes gliding of the head easier. The method to use hydrogel sheets for transmission is as follows:

1. Place the dressing over the superficial to full-thickness open area, ensuring that no air is trapped beneath the dressing.
2. Coat the surface of the dressing lightly with US transmission gel or lotion to ease the movement of the applicator head over the dressing surface.

Underwater application is a useful method for transmission of US. A metal whirlpool tank is a poor choice to hold the water because the metal reflects sound energy and increases the intensity in the body area near the metal. A plastic

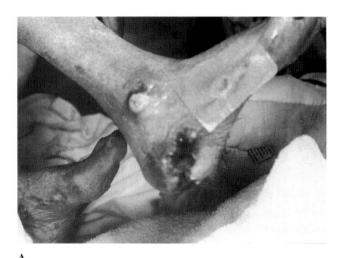

A

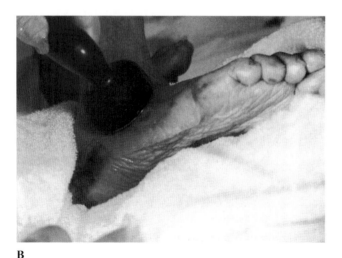

B

Figure 24–1 A and **B**. Application of US through a Hydroscan. Courtesy of CIVCO Medical Instruments, Kalona, Iowa.

or rubber basin or tub would be acceptable. Air bubbles need to be eliminated by running the water and letting it stand for a few minutes before using it for US transmission. Underwater application is a good choice if the region to be treated is irregular and the area to be treated can be conveniently placed in the container. This includes foot, ankle, hand, and elbow. Infection control requires proper disinfection of the water basin between uses. The applicator and the body part must be submerged throughout the treatment, and the applicator should not touch the skin. This would be advantageous if the area of treatment is painful. If possible, select a large container, such as a baby's plastic bathtub, where the target tissues can be placed a significant distance from the applicator. At that distance, the target tissues will be in the far field, where the spatial intensity is more uniform. It is recommended that the PT wear waterproof gloves that trap US reflecting air, so as to minimize exposure to the sound energy. US at the kHz frequency is often delivered via a water bath so that the wound can be cleaned and debrided by it. Kilohertz US applied in a water bath stimulates the healing of chronic venous ulcers[53] and facilitates the debridement of bacteria- and particulate-contaminated wounds.[61]

Manipulation of the Applicator

Movement of the MHz applicator throughout treatment is essential to avoid exposure of units of tissue to regions of high intensity; in the near field, where most treatments occur, the spatial peak intensity can be more than three times the SA. It is also essential to avoid excessive exposure to the peaks of pressure variation that occur in *standing wave fields* produced by the interaction of incident and reflected waves of US. Standing waves can damage tissue components, endothelial cells in particular, and exposure to them must, therefore, be avoided.

The applicator should be moved either in short linear strokes a few cm long, ensuring that they overlap, so that the entire region is treated or in small circular movements, also overlapping, so that the movement is essentially spiral.

Setup for Treatment (Figure 24–2)

1. Explain the procedure to the patient and the caregiver.
2. Position the patient for comfort in a position that can be maintained for up to 15 minutes.
3. Remove clothing from the area to be treated.
4. Warm US gel by placing it in a warmer or between folds of a hot pack—always test a drop for temperature before applying to the patient.
5. Remove the wound dressing, unless it is a film or hydrogel sheet that is to be left in place. Check for bubbles under the dressing and bleed them from the edges, if present.

6. Use either as a periwound treatment or direct application over a film or hydrogel sheet, as described above.
7. Treat deep wounds by a periwound application around the margins of the wound.
8. Keep the sound head perpendicular to the surface in complete contact with the surface area throughout the treatment.

Clinical Wisdom: *Use US for Blisters*

Treating blisters with US promotes absorption of the hemorrhagic material beneath the blister and healing of superficial and partial-thickness wounds. Absorption of hemorrhagic material may be due to enhanced macrophage activity via acoustic streaming and/or stable cavitation. Use the protocol for acute inflammation and apply as a periwound application or in a water bath. Continue after the blister roof is removed as long as hemorrhagic material is absorbed. Hemorrhagic material should shrink in size daily; when it is no longer shrinking, it has probably necrosed and will need to be debrided. *Color Plates 77–80* and *Case Study 2* demonstrate a case in which US was the only treatment intervention, besides a transparent film dressing, until it was determined that focal area of necrosis needed debridement.

Clinical Wisdom:
Sonation of Undermined/Tunneled Areas

One-MHz US is a very useful means to treat undermined/tunneled areas surrounding wounds. These areas can be "mapped" on the skin surface with a marker pen (see Chapter 5, Wound Measurements, about measuring undermining and tunneled areas) to guide the treatment. Imagine the wound with a grid over the area or use a plastic screen with cm markings and divide the wound into quarters at the 12-, 3-, 6-, and 9-o'clock positions. Depending on the size of the applicator, sound at the rate of 1 min/cm². For example, a 5-cm² applicator would be used to stimulate a 25-cm² wound area for 5 minutes. Undermined/tunneled regions can be visualized in high-resolution US B-scans.

Aftercare

If the dressing is left intact, all that is required is to clean off excess US transmission gel/lotion. If a new dressing is to be applied, this should be done as soon as possible to avoid

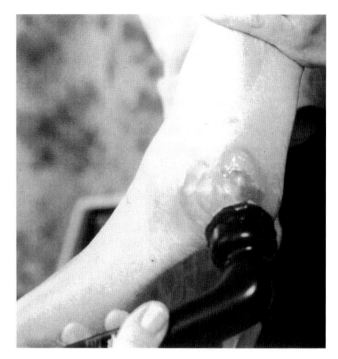

Figure 24–2 Periblister application of US gel.

chilling of the wound tissues and slowing of epithelial migration and mitotic cell activity.

The US applicator must be handled carefully after use to avoid environmental contamination. After use, place the applicator in a rubber glove and transport it to a dirty sink area for cleansing with cold tap water and soap. Then place it in a cold disinfecting solution for the specified time, depending on the product used. This is usually from 5 to 20 minutes. It is useful to have two applicators, so that one can be used while the other is being disinfected, thus reducing down time.

Adjunctive Treatments

It is an essential part of the clinical decision making to consider adjunctive treatments that may be given. Ultrasound may be the primary physical agent or it may be an adjunctive treatment, along with another physical agent or electrotherapeutic modality. For example, for a deep wound, HVPC may be the treatment for the wound bed and US for the undermined periwound area. If this is done, do the HVPC treatment first and leave the packing in the wound bed to keep it warm and clean while the US treatment is given.

Ultrasound may be given as an adjunctive treatment to whirlpool, when the whirlpool is used to soften necrotic tissue and the US is used to stimulate at the cellular level. Do the whirlpool first, then any debridement; flush out debris and any topical agents that could possibly be phonophoresed through the skin by the US. Ultrasound should follow the whirlpool because cells are stimulated by US to release chemotactic agents; those chemicals should not be washed out of the wound. As in the Nussbaum et al[50] study, US can be alternated with UVC (see Chapter 23).

Wound care products are part of the treatment regimen also and should be considered in the treatment planning. Will the dressing be part of the US treatment, as described above, or will the dressing be removed and replaced when the US treatment is given? Will the dressing be changed every other day? Can it be changed in conjunction with the US treatment to minimize disruption of the wound healing environment? PTs need to check with nurses about the application of topical agents, such as petrolatum or petrolatum-based products, which will interfere with the US transmission. This is another example of the importance of collaboration between nurses and PTs about treatment regimens to avoid conflicting treatment approaches and to improve utilization management of services for the patient.

SELF-CARE TEACHING GUIDELINES

Ultrasound should *not* be taught to a patient or a caregiver as a home treatment. Although it appears very innocuous, harm can be done by improperly trained and unsupervised individuals. To avoid harm, the many precautions listed earlier must be carefully considered. There are definite risks that are not readily apparent to the unskilled individual.

DOCUMENTATION

The functional outcome report (FOR)[62] is an acceptable method to meet Medicare and other third-party payer guidelines for documentation of the need for physical therapy intervention for wound healing. The cases presented here are examples of how to use the FOR methodology. More information on the method is available in Chapter 1. Documentation of US treatment outcomes is extremely valuable. The cases documented below are examples of the value of recording on film those changes in wound healing that are produced by selected interventions. In both cases, US was the only intervention given. For example, it would be difficult to do a controlled, double-blind study of patients with new hematoma formation, as in Case Study 1. A single-subject design study would be one method of developing a body of knowledge about clinical outcomes. Case Study 2 was done as part of a student clinical affiliation project to see how US affects hematoma formation under a blister. Photography was done every 2 days to track the change in the hematoma. There are many ways that the thoughtful clinician can present information about treatment interventions and advance clinical practice as part of the documentation process.

REVIEW QUESTIONS

1. Explain the physical properties of US with respect to frequency and intensity as it relates to clinical use.
2. Explain the physiologic and physical properties of US that make it useful for wound healing.
3. Describe three factors that could interfere with achieving the expected results.
4. Describe how the coupling agent can effect the transmission of the sound energy.
5. Review the clinical reasoning for choosing an intervention with US.
6. What are the new uses for diagnostic US?

Case Study 1: Venous Ulcer Treated with US

Patient: E.F.   Age: 82 years

Functional Outcome Report: Initial Assessment

Reason for Referral

The patient was referred to physical therapy for evaluation of ulceration of her left leg. The patient had a long history of Alzheimer's disease and was noncompliant with all attempts to keep the wound dressed. Nurses in the nursing home where she lived were concerned about infection and healing of the ulcer and wanted a physical therapist's opinion.

Medical History

The patient had a cardiac pacemaker and venous insufficiency. As a consequence of her neurologic system changes associated with Alzheimer's disease, she was hyperactive and would not stay still for more than a couple of minutes at a time. Wound onset was 24 hours prior to referral.

Functional Diagnosis and Targeted Outcomes

Wound Examination. The wound is located above the left medial malleous. The surrounding skin is very friable, with extensive subcutaneous hemorrhaging and epidermal necrosis; petechiae surround the open area. There is mild edema, which is reactive to touching. The wound tissue is pink, with partial-thickness loss of the skin surface area (see *Color Plate 74*).
    Functional diagnosis: impairment of the integumentary system; targeted outcome: wound closure; due date: 4 weeks.
    Functional diagnosis: impairment of the venous system (venous insufficiency); targeted outcome: absorption of hematoma; due date: 2 weeks.
    Functional diagnosis: acute inflammatory phase; targeted outcome: rapid wound contraction; due date: 4 weeks.

Psychosocial Examination. The patient removed dressings and would not tolerate any topical medications, compression stockings, or staying off her feet. She walked all day long and was very accomplished at removing passive restraints in a flash. She was totally noncompliant during the last episode of wounding.

Functional diagnosis: impairment of mental functions. The functional loss causes undue susceptibility to venous ulceration of the legs and inability to heal without integumentary intervention. The patient has improvement potential and will heal after intervention, but she may continue to be at risk for venous ulceration.

Need for Skilled Services: The Therapy Problem

The patient has a history of recurrent ulceration above the left medial malleolus and impaired healing due to impairment of the venous system and impaired mental status. US is indicated during the first 72 hours after injury during acute inflammation. US would promote absorption of the hemorrhagic material and stimulate acceleration of the inflammatory phase, leading to rapid wound contraction.

Treatment Plan

Periwound ultrasound will be applied at 1 MHz, at 0.5 W/cm^2 (SATP), 20% pulsed for 5 minutes five times per week for 4 weeks. The nurses will attempt to do a wound dressing with a transparent film as tolerated.

Discharge Outcomes

Hemorrhagic material was significantly absorbed within 3 days. There was a change in wound shape and a reduction in size after 2 weeks. There was an 85% reduction in wound size at 4 weeks (see *Color Plates 65–67* for a pictorial review of the case).

Discussion

Behavioral information as well as medical history were important considerations in choosing the intervention. From all perspectives, US was the most practical choice for this patient. However, because of her noncompliance with any other treatment, it was also an opportunity to evaluate the effects of the US. The absorption of the hemorrhagic material was unquestionable. The patient required constant engagement and diversionary activities by a physical therapy aide to tolerate the US by the physical therapist for even 5 minutes. By the end of 4 weeks she refused to comply further. Since the wound was closing, physical therapy was discontinued.

Case Study 2: Blood Blister on the Heel Treated with US

Patient: M.M.   Age: 83

Functional Outcome Report: Initial Assessment

Reason for Referral

The patient was referred to the physical therapist because the nursing staff had identified a blood blister on a heel.

Medical History

The patient had had a below-the-knee amputation on the other leg due to peripheral vascular disease. The limb was at risk for amputation, and early intervention was requested for limb salvage. Patient was alert/confused and nonambulatory. She could reposition but not consistently. She had had a prior episode of a cerebrovascular accident. The following medical problems are associated with this request for service.

Functional Diagnosis and Targeted Outcomes

Integumentary Examination. The surrounding skin was erythematous, edematous, and tender.

Functional diagnosis: loss of function due to integumentary impairment; targeted outcome: accelerate the inflammatory response; due date: 2 weeks.

Wound Tissue Examination. The wound was covered with a bloody, fluid-filled blister. Bloody fluid suggests rupture of vessels beneath the blister.

Functional diagnosis: wound in acute inflammatory phase; targeted outcome: debridement of blister, conservation of healthy tissue under the blister; due date: 2 weeks.

Associated impairment: possibility of necrotic tissue beneath blister; targeted outcome: clean wound bed; due date: 4 weeks.

Functional diagnosis: impairment of integument, depth to be determined; targeted outcome: exhibits granulation tissue; due date: 6 weeks.

Vascular Examination. Visual examination showed an inflammatory response to wounding. Palpation indicated weak but palpable pulses. Because of the prior vascular history the presence of peripheral vascular disease was assumed.

Functional diagnosis: vascular impairment; targeted outcome: enhanced perfusion; due date: 2 weeks.

Musculoskeletal Examination. The patient is nonambulatory, has limited mobility in bed, and needs verbal cues to reposition. Motor impairment from the stroke limits

her mobility. Her Braden Risk Score is 15, indicating risk for pressure ulcers.

Functional diagnosis: undue susceptibility to pressure ulceration; targeted outcome: pressure elimination; due date: immediately.

Evaluation

The patient's loss of function in these systems is responsible for the undue susceptibility to skin breakdown on the legs and inability to heal without integumentary intervention. The patient has improvement potential, and the wound will heal with intervention to bring perfusion to tissues and relieve pressure.

Need for Skilled Services

The patient has a prior history of failed wound healing leading to amputation. Intervention that will enhance wound tissue perfusion to conserve tissues underneath the blister and stimulate healing will be required. Wound dressings will not address these issues. The blister needs to be debrided to assess tissue damage. Absorption of hemorrhagic materials will conserve healthy tissues and result in a healed wound. Pulsed nonthermal US is the choice for tissue perfusion in the presence of peripheral vascular disease and for stimulation of macrophage activity to absorb clotted blood in the tissues.

Treatment Plan

- Apply periwound nonthermal US to accelerate the inflammatory phase and promote absorption of hemorrhagic material (0.5 W/cm^2 [SATP], 1 MHz, 20% pulsed for 5 minutes).
- Sharply debride the blister roof.
- Continue US until the extent of the wound depth is determined.

Outcomes

Periwound US and debridement were begun on August 26. On August 31 the blister was debrided, and a large hemorrhagic/necrotic area was seen under the tissues; inflammation in the surrounding tissues was subsiding. On September 2, there was a 50% reduction in the size of the hemorrhagic area and resolution of the inflammation in the surrounding tissues. Minimal reduction in the area of the hematoma in next 2 weeks indicated that the tissues had necrosed and debridement had begun. On October 8 the wound was progressing to the proliferative phase; there was a small area of necrosis (see *Color Plates 77–80*). The US seemed to have had maximum benefit and treatment was changed to HVPC.

continues

Case Study 2 continued

Discussion

Removal of the blister roof identified an area of focal necrosis or hematoma. The only other treatment intervention was transparent film dressing. The size of the hematoma was reduced 50% with seven US treatments. Inflammation was accelerated, and the wound progressed to the proliferative phase. At this point treatment was changed to HVPC. Closure was achieved on November 2.

REFERENCES

1. Gam AN, Johannsen F. Ultrasound therapy in musculoskeletal disorders: A meta-analysis. *Pain.* 1995;63:85–91.

2. Johannsen F, Gam AN, Karsmark T. Ultrasound therapy in chronic leg ulceration: A meta-analysis. *Wound Repair Regeneration.* 1998;6:121–126.

3. Falconer J, Hayes KW, Chang RW. Therapeutic ultrasound in the treatment of musculoskeletal conditions. *Arthritis Care Res.* 1990;3(2):85–90.

4. Sackett D. Rules of evidence and clinical recommendations on the use of antithrombotic agents. *Chest.* 1989;95(2):2s–4s.

5. Ovington LG. Dressings and adjunctive therapies: AHCPR guidelines revisited. *Ostomy/Wound Manage.* 1999;45(Suppl 1A):94s–106s.

6. Bergstrom N, Allman RM, Alvarez OM, Bennett MA, Carlson CE, Frantz R. *Clinical Practice Guideline: Treatment of Pressure Ulcers.* U.S. Department of Health and Human Services (DHHS), Public Health Service (PHS) Agency for Health Care Research and Quality (AHRQ), formerly known as the Agency for Health Care Policy and Research (AHCPR). Rockville MD: AHRQ; 1994.

7. Ziskin MC, Michlovitz SL. Therapeutic ultrasound. In: Michlovitz SL, ed. *Thermal Agents in Rehabilitation.* Philadelphia: F.A. Davis; 1990.

8. Cameron MH, ed. *Ultrasound* in *Physical Agents in Rehabilitation.* Philadelphia: WB Saunders; 1999:275–276.

9. Simpson SL, Hertzog MS, Barja RH. The plantaris tendon graft: An ultrasound study. *J Hand Surg.* 1991;16:708–711.

10. O'Reilly MAR, Massouh H. Pictorial review: The sonographic diagnosis of pathology in the Achilles tendon. *Clin Radiol.* 1993;48:202–206.

11. Karim A, Young SR, Lynch JA, Dyson M. A novel method of assessing skin ultrasound scans. *Wounds.* 1994;6:9–15.

12. Lynch JA, O'Reilly MAR, Massouh H. A robust and accurate method for calculating the fractal signature of texture in macroradiographs of osteoarthritis knees. *Med Inf.* 1991;2:241–251.

13. Williams PL, Bannister LH, Berry M, et al. *Gray's Anatomy.* 38th ed. Edinburgh, Scotland: Churchill-Livingstone; 1995:417.

14. Gonzalez RC, Wintz P. Digital image processing. In: Gonzalez RC, Winter P, eds. *Digital Image Fundamentals.* Reading, MA: Addison-Wesley; 1987:13–59.

15. Bamber JC, Tristam M. The physics of medical imaging. In: Webb S, ed. *Diagnostic Ultrasound.* Bristol, England: Adam Hilgerl; 1988:319–386.

16. Fornage BD, Deshayes JL. Ultrasound of normal skin. *J Clin Ultrasound.* 1986; 14:619.

17. Whiston RJ, Young SR, Lynch JA, Harding KG, Dyson M. Application of high frequency ultrasound to the objective assessment of healing wounds. In: *Proceedings of the 2nd Conference on Advances in Wound Management.* London: Macmillan Press; 1992:26–29.

18. Young SR, Lynch JA, Leipins PJ, Dyson M. Ultrasound imaging: A non-invasive method of wound assessment. In: *Proceedings of the 2nd Conference on Advances in Wound Management.* London: Macmillan Press; 1992:29–31.

19. Miller M, Dyson M. *Principles of Wound Care: A Professional Nurse Publication.* London: Macmillan Magazines Ltd; 1996:72–73.

20. Liong JL. *High Frequency Diagnostic Ultrasound as an Adjunct to Irritant Patch Assessment.* Thesis. London: University of London UMDS; 1996.

21. Van Holsbeek M, Introcaso JH. Sonography of muscle. *Musculo-Skeletal Ultrasound.* Chicago, IL: Mosby-Yearbook; 1990:13.

22. Shafir R, Itzchak Y, Heyman Z, et al. Preoperative ultrasonic measurements of the thickness of cutaneous malignant melanoma. *J Ultrasound Med.* 1984;3:205.

23. Breslow A. Thickness, cross-sectional areas and depth of invasion in the prognosis of cutaneous melanoma. *Ann Surg.* 1970;172:902.

24. Graves D. Stage I pressure ulcer in ebony complexion. *Decubitus.* 1990;3:4.

25. Bennett M. Report of the task force on the implications for darkly pigmented intact skin in the prediction and prevention of pressure ulcers. *Adv Wound Care.* 1995;8:34–35.

26. Lyder C. Examining the inclusion of ethnic minorities in pressure ulcer prediction studies. *JWOCN.* 1996;23:257–260.

27. Henderson C, Ayello C, Sussman C. et al. Draft definition of stage I pressure ulcers: Inclusion of person with darkly pigmented skin. *Adv Wound Care.* 1997;10:34–35.

28. Dyson M, Lyer C. Wound management with physical modalities. In: Morison M, ed. *The Prevention and Treatment of Pressure Ulcers.* Harcourt Health Sciences; 2000.

29. Sussman C. *Ultrasound for Wound Healing.* Monograph. Houston, TX: The Chattanooga Group; 1993.

30. Dyson M. Mechanisms involved in therapeutic ultrasound. *Physiother J Chartered Soc Physiother.* 1987;73(3):8.

31. Dyson M. Role of ultrasound in wound healing. In: McCulloch JM, Kloth LC, Feedar JA, eds. *Wound Healing: Alternatives in Management.* 2nd ed. Philadelphia: FA Davis; 1995:318–346.

32. Dyson M, Young SR. Acceleration of tissue repair by low intensity ultrasound applied during the inflammatory phase. Presented at the meeting of American Physical Therapy Association and Canadian Physical Therapy Association; 1988.

33. Hart J. The effect of therapeutic ultrasound on dermal repair with emphasis on fibroblasts activity. Thesis. London: University of London; 1993.

34. Gillet JH, Mitchell JLA. Acceleration of tissue repair of damaged skeletal muscle using ultrasound. *Orthop Prac.* 1989;2(4):36.

35. Harding K. Wound care: Putting theory into clinical practice. In: Krasner D, ed. *Chronic Wound Care: A Clinical Source Book for Health Care Professionals.* Wayne, PA: Health Management Publications; 1990:19–30.

36. Hardy M. The biology of scar formation. *Phys Ther.* 1989;69:1014–1024.

37. Frieder S, Weisberg J, Flemming B, Stanek A. The therapeutic effects of ultrasound following partial rupture of Achilles tendons in male rats. *J Orthop Sports Phys Ther.* 1988;10:39–46.

38. Jackson BA, Schwane JA, Starcher BC. Effect of ultrasound therapy on the repair of Achilles tendon injuries in rats. *Med Sci Sports Exerc.* 1991;23:171–176.

39. Consentino AB, Cross DL. Ultrasound effects on electroneuromyographic measures in sensory fibers of the median nerve. *Phys Ther.* 1983;63:1788–1792.

40. Byl N, Hopf H. The use of oxygen in wound healing. In: McCulloch J, Kloth L, Feedar JA, eds. *Wound Healing: Alternatives in Management,* 2nd ed. Philadelphia: FA Davis; 1996:365–404.

41. Knighton DR, Halliday B, Hunt TK. Oxygen as an antibiotic. *Arch Surg.* 1984;119:199–204.

42. McDiarmid T, Burns P. Clinical applications of therapeutic ultrasound. *Physiother J Chartered Soc Physiother.* 1987;73(4):14–21.

43. Parish L, Witkowsky J. Decubitus ulcers: How to intervene effectively. *Drug Ther.* 1983.

44. Shamberger RC, Talbot TL, Tipton HW, Thibault LE, Brennan MT. The effect of ultrasonic and thermal treatment on wounds. *Plast Reconstr Surg.* 1981;68(6):860–869.

45. Cambier DC, Vanderstraeten GG. Failure of therapeutic ultrasound in healing burn injuries. *Burns.* 1997;23(3):248–249.

46. Byl N, McKenze A, Wong T, West J, Hunt T. Incisional wound healing: A controlled study of low and high dose ultrasound. *Orthop Sports Phys Ther.* 1993;18:619–628.

47. Taskan I, Ozyazgan I, Tercan M, et al. A comparative study of the effect of ultrasound and electrostimulation on wound healing in rats. *Plast Reconstr Surg.* 1997;100(4):966–972.

48. Paul BJ, Lafratta CW, Dawson RA, Baab E, Bullock F. Use of ultrasound in the treatment of pressure sores in patients with spinal cord injury. *Arch Phys Med Rehabil.* 1960;41:438–440.

49. McDiarmid T, Burns PN, Lewith GT, Machin D. Ultrasound and the treatment of pressure sores. *Physiotherapy.* 1985;71(2):66–70.

50. Nussbaum EL, Biemann I, Mustard B. Comparison of ultrasound/ultraviolet C and laser for treatment of pressure ulcers in patients with spinal cord injury. *Phys Ther.* 1994;74:812–825.

51. ter Riet G, Kessels AGH, Knipschild P. A randomized clinical trial of ultrasound in the treatment of pressure ulcers. *Phys Ther.* 1996;76:1301–1312.

52. Dyson M, Frank C, Suckling J. Stimulation of healing of varicose ulcers by ultrasound. *Ultrasonics.* September 1976:232–236.

53. Peschen M, Weichenthal M, Schopf E, Vanscheidt W. Low frequency ultrasound treatment of chronic venous leg ulcers in an outpatient therapy. *Acta Dermatol Venereol.* 1997;77(4):311–314.

54. Roche C, West J. A controlled trial investigating the effect of ultrasound on venous ulcers referred from general practitioners. *Physiotherapy.* 1984;70(12):475–477.

55. Lundeberg T, Nordstrom F, Brodda-Jansen G, Eriksson S, Kjartansson J, Samuelson U. Pulsed ultrasound does not improve healing of venous ulcers. *Scand J Rehabil Med.* 1990;22(4):195–197.

56. Callam M, Harper D, Dale J, Ruckley C, Prescott R. A controlled trial of weekly ultrasound therapy in chronic leg ulceration. *Lancet.* 1987;2(8552):204–206.

57. Eriksson S, Lundberg T, Malm M. A placebo controlled trial of ultrasound therapy in chronic leg ulceration. *Scand J Rehabil Med.* 1991;23(4):211–213.

58. Ward RS, Hayes-Lundy C, Reddy R, Brockway C, Mills P, Saffle JR. Evaluation of topical therapeutic ultrasound to improve response to physical therapy and lessen scar contracture after burn injury. *J Burn Care Rehabil.* 1994;15(1):74–79.

59. Sicard-Rosenbaum L, Danoff JV, Guthrie JA, Eckhaus MA. Effects of energy-matched pulsed and continuous ultrasound on tumor growth in mice. *Physther.* 1998;78:271–277.

60. Klucinec B, Scheidler M, Denegar C, Domholdt E, Burgess SS. Effectiveness of wound care products in the transmission of acoustic energy. *Phys Ther.* 2000;469–476.

61. McDonald W, Nichter L. Debridement of bacterial and particulate contaminated wounds. *Ann Plast Surg.* 1994;33(2):142–147.

62. Swanson G. Functional outcome report: The next generation in physical therapy reporting. In: Stuart D, Ablen S, eds. *Documenting Physical Therapy Outcomes.* St. Louis, MO: Mosby-Year Book; 1993:101–134.

CHAPTER 25

Whirlpool

Carrie Sussman

CHAPTER OBJECTIVES

At the end of this chapter, the reader will be able to:

1. Describe evidence about the putative effects of whirlpool for wound healing
2. Identify the conditions that are suitable for application of whirlpool
3. Discuss negative aspects of whirlpool therapy
4. Discuss alternative methods of using whirlpool that affect wound healing

INTRODUCTION

Hydrotherapy and use of warmth for wound healing is reported in the literature back to ancient times. In current physical medicine practice, whirlpool is often the hydrotherapy method selected. The rationale for selecting whirlpool to treat wounds includes the putative effects of:

1. Mechanical debridement:
   • to reduce wound contamination and infection by softening and removal of debris and exudate
2. Thermal effects:
   • to increase local tissue perfusion to transport oxygen and nutrients to the tissues and remove waste products
   • to stimulate cellular activities for regeneration to facilitate neuronal mechanisms of analgesia for pain relief and increased mobility
   • to facilitate neuronal mechanisms of analgesia for pain relief and increased mobility

The putative effects and the efficacy of whirlpool for wound healing will be discussed.

EVALUATING THE EVIDENCE

Whirlpool—hydrotherapy—has been a standard treatment for chronic wounds and burns for many years. In 1994, the Agency for Health Care Policy and Research, now known as the Agency for Health Care Research and Quality (AHRQ) panel considered the evidence and, based on an absence of clinical trials, recommended a level "C" grade for this therapy (see the book, *Introduction for the AHCPR Evidence Grading System*). The AHCPR recommendation was "to consider whirlpool treatment for pressure ulcers that contain thick exudate, slough, or necrotic tissue and to discontinue whirlpool when the ulcer is clean.[1(p52)] Feedar and Kloth recommended twice daily (BID) hydrotherapy for most necrotic wounds and daily if used in conjunction with other methods, such as wet to dry dressings to facilitate debridement of wounds with slough.[2] The author published evidence in this chapter.

Debridement, Cleansing, Wound Decontamination, and Infection

Debridement is the process for removal of devitalized tissue. It is now recognized as a key component for the management of chronic wounds and, as such, has become a standard of care to speed and achieve optimal wound healing. Debridement is differentiated from wound cleansing. The process of wound cleansing involves selecting a wound cleansing solution and a method of delivery that cleanses the wound with minimum chemical or mechanical trauma.[1] Whirlpool is both a method of mechanical debridement and wound cleansing. Other methods of debridement to manage necrotic tissue are discussed in Chapters 8 and 26. Devitalized tissue in the wound prolongs the inflammatory process, and delays the onset of the healing cascade and the healing process. When the body cannot rid itself of the bioburden of dead tissue and debris efficiently and effectively, due to compromised body systems or an excessive amount of debris, an intervention to speed the process must be considered. By performing a debridement procedure, the clinician minimizes the body's inflammatory response and removes a staging place for bacteria and fungi.

Use of mechanical force, such as turbulent water, to remove nonviable tissue is an invasive procedure that is nonselective and may cause damage to healthy as well as nonviable tissues. Trauma to granulation tissue and epithelial cells may occur if the wound is positioned too close to the high-pressure jets of the whirlpool.[2] Trauma from mechanical force prolongs inflammation and delays healing.[3] Therefore, care must be exercised during delivery of the whirlpool treatment to minimize trauma to healthy granulation tissue, as well as to surrounding soft tissues, because even trauma distant from the wound site can influence the occurrence of local wound infection.[4] Trauma from shearing forces and turbulence can be avoided by adjusting the level of aeration from the jet to minimal or by turning off the aerator if tissues are very fragile, such as new skin grafts.[5]

The physical effects of immersion in water are soaking, saturating, loosening, and softening of loosely adherent necrotic tissues, which aids phagocytosis and deodorization. Whirlpool has little or no effect on densely adherent fibrous tissue, and other methods of debridement should be considered. Whirlpool as a debridement intervention is often followed by other debridement methods, eg, sharp, enzymatic, or autolytic.

Whirlpool Associated Risks

Surface environment of the skin is normally unfavorable to most microflora because its body surface pH is between 5 and 6.[6] Prolonged soaking supersaturates the wound tissue and surrounding skin, which may result in maceration, or the breaking down of the fibers of the skin and a change in the pH. During immersion, exudate is cleansed from the wound along with sweat and oils from the surrounding skin. Autonomic neuropathy impairs function of sweat and sebaceous glands, resulting in dry skin. Therefore, soaking of the neuropathic foot that has already impaired sweat and oil production and risk of maceration is not recommended.[7] Agitation is used to cleanse and debride the wound tissue by scrubbing it. The mechanical effects on circulation caused by agitation of the whirlpool are small.[8] It has been postulated that the mechanical stimulation of the cells stimulates granulation tissue formation.

There is evidence that wounds treated in hydrotherapy are at risk for waterborne contamination and other complications. Reports in the literature demonstrate *Pseudomonas aeruginosa*-associated skin disease after immersion in whirlpool.[9–11] Factors that influence host susceptibility include the anatomic and physiologic defenses of the skin, the skin surface microecology where the skin humidity is altered, and intrinsic factors, including disease and age. The skin's relative dryness may be a defense mechanism to resist infection. The immersion in the whirlpool may negate the normal skin defenses. Chronic antibiotic therapy changes the normal flora of the skin and can lead to colonization and superinfection with organisms such as *P. aeruginosa*.[9]

A variety of intrinsic facts, such as diabetes, appear to increase the host susceptibility to infection through the skin. Traumatic injuries such as burns and immunosuppressive therapies also increase host susceptibility to skin infection with *P. aeruginosa*.[9] Hydration of the skin and increased skin tissue temperature have been associated with *P. aeruginosa* infections and most likely negates many of the skin's normal defenses. In experimental models, supererhydration of the skin must be continued for several days before symptoms occur and whirlpool ususally offers considerably shorter exposure periods. Repeated immersion and exposure to the whirlpool water may lead to colonization of the *P. Aeruginosa* despite drying of the skin surface between sessions. There is potential for the bacteria to be harbored in the invaginations of the skin appendages where they release proteolytic enzymes and exotoxins that result in an inflammatory reaction of the surrounding tissues.[8]

Wound decontamination and controlling infection are cited as reasons to use hydrotherapy. Evidence to support use of whirlpool as a means of achieving wound decontamination and prevention of infection is mixed. Two studies compared the effects of whirlpool treatment and whirlpool treatment followed by vigorous rinsing. Neiderhuber et al[12] studied removal of bacterial load from the soles of the feet of 76 normal adults with intact skin. Factors considered in their investigation included temperature of the water, immersion time, agitation of the water versus soaking, spraying the part with clean water for 30 seconds, and agitation of the water during immersion, followed by spraying of the part with clean water for 30 seconds.[12] Findings of the study were that temperature of the water was not a significant factor. There was a steady removal of bacterial load with longer duration treatment, 10–20 minutes being optimal. Agitation was best, compared with either soaking or spraying, in removal of skin surface bacteria, but the combination of immersion with agitation and spraying rinsed away 70% of the remaining contaminants, providing the best outcome. Bohannon[13] studied a single subject with a venous ulcer and compared bacterial load following whirlpool with low concentration of povidone-iodine without and with rinsing for 30–90 seconds at the maximum pressure tolerated by the subject. More than four times as many bacteria were removed with rinsing added than without. Both studies support the use of whirlpool with rinse to reduce bacterial colonies present on skin and wound surface. There is considerable documentation in the literature that, when the bacterial content of an ulcer exceeds 10^5 organisms per gram of tissue, healing is impaired.[1] However, neither the Neiderhuber nor the Bohannon study identifies the organisms isolated, nor do they use the threshold standard of an infected wound as 10^5 organisms per gram of tissue measured by wound biopsy or culture.[14] Only one patient with a wound was evaluated. The strength of evidence based on these studies that whirlpool controls infection is poor.

Risk of infection for the patient who has a burn or wound has been documented. Shankowsky et al[11] surveyed 202 burn units in the United States and Canada with 158 (75.7%) responding and found that these facilities regularly use hydrotherapy as part of burn care. Whirlpool was implicated as a cause of nosocomial infection leading to sepsis with *P. aeruginosa* (52.9%), *Staphylococcus aureus* (25.5%), and *Candida albicans* (5.2%).[11] Cardany et al[15] found that hydrotherapy did not reduce bacterial load on burned or normal skin, but the water contained heavy contamination with viable organisms that have the potential for contaminating clean wounds and for patient cross-contamination. A further documented complication is superhydration of the skin, which allows penetration of bacteria.[9,11] Water content of the skin may increase to 55–70% following a 20-minute immersion.[9] Intrinsic factors, such as immunosuppression, and diseases, such as diabetes, are known to increase susceptibility to infection. Hospitalized individuals, compared with healthy individuals, have a decreased resistance to infection and have the highest risk of secondary health effects.

Exposure to pathogens has been associated with many sources, including whirlpool tanks. Infectious organisms, particularly *P. aeruginosa*, have been identified in hydrotherapy equipment, despite rigorous efforts to disinfect properly and to monitor for cultures. For instance, Shankowsky et al[11] reported a lethal outbreak of aminoglycoside-resistant *P. aeruginosa* in a newly constructed burn center where stringent methods of disinfection were used and despite routine bacterial surveillance. Control of the outbreak was achieved when the hydrotherapy tanks were used for closed wounds during rehabilitation.[11] The following reports show how different settings interpreted and responded to data collected from studies of infectious organisms in hydrotherapy tanks.

Over a 4-week period, cultures were taken in the morning before treatment and at the end of the day from whirlpools in two institutions in a university medical center commonly used by diabetic dysvascular patients. Special attention was directed toward recovery of *S. aureus*, *P. aeruginosa*, and *Escherichia coli* organisms. Results of the testing were that only 11 of 96 cultures (11.5%) were positive for these prospective pathogens. The opinion of the study authors was that immersion in these whirlpool tanks was not likely to

expose patients with open wounds to potential iatrogenic contamination.[16] Seventeen whirlpool baths in 16 nursing homes were examined for presence of *P. aeruginosa*. There were findings of large numbers of these organisms in water samples taken from whirlpool baths after agitation, but only one patient out of 253 residents was known to have a *P. aeruginosa* wound infection. Results of these findings led the Health Commission to advise the local survey team that, although the prevalence of known *P. aeruginosa* infection was low, the whirlpool baths should continue to be used only by continent residents with intact skin to avoid an infection hazard to the residents.[17]

Although the reports in the literature provide considerable evidence of risk of wound contamination, hydrotherapy is used in 94.8% of the surveyed institutions. Despite the reported high incidence of infection, hydrotherapy immersion continues to be used in 118 burn units. Only 27 respondents to the survey have discontinued immersion in favor of showers. Patients who are mechanically ventilated and/or invasively monitored are regularly immersed at 47.6% of the responding burn units.[11] Local treatment appears to reduce risk of lethal sepsis. Alternative measures of controlling wound infection with hydrotherapy using irrigation with sterile solution applied by a syringe or pulsatile lavage with suction are described in Chapters 8 and 26. Risk of infection due to immersion in hydrotherapy is becoming more widely recognized but has not yet significantly changed clinical practice.

THEORY AND SCIENCE OF THE THERAPY

Thermal Effects

Heat Transfer

The body's ability to transfer heat is dependent on four factors: the area of body surface immersed, the temperature of the water, the duration of the application, and the ability to dissipate internal heat and maintain proper core temperature. Heat is transferred from the water to the body by conduction and convection. Conduction is the exchange of thermal energy between two surfaces. If there is a temperature gradient, the heat will be transferred from the warmer to the cooler surface, eg, from the water to the body.[5] Body fat will lessen and slow the conduction of heat to the body core. At the same time, high body fat content reduces the body's ability to dissipate heat and can cause body core temperature to rise to a dangerously high level. Obese persons may not be candidates for immersion of a large body area in the whirlpool because they are unable to dissipate heat well, and other methods of treatment should be considered.[5] Submerged skin does not transfer heat from the surface; therefore, heat dissipation is shifted to the exposed body areas that can sweat and to the lungs. The greater the body surface area immersed, the less transpiration can take place on the skin surface. Respiration and heart rates increase as temperature of the water increases, most likely due to enhanced requirements for skin blood flow,[7] resulting in dehydration and increased cardiac output. Individuals with cardiopulmonary impairments or peripheral vascular disease are at risk in this situation.

Convection is a transfer of heat that occurs when there is circulation of a fluid, such as when water flows over the skin.[5] Heating occurs more rapidly by convection than by conduction. Surface body heat warms venous blood that is then carried toward the core, thus potentially raising core body temperature. As with conduction, this method of heat transfer stresses the cardiopulmonary system and peripheral vascular system. Again, caution should be used when considering immersion of persons with those impairments. Together, conduction and convection bring the heat into and out from the body core to the surface. Radiation transfers the heat from the body surface to the atmosphere but cannot take place from immersed body areas, limiting heat dissipation and increasing risk of hyperthermia.[5]

Thermal Regulation

The human body thermoregulatory system is centrally controlled by the hypothalamus to maintain a core temperature of about 98.6° F (37° C). Because of the effectiveness of the thermoregulatory defenses, the body temperature rarely deviates more than a few tenths of a degree. The range of core temperature that does not trigger thermoregulatory responses is termed the *interthreshold range*.[8] Information from the skin surface, deep abdominals, thoracic tissue, spinal cord, and nonhypothalamic portions of the brain, as well as the temperature of the hypothalamus itself each contribute roughly 20% of the information used by the hypothalamus for thermoregulatory control. The range of temperatures that do not trigger any thermoregulatory responses is only 0.2° C. Autonomic thermoregulatory defenses are not triggered unless the body temperature moves out of this interthreshold range. Under normal conditions, the body maintains a temperature gradient between the core and periphery of 2–4° C.[18] Both systemic and local tissue temperatures are of considerable importance. If the hypothalamus receives a signal from the skin that there is a rise in temperature, the response is sweating. If the signal from the skin is cold, response would be vasoconstriction and shivering. The object is a redistribution of body heat from the core to the periphery. All thermoregulatory responses are neuronally mediated. Nerve blocks prevent the normal activation of thermoregulatory defenses, such as sweating, vasoconstriction, and shivering. Peripheral inhibition of thermoregulatory defenses is a major cause of hypothermia during regional anesthesia.[18] Spinal cord-injured individuals and those with peripheral neuropathy also have peripheral inhibition of thermoregulatory defenses and are at risk

for both mild hypothermia and thermal injury from immersion.

Nineteen percent of 104 control group postsurgical patients who experienced mild hypothermia during surgery developed postsurgical wound infection. Mild hypothermia impairs the oxidative killing by neutrophils and decreases cutaneous blood flow, which reduces tissue oxygen and contributes to decreased wound strength by reducing the deposition of collagen. Heating core body temperature to 37° C, normothermia, during surgery in the experimental study group of 96 patients was found to reduce significantly the incidence of postsurgical wound infection and to increase significantly collagen deposition near the wound.[19] Mild hypothermia also reduces platelet function and increases coagulation time.[20] These inhibitory effects were found to be completely reversible by rewarming the blood to 37° C.[21,22] There is a linear relation near 20% between mean skin temperature and core temperatures at the vasoconstriction and shivering thresholds; however, there is individual variability.[23] This function is accomplished by the shunting of blood from the arterioles to the venules and venous plexuses located in the hands, feet, and face.

Clinical Wisdom:
Monitor Temperature

Use a thermometer to record tympanic membrane temperature during whirlpool treatment to monitor for changes in core body temperature.

Circulatory Effects

Heat is used to increase blood flow to the tissues.[24,25] Infection rates of tissues are inversely proportional to blood flow, and oxygenation of tissues is totally dependent on perfusion.[26,27] Application of heat for 20 minutes produces an immediate increase in blood flow but the increase in blood flow is greater in the posttreatment period, with peak blood flow achieved an average of 46 minutes after terminating the application of the heat. Longer exposure of up to 2 hours had no real effect on increasing the peak rise.[24] Local heating can increase local perfusion an average of threefold and is the simplest and most effective way of enhancing blood flow and increasing subcutaneous oxygen tension that is sustained, even after the heat source is removed.[26,28] Tissues are totally dependent on blood flow to meet metabolic demands of inflammation. Increased oxygen tension makes tissue more resistant to infection.[28] Decreased tissue oxygen tension impairs the deposition of collagen and oxidative killing by the neutrophils.[27] Three different temperatures (38, 42, and 46° C) were tested in healthy adults to determine effects on local subcutaneous oxygen. Results of 100% increase in blood flow and 50% increase in subcutaneous oxygen were comparable for all three temperatures.[29] Local warming influences wound healing.

Methods of applying heat are through general body heating, local heating, and indirect heating. General body heating can be used to raise core body temperature if there is mild core hypothermia but can overtax the system if the patient is febrile. Mild core hypothermia can impair immune functions by vasoconstriction-induced hypoxia. Vasoconstriction-induced tissue hypoxia may decrease the strength of the healing wound because the process of collagen deposition and cross-linkages between strands of collagen is dependent on oxygen tension.[19] Full body immersion in a whirlpool at normothermia could be used as an active way to raise core body temperature, induce peripheral vasodilation, increase blood flow and oxygen tension, and accelerate healing.[30] Exposure of a large body area to heat will also have systemic effects on the cardiovascular and other organ systems. Initially, there will be a rise in blood pressure, followed by a decrease as peripheral vasodilation occurs. At 40° C, mean cardiac output and oxygen consumption increase, but not significantly, after a 20-minute session. Pulse rate increased 1.3–1.5 times over the sitting or supine resting level, and mean blood pressure increased 1.1 times over the supine resting values. Patients should be monitored closely for dizziness or changes in mental status. Direct heating has a direct relationship with increasing both superficial and deep tissue temperatures.[5] In many situations, localized direct heating may have more advantages than generalized direct or indirect heating. In Chapter 12, Management of the Wound Environment with Advanced Therapies, the Warm Up Therapy System section discusses another strategy for delivering localized direct heat to the tissues.

Indirect heating, also referred to as *reflex heating*, involves heating a distant body area. Local cutaneous thermoreceptors are stimulated by heat and carry impulses to the spinal cord and the thermoregulatory mechanisms of the hypothalamus. Core body temperature is also elevated when the lower body is warmed.[31] The warmed blood acts on constricted blood vessels of the skin, where a vasoactive mediator is released that stimulates vasodilatation. Vasodilation produces a mild inflammatory reaction through the release of histamine and prostaglandins. Bradykinin, which is a byproduct of an enzyme from sweat, is also released. Together, these chemical mediators enhance the permeability of the blood vessels. Increased blood flow following vasodilatation increases capillary hydrostatic pressure, producing fluid shift from the vessels into the interstitial spaces and resulting in mild edema and mild inflammation.[5] Mild inflammation can stimulate the biologic cascade of wound healing and restart healing.

Direct heating of an ischemic extremity presents risk of thermal injury, due to the rapid increase of tissue temperature and lack of adequate blood supply to dissipate and remove the heat. Indirect heating has been shown to increase blood flow and pulse rate at a distant area.[25] Application of heat to an extremity with impaired sensation likewise presents risk of burns because of lack of sympathetic nervous system input to mediate vasodilation needed to dissipate and remove the heat and/or lack of sensory input to warn of overheating[32] (Figure 25–1). Immersion of one upper extremity to produce indirect heating can be a useful way of applying heat and producing generalized vasodilatation. This will cause increased perfusion to the lower extremities with minimal fluid shift and is an alternative approach that can be used to treat a wound in a patient with peripheral vascular disease or impaired lower extremity sensation. Indirect application of heat would also minimize exposure of an open wound to contamination and the risk of infection.

Vasodilatation is a benefit for a patient with reduced perfusion, but it can be disastrous for a patient with venous insufficiency, whose venous system has difficulty managing tissue fluids.[33] Fluid shifts also occur within the wound, with a loss of proteins, electrolytes, other nutrients, and growth factors found in wound fluid that pass out into the water. If the wound surface area is large, fluid shifts can lead to dehydration and depletion of nutrients needed for healing.[34] Use of saline instead of tap water will prevent loss of fluids. A saline whirlpool can be made by adding salt to the water. If fluid shift is of concern, perhaps another intervention would better meet the goals of treatment.

Research Wisdom:
Whirlpool Implications for Venous Congestion

McCulloch and Boyd[33] reported that whirlpool treatment of a dependent leg resulted in increased hypotension and lower extremity vascular congestion, even in healthy individuals. The implications for the patient with a compromised venous system are very serious.

A further benefit of increased blood flow is improved delivery of oxygen, nutrients, antibodies, leukocytes, and systemic antibiotics to the tissues, and removal of metabolites. In patients with comorbidities, such as diabetes, arterial occlusive disease, and limited mobility, there is a reduction of blood flow to the tissues. The impaired circulation compromises the effectiveness of antibiotics to control wound infection. Timing treatment to enhance perfusion and delivery of antibiotics to wound tissue is being tested with transcutaneous electrical stimulation.[35] Heat-induced perfusion in the whirlpool may be another way to enhance the delivery of antibiotic therapy. The physical therapy department and nurses who administer the antibiotics should consider collaborating

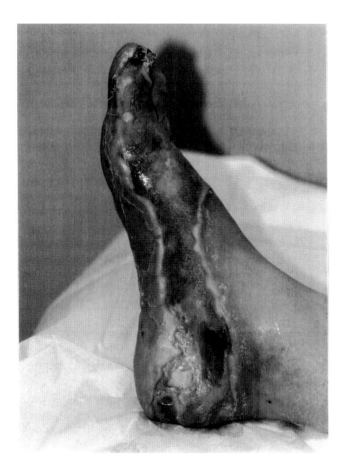

Figure 25–1 Burn resulting from putting neuropathic foot in hot water. *Source:* Copyright © Nancy Elftman.

in scheduling whirlpool treatment time to coincide with optimal delivery of antibiotics circulating in the bloodstream to the tissues, because it could enhance the benefits of both treatments. A clinical trial would test this hypothesis.

Cellular Effects

Studies on the effect of temperature on cells of tissue repair show contrasting results that may be cell-specific. Warmth stimulates cell mitosis and enhances leukocytic activity. Research on pigs has shown experimentally that the speed of production of new epidermal cells is enhanced if the temperature is maintained at 37° C. Similar results have been reported following in vitro testing of human skin cultures. Leukocyte activity may fall to zero when wound temperature is cooled, such as during a dressing change. This will impair the phagocytic activity of the leukocytes.[36] It has been observed that it takes 40 minutes for a freshly cleaned wound to return to normal temperature and 3 hours for mitotic cell division to resume.[37,38]

Clotting factor activity is prolonged at temperatures below 35° C, resulting in decreased activation of the coagulation cascade. More bleeding could be expected during debridement if a tepid whirlpool is used. Clotting function is restored with warming.[20] However, at 33° C, the proliferative capacity of endothelial cells was potentiated.[39] Fibroblasts treated with heat at 38° C have increased cell division and metabolic activity.[40] Chronic wound fluid is known to inhibit fibroblast activity. Heating of chronic wound fluid in a water bath showed that there was a temperature-dependent reduction in the inhibitory effect on fibroblasts. When the heated chronic wound fluid was added to fetal and adult fibroblasts, the heated wound fluid assisted in the growth of both fetal and adult fibroblasts.[41] Heating of wound fluid during whirlpool treatment may have a significant effect on restarting the growth of fibroblasts in chronic wounds.

Delayed phagocytosis and wound healing may be attributed to frequent changes in wound temperature. Therefore, the effect of temperature on cellular activity is an important consideration when choosing a treatment temperature for the whirlpool and in prompt aftercare. The effect of temperature changes on the cells of repair should also be considered an important factor when selecting the frequency of hydrotherapy treatment.

Neuronal Effects

Neural receptors for heat and cold are distributed all over the body. Signals from cold receptors travel along A delta fibers and from warm receptors along C fibers. Neuronal mediation of thermoregulatory responses is the primary means of activation. The warm water has mild analgesic effects, reduces inflammation, is soothing, and relaxes muscle tension.[30,42,43] Patients experiencing severe pain or anxiety may find these effects soothing and analgesic. However, patients who are lethargic or semicomatose with already suppressed central nervous system function would be neurosuppressed to a point where they could become totally unresponsive. These patients should not be put in the whirlpool. Analgesia from the warm water is often reported, but some wound patients, especially those with ischemic limbs or burns, find that the agitation stimulates pain receptors. Treatment at a very gentle agitation level directed away from the wound tissue can be used to soothe, rather than stimulate, the nerves. Patient tolerance should be evaluated and treatment modified as required.

During the whirlpool treatment, the patient should be encouraged to perform gentle exercise for muscle pump functions and strengthening. Both skin blood flow and sweating during exercise increase with a rise in water temperature and are notable at 35° C.[7] If exercise is to be performed during the wound treatment, consider the physiologic effects when choosing the water temperature and the extent of body area to be immersed. Joint range of motion extensibility is usually performed more easily and less painfully in the warm water. The gentle stretching forces around the wound may stimulate tissue regeneration. Of course, stretching and exercise of a newly sutured wound should be avoided until the sutures are removed.

Clinical Wisdom: *Fluids*

Provide patients with fluids during hydrotherapy to compensate for loss of fluids.

Effects at Different Temperatures

The average skin temperature of the body is 93° F (34° C). The range of body indifference to temperature is 93–100.4° F (34–38° C). At 80–92° F (27–33.5° C), the temperature is tepid or nonthermal. At this temperature range, chilling with local vasoconstriction, decreased oxygen uptake, and tissue cooling that affects the cells of repair occurs.[24,40] Avoid mild core hypothermia at this thermal range by treating only a limited body area for a very short duration (eg, 5 minutes) for cleansing or to soften dry tissue; keep the rest of the body and surrounding air temperature warm and slightly humid. Use a normothermic tap water rinse (35–37° C) immediately following the whirlpool to raise local wound temperatures.

Consider the tepid temperature choice for patients with venous disease where wound debridement and cleansing is the objective and where vasodilation would add blood volume and overload incompetent veins. The warm rinse would reduce shock to local cells of repair.

Neutral warmth is 92–96° F (33.5–35.5° C). Consider this temperature range for the patient with peripheral vascular disease, sensory impairment, or full body immersion. Possibly the best choice of temperature to optimize cellular functions and enzymatic and biochemical reactions is at normal body temperature, or normothermia, defined as 98.6° F or 37° C ± 1° C.[44] The temperature range of 35.5–37° C is best when treating the patient with cardiovascular or pulmonary disease who would be stressed at a higher temperature.[5] At neutral warmth and normal body temperatures, tissues will be soaked, softened, and cleansed, and perfusion of the tissues will be increased.

Clinical Wisdom: *Avoid Chilling*

When using lower temperatures, avoid chilling by maintaining warm room temperature and use only for single limbs, not the whole body. Reduce treatment duration from 20 minutes to 5 or 10 minutes.

Temperatures of 98–104° F (36.5–40° C) are acceptable for therapeutic heating.[5] Above 98° F or 37° C is classified as hot. Significant physiologic stress in the circulatory, nervous, and cardiopulmonary systems may occur under these conditions.[45] Water temperature choices are summarized as follows: [5]

- Nonthermal/tepid: 80–92° F or 27–33.5° C
- Neutral: 92–96° F or 33.5–35.5° C
- Normothermal: 98.6° F or 37° C
- Hot: 98–104° F or 36.7–40° C

Higher temperature levels are *not* recommended because of physiologic stress.

A tissue temperature rise of as much as 4° C at temperatures ranging from 37° to 42° C has been measured after immersion for 20 minutes in a whirlpool. As mentioned earlier, in a study of effects of the whirlpool on circulation, pulse rates increased 1.3–1.5 times over the sitting or supine resting level, and the mean blood pressure increased 1.1 times over the supine resting values.[5] Autonomic neuropathy and pulmonary dysfunction, which are common comorbidities with wounds, interfere with evaporative cooling. Limit the body surface area, lower the water temperature, and reduce the treatment time in the whirlpool for patients with cardiopulmonary and neuropathic diseases, so that they are less physiologically challenged. If this is not practical, choose another treatment modality.

Temperature Precautions

As reviewed, water temperature modifies circulatory responses. Some precautions that the physical therapist should use to modify the heating effects of treatment are included in this list:

- Water temperature should not exceed local skin temperature (usually 34° C) in the presence of peripheral vascular disease.
- Water temperature should not exceed 38° C in the presence of cardiovascular and pulmonary disease. The heat stimulates peripheral vasodilatation, with subsequent increased return of blood to the heart and increased cardiac output. The added load of blood volume can overtax a weak or decompensated heart muscle.[2]
- Water temperature of 32° C increases blood flow of 2.3 mL/dL of limb volume but will chill the wound and slow clotting and healing.[5,45]
- Extremes of temperature should be avoided in patients with sensory loss, such as those with alcoholic or diabetic-related neuropathy or spinal cord injury, who cannot feel the temperature and respond to the heat. Loss of sensation can result in severe burns. Temperature sensation testing in a neuropathic patient is recommended before immersion in warm water. The procedure for testing is described in Chapter 4.

Clinical Studies

Many clinicians have moved away from use of the whirlpool since the release of the AHRQ *Pressure Ulcer Treatment Guidelines* because of a lack of evidence and cautions received from experts. The review of literature for other treatment interventions brought to light a number of studies where whirlpool was used as either a co-treatment modality or as the standard care treatment. Since the guidelines were published in 1994, one randomized controlled clinical trial of clean surgically debrided pressure ulcers treated with whirlpool has been published.[46] Like most treatment intervention studies, the data from these studies often has gaps such as treatment parameters used or the percentage of healing. The purpose of this review of the whirlpool reports is to look at which data have been reported and the evidence they provide for choosing an intevention with whirlpool hydrotherapy. Table 25–1 summarizes the data derived from the review and the following outlines the studies more extensively.

A randomized clinical trial was performed to test the effect of whirlpool on surgically debrided, clean granulating, stage III and IV pressure ulcers.[46] Group A was treated with moist wound dressings and whirlpool hydrotherapy (N = 24) at 96–97° F and the control group B with moist wound dressings (N = 18). One 20-minute session was given daily. The whirlpool group showed significantly faster rate of wound healing, mean rate 0.39 cm/week, in 58.33% of the whirlpool-treated ulcers, compared with mean healing rate of 0.169 cm/week for 27.78% of the nonwhirlpool controls. Fewer wounds in the whirlpool group (9 versus 11) deteriorated during the course of treatment. However, the investigators were concerned that there were so many deteriorating wounds in both groups that could not be explained.

Whirlpool with povidone-iodine was chosen as the standard treatment for all patients in the two reports from Gogia. In a clinical report, two patients were treated with whirlpool and low-energy infrared cold laser (CL).[47] The patient in case study 1 had a 1.42 cm/week or 7.12% per week (99.7% healing) reduction in size after 14 weeks of therapy. Patient in case study 2 had weekly reduction in size of 1.5 cm/week or 5% per week (90% healing) in 18 weeks. Broad conclusions cannot be reached about use of these combined interventions.The second study was in a small controlled clinical trial (N = 12) of patients with pressure ulcers. The investigators followed a daily 20-minute whirlpool with povidone-iodine intervention with 20-minute electrical stimulation (ES) in half the patients, and the control half of the study received only a 20-minute treatment of whirlpool with povidone-iodine.[48] Both groups received aftercare with saline wet-to-dry dressings. The whirlpool control group in the ES study had a 5.23% per week reduction in wound area and 28.37% per week reduction in depth. Gault and Gatens[49] found that a whirlpool control group had a 14.7% per week rate of healing. They designated one ulcer on each of six patients as a control and assigned that ulcer to a whirlpool control group. Results for those ulcers were a 14.7%/week healing rate.[49] However, the electrotherapy that was administered to the other ulcer may have had some systemic effect that influenced the rate of healing in the control ulcer.

Akers and Gabrielson[50] compared three treatment regimens: (1) whirlpool; (2) whirlpool with high-voltage pulsed current (HVPC); and (3) HVPC alone in the healing of pressure ulcers of 14 spinal cord-injured individuals. This controlled clinical trial reported that the whirlpool treatment was given once daily (QD), the HVPC was given twice daily (BID), and the whrilpool given QD and HVPC BID. The treatment parameters and the rate or percentage of healing were not reported. Results reported that there was no statistical significance between the three groups. The best outcomes were achieved by the HVPC BID group, followed by the whirlpool QD group and the HVPC BID, and last, the whirlpool QD group. The study reported that numerous interval variations existed.

Thurman and Christian[51] reported a case study of a patient with diabetes who was scheduled for surgical amputation of a foot with an infected abscess. The ulcerated foot was treated with a mixture of interventions including whirlpool and hexachlorophene for 10 minutes daily, followed by treatment with HVPC and other disinfecting agents and antimicrobials. Results were limb salvage, decreased infection, and exudate leading to closure in 4 months.

Carley and Wainapel's control group had a multitude of conventional dressing treatments, including mainly wet to dry dressings, gauze with Dakin's solution, or povodone iodine.[52] Four were treated in the whirlpool. Results were not separated from the rest of the controls.

Wood et al[53] reported on results of a randomized controlled trial of 31 patients treated with whirlpool, saline wet to moist dressings, and compared the results to a group of 43 patients treated with low-intensity direct current. The whirlpool and dressing group had 3% healing or had increased wound size while the low voltage microamperage direct current group had 58% healing. Perhaps some of the poor results in the whirlpool/saline wet to moist dressing group were due to the dressings drying out, resulting in repeated trauma during dressing changes.

In another study, whirlpool efficacy was compared to pulsed lavage by measuring the rate of formation of granulation tissue in a variety of chronic wounds.[54] Although the rate of granulation tissue formation was greater, 12.2% per week, for the pulsed lavage group, the whirlpool group had a granulation rate of 4.8% per week. Whirlpool and collagenase were both used throughout the course of treatment

Table 25–1 Clinical Studies Using Whirlpool

Investigators and Type of Study	Disease States Treated	Whirlpool	Electrical Stimulation	Other Treatments	Effects on Healing
Akers and Gabrielson[50] (N = 14) Controlled Clinical Trial	Pressure (full or partial denervation of spinal cord)	Once daily	HVPC b.i.d. WPL once and HVPC b.i.d.	Not reported	ES only best ES with whirlpool second best Whirlpool only least No statistical significance between 3 groups. Lots of internal variation
Burke et al[46] (WPL N = 24 nonWPL N = 18) RCT	Pressure	Once daily, 20 min 96–98°F	N/A	Surgical debridement Saline wet-to-dry dressings	WPL group * 58.33% (14) mean 0.39 cm/week reduction in size 4.17% (1) no change 37.5% (9) deterioration Non-WPL Group * 27.78% (5) mean° .169 cm/week reduction in size 11.11% (2) no change 61.11% (11) deterioration
Carley and Wainapel[71] (WPL N = 4 LIDC N = 30) RCT		4–5 ×/week	LIDC Direct, 2 hours b.i.d., 5 ×/week	Wet-to-dry dressings Dakin's or povidone-iodine, or hydrogel	WP group 45% healing (9%/week) * LIDC group 98.95% (19%/week) * healing in 5 weeks
Gault and Gatens[49] (WPL N = 6 (LIDC N = 6 Subgroup) Controlled Trial	Mixed	Once daily	LIDC Direct, 2 hours b.i.d. or t.i.d.		LIDC 30%/week WP 14.7%/week, 2/6 increased in size
Gogia et al[48] (N = 6) Controlled Trial	Mixed	Once daily 20 min with povidone-iodine, 100°F	HVPC 20 min Direct, 5 ×/week	Saline wet-to-dry dressings	WPL 20 days 27.19% reduction in area (9.51%/week)* 56.76% reduction in depth (19.86%/week) WPL and HVPC 20 days 34.73% reduction area (12.15%/week) 30.30% reduction in depth (10.6%/week) *
Gogia, Hurt and Zirn[47] (N = 2) Case Studies		Whirlpool with povidone-iodine	N/A	Infrared cold laser	Granulation, significant healing

continues

Table 25–1 continued

Investigators and Type of Study	Disease States Treated	Whirlpool	Electrical Stimulation	Other Treatments	Effects on Healing
Haynes et al[54] (WPL N = 15) (PL N = 15) Controlled Trial	Mixed	Whirlpool	N/A	Pulsed lavage / Varied	PL 12.2% healing/week / WP 4.8% healing/week
Juve[30] (N = 63) Controlled Trial	Major abdominal surgery	Whirlpool daily Three days postoperative	N/A	Probably dressings (type unstated)	Pain reduction / Reduced wound inflammation / Positive signs of wound healing
Thurman and Christian[51] (N = 1) Case Study	Abscess, diabetes	Whirlpool with hexachlorophene detergent cleanser (pHisohex) 10 min	HVPC daily	Debridement / Hydrogen peroxide soaks / Antibiotic medication	Decreased infection, exudate, and wound size / 6 months to closure
Vetra and Whittaker[55] Uncontrolled Clinical Trial (N = 140)	Mixed	Whirlpool 40°C daily		Collagenase daily	80% closure / Mean time 37.0 days (SD 27.5 days) / 7% good granulation and epithelialization / 3% healthy granulation / 10% reduction or cessation of drainage
Wood et al[53] (WPL N = 31) (PLIDC N = 43) Randomized Controlled Trial	Pressure and venous	Whirlpool	PLIDC Brackets, 3 ×/week	Cleansing / Saline wet-to-dry dressings	Whirlpool and dressing group / 3% healed or increased in size / PLIDC 58% healed / Data for whirlpool only, ulcers not reported

WPL = whirlpool, HVPC = high-voltage pulsed current, LIDC = low-intensity direct current, PLIDC = pulsed low-intensity direct current, b.i.d. = twice daily, t.i.d. = three times daily.
* Percentage healing per week calculated study data to transform data for comparison.

Source: Data from reference #'s 30, 46, 47, 48, 49, 50, 51, 53, 54, 55, and 71.

for ulcers of mixed etiologies, and 80% reached closure in a median time of 37 days (SD 27.5 days).[55]

Major abdominal surgery is often followed by pain due to increased tension on muscles and tissues. Results of these events have been attributed to causing anxiety, stress, and altered tissue regeneration. Findings of a controlled clinical trial of postoperative patients (N = 63) who had major abdominal surgery and who received an intervention with whirlpool after surgery showed reduced pain behavior, less signs of wound inflammation, and positive signs of healing over a 3-day period following surgery.[30]

Review of the results suggest that there were extrinsic factors that may have influenced the results of the treatment interventions, such as use of cytotoxic agents like povodone iodine,[47,48,52] and hexachlophene and hydrogen peroxide.[51] Two studies[46,53] reported conscientiously avoiding chemical and mechanical trauma to the wounds treated with whirlpool, yet both reported significant deterioration of the whirlpool groups that were not explained.

CHOOSING AN INTERVENTION: CLINICAL REASONING

Applying Theory and Science to Clinical Decision Making

The previous sections reviewed the theory and science of intervention with whirlpool. The physical therapist would review the patient's medical history and do a systems review as guidelines for selection of an intervention with whirlpool.

Evaluation of study reports reviewed produced no evidence that whirlpool is harmful to granulation tissue. Good practice would be to take care that fragile granulation tissue or a new skin graft is protected from direct force of the whirlpool jet and that the force of the aeration is modified to avoid any problems. Whirlpool therapy will increase local blood flow for a sustained period of time after cessation of the treatment, will increase subcutaneous oxygen, and will stimulate the cells needed for healing. It is safe and effective to use, even after the wound is clean and free of exudate and necrotic debris.

Evidence of wound healing efficacy in treatment of patients with whirlpool is reported in two controlled clinical trials on pressure ulcers and surgical wounds,[30,46] as is evidence from studies where it was the control treatment. Whirlpool may be the most efficient way to treat multiple or extensive wounds. It can be used to heat a large body area or a limited body area and raise core body temperature; it is useful to relax tissue tension and provide relief for painful wounds. Although the evidence is still limited, additional study would be helpful to identify the best frequency of treatment and temperature that best speed healing.

Candidacy

AHCPR *Pressure Ulcer Treatment Guidelines* state: "Heel ulcers with dry eschar need not be debrided if they do not have edema, erythema, fluctuance, or drainage. Assess these wounds daily for pressure ulcer complications."[1(p49)] It is the AHCPR panel's opinion that these findings indicate wound stability. The guidelines acknowledge that there is no research reported in the literature to support this recommendation. The recommendation does not take into consideration several issues. The expectation that eschar will be assessed daily is not realistic or practical in most care settings. The wound may appear stable, but the wound has an absence of inflammatory phase. Inflammatory phase may be suppressed for many reasons. Shouldn't the reason for suppressed inflammation be determined before deciding whether to debride the eschar? Functional mobility is a key indicator of risk for pressure ulcers. Eschar on a heel limits the functional activity of the patient who is otherwise able, by limiting weight bearing on the eschar surface for transfers or ambulation. The patient with eschar on the heel cannot wear shoes and requires a special orthosis to remove pressure from the eschar. This precaution would be necessary until the wound heals. Leaving the eschar intact also means that the extent of the soft tissue injury cannot be determined. Wounds with eschar have the potential for healing or for deterioration. For example, documentation in the literature supports the potential for complete ulcer closure of heel wounds with eschar following debridement with hydrotherapy and collagenase.[55] When should the eschar be left intact? When the patient has inadequate circulation or is in a state of health that will fail to support healing, eschar should not be soaked or debrided. For example, wounds and adjacent tissues that look like those in *Color Plate 52* should not be debrided of eschar. If there is no report of vascular studies in the medical record, the physical therapist or nurse would consider performing noninvasive vascular testing or the patient should be referred to a vascular lab; then candidacy for healing would be determined. For candidates, whirlpool is a quick and efficient way to soften eschar on the heels and enhance local tissue perfusion to facilitate debridement. In the case study used to illustrate clinical decision making at the end this chapter, circulatory status was evaluated in a patient with eschar on both heels and found to be adequate for healing. The patient was being positioned up in wheelchair, and significant pressure was being supported on the heels during transfer, creating risk of trauma to tissues already compromised. Whirlpool was used to soften and debride the eschar. As it turned out, the outer eschar concealed two smaller eschar areas, and these two needed to be softened and debrided, revealing deep tissue damage. Once that was accomplished, the wounds were treated by other means to closure. The patient's functional outcome after heels were healed was the ability to do a standing pivot transfer with one person to assist while weight bearing on both feet.

Patients with large amounts of necrotic tissue have a body system impairment of autolytic debridement and phagocytosis, and they need help from an intervention to hasten the process of removing the bioburden from the body. Whirlpool will hasten the softening of necrotic tissue and debridement. Wounds that contain debris, foreign bodies, and slough or that are highly exudative or malodorous and need intensive cleaning would benefit from whirlpool. Wounds of all tissue depths are treated in the whirlpool, but those that are deep, with undermining and tunneling would be at greater risk for transmitting infection into the body. All wounds and surrounding skin should be vigorously rinsed with clean, warm tap water following removal from the whirlpool water to remove deposits of debris and bacteria.

Patients with impaired vascular perfusion of the lower extremities have risk for impairment of healing and undue susceptibility to pressure ulceration. These individuals may be candidates for whirlpool intervention as a prevention strategy because of induced vasodilatation by direct and reflexive stimulation, as well as the enhanced perfusion by gravitational pull in the dependent position. A suggested method of preventive treatment strategy for individuals who have high risk of pressure ulcers or those with intact stage I pressure ulcers includes daily whirlpool at 38–40° C to stimulate peripheral circulation. The improved circulation to the skin encourages skin growth and replacement, which makes the skin more elastic and less susceptible to shearing and pressure.[55,56] Patients with circulatory impairment who have wounds with extensive necrotic tissue to soften for debridement may benefit from this treatment. Vetra and Whittaker[55] found that patients with limited circulation and extensive necrotic tissue who most likely would have had to have amputation of the affected limb received benefit from the enhanced perfusion associated with heating in the whirlpool, combined with enzymatic debridement using collagenase.

In summary, the physical and mechanical effects of whirlpool are:

Benefits

- Mechanical debridement:
  - Soaking and softening of eschar and other necrotic tissue
  - Scrubbing and loosening of necrotic tissue
  - Debriding by mechanical action of turbulence
  - Deodorizing the wound through cleansing
  - Soaking to remove dried dressings
- Removing excess antibacterial creams
- Increasing blood flow and tissue oxygen
- Increasing core body temperature
- Cellular effects:
  - Stimulating cell mitosis

  - Enhancing leukocytic activity
  - Speeding epidermal cell production
  - Bringing antibodies to wound area
- Fighting infection by improved oxygenation of tissue and removal of bacteria and debris
- Reducing pain through mild analgesia

Disadvantages

- Superhydrating and macerating skin
- Changing of skin pH changes skin surface environment
- Increasing risk of skin infection and wound infection
- Changing of mental status and possible dizziness
- Increasing heart and respiratory rates
- Increasing edema in the dependent position
- Shifting fluids away from the body may lead to dehydration and nutrient depletion
- Traumatizing the wound or surrounding tissues by mechanical forces
- Traumatizing the tissues by overheating (burns) of insensate skin or ischemic tissue

Precautions

Historically, wounds of nearly every type are referred for hydrotherapy. Appropriate use versus overuse of whirlpools is an issue. There has been a definite pendulum swing from treating every wound in the whirlpool to avoiding whirlpool entirely or limiting use to only necrotic wounds. Whirlpool benefits for treating some specific wound-related problems (eg, necrosis, thick exudate, circulation) have been described. The benefits and disadvantages must be carefully weighed. Whirlpool treatment can and should be modified to meet the intentions of the therapy. Patients with venous impairment already have more circulation to the area than the venous system can handle. Changing parameters are required if whirlpool is used. For example, if cleansing is the intention, tepid or neutral warmth (92–96° F or 33.5–35.5° C) will cleanse an ulcer in a patient with venous disease. Minimize the time in the dependent position (eg, treat for 5 minutes, not 20 minutes). Follow with a warm water rinse, then apply compression therapy.[57] If the wounded limb is edematous or has friable skin around the wound and should not be immersed, perfusion can be enhanced by reflexive vasodilatation through immersion of the opposite lower extremity or an upper extremity.

Additional precautions should be considered to avoid potentially harmful effects when the following wound situations are present:

- Clean, granulating wounds: Clean, granulating wounds are easily traumatized by the force of mild agitation. Reduce aeration.
- Epithelializing wounds: Migrating epidermal cells may be damaged by even the least force. Shut off aeration.

- New skin grafts: Skin grafts will not tolerate high shearing forces and turbulence. Shut off aeration.
- New tissue flaps: New tissue flaps are very sensitive to shearing forces and vasoconstriction that may occur if the water or air temperature causes chilling. Shut off aeration, use normothermal temperature.
- Nonnecrotic diabetic ulcers: Callus often surrounds diabetic ulcers and will be softened and macerated. Macerated tissue will not tolerate pressure, and the wound will be enlarged. Moisture retention under the callus may become a source of infection.

Contraindications

Contraindications to use of whirlpool include the presence of any of the following:

- Moderate to severe extremity edema
- Lethargy
- Unresponsiveness
- Maceration
- Febrile conditions
- Compromised cardiovascular or pulmonary function
- Acute phlebitis
- Renal failure
- Dry gangrene (evaluate for ischemia)
- Incontinence of urine or feces (if whirlpool will be contaminated)

Patients who are noncandidates for whirlpool therapy are those who are febrile, who have cardiac or ventilatory pump failure or renal failure, who are lethargic, or who have venous system impairment. Even heating a single limb will raise core body temperature, which is already a problem with febrile patients. Local heating will increase cardiac output and respiration rate, and can overload the cardiopulmonary system and renal system in those with impaired function.[5,34]

Patients with fetal posture contractures may not be able to be safely positioned in the whirlpool. Diabetics and spinal cord-injured individuals who have insensitivity of the feet may experience burns because of the inability to respond neurologically to thermal changes. Diabetics with callus formation on the plantar surfaces of the feet should *not* be treated in the whirlpool because the integumentary system is impaired, calluses will be softened, and subsequent exposure to pressure from standing on the foot will result in skin breakdown. The break in the skin will become a portal for infection.

Patients with dry gangrene should not have the tissues softened because the dry gangrene is nature's method of walling off the tissues and encapsulating the area. Softening of the tissue will reduce the barrier and allow infectious organisms to enter the body. Autoamputation of necrotic digits usually occurs anyway (see Chapter 8).

Personnel Safety

Universal precautions should, of course, be followed by hydrotherapy personnel. The hydrotherapy personnel are exposed to airborne water vapor. Inhalation or contact dermatitis of water droplets containing bacteria and antiseptic or disinfection products presents health risks. Isolation of the patient with an open wound during treatment in the whirlpool may be beneficial because of aerosolization of infectious organisms and production of respirable droplets from the agitation of the water.[58,59] Staff should also use protective gear. Policies and procedures should be developed for each health care facility to minimize staff exposure.[58] Masks, gowns, and goggles are appropriate attire to use as barriers (see Chapter 26, Figure 26–2).

> **Clinical Wisdom:** *Whirlpool Bathing*
>
> One situation that needs clarification is the common referral of patients with wounds for whirlpool treatment and the expectation that this will serve as the patient's bath. The whirlpool is not a bathing pool or shampoo basin. The water in the tank is dirty with wound exudate and debris. Soap, shampoo, and disinfectants have ingredients that are harmful to wounds and may irritate delicate skin during soaking. For personal hygiene, a shower is preferable because all substances are flushed away from the wound and the skin.

Delivery of Care

The survey of Thomson et al[60] found that, in most burn units (100 units polled), nurses perform hydrotherapy procedures, although there is no consensus on who does it. Shankowsky et al[11] found that, in most of the responding 118 burn units using immersion hydrotherapy, both debridement and rehabilitation/physical therapy treatments were included in a single hydrotherapy session (71.7%) and that hydrotherapy continued throughout the patient's length of stay. According to Medicare guidelines, whirlpool is considered a skilled physical therapy procedure when the patient's condition is complicated by disease processes, such as impaired circulation, areas of desensitization, open wounds (eg, stage III and IV pressure ulcers), or other complications that require the skills, knowledge, and judgment of a physical therapist. Diagnosis or prognosis is not the sole factor in deciding whether the service is skilled or not.[61] Recently, some Medicare contractors have issued specific guidelines for physical therapy skilled services for wound care. The guidelines state that interventions that will increase function using treatment modalities specific to physical therapy require the skills of the physical therapist (eg, treatment of an open wound or burn over a joint while undergoing functional mobility training in the whirlpool). Wound care alone does not require the skills of the physical therapist.[62] There is no consensus on who should deliver the hydrotherapy procedure. Whirlpool has long been considered a physical therapy procedure for patients with burns and wounds. Delivery of hydrotherapy services requires professional skills to select the appropriate method of application of the therapy. As a health care professional licensed in the use of physical agents, the physical therapist would be expected to know the effects of hydrotherapy and thermal agents on the different body systems and the appropriate precautions.

EQUIPMENT

Whirlpool Tanks

Whirlpool tanks are used for immersion of either the full body or extremity and are sized accordingly. Large hydrotherapy tanks are called *Hubbard tanks* and may be used for aquatic exercise, as well as for wound healing. They have either an attached turbine or a built-in turbine, or the turbine may be suspended from the side of a bathtub. The whirlpool is created by a mixture of water and air to create controlled turbulence. The more aeration, the greater will be the turbulence and pressure at the surface of the water.[5] The mixture is adjustable but varies from one piece of equipment to another. Force and directions of the agitation are usually adjustable. The tank may be made of stainless steel, Plexiglas, or tile (Figure 25–2).

Tank Selection

Select a whirlpool tank sized for the wound or body area to be treated. If a patient has multiple wounds, the water should cover those that need soaking, cleansing, or debriding. The full body tank or tub will allow the patient to extend the legs fully and may be more comfortable. If the patient is contracted, select a tank in which the patient can be comfortably positioned. Hydraulic lift chairs and chaises or Hoyer lifts can be used to transfer a patient into the tank if the tank is too high or if the patient is nonambulatory. If the patient is seated on a chair for a leg whirlpool treatment, be sure there is no pressure under the thigh.

PROCEDURE

Frequency and Duration

Frequency of hydrotherapy treatment has been traditionally tied to washing of burn wounds to remove topical creams

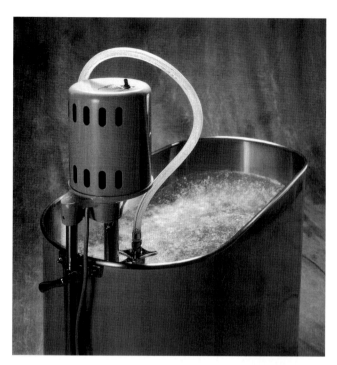

Figure 25–2 Whirlpool tank. Courtesy of Whitehall Manufacturing/Acorn Engineering, City of Industry, California.

used almost universally for patients in burn units. Protocols in burn facilities mandate washing the wound between each application of the topical agent. Soaking is also used to facilitate dressing changes. Topical agents commonly used to treat burns include silver sulfadiazene (Silvadene, Thermazene, SSD), sulfamylon suspension, and silver nitrate used for bactericidal effects. Survey results of burn units[11] show that hydrotherapy treatment is carried out at least daily (56.6%) and bidaily (33.8%). Although the same topical agents are used for other acute or chronic wounds, this is not universally the case. Therefore, the frequency of hydrotherapy treatment to cleanse the wound of topical agents should be modified to correspond to a different rationale of wound management. For instance, once daily 10- to 20-minute treatment for indicated wounds would be preferable in most cases to twice-daily 20-minute whirlpool treatments, which are still common. Once-daily or three-times-weekly whirlpool treatments minimize the frequency of dressing changes and exposure to infection, and maintain the wound temperature and the healing environment. Discontinue treatment when target outcomes are met, if the wound is not responding, or if other treatment options would better meet the needs of the wound and the patient.

Many whirlpool treatments are ordered twice daily. If wound cleansing and debridement are the reasons for selecting this intervention, once-daily treatment followed by application of moisture retentive wound dressings or enzymes would be a good treatment protocol. Prompt wound dressing following the whirlpool/rinse treatment is needed. However, if enhancement of circulation and cellular effects are the reasons, a twice-daily treatment could be desirable. Intermittent heating at normothermia has been demonstrated to increase subcutaneous oxygen tension and presumably reduce infection.[28] Twice-daily treatments to the wound require twice-daily dressing changes and disrupts the wound environment twice. Dressings need to be selected that can safely and cost-effectively be removed that frequently. Wound dressing technology can now provide the healing wound with a scientifically controlled environment of temperature and wound fluid to promote healing. Infrequent dressing changes are now considered the method of choice to promote healing. Reimbursement should also be considered when selecting specialized dressings because they are expected to be left in place longer than gauze. Obviously, the physical therapist, nurse, and physician must collaborate on making a dressing selection that will provide the best wound environment and that is appropriate for twice-daily removal.

Water Temperature

Select water temperature based on the medical condition of the patient and the clinical objective of the treatment. All temperature ranges will soak, soften, and loosen necrotic tissue and cleanse the wound. Keep in mind that the temperature of 37° C is considered optimal for epithelial cell migration, mitotic cell division, and leukocytic activity.[9] Use the temperature closest to the optimal that will be consistent with the medical status of the patient.

Monitoring Vital Signs

Patients who have a medical history of cardiopulmonary or cardiac disease, cerebrovascular accident, or hypertension should have vital signs monitored while in the whirlpool. Record the patient's respiration and pulse rate, and take blood pressure. Observe for change in mental status and report of being lightheaded. The latter is common with immersion of large body areas. The feeling of being lightheaded should go away after the patient sits for 5–10 minutes outside the hydrotherapy area.

Infection Control

Use of Antiseptics

There remains controversy about the use of antiseptic agents in the whirlpool. Most burn facilities use a disinfecting solution for hydrotherapy.[11,60] Bacterial resistance to antiseptics is documented. In addition, antiseptics have limited effectiveness in reducing bacteria when high bacterial counts are measured and are inactivated by organic matter, such as pus and wound exudate.[11,38] Research shows that the most commonly used antiseptic agents are harmful to the cells of tissue repair. AHCPR treatment guidelines for pressure ulcers state that antiseptic agents (eg, povidone-iodine, iododophor, sodium hypochlorite solution (Dakin's solution), hydrogen peroxide, and acetic acid) should not be used to clean ulcers because of their cytotoxicity to fibroblasts.[1,63] No controlled studies document that repeated application of antiseptics to chronic wounds significantly reduces the level of bacteria in wound tissues.[1,63] All commonly used antiseptic agents that are used in the whirlpool have cytotoxicity, even at very low dilutions.[64]

Successful wound healing is detained by bacterial counts greater than 10^5 per gram of tissue. Bacterial counts were reduced to 10^5 or less per gram of tissue within a 3-week test period for 100% of ulcers treated with silver sulfadiazine cream, compared with 78.6% in those treated with saline and 63.6% in those treated with povidone-iodine solution. In addition, the ulcers treated with the silver sulfadiazine cream responded more rapidly to reach these lowered bacterial counts than did either of the others.[65] Chemicals in antiseptics are absorbed through the wound tissue, and some patients develop toxicity or allergic responses to the chemical agents. As described above in the personnel safety section, water vapor dispersed into the atmosphere during the agitation process contains droplets of the antiseptic and are inhaled by both patients and staff.

Although an antiseptic's use in the whirlpool is not encouraged, there are times when they should be used, such as for necrotic, heavily exudating wounds. Sodium hypochlorite solutions dissolve blood clots and may be useful in solubilizing the clotted material that constitutes a considerable portion of necrotic tissue but, as a consequence, delayed clotting may occur, and the wound exudate will become sanguineous. There are times when antibiotic-resistant organisms, such as *P. aeruginosa*, are found in a wound, and wound decontamination is required. A hydrotherapy burn unit tested different concentrations of chloramine-T (Chlorazene) to determine its affect on Gram-negative organisms.[66] Chloramine-T is an aqueous hypochlorite with a molecular structure that allows for slower release of free chlorine into the water, and this increases the bactericidal effects for a longer time.[67] Findings included negative cultures from patients and from the equipment after a 5-day treatment regimen using chloramine-T at a concentration of 200 parts per million (ppm). Patients' wounds, surrounding tissues, and staff reactions to the chloramine-T additive were carefully monitored, and no adverse side effects were found. Tank decontamination was achieved by running the turbine in the tank with the same solution after the treatment of the patients. This reduced staff cleaning and disinfection time.

There has been heightened awareness of cytotoxicity to the cells of wound repair from antiseptics. Guinea pigs with an induced full-thickness wound were inoculated with *P. aeruginosa* to study the effects of chloramine-T on wound healing and wound decontamination.[68] One group of animals was immersed in tap water and the other set in water containing 300 ppm of chloramine-T solution at 36° C for 20 minutes. Results showed that, within 8–10 minutes of exposure to the chloramine-T solution, all microorganisms were killed. After immersion of the infected wounds in tap water on days 6–7 after wounding, there were a number of colony-forming units cultured from the water. There was no evidence of skin irritation in the chloramine-T group. Rates of wound healing of the full-thickness inoculated skin wounds were comparable in both the tap water and chloramine-T groups. After the 5 days, a wound culture, or clinical signs that show significant wound decontamination, the treatment should be changed to clear water, followed by vigorous rinse to rid the tissues of deposits of debris and bacteria. Longer use of the antiseptic agent may retard the healing process, due to the cytotoxic effects on the cells of repair. Also consider other methods of wound decontamination, such as ultraviolet light (described in Chapter 23) or electrical stimulation (described in Chapter 21). Appendix A and Chapter 11 have additional information on the use of antiseptics, their actions, indications, precautions, directions for use, packaging, and the effect on wound healing.

Be sure that the intention for using the antiseptic is clear, monitor carefully, and stop when the desired outcome is met (eg, the wound is exudate free or necrosis free). Use at low concentrations. Some commonly used antiseptics in the whirlpool are as follows:

- povidone-iodine
- sodium hypochlorite
- chlorhexidine gluconate (Hibiclens)
- chloramine-T (Chlorazene)

Clinical Wisdom

Chloramine-T could be put into the water at the manufacturer-recommended dilutions and agitated for 10 minutes *following* removal of the wound to disinfect the tank. Then the tank can be emptied, scrubbed with a disinfectant, and refilled with fresh water.[5]

Use of Tap Water

Questions arise about the safety and efficacy of using plain tap water for wound cleansing and decontamination. A comparison study on 705 wounds looked at infection rates following wound cleansing with tap water and saline. It was found that less infection occurred in wounds cleaned with tap water than with saline, and no bacteria were transferred to the wounds.[38] A comparison of normal saline and clean tap water wound irrigation used to remove bacteria from simple skin lacerations showed that both substances were comparable in reduction of bacterial counts.[69] Monitoring of local water supply for organisms has been useful in controlling nosocomial infection.[11]

Vigorous Rinsing

When a body or extremity is removed from the whirlpool, a layer of residue remains on the surfaces exposed to the water, just like the bathtub ring residue after a tub bath. This residue has many contaminants associated with it. A proven, safe method to reduce bacterial count is to follow whirlpool treatment with vigorous rinsing of the patient's skin and wound tissue with clean, warm water to remove the residue. A shower may be the best method to cleanse a large body surface.

Aftercare

After the patient is removed from the whirlpool and rinsed with warm water, the wound should be debrided of any softened and loosened necrotic tissue, then rinsed again with warm tap water to remove loosened debris. After the final warm water rinse, the wound should be protected from cooling, contaminants, and desiccation. The best approach would be for the wound to be dressed immediately in the hydrotherapy area. If the setting does not allow for a complete dressing application while the patient is in hydrotherapy, a protective moist dressing, such as warm, saline-soaked gauze, should be placed in the wound and covered with a secondary dry dressing.

Infection Control for Whirlpool Equipment

The Centers for Disease Control and Prevention and the American Physical Therapy Association (APTA) reviewed procedures for infection control in hydrotherapy and prepared a guide that is available through the APTA.[70] The procedures described are adapted from the APTA guide. A copy of the guide would be valuable to all hydrotherapy departments.

Patients using whirlpools and other hydrotherapy tanks are often referred because of active infections. The infectious organisms and the organic debris are then deposited into the water. In the warm water, steady temperature and agitation make it easy for bacterial pathogens to become harbored in the hydrotherapy equipment water pipes, drains, and other steel components associated with the device. These regions are difficult to clean and to disinfect or sterilize. In addition, the *Pseudomonas* bacteria has the ability to assume a sessile form, secreting a thick protective glycocalyx that colonizes the components described.[11] This increases the likelihood that highly contaminated water will contact the sites of open wounds, Foley catheters, and other percutaneous devices. Besides the whirlpool tank and attached equipment, other equipment commonly used in the hydrotherapy department, such as Hoyer lifts, wheelchairs, and other transfer equipment, should be considered to be potential sources for colonization and transfer of infectious organisms.[70]

Procedure for Basic Cleaning of Hydrotherapy Equipment

1. Hydrotherapy equipment must be thoroughly cleansed to remove all foreign and organic materials from the object. Cleansing by vigorous manual scrubbing with detergents should precede disinfection procedures. The scrubbing should include the inside tank surfaces, the overflow pipes, the drains, the turbine shaft, and the thermometer shaft. The product chosen for cleaning should be an Environmental Protection Agency (EPA)-registered disinfectant.
2. Because the cleaning procedures often involve actions that may cause splattering, the cleaner should wear gloves and goggles while cleaning. Follow universal precautions.
3. Drain the hydrotherapy tank after each use.
4. Rinse all inside tank surfaces with clean water.

Procedure for Disinfection of Hydrotherapy Equipment

1. An intermediate level of disinfection is recommended for all hydrotherapy equipment after treatment of patients with open wounds. Be sure that the exposure time to the disinfectant at label-recommended dilutions is equal to or not less than 10 minutes. Check with the housekeeping department for different choices of disinfection products that are in this category.
2. After the cleansing and rinsing of the tank, the disinfection process can precede. Fill the tank with hot water, then add the disinfection product at the recommended dilutions. Expose all inside tank surfaces.
3. The agitator needs to be disinfected also, which may be done separately by immersing it in a bucket with a solution of the disinfectant and running the agitator in the solution for 10 minutes.
4. Following disinfection, drain and rinse the tank.
5. *Dry* inside the tank with clean towels and keep the tank dry and covered until it is used again.
6. Wipe all related hydrotherapy equipment surfaces with germicide after *each use*.[70]

Disinfection Products. A great variety of disinfection products are on the market, and each formulation must be EPA-registered. These disinfectants are not interchangeable and should be reviewed for the varying performance characteristics of each.

Cleaning and Disinfection of Whirlpools with a Built-in Turbine Agitator. The procedure for cleaning and disinfection of whirlpools with built-in turbines/agitators differs slightly from the above procedures. The manufacturers of these whirlpools have specific instructions for spraying the internal turbine with a disinfecting solution. This disinfecting solution would need to remain in contact with the turbine for the time required, based on the product used. In all other respects, the cleaning procedure would be the same as that for other whirlpool tanks.

Culturing the Whirlpool and Related Equipment

Culturing is a controversial topic in the hydrotherapy area. One rationale for culturing is to prevent infection. To contribute to the prevention of infection, the results must be interpretable. The best definition of *interpretable* is that certain results lead to specific actions.[70] One school of thought is that, if the best methods of disinfection are already accepted procedures, routine culturing of whirlpool and associated equipment is not going to cause a change in procedure and, therefore, is superfluous. On the other hand, there are reports that careful monitoring of equipment and the water supply to identify potential sources of bacteria is useful in preventing outbreaks.[11]

EXPECTED OUTCOMES

Prognosis for wounds treated by whirlpool is a change in tissue function in 2–4 weeks. Expect a wound treated for exudate and odor to be odor and exudate free in 2 weeks. Wounds that are treated for debridement should be necrosis free in 2–4 weeks, depending on volume of necrotic tissue present. Wounds that have a wound healing phase diagnosis of chronic inflammatory phase or absence of inflammatory phase should progress toward a wound healing phase of *acute inflammatory phase* in 2 weeks and to a wound acute proliferative healing phase in 4–5 weeks. The signs and symptoms of acute inflammation would include hyperemia, increased temperature of the skin, and mild edema, followed by a decrease in temperature by the end of the inflammatory phase and return to skin color to that of adjacent skin or comparable area on the opposite side of the body, progressing to a granulating, contracting wound in the proliferative phase, as seen in *Color Plates 1* and *2*. The reported mean weekly healing rate from four studies where whirlpool was used is 9.5% per week.[48,49,54,71] Burke et al[46] reported a 0.39 cm/week reduction in size but did not state the size of wounds; they also reported a 37.5% deterioration in the whirlpool group, with an overall outcome of healing for the treatment group and a 28% improvement and 61% deterioration in the nonwhirlpool group.[46] Payer data from 1989 showed that wounds treated with whirlpool were usually treated for 3 months, with presumed outcome of a clean wound.[72] Wounds treated with other physical therapy technologies and advanced therapies have average lengths of treatment that range from 7.5 to 10.5 weeks, with closure as the reported outcome (see Chapters 12, 21, 22, 24). To be competitive, treatment with whirlpool must have comparable outcomes. If the wound is not progressing on the trajectory of healing, another intervention should be considered (see Table 25–1).

SELF-CARE TEACHING GUIDELINES

After completing the diagnostic process, the physical therapist may determine that hydrotherapy can be performed at home with a portable whirlpool unit attached to a bathtub. Grossly necrotic or purulent wounds are probably best not self-treated until the necrosis and purulence are reduced to a level where the patient and/or caregiver can manage them comfortably. Careful selection of the patient and caregiver must be made to have successful, noninjuring treatment results. The ability to understand and follow directions is critical. Bathtub cleansing and disinfection of the portable whirlpool is extremely important to avoid infection and sepsis.

Clinical Wisdom

Instruct patients and caregivers to turn the home hot water heater down to 120° F and always to use a thermometer to test the water temperature before immersion to avoid burn injury.

- The patient and/or caregiver should be instructed in the correct water temperature, the duration of the immersion, how to rinse the wound after immersion, and the proper aftercare. A thermometer to take the water temperature should be used for safety to prevent burns. Some people believe that the water must be as hot as tolerable to be beneficial, and scald burns are common—especially in the elderly. Proper cleaning and disinfection procedures also must be taught for the tub and the portable agitator and thermometer.

- Patients with neuropathy should be instructed *never* to do home foot soaks or whirlpool because of the high risk of self-inflicted injury.
- Patients who are lethargic should have minimal soaking in tepid water, primarily for cleansing and softening of tissue, and this should be limited to single limb immersion. Instruct all patients and caregivers to monitor vital signs during the whirlpool treatment. Teach the side effects of the treatment and how to respond to symptoms such as lightheadedness, dizziness, or lethargy.
- Explain the desired effects of the treatment and any symptoms that are undesirable. If the patient is being seen through a home care agency, a demonstration and return demonstration in the home, including repetition of instructions, is essential to ensure the correct care delivery. If this is not possible, perhaps a mock setup can be simulated in the hospital or clinic.
- Accountability is essential and encourages compliance. Set up a regular reporting schedule. A tracing of the wound by the therapist can be left with the patient, then laid over the wound for the patient or caregiver to compare changes in size and shape. It will also help to reinforce compliance with the treatment regimen. The changes can be reported to the physical therapist by phone with periodic visits to monitor outcomes.

REVIEW QUESTIONS

1. What are three benefits of using whirlpool hydrotherapy?
2. How can temperature be used to modify therapeutic results?
3. How can risks of infection be mitigated?
4. What are the negative effects of using whirlpool hydrotherapy?
5. A patient has a neuropathic plantar ulcer over the fifth metatarsal head. Wound has callus of periwound tissue, granulation tissue in the wound bed with moist environment. There is no necrotic tissue or signs of reepithelialization or infection. Ankle-brachial index is 1.0. Is this patient a candidate for whirlpool?
6. A patient has chronic venous insufficiency with ulceration of the left tibia area proximal and superior to the medial malleolus. Wound originated following trauma. There is edema present and a grade II ulceration. There is minimal to no exudate, 100% granulation, no epithelialization, and no signs of infection. Ankle/brachial index is 1.0. Is this patient a candidate for whirlpool?

Case Study: Patient with Eschar on Both Heels

Functional Outcome Report

Patient Name: G.W.   **Start of Care Date:** 9/27

Medical History

84-yr-old, alert, confused black female. Nonambulatory resident of long-term care facility. Sits up in wheelchair and attends activity program. Medical diagnosis of Alzheimer's disease, prior history of cerebrovascular accident (CVA). No prior history of pressure ulceration.

Reason for Referral

1. Dry, leathery eschar on both heels not responding to treatment with occlusive dressings. Indicates loss of healing capacity.
2. Need to determine severity of pressure ulcers on the heels.
3. Severely limited mobility and activity levels.

Systems Review and Exam

Circulatory System

Circulatory perfusion adequate for healing indicated by palpable pulses, warm feet, no significant leg edema, and ankle-brachial index (ABI) of 0.8, but produces inadequate response to wounding due to motor and joint impairment of lower extremities (loss of muscle pump function for circulation).

Musculoskeletal System

Musculoskeletal impairments of the lower extremities due to weakness, joint pain, and stiffness with contractures (10º) at the knees. Patient being positioned upright in wheelchair. Requires minimum assist to perform pivot transfer from bed to wheelchair. Weightbearing during transfer places stress on eschars. Unable to retain upright posture to ambulate and unable to reposition in wheelchair or bed for pressure relief. Braden risk assessment scores each for activity and for mobility 2/4.

Neuromuscular System

Loss of volitional movements due to impaired neuromotor system. Loss of cognitive awareness of position. Loss of protective sensation to reposition (sensory impairment).

Cardiopulmonary System

No clinical signs of cardiopulmonary impairment. Probable diminished oxygenation due to inactive mobility status.

Integumentary System

Adjacent and surrounding skin has normal skin color tones and turgor, compared to adjacent areas. No pain responses in wounded tissues.

Wound Healing Tissue Assessment: Bilateral heels crusted with hard dry eschar; impairment of integumentary integrity. No thermal changes at the margins of the eschars compared to adjacent tissues. No edema or erythema (color changes) signifies impairment of inflammation response. Unable to see the tissue status under the eschar; unable to determine extent/severity of tissue loss.

Size: 25 cm^2 area of eschar on each heel.

Psychosocial

Patient unable to understand directions to reposition or exercise independently. Will follow guided movements. Needs caregiver intervention for repositioning, exercise, and transfers.

Functional Impairments and Functional Diagnosis

Loss of function in above systems causes the following:

1. Wound Severity Diagnosis unable to stage: impaired integumentary integrity associated with eschar on both heels. Removal of eschar needed to determine extent of wound depth.
2. Wound Healing Phase Diagnosis: absence of inflammatory phase and absence of proliferative phase. Needs restart of the inflammatory phase of healing after conversion to a clean wound that will progress through phases of healing.
3. Associated impairment of mobility and activity secondary to neuromuscular disability (Alzheimer's disease and CVA).
4. Undue susceptibility to pressure ulceration on the feet due to motor and sensory impairment.
5. Low blood flow state but has adequate circulation to predict healing.

Short-Term Target Outcomes:		**Due Date**
Wounds:	Softening of eschar	3 days
	Debridement of eschar	7 days
	Shows evidence of inflammatory phase	14 days
	Shows evidence of proliferative phase	28 days

continues

Case Study continued

Mobility:　Nursing assistant will
　　　　　　perform range of motion
　　　　　　and guided exercise　　3 days
　　　　　　Therapeutic positioning in
　　　　　　bed and wheelchair will
　　　　　　be performed by nursing
　　　　　　assistants all shifts　　7 days
　　　　　　Transfers with multipodus-
　　　　　　type splint　　　　　　5 days

Prognosis: A clean stable wound with potential for closure in　28 days. Undue susceptibility to pressure ulcers on the feet due to impaired mobility and cognition will continue after wounds are healed. Wound closure in 90 days both heels.

Plan of Care with Rationale for Skilled Services

1. Multiple debridement methods required to hasten progression to clean wound bed

   Procedures:
   • Score eschar—to allow penetration of moisture
   • Whirlpool to soak and soften tissue, enhance circulation daily
   • Sharp debridement—incremental as tissue softens and loosens PRN
   • Electrical stimulation—enhance microcirculation and stimulate cells leading to progression through phases of healing daily
   • Enzymatic debridement daily—to hasten solubilization of necrotic tissues
   • Autolysis with transparent film—to maintain moist wound environment to soften eschar

2. Therapeutic positioning to reduce risk of pressure and shearing to feet during transfers, in wheelchair, and in bed

3. Instruction of nurses' aides in range of motion and exercises to stimulate delivery of circulation to the tissues

4. Therapeutic exercise performed while in the whirlpool

5. Fitting of multipodus-type splint

Target Outcomes Achieved at First Reassessment 10/1

Wound status:
1. Eschar softened, partially debrided by day 4
2. Removal of outer eschar revealed two focal areas of necrosis covered by eschar
3. Wound has evidence of inflammatory phase: edema, increased warmth in surrounding tissues

Mobility:
1. Patient lying on pressure relief support surface with pillows and multipodus splint to relieve pressure
2. Patient sitting up in wheelchair with feet supported with multipodus-type splint to relieve pressure during transfers
3. Range of motion and guided exercises by nurses' aide performed daily
4. Guided lower extremity exercise performed in the whirlpool

Reassessment 11/9

Wound status:
1. Eschar free, yellow slough
2. Wound depth greater than 0.2 cm
3. Two interconnecting wounds (medial and lateral sides of heel with viable tissue connecting)
4. Wound healing phase progressed to proliferation phase—presence of contraction and granulation tissue

Mobility:
1. Patient is participating in daily exercise and range of motion regimen
2. Therapeutic positioning is in place for all shifts

Functional Impairments

1. Integumentary impairment secondary to full-thickness pressure ulcer on the heels.
   Target outcome: clean proliferating and contracting wound—due date 21 days.
2. Absence of epithelialization phase and sustained contraction
   Target outcome: Progress to epithelialization phase and sustained contraction—due date 21 days.

Revised Prognosis

Wound will heal to closure in 60 days.

Revised Treatment Plan and Target Outcomes

Need for Continuation of Skilled Services

Patient failed to respond to routine dressing and conservative management, is now responding to the treatment program. Treatment is done as a collaborative effort between the physical therapist and nurse. Change in treatment interventions required due to change in wound status. Patient has demonstrated potential for healing

continues

Case Study continued

following interventions but will continue to be at risk for pressure ulceration.

Plan of Care (Intervention) with Rationale

- Discontinue whirlpool and sharp debridement tissue—neither needed to debride slough
- Continue electrical stimulation for microcirculation and stimulation of healing
- Discontinue enzymatic debridement—not needed to debride slough
- Change dressing to hydrogel and secondary dressing—to debride slough, for moist wound healing

environment compatible with ES treatment regimen

Target Outcomes:
Clean wound bed	7 days

Proliferative phase: sustained contraction	14 days
Progress to epithelialization phase	21 days

Discharge Outcome

Wounds on both heels healed in 90 days from start of care.

Source: Functional Outcome Reporting System methodology used with permission of Swanson and Co., Long Beach, CA.

REFERENCES

1. Bergstrom N, Bennett MA, Carlson C, et al. *Treatment of Pressure Ulcers.* Clinical Practice Guideline No. 15. Rockville, MD: Agency for Health Care Research and Quality (AHRQ), formerly known as the Agency for Health Care Policy and Research (AHCPR), U.S. Public Health Service (PHS), U.S. Department of Health and Human Services (DHHS); AHRQ Publication No. 95-0652. December 1994:45–65.

2. Feedar JA, Kloth LC. Conservative management of chronic wounds. In: Kloth LC, McCulloch JM, Feedar JA, eds. *Wound Healing: Alternatives in Management.* Philadelphia: FA Davis; 1990:135–172.

3. Rodeheaver GT, Smith SL, Thacker JG, Edgerton MT, Edlich RF. Mechanical cleansing of contaminated wounds with a surfactant. *Am J Surg.* 1975;129(3):241–245.

4. Conolly WB, et al. Influence of distant trauma on local wound infection. *Surg Gynecol Obstet.* 1969;128(4):713–717.

5. Walsh M. Hydrotherapy: the use of water as a therapeutic agent. In: Michlovitz S, ed. *Thermal Agents in Rehabilitation.* Philadelphia: FA Davis; 1990:109–132.

6. Highsmith AK, Kaylor BM, Calhoun MT. Microbiology of therapeutic water. *Clinical Management.* 1991;11(1):34–37.

7. Shimizu T, Kosaka M, Fujishima K. Human thermoregulatory responses during prolonged walking in water at 25, 30 and 35 degrees C. *Eur J Appl Physiol Occup Physiol.* 1998;78(6):473–478.

8. Lopez M, et al. Rate and gender dependence of the sweating, vasoconstriction and shivering thresholds in humans. *Anesthesiol.* 1994;80(4):780–788.

9. Solomon SL. Host factors in whirlpool-associated *Pseudomonas aeruginosa* skin disease. *Infect Control.* 1985;6:402–406.

10. Jacobson JA. Pool-associated *Pseudomonas aeruginosa* dermatitis and other bathing-associated infections. *Infect Control.* 1985;6:398–401.

11. Shankowsky HA, Callioux LS, Tredget EE. North American survey of hydrotherapy in modern burn care. *J Burn Care Rehabil.* 1994;15:143–146.

12. Neiderhuber SS, Stribley RF, Koepke GH. Reduction of skin bacterial load with use of the therapeutic whirlpool. *Phys Ther.* 1975;5(5):482–486.

13. Bohannon R. Whirlpool versus whirlpool and rinse for removal of bacteria from a venous stasis ulcer. *Phys Ther.* 1982;62:304–308.

14. Swanson G. *Hydrotherapy Use in Standard Physical Therapist Practice Project.* Presented at class, University of Southern California, BKN 599. Los Angeles, CA; July 1997.

15. Cardany CR, Rodeheaver GT, Horowitz JH. Influence of hydrotherapy and antiseptic agents on burn wound bacterial contamination. *J Burn Care Rehabil.* 1985;6:230–232.

16. Stanwood W, Pinzur M. Risk of contamination of the wound in a hydrotherapeutic tank. *Foot Ankle Int.* 1998;19(3):173–176.

17. Hollyoak V, Boyd P, Freeman R. Whirlpool baths in nursing homes: Use, maintenance and contamination with *Pseudomonas aeruginosa*. *Burn.* 1995;5(7):R102–R104.

18. Sessler DI. Mild perioperative hypothermia. *New Engl J Med.* 1997;336(24):1730–1736.

19. Kurz A, Sessler DI, Lenhart R. Perioperative normothermia to reduce the incidence of surgical-wound infection and shorten hospitalization. *New Engl J Med.* 1996;334(19):1209–1215.

20. Reed RL 2d, et al. Hypothermia and blood coagulation: Dissociation between enzyme activity and clotting factor levels. *Circ Shock.* 1990;32(2):141–152.

21. Valeri CR, et al. Effect of skin temperature on platelet function in patients undergoing extracorporeal bypass. *J Thoracic Cardiovasc Surg.* 1992;104(1):108–116.

22. Michaelson AD, et al. Reversible inhibition of human platelet activation by hypothermia in vivo and in vitro. *Thromb Haemost.* 1994;71(5):633–640.

23. Lenhart R, et al. Relative contribution of skin and core temperatures to vasoconstriction and shivering thresholds during isoflurane anesthesia. *Anesthesiol.* 1999;91(2):422–429.

24. Abramson D, et al. Changes in blood flow, oxygen uptake and tissue temperatures produced by the topical application of wet heat. *Arch Phys Med Rehabil.* 1961;42:305–317.

25. Wessman HC, Kottke FJ. The effect of indirect heating on peripheral blood flow, pulse rate, blood pressure and temperature. *Arch Phys Med Rehabil.* 1967;48:567–576.

26. Rabkin JM, Hunt TK. Local heat increases blood flow and oxygen tension in wounds. *Arch Surg* 1987;122:221–225.

27. Hopf H. *The Role of Warming and Oxygen Tension in Wounds.* Symposium on thermoregulation in wound care. Oxford, England: 1999.

28. Ikeda T, et al. Local radiant heating increase subcutaneous oxygen tension. *Am J Surg.* 1998;175:33–37.

29. Ikeda T, et al. The effect of three different local temperatures on subcutaneous oxygen tension. *Anesthesiol Analg.* 1997;84(2S).

30. Juve MB. Whirlpool therapy on postoperative pain and surgical wound healing: An exploration. *Patient Educ Couns.* 1998;33(1):39–48.

31. Kurz A, et al. Thermoregulatory response thresholds during spinal anesthesia. *Anesthesiol Analg.* 1993;77(4):721–726.

32. Hwang J, Himel H, Edlich R. Bilateral amputations following hydrotherapy tank burns in a paraplegic patient. *Burns.* 1995;21(1):70–71.

33. McCulloch JM, Boyd VB. The effects of whirlpool and the dependent position on lower extremity volume. *J Orthop Sports Phys Ther.* 1992;16:169.

34. Guyton AC, ed. *Textbook of Medical Physiology.* 6th ed. Philadelphia: WB Saunders; 1981.

35. Alon G. *Antibiotics Enhancement by Transcutaneous Electrical Stimulation.* Presented at the Future Directions in Wound Healing Symposium; American Physical Therapy Association Scientific Meeting; June 1997.

36. Lock PM. The effect of temperature on mitosis at the edge of experimental wounds. In: Lundgren A, Soner AB, eds. *Symposia on Wound Healing: Plastic, Surgical and Dermatologic Aspects.* Sweden: Molndal; 1980:103–107.

37. Myers JA. Wound healing and the use of modern surgical dressing. *Pharm J.* 1982;229(6186):103–104.

38. Miller M, Dyson M. *Principles of Wound Care.* London: Macmillan Magazines Ltd; 1996:29–36.

39. Yang Q, Berghe D. Effect of temperature on in vitro proliferative activity of human umbilical vein endothelial cells. *Experientia.* 1995;51(2):126–132.

40. Xia Z, et al. Stimulation of fibroblast growth in vitro by intermittent radiant warming. *Wound Repair Regen.* 2000;8(2):138–144.

41. Park H-Y, Shon K, Phillips T. The effect of heat on inhibitory effects of chronic wound fluid on fibroblasts in vitro. *Wounds.* 1998;10(6):189–192.

42. Rush J, et al. The effects of whirlpool baths in labor: A randomized controlled trial. *Birth.* 1996;23(3):136–143.

43. Lenstrup C, et al. Warm tub bath during delivery. *Acta Obstet Gynecol Scand.* 1987;66(8):709–712.

44. Kloth LC, et al. Effects of normothermic dressing on pressure ulcer healing. *Adv Wound Care.* 2000;13(2):69–74.

45. Sussman C. The role of physical therapy in wound care. In: Krasner D, ed. *Chronic Wound Care: A Sourcebook for Health Care Professionals.* Wayne, PA: Health Management Publications; 1990:327–366.

46. Burke DT, et al. Effects of hydrotherapy on pressure ulcer healing. *Am J Phys Med Rehabil.* 1998;77(5):394–398.

47. Gogia PP, Hurt BS, Zirn TT. Wound management with whirlpool and infrared cold laser. *Phys Ther.* 1988;68(8):1239–1242.

48. Gogia P, Marquez R, Minerbo G. Effects of high voltage galvanic stimulation on wound healing. *Ostomy/Wound Manage.* 1992;38(1):29–35.

49. Gault W, Gatens PF. Use of low intensity direct current in management of ischemic skin ulcers. *Phys Ther.* 1976;56(3):141:145.

50. Akers T, Gabrielson A. The effect of high voltage galvanic stimulation on the rate of healing of decubitus ulcers. *Biomed Sci Instrum J.* 1984;20:99–100.

51. Thurman B, Christian E. Response of a serious circulatory lesion to electrical stimulation. *Phys Ther.* 1971;51(10):137–140.

52. Carley PJ, Wainapel S. Electrotherapy of acceleration of wound healing: low intensity direct current. *Arch Phys Med Rehabil.* 1985;66:443–446.

53. Wood JM, Evans PE III, Schallreuter KU, Jacobson WE, Sufit R. Newman J, et al. A multicenter study on the use of pulsed low intensity direct current for healing chronic Stage II and Stage III ulcers. *Arch Dermatol.* 1993;130(5):660–661.

54. Haynes L, et al. Comparison of Pulsavac and sterile whirlpool regarding the promotion of tissue granulation (abstract). *Phys Ther.* 1994;74(Suppl):S4.

55. Vetra H, Whittaker D. Hydrotherapy and topical collagenase for decubitus ulcers. *Geriatrics.* 1975;30:53–58.

56. Novotne J. Efficient bathing systems benefit patients and care givers. *DON.* July 1987:28–30.

57. McCulloch J. *Physical Modalities in Wound Management.* Preconference course. Presented at the Symposium on Advanced Wound Care; April 1995; San Diego, CA.

58. Baron R, Willeke K. Respirable droplets from whirlpools: Measurement of size, distribution and estimation of disease potential. *Environ Res.* 1986;39:8–18.

59. Loehne HB, et al. *Aerosolization of Microorganisms during Pulsatile Lavage with Suction.* In Combined Sections Meeting, American Physical Therapy Association; 2000; New Orleans, LA: APTA.

60. Thomson PD, Bowden ML, McDonald DK, Smith DJ Jr, Prasad JK. A survey of burn hydrotherapy in the United States. *J Burn Care Rehabil.* 1990;11(2):151–155.

61. Health Care Financing Administration. Coverage of Services, 3132.4. Woodlawn, MD: December 1987.

62. Blue Cross of North Carolina. Medicare Bulletin Number 98-9. December 1996, Part A Office, Durham, NC: 2–3.

63. Lineaweaver W, Howard R, Soucy D, et al. Topical antimicrobial toxicity. *Arch Surg.* 1985;120:267–270.

64. Kozol MD. Effects of sodium hypochlorite on cells of the wound module. *Arch Surg.* 1988;123:420–423.

65. Kucan JO, Robson MC, Heggers JP, Ko F. Comparison of silver sulfadiazine, povidone-iodine and physiologic saline in the treatment of chronic pressure ulcers. *J Am Geriatr Soc.* 1981;29:232–235.

66. Steve L, Goodhart P, Alexander J. Hydrotherapy burn treatment: Use of chloramine-T against resistant microorganisms. *Arch Phys Med Rehabil.* 1979;60:301–303.

67. Marquez RR. Wound debridement and hydrotherapy. In: Gogia P, ed. *Clinical Wound Management.* Thorofare, NJ: Slack; 1995:122–126.

68. Henderson JD, Leming JT, Melon-Niksa DB. Chloramine-T solutions: Effect on wound healing in guinea pigs. *Arch Phys Med Rehabil.* 1989;70(8):628–631.

69. Moscati R, et al. Comparison of normal saline with tap water for wound irrigation. *Am J Emerg Med.* 1998;16(4):379–381.

70. American Physical Therapy Association. *Hydrotherapy/Therapeutic Pool Infection Control Guidelines.* Alexandria, VA: American Physical Therapy Association; 1995:8–11.

71. Carley PJ, Wainapel S. Electrotherapy of acceleration of wound healing: Low intensity direct current. *Arch Phys Med Rehabil.* 1985;66:443–446.

72. Swanson G. Use of cost data, provider experience, and clinical guidelines in the transition to managed care. *J Insurance Med.* 1991;23(1):70–74.

CHAPTER 26

Pulsatile Lavage with Suction

Harriett Baugh Loehne

CHAPTER OBJECTIVES

At the completion of this chapter, the reader will be able to:

1. Know the indications and precautions of treatment with pulsatile lavage with suction
2. Know the benefits and outcomes expected with pulsatile lavage with suction
3. Be aware of Occupational Safety and Health Administration guidelines and infection control issues
4. Know policies and procedures for treatment with pulsatile lavage with suction
5. Be familiar with the features of the products made by the three different manufacturers of pulsatile lavage with suction equipment.

DEFINITION

Pulsatile lavage with suction (PLWS) is a method of wound care that provides cleansing and debridement with pulsed irrigation combined with suction. Therefore, it provides negative pressure to remove the irrigant and debris to help reduce infection and to enhance granulation. This ultimately provides an improved foundation for wound healing.

Both console and battery-powered units are available, along with a selection of tips for cleansing and debridement of different wound configurations. Physicians have used these systems in the operating room since the early 1980s for irrigation in surgical procedures and to clean wounds of debris. Physical therapists (PTs) have used the systems since the late 1980s for irrigation and debridement to enhance healing of soft tissue wounds.

THEORY AND SCIENCE OF THE THERAPY

Whirlpools traditionally have been the most common choice for hydrotherapy, with jet lavage and bulb syringes also being used. Just as with whirlpool, there is limited research to support the use of PLWS for wound healing. There are numerous anecdotal reports and case studies of benefits.[1,2]

Haynes et al[1] reported that the rate of granulation tissue formation was 12.2% per week for wounds treated with PLWS and 4.8% per week for those treated with whirlpool. This study included six subjects as a control, using sterile whirlpool at one hospital, and seven subjects as an experimental group, using the Pulsavac (Zimmer Patient Care Division, Dover, Ohio) at another hospital. Photographs taken at initial evaluations and at discharge were entered into a computer for calculation of wound area and rate of wound closure. Data analysis used analysis of covariance. The increase in mean wound closure rate for all patients treated with whirlpool was 766.139 mm^2 per length of stay and for those treated with Pulsavac was 3373.690 mm^2. With the rate of wound closure significantly higher for those treated with Pulsavac versus sterile whirlpool, the authors state that PTs should consider that Pulsavac can decrease the healing time for a wound, as well as the time required for the patient to be in the hospital for treatment of the wound. The study concludes that, although there were many factors—both physiologically and environmentally—that could affect the rate of wound closure, the research suggested that treatment with PLWS promoted wound closure at a faster rate than did sterile whirlpool.

Other scientific and theoretic rationales for use of the therapy are as follows:

- It cleanses via gentle pulsatile lavage to stronger irrigation and debridement.
- It reduces bacteria and infection.
- It promotes granulation and epithelialization.
- Theory: The negative pressure of the suction stimulates granulation of clean wounds.

Management of Infection

Wound infection is a major concern in management of wounds. Dead and dying tissue, debris, clotted blood, and foreign bodies are predisposing conditions to wound infection. Rapid removal of these contaminants has been demonstrated to speed healing. Studies in the literature report that high-pressure pulsating irrigation decreases the presence of these contaminants and results in a lower incidence of wound infection.

Debridement and irrigation are important methods for controlling infection in wounds. Different methods are described for irrigation of wounds, including bulb syringe, Water Pik, shower spray, spray bottles, and pulsatile irrigation/lavage. Irrigation pressures vary with use of these different devices. If the impact pressure is too low, below 4 pounds per square inch (psi), the lavage will not cleanse effectively. Safe, effective irrigation pressures range from 4 to 15 psi. Exhibit 26–1 indicates the irrigation pressures obtained with these commonly used clinical devices.[3(p52)] A pressure of 8 psi has been found to be significantly effective in removing bacteria and infection.[4] Irrigation at 13 psi has been attributed to reduction of inflammation in traumatic wounds. Irrigation pressures exceeding 15 psi may traumatize tissue and drive bacteria into the wound tissues.[5,6] Stevenson et al[4] reportedly calculated and tested combinations of syringe and needle sizes to determine wound irrigating pressure. The pressure produced by a 35-mL syringe and a 19-gauge needle combination produced 8 psi. Irrigation pressure of a bulb syringe is 2 psi, which is not adequate to cleanse a wound.[3] The Water Pik ranges from 6 to more than 50 psi, which may cause trauma to a wound and drive bacteria into it.[5]

Comparison studies among gravity flow irrigation, bulb syringe, and jet lavage on removal of bacteria and foreign bodies in wounds showed that the number of bacteria in the jet lavage group was comparable to the 10^5 levels attributed to the body's ability to manage infection.[7] The pulsatile lavage systems, described later in this chapter, allow the psi to be adjusted. The psi treatment setting chosen will depend on the amount of necrotic tissue/exudate, the location of the wound, and the patient's comfort. Pulse rate, as well as psi, has been demonstrated clinically to effect granulation formation and epithelialization of clean wounds.[2]

The medical community has been concerned that high-pressure irrigation may drive bacteria and contaminants into

Exhibit 26–1 Irrigation Pressures Delivered by Various Devices

Device	Irrigation Impact Pressure (PSI)
Spray bottle—Ultra Klenz	1.2
Bulb syringe	2.0
Piston irrigation syringe (60 mL) with catheter tip	4.2
Saline squeeze bottle (250 mL) with irrigation cap	4.5
Water Pik at lowest setting (1)	6.0
Irrijet DS syringe with tip	7.6
35-mL syringe with 19-gauge needle or angiocatheter	8.0
Water Pik at middle setting (3)	42
Water Pik at highest setting (5)	> 50
Pressurized cannister—Dey-Wash	> 50

Source: Reprinted from N. Bergstrom, M.A. Bennett, C.E. Carlson, et al., *Treatment of Pressure Ulcers*, Clinical Practice Guideline No. 15, December, 1994, U.S. Department of Health and Human Services, Public Health Service, Agency for Health Care Policy and Research, AHCPR Publication No. 95-0652.

a wound and adjacent tissues. Bierbaum[7] reviewed several studies that looked at this problem. A high pressure of 70 psi delivered 3 cm from the surface in moderately contaminated wounds was found to spread the fluid laterally, rather than beneath the wound surface; however, it also impaired tissue defenses. In heavily contaminated wounds, there was a 100-fold reduction in bacterial count after high-pressure irrigation. Part of clinical decision making involves weighing the risk/benefit ratio. Sometimes multiple risks have to be considered when selecting a treatment intervention. For example, will the benefit of high-pressure cleansing of a highly contaminated wound outweigh the known risk of tissue trauma and have a better outcome than an inadequate response? Physical therapists would not use high-pressure irrigation unless under the direct supervision of a physician. If the assessment indicates that high-pressure irrigation needs to be considered, it is a criterion for referral to the physician.

Pulsed jet lavage has been used for treatment of traumatic wounds in operating rooms and in the military for decades.[8] Delivery of vancomycin-, streptomycin-, and tetracycline-water solutions with pulsating jet lavage eliminated or reduced bacteria as early as the second day, with earlier healing, less tissue loss, and reduced scarring. Infected diabetic foot lesions treated with pulsatile lavage and topical antibiotics had infection controlled, and the wounds were able to be closed surgically with grafts or flaps. Reduced inflammation has been reported following pulsed lavage treatment and was correlated to the extent of foreign material remaining in the tissues. Early cleansing with this therapy accelerated wound healing.[7]

Wound cleansing with battery-powered, disposable pulsatile, irrigation devices modeled after operating and emergency room equipment received favorable mention as an alternative to whirlpool therapy to minimize cross-contamination, decrease treatment time, speed healing, and shorten length of hospital stays. Additionally, these devices were recommended for their versatility and the ability to personalize treatment to provide a best outcome for the patient and the wound.[9] However, in a review of evidence, there were no controlled clinical trials to support efficacy for wound healing.[9]

Luedtke-Hoffmann and Schafer[10] reviewed the literature for effects of PLWS on wound cleansing and attempted to compare it with more traditional methods. Research comparing the effectiveness was scant. Pulsed lavage following whirlpool was more effective at removing bacterial contamination than was pulsed lavage alone.[11,12] They concluded that PLWS is a safe method of cleansing. Research shows no evidence of bacteremia after lavage applications, regardless of pressure, but and until more research is done, impact psi should remain between 4 and 15 psi.[10]

Mechanical Debridement

Irrigation is an effective mechanical debridement method to loosen and flush out debris and bacteria from contaminated wounds. Fluid dynamics play an important role in expelling the loosened debris with the high-flowing irrigation stream. The incidence of wound infection is decreased as the amount of irrigation fluid increases.[7]

Pulsed stimulation of the tissue is also thought to affect wound debridement. The pulse phase rapidly compresses the tissue; then, during the interpulse phase, the tissue decompresses. This may be a mechanism for mechanically loosening debris. There is increased ease of sharp debridement after the treatment, due to the loosened and softened necrotic tissue.

PLWS is considered a strategy of debridement. There are no licensing boards in the United States that prohibit PTs from performing debridement. PT assistants should get a ruling from their state boards as to the legality of their using PLWS.

Clinical Wisdom: *CPT Code*

A new CPT code for wound debridement 97601 includes PLWS and is effective in 2001.

Negative Pressure

Concurrent suction with pulsatile lavage appears to stimulate production of granulation tissue in "clean" wounds as a result of the negative pressure.[13] Negative pressure applies noncompressive mechanical forces to the tissues and dilates arterioles. Dilatation allows increased blood flow and transcutaneous oxygen delivery to the tissues.[14] Suction also removes debris, bacteria, and irrigant.

INDICATIONS FOR THERAPY

The author's clinical experience includes use of PLWS for both clean and infected wounds of many etiologies. Wounds that have benefited from this therapy are included in the list shown in Exhibit 26–2.

Benefits to the Patient

There are many benefits to the patient with treatment by PLWS. Frequently, the patient can be treated by the PT instead of the physician in the operating room, with significant cost savings. Treatment has contributed to the salvage of limbs.[2] There is improved safety with no transfers into/out of the whirlpool, as well as improved comfort with no change in temperature and the ability to control the pressure of the fluid on the wound. Periwound maceration is avoided with site-specific treatment. Benefits to the patient are summarized as follows:

- PLWS offers cost savings if operating room is not needed.
- It has contributed to salvage of limbs.
- It has improved safety.
- It offers improved comfort.
- Periwound maceration is avoided.
- It can be used for treatment of tunnels and undermining (Figure 26–1).
- Treatment is possible if whirlpool treatment is contraindicated.
- Treatment is possible if whirlpool treatment is inaccessible.

Clinical Wisdom:
Irrigation and Debridement of Tunnels

Pulsatile irrigation is an excellent choice for irrigation and debridement of tunnels and/or undermining.

Patients who would benefit from hydrotherapy but are contraindicated for whirlpool should be considered for pulsatile lavage, such as those who are unresponsive, those with

Exhibit 26–2 Examples of Indications for Pulsed Lavage

Type or Wound/Patient History	Rationale
Venous insufficiency ulcer A patient with a history of chronic leg wounds hit the pretibial area of his right lower extremity on a table leg 6 months ago. He has had open wounds on the lower extremity since then. The lower extremity is also edematous and there is periwound maceration. The patient is using a compression stocking.	If pulsed lavage with suction is used, the wounds can be treated with the lower extremity elevated to avoid increased edema. Treatment is site-specific so periwound maceration is not increased. Granulation and epithelialization can be stimulated, possibly by negative pressure of the suction.
Neuropathic ulcer A patient with diabetes and loss of protective sensation in both feet has an ulcer on the plantar surface of his left heel. He has a callus with a fragile area in the center at the head of the fifth metatarsal.	Instead of soaking the foot in a whirlpool, pulsed lavage with suction will offer site-specific treatment that will not compromise the callus and fragile area. In addition, the patient's lower extremity will not be in a dependent position, thereby avoiding edema, and the patient's skin will not be burned due to loss of sensation (a risk with whirlpool).
Pressure ulcer A paraplegic patient with bowel and bladder incontinence has a large sacral pressure ulcer.	An incontinent patient cannot be immersed in a whirlpool, but incontinence is not a contraindication to pulsed lavage with suction. Even if the patient were not incontinent, his wound would be difficult to treat in a whirlpool because he would have to lie on his sacrum, putting pressure on the wound site. In addition, he would have to be transported to physical therapy on a hard stretcher. This is not necessary with pulsed lavage because it is a bedside procedure.
Sternal wound Following coronary artery bypass graft surgery, a patient develops a wound infection and dehiscence. She is on a cardiac monitor and ventilator in the intensive care unit.	This patient's wound can be irrigated and debrided at the bedside using pulsed lavage with suction. Whirlpool immersion is not an option because of her medical equipment—cardiac electrodes cannot be placed in water.
Perineal wound A patient has Fournier's gangrene with multiple deep, narrow tunnels; there is purulent drainage with a foul odor. The patient is septic with a temperature of 105° F.	Whirlpool is contraindicated for a febrile patient. Pulsed lavage with suction is the alternative, using a product with a flexible tip to allow irrigation and debridement of the tunnels and to decrease the bacterial count.
Partial-take split-thickness skin graft A patient with pyoderma gangrenosum has had a split-thickness skin graft on the right lower extremity. There has been only partial take, with eschar and necrotic slough at the failed site.	Because pulsed lavage with suction is site-specific, it can be used to treat only the failed portion of the graft without compromising the remainder of the graft. Eschar will be hydrated enough to allow sharp debridement (escharotomy) following pulsed lavage.
Fasciotomies A patient with multiple fractures to his left lower extremity secondary to a motor vehicle accident is in skeletal traction. Medial and lateral fasciotomies have been performed, due to edema, and now there is periwound erythema and purulent drainage from tunnels and undermining.	Traction can be maintained and the wounds can be treated without disturbing the hardware if pulsed lavage with suction is used. The tracts can be irrigated using a device with a long, flexible tip.

Source: Used with permission from *Advances in Skin and Wound Care* 2000 May/June 13 (3): 133–134, © Springhouse Corporation/ www.springnet.com.

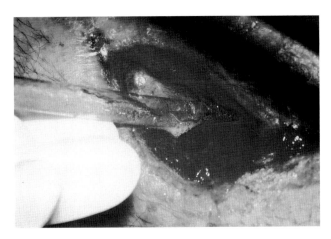

Figure 26–1 Gunshot wound with tunnel.

cardiopulmonary compromise or venous insufficiency, and those who are febrile or incontinent. Pulsatile lavage also can be offered to patients who cannot be placed in the whirlpool because of contractures; ostomies; incisions with intact sutures; IV placement; skeletal traction; casted extremities; obesity; confinement to the intensive care unit (ICU), intermediate care unit (IMCU), burn unit, or isolation (negative pressure room); or combativeness/restraints.

Treatment is possible for the following conditions if whirlpool treatment is contraindicated:

- Unresponsiveness
- Cardiopulmonary compromise
- Venous insufficiency
- Fever
- Incontinence if body whirlpool is required

Treatment is possible in the following circumstances if whirlpool treatment is inaccessible:

- Contractures—difficult body placement
- Ostomies
- Closed incisions with sutures intact
- IV placement
- Skeletal traction
- Casted extremities
- Obesity exceeding weight limit for stretcher/whirlpool
- Patient combative/restrained
- Patient in ICU, IMCU, burn unit, or isolation (negative pressure room).

Benefits to the Physical Therapist

The PT is able to use time more efficiently and effectively when performing PLWS compared to whirlpool. A pulsatile lavage treatment can take 15–30 minutes, compared with 45–60 minutes of the therapist's time for a whirlpool treatment. It is convenient since there is no need to fill, drain, and clean a whirlpool. Cleanup is minimized since all supplies are disposable. This makes it possible for the PT to schedule more treatment visits. The design of the devices used for PLWS provides the PT with the ability to control the intensity of the treatment, in pounds per square inch, and to select the correct tip for specific effects, leading to optimal results while safeguarding tissue. Some units allow greater control than others. Therefore, it is important for the PT to be aware of parameters and the limitations of the available equipment. Sharp debridement is significantly easier after PLWS treatment because of the presence of loosened, softened debris and necrotic tissue. Benefits to the PT are summarized as follows:

- There is no destruction of granulation tissue if 4–15 psi impact pressure is used.
- There is increased efficiency with increased productivity.
- The PT has the ability to control psi.
- Ease of sharp debridement is increased after treatment.
- Treatment is convenient.
- Cleanup is minimized.

Benefits to the Facility

In an acute care facility, PLWS contributes to a decreased length of stay because of the rapid rate of granulation and epithelialization. Physician and staff time is saved if the patient does not have to be taken to the operating room for treatment. Cross-contamination is virtually eliminated, because all supplies are disposable. This is especially important with infection control issues for bloodborne pathogens (BBP) and the spread of methicillin-resistant *Staphylococcus aureus* (MRSA) and vancomycin-resistant enterococci (VRE). There are cost savings with no need to buy whirlpools, the disinfectant to clean them, the water and the power to heat the water, and the staff to maintain them. Benefits to the facility are summarized as follows:

- The length of stay is decreased because of the rapid rate of granulation and epithelialization.
- Physician and operating room staff time is saved.
- Cross-contamination is eliminated.
- Cost savings are gained with elimination of whirlpools.

PRECAUTIONS

The most important three words to remember when treating a patient with PLWS are: ***know your anatomy!*** As with any method of debridement, it is imperative to have a strong anatomy background, enhanced by cadaver dissection, and to have an illustrated textbook in close proximity. Just as important is awareness of the possibility of anomalies. When unsure of specific anatomy, it is recommended that the patient's surgeon be contacted for edification as to exposed and nearby structures. This is especially true when irrigating tracts and undermining.

There are no known absolute contraindications to treatment with PLWS. As with any wound care treatment, however, certain precautions should be observed. These precautions apply to treatment of the following:

- Insensate patients
- Those taking anticoagulant medication
- Those with wounds with tunnels and/or undermining.

Experienced therapists will treat wounds that require extra attention to the entire procedure (see *Color Plate 83*). These include the following:

- Wounds near major vessels (eg, in the groin or axilla)
- Wounds near a cavity lining (eg, pericardium or peritoneum)
- Bypass graft sites, anastomoses
- Exposed vessel, nerve, tendon, bone
- Grafts, flaps
- Facial wounds

Certain wounds should be assessed carefully before being treated in a facility or home where a physician and emergency medical aid is not immediately available. Careful decision making is needed before treating wounds near major vessels, cavity linings, and bypass graft sites outside of an acute care hospital or hospital outpatient setting.

OUTCOME MEASURES

Clinical decision making involves evaluation of intervention choices to achieve a desired outcome. PLWS is a very versatile treatment choice. As discussed earlier, it can be used for all wounds where the expected functional outcome is infection free, necrosis free, inflammation free, exudate free, and good granulation base, in preparation for closure by secondary intention or surgery.

Wound closure by secondary intention or preparation for surgical closure and limb salvage with an intention of PLWS are reported in case studies.[2,7] Surrounding skin is protected from maceration. Because there are no controlled clinical trials of this therapy to compare, they cannot be used as a guide to length of time to achieve an expected outcome. Clinical judgment of the author suggests that the clinician should expect a decrease in necrotic tissue in 1 week and an increase in granulation/epithelialization in 1 week (see *Color Plates 82* and *83*). Following are some additional expected clinical outcomes:

- Odor and exudate free: 3–7 days
- Necrosis free: 2 weeks
- Progression from chronic inflammatory phase to acute inflammatory phase: 1 week
- Progression from acute inflammatory phase to proliferation phase: 2 weeks

A clinical outcome is one type of expected outcome. Another type of outcome to be considered is cost outcome. The cost of an outcome includes many factors, such as labor, supplies, and length of stay. For example, the average treatment time with pulsatile irrigation is 15–30 minutes, compared with 45–60 minutes for a whirlpool treatment. Infection control costs are minimal because of single-use, disposable components. Cross-contamination is virtually eliminated. These are very important cost-management factors in facilities that must work continuously to control contamination with BBP, MRSA, and VRE. Debridement with pulsatile irrigation with suction can be performed as a physical therapy procedure, rather than as a surgical procedure. This reduces surgeon and operating room costs.

Patient and caregiver satisfaction surveys monitor perceptions of how patients feel about the treatment they received and how it has affected function. Patients want to feel safe, secure, and comfortable during the treatment procedure. They may be scared about the consequences of failure to heal. Some are unable to attend a therapy session in the PT department. Treatment with pulsatile lavage can be given at the bedside with no need for lifts and transfers. Because of its portability and disposable components, it is an ideal modality for home treatment.

FREQUENCY AND DURATION

Patients are usually treated once a day. If the wound has more than 50% necrotic/nonviable tissue with purulent drainage/foul odor, and especially if sepsis is present, treatment twice a day is reasonable. Treatment two or three times a week is recommended if there is a full granulation base, no odor, and no purulent drainage. If the wound is being treated with the Vacuum-Assisted Closure (VAC, Kinetic Concepts, San Antonio, TX [described further later] device), PLWS is used with each VAC change, usually three times a week. PLWS should be discontinued when the wound is closed, there is no increase in granulation/epithelialization in 1 week, or there is no decrease in necrotic tissue in 1 week (Exhibit 26–3).

CAUTIONS

Treatment should be stopped if the patient complains of increased pain or is unable to tolerate treatment because of pain. A premedication order may be needed from the patient's physician. With an arterial bleeder, treatment must be

Exhibit 26–3 Frequency and Duration of Treatment

Frequency	Daily	Twice Daily	Three Times per Week	Discontinue
Most wounds	X			
> 50% Necrotic		X		
Purulent drainage		X		
Sepsis		X		
Full granulation base			X	
VAC being used			X	
Duration				
No increased granulation for 1 week				X
No decreased necrotic tissue for 1 week				X
Wound closed				X

stopped immediately and the physician called immediately. Any other bleeding not stopped with pressure within 10 minutes requires a physician consultation. If an abscess other than the one being treated is opened or a bone/joint disarticulation occurs, the physician also should be notified. Cautions are summarized as follows:

- Stop treatment when the following occurs:
  1. Patient complains of increased pain.
  2. Patient is unable to tolerate treatment because of pain.
- Stop and call physician in any of the following circumstances:
  1. Patient has an arterial bleeder: notify physician immediately.
  2. Bleeding has not stopped after 10 minutes of pressure.
  3. Abscess is opened.
  4. Joint is disarticulated.

Clinical Wisdom: *Prevent Disruption of Clot following Pressure To Stop Bleeding*

After applying pressure over gauze packing to stop bleeding and bleeding has stopped, leave the bottom layer of gauze in place to avoid disruption of the clot and restarting of the bleeding. Cover with the prescribed dressing.

VACUUM-ASSISTED CLOSURE

KCI's VAC is a device that uses a pump, attached by tubing to a foam dressing placed in the wound, to create a vacuum to remove fluid. The negative pressure on the wound helps to reduce edema, increase blood supply, and decrease bacterial colonization. The procedure increases tension among the surrounding cells, which encourages cell growth and division, drawing the edges of the wound to the center and assisting wound closure. It provides a moist wound environment to promote more effective cellular activity; it also helps to prevent contamination of the wound site from outside bacteria.

Details and use of the VAC are described in Chapter 12. There is frequently confusion among patients and clinical personnel due to the similarity in the names *VAC* (originally called *Decubivac* and *Dvac*) and *Pulsavac*. These are two entirely different interventions for wound management, and, indeed, they complement each other. The combination of the VAC and pulsed lavage has healed wounds four times faster than nontreated wounds, producing extraordinary cost savings.

Clinical Wisdom: *The VAC and PLWS*

The VAC and PLWS, used in conjunction with each other, provide an optimal intervention for management.

PERFORMANCE OF PLWS

Procedures for PLWS

Procedure Setup

Most patients ideally are treated on a high-low stretcher, bed, or treatment table adjusted to a height that ensures the therapist's proper body mechanics. Treatment may be delivered in a private treatment room in the physical therapy department or elsewhere, or at bedside in the patient's private room. A fluid-proof or fluid-resistant pad is placed under the body part with the wound, and towels are strategically placed around the wound and covering adjacent body parts, IV sites, and other portals of entry. A sterile field is set up, with treatment and dressing supplies in easy reach. A strong light source is important during pulsatile lavage and debridement.

Outpatients with foot wounds can be treated while seated in a wheelchair with an elevating footrest, with towels padding the footrest. The therapist sits on a low footstool in front of the patient and in easy reach of the sterile field setup of treatment and dressing supplies. A basin may be placed under the foot to catch any overflow of irrigant.

An aide is invaluable for efficiency and assistance with difficult body placement in treatment of some wounds. Duties vary, depending on the system used. Connecting the tubing to the power source and suction source, spiking the bags of fluid, turning the unit off and on, adjusting the psi at the therapist's direction, and emptying and replacing the filled suction canisters and new fluid bags are common procedures that can be done by the aide, saving the therapist time and from having to change gloves during treatment. After the treatment is completed, the aide also can dispose of the personal protective equipment, old dressings, and disposables while the therapist completes the documentation.

Infection Control

Standard Precautions. Protocols should adhere to each facility's policy, which can be more, but not less, stringent than Occupational Safety and Health Administration (OSHA) guidelines.[15]

Due to aerosolization of microorganisms during treatment, as evidenced in a study by Loehne et al[16] the patient should be treated in a private room with walls and doors, not curtains. On admission to the facility, if wound management with PLWS is anticipated and PTss provide the treatment at bedside, the patient should be assigned a private room as a medical necessity. This should be included in the facility's policies and procedures.

If the patient is treated at the bedside, all visitors should leave the room during treatment. If treated at home, family members/visitors should leave the room during treatment. All IV sites and other portals of entry on the patient should be covered with a clean towel.

All exposed linen used to control splash should be placed in a clear plastic biohazard bag after treatment for transport to the laundry. Clean the stretcher/wheelchair after each treatment if it is used to transport and treat the patient. Do not use a mattress or cushion with tears in the protective covering. Use basins to contain the irrigant overflow with treatment of extremity wounds. Disinfect the basin after each use.

Clean the dressing cart with an approved disinfectant solution after each use. Reusable face shields should be cleaned with a disinfectant that has been approved as effective against HIV, hepatitis B, and tuberculosis. Dispose of all disposables in the appropriate waste stream per OSHA guidelines.

Personal Protective Equipment. Secondary to aerosolization and splashing, all staff present during treatment must wear personal protective equipment, consisting of the following[17] (see Figure 26–2):

- Surgical masks
- Hair covers (with ears covered)
- Face shields
- Fluid-proof gowns
- Fluid-resistant knee-high boots (at the therapist's discretion for the aide)
- Nonsterile/sterile gloves

Single Use Only. All disposables except two discussed below are marked for single use only. The U.S. Food and Drug Administration (FDA) and OSHA mandate compliance. In fact, if used more than one time, Medicare and other payers consider the occurrence investigational and not reimbursable. Legal liability is possible if disposables are reused.

Davol (Figure 26–3) and Stryker each have a suction diverter tip that allows the same hand piece to be used multiple times with the *same* patient, with a new tip being utilized at different treatment times. This is due to the fact that the suction mechanism is diverted from the interior mechanism of the product. Otherwise, units cannot be cleaned without damaging the product or being assured that all contaminants and/or disinfection material is removed.

Even with FDA approval, this author has reservations about the ability to disinfect the external components of the product, such that the device can be stored and reused without concern for contamination. It also requires time, products, and space to disinfect and store. It precludes sterile procedure except for the first usage.

Clinical Wisdom: *Single Use Only*

Use of PLWS products only one time with disposal after use ensures no cross-contamination between patient treatments.

Latex Content

The latex content of the product used (see Exhibit 26–4) is important for latex-sensitive and latex-allergic patients, especially those with myelodysplasia, who must be treated in a latex-free environment.[18]

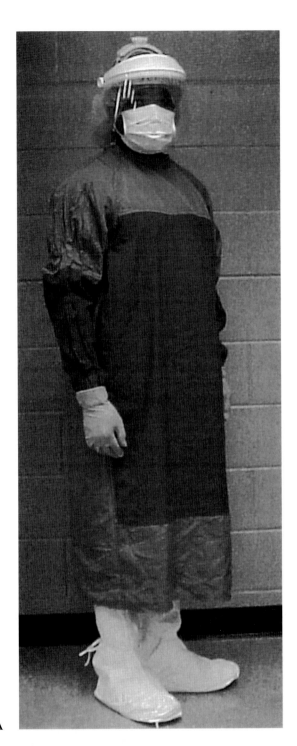

A

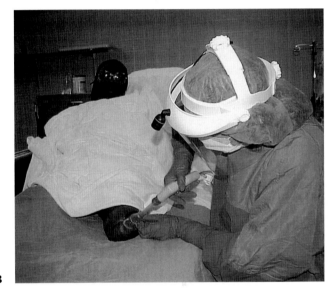

B

Figure 26–2 Personal protective equipment for hydrotherapy treatment.

Equipment Needed

Power Unit. Units are available powered by three sources (Exhibit 26–5). A machine console unit is electrically driven and is attached to a mobile operating room base and stand or a mobile wound care cart. Another product is driven by nitro-gen or medical air tanks, which can be attached to a wound care cart. All product manufacturers have a battery unit that is completely disposable.

Sterile debridement tips include a small splash shield for soft tissue debridement and general irrigation, and open tract tips for undermining, tracts, and tunnels (Exhibit 26–6).

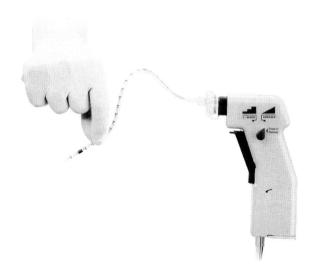

Figure 26–3 Simpulse Plus System by Davol, Inc., Cranston RI. Courtesy of Davol, Inc., Cranston, Rhode Island.

Exhibit 26–4 Latex Content of Products

Latex	Davol	Stryker	Zimmer
Present	Simpulse Plus	N/A	Pulsavac
Not present	VariCare	SurgiLav InterPulse	Pulsavac III Var-A-Pulse

Multiple other tips are available, depending on the manufacturer; however, these are utilized by physicians in the operating room. The PT needs only the small splash shield and the long, narrow, flexible tips, although new tips are in product development. The small splash shield placed in total contact with the tissue is recommended to obtain adequate suction for negative pressure, unless in undermining or tunnels. The same tip can be used for treating multiple wounds on the same patient in the same treatment session, if the least necrotic wounds are treated first. Figure 26–4 shows a wound view with an irrigation tip.

Exhibit 26–5 Products Available and Power Sources

Power Source	Davol	Stryker	Zimmer
Electrically driven console	None	None	Pulsavac Pulsavac III
Medical air/nitrogen tanks	Simpulse Plus	None	None
Batteries—unit disposable	VariCare	SurgiLav Plus InterPulse	Var-a-Pulse Pulsanic Plus for PT available 2001

Exhibit 26–6 Most Often Used Tips for Soft Tissue Wound Care

Tip	Davol	Stryker	Zimmer
Fan spray with splash shield	Yes	Yes	Yes
Retractable splash shield	Yes	No	No
Open tract	Yes	Yes	Yes
Narrow open tract	Yes	No	Yes
Retractable splash shield	No	No	Yes
Flexible, narrow open tract	Yes	No	Yes
Suction Diverter	Yes	Yes	No

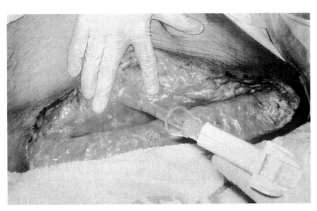

Figure 26–4 Wound view with a tip. Photo used courtesy of Zimmer, Inc.

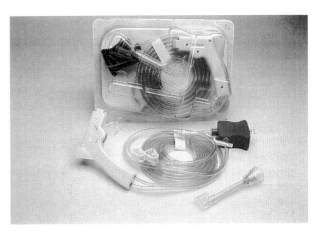

Figure 26–5 Hand controls and tubing pack. Photo used courtesy of Zimmer, Inc.

All products have hand controls and tubing for spiking the saline bag (see Figure 26–5).

Irrigation Fluid. Normal saline (0.9% sodium chloride) is preferred. Antibiotics can be added with a physician's order. Water is not recommended because it is not physiologic. Antiseptic agents or skin cleansers (povidone-iodine, iodophor, sodium hypochlorite, hydrogen peroxide, acetic acid) should not be used due to cytotoxicity to normal and/or wound tissue.[5]

Saline bags should be warmed to 39–41° C with a fluid warmer or in hot tap water. The number of bags used depends on the number and size of the wounds, the amount of necrotic tissue and exudate, and the patient's tolerance of the procedure.

Suction. Either a wall suction or portable pump is necessary for this modality. Equipment includes canisters, a regulator, and connecting tubing, which is required if the suction source is too far away from the wound with the tubing provided.

The suction removes debris, bacteria, and the irrigant, and provides negative pressure to increase the rate of granulation tissue.[3] Parameters are usually 60–100 mm Hg of continuous suction. It should be decreased if there is bleeding, if the wound is near a vessel or cavity, or if the patient complains of pain.

Clinical Wisdom: *Importance of Impact Pressure*

It is very important for the therapist to control and to know the impact pressure at all times during the treatment.

Pressure

Pressure is measured in psi. If the pressure is too high, bacteria and foreign matter can be forced into viable tissue, and granulation and epithelial tissues can be damaged. The Agency for Health Care Research and Quality, formerly known as the Agency for Health Care Policy and Research guidelines recommend a treatment range of 4–15 psi.[3]

Initiation of treatment is usually 4–6 psi, with a typical range of 8–12 psi. A setting of 4–6 psi is advised for tracts and undermining, due to inability to visualize the wound base and nearby structures. Treatment with greater than 15 psi should be undertaken only if the physician is present and with a specific written order (Exhibit 26–7).

During treatment psi should be increased in the presence of tough eschar and excessive necrotic tissue. It should be decreased if the patient complains of pain, if bleeding occurs, or if the tip is near a major or exposed vessel, nerve, tendon, or cavity lining. Exhibit 26–8 gives the pressure range and control available on various pressure products.

CONCLUSION

PLWS is an optimal strategy for debridement and irrigation for all wounds. With control of impact psi; site-specific treatment; the ability to treat tunnels, tracts, and undermining; enhancement of sharp debridement; avoidance of cross contamination; and an increased rate of granulation and epithelialization, PLWS offers the PT a valuable intervention for wound management. Treatment with PLWS, resulting in decreased length of stay and avoidance of facility-acquired infections with increased rate of wound closure, contributes to cost-effective treatment.[1]

Exhibit 26–7 Pressure Used

Pulsatile Lavage with Suction					
PSI	**4–6 psi**	**4 psi**	**8–12 psi**	**15 psi**	**16+ psi**
Initiation	X				
Tracts/undermining	X				
Minimum effective		X			
Typical range			X		
Maximum—PT				X	
With physician present					X

Exhibit 26–8 Pressure Range and Control Available (On/Off Control on All Hand Pieces)

Product	PSI Range	Gauge on Power Source	Digital Readout LED	Adjust at Source	Vary at Hand Control
Davol					
Simpulse Plus	3.6–12.3 psi (Flexible open tract tip 1.3–5.1 psi)	Yes	No	Source gauge	Yes
VariCare	3–11.3 psi (Open tract tip 1.7–11.5 PSI)	N/A	No	Dial control— three settings	Yes
Stryker					
Interpulse	0.8–9.0 psi (Varies with tip used)	N/A	No	No	Switch with two settings
Zimmer					
Pulsavac	0–28 psi	Yes	No	Dial control	Yes
Pulsavac III	0–60 psi 0–30 psi switch	Yes	Yes	Dial control	Yes
Var-A-Pulse	0–60 psi	N/A	No	Dial control— six settings	Yes

HOW TO USE DIFFERENT EQUIPMENT MODELS

Davol Simpulse Plus Procedure

Begin Treatment

1. Attach the suction canister to the regulator on suction source.

2. Adjust suction to the appropriate mm Hg continuous.
3. Hang the saline bag(s) on an IV pole.
4. Remove the hand piece, tubing, tip, and dual spike adapter from the package; place on sterile field.
5. Connect the dual spike adapter to the pump spike, if desired.
6. Remove the blue lock pin on the hand piece to release the trigger, and the blue retaining ring, if the tip with the large splash shield is used. Discard blue items.

7. Insert the tip into the hand piece.
8. Attach the suction tubing onto the suction tubing connector and suction canister.
9. Spike the irrigation bag.
10. Prime the unit by squeezing the trigger until irrigant exits the tip. The bag may be squeezed to facilitate priming.
11. With the gas source (nitrogen or medical air) pressure at zero, insert the gas connector into a Schrader-style connector until a click is heard. Do not connect clamp or obstruct the exhaust line.
12. Set the source pressure to the desired psi. Do not exceed 80 psi source pressure for open tract tips or 60 psi for the splash shield, so as not to exceed 15 psi impact pressure. Pressure may be adjusted from 2 to 15 psi impact pressure.
13. Place the tip in/on the wound as you squeeze the hand piece trigger to irrigate.
14. The trigger lock button may be used to lock at maximum flow. While squeezing the trigger, push the lock button to engage; to release, squeeze the trigger.

When Treatment Is Completed

1. Reduce the pressure regulator to 0 psi at the gas source.
2. Detach the unit from the source.
3. Turn off suction and remove the tubing from the suction source.
4. Dispose of all equipment in a white biohazard bag.
5. Empty the suction canister into a hopper or commode.
6. If disposable, place the empty canister in a white biohazard bag. If glass, place in a clear biohazard bag to be sent for reprocessing.

Davol Simpulse VariCare Procedure

Begin Treatment

1. Attach the suction canister to the regulator on suction source.
2. Adjust suction to the appropriate mm Hg continuous.
3. Hang the saline bag(s) on an IV pole.
4. Remove the hand piece, tubing, and the tip from the package; place on sterile field.
5. Attach the tip to the hand piece.
6. Spike the irrigation bag; a dual spike adapter is available.
7. Connect the tubing to the suction connection on the hand piece and to the suction source.
8. Remove the blue lock pin on the hand piece to release the trigger, and the blue retaining ring, if the tip with the large splash shield is used; discard blue items.

9. Squeeze the trigger with the mode selection switch set to continuous variable mode to fill the tubing with solution. The bag may be squeezed to facilitate priming.
10. Place the tip in/on the wound and pull the trigger. The delivered pressure varies with the amount of pressure on the trigger.
11. Two modes of use are available: continuous variable control or three-step variable control for low, medium, or high psi.

When Treatment Is Completed

1. Turn off suction and remove the tubing from the suction source.
2. Release the latch on the bottom of the hand piece, pull out the battery compartment, and remove the batteries. Batteries can be recycled if not contaminated.
3. Follow manufacturer's directions for disinfecting and storage of reusable equipment if suction diverter tip is used.
4. Dispose of all other equipment in a white biohazard bag.
5. Empty the suction canister into a hopper or commode.
6. If disposable, place the empty canister in a white biohazard bag. If glass, place in a clear biohazard bag to be sent for resterilization.

Stryker SurgiLav Plus and InterPulse Procedure

Begin Treatment

1. Attach the suction canister to the regulator on suction source.
2. Adjust suction to the appropriate mm Hg continuous.
3. Hang the bag of saline on an IV pole.
4. Remove the hand piece, tubing, and the tip from the package; place on sterile field.
5. Insert the tip into the hand piece.
6. Spike the bag of saline.
7. Connect the suction to the suction canister.
8. Squeeze the trigger to fill the tip with solution.
9. Place the tip in/on the wound and pull the trigger.
10. Adjust speed for desired psi—varies with the tip; only two pressures are available with each tip.

When Treatment Is Completed

1. Turn off suction and remove the tubing from the suction source.
2. Break open the hand piece to remove the batteries. If using disposable batteries, they can be recycled if not contaminated. Recharge batteries if using rechargeable hand piece and batteries.

3. Follow manufacturer's directions for disinfecting and storage of reusable equipment if suction diverter tip is used.
4. Dispose of all other equipment in a white biohazard bag.
5. Empty the suction canister into a hopper or commode.
6. If disposable, place the empty canister in a white biohazard bag. If glass, place in a clear biohazard bag to be sent for reprocessing.

Zimmer Pulsavac Procedure

Begin Treatment

1. Attach the suction canister to the regulator on suction source.
2. Adjust suction to the appropriate mm Hg continuous.
3. Hang the saline bag(s) on the suspension support on the solution support pole.
4. Remove the hand piece, tubing, and tip from the package; place on sterile field.
5. Attach the tip to the hand piece.
6. Connect the hand control suction tube to the wall suction canister.
7. Insert the fluid pump; close and secure the door to the unit.
8. Push the transducer connector onto the barbed fitting on the side of the unit.
9. Push the tubing into the retainer clip.
10. Move the clamps to "Y" and close.
11. Spike the irrigation bag; the unit is dual spike capable.
12. Remove the dust covers from the tubing and connect the hand control to the fluid set.
13. Plug in the unit with the power switch in the *off* position and the pressure control at zero setting.
14. Depress the power switch to the *on* position.
15. Rotate the pressure control setting to 10 to prime; return to the appropriate setting for desired psi.
16. Place the tip in/on the wound.
17. Pull or push on the trigger available to turn the unit on.

When Treatment Is Completed

1. Reduce the pressure control to zero.
2. Turn off suction and remove the tubing from the suction source.
3. Remove the tubing from the retainer clip and the transducer connector from the barbed fitting.
4. Open the door to the unit and remove the fluid pump.
5. Dispose of all equipment in a white biohazard bag.

6. Empty the suction canister into a hopper or commode.
7. If disposable, place the empty canister in a white biohazard bag. If glass, place in a clear biohazard to be sent for reprocessing.

Zimmer Pulsavac III Procedure

Begin Treatment

1. Attach the suction canister to the regulator on suction source.
2. Adjust suction to the appropriate mm Hg continuous.
3. Hang the saline bag(s) on the IV hanger on top of the Pulsavac III console.
4. Empty the sterile packages of Pulsavac supplies onto a sterile field.
5. Attach the appropriate tip to the hand control.
6. Plug the console into the electricity source.
7. Turn the machine to *on*.
8. Depress the *load/unload* switch; the cassette platform will recede into the unit.
9. Securely snap the blue fluid pump cassette onto the platform, pressing gently *one* time until clicks are heard; the platform will slide out automatically.
10. Move the clamps to "Y" and close.
11. Connect the suction tube, and the connecting tubing, if needed, to the suction canister.
12. Spike the irrigation bag.
13. With the hand control in the *on* position, open the clamp compressing the spike tubing.
14. To prime the fluid, depress the *run/stop* switch and turn the pressure setting to maximum psi until fluid flows freely. The half-power switch, located on the back of the console, should be used.
15. Decrease the psi setting to the desired pressure.
16. Place the top in/on the wound.
17. Pull on or push on the trigger.

When Treatment Is Completed

1. Depress the *run/stop* switch.
2. Depress the *load/unload* switch; the plate will slide in.
3. Remove the tubing and the hand control by removing the cassette, squeezing on the concave sides of the cassette body, then lifting up.
4. Depress the *on/off* switch to the *off* position.
5. Turn off suction and remove the tubing from the suction source.
6. Dispose of all equipment in a white biohazard bag.
7. Empty the suction canister into a hopper or commode.

8. If disposable, place the empty canister in a white biohazard bag. If glass, place in a clear biohazard bag to be sent for reprocessing.

Zimmer Var-A-Pulse Procedure

Begin Treatment

1. Attach the suction canister to the regulator on suction source.
2. Adjust the suction to the appropriate mm Hg continuous.
3. Hang the saline bag(s) on an IV pole.
4. Remove the hand piece, tubing, and tip from the package; place on sterile field.
5. Attach the tip to the hand piece.
6. Spike the irrigation bag; a dual spike is available.
7. Connect the tubing to the suction source.
8. Set the dial at the hand piece's base for the desired psi.
9. Place the tip in/on the wound and turn the hand piece on.

When Treatment Is Completed

1. Turn off suction and remove the tubing from the suction source.
2. Open the latch at the base to separate the handle to remove the batteries (can be recycled if not contaminated).
3. Dispose of the entire unit in a white biohazard bag.
4. Empty the suction canister into a hopper or commode.
5. If disposable, place the empty canister in a white biohazard bag. If glass, place in a clear biohazard bag to be sent for reprocessing.

DOCUMENTATION

The following case study uses the diagnostic process described in Chapter 1, The Diagnostic Process, to document the need for skilled PT intervention using PLWS. The methodology of the functional outcome report is provided.[1]

REVIEW QUESTIONS

1. A patient three weeks s/p coronary artery bypass graft (CABG) has a dehisced, infected sternal wound and has undergone a sternectomy. The pericardium is exposed and there is undermining at the margins. What is the treatment strategy of choice for PT wound management?
   - Treatment with PLWS is ideal, as the patient can be treated bedside with all monitors in place. The treatment is site specific, the open area of the wound can be treated with the small splash shield tip, and the undermining can be irrigated and debrided with the open tract tip. Suction should be at 80 mm Hg, with the therapist's gloved fingers on the tip at all times.

2. A patient is readmitted from an extended care facility, 4 weeks s/p right total hip replacement. The dehisced wound has purulent drainage with a foul odor, from a narrow tunnel that probes to the joint. How is this wound best treated by physical therapy?
   - With PLWS, use of a flexible long, narrow tip to irrigate and debride the tunnel is efficacious in reducing bacteria and allowing an optimal environment for granulation from the base of the tunnel toward the surface of the wound. The impact psi should be 4–6, as the base of the tunnel cannot be visualized

3. A patient with paraplegia is admitted with a stage III –IV? sacral pressure ulcer. What is the treatment of choice for wound management?
   - Optimizing nutrition and providing pressure relief are mandatory. The patient's eschar should be treated cross hatched and treated with PLWS to hydrate the eschar, to allow for ease of an escharotomy. The wound can then be evaluated for the actual depth and staging of the wound. Treatment with PLWS will irrigate and debride necrotic slough, and promote granulation and epithelialization.

4. An outpatient who is a heavy smoker is referred to physical therapy for treatment of venous insufficiency ulcers on both lower extremities. He cannot tolerate sharp debridement of the necrotic tissue in the wounds. What is the ideal treatment plan?
   - The patient should be encouraged to quit all use of and exposure to tobacco, and be encouraged with proper nutrition. Lower extremities should be elevated above the level of the heart when not ambulatory. He should avoid long periods of being on his feet.
   - The wounds can be treated with PLWS with impact psi 10–12, with the small splash shield in contact with the wound and periwound tissue at all times. The tip can be lifted from the surface and moved if the patient cannot tolerate it being slid along the wound surface. The PLWS will debride the necrotic tissue without the pain of sharp debridement.
   - An ABI that is WNL allows for bilateral gradient compression wraps while wounds are open. If the wound is heavily draining, a foam dressing under the wraps, with moisture barrier ointment periwound is appropriate. After closure, the patient should be fitted with compression stockings; to prevent future ulcers they must be worn at all times when out of bed for the rest of his life.

Case Study: Gunshot Wound Treated with Pulsatile Lavage with Suction

Patient ID: W.S.   Age: 29   Onset: January 2

Initial Assessment

Reason for Referral

The patient was referred for a blasted shoulder wound with buckshot, necrotic tissue, tunnels, and undermining in the wound.

Medical History and Systems Review

The patient, previously fully functionally independent with no prior medical history, suffered a self-inflicted gunshot wound to the left shoulder. On the day of the injury and admission to the hospital, January 2, 1995, he had surgical exploration of the blasted shoulder wound. The humeral head was resected; fragments were resected from the laterally pulverized clavicle. There was no injury to the brachial plexus or axillary vasculature. The left upper extremity was placed in traction with pins. He had subsequent surgical incisions and drainage of the wound in the operating room on January 3, 4, 5, and 6, with closure of the shoulder capsule on January 6 (see Figure 26–4).

Evaluation

The patient was admitted to the burn unit after the initial surgery because of the severity of the wounds and the complicated dressing changes required. The presence of necrotic tissue, purulent exudate, buckshot, and numerous tunnels and undermining were indications for treatment with pulsatile lavage with concurrent suction.

Examination—January 13

Joint Integrity

The left humeral head has been resected. The left upper extremity is in skeletal traction with pins, with shoulder abducted to 90°. The lateral clavicle is pulverized.

Circulation

There is no injury to the axillary vasculature; there is edema in the left upper extremity.

Sensation

There is no injury to the brachial plexus.

Mobility

The patient is restricted to the supine position.

Integumentary

The left shoulder has a through-and-through wound, with the shotgun entrance wound on the anterior and the exit wound on the posterior.

Size.

- Anterior border—118.75-cm surface open area
- Posterior border—50.0-cm surface open area
- Medial depth—2.0 cm
- Lateral depth—1.75 cm
- Tunneling and undermining cannot be measured because of proximity of vessels.

Tissue Assessment. The wound has red granulation with scattered areas of yellow and brown necrotic tissue; there is buckshot present. The periwound tissue is erythematous and edematous.

Wound Healing Phase. The wound is in acute inflammatory phase.

Functional Diagnosis

- Soft tissue injury
  1. Absence of proliferative phase
  2. Absence of epithelialization phase
  3. Undue susceptibility to infection caused by debris in wound
- Functional loss of mobility associated with shoulder injury leading to inability to perform self care and undue susceptibility to pressure ulcers.

Need for Skilled Services

Pulsatile lavage with suction by physical therapist is indicated in an attempt to avoid another surgical incision and drainage and to prepare the wound for a subsequent skin graft. Increased mobility will be allowed with an accelerated healing process. Therapeutic positioning is necessary to avoid pressure ulcers.

Targeted Outcomes

- The wound bed will be clean, including tunnels and undermining.
- The wound will progress through the phases of healing from inflammatory to epithelialization.
- The patient will be properly positioned to remove pressure.

Treatment Plan

- Irrigate and mechanically debride the wound with the Pulsavac System, including tunnels and undermining. Remove the buckshot. Treat with 1 L of normal saline, 4 to 12 psi, 80 mm Hg suction.

continues

Case Study continued

- Perform sharp debridement of necrotic tissue with forceps and scissors.
- Maintain moist wound bed and obliterate dead space with dressing changes of wet to damp Dakin's solution–soaked gauze; cover with a 5 × 9-inch gauze pad and secure with dry gauze and paper tape. Tunnels and undermining will be loosely packed.
- Perform therapeutic positioning.

Prognosis

There will be no necrotic tissue and no debris. The wound will have a red granulation base and be ready for skin grafting by the physician.

Target Date. Two weeks.

Frequency. Once a day, 6 days per week.

Reexamination by Physical Therapy on January 20

Size.

- Anterior wound—68.25-cm surface open area
- Posterior wound—28.75-cm surface open area
- Medial depth—1.5 cm
- Lateral depth—1.0 cm

Tissue Assessment. The wound has no necrotic tissue. There is a full red granulation base and increased epithelialization. There is no periwound erythema. Tunneling and undermining are present only in the proximal portion of the anterior wound.

Wound Healing Phase. Proliferative phase.

Intervention

Physical Therapy. Six treatments of pulsatile lavage with suction, followed by sharp debridement as needed.

Physical Therapy and Nursing. Dressing changes.

Physicians. On January 19 the pins are removed and traction is discontinued. The patient is transferred from the burn unit to a regular room.

Revised Prognosis

Closure of the wound by secondary intention.

Discharge Outcome

The patient's wounds not only required no further surgical incisions and drainage, but also had a significant increase in granulation and epithelialization with no necrotic tissue present. Anterior and posterior wounds had a decreased surface open area of 42%. Medial depth decreased 25% and lateral depth decreased 43% within 7 days. The physicians decided to allow the wound to close by secondary intention rather than a skin graft. The patient was discharged home January 21, to continue dressing changes by his mother. Future surgical procedures were anticipated to replace the shoulder joint. He was lost to follow-up.

REFERENCES

1. Haynes LJ, Handley C, Brown MH, Ho L, Merrifield HH, Griswold JA. *Comparison of Pulsavac and Sterile Whirlpool Regarding the Promotion of Tissue Granulation.* Lubbock, TX: University Medical Center and Methodist Hospital; 1994.

2. Loehne HB. Enhanced wound care using Pulsavac System: Case studies. *Acute Care Perspect.* 1995;9:13–15.

3. U.S. Department of Health and Human Services. Treatment of pressure ulcers. *AHCPR Clin Pract Guideline.* 1994;15:50–53.

4. Stevenson TR, Thacker JG, Rodeheaver GT, Bacchetta C, Edgerton MT, Edlich RF. Cleansing the traumatic wound by high pressure syringe irrigation. *JACEP.* 1976;5(1):17–21.

5. Bhaskar SN, Cutright DT, Gross A. Effect of water lavage on infected wounds in the rat. *J Periodont.* 1969;40:671.

6. Wheeler CB, Rodeheaver GT, Thacker JG, Edgerton MT, Edlich RF. Side effects of high pressure irrigation. *Surg Gynecol Obstet.* 1976;143:775–778.

7. Bierbaum B. *High Pressure, Pulsatile Lavage in Wound Management: A Literature Review.* Cranston, RI: Davol, Inc.; 1986.

8. Bhaskar SN, Cutright DE, Hunsuck EE, Gross A. Pulsating water jet devices in debridement of combat wounds. *Milit Med.* 1971;136:264–266.

9. Rodeheaver GT. Pressure Ulcer Debridement and Cleansing: A Review of Current Literature. *Ostomy/Wound Manage.* 1999;45(Suppl):80S–85S.

10. Luedtke-Hoffmann KA, Schafer DS. Pulsed lavage in wound cleansing. *Phys Ther.* 2000;80:292–300.

11. Niederhuber SS, Stribley RF, Koepke GH. Reduction of skin bacterial lead with use of the therapeutic whirlpool. *Phys Ther.* 1975;55:482–486.

12. Bohannon R. Whirlpool versus whirlpool and rinse for removal of bacteria from a venous stasis ulcer. *Phys Ther.* 1982;62:304–308.

13. Morykwas MJ, Argenta LC. Use of negative pressure to increase the rate of granulation tissue formation in chronic open wounds. Presented at the annual meeting of the Federation of American Societies of Experimental Biology; March 28–April 1, 1993; New Orleans, LA.

14. Argenta LC, Morykwas M, Rouchard R. The use of negative pressure to promote healing of pressure ulcers and chronic wounds. Presented at the joint meeting of the Wound Healing Society and the European Tissue Repair Society; August 22–25, 1993; Amsterdam, Netherlands.

15. Occupational Safety and Health Administration. Bloodborne pathogen standard. *Federal Register.* 1991;56(235):64175–64182.

16. Loehne HB, Streed SA, Gaither B, Sherertz RJ. Aerosolization of microorganisms during pulsatile lavage with suction. Presented at Com-

bined Sections Meeting/American Physical Therapy Association. February 2000; New Orleans, LA.

17. Goodman CC, Boissonnault WG. *Pathology: Implications for the Physical Therapist.* WB Saunders. 2nd ed. In press.

18. U.S. Food and Drug Administration. Allergic reactions to latex-containing medical devices. *FDA Med Bull.* 1991;July 2–3.

Guide to Topical Antiseptics, Antifungals, and Antibacterials

Source: Adapted with permission from *Topical Agents for Open Wounds: Antibacterials, Antiseptics, Antifungals,* G. Gilman, ed., reviewed by G. Rodeheaver, J.W. Cooper, D.R. Nelson, and M. Meehan, © 1991, Hill-Rom International.

INDEX TO TOPICAL ANTISEPTICS

Generic Name	Product Name(s)
Acetic acid irrigation	
Aluminum salts	Burow's solution, Domeboro
Chlorhexidine gluconate	Hibiclens, Exidine skin
Hexachlorophene	pHisoHex
Hypochlorites	Dakin's solution, chloramine-T
Oxidizing agents	Hydrogen peroxide, 1.5%, 3%
Povidone-iodine	Betadine, Efodine
Quaternary ammonium compound	Zephiran

ACETIC ACID IRRIGATION

Description

A sterile solution of glacial acetic acid in water is used for irrigation. The pH range is between 2.9 and 3.3.

Action

The exact mechanism of action is unknown. Microorganisms will not proliferate at low pH, and all acids are bacteriostatic at low concentrations and bactericidal at higher concentrations.

Indication

Acetic acid is used to discourage bacterial infections in surgical wounds and to suppress growth by *Pseudomonas aeruginosa* in extensive burns; it is also a component in several dermatologic preparations.

Adverse Reactions

Acetic acid can cause irritation and inflammation. A solution of 0.25% acetic acid decreased bacterial survival by only 20% in cultured human fibroblasts.[1] The 0.25% acetic acid solution proved to be more damaging to fibroblasts than to bacteria whenever a difference in toxicity was observed.[1]

Dosage

Most physicians use acetic acid irrigant for wet-to-dry dressings. Acetic acid irrigant of a 0.25% solution is commonly used for bladder irrigation.

Packaging

Most institutional pharmacists prepare as a 1% surgical dressing.

Dermatologic lotion 0.1%
Irrigant 0.25%, 60 mL
Vosol 2% (Wallace Labs), 15 mL (multipack), 30 mL (multipack)

Other manufacturers of acetic acid: Kendall McGaw; Baxter Labs; Abbott Labs.

ALUMINUM SALTS (BUROW'S SOLUTION, DOMEBORO)

Description

Aluminum salts have strong antibacterial effects. The general solutions containing aluminum salts are 1% aluminum chlorhydrate, 10% aluminum acetate, 30% aluminum chloride hexahydrate, and 5% aluminum diacetate.

Action

A mild astringent solution is made with Domeboro tablets or powder.

Indications

Relief of inflammatory condition. One percent aluminum chlorhydrate, 10% aluminum acetate, and 30% aluminum chloride hexahydrate completely inhibit representative dermatophytes, yeasts, and gram-positive and gram-negative bacteria in vitro. Twenty percent aluminum chlorhydrate, 10% to 20% aluminum acetate, and 20% to 30% aluminum chlorhydrate salt are the most potent in vivo. The recommended concentrations (1:20 and 1:40) of 5% aluminum diacetate (Burow's solution) exert no in vivo bacteriostatic or bactericidal effects.

Precautions

Do not use plastic or other impervious material to prevent evaporation. For external use only. The enzyme activity of topical collagenase may be inhibited by aluminum acetate solution because of the metal ion and low pH. Cleanse the wound thoroughly with normal saline before applying enzymes.

Directions

Thirty milliliters of USP solution are diluted to 1 or 2 L with water, *or* Domeboro tablets or powder may be dissolved in 0.5–1 L of water. Domeboro tablets make a modified Burow's solution equivalent to 1:40.

Packaging

Pharmacy prepares Burow's solution.

Domeboro 2.2-g packets of powder or tablets (Miles, Inc.)
Blue Boro 2.2-g packets of powder or tablets (Herbert)
Burow's solution
    (J.J. Balan, Inc.), 480-mL solution
    (Paddock Labs), 480-mL solution, 3,840-mL solution
    (Wisconsin Pharm.), 480-mL solution, 3,840-mL
    solution

CHLORHEXIDINE GLUCONATE (HIBICLENS, EXIDENE SKIN)

Description

Chlorhexidine gluconate was introduced in the United States from Europe in 1977 as Hibiclens, which is 4% chlorhexidine gluconate with 4% isopropyl alcohol in a sudsing base. Hibitane is a chlorhexidine tinction for use as a skin preparation. It is an antiseptic and antimicrobial.

Action

Bactericidal on contact. Antiseptic activity and a persistent antimicrobial effect with rapid bactericidal activity against a wide range of microorganisms, including gram-positive bacteria and gram-negative bacteria as *Pseudomonas aeruginosa*.

Indications

Effective against a wide variety of gram-positive and gram-negative bacteria, molds, yeasts, and viruses. Sporicidal only at elevated temperatures. Rapid acting—the reduction of bacterial flora on the skin occurs immediately. Repeated use produces further reductions. Safe to use on the skin. No significant problems with irritation, allergy, or photosensitivity. No evidence of toxicity if absorbed; does not appear to be absorbed due to the protein-binding characteristic, which causes retention in the stratum corneum. It does not lose its effectiveness in the presence of whole blood.

Precautions

For external use only. Avoid contact with the meninges. Not recommended for full-thickness wounds.

Directions

Thoroughly rinse wound with sterile water. Apply sufficient Hibiclens and wash gently. Rinse thoroughly.

Packaging

Hibiclens skin cleanser (Stuart Pharm.) (4% chlorhexidine gluconate in a sudsing base), 120 mL
Hibistat germicidal hand rinse (Stuart Pharm.) (0.5% chlorhexidine in 70% isopropyl alcohol), 120 mL
Hibiclens antiseptic antimicrobial skin (Stuart Pharm.) (4% in sudsing base), 120 mL, 240 mL, ½ gal, 1 gal
Exidine skin (yttrium) (4% with 4% isopropyl alcohol)

HEXACHLOROPHENE (pHISOHEX)

Description

Hexachlorophene is a chlorinated phenolic compound.

Action

Antibacterial cleanser. Its antibacterial action is unknown.

Indications

Active primarily against gram-positive bacteria, including staphylococci. Peak antibacterial effect of hexachlorophene is obtained only by repeated scrubs on successive days. It has very little effect on gram-negative bacteria or spores.

Precautions

Tends to leave a residual film on the skin that can persist for several days. Protective film can be easily disrupted by alcohol. It can be absorbed through the skin. Once in the blood stream, there is potential for toxicity to the central nervous system. Up to 3.1% of topically applied hexachlorophene could be absorbed through the skin.

Hexachlorophene contamination with gram-negative bacteria, *Klebsiella* species, *Pseudomonas aeruginosa*, *Escherichia coli*, and *Candida albicans* is possible.

Contraindicated for use on burned or denuded skin as an occlusive dressing, wet pack, or lotion, or on any mucous membrane. Do not use in deep wounds.

Directions

Clean area for 3 minutes with pHisoHex and rinse thoroughly.

Packaging

pHisoHex 3% (Winthrop-Breon), 5-oz bottle, 1 pt, 1 gal
Septi-Soft 0.25% (Vestal), liquid, 240 mL
Septi-Sol 0.25% (Vestal), solution, 240 mL

HYPOCHLORITES (DAKIN'S SOLUTION, CHLO-RAMINE-T)

Description

Sodium hypochlorite has germicidal, deodorizing, and bleaching properties. Henry D. Dakin, U.S. chemist, 1880–1952, developed this solution for cleansing wounds during World War I as a very dilute neutral solution (0.45–0.5%) of sodium hypochlorite and 0.04% boric acid.

Action

The exact mechanism of action by which free chlorine destroys microorganisms has not been established. The postulated mechanism is inhibition of some key enzymatic reactions within the cell, protein denaturation, and inactivation of nucleic acids.

Indications

For prophylaxis of epidermophytosis, diluted sodium hypochlorite solution is sometimes employed as a foot bath. It is employed in full strength, as a freshly prepared solution, in the management of suppurating wounds, often by continuous irrigation (Carrel technique). It is useful in the dissolving of necrotic tissue.

Precautions

Cellular damage occurs at concentrations of Dakin's solution formerly thought to be safe for use in open wounds (0.05%). Even at lower concentrations (0.025%), significant damage is seen in fibroblasts and endothelial cells.[2] Significant damage occurs at more dilute concentrations of 0.001% and 0.00001%.

In experiments done by Robert Kozol, cultured fibroblasts and endothelial cells exposed to Dakin's solution (2.5×10^{-2} or 2.5×10^{-3}) for 30 minutes showed a marked increase in cell injury characterized by convoluted nuclei, cytoplasmic vacuolation, dilated endoplasmic reticulum, and swollen mitochondria. They also found Dakin's solution to have an inhibitory effect on random and stimulated migration of neutrophils, a functional response rather than as a result of cellular damage.[2]

Chloramine-T, an aqueous hypochlorite antiseptic agent, retards the development of collagen in healing skin defects and prolongs the acute inflammatory response; therefore, healing is delayed. It is toxic to granulation tissue, leading to complete and irreversible capillary shutdown. Reepithelialization at wound edges is delayed in wounds treated with hypochlorite solutions.

Sodium hypochlorite solutions dissolve blood clots, delay clotting, and are irritating to the skin. It has been suggested that the use of hypochlorites can cause endotoxins to be released from gram-negative bacteria in chronic wounds such as pressure ulcers, which can initiate a clinical response varying from mild pyrexia to acute oliguric renal failure.

Directions

Most physicians order wounds packed with Dakin's solution and gauze three or four times daily.

Packaging

Most pharmacists prepare Dakin's solution as a 0.5% sodium hypochlorite solution. Even at this concentration, the solution is toxic to native cells. **There is *no* safe concentration of Dakin's solution for use in open wounds.**

Dakin's solution is prepared as a topical solution containing 0.15–0.5% of NaOCL. The full-strength solution contains 0.5% NaOCL. To prepare the 0.15% solution, it should be diluted 1:3.

Dakin's solution (Century Pharm.), 5% gallon solution
Chloramine-T (A.A. Spectrum), 250 g, 1,000 g, 2,500 g

OXIDIZING AGENTS

Hydrogen Peroxide Solution USP

Contact with tissues releases molecular oxygen, and there is a brief period of antimicrobial action. There is no penetration of tissues. It has been reported that the instillation of peroxide into wound cavities under pressure can result in oxygen passing into the bloodstream, causing a life-threatening embolus.[3] Hydrogen peroxide has been documented to liberate oxygen that can spread along fascial planes, which causes swelling and crepitation and is frequently misdiagnosed as invasion by gas-forming bacteria.[3,4] It is toxic to exposed fibroblasts unless it is diluted more than 1:100.[4]

Packaging

A.A. Spectrum, 3% solution in water, 500 mL, 4,000 mL
J.J. Balan, 3% solution in water, 480 mL

Hydrous Benzoyl Peroxide USP

Can be bactericidal to microorganisms. When applied as a lotion, it is also keratolytic, antiseborrheic, and an irritant. May produce contact dermatitis. Its principal use is in the treatment of acne and seborrhea.

Potassium Permanganate USP

Consists of purple crystals that dissolve in water to give deep purple solutions. Tends to stain tissue and clothing brown. A 1:10,000 dilution applied in inert surfaces kills many microorganisms in 1 hour. Higher concentrations are irritating to the tissues. Its principal use is in treatment of weeping skin lesions with questionable justification.

Packaging

A.A. Spectrum, granules, 454 g
Humco Lab, Inc., granules, 120 g, 420 g, 454 g, 2,270 g

POVIDONE-IODINE

Description

Yellow-brown acidic water-soluble solution made of the polymer polyvinylpyrrolidone and iodine, creating a water-soluble agent that slowly releases free iodine.

Action

Potent antiseptic with a broad spectrum of antimicrobial activity, although its exact mechanism of action is unknown. Povidone-iodine is inactivated in the presence of blood and organic matter.

Indications

Povidone-iodine kills gram-positive and gram-negative bacteria, fungi, viruses, protozoa, and yeasts. Spore destruction is achieved only with moist contact for more than 15 minutes.[5] A 10% solution of povidone-iodine (1% of available iodine) kills 85% of cutaneous bacteria. Clinically indicated for prevention and treatment of surface infections, as well as to degerm the skin prior to invasive procedures.

Precautions

Stinging and burning of the tissue is a common side effect. One percent povidone-iodine is indiscriminate in toxic effects at full strength. A dilution of 1:1,000 is identified where no fibroblast toxicity occurs, while remaining bactericidal in in vitro studies.[1]

In vivo studies showed that povidone-iodine surgical scrub solution significantly potentiated ($p < 0.002$) the development of wound infection when compared with the incidence of infection in wounds treated with 0.9% saline solution.[6]

It is important to know that the Food and Drug Administration (FDA) has not approved povidone-iodine antiseptic solution or povidone-iodine surgical scrub solution for use in wounds.[6]

For an antimicrobial agent to eliminate bacterial contamination, it must reach the bacteria in an active form. Because of the insolubility of iodine in water and its rapid complex formation with tissue and body fluids, its ability to reach and kill bacteria in a wound or tissue is highly suspect.[6]

Adverse Reactions

A continuous irrigation with Betadine in a 72-year-old woman, postsurgical debridement of a hip wound resulted in death 10 hours later. Her serum total iodine level at autopsy was 7,000 μg/100 mL, while the normal value is 5 to 8 μg/dL.[7]

Povidone-iodine has been reported to cause acidosis in burn patients. Lasting systemic side effects identified include cardiovascular toxicity, renal toxicity, hepatoxicity, and neuropathy.[8]

Povidone-iodine's toxicity directly interferes with wound healing at the cellular level and places the patient at a greater risk for wound infection.[9] Rodeheaver's studies showed that both aqueous iodine and povidone-iodine solutions significantly impair the wound's ability to fight infection.[6]

In separate studies it was found that povidone-iodine inhibits wound healing at the cellular level, and that the incidence and potential for infection are greater than if wounds are irrigated only with normal saline.[9]

Rodeheaver found that even though povidone-iodine solution significantly lowered contaminants in the wound, the wound was still heavily contaminated. He also found that povidone-iodine surgical scrub did not reduce the level of bacteria in the wound.[6]

Dosage

Topical: 0.5–10% to the skin
Solution: 0.5–1% to the skin

Packaging

Purdue Frederick, 10% solution, 8 oz
Generic, 10% solution, 8 oz, 480-mL, 3,840-mL

QUATERNARY AMMONIUM COMPOUND (ZEPHIRAN)

Description

Benzalkonium chloride (BAC) is a quaternary ammonium compound commonly known as Zephiran. It is a cationic surfactant. The quaternaries are organically substituted ammonium compounds in which the nitrogen atom has a valence of 5.

Action

The bactericidal action has been attributed to the inactivation of energy-producing enzymes, denaturation of essential cell proteins, and disruption of the cell membrane.

Indication

Effective against some gram-positive and gram-negative bacteria, some fungi, and protozoa. Many bacteria grow in its presence. It is not effective against *Mycobacterium tuberculosis*, *Pseudomonas aeruginosa*, spores, and viruses.

Precautions

It is inactivated by anionic compounds such as soaps and detergents. Any residual detergent on the skin will neutralize the antiseptic effect. It is inactivated by blood and other organic matter. There are reports of contamination with *Pseudomonas cepacia*, *Enterobacter cloacae*, *E. agglomerans*, and *Serratia marcescens*.

Directions

Rinse anionic detergents and soaps from the area first so that the antibacterial activity of BAC will not be reduced. Minor wounds and lacerations use 1:750 tincture or spray. Deep, infected wounds use 1:30,000–1:20,000 aqueous solution. Wet dressings use 1:5,000 or less solution.

Packaging

Germicin (CMC), 50% solution, 1 pt, 1 gal
Benza (Century Pharm.), 1:750 solution, 60 mL, 120 mL
Zephiran (Winthrop-Breon)
  Aqueous solution 1:750, 240 mL, 1 gal
  Disinfectant concentration 17%, 120 mL, 1 gal
  Tincture spray 1:750, 30 g/gal, 80 g/gal
  Tincture 1:750, 1 gal

INDEX TO TOPICAL ANTIFUNGALS

Generic Name	Product Name(s)
Amphotericin B	Fungizone
Ciclopirox olamine	Loprox
Clotrimazole	Lotrimin, Mycelex
Econazole nitrate 1%	Spectazole
Haloprogin	Halotex
Ketoconazole	Nizoral
Miconazole nitrate	Monistat-Derm
	Micatin, Monistat
Nystatin	Mycostatin, Nilstat
Tolnaftate	Tinactin

AMPHOTERICIN B (FUNGIZONE)

Description

Yellow-orange, odorless; may stain skin. A polyene antifungal for topical use, produced by a stain of *Streptomyces nodosus*.

Action

Amphotericin B binds sterols in the cell membrane with an alteration in permeability that results in leakage of intracellular materials.

Indications

Superficial *Candida albicans*, histoplasmosis, coccidiomycosis, and crytococcocis. It has no significant effect against gram-positive or gram-negative bacteria or viruses.

Precautions

Ineffective against dermatophytes. May stain skin. Rash may develop. Lotion may have a drying effect on some skin.

Vehicle

Cream: aqueous base containing titanium dioxide, thimerosal propylene glycol, cetyl alcohol, ceteareth-20, white petrolatum, methylparaben, propylparaben, sorbitol solution, glycerylmonostearate, polyethylene glycol monostearate, simethicone, and sorbic acid.

Lotion: aqueous base containing thimerosal, titanium dioxide, guargum, propylene glycol, cetyl alcohol, stearyl alcohol, sorbitan monopalmitate, polysorbate 20, glyceryl monostearate, polyethylene glycol monostearate, simethicone, sorbic acid, sodium citrate, methylparaben, and propylparaben.

Ointment: Plastibase (plasticized hydrocarbon gel). A polyethylene and mineral oil gel base with titanium dioxide.

Dosage

Apply two to four times a day. Apply liberally to candidal lesions. Duration of therapy depends on individual response to treatment. May require 2–4 weeks of therapy.

Packaging

Fungizone (Squibb Pharm.)
   3% cream and ointment, 20 g
   3% lotion, 30 mL

CICLOPIROX OLAMINE (LOPROX)

Description

Effective broad-spectrum hydroxpyrimidinone antifungal agent that inhibits the growth of pathogenic dematophytes, yeasts, and *Malassezia furfur*.

Action

Inhibits the uptake of precursors of macromolecular synthesis. Acts by impairing transmembrane transport, thus preventing essential amino acids and electrolytes from entering the cell.

Indications

Tinea pedis, cruris, corporis due to *Trichophyton rubrum, T mentagrophytes, Epidermophyton floccosum*, and *Microsporum canis*. Cutaneous candidiasis (moniliasis) caused by *Candida albicans* and pityriasis (tinea) versicolor, due to *Microsporum canis*.

Adverse Reactions

Burning, stinging, pruritis, and erythema are reported side effects. Avoid eye contact.

Dosage

Gently massage into affected area and surrounding skin. Use twice-daily application (morning and evening). Treatment should last from 2 to 4 weeks. Avoid use of occlusive wrappings or dressings. There is only minimal absorption (1.3%) when applied topically to intact or broken skin.

Vehicle

Lotion: water-miscible lotion base consisting of purified water USP, cocamide DEA, octyldodecanol NF, mineral oil USP, stearyl alcohol NF, cetyl alcohol NF, polysorbate 60 NF, myristyl alcohol NF, sorbitan monostearate NF, lactic acid USP, and benzyl alcohol NF (1%) as preservative.

Cream: water-miscible vanishing cream base consisting of purified water USP, octyldodecanol NF, mineral oil USP, stearyl alcohol NF, cetyl alcohol NF, cocamide DEA, polysorbate 60 NF, myristyl alcohol NF, sorbitan monostearate NF, lactic acid USP, and benzyl alcohol NF (1%) as preservative.

Packaging

Loprox (Hoechst-Rousell Pharm.)
   1% cream, 15 g, 30 g, 90 g
   1% lotion, 30 mL

CLOTRIMAZOLE (LOTRIMIN, MYCELEX)

Description

Synthetic imidazole agent that is an odorless, white crystalline and practically insoluble in water.

Action

Mechanism of action is unclear but probably involves damage to the cell wall, resulting in loss of intracellular electrolytes, similar to that of the polyene antibacterials.

Indications

Indicated for superficial fungal infections, *Candida albicans* infections, yeasts, and *Malassezia furfur*. Inhibits growth of most dermatophyte species as well as of some gram-positive bacteria. In high concentration clotrimazole is active against *Trichomonas* species. Also active against tinea pedis, cruris, corporis caused by *Trichophyton rubrum, T mentagrophytes, Epidermophyton floccosum*, and *Microsporum canis*.

Adverse Reactions

Occasional erythema at site of application has been reported along with urticaria, burning, edema, peeling, blistering, and stinging. Do not use in first trimester of pregnancy.

Note: Lotrisone is not the same as Lotrimin. Lotrisone contains a steroid.

Vehicle

Cream: vanishing cream base of sorbitan monostearate, polysorbate 60, cetyl ester wax, cetyl alcohol, 2-octyl-dodecanol, purified water, and, as preservative, benzyl alcohol (1%).

Lotion: emulsion composed of sorbitan monostearate, polysorbate 60, cetyl ester wax, cetyl alcohol, 2-octyl-dodecanol, purified water, benzyl alcohol (1%), and, as preservative, sodium phosphate dibasic sodium biphosphate to adjust pH.

Solution: nonaqueous vehicle of polyethylene glycol 400.

Dosage

Twice daily until eruption clears. Gently rub into the affected areas morning and evening. Clinical improvement should be evident in 1 week. Continue treatment for 4 weeks. Reevaluate after 4 weeks if no improvement. Use the solution four times daily.

Packaging

Lotrimin (Shering Corp.)
    1% cream, 15-g tube, 30-g tube, 45-g tube, 90-g tube
    1% solution, 10 mL, 30 mL
Mycelex (Milex, Inc.)
    1% cream, 15-g tube, 30-g tube, 90-g tube

ECONAZOLE NITRATE 1% (SPECTAZOLE)

Description

Synthetic imidazole.

Action

Interferes with the biosynthesis of ergosterol (chemical needed by fungi to maintain cell wall integrity), resulting in the disorganization of the fungal plasma cell membrane.

Indications

For the topical treatment of tinea pedis, tinea cruris, tinea corporis (ringworm of the body), cutaneous candidiasis (caused by *Candida albicans*), and pityriasis (tinea) versicolor; effective against *Microsporum gypseum.* Effective against *Trichophyton rubrum, T. mentagrophytes, T. tonsurans, Microsporum canis, M. audouinii*, and *Epidermophyton floccosum.*

Adverse Reactions

Three percent of patients complain of burning, stinging, pruritus, and erythema after 3–4 days of treatment. Avoid eye contact.

Vehicle

Cream: water-miscible base consisting of pegoxol F stearate, peglicol 5 oleate, mineral oil, benzoic acid, butylated hydroxyanisole, and purified water.

Dosage

Twice daily (morning and evening) for 2 or more weeks. There is only minimal absorption when applied topically to intact or broken skin. Occlusive dressings slightly increase the amount of absorption.

Packaging

Spectazole (Ortho Pharm., Dermatological Division), 1% cream, 15 g, 30 g, 85 g

HALOPROGIN (HALOTEX)

Description

Synthetic chlorinated ildopropynyl trichlorophenyl ether.

Action

The exact mechanism of action is unknown.

Indications

Topical treatment of dermatophyte infections and tinea vesicolor caused by *Malassezia furfur*. Active in vitro against staphylococci, streptococci, and *Candida albicans*. Indicated for tinea pedis, tinea cruris, tinea corporis, and tinea manuum caused by *Trichophyton, Epidermophyton floccosum.*

Adverse Reactions

Local irritations, burning sensation, pruritus, erythema, scaling, folluculitis, and vesicle formation are reported.

Vehicle

Cream: water-dispersible base composed of polyethylene glycol 400, polyethylene glycol 4,000, diethyl sebacate, and polyvinylpyrrolidone.
Solution: 75% alcohol and diethyl sebacate.

Dosage

Twice daily gently massage the 1% cream liberally onto the affected area for 2–3 weeks' duration. Interdigital lesions may require 4 weeks.

Packaging

Halotex (Westwood Pharm., Inc.)
1% cream, 15 g, 30 g
1% solution, 10 mL, 30 mL

KETOCONAZOLE (NIZORAL)

Description

Water-soluble imidazole derivative.

Action

Affects fungi by mechanisms involving increased membrane permeability, inhibition of uptake of precursors of RNA and DNA, and synthesis of oxidative and perioxidative enzymes.

Indications

Highly effective in chronic dermatophyte infections, including those resistant to *Candida* species*, Cryptococcus neoformans, Coccidioides immitis, Histoplasma capsulatum, Blastomyces dermatitidis*, and pathogenic dermatophytes. Effective for treatment of mucocutaneous candidiasis. Used in the treatment of tinea corporis, tinea cruris, and tinea versicolor.

Adverse Reactions

Stinging, irritation, and pruritus are reported.

Vehicle

Propylene glycol, stearyl and cetyl alcohols, sorbitan monostearate, polysorbate 60, isopropyl myristate, sodium sulfite anhydrous, polysorbate 80, and purified water.

Dosage

Apply 2% cream over affected area and the immediate surrounding area once daily for 2 weeks.

Packaging

Nizoral (Janssen Pharm.), 2% cream, 15-g tube, 30-g tube, 60-g tube

MICONAZOLE NITRATE (MONISTAT-DERM, MICATIN, MONISTAT)

Description

Synthetic imidazole antifungal.

Action

Destroys fungi presumably by inhibiting cell wall synthesis.

Indications

Effective against most dermatophyte species and against cutaneous candidiasis caused by *Candida albicans*. Effective against tinea pedis, cruris, and corporis caused by *Trichophyton rubrum, T. mentagrophytes*, and *Epidermophyton floccosum*, the yeastlike fungus. Effective against *Malassezia furfur*, the organism responsible for tinea versicolor.

Adverse Reactions

May cause irritation, burning, erythema, maceration, and allergic contact dermatitis. Avoid eye contact.

Vehicle

Cream and lotion: water-miscible base consisting of pegoxol 7 stearate, peglicol 5 oleate, mineral oil, benzoic acid, and butylated hydroxyanisole, and purified water.

Dosage

Apply twice daily until eruption clears. Cream should be gently rubbed in thoroughly (to avoid maceration) on the affected areas and surrounding skin morning and evening. Clinical improvement should be evident (relief of pruritis) within 1 week. Continue treatment for 2–4 weeks.

Packaging

Monistat-Derm (Ortho Derm. Div.), 2% cream, 15 g, 28 g, 85 g

Micatin (Ortho), 2% cream, 15 g, 30 g

Monistat-7 (Ortho Pharm), lotion, cream, 45-g/tube with applicator

NYSTATIN (MYCOSTATIN, NILSTAT)

Description

Polyene antimicrobial derived from a species of the order Actinomycetales, *Streptomyces noursei*.

Action

Binds to sterols in fungal cell membranes, causing a change in the permeability of cell membranes and leakage of cell components.

Indications

Candidal infections of skin and mucous membranes.

Adverse Reactions

None known.

Vehicle

Nilstat's vehicle is composed of light mineral oil and Plastibase 50W.

Dosage

Apply twice daily and gently massage into affected area.

Packaging

Ointment and cream, 100,000 U/g
   Mycostatin (Squibb), 15 g
   Nilstat (Lederle), 15 g
   Generic, 15 g
Nilstatin (Lederle), 0.1% triamcinolone acetonide cream and ointment
   Mycolog (Squibb), 15 g
Generic, 15 g

TOLNAFTATE (TINACTIN)

Description

Fungistatic and fungicidal agent.

Action

Mechanism of action is unknown.

Indications

Effective against *Trichophyton rubrum, T. mentagrophytes, T. tonsurans*, and various *Microsporum* and *Aspergillus* species. Effective against intradermal dermatophytic infections. Commonly used to treat tinea pedia (athlete's foot), tinea cruris (jock itch), tinea corporis (ringworm of the body), and tinea manuum when caused by the above fungal pathogens.

It is ineffective against *Candida albicans, Cryptococcus neoformans*, and *Aspergillus fumigatus*, and against bacteria, protozoa, and viruses.

Adverse Reactions

Essentially none, although local irritation and burning have been reported when applied to excoriated skin or lesions caused by multiple pathogens. Avoid eye contact.

Dosage

Dry the affected area first, then apply a small amount and gently massage into the area until the medication disappears. Apply twice daily for several weeks (may be required over 6 weeks with long-standing infections). Clinical improvement should be noted in 2 or 3 days. Only small amounts of the cream are necessary for therapy.

Packaging

Tinactin (Sherring-Plough Healthcare Products)
   1% cream, 15-g tube
   1% powder, 45-g container
   1% powder, 120-g aerosol container
   1% solution, 10-mL container
Generic
   1% cream, 15-g tube
   1% powder, 45-g container

INDEX TO TOPICAL ANTIBACTERIALS

Generic Name	Product Name(s)
Bacitracin	Baciguent
Gentamicin sulfate	Gentamicin, Garamycin
Metronidazole	Metrogel
Mupirocin	Bactroban
Neomycin sulfate	Myciguent, Neosporin
Nitrofurazone	Furacin
Polymyxin B	Aerosporin
Silver sulfadiazine	Silvadene, SSD
Zinc bacitracin	Zinc bacitracin

BACITRACIN (BACIGUENT)

Description

Bacitracin is a polypeptide antibiotic produced from the Tracy I strain of *Bacillus subtilis* and licheniformin discovered in 1954. Bacitracin is stable in petrolatum and is available as an ointment or as a component of antibiotic mixtures.

Action

Bacitracin interferes with cell wall synthesis and has a wide antibacterial spectrum.

Indications

Topical bacitracin will eradicate susceptible bacteria in open infections such as infected dermatosis and cutaneous ulcers. Gram-positive cocci and bacilli, *Neisseria, Haemophilus influenzae,* and *Treponema pallidum* are sensitive to bacitracin 0.1/mL or less. *Actinomyces* and *Fusobacterium* are sensitive to 0.5 U/mL. Resistant strains are *Pseudomonas, Candida, Norcardia, Enterobacteriaceae,* and *Cryptococcus* (formerly called *Torula*). Although bacitracin ointment has been applied to the nose of subjects colonized with methicillin-resistant *Staphylococcus aureus,*[10] two studies found it ineffective in eradicating nasal carriage.[11,12]

Precautions

Bacitracin patch tests may not show positive results for 96 hours after the usual 48 hours. Anaphylaxis (type I hypersensitivity) occurs almost exclusively in settings of topical application to sites of venous stasis dermatitis and ulcers, and presumably arises from systemic absorption of the drug. A patient sensitive to neomycin is probably sensitive to bacitracin. Local application of bacitracin has been associated with severe allergic disorders.[13]

Vehicle

Anhydrous ointment base, mineral oil, and white petrolatum.

Directions

Apply four to six times daily directly to the wound.

Packaging

Generic, 15-g tube (500 U/g), 30-g tube
Baciguent (The Upjohn Co.), 15-g tube, 30-g tube, 120-g tube

GENTAMICIN SULFATE (GENTAMICIN, GARAMYCIN)

Description

Gentamicin is a combination of three related aminoglycoside agents obtained from cultures of *Micromono-spora purpurea.*

Action

Gentamicin is active against gram-negative organisms, including *Escherichia coli* and a high percentage of strains of species of *Pseudomonas* and other gram-negative bacteria. *Proteus* organisms show a variable degree of sensitivity. Some gram-positive organisms are affected, such as *Staphylococcus aureus* and group A ß-hemolytic streptococci. In general, higher concentrations are needed to inhibit streptococci than are needed to inhibit staphylococci and many gram-negative bacteria. The most important use of gentamicin is in the treatment of systemic gram-negative infections, particularly those due to *Pseudomonas* organisms.

Precautions

Gentamicin's antibiotic spectrum is similar to that of neomycin, and cross-resistance does occur. Widespread use is especially unwarranted because of the risk of increasing gentamicin-resistant organisms (because this drug may be very useful in eradicating *Pseudomonas*) and because equally effective drugs are available. Allergic reactions to gentamicin are unusual. As with any aminoglycoside, gentamicin should be avoided in patients with kidney disease or renal failure.

Vehicle

Cream: bland emulsion-type base consisting of stearic acid, propylene glycol stearate, isopropyl myristate, propylene glycol, polysorbate 40, sorbitol solution, and purified water.
Ointment: bland, unctuous petrolatum base.

Directions

Apply four to six times daily directly to the wound.

Packaging

Generic, 3.5-g cream or ointment, 15-g cream or ointment
Gentamicin (Schering, Fougera), 15-g tube
Garamycin (Schering), 3.5-g tube, 15-g tube
Jenamicin (Hauck), 2-mL vial

METRONIDAZOLE (METROGEL)

Description

Contains metronidazole USP at a concentration of 7.5 mg/g. Classed as both antibacterial and antiprotozoal. The 0.75% topical gel, which is bactericidal, amebicidal, and trichomonacidal, is used for acne rosacea.

Action

The mechanisms by which Metrogel acts to reduce inflammation are unknown, but may include an antibacterial and/or an antiprotozoal effect.

Indications

Topical application for the treatment of inflammatory papules, pustules, and erythema of rosacea. In the United Kingdom, it has been used on pressure ulcers, fungate tumors, and malodorous lesions with success.[14]

Precautions

Use with care in patients with evidence of, or history of, blood dyscrasia. Use care in administration to patients receiving anticoagulant treatment.

Vehicle

Gelled, purified water solution containing methylparaben and propylparaben, propylene glycol, carbomer 940, and edetate disodium.

Directions

Apply and rub in a thin film of Metrogel twice daily (morning and evening) to the entire affected area after washing. Significant therapeutic results should be noticed within 3 weeks.

Packaging

Metrogel (Curatek Pharm.), 30-g tube

MUPIROCIN (BACTROBAN)

Description

Mupirocin 2% ointment is in a water-miscible, nonocclusive polyethylene glycol base. Mupirocin, or pseudomonic acid A, is produced by fermentation of the organism *Pseudomonas fluorescens*.

Action

Apparently exerts its antimicrobial activity by reversibly inhibiting isoleucyl–transfer RNA, thereby inhibiting bacterial protein and RNA synthesis.

Indications

For topical treatment of impetigo due to *Staphylococcus aureus*, *ß-hemolytic streptococcus*, and *Streptococcus pyogenes*. Highly active against all species of *Staphylococcus*, including methicillin-resistant *S aureus* (MRSA), *S. aureus*, and most species of *streptococci*. It is ineffective against most gram-positive bacilli, anaerobes, and aerobic gram-negative bacilli, such as *Pseudomonas* species. In the treatment of MRSA and impetigo, mupirocin is usually used in combination with suitable systemic antibiotics.

Precautions

Caution should be used in pregnant and nursing women. Burning, itching, contact dermatitis has been reported. Prolonged use may result in overgrowth of nonsusceptible organisms, including fungi.

Vehicle

Bland, water-miscible ointment base consisting of polyethylene glycol 400 and polyethylene glycol 3,350.

Directions

Mupirocin 2% is usually applied topically two or three times per day for 5 to 14 days in adult and pediatric patients with primary or superficial skin infections.

Packaging

Bactroban (Beecham Labs), 15-g tube

NEOMYCIN SULFATE (MYCIGUENT, NEOSPORIN)

Description

Neomycin is an active aminoglycoside against staphylococci, but less so against streptococci. Neomycin sulfate is obtained from species of the actinomycete *Streptomyces*.

Action

Neomycin acts by inhibiting protein synthesis, as do all aminoglycosides.

Indications

Neomycin is effective against most gram-negative organisms, except *Pseudomonas aeruginosa* and obligate anaerobic bacteria. Group A streptococci are relatively resistant.[15] Neomycin is active against staphylococci. Often neomycin is combined with bacitracin, which inhibits staphylococci and streptococci, as well as gram-negative bacilli.

Precautions

Neomycin is responsible for a greater incidence of allergic sensitivity and cross-sensitivity to other aminoglycosides than any other topical antibiotic, especially in wounds, because they have lost their epidermal barrier and cannot resist penetration.[16,17]

Directions

Apply four to six times daily to the wound.

Packaging

Generic, 15-g ointment, 30-g ointment
Neomycin (Burroughs-Wellcome)
Neomycin (various other manufacturers)

Neomycin-Containing Ointments and Creams

- Neodecadron topical cream (Merck & Co., Inc.)
  Contents per gram: 3.5 mg neomycin sulfate and 1 mg dexamethasone sodium phosphate

- Campho-Phenique triple antibiotic plus pain reliever (Winthrop)
  Contents per gram: 400 U bacitracin, 5 mg neomycin sulfate, 5,000 U polymyxin B sulfate, and diperodon hydrochloride

- Myciguent ointment or cream (Upjohn)
- Neosporin ointment (Burroughs-Wellcome)
  Contents per gram: 5,000 U polymyxin B sulfate, 400 U zinc bacitracin, and 3.5 mg neomycin sulfate (as base)
  Directions: Apply four to six times daily directly to the wound.
  Packaging:
    Generic, 15-g tube
    Neomycin (Burroughs-Wellcome), 15-g tube, 30-g tube

- Neo-Polycin ointment (Merrell Dow)
  Contents per gram: 8,000 U polymyxin B sulfate, 400 U zinc bacitracin, 3 mg neomycin sulfate (base)
  Directions: Apply four to six times daily directly to the wound.
  Packaging:
    Generic, 15-g tube
    Neo-Polycin (Lakeside), 15-g tube

NITROFURAZONE (FURACIN)

Description

Odorless, lemon-yellow, crystalline powder; pH between 5 and 7.5.

Action

The exact mechanism of action is unknown.

Indication

Effective against *Staphylococcus aureus, streptococcus, Escherichia coli, Clostridium perfringens, Enterobacter aerogenes,* and *proteus.* It has a broad spectrum of activity. Most bacteria of surface infections of the skin and mucosal surfaces are sensitive.

It has not been shown to be effective in the treatment of minor burns, wounds, or cutaneous ulcers that are infected. It has been successfully used in the treatment of second- and third-degree burns and in skin grafting where there are complications from bacterial infections that are refractory to the usual drugs of choice, but in which sensitivity to nitrofurazone is demonstrated by culture and sensitivity.

Nitrofurazone's antibacterial activity is inhibited in blood, serum, pus, and animobenzoic acid.[18] Phagocytosis is not inhibited, but animal studies have shown nitrofurazone to delay wound healing.[19]

Precautions

Burning, stinging, dryness, itching, local irritation, and erythema are reported side effects. Use with caution on patients with known or suspected renal impairment, because it contains polyethylene glycols, which may be absorbed and may produce adverse effects.

Vehicle

Water-miscible base consisting of glycerin, cetyl alcohol, mineral oil, an ethoxylated fatty alcohol, methylparaben, propylparaben, and purified water.

Directions

Nitrofurazone is a slow-acting drug, and at least 24 hours are required for it to take effect properly. Treatment should last at least 2 or 3 days. Only about 6% is absorbed.

The dosage interval and duration of treatment vary with the particular use and dosage form. Five days is the usual duration except in severe burns. The use in burn therapy is generally less than 1 week to avoid sensitization. Gently massage cream (1%) into affected and surrounding skin daily.

Packaging

Furacin topical cream (Norwich Eaton Pharm. Inc.)
  0.2% cream, 28 g
  0.2% ointment, 28 g, 454 g
Generic, 0.2% ointment, 30 g

POLYMYXIN B (AEROSPORIN)

Description

Polymyxin B is one of a group of cyclic polypeptides. The B represents *Bacillus polymyxa,* in which the polypeptides were derived from this organism found in the soil.

Action

Polymyxin B is a surface-active agent and is thought to alter the lipoprotein membrane of bacteria so that it no longer functions as an effective barrier, and thereby allows the cell contents to escape.

Indications

Polymyxin B is effective against *Pseudomonas* and other aerobic gram-negative bacilli, including *Pseudomonas aeruginosa,* but not against the *Proteus* and *Serratia* species. Polymyxin B has little to no effect on gram-negative bacteria. Polymyxin B is often used with neomycin and bacitracin. The triple combination is effective against a broad variety of gram-positive and gram-negative bacilli.

Precautions

Sensitization can occur after long-term usage.

Directions

Apply three to four times daily directly to the wound.

Packaging

Generic
Aerosporin (Burroughs-Wellcome), 15 g

Polymyxin B–Containing Ointments

- Topisporin (Pharmafair)—neomycin, polymycin B sulfate, bacitracin zinc

- Neosporin (Burroughs-Wellcome)—polymyxin B sulfate, bacitracin zinc, neomycin sulfate
- Cortisporin (Burroughs-Wellcome), 5,000 U polymyxin B sulfate, 400 U bacitracin zinc, 3.5 mg neomycin sulfate, and 10 mg (1%) hydrocortisone
- Campho-Phenique triple antibiotic plus pain reliever (Winthrop)

Contents per gram: 400 μ bacitracin, 5 mg neomycin sulfate, 5,000 u polymyxin B sulfate, and diperodon hydrochloride

POLYSPORIN OINTMENT

Description

Polysporin was introduced to leave out Neomycin which may cause sensitivity to aminoglycosides.

Contains

Per gram: 10,000 units Polymyxin B sulfate
               500 units zinc Bacitracin

Directions

Apply 4 to 6 times daily directly to the wound.

Packaging and Costs*

generic	30 gram tube	$2.50
Polysporin	15 gram tube	$2.66
(Burroughs-Wellcome)	30 gram tube	$4.39

*These costs are average wholesale prices according to *American Druggist First Data Bank Directory of Pharmaceuticals*, 1990-1991 Edition.

SILVER SULFADIAZINE (SILVADENE, SSD)

Description

White, odorless cream. Less than 1% of the silver content is absorbed, and up to 10% of the sulfadiazine may be absorbed.

Action

Acts only on the cell membrane and cell wall to produce its bactericidal effect. Silver, which is selectively toxic to bacteria, is slowly released. Both components in the complex are active.

Indications

Micronized silver sulfadiazine (1%) has a broad antibacterial spectrum, including many strains found in soft tissue infections: *Staphylococcus aureus, Escherichia coli, Pseudomonas aeruginosa, Proteus mirabilis,* and *ß-hemolytic streptococci*[20]; it is also effective against yeasts such as *Candida albicans.*

Although silver sulfadiazine is used commonly in chronic wound management, it has never been approved by the FDA for such application.

Precautions

Patients with known sensitivity to sulfa drugs should not utilize silver sulfadiazine. Do a patch test prior to using. Silver may inactivate topical proteolytic enzymes. Silver sulfadiazine should not be used at term pregnancy. Avoid use of silver sulfadiazine in the presence of hepatic and renal impairment because of poor drug elimination.

Vehicle

The cream vehicle consists of white petrolatum, stearyl alcohol, isopropyl myristate, sorbitan monooleate, polyoxyl 40 stearate, propylene glycol, and water, with 0.3% methylparaben as preservative.

Directions

Apply with a sterile applicator once or twice daily in the amount of $1/16$-inch thickness to a clean, debrided wound. Because the vehicle is water soluble, it will be miscible in wound fluid; therefore, in most cases, less than 1 g is sufficient.

Packaging

Flint SSD (Boots-Flint), 50-g jar, 400-g jar, 1,000-g jar
Silvadene cream 1% (Marion), 20-g tube, 50-g jar, 85-g jar, 400-g jar, 1,000-g jar
Both are creams, 10-mg/g, in a water-miscible base.

ZINC BACITRACIN

Description

Zinc bacitracin (7% zinc) is prepared by the action of zinc salts on bacitracin broth. Zinc bacitracin is less water soluble than bacitracin and is more stable than bacitracin at room and elevated temperatures (shelf life may be 5 years). Zinc bacitracin and bacitracin have different degrees of sensitizing potential.

Action

Zinc bacitracin is a cell wall synthesis inhibitor. Zinc increases the potency of bacitracin and also enhances its stability.

Precaution

May cause a generalized itching.

Vehicle

Special white petrolatum base.

Directions

Apply directly to the wound four or five times daily.

Packaging

Zinc bacitracin (Pharma-Tek, Inc.), 500 mμ

Zinc Bacitracin–Containing Ointments

Costs and package size are very similar among manufacturers.
Cortisporin (Burroughs-Wellcome), 3.75 g
Neo-Polycin (Merrell Dow), 15 g
Neosporin (Burroughs-Wellcome), 30 g
Polysporin (Burroughs-Wellcome), 15 g
Topisporin (Pharmafair), 30g

REFERENCES

1. Lineaweaver W. Cellular and bacterial toxicities of topical antimicrobials. *Plastic Reconstr Surg.* 1985;75(3):394–396.

2. Kozol RA. Effects of sodium hypochlorite on cells of the wound module. *Arch Surg.* 1988;123(4):420–423.

3. Schneider D, Herbert L. Subcutaneous gas from hydrogen peroxide administration under pressure. *Am J Dis Children.* 1987;141:10–11.

4. Oberg MS, Lindsey D. Do not put hydrogen peroxide or povidone iodine into wounds! *AJDC.* 1987;141:27–28.

5. Strachan C. Antibiotic prophylaxis in "clean" surgical procedures. *World J Surg.* 1972;6:273–280.

6. Rodeheaver G, et al. Bactericidal activity and toxicity of iodine-containing solutions in wounds. *Arch Surg.* 1982;117:181–185.

7. D'Auria J, Lipson S, Garfield JM. Fatal iodine toxicity following surgical debridement of a hip wound: case report. *J Trauma.* 1990;30(3):353–355.

8. Aronoff TG, Friedman S, Doedens D, Lavelle K. Increased serum iodine concentration, serum iodine absorption through wounds treated topically with povidone-iodine. *Am J Med Sci.* 1980;279(3):173–176.

9. Thomas C. Nursing alert: wound healing halted with the use of povidone-iodine. *Ostomy/Wound Man.* Spring 1988:30–33.

10. O'Keefe JP, et al. Eradication of resistant *Staphylococcus aureus* on a surgical unit. *N Engl J Med.* 1985;312:858.

11. McAnally TP, et al. Antimicrobial agents. *Chemo.* 1984;25:422.

12. Yu VL, et al. *Staphylococcus aureus* nasal carriage and infection in patients on hemodialysis. *N Engl J Med.* 1986;315:91.

13. Vale MA, et al. Bacitracin-induced anaphylaxis. *Arch Derm.* 1978;114:800 (letter).

14. McMullen D. Topical metronidazole use in malodorous ulcerating skin lesions. IAET Conference Bulletin Abstract, 1990.

15. Reynolds JEF, ed. *Martindale the extra pharmacopoeia*, 29th ed. London, England: The Pharmaceutical Press; 1989.

16. Hirschman JV. Topical antibiotics in dermatology. *Arch Derm.* 1988;124:1691–1700.

17. Leyden JJ, Klingman AM. Rationale for topical antibiotics. *Curtis.* 1978;22:515–526.

18. Gennaro AR. *Remington's pharmaceutical sciences*, 18th ed. Mack Publishing Company; 1990.

19. Geronemus RG, Mertz PM, Eaglestein WH. Wound healing—the effects of topical antimicrobial agents. *Arch Derm.* 1979;115:1311–1314.

20. Kucan O, et al. Comparison of silver sulfadiazine, povidone-iodine and physiologic saline in the treatment of chronic pressure ulcers. *J Am Ger Soc.* 1981;29:232–235.

A Quick Reference Guide to Wound Care Product Categories

Diane L. Krasner

This listing of wound care products highlights the importance of generic product categories. Under each generic product category, *up to four product examples are given (a mix of old and new products)*, to help familiarize the reader with each category. No endorsement of any product or manufacturer is intended. Within each category, products must be individually evaluated. Products within a category do not necessarily perform equally. Combination products may be listed in more than one category. Refer to manufacturers' instructions for specifics regarding product usage. All product names should be considered copyrighted or trademarked.

1. Antimicrobial Dressings

Product	Manufacturer
Acticoat	Westaim Biomedical
Arglaes Film/Island	Medline Industries
Iodosorb/Iodoflex Gel Pad	Healthpoint
Kerlix AMD	Kendall

2. Alginate Dressings

Product	Manufacturer
AlgiCell	Dumex Medical
Cutinova alginate	Beiersdorf-Jobst
Restore CalciCare	Hollister
Sorbsan	Dow Hickam Pharmaceuticals

3. Biosynthetic Dressings

Product	Manufacturer
BiobraneII	Dow Hickam Pharmaceuticals
Silon	BioMed Sciences

4. Cleansers

Product	Manufacturer
SALINE	Multiple
SKIN CLEANSERS	
CliniClens	Dumex Medical
Peri-Wash	Sween
Sensi-Care	ConvaTec
Skin Cleanser	Mentor
WOUND CLEANSERS	
Clinical Care	Care-Tech Laboratories
Curasol	Healthpoint Medical
Dermagran Spray	Derma Sciences
RadiaCare Klenz	Carrington Laboratories

5. Collagen Dressings

Product	Manufacturer
BGC Matrix (Collagen/ Beta-glucan)	Brennen Medical
ChroniCure	Derma Sciences
Fibracol (Collagen/Alginate)	Ethicon
Medifil/SkinTemp	BioCore

6. Composite Dressings

Product	Manufacturer
Alldress	Mölnlycke
CombiDERM ACD	ConvaTec
CovaDerm/CovaDerm Plus	DeRoyal Industries
OsmoCyte Island	ProCyte Corporation

Source: © Diane L. Krasner 2001. Used with permission.

7. Compression Bandages/Wraps

Product	Manufacturer
Coban	3M Health Care
Dome Paste	Miles
Elastoplast	Beiersdorf-Jobst
Setopress	ConvaTec

Multilayered Systems	Manufacturer
Circulon System	ConvaTec
Dufore	Dumex Medical
Dyna-Flex	Johnson & Johnson Heritage
Profore	Smith & Nephew

8. Conforming/Wrapping Bandages

Product	Manufacturer
Duform/Durlix	Dumex Medical
Elastomull	Beiersdorf-Jobst
Kerlix/Kerlix Lite	Kendall Healthcare
Kling Fluff/ Sof-Kling	Johnson & Johnson Heritage

9. Contact Layers

Product	Manufacturer
Mepitel	Mölnlycke
Profore	Smith & Nephew
Tegapore	3M Health Care
Ventex Vented Dressing	Kendall Healthcare

10. Creams/Oils

Product	Manufacturer
Biafine	Medix Pharmaceuticals Americas
Decubitene Oxygenated Oil	Ferndale Labs
Eucerin Cream	Beiersdorf-Jobst
Sween Cream	Coloplast Sween

11. Devices

Product	Manufacturer
Derma-Wand UVC Lamp	National Biological Corporation
THBO (topical hyperbaric oxygen)	GWR Medical LLP
The VAC/Mini-VAC	KCI
Warm-Up (Wound Therapy System)	Augustine Medical

12. Enzymes/Debriding Agents

Product	Manufacturer
Accuzyme (Papain-Urea)	Healthpoint
Panafil Ointment (Papain-Urea-Chorophyllin Copper)	Healthpoint
Santyl (Collagenase)	Smith & Nephew

13. Foam Dressings

Product	Manufacturer
Allevyn	Smith & Nephew
Cutinova Foam	Beiersdorf-Jobst
Lyofoam/Lyofoam C/Lyofoam T	ConvaTec
Mepilex	Mölnlycke

14. Gauze Dressings (see also Composite Dressings)

Product	Manufacturer
a. Woven	Multiple
b. Nonwoven	Multiple
c. Packing/Packing Strips (Nonimpregnated)	Multiple
d. Debriding	Multiple
e. Impregnated—Sodium Chloride	Multiple
f. Impregnated—Other	Multiple
g. Nonadherent gauze	Multiple
h. Specialty Absorptive Gauze	Multiple

15. Growth Factors

Product	Manufacturer
Procuren (autologous)	
Regranex Gel (becaplermin 0.01%)	Ortho-McNeil Pharmaceutical

16. Human Skin Equivalents (HSE)/Skin Substitutes

Product	Manufacturer
Apligraf (Graftskin)	Organogenesis/Novartis
Dermagraft	Advanced Tissue Sciences/Smith & Nephew
Integra Artificial Skin	Ethicon
Oasis	Cook

17. Hydrocolloid Dressings

Product	Manufacturer
DuoDERM/CGF/Extra Thin	ConvaTec
Hydrocol	Bertek Pharmaceuticals
Restore/CX/Extra Thin	Hollister
Tegasorb/Extra Thin	3M Health Care

18. Hydrofiber

Product	Manufacturer
Aquacel	ConvaTec

19. Hydrogel Dressings (see also Impregnated Gauze Dressings)

Product	Manufacturer
SHEET	
CarraSorb M	Carrington Laboratories
Elasto-Gel	Southwest Technologies
Gentell	MKM
Vigilon	Bard

AMORPHOUS

AquaSite	Dumex Medical
Comfeel Purilon Gel	Coloplast
DuoDERM Hydroactive Gel	
(Hydrogel/Hydrocolloid)	ConvaTec
IntraSite Gel	Smith & Nephew

STRANDS

FlexiGel Strands	Smith & Nephew

---

20. Skin Sealants

Product	*Manufacturer*
Preppies	Kendall Healthcare
Skin Prep	Smith & Nephew United
Skin Shield	Mentor
3M No Sting Skin Protectant	3M Health Care

---

21. Transparent Film Dressings

Product	*Manufacturer*
BIOCLUSIVE/MVP	Ethicon
ClearCell	Dumex Medical
OpSite/Flexifix/Flexigrid/3000	Smith & Nephew
Tegaderm/HP	3M Health Care

---

22. Wound Fillers: Pastes, Powders, Beads, Strands

Product	*Manufacturer*
Bard Absorption Dressing	Bard
FlexiGel Strands	Smith & Nephew
OsmoCyte Pillow Wound Dressing	Procyte
Multidex	DeRoyal Industries

---

23. Wound Pouches

Product	*Manufacturer*
Wound Drainage Collector	Hollister
Wound Manager	ConvaTec
Adult & Pediatric Sized Ostomy Pouches	Multiple

Not Otherwise Classified (NOC) Product Categories

24. Adhesives
25. Adhesive Removers
26. Adhesive Skin Closures
27. Adhesive Tapes
28. Antibiotics
29. Antimicrobials
30. Antiseptics
31. Bandages
32. Dressing Covers
33. Health Care Personnel Hand Rinses
34. Lubricating/Stimulating Sprays
35. Moisture Barrier Ointments/Creams/Skin Protectant Pastes
36. Moisturizers
37. Ointments
38. Perineal Cleansing Foams
39. Sterile Fields
40. Surgical Scrubs
41. Surgical Tapes
42. Miscellaneous

Index

Q

R

surgical dissection, Color Plate Page 12
ultrasound, 615

U

Ulcerating malignant tumor. *See* Malignant cutaneous wound
Ultrasound, 596–619
  absence of inflammatory phase, Color Plate Page 30
  acoustic streaming, 600
  acute inflammatory phase, Color Plate Page 29, Color
    Plate Page 30
  acute wound, 612, 613
  adjunctive treatments, 615–616
  aftercare, 615
  animal studies, 605–606
  applicator manipulation, 614
  attenuation, 597
  blister, Color Plate Page 30, 615
  candidacy for intervention, 610–611
  case studies, 617–618
  chronic leg ulcer, 608, 609
  chronic wound, 612
  circulation, 605
  contraindications, 610
  coupling media, 613–614
  defined, 597
  documentation, 616
  ecchymosis, Color Plate Page 29
  edema, 604–605
  epithelialization phase, Color Plate Page 29, 604
  equipment for generation, 598
  equipment selection, 599
  erythema, Color Plate Page 30
  expected outcomes, 611–612
  frequency, 597, 612–613
  half-value thickness, 597–598
  hematoma, Color Plate Page 30, 605
  high-voltage pulsed current, 604
  human studies, 606–608
  hydration, 605
  inflammatory phase, 603
  intensity, 599–600
    nonthermal effects, 599–600
    terminology, 599
    thermal effects, 599–600
  intervention selection, 608–611
  maturation phase, 604
  microstreaming, 600
  necrosis, Color Plate Page 30
  oxygen, 605
  pain, 604–605
  partial-thickness skin loss, Color Plate Page 29

  precautions, 610
  pressure ulcer, 606–607
  procedures, 611–616
  proliferative phase, Color Plate Page 30, 603–604
  protocol considerations, 611
  remodeling phase, 604
  scar, 608
  self-care teaching guidelines, 616
  setup for treatment, 614–615
  skin tear, 604
  stable cavitation, 600
  terminology, 597–600
  ultrasonic field, 598–599
  undermined/tunneled area, 615
  venous ulcer, Color Plate Page 29
  wavelength, 598
  wound edge, Color Plate Page 29
  wound healing
    healing phase, 603–604
    theory and science, 602–608
Ultraviolet light, 580–594
  administration, 588–592
  bactericidal effects, 584–586
  biologic effects, 582–587
  case study, 593–594
  clinical studies, 586–587, 588
  contraindications, 592–593
  debridement, 583
  definitions, 580
  depth of penetration into integument, 581–582
  documentation, 593
  early cutaneous effects, 583–584
  epithelialization phase, 532
  equipment selection, 588–590
  historical perspective, 580
  indications, 592
  late cutaneous effects, 583, 584
  physical science, 581–587
  preclinical studies, 586, 587
  self-care and teaching guidelines, 593
  spectrum, 580, 581
  treatment, 587–593
    algorithm, 587–588, 589
  treatment distance, 592
  treatment times, 588, 591–592
  UVA application, 592
  UVB application, 592
  UVC application, 592
  wound and periwound area preparation, 590–591
Undermining, Color Plate Page 13, 105–106, 126–128,
  146
  ultrasound, 615
Urinary incontinence, wound diagnosis, 9

About the Editors

Carrie Sussman, PT, is President of Sussman Physical Therapy, Inc. and Wound Care Management Services, and an alumni of the University of Southern California. Of her more than 35 years experience as a physical therapist, 20 years have been spent working to rehabilitate geriatric patients in long-term and subacute settings as both clinician and rehab director. As a geriatric physical therapist, she has had serious concern for the problems and issues of trying to rehabilitate patients with musculoskeletal problems who also have problems with chronic wounds. Her innovative and successful wound treatment program incorporating rehabilitation and use of physical therapy technologies for wound healing has been of interest to the medical, therapy, and payer community for many years.

Sussman is a strong advocate of public policy issues and education for the prevention and healing of chronic wounds. Her advocacy has led to involvement in groups, organizations, and research and writing projects that promote those interests. In 1986, she became an advisor to Blue Cross of California on matters relating to appropriate wound care guidelines and reimbursement issues. For 9 years she served as a member of the Multidisciplinary Advisory Board of the University of Southern California Enterostomal Therapy Program. The American Physical Therapy Association (APTA) selected her to serve as an expert panelist for the APTA Integumentary Panel that has developed *A Guide for Physical Therapist Practice:* Vol. I, Part II, Preferred Practice Patterns for the Integument. She served on the founding committee and practice committee for the APTA Section on Clinical Electrophysiology Wound Management Special Interest Group.

Elected to the Board of Directors of National Pressure Ulcer Advisory Panel (NPUAP), Sussman served for 5 years (1995–2000) and had the distinction of being the first physical therapist elected to the board. During her years of service she was chair of the NPUAP public policy committee, vice president, and chair of the Challenge 2000 Task Force. Major public policy successes during that period include testifying on behalf of NPUAP at a public hearing on including prevention of pressure ulcers as a major health objective for the United States for the next decade. In January 2000, an objective to reduce pressure ulcers over the next decade was included in the national health prevention program, *Healthy People 2010.* A second success was the research and preparation of a monograph by the Challenge 2000 Task Force and entire NPUAP panel: *Pressure Ulcers in America: Prevalence, Incidence, and Implications.*

For 9 years Sussman sponsored and chaired the Annual Physical Therapy Wound Care Management Services conference to educate clinicians and educators in the prevention and management of chronic wounds. To reach more clinicians, educators, and patients, she has changed her focus to lecturing nationally and internationally, publishing articles, chapters and books, including this text, on topics relating to wound prevention and management issues. Sussman, along with James Wethe, MD, and Evonne Fowler, RN, MN, CNS, CWOCN, developed and produced a three-part video series, *Sharp Debridement of Wound.* From these many activities she has learned the value of collaboration among the disciplines involved in wound healing. In collaboration with an expert panel of wound healing clinicians, Sussman has edited and produced the *Wound Care Patient Education and Resource Manual* to help educate clinicians, who are not experts, and patients about wound prevention, treatment options, and wound clinic operations.

Barbara M. Bates-Jensen, PhD, RN, CWOCN, received her doctoral degree and master's degree in nursing from UCLA and her bachelor of science in nursing degree from the University of Nebraska. As a part of her coursework at UCLA she completed a methodological study developing the Pressure Sore Status Tool, or PSST, and her doctoral dissertation further evaluated the PSST instrument. The PSST has been translated into many languages and used globally in countries such as Canada, Japan, Brazil, Finland, France, and Italy.

Bates-Jensen's experience includes an independent practice as a wound care consultant for acute care hospitals, home health care agencies, and long-term care facilities. As a certified wound, ostomy, and continence nurse, she has acquired a wealth of information and experience with chronic wounds and pressure sores in particular, which she shares enthusiastically as an international and national lecturer and author.

Bates-Jensen is a member of the National Pressure Ulcer Advisory Panel. She was the recipient of the 1997 Baranoski Founder's Award in recognition of creative practice strategies that have enhanced the care of wound care clients, the 1997 University of Southern California Department of Nursing Bullough Award for faculty excellence, and the 2001 University of Southern California Department of Nursing Theory Instructor of the Year. She was the director of the graduate Wound, Ostomy, Continence Nursing Program and assistant professor of nursing at the University of Southern California for 9 years. She is currently Adjunct Assistant Professor in Residence with the University of California Los Angeles School of Medicine, Division of Geriatrics, and the Borun Center for Gerontological Research.